LOGAN TURNER'S

DISEASES OF THE NOSE, THROAT AND EAR

HEAD AND NECK SURGERY

ELEVENTH EDITION

LOGAN TURNER'S

DISEASES OF THE NOSE, THROAT AND EAR HEAD AND NECK SURGERY

Edited by

S Musheer Hussain MBBS MSc (Manc) FRCS (Ed & Eng) FRCS (ORL-HNS) FRCP (Ed)
Consultant ENT Surgeon and Honorary Professor of Otolaryngology, Ninewells Hospital and the University of Dundee School of Medicine, Dundee, UK

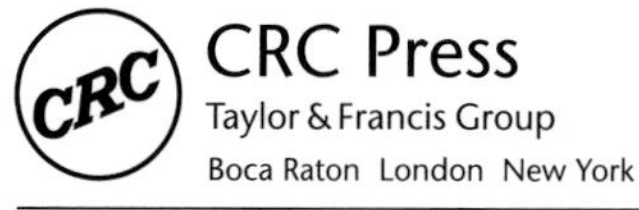

CRC Press is an imprint of the
Taylor & Francis Group, an **informa** business

CRC Press
Taylor & Francis Group
6000 Broken Sound Parkway NW, Suite 300
Boca Raton, FL 33487-2742

Printed and bound in India by Replika Press Pvt. Ltd.

Printed on acid-free paper
Version Date: 20150708

International Standard Book Number-13: 978-0-340-98732-2 (Paperback)

Library of Congress Cataloging-in-Publication Data

Logan Turner's diseases of the nose, throat and ear : head and neck surgery / [edited by] S. Musheer Hussain. -- 11th edition.
p. ; cm.
Preceded by Turner, A. Logan (Arthur Logan), 1865-1939. Logan Turner's diseases of the nose, throat, and ear. 10th ed. London ; Boston : Wright, 1988.
Includes bibliographical references and index.
ISBN 978-0-340-98732-2 (pbk. : alk. paper)
I. Hussain, S. Musheer, editor.
[DNLM: 1. Otorhinolaryngologic Diseases. 2. Otorhinolaryngologic Surgical Procedures. WV 140]

RF46
617.5'1--dc23 2015026103

Visit the Taylor & Francis Web site at
http://www.taylorandfrancis.com

and the CRC Press Web site at
http://www.crcpress.com

Contents

Foreword

Two years before the First World War began in 1914, Dr Porter, an Edinburgh otolaryngologist, wrote a book that became a 'best-seller'. We do not know how his career would have progressed, nor how his book would have developed, because he, like so many other young professional men, was killed before the end of the war.

Fortunately his Edinburgh colleagues revived the book the year after the war ended in 1919 under the editorship of Dr Arthur Logan Turner, who became President of the Royal College of Surgeons of Edinburgh. Between then and 1982 there were nine editions; the contributing authors traditionally were the consultants in post at the time in the Edinburgh department of otolaryngology. The tenth edition in 1988 was edited by Professor Arnold Maran who, like Dr Logan Turner, became a President of the Royal College of Surgeons of Edinburgh, and the edition he edited was also written by Edinburgh laryngologists.

Many plans for further editions were discussed, but they were in the years during which written works were being replaced by electronic publishing, and there was doubt about the value of an 'old-fashioned' text book. During this period of uncertainty there were many 'false starts', and for a time it looked as if this historic book would disappear. However, we are grateful to Musheer Hussain, who has had the perseverance to create a team of contributors to complete this eleventh edition.

So much time has passed and so many changes have occurred in the delivery of health care in Scotland that the authors of the chapters are now no longer confined to Edinburgh. That in itself is a marker of the development of the delivery of health care in Scotland, where now every centre has a standard of excellence that was once confined to the big cities.

This new edition reflects the huge change that has occurred in the specialty since the last century. Although otolaryngology was originally a specialty that was created in order to remove pus from bony boxes in the skull to avoid intracranial complications, it has morphed into a form that would be unrecognisable to the original innovators. These changes are elegantly presented in this book, which now covers neuro-sensory deafness, head and neck cancer, paediatric airway disease, skull base surgery and the rhinological revolution brought about by the endoscope.

Should there still be a place for the printed word? My answer would be in the affirmative, because electronic publishing has not reached the point where instant access to a single topic is as easy as it is with the printed word.

Is there still a place for a single work on a whole specialty? My answer would again be in the affirmative, because 95% of that specialty is between these hard covers. The more specialised areas are the domain of single-subject volumes, but in this book, the jobbing otolaryngologist will find most of the answers to everyday problems.

Professor Arnold A G Maran

Preface

When I was asked to edit the eleventh edition of *Logan Turner's Diseases of the Nose, Throat and Ear: Head and Neck Surgery,* I felt deeply honoured but did not quite grasp the magnitude of the task. It is a great privilege to edit this famous textbook in its centenary year. Not many medical books have been in continuous publication for 100 years.

The response I received from the chapter authors, all leaders in their field who un-hesitantly completed their chapters, was overwhelming. Many mentioned their feelings about the textbook. 'I still keep my copy of the ninth edition', said one. 'It was the book that got me through the exams', said another. 'It was my introduction to otolaryngology' was another comment. The last three editions of this book were popular not only in the British Isles, but also in South Asia, the Far East and the Middle East. The fifth edition was sold in North America and was well received.[1]

This edition has been completely revised to meet the needs of aspiring otolaryngologists. All four sub-specialities are represented in the chapters, along with a fifth section on radiology.

I must acknowledge the previous editors of the book: Dr Proctor, who first published the book in 1914 but died in the service of his country; and Dr Logan Turner, who edited Dr Proctor's book and contributed additional material.

Several editions followed. The ninth and tenth editions were prepared by Professor Arnold Maran, an acknowledged leader in field of otolaryngology who has very kindly written the Foreword to the book.

I would like to thank my former colleague, Robin Blair, and my colleague Brian Bingham for their trust.

If there are errors in the text, the responsibility is entirely mine. The publishers Taylor and Francis, and in particular Henry Spilberg and Linda Van Pelt, were unfailingly helpful, and this book would not have been completed without their support.

S Musheer Hussain
Editor

[1] Hussain SM: Three textbooks and the 'Edinburgh Brand'. ENT and Audiology News 2010; 19 (3): 52-53.

Contributors

Aanand Acharya FRCS (ORL)
Specialist Registrar in Otorhinolaryngology
Department of Otorhinolaryngology
Queen Elizabeth University Hospital
Birmingham, UK
Chapter 43: Acute otitis media

Richard M Adamson FRCS (ORL)
Consultant Otolaryngologist Head and Neck Surgeon
Honorary Senior Lecturer
University of Edinburgh
Edinburgh Royal Infirmary
Edinburgh, UK
Chapter 17: Anatomy of the larynx and pharynx

Kim W Ah-See MBChB, FRCS, FRCS (ORL-HNS), MD
Consultant ENT Head and Neck Surgeon
Aberdeen Royal Infirmary
Aberdeen, UK
Chapter 14: Tumours of the nose and sinuses

David Albert FRCS, MBBS
Senior ENT Surgeon
Great Ormond Street Hospital
London, UK
Chapter 58: Stridor and airway endoscopy

Safina Ali FRCS (ORL)
Head and Neck Fellow
Department of Otolaryngology
Head and Neck Surgery
St Georges Hospital
London, UK
Chapter 17: Anatomy of the larynx and pharynx

C Martin Bailey BSc, FRCS, FRCSEd
Honorary Consultant Otolaryngologist
Department of Paediatric Otolaryngology
Great Ormond Street Hospital
London, UK
Chapter 65: Chronic otitis media

Yogesh Bajaj MD, FRCS (ORL)
Consultant Otolaryngologist
The London Hospital
London, UK
Chapter 58: Stridor and airway endoscopy

Anil R Banerjee MBBS, FRCS, FRCS (ORL-HNS)
Clinical Director
Department of ORL/HNS and the Leicester Balance Centre
University Hospitals of Leicester
Leicester, UK
Chapter 54: Tumours of the middle ear

David E C Baring FRCSEd (ORL-HNS)
Consultant Otolaryngologist
Honorary Senior Clinical Lecturer
University of Edinburgh
Edinburgh, UK
Chapter 46: Otosclerosis

Martyn L Barnes FRCS (ORL), MD, MSc
Consultant Rhinologist
Southend University Hospital
Director
SurgTech.net
Westcliff-on-Sea, UK
Chapter 8: Allergic rhinitis

Neil Bateman BMedSci, BM, BS, FRCS (ORL-HNS)
Consultant Paediatric Otolaryngologist
Royal Manchester Children's Hospital
Clinical Senior Lecturer
University of Manchester
Manchester, UK
Chapter 60: Subglottic stenosis

Brian Bingham MBBS, FRCS
Consultant Rhinologist and ENT Surgeon
Southern General and Victoria Hospitals
Glasgow, UK
Chapter 3: Epistaxis

Duncan Bowyer FRCS (ORL-HNS)
Consultant ENT Surgeon
Shrewsbury and Telford Hospital NHS Trust
Shrewsbury, UK
Chapter 45: Complications of otitis media

Patrick J Bradley MBA, FRCSEd, FRCS (Hon), FRACS (Hon), FRCSLT (Hon)
Emeritus Honorary Professor
School of Medicine
The University of Nottingham
Nottingham, UK
Chapter 28: Salivary gland disease

Peter D Bull MB BCh, FRCS
Retired Paediatric Otolaryngologist
Sheffield Children's Hospital
Sheffield, UK
Chapter 60: Subglottic stenosis

Sean Carrie MB BCh, FRCS (ORL)
Honorary Senior Clinical Lecturer
Institute of Health and Society
University of Newcastle upon Tyne
Consultant Rhinologist / ENT Surgeon
Newcastle upon Tyne City Hospitals NHS Foundation Trust
President of British Rhinological Society
Newcastle upon Tyne, UK
Chapter 12: Pituitary surgery; Chapter 13: Smell and anosmia

Emma C Cashman FRCS (ORL)
Senior Registrar
Otolaryngology Head and Neck Surgery
St James Hospital
Dublin, UK
Chapter 33: Vocal cord paralysis

Ray Clarke BA, BSc, DCH, FRCS, FRCS (ORL)
Senior Lecturer and Associate Dean
University of Liverpool
Consultant Paediatric Otolaryngologist
Alder Hey Children's Hospital
Liverpool, UK
Chapter 68: Obstructive sleep apnoea

John Crowther FRCS
Consultant Otolaryngologist and Skull Base Surgeon
Institute of Neurological Sciences
Southern General Hospital
Glasgow, UK
Chapter 51: Otological trauma

John Dempster MBChB, FRCS
Otolaryngology Department
Crosshouse Hospital
Kilmarnock, UK
Chapter 35: Tracheostomy

Adam J Donne FRCS (ORL-HNS)
Consultant Paediatric Otolaryngologist
Alder Hey Children's NHS Foundation Trust
Honorary Senior Lecturer
University of Liverpool
Liverpool, UK
Chapter 4: Acute rhinosinusitis and its complications

Stephen R Ell BSc (Hon), MBBS, FRCSEd, FRCS (ORL-HNS), MD
Honorary Professor of Otolaryngology
University of Hull
Consultant ENT Surgeon
Hull and East Yorkshire NHS Trust
Hull, UK
Chapter 19: Benign disease of the pharynx

Liam M Flood FRCS, FRCSI
Consultant Otolaryngologist
James Cook University Hospital
Middlesbrough, UK
Chapter 39: Anatomy and physiology

Quentin Gardiner FRCS (Eng & Edin), FRCS (ORL)
Consultant Rhinologist
Honorary Senior Lecturer
Ninewells Hospital and Medical School
Dundee, UK
Chapter 8: Allergic rhinitis

Julian A Gaskin FRCS (ORL-HNS) Edin, CCT Otol (UK), MBChB, DOHNS
Consultant ENT Surgeon (Paediatric)
University of Leicester Medical School Examiner
University Hospitals of Leicester
Leicester Royal Infirmary
Leicester, UK
Chapter 48: Tinnitus

Charles E B Giddings FRCS (ORL-HNS)
Consultant ENT/Head and Neck Surgeon
Monash Health
Honorary Lecturer
Monash University
Melbourne, Australia
Chapter 37: Dysphagia

Joe Grainger BMBS, MMedSci, DCH, FRCS (ORL-HNS)
Consultant Paediatric ENT Surgeon
Birmingham Children's Hospital
Birmingham, UK
Chapter 59: Tracheostomy

Meredydd Harries FRCS, MSc
Consultant Laryngologist
Brighton NHS Trust
Brighton, UK
Chapter 21: Investigations of laryngeal disease

Andrew Harris FRCS (ORL), BSc (Hon), MBChB (Hon), DOHNS, MRCS (Eng), PhD
Clinical Lecturer in Otorhinolaryngology - Head and Neck Surgery
Department of Molecular and Clinical Cancer Medicine
University of Liverpool
Aintree University Hospital
Liverpool, UK
Chapter 34: Laryngo-tracheal trauma

Katherine Harrop-Griffiths MSc, FRCS
Consultant in Audiovestibular Medicine
Nuffield Hearing and Speech Centre
Royal National Throat, Nose and Ear Hospital
London, UK
Chapter 66: Balance disorders in children

John Hill MBBS, FRCS, FRCSEd, FCSHK
Consultant Otolaryngologist
Freeman Hospital
Newcastle upon Tyne, UK
Chapter 12: Pituitary surgery

Omar J Hilmi FRCS (ORL-HNS), FRCSEd
Honorary Senior Lecturer
University of Glasgow
Consultant Otolaryngologist
Glasgow Royal Infirmary
Glasgow, UK
Chapter 29: Thyroid disease

S Musheer Hussain MBBS, MSc (Manc), FRCS (Ed & Eng), FRCS (ORL-HNS), FRCP (Ed)
Consultant ENT Surgeon
Honorary Professor of Otolaryngology
Ninewells Hospital
University of Dundee School of Medicine
Dundee, UK
Chapter 31: Neck space infections; Chapter 42: Diseases of the external ear; Chapter 53: Otitis externa; Chapter 69: Drooling

Richard Irving MD, FRCS
Consultant in Otology, Neurotology and Skull Base Surgery
Birmingham Children's Hospital and
Queen Elizabeth Hospital
Birmingham, UK
Chapter 52: The facial nerve

Jean-Pierre Jeannon MBChB, FRCS, FRCS (ORL)
Consultant ENT and Head and Neck Surgeon
Guy's and St Thomas' NHS Foundation Trust
Honorary Senior Lecturer
Kings College
London, UK
Chapter 25: Tumours of the hypopharynx

Nick S Jones MD, FRCS
Retired Consultant Rhinologist
Honorary Professor
Queen's Medical Centre
University of Nottingham
Nottingham, UK
Chapter 9: Facial pain

Owen Judd MRCP (Glas), FRCSEd, FRCS (ORL-HNS), FRSA, PGDipClinEd, DCH
Consultant Neurotologist
Ear, Nose and Throat Surgeon
Royal Derby Hospital
Derby, UK
Chapter 48: Tinnitus

Tawakir Kamani MD, MSc, FRCS, FRCS (Otol)
Paediatric ENT Fellow
Royal Children's Hospital
Melbourne, Australia
Chapter 1: Anatomy and physiology of the nose and paranasal sinuses

Rahul Kanegaonkar MBBS, BSc (Hon), MRCS, DLO, FRCS (ORL-HNS)
Consultant ENT Surgeon
Medway NHS Foundation Trust
Visiting Professor in Otorhinolaryngology
Medway Campus
Canterbury Christ Church University
Canterbury, UK
Chapter 49: Disorders of balance

Bhik Kotecha MB BCh, MPhil, FRCS, DLO
Consultant Otolaryngologist
Royal National Throat, Nose and Ear Hospital
London and Queens Hospital
Essex, UK
Chapter 16: Snoring and OSA in adults

Haytham Kubba MBBS, MPhil, MD, FRCS (ORL-HNS)
Consultant Paediatric Otolaryngologist
Royal Hospital for Sick Children
Glasgow, UK
Chapter 67: Choanal atresia

Thushitha Kunanandam FRCS (ORL-HNS)
Consultant Paediatric Otorhinolaryngologist
Royal Hospital for Sick Children
Glasgow, UK
Chapter 3: Epistaxis

Michael S W Lee MBChB, FRCSEd, FRCS (ORL-HNS) Eng
Consultant ENT Head and Neck Surgeon
Honorary Senior Lecturer
St. George's Hospital
St. George's University of London
London, UK
Chapter 22: Infections of the larynx

Valerie J Lund CBE, MS, FRCS, FRCSEd
Professor of Rhinology
University College London
Honorary Consultant ENT Surgeon
Royal National Throat Nose and Ear Hospital
London, UK
Chapter 5: Granulomatous conditions of the nose

Fiona B MacGregor MBChB, FRCS, FRCS (ORL)
Consultant Otolaryngologist, and Head and Neck Surgeon
Gartnavel General Hospital
Glasgow, UK
Chapter 61: Tumours and cysts of the head and neck

Kenneth Mackenzie FRCSEd
Visiting Professor
University of Strathclyde
Honorary Clinical Senior Lecturer
University of Glasgow
Glasgow, UK
Chapter 27: Tumours of the larynx

Samit Majumdar BM BS, BMedSci (Hon), FRCSEd, FDS RCPS, MFST Ed, FRCSEd (ORL-HNS)
Honorary Senior Lecturer
Consultant Ear, Nose and Throat Surgeon
Ninewells Hospital and Medical School
Dundee, UK
Chapter 32: Disorders of voice

Ann-Louise McDermott BDS, FDSRCS, MBChB, FRCS (ORL-HNS), PhD
Consultant Paediatric Otolaryngologist
The Birmingham Children's Hospital
Birmingham, UK
Chapter 59: Tracheostomy

Simon A McKean MBChB, BSc, DOHNS, FRCS (ORL-HNS) Glasg
Consultant ENT Surgeon
Raigmore Hospital
Inverness, UK
Chapter 53: Otitis externa

Philip McLoughlin MBBS, FDSRCS, FRCS
Consultant Oral and Maxillofacial Surgeon
NHS Tayside
Associate Medical Director Surgical Directorate
Consultant Maxillofacial Surgeon
Ninewells Hospital
Dundee, UK
Chapter 26: Tumours of the oral cavity

Emma McNeill MBBS, MSc, FRCS (ORL-HNS)
Consultant
Sunderland Royal Hospital
Sunderland, UK
Chapter 13: Smell and anosmia

Hisham Mehanna PhD, BMedSci (Hon), MBChB (Hon), FRCS, FRCS (ORL-HNS)
Chair of Head and Neck Surgery
School of Cancer Sciences
Director
Institute of Head and Neck Studies and Education
University of Birmingham
Birmingham, UK
Chapter 36: Neck masses

Mary-Louise Montague MBChB (Hon), PG, Dip Clin Ed, FRCS (ORL-HNS)
Consultant Paediatric Otolaryngologist
The Royal Hospital for Sick Children
Honorary Senior Clinical Lecturer
University of Edinburgh
Edinburgh, UK
Chapter 57: Acute rhinosinusitis and complications

Gavin Morrison MA, FRCS
Consultant Otolaryngologist
Guy's and St Thomas' NHS Foundation Trust
Evelina London Children's Hospital
London, UK
Chapter 63: Acute otitis media and mastoiditis

Salil Nair MD, FRCS (ORL-HNS)
Consultant Rhinologist and Anterior Skull Base Surgery
Honorary Senior Lecturer
Auckland University Hospitals (ADHB & CMDHB)
Auckland, NZ
Chapter 15: Specific chronic nasal infections

Antony A Narula MA, FRCS, FRCSEd
Visiting Professor
Middlesex University
Formerly ENT Consultant
Imperial Healthcare
London, UK
Chapter 64: Otitis media with effusion

Desmond A Nunez MBBS, MD, FRCS (ORL), FRCSC
Associate Professor
Head
Division of Otolaryngology
Department of Surgery
The University of British Columbia
Diamond Health Care Centre
Vancouver, Canada
Chapter 40: Tests for hearing

Graham R Ogden BDS, MDSc, PhD, FDS RCPS, FDS RCS Eng, FHEA, FRSA
Head of Division of Oral and Maxillofacial Clinical Sciences
University of Dundee Dental Hospital and School
Dundee, UK
Chapter 30: Benign diseases of the oral cavity

Nashreen Banon Oozeer FRCSEd (ORL-HNS)
Head and Neck Surgeon
City Hospitals Sunderland NHS Foundation Trust
Sunderland, UK
Chapter 51: Otological trauma

Vinidh Paleri MS, FRCS (ORL-HNS)
Consultant Head-Neck and Thyroid Surgeon
Otolaryngology—Head and Neck Surgery
Newcastle upon Tyne Hospitals NHS Trust
Honorary Professor of Head and Neck Surgery
Northern Institute for Cancer Research
Newcastle University
Newcastle upon Tyne, UK
Chapter 36: Neck masses

Nimesh Patel FRCS (ORL)
Consultant ENT Head and Neck Surgeon
Honorary Senior Lecturer
University of Southampton
Southampton General Hospital
Southampton, UK
Chapter 18: Investigation of pharyngeal disease

Henry Pau MD, MBChB, FRCSEd, FRCSEd (ORL-HNS), FRCS (ad eundem)
Consultant Otorhinolaryngologist
University Hospitals of Leicester
Visiting Professor
Department of Healthcare Engineering
Loughborough University
Loughborough, UK
Chapter 48: Tinnitus

Carl Philpott MBChB, DLO, FRCS (ORL-HNS), MD, PGCME
Anthony Long Senior Lecturer
Norwich Medical School
University of East Anglia
Honorary Consultant ENT Surgeon and Rhinologist
James Paget University Hospital
Norwich, UK
Chapter 2: Investigation of nasal diseases

Paul Pracy BSc, MBBS, FRCS (Glas), FRCS, FRCS (ORL-HNS)
ENT - Consultant Surgeon
Queen Elizabeth Hospital, Queen Elizabeth Medical Centre
Birmingham, UK
Chapter 24: Tumours of the oropharynx

S J Prowse BSc, MB BCh, FRCS (ORL-HNS)
Specialist Registrar
Bradford Royal Infirmary
Bradford, UK
Chapter 62: The deaf child

Li Qi PhD, MSc, RAUD (C)
Senior Audiologist
Audiology Practice Lead
Neuro-otology Unit
Vancouver General Hospital
Vancouver, Canada
Chapter 40: Tests for hearing

Muhammad Shahed Quarishi FRCS, FRCS (ORL-HNS)
Consultant Otolaryngologist
Thyroid and Parathyroid Surgeon
Director
ENT Masterclass®
Honorary Senior Lecturer in Surgical Oncology
University of Sheffield
Doncaster Royal Infirmary
Sheffield, UK
Chapter 38: The parathyroid

C H Raine MBE, BSc, MBBS, ChM, FRCS (Otol)
Consultant ENT Surgeon
Bradford Royal Infirmary
Bradford, UK
Chapter 62: The deaf child

Peter A Rea MA, FRCS
Consultant ENT Surgeon
Chairman British Society of Neuro-otology
Secretary British Society of Otology
Leicester, UK
Chapter 41: Tests for balance

Andrew Reid MBChB (Birm), FRCSEd
University Hospitals Birmingham NHS Trust
Birmingham, UK
Chapter 43: Acute otitis media

Joanne Rimmer MA, FRCS (ORL-HNS)
Consultant ENT Surgeon/Rhinologist
Monash Health
Honorary Senior Lecturer
University of Monash
Melbourne, Australia
Chapter 5: Granulomatous conditions of the nose

Peter J Robb BSc (Hon), MBBS, FRCS, FRCSEd
Consultant ENT Surgeon
Epsom and St Helier University Hospitals NHS Trust
Epsom, UK
Chapter 56: Tonsils and adenoids

Andrew Robson FRCS (ORL)
Consultant Otolaryngologist
North Cumbria University Hospitals NHS Trust
Carlisle, UK
Chapter 20: Infections of the pharynx

Matt Rollin FRCS (ORL-HNS)
Dept of ENT/Head and Neck Surgery
Imperial College Healthcare
London, UK
Chapter 64: Otitis media with effusion

Peter D Ross MBChB (Dundee), FRCS (ORL-HNS) Glas, FRCS Edin
Consultant Otolaryngologist
NHS Tayside
Honorary Senior Clinical Tutor
University of Dundee
Dundee, UK
Chapter 10: Nasal and facial trauma

Shakeel R Saeed MD, FRCS (ORL)
Professor of Otology/Neuro-otology
University College London Ear Institute
Consultant ENT and Skullbase Surgeon
Clinical Director
The Royal National Throat, Nose and Ear Hospital and National Hospital for Neurology and Neurosurgery
London, UK
Chapter 50: Cerebellopontine angle tumours

Anshul Sama BMedSci, BMBSc, FRCS (Gen Surg), FRCS (Otol)
Consultant Rhinologist
Nottingham University Hospital
Nottingham Woodthorpe Hospital
Visiting Professor
Loughborough University
Associate Director
Trent Simulation and Clinical Skills Centre
Loughborough, UK
Chapter 1: Anatomy and physiology of the nose and paranasal sinuses

Jaswinder S Sandhu MPhys, MBChB, MSc, CS (Aud), PhD
Clinical Research Fellow in Neurotology
Royal Hallamshire Hospital Sheffield Teaching Hospitals
Sheffield, UK
Chapter 41: Tests for balance

David K Selvadurai MD, FRCS, FACS
Director
Auditory Implant Service
St Georges Hospital
London, UK
Chapter 47: Sensorineural hearing loss

Muhammad Shakeel MBBS, FRCS (ORL)
Fellow
Otolaryngology Head and Neck Surgery
Counties-Manukau Health Hospitals
Auckland, NZ
Chapter 31: Neck space infections; Chapter 69: Drooling

E Mary Shanks FRCS
Consultant ENT Surgeon
Department of Otolaryngology
Cross Hospital
Kilmarnock, UK
Chapter 55: Implants in otology

Somiah Siddiq MRCS, DOHNS
ENT Registrar
University Hospitals Coventry and Warwickshire NHS Trust
Coventry, UK
Chapter 52: The facial nerve

Christopher J Skilbeck MPhil (Cantab), FRCS (ORL-HNS)
Locum Consultant ENT Skull Base Surgeon
Guy's and St Thomas' Hospitals
NHS Foundation Trust
London, UK
Chapter 50: Cerebellopontine angle tumours

Sanjai Sood MBChB, FRCS (CSiG), FRCS (ORL-HNS)
Consultant Otorhinolaryngologist - Head and Neck Surgeon
Bradford Teaching Hospitals
Bradford, UK
Chapter 34: Laryngo-tracheal trauma

Patrick M Spielmann MBChB, FRCS (ORL-HNS)
Consultant Otolaryngologist
University Department of Otolaryngology
Ninewells Hospital and Medical School
Dundee, UK
Chapter 42: Diseases of the external ear

Nicholas D Stafford MB, FRCS
Professor of Otolaryngology/Head and Neck Surgery
Hull York Medical School
Kingston upon Hull, UK
Chapter 23: Tumours of the nasopharynx

Thiru Sudarshan MBBS, DMRD, FRCR, EBHNR
Consultant Radiologist
Department of Clinical Radiology
Ninewells Hospital and Medical School
Dundee, UK
Chapter 70: ENT head and neck radiology

Iain R C Swan MBChB, MD, FRCS
Senior Lecturer in Otolaryngology
University of Glasgow
Honorary Consultant Otologist
Glasgow Royal Infirmary
Consultant Otologist
MRC/CSO Institute of Hearing Research
Glasgow, UK
Chapter 46: Otosclerosis

Andrew C Swift MBChB, ChM, FRCS, FRCSEd
Consultant ENT Surgeon and Rhinologist
Aintree University Hospital
Liverpool
Honorary Senior Lecturer
Edge Hill University
Ormskirk, UK
Chapter 4: Acute rhinosinusitis and its complications

Conrad Timon MD, FRCS (Ire), FRCS (ORL)
Clinical Professor of Otolaryngology
Head and Neck Surgeon
Trinity College
St James Hospital
Dublin, UK
Chapter 33: Vocal cord paralysis

Joseph G Toner MB, MA, FRCS
Consultant ENT Surgeon
Hone Senior Lecturer
Queen's University and The Victoria Infirmary
Belfast, UK
Chapter 44: Chronic otitis media

Francis M Vaz FRCS
Consultant ENT and Head and Neck Surgeon
University College London Hospitals
London, UK
Chapter 37: Dysphagia

Peter Wardrop FRCSEd (ORL-HNS)
Consultant ENT Surgeon
Scottish Cochlear Implant Centre
Crosshouse Hospital
Kilmarnock, UK
Chapter 55: Implants in otology

Paul S White MBChB, FRCSEd, FRACS
Consultant ENT Surgeon and Rhinologist
Ninewells Hospital and Medical School
Dundee, UK
Chapter 7: The blocked nose

Tim J Woolford MD, FRCS (ORL-HNS)
Consultant Ear, Nose and Throat Surgeon
University Department of Otolaryngology - Head and Neck Surgery
Manchester Royal Infirmary
Manchester, UK
Chapter 11: Facial plastic surgery

Robin Youngs MD, FRCS
Consultant Otolaryngologist
Gloucestershire Hospitals NHS Foundation Trust
Gloucester, UK
Chapter 6: Chronic rhinosinusitis

SECTION I

The Nose

1

Anatomy and physiology of the nose and paranasal sinuses

TAWAKIR KAMANI AND ANSHUL SAMA

EMBRYOLOGY OF THE NOSE AND PARANASAL SINUSES

The nose and paranasal sinuses are interlinked during development. At the end of the gestational fourth week, branchial arches, branchial pouches and primitive gut make their appearance. This is when the embryo gets its first identifiable head and face with an orifice in its middle known as the stomodeum (primitive mouth). The stomodeum is surrounded bilaterally by mandibular and maxillary prominences, which are derivatives of the first arch. The stomodeum is limited superiorly by the presence of the frontonasal eminence and inferiorly by the mandibular arch. Inferiorly, the frontonasal process gives two projections, the nasal placodes. These fuse to form the nasal cavity and primitive choana. The primitive choana forms the point of development of the posterior pharyngeal wall and the various paranasal sinuses.[1]

DEVELOPMENT OF THE NOSE AND NASAL CAVITY

Development of the nasal cavity

The primitive nasal cavity forms as the maxillary process of the first branchial arch and grows anteriorly and medially, fusing with the medial nasal folds and the frontonasal processes. The bucconasal membrane initially separates the primitive nasal cavity from the mouth, but it eventually breaks down, forming the primitive choanae. The palatal processes derived from the lateral maxillary mesoderm grow medially, fusing in the midline with each other and the septum to separate the nasal and oral cavities anteriorly. Posteriorly, this midline floor separates the nasopharynx and oral cavities and forms the soft palate.[1]

Development of the external nose and nasal septum

The lateral nasal folds form the nasal bones and the upper and lower lateral cartilages during the tenth to eleventh weeks. The nasal septum arises from a dorsal extending midline ridge from the posterior end of the frontonasal processes. This is continuous with the partition of the primitive nasal cavities anteriorly. The superior and posterior part of the primitive nasal septum ossifies to form the perpendicular plate and vomer, respectively. The anterior and inferior portions remain cartilaginous to form the quadrilateral cartilaginous septum.

DEVELOPMENT OF THE PARANASAL SINUSES

Development of the maxillary sinus

The maxillary sinus is the first to develop, appearing as a shallow groove in the primitive ethmoidal infundibulum into the maxilla at 7–10 weeks. At birth it measures 7 × 4 × 4 mm. It shows a biphasic growth at 3 and 12 years of age.

Development of the ethmoid sinus

The fetus develops six to seven folds in the lateral nasal wall at the ninth and tenth weeks. These folds fuse, forming crests termed *ethmoturbinates* from which the permanent ethmoidal structures develop. The first crest gives rise to the agger nasi and the uncinate process. The ethmoidal bulla arises from the second crest. The third crest is the basal lamella of the middle turbinate that divides the ethmoidal air cells in the anterior and posterior groups. The other structures that arise from these crests include the middle, superior and supreme turbinates, and all are seen to be attached to the lateral nasal wall by their basal lamella.

Development of the sphenoid sinus

The sphenoid sinus appears at the third intrauterine month as an evagination from the sphenoethmoidal recess and is about 2 × 2 × 1.5 mm at birth, to reach adult size at the age of 12–18 years.

Development of the frontal sinus

The frontal sinus starts developing at the fourth intrauterine month. The frontal sinus, the anterior ethmoidal complex and the complex array of the frontoethmoidal cells develop from five or so pits that lie between the first and second ethmoturbinates. The frontal bone is very poorly pneumatized at birth and the frontal sinuses not distinguishable from the anterior ethmoid complex. The fetal pits start to pneumatize the frontal bone and can be noted at the end of the first year of life. One of these fetal pits continues to pneumatize both plates of the frontal sinus such that by the twelfth year of life the frontal sinuses have largely developed.

ANATOMY OF THE NOSE AND PARANASAL SINUSES

THE EXTERNAL NOSE

The external nose is a pyramidal structure with a framework of bone and cartilage, covered by connective tissue and skin. The bony structure is made of the nasal bones, which unite superiorly with the frontal bone at the nasion and laterally with the frontal processes of the maxilla. The distal two-thirds of the nose is formed by the upper and lower lateral cartilages, which overlap each other at the margins. The upper lateral cartilages fuse medially with the quadrilateral cartilage, forming the cartilaginous part of the nasal dorsum. The lower lateral cartilages, also called the *alar cartilages*, are each composed of the medial and lateral crus connected by the intermediate crus. The latter forms the dome of the nostril and the tip-defining points. The medial crus contributes to the columella attached posteriorly with the membranous septum. The lateral crus forms the alar or nostril rim.

Branches of the facial artery supply the alar region, and branches of the ophthalmic and maxillary artery supply the dorsum and lateral walls. The venous drainage is to two units: the angular vein and the ophthalmic veins. The latter interlinks with the anterior ethmoid system and thence into the cavernous sinus. The submandibular and submental nodes provide the main lymphatic drainage to the external nose.[2]

THE NASAL CAVITY AND PARANASAL SINUSES

The nasal cavity extends from the nostrils anteriorly to the choanae posteriorly, where it becomes continuous with the nasopharynx. The nasal cavity is divided in the midline by the nasal septum, which forms the medial wall of the nasal passages. The roof is formed anteriorly by the undersurface of the upper lateral cartilages and nasal bones, and posteriorly by the cribriform plate, which houses the olfactory epithelium. The rest of the nasal cavity is lined by respiratory epithelium. The nasal floor is made up of the palatine process of the maxillary bone anteriorly, fused with the horizontal process of the palatal bones posteriorly.

Nasal septum

The nasal septum is composed of a small anterior membranous portion, the cartilaginous portion called *quadrilateral cartilage* and the bony portions of the perpendicular plate of the ethmoid, the vomer and the nasal crests of the maxilla and palatine bones. These components articulate as shown in Figure 1.1. The medial crura of the lower lateral cartilages attach to the thin membranous septum anteriorly, forming one of the major tip support structures. At its upper margin, the quadrilateral cartilage is connected to the upper lateral cartilages, contributing to the projection and height of the mid-third of the nose. The keystone area represents the attachment of the quadrangular cartilage to the bony septum and nasal bones at the rhinion. Continuity and fixation at this point are important both aesthetically and functionally because it supports the projection of the upper third to mid-third of the nose.

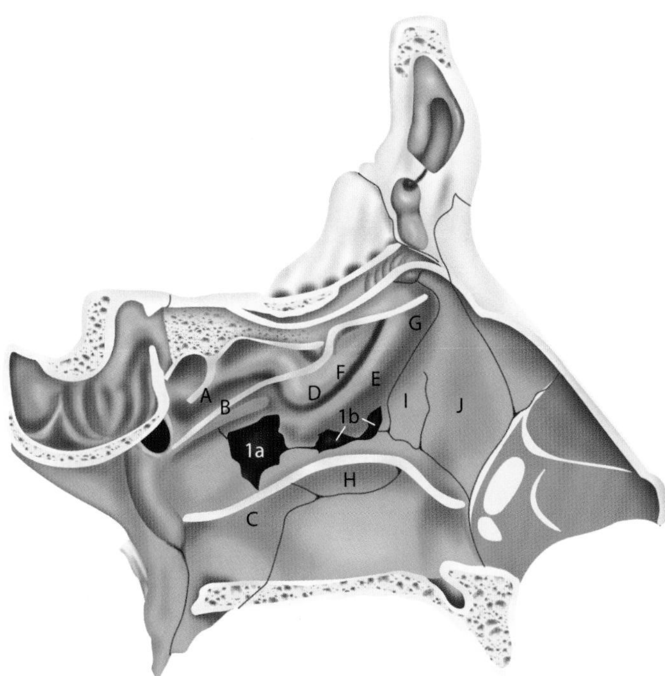

Figure 1.1 Left lateral nasal wall on removal of the turbinates. A, sphenoethmoidal recess; B, basal lamella; C, palatine bone; D, ethmoid bulla; E, uncinate process; F, hiatus semilunaris; G, aggar cell; H, maxillary process of inferior turbinate; I , lacrimal bone; J, frontal process of maxillary bone; 1a, posterior fontanel; 1b, anterior fontanels.

Lateral nasal wall

The lateral wall of the nasal cavity is predominantly composed of the maxilla, with contribution from the perpendicular plate of the palatine bone and the medial pterygoid plate posteriorly. The anterior aspect of the lateral wall has contributions from the nasal bones and upper lateral cartilage, the latter forming the internal nasal valve at its junction with the nasal septum. There are three prominences on the lateral nasal wall termed *inferior, middle,* and *superior turbinates*, respectively. Occasionally, there may be a fourth turbinate called the *supreme turbinate.* The spaces lateral to the turbinates are called *meati.* Figure 1.2 illustrates this anatomy.

The inferior turbinate develops as a separate bone whilst the middle, superior and supreme turbinates are medial projections of the ethmoid complex. Lateral to the inferior turbinate is a recess called the *inferior meatus* into which the nasolacrimal duct opens.[3]

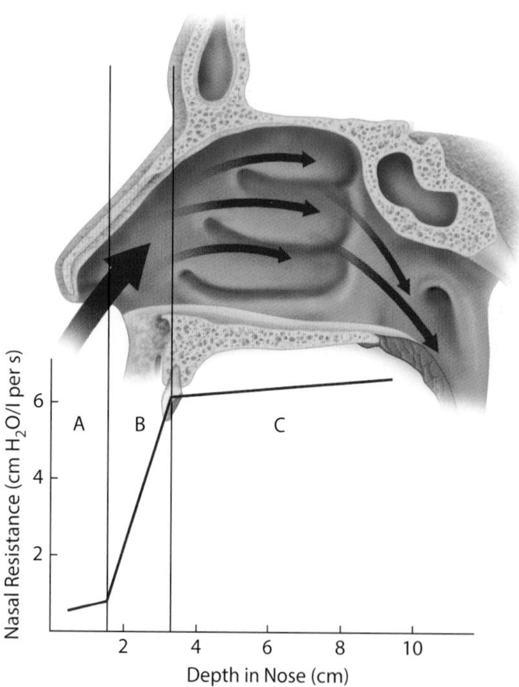

Figure 1.2 Nasal resistance and laminar airflow within the nasal cavity.

The middle turbinate has a complex configuration and attachment. Anterosuperiorly it is attached to the skull base, and posteriorly it curves laterally to attach to the lamina papyrecea forming a lamella termed the *basal lamella.* The basal lamella divides the ethmoidal complex into an anterior and a posterior group. Lateral to the middle turbinate is a recess termed the *middle meatus.* The middle meatus is a recess into which drain the frontal, maxillary and anterior ethmoid sinuses.

Two distinct bony prominences are seen laterally on removal of the vertical portion of the middle turbinate: the uncinate process and the ethmoid bulla. The uncinate process is a thin, boomerang-shaped bone anterior to the ethmoid bulla. It attaches to the lacrimal bone anteriorly and to the inferior turbinate inferiorly. The posterior margin of the uncinate process is unattached and forms a sickle-shaped cleft between its free margin and the anterior face of the ethmoid bulla, called *hiatus semilunaris.* The hiatus semilunaris communicates laterally with a three-dimensional space, the ethmoidal infundibulum, bounded anteriorly by the aggar nasi and frontoethmoidal cells, medially by the uncinate process, posteriorly by the bulla ethmoidalis and laterally by the lamina papyracea.[4] See Figure 1.3.

The blood supply to the lateral nasal wall and septum is mainly provided by the branches of the sphenopalatine artery with contribution from the anterior and posterior ethmoid artery, the greater palatine artery and the facial artery. Nerve supply is from the nasociliary branch of the anterior ethmoidal nerve, branches of the pterygopalatine ganglion and anterior palatine nerves. Lymphatic drainage is to the submandibular nodes anteriorly and to the retropharyngeal and upper deep cervical nodes posteriorly.

The ethmoid sinus

The ethmoid sinuses are the most variable of the sinuses and develop from pneumatization of the ethmoid bone. When this pneumatization extends to the middle turbinate, it is termed a *concha bullosa.* Occasionally, the pneumatization of the ethmoid bone can extend beyond the ethmoid bone. These extra-ethmoidal pneumatizations

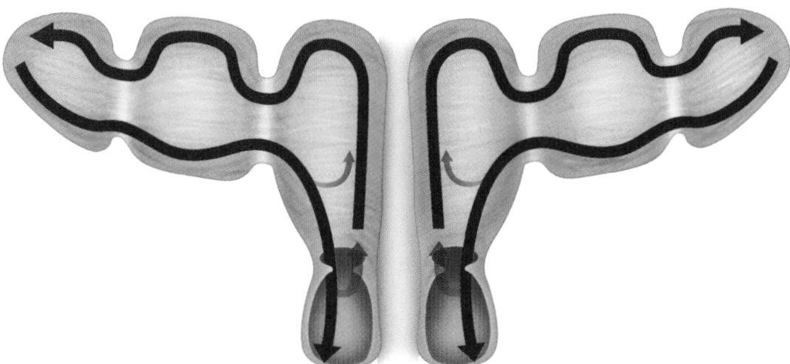

Figure 1.3 Direction and movement of mucociliary activity within the frontal sinus.

are often allocated with specific terms: orbit bone (supraorbital cell), roof of the maxillary sinus (Haller cell), floor of the frontal sinus (fronto-ethmoidal cell) and superolateral to the sphenoid sinus (onodi cell).

The ethmoid roof is seen to slope medially and posteriorly. Medially, it forms the fovea ethmoidalis and the cribriform plate. The lamina papyracae separates the ethmoid sinus laterally from the orbit. The sphenoid sinus forms the posterior boundary of the ethmoid sinuses.

A number of bony septa divide the ethmoidal sinus into up to 18 air cells, and these are grouped to form the anterior and posterior ethmoid air cells depending on their relationship to the basal lamella. The attachment of the basal lamella of the middle turbinate divides the anterior and posterior ethmoid systems.

The largest of the anterior ethmoid air cells is the ethmoid bulla. This is the most consistent surgical landmark. It may be unpneumatized in 8 per cent of patients. The ground lamella constitutes the posterior boundary of the bulla ethmoidalis. Suprabullar and retrobullar recesses may be formed when the ethmoid bulla does not extend to the skull base. The suprabullar recess is formed when there is a cleft between the roof of the ethmoid bulla and the fovea. The retrobullar space is formed when there is a cleft between the basal lamella and the bulla. These spaces are collectively called the *lateral sinus*. The ostia of the anterior ethmoid cells open into the ethmoid infundibulum in the middle meatus. The most anterior ethmoid air cell is called the *agger nasi cell*. The face of the bulla attaches to the skull base immediately anterior to the anterior ethmoid artery. The anterior ethmoid artery exits the orbit through the lamina papyracae and courses horizontally across the roof of the ethmoid sinus in a thin bony mesentery (dehiscent inferiorly in 40 per cent of patients) to enter the cribriform plate and anterior cranial cavity through the fovea ethmoidalis. It then vertically penetrates the most anterior aspect of the cribriform plate to enter the nasal cavity to supply the septum and the anterosuperior nasal cavity as the terminal septal branch. The posterior cells drain into the superior or supreme meatus. The most posterior ethmoidal air cell may extend superiorly and laterally to the sphenoid in 10 per cent of cases (the onodi cell) and may have the optic nerve and internal carotid artery bulging into it.

The blood supply to the ethmoid sinus is from branches of the anterior and posterior ethmoidal and sphenopalatine arteries. Venous drainage follows the arterial supply. Lymph drainage is to submandibular and retropharyngeal nodes. The innervation is from the supraorbital, anterior ethmoidal and orbital branches from the pterygopalatine ganglion.

The maxillary sinus

The maxillary sinus lies within the maxillary bone and is pyramidal in shape, with its base forming part of the lateral nasal wall and its apex pointing towards the zygomatic process. The roof of the sinus constitutes the orbital floor and contains the infraorbital nerve, which may be dehiscent in 14 per cent of cases. The alveolar process of the maxilla and the hard palate form the floor of the maxillary sinus. The thinnest part of the anterior wall corresponds with the canine fossa. The posterior wall separates the maxillary sinus from the pterygomaxillary fossa and its contents, i.e. the internal maxillary artery, sphenopalatine ganglion and greater palatine nerve.

At the superior aspect of the medial wall of the sinus, opening into the region of the inferior aspect of the ethmoid infundibulum, is the natural ostium. This is normally hidden from view by an intact uncinate process and therefore cannot be visualized endoscopically. The nasolacrimal duct runs 4–9 mm anterior to the ostium. The medial wall of the maxillary sinus has areas of bony dehiscence usually covered by mucosa called the *anterior and posterior fontanels*. In up to 30 per cent of cases these may be patent, usually at the posterior fontanel, to form an accessory ostium. The accessory ostia are nonfunctional.

Branches of the internal maxillary artery, i.e. the infraorbital and greater palatine arteries, provide the blood supply, and venous drainage is through the pterygoid plexus and facial vein. Lymphatic drainage is to the submandibular lymph nodes. The infraorbital, greater palatine and superior alveolar nerves provide the nerve supply to the maxillary sinus mucosa.

Frontal sinus

Frontal bone pneumatization to develop the frontal sinus is variable, with approximately 5 per cent of the population demonstrating no frontal sinuses. Being a midline sinus, the two sides are usually separated by intersinus septa, with both frontal sinuses draining independently at the lowest medial portion of the cavity. The frontal sinus drains into the superior aspect of the ethmoid infundibulum via the frontal recess.

The anterior and posterior walls of the frontal sinus are composed of diploeic bone. The posterior wall separates the frontal sinus from the anterior cranial fossa and is much thinner. The floor of the sinus also functions as a portion of the orbital roof. The supraorbital and supratrochlear branches of the ophthalmic artery provide its blood supply, but venous drainage is to the cavernous sinus via the superior ophthalmic veins and to the dural sinuses through the posterior wall venules. The supraorbital and supratrochlear nerves provide its innervation.

Sphenoid sinus

The sphenoid sinuses are the deepest of the paranasal sinuses pneumatizing the sphenoid bone. The sinus can be absent in about 1 per cent of the population. Like the frontal sinus, sphenoid sinuses are divided, often asymmetrically, by a septum in the paramedian position. Anteroinferiorly, the sphenoid rostrum articulates with the perpendicular plate and vomer of the nasal septum. The sphenoid sinus ostium lies in the anterior medial wall of the sinus and drains medial to the superior turbinate into the sphenoethmoidal recess.

Several important vascular and neural structures lie in the walls of the sphenoid sinus and can indent the walls to a variable degree depending on the degree of pneumatization. The posterior wall is formed by the sella turcica superiorly and clival bone inferiorly. The clival carotid artery traverses vertically in the clival portion of the posterior wall and loops forward in the cavernous portion. Together with the optic nerve, these are prominences evident in the superolateral wall of the sphenoid sinus, with an indentation separating the two called the *lateral oculo-carotid recess*. The maxillary part of the trigeminal nerve traverses the lateral wall and the vidian nerve of the floor of the sphenoid sinus. Some bony dehiscence over structures such as the optic nerve (6 per cent of the population) and carotid arteries (8 per cent of the population) are not infrequent. Intersinus septa can often be in continuity with the carotid and the optic canal, and uncontrolled avulsion can result in a catastrophic bleed or blindness.[4]

Apart from the roof, which is supplied by the posterior ethmoid artery, the rest of the sphenoid receives its blood supply from the sphenopalatine artery. Venous drainage is via the maxillary veins to the jugular and pterygoid plexus systems. The nasociliary nerve supplies the roof, whilst the floor receives its innervations from branches of the sphenopalatine nerve.

PHYSIOLOGY OF THE NOSE AND PARANASAL SINUSES

The two main functions of the nose are respiration and olfaction.

RESPIRATION

The nose is solely responsible for the warming and humidification of air that reaches the lungs. Humidification is facilitated by evaporation of the secretions of the numerous serous glands found in the mucosal blanket and condensation of expired air at the anterior nose. Air is humidified to 75–80 per cent.

Warming occurs as cool, inspired air creates a temperature gradient as it comes into contact with the counterflowing rich arterial blood from the sphenopalatine artery, especially the inferior turbinate mucosa, such that the air reaching the postnasal space is approximately 31°C. Although this countercurrent exchange creates a more efficient heat exchange, this process remains imperfect, with as much as 10 per cent of total body heat being lost through the nose with expired air. Filtration of inspired air occurs first in the nose. The vibrissae filter the largest particles, and the mucous blanket filters the rest. The mucous membrane is enriched with immunoglobulin A (IgA), providing the first line of immunological defence.[5]

OLFACTION

Olfaction is the perception of smell and is a primal sense for humans and animals, allowing receptors to identify food and mates, and provide warnings of danger (such as fires or chemical dangers) as well as sensual pleasures (such as perfumes). For an odorant molecule to reach the olfactory area, turbulent airflow from the anterior nares is required. About 15 per cent of inspired air reaches the olfactory area within the nose, where it interacts with the mucus secreted by the Bowman's glands in the lamina propria and respiratory epithelium. To reach the olfactory receptors, the odorant molecules must be soluble in the mucus and need high water and lipid solubility. These molecules react with the lipid bilayer of the receptor cells at specific sites, which causes an efflux of K+ and CI–, resulting in depolarization of the cells. This process is mediated by G-protein coupled receptors in the cells that interact with a specific adenyl cyclase within the neuroepithelium.

Olfactory responses show variations in both thresholds and adaptation depending on the chemical nature of the stimuli. Thresholds of perception are lower than identification, because smells are sensed before they are recognized. Changes in the composition of the mucus can influence the diffusion time required for odorant molecules to reach the receptor sites. The beta-adrenergic, cholinergic, and peptidergic agents' effect on the sensory perception of smell is through their effect on the secretory activities of the mucosal layer.

These functions are facilitated by a number of physiological systems, which are described in the following sections.

Airflow

The biomechanics of airflow and nasal resistance is described by Bernoulli's and Raymond's equations, given below. Based on laminar flow equations, decreases in *r*, or the nasal airway radius, cause four-fold decreases in flow, as described by Bernoulli's equation.

$$Q = (\Delta P \pi r^4)/(8 \eta L)$$

Reynolds number = $2rQ \rho/\eta$ (Reynolds number greater than 2000 is equated with turbulent flow)

where L = length, r = radius, P = pressure, η = viscosity, and ρ = density.

The presence of laminar or turbulent flow is pertinent to the physiology of air exchange. The cross section within the nose is variable, and this continuously alters the pressure and velocity within the system. During inspiration, the airflow is directed upwards and backwards from the nasal valve mainly over the anterior part of the inferior turbinate, below and over the middle turbinate and then into the posterior choana. Air reaches the other parts of the nose to a lesser degree. The

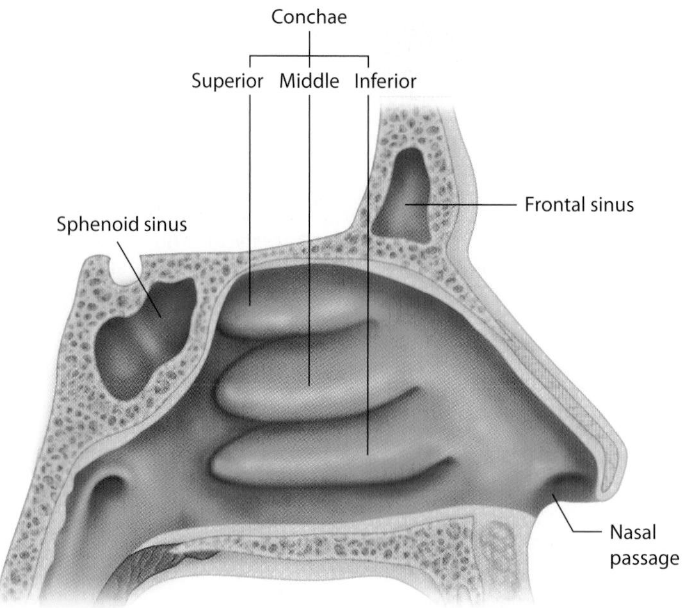

Figure 1.4 Lateral nasal wall with the superior, middle and inferior turbinates.

velocity at the anterior valve is 12–18 m/s during quiet respiration, and it is considered laminar, although in practice it is turbulent even in quiet respiration, producing eddies in the olfactory region. Turbulent flow results when the velocity of nasal flow is increased. Expiration lasts longer than inspiration, and flow is more turbulent. A sniff is required to facilitate olfaction with turbulent airflow. Narrowing or alterations at the nasal valve area (septal perforations, septal deviations) result in turbulent flow within the nose, which can cause a sensation of obstruction regardless of nasal passage patency.[6] See Figure 1.4.

The nasal cycle

This feature of normal nasal physiology is a cyclical alteration in nasal resistance between the two nostrils secondary to alteration in vascular activity that regulates the volume of venous sinusoids (capacitance vessels) in the nasal erectile tissue (located primarily in the inferior turbinate and to a lesser extent in the anterior septum). These changes occur between 4 and 12 hours and enhance humidification, warming and mucociliary clearance. The nasal cycle is affected by factors such as allergy, infection, exercise, hormones, pregnancy, emotions, sexual activity and recumbent position.

The mucociliary system

The mucociliary system is a vital component of the normal sinonasal function of humidification, filtering of inspired air, and elimination of secretions and debris from the paranasal sinuses and nasal airway. This system consists of three components:

a. *Ciliated, pseudostratified columnar epithelium lines nasal and paranasal sinuses.* Cilia on the surface of these cells propel mucus backwards in the nose towards the postnasal space. Each cilium has a surface membrane and encloses an organized ultrastructure of nine paired outer microtubules that surround a single inner pair of microtubules. Outer-paired microtubules are linked together by nexins and to the inner pair by central spokes. Outer pairs also have inner and outer dynein arms.
b. *Double-layered mucous blanket* has a less viscous, watery layer (sol phase) in which cilia move freely as well as a superficial, more viscous mucous fluid (gel phase) into which the tips of the cilia enter to move it.

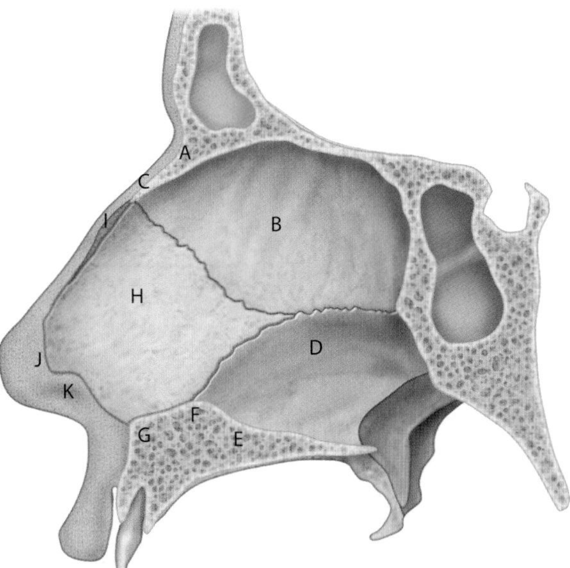

Figure 1.5 Nasal septum and its components. A, nasal spine of frontal bone; B, perpendicular plate of ethmoid; C, nasal bones; D, vomer; E, palatine process of maxillary bone; F, maxillary crest; G, anterior nasal spine; H, quadrilateral cartilage; I, upper lateral cartilage; J, lower lateral cartilage; K, columella.

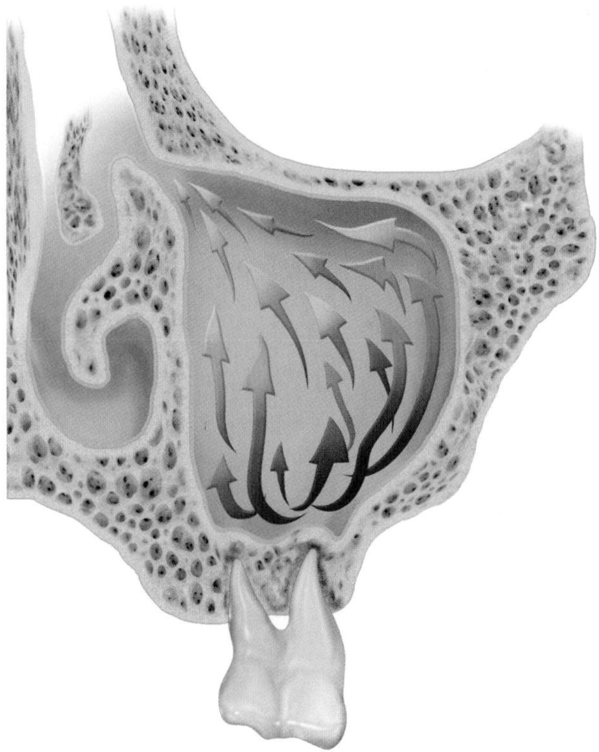

Figure 1.6 Direction and movement of mucociliary activity within the maxillary sinus.

c. *Mucous-producing glands* include goblet cells, seromucinous glands and intraepithelial glands. The major composition of nasal mucus is water (95 per cent), glycoproteins or mucin (3 per cent), salts (2 per cent), immunoglobulins (IgA), lysozymes (bacteriolytic) and lactoferrin (bacteriostatic).

The ciliated cells beat in a specific direction, resulting in a pattern of mucus flow. The cilia actively beat to propel mucus to the nasopharynx. This mucociliary flow occurs at 1 cm/min, and mucus stasis as a result of decreased beat frequency may allow noxious substances to penetrate the mucosa, resulting in disease. Pathological processes such as bacterial and viral infections impede ciliary beating by altering the ultrastructure or the viscosity of the mucous blanket.[7]

In the paranasal sinuses, the cilia beat such as to move material towards the sinus ostia. This means that cilia often move mucus against gravity to drain the sinus at its ostium. See Figure 1.6.

KEY LEARNING POINTS

- Continuity and fixation at the keystone area are important because this supports the projection of the upper third to mid third of the nose.
- The frontal, maxillary and anterior ethmoid sinuses drain into the middle meatus.
- Intersinus septa within the sphenoid sinus can often be in continuity with the internal carotid artery and the optic canal.
- Turbulent airflow within the nose can cause a sensation of obstruction regardless of the patency of the nasal passage.
- The nasal cycle is affected by allergy, infection, exercise, sexual activity and recumbent position.

REFERENCES

1. Moore KA. *The Developing Human.* Philadelphia: W.B. Saunders, 1982: 197–206.
2. Lund V, Stammberger H. *Anatomy of the Nose and Paranasal Sinuses.* In: *Scott-Brown's Otorhinolaryngology, Head and Neck Surgery.* Eds. Gleeson M, Browning G, Burton MJ, et al. London: Hodder Arnold, 2008: 1313–43.
3. Dharmbir S. *Applied Surgical Anatomy of the Nasal Cavity and Paranasal Sinuses.* In: Jones N. *Practical Rhinology.* London: Hodder Arnold, 2010: 1–14.
4. Stammberger H. *The Messerklinger Technique.* In: *Functional Endoscopic Sinus Surgery.* Ed. Stammberger H. Philadelphia: B.C. Dekker, 1991: 17–46.
5. Cole P. *Modification of Inspired Air.* In: *The Nose: Upper Airway Physiology and the Atmospheric Environment.* 1st ed. Eds. Proctor DJ, Andersen I. Amsterdam: Elsevier, 1982: 351–73.
6. Cole P. Nasal and oral airflow resistors site, function, and assessment. *Archives of Otolaryngology – Head and Neck Surgery.* 1992; 118(8): 790–3.
7. Drake-Lee A. *Physiology of the Nose and Paranasal Sinuses.* In: *Scott-Brown's Otorhinolaryngology, Head and Neck Surgery.* Eds. Gleeson M, Browning G, Burton MJ, et al. London: Hodder Arnold, 2008: 1355–71.

2

Investigation of nasal diseases

CARL PHILPOTT

INTRODUCTION

Rhinological diseases are very common, and whilst an array of investigative tools exists for them, many of these are not common practice in routine ear, nose and throat (ENT) clinics. The advent of the endoscope and the significant improvements seen in the imaging and image capture technology have allowed us to better see inside the nose and beyond. This not only gives the clinician a much more comprehensive assessment of the nose and sinuses, but also facilitates education and engagement of the patients themselves as they too can see the effects of their disease and the response to any treatments. The 'European Position Paper on Rhinosinusitis and Nasal Polyps' (EPOS) has been a key document for guiding clinicians involved in managing chronic rhinosinusitis, and it brings guidance as to the logical flow of investigation in this condition. This chapter will lay out the full armoury of investigations available for rhinological disease that are suitable both in clinical practice and in the research domain, or even in tertiary centres. It will also give some direction as to how these fit with the EPOS guidance and a framework for investigating rhinological disease.

HISTORY AND EXAMINATION

As with any part of medicine, history taking is the crucial step that should ideally precede all investigations, but symptom scores filled in by patients in the waiting room can certainly help to focus both the patient's and clinician's mind on the key symptoms that have brought the patient to the clinic. These questionnaires are discussed in further detail later, but the key is to utilize a validated questionnaire that is relevant to the patient's presenting complaint. Use of open questions initially will allow patients to address their concerns and the reason they believe they are sitting in front of you (which may not always be the reason they were referred). Following this, closed questions may be needed to checklist key rhinological symptoms that the patient may not have covered. These include:

- Congestion/blockage/obstruction
- Rhinorrhoea – anterior and posterior
- Olfactory disturbances – quantitative (reduced or absent) and qualitative (distorted)
- Facial pressure/pain
- Epistaxis and crusting

Other related symptoms include sneezing, itching, cough, fever, dental pain, otalgia/aural fullness, snoring, visual disturbances and nasal deformity, but this list is not exhaustive. It is also crucial to explore what patients actually mean because 'congestion' and 'facial pressure' often overlap for many, and it is common for patients to say, 'I've got sinus, doc' or something to that effect. Because the symptoms and their duration are the centre point to making the diagnosis of both rhinitis and rhinosinusitis, it is important to have focused on this in order to proceed with the appropriate investigations. When faced with olfactory disorders, it is equally important to listen to the patient carefully and explore exactly what his or her prime complaints are. Many patients will talk about loss of taste without there being any true gustatory disturbance. Also, patients may be significantly affected by olfactory distortions such as parosmia and phantosmia, which may even outweigh any actual loss of olfactory acuity.

The social and occupational history of many patients will also be relevant, especially in the presence of atopy, and may influence the subsequent management of the patient. Thus exploration of the presence of any animal contacts, work environment and smoking status is needed, and alcohol intake may also influence symptoms and may give a key to salicylate sensitivity. This leads to key factors in the medical history such as any adverse effects of aspirin and nonsteroidal anti-inflammatory drugs (NSAIDs) as well as other drugs that may influence nasal physiology such as β-blockers. Many patients will have concomitant respiratory disease, and the severity of this should be quantified along with an understanding of any key areas of interaction between the two (e.g. common triggers, exacerbations linked to upper airways).

Examination of the external nose can easily be achieved by carefully viewing the nose from in front of the patient as well as from above and underneath and finally from the side (profile view). Traditionally, using a head mirror and Mills lamp along with a Thudicum's forcep allowed a clinician to perform anterior rhinoscopy. Most modern ENT clinics provide a battery-operated headlight, and this can be used to perform anterior rhinoscopy, which is useful in assessing the nasal vestibule, nasal valve and anterior nasal septum, especially the position of the columella. Internal examination of the nose is best achieved with a rigid nasendoscope connected to a monitor and image capture device, and this should be considered the gold standard. In the face of most rhinological symptoms, this is the only sure way to carefully assess the nasal cavity and the relevant meati. Use of a flexible nasendoscope will reduce the ability to use suction or take biopsies. A common approach with the rigid endoscope is to use the three-pass technique, working from inferior to superior in the nose and identifying the three meati, the three turbinates and the postnasal space (Fig. 2.1). In this method a 0° endoscope is passed first along the nasal floor towards the postnasal space and if possible underneath the inferior turbinate. The second pass is into the middle meatus lateral to the middle turbinate allowing identification of the ethmoid bulla and uncinate process. The third pass is medial to the middle turbinate and into the sphenoethmoidal recess to identify the superior turbinate, superior meatus and sphenoid ostium. However, an alternative strategy is to use a 30° endoscope inserted into the nose with the bevel facing superiorly and insert the scope into the middle meatus. By rotating the light post, the endoscope can then be turned

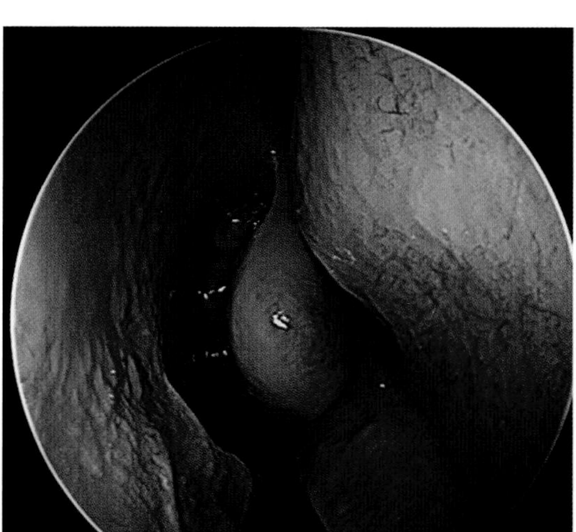

Figure 2.1 Endoscopic view of nose.

to visualize the middle meatus both laterally and then inferiorly and then passed under the middle turbinate towards the postnasal space. Here, rotation of the light post again will allow visualization of the superior meatus and sphenoid ostium. In a post-operative patient (after sinus surgery), the 30° endoscope should be mandatory to allow visualization of the sinus cavities, with a 70° endoscope in reserve if needed.

There are two schools of thought on the use of decongestant preparations prior to endoscopy. Some clinicians will routinely apply a spray such as co-phenylcaine to the nose before any examination, whereas others will choose to examine the nose without the influence of any vasoconstrictor. The latter approach gives the physician the advantage of being able to view the diseased mucosa in the nose in its current state as relevant to the patient's symptoms; this may be distorted by decongestants. Endoscopy requires a careful hand to avoid discomfort to the patient but can be seen as an extension of endoscopic sinus surgery where avoiding contact with the nasal mucosa reduces trauma to the mucosa and the need to clean the endoscope tip frequently. Nonetheless, some patients will need a local anaesthetic to tolerate the procedure or decongestant to enable visualization where anatomical variations such as a septal deviation are present.

MICROBIOLOGY

In chronic sinusitis without nasal polyps (CRSsNPs) identification of mucopus on endoscopy is one of the two ways in which the diagnosis based on the symptoms can be confirmed, and in the current EPOS guidelines indicates the potential use of long-term antibiotics (macrolides). However, retrieval of this material can also help to guide the clinician further in the appropriate choice of antibiotics because it will yield information on the bacterial sensitivity and resistance profiles. In the case of chronic sinusitis with nasal polyps (CRSwNPs), retrieval of thick eosinophilic mucin may be important in the process of defining a case of allergic fungal rhinosinusitis. This material should be sent for fungal smear and culture alongside the usual culture and sensitivity. Collection of such material can be achieved either by using a swab or by using one of a variety of suction traps such as a Leukens trap or a Xomed sinus secretion collector (Fig. 2.2). The latter has a more significant advantage in a post-operative patient in whom use of a curved suction tip can allow retrieval of mucus from sinus cavities. Although the evidence for the use of topical antibiotics is at present limited with formal randomized control trials (RCTs) lacking, culture-directed management can still be implemented so that any antibiotics given either orally or topically can be based on material sampled directly from the site of the disease process. This

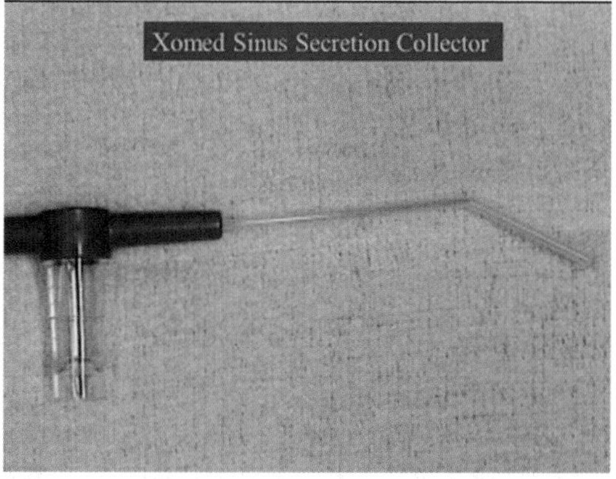

Figure 2.2 Xomed sinus secretion collector.

has the advantage of ensuring that antibiotic use is appropriate and helps to avoid resistant strains in common pathogens such as methicillin-resistant *Staphylococcus aureus* (MRSA). Liaison with colleagues in microbiology will also help to ensure that they understand your requirements, especially with respect to fungal specimens, for which it can be notoriously difficult to yield positive results.

BLOOD AND ALLERGY TESTS

The choice of chemical pathology testing will be largely influenced by the history. Investigation of atopy can be undertaken by either skin prick testing (SPT) or radioallergosorbent test (RAST), with the former considered the gold standard. However, this is dependent on staff availability to perform the skin prick. RASTs, on the other hand, are less involved in terms of staff resources in the clinic but are more costly to perform owing to the analysis required in the laboratory. RASTs do provide the option to test for allergens not available in routine sets of aeroallergens available for SPT, which may be useful for specific patient exposures or patients with suspected allergic fungal rhinosinusitis. The prevalence of atopy in chronic rhinosinusitis (CRS) varies in the literature but probably accounts for 50 per cent of CRS with nasal polyps (CRSwNPs). Detection of atopy in rhinitis will influence medical management and should be checked for if the history is unclear and initial medical measures have failed; in fact rhinitis cannot ultimately be classified as allergic or non-allergic without formal testing.

When considering blood tests, a total IgE level may indicate a patient's overall level of allergic response; in the latest EPOS guidelines, this is recommended in CRS without nasal polyps (CRSsNPs) to determine a patient's suitability for the use of macrolides. Other blood tests to be considered include:

- Full blood count (eosinophilia seen in allergic fungal rhinosinusitis and Churg-Strauss Syndrome, anaemia from epistaxis)
- Clotting screen – for epistaxis where anticoagulants used or deficiency suspected from history
- Immunoglobulin screening
- Blood markers of systemic diseases such as anti-neutrophil cystoplasmic antibody (ANCA), angiotensin-converting enzyme (ACE)
- Exclusion of potential underlying medical comorbidities (e.g. renal/hepatic dysfunction, hypothyroidism, Cushing's disease, sarcoidosis) in cases of suspected idiopathic anosmia

In patients with recurrent sinusitis or with CRS refractory to combined medical and surgical therapy, immunodeficiency should be considered (e.g. common variable immunodeficiency). An array of specific and complete immunodeficiencies is possible, with the most common ones found in the immunoglobulin G subclasses such as 2 and 3, which confer protection against common encapsulated nasal pathogens such as *Haemophilus influenzae*. The relevance of specific deficiencies should be assessed by referral to an immunology specialist; this may simply result in additional vaccinations being given. Severe combined immunodeficiencies will need much greater input from an immunologist.

If factors in the history or clues from examination suggest the possibility of systemic diseases such as sarcoidosis, these should be investigated on their own merit and, where appropriate, further corroborated with nasal biopsies.

CYTOLOGY AND HISTOLOGY

NASAL BRUSHINGS

Patients with rhinitis can grossly be divided into those with atopy (persistent or intermittent allergic rhinitis) and those who are not atopic. In a subset of those with non-allergic rhinitis, entopy may be present. This implies a local allergic response in the nasal mucosa that is not associated with a systemic atopic response seen on positive SPT/RASTs. This can be determined by taking a nasal brushing and sending it for cytological examination to look for eosinophilia. A positive result suggests a diagnosis of non-allergic rhinitis eosinophilia syndrome (NARES), which can be treated much the same as allergic rhinitis, although it may require a nasal allergen challenge to confirm this. A nasal brushing can be performed easily with a bronchial brush rubbed along the anterior inferior turbinate.

HISTOLOGICAL EXAMINATION

Unilateral nasal masses should always be viewed with suspicion, especially in the older patient, and consideration should be given to performing a biopsy. This decision will be taken on a case-by-case basis influenced by any sinister symptoms in the history such as unilateral epistaxis, crusting, orbital symptoms, numbness or cranial neuropathies. In certain cases it may be prudent to arrange imaging before a biopsy is undertaken, as follows:

- Possibility of the lesion arising from the skull base with intracranial extension (e.g. meningo-encephalocoele)
- Posterior unilateral nasal mass in a juvenile male patient (juvenile angiofibroma)

Other circumstances for taking a biopsy will include suspicion of systemic diseases such as Wegner's granulomatosis or as part of investigation of a septal perforation. The location in which the biopsy is performed will be influenced by patient suitability for local anaesthesia, equipment available in the clinic and the nature of the lesion/condition being investigated, but biopsy of many lesions can be appropriately performed in the clinic.

RADIOLOGICAL INVESTIGATIONS

In the modern era the use of plain film radiography is negligible, and it has no real place in the investigation of rhinological diseases, with perhaps the occasional exception of a lateral film in the case of a young child in whom adenoidal hypertrophy is suspected but who will not tolerate endoscopic examination. The use of computed tomography (CT) imaging in patients who are due to undergo any form of nasal polypectomy or sinus surgery should be considered mandatory because this allows the clinician to assess any unfavourable anatomic features and provide a targeted approach to the affected sinuses as part of careful preoperative planning. CT scans in the presence of nasal polyposis can also give a clearer picture of the likelihood of an adequate response to medical and surgical treatment. For instance, a scan showing a Lund-Mackay score of 24 out of 24 and double-density signs would alert the clinician to the possibility of allergic fungal rhinosinusitis. A guide to the timing of imaging in the management of CRS can be found in the EPOS guidelines. As mentioned earlier, any case of suspected neoplasia will require imaging to assess and stage the lesion and will often require both CT and magnetic resonance imaging (MRI). Asymmetrical symptoms, even in the absence of endoscopic findings, usually warrant radiological investigation to ensure that no sinister pathologic organism is responsible. Liaison with radiological colleagues for unusual cases and neoplasia is important to ensure that the imaging is relevant and, when performed, answers the clinical question intended. However, clinicians should always aim to review all imaging personally to ensure that patient symptoms are carefully correlated with the findings. In cases proceeding to surgery, review of the imaging should be mandatory.

NASAL AIRWAY MEASUREMENTS

SPATULA MISTING

A simple test of the nasal airway is to place a cold metal spatula underneath the nose to look for any signs of unequal misting relating to each nasal cavity. It is a crude test but will demonstrate any gross asymmetry.

PEAK INSPIRATORY NASAL FLOW

This is performed using a peak flowmeter similar to the expiratory one used for lower airway function. The device has a mask that is placed over the nose and mouth. With the mouth closed, the patient is asked to take a deep breath in through the nose. The measurement is repeated twice more, and the best of the three readings is taken as the final result. Limitations to the test include the presence of alar collapse and lower respiratory tract disease. A guide to interpreting the results is as follows:

<50 L/min = severe nasal obstruction
50–80 L/min = moderate nasal obstruction
80–120 L/min = mild nasal obstruction
>120 L/min = normal

ACOUSTIC RHINOMETRY

In what is effectively sonar of the nose, acoustic rhinometry relies on the reflection of a sound wave to measure the cross-sectional area of the nose and estimate volume. A frequency of 150–10,000 Hz in the form of an audible sound pulse is used by propagating the sound from a click in a tube positioned under the nostril. The differing cross-sectional areas of the nose created by the anatomical structures of the nasal valve and beyond create reflected sound waves that are picked up by the microphone. These are then plotted by the attached computer software as a trace. This is largely a research tool because it is cumbersome to perform and the user needs practice to get a meaningful reading. However, a standardization committee has written guidelines for the application and interpretation of the results.

RHINOMANOMETRY

Similar to acoustic rhinometry, rhinomanometry is generally performed in a research setting but may provide a useful tool in selected patients who complain bitterly about nasal obstruction in the absence of objective blockage. Nasal airway resistance is measured using a combination of flow and pressure readings from the nose. The technique can be performed actively or passively via anterior or posterior approaches. Typically, active anterior rhinomanometry is the choice. One nostril is blocked, and a mask is placed over the mouth and nose with a firm seal created on the face. One nostril is blocked using a sponge seal or tape, but within this is a catheter that will measure the pressure. With the patient breathing in and out moderately through the other nostril and with the mouth closed, the mask will measure the flow rate in the attached pneumotachograph. The combined readings produce a sigmoid-shaped curve on the attached computer software. This is repeated on the opposite nostril by switching the catheter over. Following the standardization protocols of the European committee, the resistance is measured at a fixed pressure of 150 pascals. Taking measurements before and after nasal decongestion is standard. Although results can vary significantly, rhinomanometry may still provide an objective before-and-after comparison in an individual subject.

RHINOSTEREOMETRY

This is a rarely performed investigation involving examination of the nasal cavity before and after an allergen challenge or mucosal moderator to assess the two-dimensional change in the inferior turbinate.

SPIROMETRY

This is traditionally a measure of lower respiratory tract function using peroral exhalation to measure forced expiratory volume; however, spirometers can be adapted with nasal prongs to provide the same function for measurement of the nasal airway, in the same way that peak inspiratory nasal flow (PINF) achieves the equivalent of peak expiratory flow rate (PEFR). Standard spirometry will usually be obtained by a respiratory department or a cardiorespiratory assessment unit and will provide measurements of forced expiratory volume in one second (FEV_1) and forced vital capacity (FVC) as well as the ratio of these two measurements.

OTHERS

PEFR is a well-recognized test of pulmonary function and simply requires a best of three peroral exhalations using a handheld flowmeter, which can be readily available in the clinic. Patients with concomitant lower respiratory disease may already be well versed in this measurement, but, nonetheless, it can provide a useful measure of the impact of upper respiratory tract (URT) disease on the lower airways.

NASAL PHYSIOLOGICAL MEASUREMENTS

MUCOCILIARY CLEARANCE TIME

A simple measure of the mucociliary train inside the nose is the saccharin test. This relies on the normal function of the nasal cilia, which pass the mucus blanket posteriorly towards the postnasal space. To perform the test, the patient is asked to identify when a sweet taste in the back of the mouth is detected. This moment is considered the end point of the test. To begin, a saccharin tablet is placed just underneath the anterior end of the inferior turbinate on one side of the nose, and a stopwatch is started. The stopwatch is then stopped when the patient experiences the sweet sensation. Normal mucociliary function is considered to be a duration of less than 20 minutes; however, the test may be used to compare function before and after treatment by looking for a decrease in the duration of the time interval. Those patients with a duration of 30 minutes or more should certainly be considered for further investigation for underlying ciliary dysfunction or dyskinesia. Clues in the history to primary ciliary dyskinesia include middle ear effusions and situs inversus, which can be seen in Kartagener's syndrome.

CILIARY BEAT FREQUENCY

This is a very specialized test to investigate ciliary dyskinesias and is performed in only three centres in the UK: Leicester, Royal Brompton (London) and Southampton. A normal-functioning sinonasal epithelium will beat at a frequency of 12–16 Hz, but if lower than 11, it is considered in keeping with ciliary dyskinesia, although ciliary beat pattern analysis may pick up some cases with a normal frequency. Abnormal responses will usually be correlated with electron microscopy of the tissue itself.

ELECTRON MICROSCOPY

As an adjunct to ciliary beat frequency and an abnormal mucociliary clearance test, electron microscopy (EM) allows detailed examination of the microstructure of the sinonasal epithelium, which may be relevant to any findings of poor function. Typical abnormalities detected include microtubule array anomalies in the cilia, such as incorrect number of pairs of microtubules, compound cilia and dynein arm irregularities.

NITRIC OXIDE

As with many of the airway parameters already discussed, measurement of nitric oxide (NO) remains largely a research tool. NO levels in the sinuses appear to have an optimum level; levels above or below can be associated with disease states. The ostiomeatal complex is believed to act as an interface controlling NO levels between the nose and sinuses. Nasal nitric oxide can be measured by inserting a probe into one nostril, and, while the patient holds her breath, a reading is taken by the attached gas analyzer. Normal levels are considered to be 450–900 parts per million (ppm); a level above 900 ppm infers inflammation, one less than 450 ppm is associated with blockage and one less than 100 ppm indicates ciliary dyskinesia. The measurement is performed for both nostrils and the mean value derived.

SWEAT TEST AND OTHER CYSTIC FIBROSIS TESTS

Many cases of cystic fibrosis (CF) are now detected perinatally, but if the family history or presentation of a paediatric patient with nasal polyps suggests the need to investigate for CF, the patient should be referred for a formal sweat test. Other clues to the diagnosis may be found in the medical history (lower respiratory tract or gastro-intestinal symptoms) or from CT imaging, because patients with CF typically have hypoplastic frontal and sphenoid sinuses in addition to the opacification associated with the apparent rhinosinusitis. Most units will have the facility to refer locally to their paediatric colleagues for sweat testing. Should this test be positive, patients will also require further testing for the CF transmembrane regulator (CFTR) gene and genetic counselling for future implications. A finding of two CFTR mutations in association with clinical symptoms is diagnostic. The pilocarpine iontophoresis sweat test remains the gold standard and will produce a chloride concentration of greater than 60 mmol/L in CF. However, this result should be found on two separate occasions when the individual is not suffering any infective exacerbations before a diagnosis of CF is confirmed. Although nasal potential difference across the epithelium is a sensitive test for CF, the equipment to perform this is rarely available; hence few centres perform this test as part of a diagnostic workup.

OLFACTORY TESTS: PSYCHOPHYSICAL

Although olfaction is a key function of the nose that most of us take for granted, it is rarely tested as a matter of routine. There are a number of commercially available kits for olfactory testing with a variety of prices, and they vary in the aspects of olfaction that they address. Validation in a local population is key to the relevance of an olfactory test because cultural influences have a significant impact on their suitability. This is particularly the case when employing an identification test, owing to the need for a subject to verbalize the odour names and to have sufficient familiarity with them for the test to be relevant. Hedonics also have a role to play in this context, because what may be a pleasant odour to one cultural group may be considered repulsive to another.

Olfactory threshold testing

This is the olfactory equivalent of determining hearing thresholds in audiology. However, in contrast to audiology, olfactory threshold testing starts by using small odour concentrations and working towards greater ones as the test progresses. Odours typically used for this purpose include phenethyl alcohol (PEA) and 1-butanol (1-BUT); the former has a rose-like smell, but the latter is a more nonspecific solvent-like smell. However, both are considered to be pure olfactory stimulants in the concentrations used for testing and therefore avoid the issue of trigeminal pathway activation. Recognition of the odour here is not relevant, because subjects are required to simply detect the presence or absence of an odour stimulus. To perform this test, the internationally recognized format is the alternative forced-choice format using a ladder progression. This can include two alternative choices, as found in the Connecticut Chemosensory Clinical Research Centre Test (CCCRCT), or three alternative choices, as found in the Sniffin' Sticks test. Subjects are asked to choose which of two or three stimuli contains an odour, even if the subjects cannot detect anything. Some subjects struggle to understand why they must name a choice regardless of definitive detection, but this avoids allowing a subject to skew the test when close to his or her threshold and tempted to give a null response. Starting with the smallest odour concentration, subjects are given two or three sets of stimuli (two for three alternative forced-choice and vice versa for two), and any incorrect response will automatically mean that the next stimulus will be from a level up on the odour concentration chart. In Sniffin' Sticks, this means a jump up of two levels during the first part of the test, allowing quicker focus on the threshold level relevant to the subject. Once a subject detects two or three correct sets for one odour concentration, the level is then moved down to a smaller concentration. This ladder approach is repeated until seven reversals have occurred; the first three reversals are excluded. The average of the final four reversals is then taken as the threshold. This test is time consuming and at present usually requires a member of staff to perform the test. However, it is considered the most sensitive indicator of overall olfactory function, especially because it avoids recognition and verbalization of odours in the test.

Olfactory discrimination

Tests of discrimination examine a subject's ability to distinguish one odour from another. For example, in the Sniffin' Sticks test, subjects are asked to identify which of three stimuli represents the 'odd one out', where two of the three stimuli are the same odour. All odours presented are suprathreshold to avoid an additional dimension to the test.

Olfactory identification

One of the most widely recognized formats of olfactory testing is identification. Its greatest advantage is that it can often be performed by subjects with little or no supervision, such as is seen with the University of Pennsylvania Smell Identification Test (UPSIT). The disadvantage is that this form of testing is culturally specific and requires verbalization of the odour in question, although research has shown some good correlation with threshold testing. In essence it is dependent on individual experience and familiarity with the odours being tested. Common formats for the test include scratch-and-sniff booklets, pens and diskettes, such as seen in the Zurich Smell Diskettes test. All identification tests include a four alternative forced-choice format with three possible distractors listed alongside the correct answer for each stimulus presented.

Retronasal testing

All of the previously discussed test modalities are orthonasal tests. In daily life we smell in two ways: orthonasally when something is in the environment around us, and retronasally when we are eating food. This is why many patients with olfactory loss may complain of taste disturbances in the absence of any true gustatory dysfunction. If there are specific issues around perceived loss of flavour, then this can be better evaluated using a retronasal test kit. This involves placing a selection of food powders on the back of the tongue using a dispenser and then asking the subject to perform an identification test, much as in the aforementioned format. This may be relevant in subjects with pathologic disorders causing blockages to the spheno-ethmoidal recesses or postnasal space.

OLFACTORY TESTING: OBJECTIVE

Most objective forms of testing currently lie in the research domain owing to the costs, manpower and time involved in performing them. A summary of those tests follows.

Olfactory event-related potentials

Akin to the electroencephalogram of smell, the olfactory even-related potentials (OERP) test is conducted using electrodes placed on the scalp, measuring a cortical response to an odour stimulus. The key apparatus involved is an olfactometer, which delivers a continuous stream of humidified air to one nostril with pulsed bursts of one of two odours that are released into the stream at varying intervals and durations. Airflow presented during the inter-stimulus interval must be odour free and warmed to body temperature and have more than 80 per cent relative humidity. Odours typically used are phenethyl alcohol (PEA) and hydrogen sulphide, to give both a pleasant and an unpleasant odour. For OERPs three midline electrodes are placed on the scalp (FZ, CZ, and PZ) referenced to linked earlobes (A1A2). In most circumstances, obtaining reliable OERPs requires the recording and averaging of 10–30 consecutive trials. The waveforms recorded are analyzed for the presence of negative-positive complexes consisting of an initial negative peak (N1) followed by a positive peak (P2) that have characteristic latencies and amplitudes. In simple terms, this is an all-or-nothing test where waveforms either exist or do not exist, but various factors can confound the result, such as signal noise and facial movements. Typically, subjects are given a distraction task and made to wear headphones producing white noise to reduce the influence of such factors. Testing takes 30–45 minutes and requires trained personnel, not to mention the cost of the olfactometer, which is typically in excess of £80,000.

The same setup can be used to deliver carbon dioxide to the nose, which produces a mildly painful response to trigger the trigeminal pathway. Then the responses can be measured as mentioned previously. The presence of an OERP implies that the olfactory apparatus is functioning, but its absence does not definitely imply a complete absence of function, although it is much less likely. Thus, in medicolegal work, it does have a limitation in dealing with malingerers.

Olfactory bulb volume and functional MRI

Using standard MRI sequences that include the entire olfactory bulbs (OBs), volumetric measurement of the right and left OB usually is performed by manual segmentation of the coronal slices through the OB. Usually, a 1.5 Tesla MRI with planimetric contouring of the bulb surface is performed, and the volume is calculated by multiplying the obtained surface by slice thickness. The OB volume has been shown to correlate well with psychophysical testing and can also indicate recovery of olfactory function when sequential imaging shows an increase in volume.

Giving a topographical representation of higher neural centres activated by odour stimuli, functional MRI (fMRI) has been correlated with both orthonasal psychophysical testing and OERPs. By using the large olfactometer needed for OERPs, subjects can be provided with stimuli whilst in an MRI scanner. Activity in the orbitofrontal and entorhinal cortex as well as the cingulate gyrus can be mapped and measured, with a ratio to total functioning brain area calculated. For obvious reasons, this remains in the domain of research in specialist centres.

Electro-olfactogram

Electro-olfactograms (EOGs) show the electrical potentials of the olfactory epithelium that occur in response to olfactory stimulation. The EOG represents the sum of generator potentials of olfactory receptor neurons. In combination with nasal endoscopy and air-dilution olfactometry, the EOG can help to provide a comprehensive picture of olfactory processing. Again, because of the intricacies involved as well as costs and resources, it remains in the research domain.

PATIENT REPORTED OUTCOME MEASURES AND SYMPTOM SCORES

A number of symptom scores have been developed for rhinological disease internationally, and all of them typically address disease-specific quality-of-life complaints. These symptom scores are now referred to as patient reported outcome measures (PROMs) and have been validated in both healthy and diseased subjects in several countries as a means of evaluating the response to interventions in affected patients. In the United Kingdom, the most widely used PROM is the SNOT-22, which is the third iteration of the original SNOT-16 questionnaire. It contains specific symptom questions that can be divided into nasal and ear/facial pain and quality-of-life topics divided between mood/affect and sleep disturbances/concentration. Each item has a scale of 0–5, with 0 indicating no problem and 5 indicating the worst problem ever. Patients are asked to rate these symptoms for the preceding 2 weeks. A score of less than 10 is considered to be normal, and the maximum possible score is 110.

Other commonly used symptom scores for CRS include the Rhinosinusitis Outcome Measure (RSOM-31), Rhinosinusitis Disability Index (RSDI) and Chronic Sinusitis Survey (CSS). For rhinitis other questionnaires are available that are more disease-specific, including the Rhinoconjunctivitis Quality of Life Questionnaire (RQLQ) and related questionnaires developed by Professor Juniper in Montreal. All these have been validated and, where appropriate, can be used for routine clinical and research purposes to monitor outcomes.

KEY LEARNING POINTS

- A careful history is crucial to accurate diagnosis of inflammatory nasal/sinus diseases.
- Objective measures often correlate poorly with subjective symptoms.
- Patient reported outcome measures such as SNOT-22 are recommended for monitoring response to treatment.
- A range of objective measurements and investigations are available for selection on a case-by-case basis.

3

Epistaxis

THUSHITHA KUNANANDAM AND BRIAN BINGHAM

BACKGROUND

Epistaxis, derived from the Greek term *epistazein*, is defined as bleeding from the nose. It is one of the most common emergencies dealt with by otolaryngologists, although its severity and management can vary significantly.

The overall incidence of epistaxis in the general population is difficult to determine because most cases are unreported minor self-limiting episodes or those controlled with simple first-aid measures. Fewer than 10 per cent of patients seek medical attention for this condition and, again, fewer than 10 per cent of those requiring hospitalization require surgical intervention for control of bleeding. However, because many cases involve the elderly population, epistaxis is a significant cause of morbidity and even mortality in general otolaryngology practice.

ANATOMY

The nose has an extremely rich blood supply with contributions from both the internal and external carotid arteries. Vessels from both these sources anastomose extensively within the nasal cavity, including the lateral wall, the septum and also across the midline. The Kiesselbach plexus, or Little's area, is the most frequently associated anastomotic site for epistaxis and is located on the anterior cartilaginous septum. Woodruff's plexus is a confluence of vessels on the lateral wall posterior to the inferior turbinate and is often implicated in 'posterior' bleeds.

The external carotid artery's contribution to the nasal cavity is via the facial and maxillary arteries. The superior labial artery is one of the terminal branches of the facial artery, and it supplies the anterior nasal septum. The lateral nasal artery and ascending palatine artery are two further branches that supply the nasal vestibule and a small area of the nasal cavity. The maxillary artery supplies the nose via the greater palatine branch to the anterior nasal floor and septum. The sphenopalatine branch of the maxillary artery is the most recognized and is a significant contributor to the vascular supply of the nasal cavity. It enters the nasal cavity through the sphenopalatine foramen and then divides into posterior, lateral and septal branches. The lateral branches give rise to the arteries for the middle and inferior turbinates whilst the septal branch supplies the posterior septum and then terminates in the Kiesselbach plexus anteriorly on the septum.

The internal carotid artery contributes to the nasal vasculature through both the anterior and posterior ethmoidal branches of the ophthalmic artery. The larger anterior ethmoidal artery and the smaller posterior one run below and above the superior oblique muscle, respectively, and exit the orbit through their named foramina. They both cross the ethmoid roof and enter the nasal cavity through the cribiform plate and then divide into branches to supply the lateral nasal wall and nasal septum.

EPIDEMIOLOGY

Epistaxis can occur at any age, but there is a notable bimodal age distribution with peaks in childhood and then in the more elderly population, between the ages of 60 and 80. It is rarely seen in infants and tends to be less common in early adulthood. There is a slight male preponderance (male:female ratio, 55:45).

CLASSIFICATION

Epistaxis can be classified in several ways. The pronounced age distribution, for example, lends itself to the classification of adult and childhood epistaxis. Descriptive parameters can also be used for classification such as recurrent or acute/severe epistaxis. The anatomical site of bleeding has also been proposed as a basis for classification into anterior and posterior epistaxis. This system, however, requires a consistent definition of the terms *anterior* and *posterior* epistaxis for it to be universally applicable, whereas in practice, these terms vary from author to author.

Perhaps the most useful classification is by aetiology, but rather than employing an exhaustive list, a broader division into primary and secondary epistaxis can be used. This has the advantage of guiding management, which can be quite different between the two groups.

AETIOLOGY

The majority of epistaxis cases (80 per cent), across the age groups, will be primary or idiopathic (Table 3.1). It is quite possible that with

Table 3.1 Table of aetiological factors and associations

Aetiological factors	
Idiopathic	(80%)
Trauma	Digital, acute facial/nasal, iatrogenic
Coagulopathy	Idiopathic thrombocytopaenia (ITP) Disseminated intravascular coagulopathy (DIC)
Drugs	Warfarin, aspirin, clopidogrel, nonsteroidal anti-inflammatories (NSAIDs)
Chronic granulomatous disease	Wegener's, sarcoidosis
Neoplastic	Angiofibroma, inverted papilloma, squamous cell cancer
Hereditary	Hereditary haemorrhagic telangiectasia (HHT), haemophilia, Von Willebrand's factor deficiency
Aetiological associations	
Septal abnormalities	Spurs, perforations
Alcohol	
Hypertension	

advancement in our knowledge of the aetiological factors involved, this percentage will decrease. Minor trauma may be implicated but not identified in many cases that are classified as idiopathic. Currently, only 20 per cent of cases will be classified as secondary epistaxis with a determined local or systemic underlying cause. Significant physical trauma, either acute maxillofacial or surgical injuries, is an important cause of secondary epistaxis. The majority of other cases of secondary epistaxis are due to underlying coagulopathy induced by either medication or systemic disease (haematological disorders, liver disease).

In a case of epistaxis it is important to thoroughly examine the nose. Such a nasal examination locates the source of bleeding and helps exclude sinister causes such as benign or malignant tumours and granulomatous conditions. Juvenile angiofibroma of the postnasal space should be considered in cases of unilateral epistaxis in the young/adolescent male population. Nasal endoscopy is required for a competent and complete examination of the nose.

Hereditary haemorrhagic telangiectasia (or Osler-Rendu-Weber disease) is an important hereditary cause of epistaxis and is discussed at the end of this chapter.

AETIOLOGICAL ASSOCIATIONS

Septal deviations and spurs may disrupt the normal nasal airflow, leading to dryness and epistaxis. The bleeding site is usually located anterior to the septal spur. The margin of a septal perforation may not be covered by epithelium. This lack of epithelium promotes granulation and crusting and is a common source of epistaxis. Alcohol will cause prolongation of bleeding time, although platelet counts and coagulation factor activity can be recorded as normal. Epistaxis patients are more likely to consume alcohol than matched control patients and, also, more likely to have consumed alcohol within 24 hours of admission for epistaxis.

The relationship between hypertension and epistaxis is often misunderstood. Patients with epistaxis commonly present with an elevated blood pressure. Epistaxis is more common in hypertensive patients, perhaps owing to vascular fragility from long-standing disease. Hypertension, however, is rarely a direct cause of epistaxis. More commonly, epistaxis and the associated anxiety cause an acute elevation of blood pressure.

Children with migraine headaches have a higher incidence of recurrent epistaxis than children without the disease. The Kiesselbach plexus, which is part of the trigeminovascular system, has been implicated in the pathogenesis of migraine.

MANAGEMENT

PRIMARY EPISTAXIS

Effective management of this condition should follow a logical sequence from simple first-aid measures and resuscitation to targeting and treating the bleeding point (Figure 3.1).

Simple first-aid measures should always be employed first because often the bleeding point is anterior and, therefore, amenable to such techniques. The soft cartilaginous portion of the nose should be pinched continuously for 10 minutes to exert pressure internally on the anterior nasal septum. The patient should sit down with head hanging forward breathing through an open mouth. If this is unsuccessful some cotton wool soaked in xylometazoline (Otrivine) can be inserted gently into the anterior nose and the 10-minute compression technique repeated. This correct technique should be reiterated to all patients seeking medical attention for epistaxis.

Any patient requiring further medical attention for epistaxis should be resuscitated appropriately after establishing intravenous access. Initial investigations should include a full blood count, coagulation screen, and group and save sample. A detailed and targeted history should be taken to elucidate the pattern and severity of bleeding and to take into account any underlying aetiological factors.

Direct therapies

The effective management of epistaxis relies on treating the underlying bleeding point, and key to this is close and careful examination with the appropriate equipment following adequate preparation of the nose (Figure 3.2). A combined local anaesthetic/vasoconstrictor solution should be applied topically to the nose and anterior rhinoscopy performed with a headlight and Thudichum's speculum. The nasal cavity should be cleared of all clots and then inspected with a view to identifying an anterior bleeding point. Chemical cautery with silver nitrate sticks or electrocautery with bipolar diathermy can then be applied to coagulate the appropriate vessel. If an anterior source is not visualized, rigid nasendoscopy should then be performed to try to identify a bleeding point more posteriorly in the nasal cavity. Even following successful identification of anterior bleeding points, nasendoscopy should be performed to exclude other posterior sources or underlying sinister pathology. Electrocautery rather than chemical cautery should ideally be used to coagulate these more posterior bleeding points to avoid inadvertent cauterization of normal nasal anatomy. Cautery by either method should always be performed cautiously and with precision to avoid complications such as chemical burns to the lips/nares or longer-term septal necrosis/perforation. Occasionally, a small localized pack (e.g. sinus pack) or an absorbable haemostatic agent such as Surgicel can be used to apply direct pressure to an identified bleeding point that is not amenable to cautery.

Indirect therapies

If after adequate inspection of the nasal cavity a bleeding point is not identified, then indirect therapies are employed to control the epistaxis. Nasal packs are the most commonly employed indirect techniques, but others such as hot water irrigation and anti-fibrinolytics are occasionally indicated. There are a variety of anterior nasal packs available; these include ribbon gauze, nasal tampons (Merocel) and balloon catheters (Brighton). Posterior packs may be required if bleeding persists despite anterior packing. In an awake patient this is most easily achieved with a Foley catheter advanced nasally past the posterior choanae of the nasal cavity in the nasopharynx. Formal posterior packing requires a general anaesthetic.

Once in place, nasal packing should be left *in situ* for 24–48 hours; in patients with prosthetic heart valves, antibiotic cover should be provided. Local complications of packs include sinusitis, septal perforation and alar necrosis.

More recently, topical haemostatic compounds have been proposed as an alternative, indirect treatment option for epistaxis. Floseal, a compound consisting of gelatin granules and human thrombin, is such an agent, and it has been shown to be effective in cases refractory to packing. These compounds are relatively easy to use and are associated with low morbidity. They are, however, much more costly when compared to simple chemical cautery, although they become much more cost effective when compared to surgical intervention.

Surgical management

Surgical intervention is required if indirect therapies fail to control the bleeding. There are several procedures that can be performed under a general anaesthetic in the management of refractory epistaxis, and they can be either facilitatory or more targeted. A general anaesthetic may be required to perform adequate packing of the nose, to apply anterior packing in an uncooperative patient or to insert formal posterior packing. In the uncooperative individual, a general anaesthetic may allow adequate endoscopic inspection and effective nasal cautery. Correction of a deviated nasal septum, under general anaesthesia, can facilitate good access to the bleeding site and permit cautery, effective packing or surgical arterial ligation.

In recent times, surgery has evolved in epistaxis management towards more formal arterial ligation. Arterial ligation should be performed at the most distal (nasal) point with a progression to more proximal ligation if the initial procedure is unsuccessful. Endoscopic sphenopalatine artery ligation is, therefore, the most commonly employed procedure. Internal maxillary artery and, thereafter, external carotid artery ligation are infrequently used. Anterior ethmoidal artery ligation is employed in cases of traumatic epistaxis (particularly nasal ethmoid fracture) or as an adjunct in the management of refractory epistaxis in combination with a sphenopalatine or internal maxillary artery ligation.

Embolization

Arterial embolization has a greater than 80 per cent success rate for severe epistaxis, but its usage depends on the availability and experience of an interventional radiologist. Arterial embolization is indicated either after failure of ligation techniques or in patients who are assessed to be unsuitable or for whom general anaesthetic carries a high risk. Transfemoral angiography is used to demonstrate the bleeding point with subsequent selective embolization of the maxillary or facial arteries performed with materials such as Gelfoam or microcoils. Complications from this technique, although relatively unusual, are more common than following surgical ligation and include facial skin necrosis, paraesthesia, cerebrovascular accident and groin haematoma.

RECURRENT EPISTAXIS

Nonsevere recurrent (primary) epistaxis is commonly seen in the paediatric population. In the adult population, recurrent epistaxis can be primary but is often secondary; therefore, a detailed history is vital to elucidate any causative factors. Examination in adults should always include nasendoscopy to fully visualize any potential bleeding points but also to rule out sinister underlying pathology. Any identified bleeding point can be treated with cautery, and areas of vestibulitis are treated with topical antiseptic creams. The efficacy of chlorhexidine and neomycin creams (Naseptin) is well established as an important part of treatment in paediatric recurrent epistaxis. These chlorhexidine and neomycin creams, together with instillation of Vaseline, are commonly used

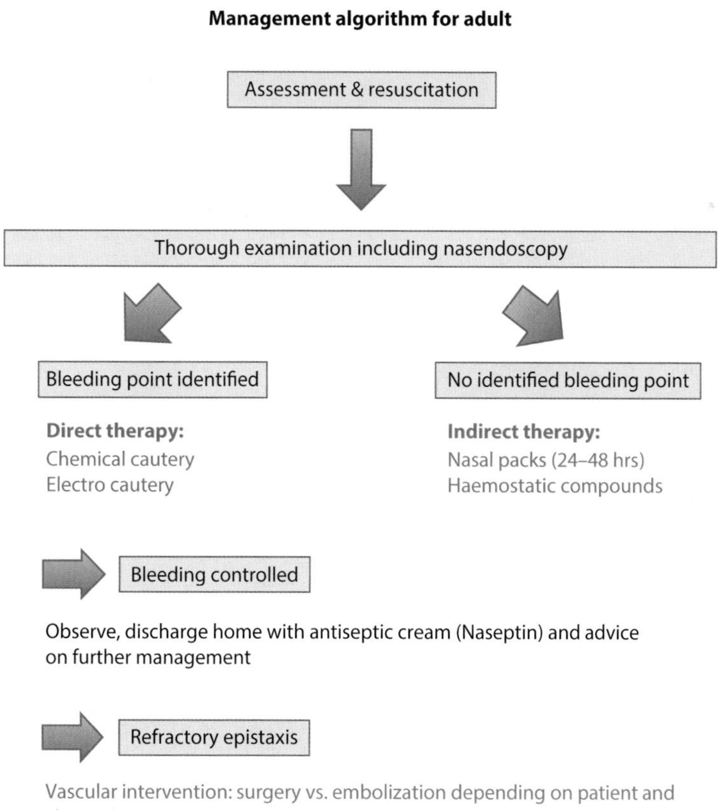

Figure 3.1 Management algorithm for adult acute idiopathic epistaxis.

in the adult population to reduce the incidence of recurrent epistaxis. In all consultations for recurrent epistaxis, it is worthwhile to reiterate the simple first-aid measures that should be employed to control each new episode.

SECONDARY EPISTAXIS

Coagulopathies

In coagulopathic cases, indirect therapies may be indicated in preference to direct measures to control the bleeding. The reason for this course of action is that the bleeding can arise from several sites and instrumentation can lead to further mucosal trauma and exacerbate the bleeding. In these coagulopathic cases haemostatic compounds and nasal packs form the mainstay of treatment, in addition to close collaboration with the haematology services to guide anticoagulant therapy or reversal. If antiplatelet therapies are implicated as a cause of epistaxis, there can be benefit in temporary cessation of this medication. In a patient using warfarin tablets, the international normalized ratio (INR) needs to be considered when managing the epistaxis. If the bleeding is easily controlled with nasal packs, then the warfarin dose may be continued. A warfarin dose can be omitted if the INR is above the

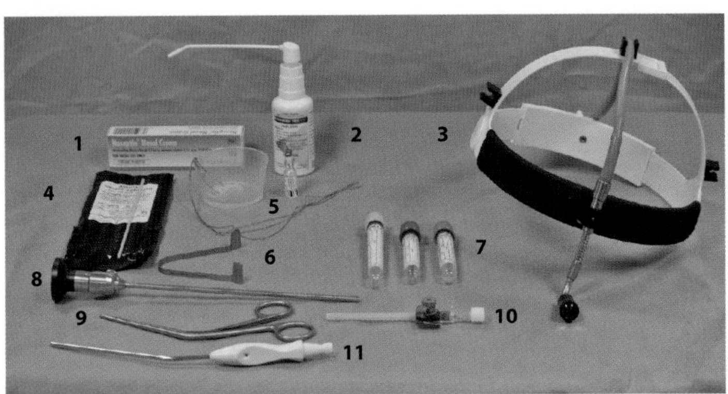

Figure 3.2 Epistaxis management: equipment and medicines.

1. Nasal cream (Naseptin).
2. Topical anaesthetic + decongestant (Co-phenylcaine).
3. Head light.
4. Silver nitrate cautery sticks.
5. Adrenaline vial + patties for application.
6. Nasal speculum.
7. Blood bottles: full blood count, coagulation, group and save.
8. Rigid nasal endoscope.
9. Tilley's dressing forceps.
10. Large bore cannula.
11. Suction.

Cautery principles: examination and silver nitrate cautery steps.

Suction clots.
Apply topical local anaesthetic/vasoconstrictor (topical spray or cotton pledget).
Identify bleeding point; anterior rhinoscopy and nasendoscopy.
Apply silver nitrate cautery (no more than 5 seconds).

therapeutic range. Unfortunately, if the bleeding is not controlled, then intravenous vitamin K can be administered to reverse the anticoagulant effect of warfarin. The INR will require close monitoring in this often difficult time for the patient.

Septal perforation

Crusting of the margin of a septal perforation should be treated with chlorhexidine and neomycin creams (Nasetin), followed by regular instillation of Vaseline. If bleeding persists despite simple measures, then options include (1) cautery of granulations and bleeding spot, (2) insertion of septal button to allow re-epithelialization of the margin or (3) surgery to the margin to trim back bare/granular cartilage and re-epithelialize the margin with a local flap.

Trauma

Epistaxis following trauma or surgery may require nasal packing but may also be amenable to direct electrocautery or arterial ligation techniques.

HEREDITARY HAEMORRHAGIC TELANGECTASIA

Hereditary haemorrhagic telangectasia (HHT) is an autosomal dominant condition associated with recurrent bleeding from vascular anomalies. The disease affects vessels – ranging from capillaries to arteries in the skin – mucous membranes and viscera, leading to the formation of telangiectasia, arteriovenous malformations and aneurysms. Although the disease is almost universally associated with recurrent epistaxis, the severity can be extremely variable. The need for blood transfusion can help to quantify the severity of HHT, which in turn can be a guide to the management of this condition. Milder cases may be simply and effectively managed with topical emollients and oestrogens with interval laser photocoagulation as required. The more severe cases warrant consideration of other measures such as septodermoplasty, arterial ligation and arterial embolization. In the most severe cases (those necessitating significant volumes of blood transfusion), an obturator or surgical closure of the nostrils (Young's procedure) should be considered. Surgical closure of the nostrils is effective in reducing the need for blood transfusion, but the patients find the loss of the sense of smell and taste a difficult side effect of this procedure.

KEY LEARNING POINTS

- Epistaxis is a common ENT emergency.
- Primary idiopathic epistaxis should be managed using a stepwise algorithm.
- Definitive treatment of primary epistaxis involves therapy directed towards an identified bleeding point.
- Refractory epistaxis may require surgery or embolization to control bleeding.
- Recurrent idiopathic epistaxis, commonly occurring in children, can be more successfully treated with topical antiseptic creams and rarely requires surgery.
- Secondary epistaxis management requires treatment of the underlying cause.

4

Acute rhinosinusitis and its complications

ANDREW C SWIFT AND ADAM J DONNE

DEFINITIONS OF ACUTE RHINOSINUSITIS

Rhinosinusitis is specifically defined in the current European Position Paper on Sinusitis and Nasal Polyps 2012 (EPOS 2012).[1] Because rhinitis and sinusitis usually coexist, the correct and accepted terminology is now rhinosinusitis. The more stringent definition includes symptoms as well as endoscopic or computed tomography (CT) findings. However, the criteria have to be adaptable to wider groups beyond otorhinolaryngologists.

The following features are necessary for a diagnosis of acute rhinosinusitis (ARS) in adults to be acceptable for epidemiological/primary care purposes where there is no ear, nose and throat (ENT) examination or imaging:

- Sudden onset of two or more symptoms, one of which must include nasal blockage/obstruction/congestion, or anterior nasal discharge/posterior nasal drip
- + Facial pain/pressure
- + Reduction of loss of smell for less than 12 weeks

This differs in children in that they should have sudden onset of two or more of the following symptoms:

- Nasal blockage/obstruction/congestion
- Or discoloured discharge
- Or cough (daytime and nighttime)

Children with adenoiditis or adenoidal enlargement/hypertrophy can have identical symptoms, but these are normally long-term and in excess of 12 weeks once seen in an ENT clinic.

Most acute episodes occur during the common cold: The duration of symptoms for ARS during the common cold/acute viral rhinosinusitis should be less than 10 days.

Extension of symptoms beyond 10 days is defined now as post-viral ARS; a small percentage of such patients will develop acute bacterial rhinosinusitis (ABRS). The criteria for ABRS require at least three of the following symptoms/signs:

- Discoloured mucus, predominantly from one side, with mucopus within the nasal cavity
- Severe local pain, mainly on one side
- Pyrexia >38°C
- Elevated C-reactive protein (CRP)/erythrocyte sedimentation rate (ESR)
- 'Double sickening', referring to deterioration after an initial milder phase of illness

THE COMMON COLD

Most people will have experienced ARS during the course of a viral upper respiratory tract infection or common cold. The common cold is in fact the most common infectious disease known to man: Adults are likely to suffer from two to five episodes of ARS per year and children seven to 10 colds per year. The prevalence of ARS is high, affecting 6–15 per cent of the population, and increases in winter months, climatic variations, damp environments and air pollution. There is good evidence to support the hypothesis that allergic inflammation and cigarette smoke are predisposing factors (EPOS 2012).

The common cold is caused by airborne viruses, mainly rhinoviruses and coronaviruses. However, other viruses include adenovirus, influenza and parainfluenza viruses, respiratory syncytial virus and enterovirus. The viruses attach to the host cells: Normal ciliary action is disrupted, the mucosa becomes very congested and mucus glands over-secrete. The mucosal congestion extends to the paranasal sinuses, and sinus ostia are likely to become blocked.

The familiar features include nasal obstruction, a mucous nasal discharge and a sense of pressure or heaviness over the cheeks. This is one condition where self-diagnosis is reasonable because we are all familiar with the symptoms and virology is not feasible. The symptoms generally start to subside after a few days, but it may take 2 to 3 weeks to resolve. Investigations such as plain radiographs and culture swabs are normally unnecessary.

The first-line treatment is generally to await natural resolution and alleviate symptoms with medication when necessary. Oral analgesics will alleviate facial discomfort; nasal obstruction is relieved by topical and/or systemic decongestants; and excess mucus discharge is treated with saline rinses or sprays.

Antibiotics are generally unnecessary, and recent Cochrane research has shown that they offer a minimal advantage and are more likely to induce a number of unwanted side effects such as nausea and vomiting, abdominal pain, diarrhoea and the risk of bacterial resistance.[1]

Topical steroid sprays have been shown to aid resolution of symptoms in moderate and severe episodes of viral ARS and in bacterial ARS in combination with antibiotics.

PURULENT RHINOSINUSITIS

Undoubtedly, some episodes of acute viral rhinosinusitis will progress to acute bacterial sinusitis. This has been estimated to occur in 0.5–2.0 per cent of patients.

The clinical features include a purulent nasal discharge and worsening of facial discomfort, often accompanied by dental neuralgia, general malaise and pyrexia.

The usual bacteria are *Streptococcus pneumonia* and *pyogenes*, *Haemophilus influenza*, *Moraxella catarrhalis* and *Staphyloccocus aureus*. Although patients with immune deficiency may well develop acute purulent bacterial sinusitis, often with more unusual organisms such as pseudomonas, there is normally an underlying chronic sinusitis.

The pathogenesis of bacterial infection has been studied for the maxillary sinus. Ostial obstruction leads to the development of low-pressure mucosal congestion and a hypoxic environment within the maxillary sinus, thus favouring bacterial proliferation and increasing ciliary disruption.

Antibiotics are certainly justified in this scenario, but resolution will often progress at the same rate even without antibiotics (EPOS 2012).[1] Amoxicillin or erythromycin is a suitable choice, but there is a lack of evidence showing a significant difference between short 5-day courses and longer courses of a week or more. Although amoxicillin is the most commonly prescribed antibiotic, bacterial resistance, particularly to *S. pneumonia* and *M. catarrhalis,* is increasing.

ACUTE RHINOSINUSITIS IN CHILDREN

Most ARS cases in children are viral and self limiting. Some understanding of sinus development is helpful in understanding the management of children with severe infection and complications of ARS.

The ethmoid and maxillary sinuses are present in small children: The frontal sinuses only begin to enlarge from the age of 4 years, and growth continues into the late teens. After the twelfth year, the floor of the maxillary sinus descends below the level of the nasal floor as the secondary dentition erupts. The sphenoid is very small at birth but has pneumatized in 85 per cent of children by the age of 8 years and continues to grow until the age of 15 years, although further aeration may occur into adulthood.

In children with ARS, it is important to exclude a foreign body and unilateral choanal atresia, and, in recurrent infection, underlying CRS and adenoiditis may be difficult to differentiate. Children with cystic fibrosis may present with exacerbations of acute sinusitis but normally have an underlying chronic sinus disorder. Examination may include rhinoscopy with an otoscope and large-diameter speculum, headlight or endoscope, according to preference and availability. A CT sinus scan is occasionally required should there be prolongation of symptoms or a suspected complication.

The main bacteria that have been implicated are *S. pneumonia, H influenza, M. catarrhalis, S. pyogenes,* and anaerobes. Although resolution will occur without antibiotics, it is likely to be faster with an antibiotic, but the advantage is modest. Antibiotics should, however, be prescribed for children with a complication of ARS, or those with concomitant chest disease such as asthma or bronchitis. There is evidence to support adding an intranasal steroid, although compliance will be an issue with younger children. There is a lack of evidence to support the use of topical and systemic decongestants, antihistamines and saline irrigation.

RECURRENT ACUTE RHINOSINUSITIS

Some patients are prone to developing recurrent episodes of ARS. It is important to differentiate these patients from those with chronic rhinosinusitis with recurrent exacerbations of their condition. By definition, patients with recurrent acute sinusitis are asymptomatic between episodes. Such episodes can become clinically significant, owing to either their severity or their frequency, and lead to frequent courses of antibiotics.

The assessment of such patients should include a search for predisposing factors such as allergic rhinitis or exposure to nasal irritants. Underlying dental disease should also be considered. Typically, nasal endoscopy shows narrow nasal cavities, especially in the region of the middle meati, and a CT scan of the sinuses normally shows osteomeatal complex obstruction with generally clear paranasal sinuses or mild mucosal thickening of the maxillary sinuses.

Daily application of a topical nasal steroid, either as a spray or sometimes as nasal drops in a head-down position, is often an effective strategy for preventing recurrent infection. If medical management fails and the CT scan confirms osteomeatal complex obstruction, endoscopic sinus surgery to open the middle meatal drainage channels is often beneficial. However, the latter can be challenging and must not be underestimated owing to the technical difficulties of operating in a narrow nose.

COMPLICATIONS OF ACUTE RHINOSINUSITIS

Fortunately, most cases of ARS resolve without the development of complications. The incidence of serious complications is low, but they are more likely in the winter months. It is also of interest to note that oral antibiotics do not necessarily protect patients from developing complications.

Acute infective complications can arise from acute or chronic rhinosinusitis: The former is more common in children and the latter in adults. Complications may affect the orbit (60–75 per cent), the intracranial tissues (15–20 per cent) or the frontal bone (5–10 per cent). In a recent UK survey, the orbit was most commonly affected (76 per cent of 78 patients), followed by intracranial infection (9 per cent) and bone infection (5 per cent).[3] Occasionally, multiple sites can be affected simultaneously.

ORBITAL COMPLICATIONS

Orbital infection secondary to sinusitis is often referred to as periorbital cellulitis, but this term lacks precision. Orbital infections have been classified into five subgroups of worsening severity.[4] Although this classification is still in common use today, it is not strictly true, and the increased escalation of infection is not necessarily sequential. However, the classification does provide a clinical aide de memoir to the possible complications that may arise with severe infection (Table 4.1).

Infections of the orbit are initially contained by the fibrous sheet of the orbital septum, and it is much more helpful to refer to preseptal cellulitis and orbital cellulitis according to whether infection is anterior or posterior to this septum.

Infection is most likely to spread from the ethmoid sinus, by direct or vascular spread across the thin lamina papyracea, although some may arise from the maxillary, the frontal or, rarely, the sphenoid sinus.

Any age group can be affected, but the incidence is much greater in children. Most cases in children are preseptal cellulitis that is relatively mild, may not be referred for an ENT opinion and may occur in the absence of sinusitis: 60–90 per cent are reported to be secondary to acute rhinosinusitis.[5] In contrast, orbital cellulitis is always secondary to acute rhinosinusitis.

Table 4.1 Complications of periorbital cellulitis as modified and described by Chandler et al.[4]

Preseptal cellulitis
Orbital cellulitis
Subperiosteal abscess
Orbital abscess
Cavernous thrombosis

Clinical features

PRESEPTAL CELLULITIS

Preseptal cellulitis presents with unilateral swelling of the eyelids, erythema, local pain and sometimes pyrexia (Figure 4.1a). There should be no proptosis and no limitation of eye movement.

Identifying clinical features in the acute stage of infection may be challenging, particularly in children, and tender, swollen eyelids may cause significant difficulty in performing a proper examination of the eye and globe. Normally, a scan is unnecessary unless there is diagnostic uncertainty or clinical progression despite adequate treatment (Figure 4.1b).

It is important to be aware that infection can progress rapidly, and spread beyond the orbital septum could lead to abscess formation and threaten vision.

ORBITAL CELLULITIS

The following are important clinical features that should be identified, documented and monitored: conjunctival oedema (chemosis), limitation of eye movement (ophthalmoplegia), painful eye movements, proptosis, pupillary reaction, visual acuity and colour vision. Colour vision as assessed by an Ishihara chart is typically impaired first, affecting particularly red colour perception, and any element of doubt should instigate an urgent opinion from an ophthalmologist. In the pre-antibiotic era, blindness following periorbital cellulitis was not uncommon, the possible causes being retinal artery occlusion, compression or inflammation of the optic nerve, panophthalmitis and corneal ulceration.

It is of paramount importance to determine whether the infection is complicated by the development of a subperiosteal abscess. These abscesses typically arise adjacent to the lamina papyracea, although some extend or arise superiorly beneath the thin floor of the frontal sinus. Displacement of the globe, proptosis and ophthalmoplegia can all arise from orbital cellulitis or a subperiosteal or orbital abscess. However, it can be very difficult to fully examine the eye in a sick, unwell, uncooperative child, and the presence of painful eye movements, chemosis and/or proptosis should instigate an urgent CT scan.

(a)

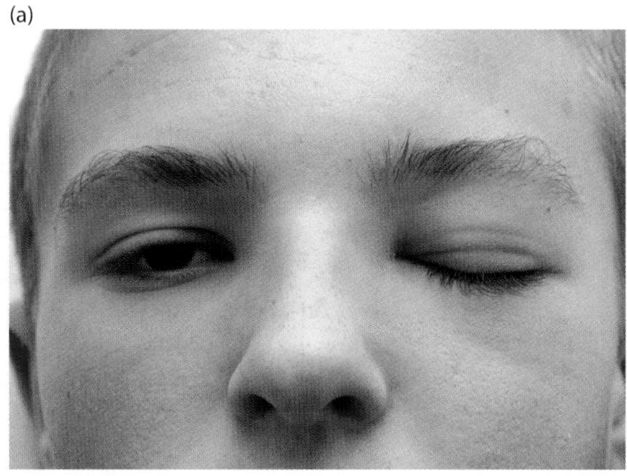

(b)

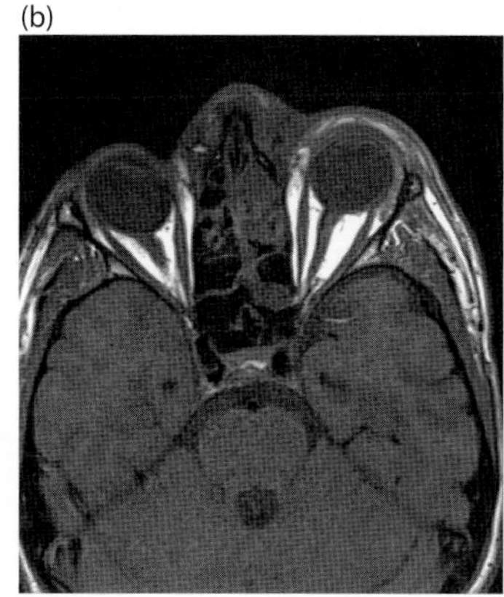

Figure 4.1 **(a)** Preseptal cellulitis in a 16-year-old male. **(b)** Axial CT scan showing ethmoid opacity and preseptal opacity in soft tissues.

Initial management

An early opinion from an ophthalmologist is wise at this stage.

Although oral antibiotics may be effective for the early stages of periorbital cellulitis, intravenous antibiotics are essential for patients with significant infection. It is generally not possible to determine the bacterial profile at the time of instigating treatment, but prior to starting an antibiotic, a blood culture should be considered, particularly if the patient is pyrexial or has rigors. Similar to acute bacterial sinusitis, the spectrum of cover should include the likely pathogens such as *Streptococcus spp.*, *Pneumococcus spp.* and *Haemophilus influenza*. It should be noted that anaerobic bacteria may cause severe infection, and the antibiotic profile should cover these virulent organisms. Early advice from a microbiologist should be sought.

Supplementary treatment with decongestant nasal drops is often practised, but there is no evidence base to support this.

Imaging

A scan is not essential in patients with preseptal cellulitis unless the condition worsens despite treatment with intravenous antibiotics.

If a subperiosteal abscess is suspected, an urgent CT scan of the sinuses and orbits should be obtained (Figure 4.2a and b). It is wise to include brain settings with this request to avoid missing a coexisting intracranial complication.

A magnetic resonance image (MRI) will provide supplementary information if there is diagnostic uncertainty, a subperiosteal abscess or suspected intracranial infection (Figure 4.3a and b).

The specific features to note on scans in patients with orbital infection include a subperiosteal abscess, oedema or bowing of the medial rectus muscle, displacement of the globe, loss of clarity of posterior extraocular muscles and optic nerve and orbital abscess formation. Gas bubbles in the soft tissues develop in anaerobic infection owing to gas-producing bacteria (Figure 4.4).

Surgical intervention

Surgery is indicated in patients who fail to improve on intravenous antibiotics after 24–48 hours, or in those with a subperiosteal or an orbital abscess. A small or early subperiosteal abscess may respond to non-operative treatment, but if this strategy is chosen, the response to treatment should be closely monitored and abscess drainage instigated if the patient fails to respond.

The standard way to explore and drain a subperiosteal abscess is by an external incision, but in the day of the endoscope, there is much discussion about endoscopic drainage. However, the latter approach is likely to be challenging in the acute

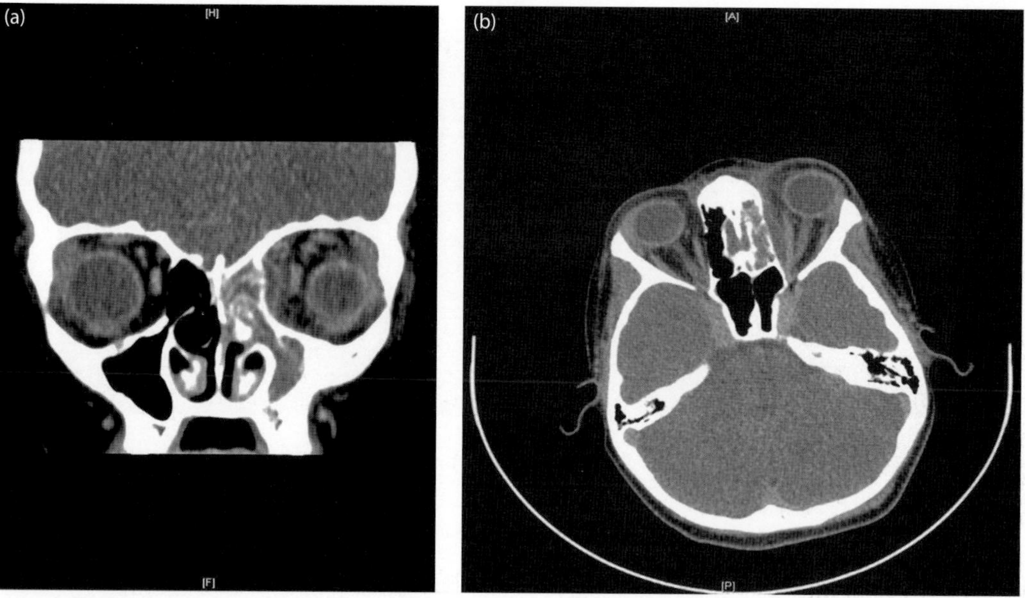

Figure 4.2 CT scan showing a left subperiosteal abscess secondary to acute sinusitis. Coronal image **(a)**, axial image **(b)**.

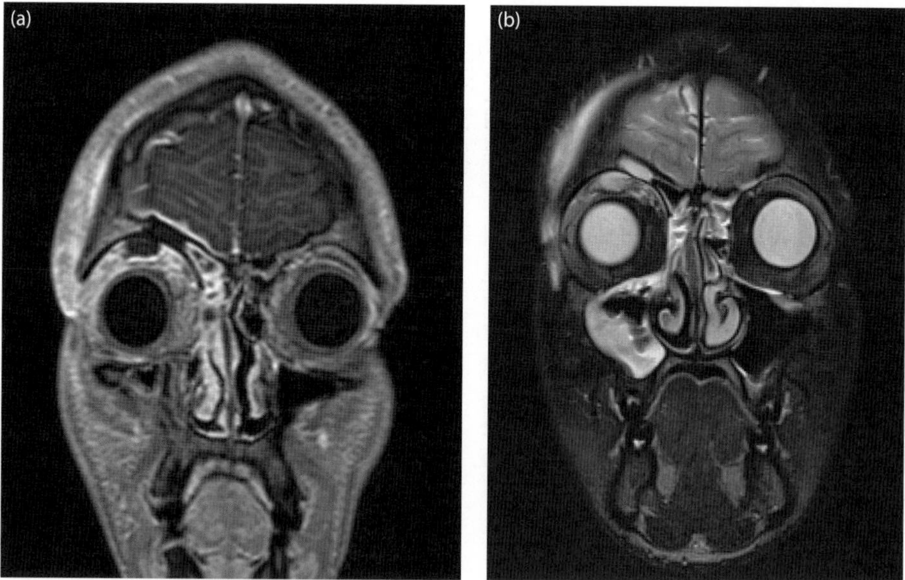

Figure 4.3 MR scan of a superior periorbital abscess with frontal sinusitis and dural inflammation secondary to localized encephalitis. T1 image **(a)**, T2 image **(b)**.

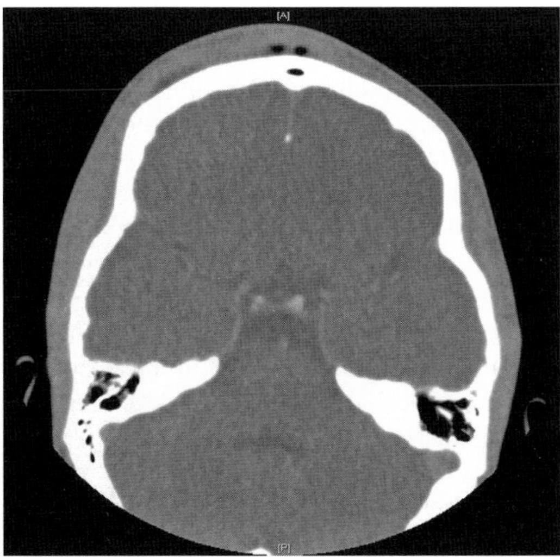

Figure 4.4 Axial CT scan showing gas bubbles in soft tissues in a child with periorbital cellulitis and frontal sinusitis.

situation, particularly in young children, and has not gained popularity within the United Kingdom. External drainage facilitates complete drainage of multilocular abscesses and access to an abscess sited superiorly above the globe (Figure 4.3a and b).

Orbital exploration should be accompanied by drainage of pus within the sinuses, by maxillary antral washout or frontal trephine. Simultaneous endoscopic drainage of the anterior ethmoid should also be considered.

INTRACRANIAL INFECTION

Fortunately, intracranial infection secondary to acute sinusitis is unusual, but the consequences are potentially very serious and include long-term morbidity: Death is reported in up to 19 per cent of cases. In contrast to otogenic intracranial infections that often develop in patients with chronic ear disease, rhinogenic brain abscesses are much more likely to occur during an episode of acute sinusitis.[6]

Infection may reach the intracranial cavity by haematogenous or direct spread. Intracranial complications of acute sinusitis include meningitis, cerebritis, extradural abscess, subdural empyema, cerebral abscess and superior sagittal and cavernous thrombosis.

Because intracranial infection is typically rapidly progressive, early recognition, rapid referral and effective treatment are essential to promote the likelihood of successful recovery.

The clinical features that should alert the clinician are an unwell patient with a persistent headache, altered level of consciousness, spiking pyrexia, nausea and vomiting. Other clinical features may include neck stiffness, photophobia, confusion, seizures, limb dysfunction, cranial nerve abnormalities and dysphasia.

MENINGITIS

Meningitis presents as a rapidly progressive illness in an acutely unwell patient who develops an incessant headache, photophobia and neck stiffness. Straight leg-raising may induce pain – Kernig's sign. The diagnosis is confirmed by performing a lumbar puncture and sending the aspirate for cellular analysis and culture. Lumbar puncture should be done only after exclusion of an intracranial abscess owing to the risk of coning.

Perhaps the most important consideration to remember in such patients is to look for a defect in the bony anterior skull base, particularly if there is a history of previous or recurrent meningitis. Significant head injuries with associated fractures of the skull or facial bones from many years ago may heal with areas of dehiscent bone and exposed dura that predispose to the development of meningitis.

INTRACRANIAL PUS

Most rhinogenic brain abscesses are sited in the cerebrum or frontal lobes, and the clinical features are determined by the site and stage of abscess formation. It is important to appreciate that some patients will have relatively few symptoms or the abscess may be silent, particularly if symptoms have been masked by the previous use of antibiotics. Eventually, meningeal irritation, raised intracranial pressure and focal deficits may occur.

In a subdural empyema, areas of the brain surface are covered by pus. The characteristics are a rapidly progressive, dramatic clinical presentation in a very ill patient. Focal features will depend on which parts of the brain are covered at any one time. Haematogenous spread of infection may result in numerous intracranial sites of pus accumulation.

An epidural abscess is normally associated with frontal sinusitis and may not be recognized until shown by a CT/MRI scan of the head (Figure 4.5a and b).

Imaging

Once the possibility of intracranial infection is considered, an urgent scan should be requested. A CT of the head with brain settings and contrast is essential: It will be helpful to include simultaneous sinus images as well (Figure 4.3a). An MRI of the head will provide important supplementary information (Figure 4.3b). Once the diagnosis has been confirmed, urgent referral to a neurosurgeon is imperative.

Management

The management priority once an intracranial infection is recognized is to seek advice from a neurosurgeon. Treatment options include long-term high-dose intravenous antibiotics, burr-hole drainage, craniotomy or image-guided aspiration.

Otorhinolaryngological intervention is based on the principle of drainage of pus and eradication of the source of infection and may include antral lavage and frontal trephine if there is frontal infection. An alternative is to open the anterior ethmoid cells with the option of draining the frontal sinus endoscopically, expertise allowing, although bleeding is likely to be an issue in the acute stage. Frontal sinus ostial drainage may be facilitated by balloon dilatation if the equipment is available. These drainage procedures can often be combined with neurosurgical drainage during the same anaesthetic administration.

THROMBOPHLEBITIS

Superior sagittal vein thrombosis

This rare complication is likely to arise with epidural or subdural sepsis. The characteristics include a severe headache and focal deficits, especially affecting the legs, because venous thrombosis spreads

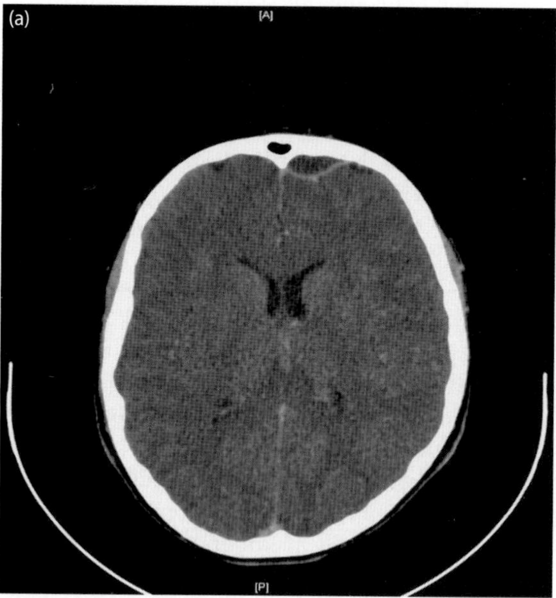

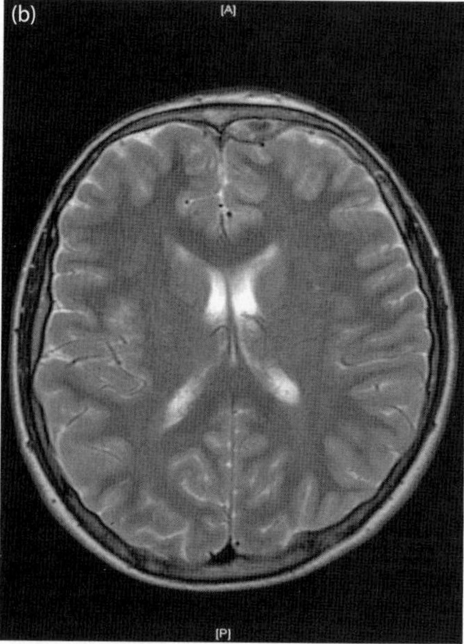

Figure 4.5 Axial images showing a left frontal epidural abscess secondary to acute sinusitis with periorbital cellulitis. CT image **(a)**, T1 MR image **(b)**.

and leads to cerebral infarction. Progression leads to raised intracranial pressure and coma.

Cavernous sinus thrombosis

Cavernous sinus thrombosis is fortunately a rare complication of acute sinusitis but is associated with a significant risk of death. It usually arises from extension of purulent sphenoid sinus infection and adjacent intracranial vein thrombosis. Cavernous sinus thrombosis secondary to acute sinusitis is associated with rapid onset of symptoms, beginning with swelling of one eye, to be followed by the other as the thrombosis progresses to the contralateral side. The clinical features include a spiking pyrexia, ptosis, deep retro-orbital pain, papilloedema and complete ophthalmoplegia due to involvement of the III, IV and VI cranial nerves. There may be corneal hypersensitivity of the affected eye to be followed by anaesthesia due to disruption of trigeminal sensation. Septic emboli may reach the brain, orbit, lungs, kidney, spleen and liver.

An MRI venogram should confirm the diagnosis by demonstrating absent venous flow from the cavernous sinus. High-resolution CT with contrast should also show a filling defect around the cavernous sinus.

Treatment includes high-dose intravenous antibiotics and drainage of purulent sinus collections, particularly from the sphenoid sinus. Systemic steroids and anticoagulants are often used, but their use remains controversial.

FRONTAL OSTEOMYELITIS

Frontal osteomyelitis is a condition that achieved notoriety when it acquired its well-known synonym of Pott's puffy tumour, described by Sir Percivall Pott, surgeon at St Bartholomew's Hospital, in 1760.

It develops as an acute frontal abscess that complicates an acute sinus infection and frontal sinusitis. The frontal bone that forms the anterior wall of the frontal sinus becomes osteomyelitic: Bone necrosis leads to a subperiosteal abscess that presents as fluctuant tender lump of the forehead. In some instances, the abscess points and bursts before surgical intervention can take place, and this may lead to a fronto-cutaneous fistula.

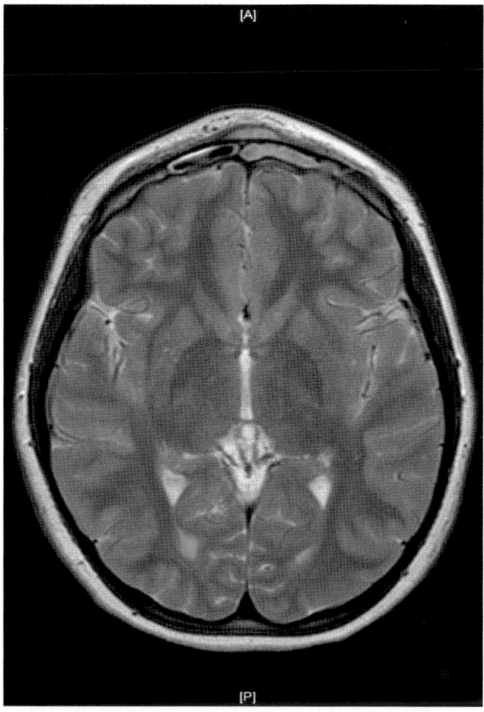

Figure 4.6 MR image showing soft tissue swelling and frontal sinusitis in acute frontal osteomyelitis (Pott's puffy tumour).

Although the condition presents as an acute purulent infection, patients often have underlying chronic rhinosinusitis, and this is important to appreciate to prevent a later recurrence.

A CT sinus scan, often combined with brain images, is necessary to assess the disease and plan operative intervention (Figure 4.6).

Treatment includes an intravenous antibiotic that is likely to cover the bacterial profile and also penetrate bone. Following microbiological advice, clindamycin is often recommended as the preferred antibiotic.

Operative intervention is normally required. Emergency procedures should be limited to simple drainage of pus. This can be achieved by placing a small incision directly over the abscess within a skin crease on the forehead. This facilitates curettage of necrotic bone and clearance of the purulent contents and loculi within the frontal sinus. A drain can be inserted into the frontal sinus to prevent recurrence of a purulent collection.

There is often infection within the other paranasal sinuses, and the maxillary antra should be checked and lavaged at the same time. Should endoscopic surgery be contemplated, this should be restricted to opening of the anterior ethmoid and frontal recess.

Oral antibiotics are often required for several weeks following acute infection. Once the patient has recovered from the acute infection, more definitive surgery can be undertaken to prevent recurrence and address any unsightly depression or scarring on the forehead. This may include performing a Draf type 3 sinuplasty median frontal drainage procedure in special cases.

KEY LEARNING POINTS

- Acute rhinosinusitis is most often viral.
- Recurrent acute rhinosinusitis may be secondary to allergy, irritants or immune deficiency.
- Complications arising from acute rhinosinusitis are uncommon but may be serious.
- Acute collections of pus within the orbit or intracranial cavity should be drained urgently.
- Purulent infections within the orbit or intracranial cavity are serious and generally require urgent additional specialist ophthalmic or neurosurgical care.

REFERENCES

1. Fokkens WJ, Lund VJ, Mullol J, Bachert C, et al. European Position Paper on rhinosinusitis and nasal polyps. *Rhinology* 2012; 50 Suppl 23: 1–299.
2. Lemiengre MB, van Driel ML, Merentstein D, Young J, De Sutter AI. Antibiotics for clinically diagnosed acute rhinosinusitis in adults. *Cochrane Database of Systematic Reviews*. 2012; 17: CD006089.
3. Baber-Craig H, Gupta Y, Lund VJ. Rhinological Society audit of the role of antibiotics in complications of acute rhinosinusitis: A national prospective audit. *Rhinology*. 2010; 48(3): 344–7.
4. Chandler JR, Langenbrunner DJ, Stevens ER. The pathogenesis of orbital complications in acute sinusitis. *The Laryngoscope*. 1970; 80(9): 1414–28.
5. Upile NS, Munir N, Leong SC, Swift AC. Who should manage acute periorbital cellulitis in children? *Journal of Pediatric Otorhinolaryngology*. 2012; 76(8): 1073–7.
6. Tandon S, Beasley N, Swift AC. Changing trends in intracranial abscesses secondary to ear and sinus disease. *Journal of Laryngology and Otology*. 2009; 123(3): 283–8.

5

Granulomatous conditions of the nose

JOANNE RIMMER AND VALERIE J LUND

A granuloma is an organized collection of macrophages, often referred to as epithelioid cells, which tend to fuse to form multinucleated giant cells. Granulomatous conditions of the nose and paranasal sinuses may be secondary to infection, inflammation, trauma or substance abuse, or may be due to an autoimmune or neoplastic condition. The disease process may be confined to the nose or be part of a systemic condition involving multiple organ systems.

GRANULOMATOSIS WITH POLYANGIITIS (WEGENER'S GRANULOMATOSIS)

HISTORY AND EXAMINATION

Granulomatosis with polyangiitis (GPA) is a systemic autoimmune disease of unknown aetiology, histologically characterized by granulomatous inflammation of the respiratory tract with necrotizing vasculitis of small and medium-sized blood vessels and focal or proliferative glomerulonephritis. It has previously been known as Wegener's granulomatosis, but its name has changed, initially to cANCA-positive vasculitis and most recently to GPA.[1] Classically, it affects the nose, lungs and kidneys, but it can affect any organ. It is also now recognized that more localized forms of the disease can occur, and up to 25 per cent of patients may only complain of sinonasal symptoms. The true incidence is therefore likely to be under-reported, but is estimated at approximately 10 per million per annum, with a prevalence of up to 100 per million in Europe. The average age at onset is 40–55 years, but it may occur at any age. Men and women are equally affected, but it is predominantly a disease of Caucasians (93 per cent).

The presenting symptoms are rhinological in 60–90 per cent of cases, including nasal obstruction, crusting, discharge, epistaxis, hyposmia or anosmia, pain, epiphora or change in shape of the nose.[2] Otological symptoms occur in up to 40 per cent, primarily conductive or sensorineural hearing loss. Approximately 16 per cent of patients have subglottic stenosis, which may prove fatal; this percentage is higher (23 per cent) in younger patients. Lower respiratory tract symptoms such as cough, haemoptysis and dyspnoea can occur, and patients may complain of constitutional symptoms such as fever, lethargy and weight loss.

Examination reveals friable granular mucosa, often with old blood and crusting or excessive adhesion formation (Figure 5.1a and b). There may be a septal perforation, and in advanced cases there may be loss of normal internal nasal architecture with a single large cavity. The classic 'saddle' deformity of the nose is seen in 5–20 per cent of patients with GPA (Figure 5.2); the only other condition that produces a similar deformity is relapsing polychondritis. Middle ear effusions may be present. The differential diagnosis of GPA includes all other nasal granulomatous conditions.

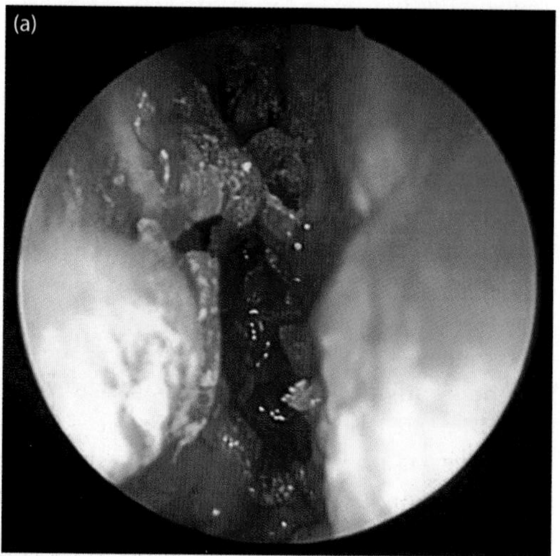

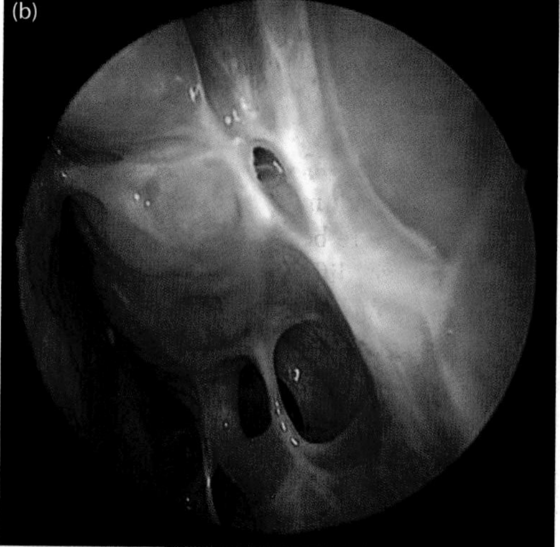

Figure 5.1 **(a)** Endoscopic photograph showing significant nasal crusting in GPA. **(b)** Endoscopic photograph showing marked adhesion formation in GPA.

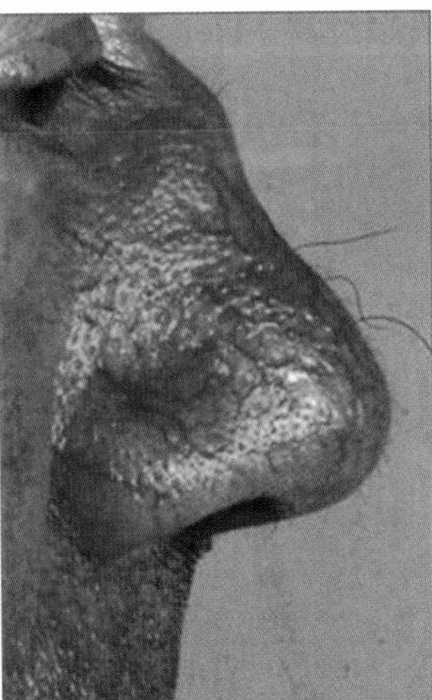

Figure 5.2 Clinical photograph showing collapse of nasal bridge in GPA.

INVESTIGATIONS

Anti-neutrophil cytoplasmic antibodies (ANCAs) are strongly associated with three vasculitides: GPA, eosinophilic granulomatosis with polyangiitis (Churg-Strauss syndrome) and microscopic polyangiitis (MPA). They are therefore not 100 per cent sensitive or specific for the diagnosis of GPA. However, cytoplasmic ANCA (cANCA) specific for proteinase 3 (PR3) is 90 per cent sensitive and 98 per cent specific for generalized GPA; the sensitivity falls to 50 per cent in localized disease. Ten per cent of patients with GPA will have a positive test for perinuclear ANCA (pANCA) against myeloperoxidase (MPO), and up to 30 per cent may have a negative ANCA test initially. This result may change over time, and cANCA may therefore be used to monitor disease activity.[3] It is often difficult to obtain a positive biopsy from nasal mucosa; lung and renal biopsies have a higher yield. Histological diagnosis of GPA requires the presence of granulomatous inflammation, vasculitis and necrosis. Computed tomography (CT) imaging of the paranasal sinuses shows non-specific mucosal thickening in more than 85 per cent of patients, but up to 75 per cent may have evidence of bony destruction, and new bone formation is seen in up to half of patients (Figure 5.3). However, sinus scans can also be normal. Chest

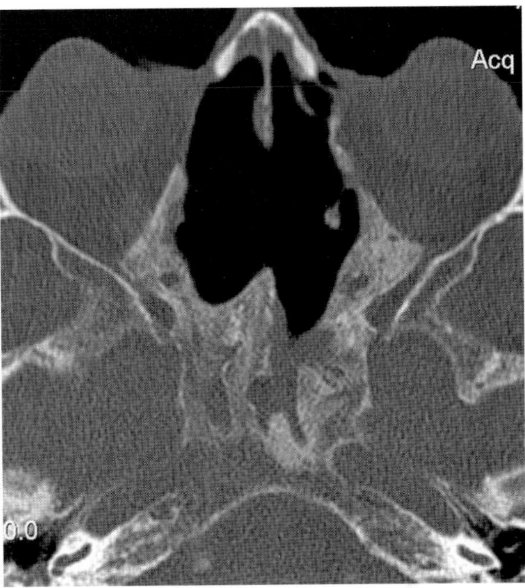

Figure 5.3 Axial CT scan of a patient with GPA showing loss of septum, ethmoids and anterior lamina papyracea together with marked sclerosis of residual bone.

x-ray (CXR) and urinalysis may be helpful in confirming the involvement of other organ systems.

MANAGEMENT

The European Vasculitis Study Group has classified GPA as *localized* (respiratory tract involvement only), *early systemic* or *generalized* disease.[4] If the disease is suspected, then a multidisciplinary approach with involvement of a rheumatologist or vasculitis specialist should begin at an early stage. Survival in generalized GPA was previously very poor, but the advent of corticosteroid treatment has reduced mortality rates to 50 per cent. The introduction of cyclophosphamide has further improved remission rates to 90 per cent, and steroid-sparing agents such as azathioprine, methotrexate and mycophenolate mofetil are then used to maintain remission. Monoclonal antibodies such as rituximab and infliximab have also been used recently with good effect. For disease localized to the nose, or for symptomatic relief of sinonasal involvement, nasal douching and topical nasal steroids are the mainstay of treatment. Nasal lubricants may also be used. Sinus surgery should be avoided if possible, as post-operative scarring can make symptoms significantly worse, but may be required in selected patients. Surgical repair of septal perforations is unlikely to be successful, but a Silastic button may be inserted in addition to the use of topical treatments. Reconstruction of a saddle deformity requires the use of cartilage or bone grafts and generally has poor results if disease is active; however, if the disease has been quiescent for at least one year, it may be considered in selected cases. Grommets should be avoided owing to the risk of chronic discharge, and hearing aids are the treatment of choice for hearing loss. Subglottic stenosis can usually be managed with regular dilatation, intralesional steroid injection and endolaryngeal laser treatment. Mortality rates remain approximately 5 per cent despite immunosuppressant treatment, and up to 10 per cent of patients will never enter remission. Of those who do, up to 50 per cent will relapse.

EOSINOPHILIC GRANULOMATOSIS WITH POLYANGIITIS (CHURG-STRAUSS SYNDROME)

HISTORY AND EXAMINATION

Eosinophilic granulomatosis with polyangiitis (EGPA) is a rare but potentially fatal systemic necrotizing vasculitis of unknown aetiology, affecting small to medium-sized vessels. It is associated with asthma, eosinophilia and extravascular eosinophilic granulomas and was previously known as Churg-Strauss syndrome.[1] The asthma is characteristically late-onset and, together with allergic rhinitis and nasal polyps, may predate the vasculitis by several years. The average time from onset of asthma to diagnosis of EGPA is 12 years (range 1–34 years). It is less common than GPA, with an incidence of 2.4–4.2 per million per year in Europe. However, it has been reported in up to 67 per million asthmatics. The mean age at onset of the vasculitis is 50 years, but it has been reported in children. Men and women are equally affected, and most patients are Caucasian (up to 98.2 per cent).[5]

Three overlapping disease phases have been described: (1) a prodromal phase that may last for several years, during which time nasal and pulmonary symptoms tend to worsen; (2) the development of peripheral eosinophilia of greater than 10 per cent, which may be associated with other organ involvement as a result of eosinophilic infiltrates; and (3) the onset of systemic vasculitis and its associated symptoms. There are peripheral nervous system (PNS) symptoms in 50–78 per cent, primarily mononeuritis multiplex; skin involvement in 40–70 per cent, with purpura and nodules; gastro-intestinal symptoms in one-third; renal disease in 21–80 per cent; and cardiac involvement, usually myocarditis, in 10–49 per cent. It has been reported to occur after treatment with zafirlukast, a leucotriene receptor antagonist, but this is thought to be due to unmasking of the vasculitis by the reduction in oral steroid treatment that zafirlukast allowed.

Nasal obstruction and rhinorrhoea are the most common sinonasal symptoms, occurring in up to 95 per cent of patients, but anosmia (90 per cent), sneezing (80 per cent), crusting (75 per cent) and epistaxis (60 per cent) are also common.

The American College of Rheumatology 1990 criteria for diagnosis of EGPA (Churg-Strauss) require at least four of the following: asthma; eosinophilia of greater than 10 per cent differential; mono- or polyneuropathy due to vasculitis; non-fixed pulmonary infiltrates; abnormalities of the paranasal sinuses; and extravascular eosinophils on biopsy. This gives a sensitivity of 85 per cent and a specificity of 99.7 per cent. The differential diagnosis includes idiopathic hypereosinophilic syndrome, GPA, MPA, sarcoidosis, allergic bronchopulmonary aspergillosis and parasite infection.

INVESTIGATIONS

EGPA is another ANCA-associated vasculitis, but pANCA (against MPO) is only positive in 31–50 per cent of cases. There is less cardiac involvement in ANCA-positive cases, but ear, nose and throat (ENT), renal and PNS symptoms are more common.[5] There is eosinophilia, and acute phase proteins are often elevated. Histological diagnosis requires the presence of extravascular eosinophilic granulomas and necrotizing vasculitis, but nasal

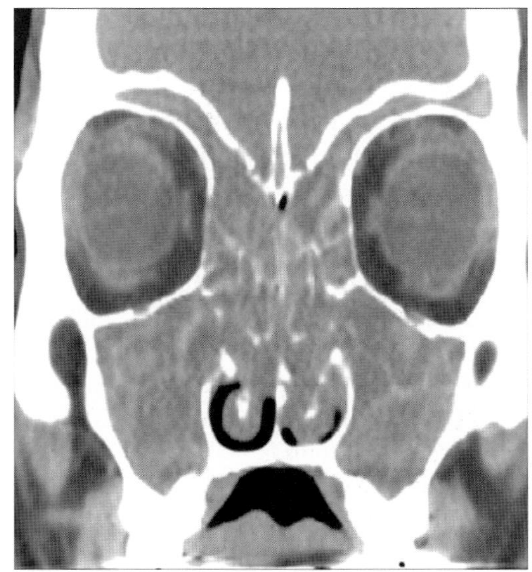

Figure 5.4 Coronal CT scan showing widespread chronic rhinosinusitis with nasal polyps in a patient with EGPA (Churg-Strauss).

biopsy is generally unhelpful. Skin, nerve, muscle or lung tissue has a higher positive yield. There is pan-opacification of the paranasal sinuses on CT, due to chronic rhinosinusitis (CRS) with nasal polyps, and there may be associated bony expansion and mucocoele formation (Figure 5.4). CXR may show nodular infiltrates.

MANAGEMENT

Again, this should be multidisciplinary, involving a respiratory physician or one with an interest in vasculitis. Outcomes have been shown to be better if patients are treated at an experienced vasculitis centre. Immunosuppression is the mainstay of treatment, with corticosteroids and steroid-sparing agents, but cytotoxic drugs such as cyclophosphamide may also be required. Rituximab has been used, and interferon-α has been tried in refractory cases with limited success. Sinonasal symptoms may be managed with topical treatments such as alkaline nasal douching and intranasal steroids, but surgery may be required for polyps or mucocoele formation. Remission is achieved in 81–92 per cent of patients, but more than a quarter will relapse. The French Vasculitis Study Group reported 5-year survival rates of 88.9 per cent, falling to 78.6 per cent at 10 years; survival was better with ANCA-positive disease.[5] Mortality rates can be as high as 46 per cent if there is cardiac involvement, which is the major cause of death in EGPA. The presence of cardiomyopathy at diagnosis, older age at diagnosis and a diagnosis of EGPA prior to 1996 were all found to be independent predictors of death in the French study.

SARCOIDOSIS

HISTORY AND EXAMINATION

Sarcoidosis is a chronic granulomatous disease of unknown aetiology, although it appears to be immune mediated.[6] It has a reported incidence of 1.2–19 per 100,000 per year but is more common in northern Europe and the southeast United States. It is significantly more common in African Americans, with an incidence of 36.5–81.8 per 100,000 per year. It can affect any age group, but its onset is most common in the third and fourth decades, and women are affected twice as often as men.

It is a multisystem disease that affects the lungs in more than 90 per cent, but cutaneous lesions are also common with a classic purple discolouration, known as lupus pernio (Figure 5.5), and

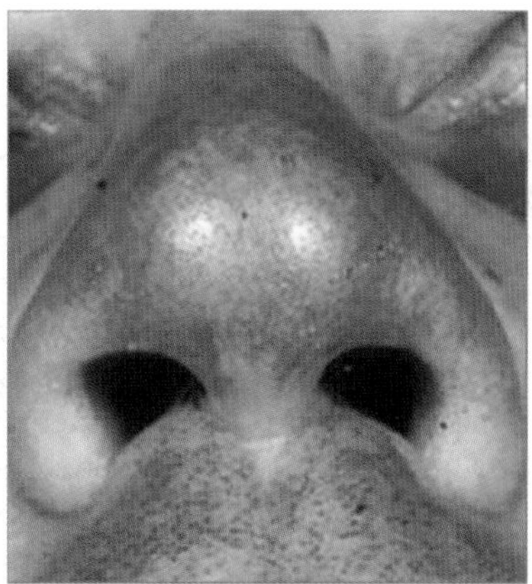

Figure 5.5 Clinical photograph showing lupus pernio affecting tip of the nose.

subcutaneous nodules. The upper respiratory tract is affected in up to 9 per cent of cases. Nasal obstruction, crusting, bleeding and facial pain are the most common symptoms. The ears and mouth may also be affected, as can the larynx, classically with supraglottic lesions. The nasal mucosa tends to have a characteristic 'strawberry' appearance of inflamed erythematous mucosa covered with pale granulomas. Crusting is often seen, and there may be an anterior septal perforation. The differential diagnosis includes all other granulomatous conditions of the nose.

INVESTIGATIONS

Sarcoidosis was previously diagnosed using the Kveim test, but this has been withdrawn in the United Kingdom due to health and safety reasons. Serum angiotensin-converting enzyme (ACE) level may be elevated, although this is also seen in other conditions such as tuberculosis (TB) and lymphoma and so is not specific. Serum calcium may be elevated in systemic disease, but only in 11 per cent of patients. Histology shows non-caseating epithelioid granulomas; nasal biopsy is usually negative if the mucosa appears normal, but a positive result is obtained in 91 per cent if it is clinically abnormal. CT of the paranasal sinuses may show changes consistent with CRS, and lacrimal gland enlargement is common. Sometimes there may be soft tissue infiltration of the nasal bones. CXR classically shows bilateral hilar lymphadenopathy.

MANAGEMENT

Management should be multidisciplinary with a respiratory physician. The Krespi staging classifies sarcoidosis into mild (stage I), moderate (stage II) or severe (stage III). The mainstay of treatment is systemic steroids and steroid-sparing agents. Topical treatment for the nose includes nasal douching, topical steroids and lubricants. Intralesional steroids may be used in cutaneous or laryngeal lesions. Surgery has only a limited role. Sarcoidosis may remit spontaneously, but severe pulmonary or cardiac involvement may be fatal.

COCAINE-INDUCED MIDLINE DESTRUCTIVE LESION

HISTORY AND EXAMINATION

Chronic intranasal cocaine abuse can cause granulomatous inflammation and destruction of the nose, sinuses and palate that may be clinically indistinguishable from GPA. This process is thought to be due to the marked vasoconstrictive effect of cocaine. A history of intranasal substance abuse should therefore be sought in all patients presenting with such symptoms.

INVESTIGATIONS

ANCA is often positive in this condition, with PR3 reactivity in more than 50 per cent, which compounds the similarity with GPA, but there are some subtle differences in capsase 3 and 9 expression and ANCA reactivity with neutrophil elastase that can distinguish the two conditions.

MANAGEMENT

Cessation of cocaine abuse is most important, and topical nasal treatments may provide symptomatic relief. Surgical reconstruction is often difficult with poor outcomes.

NATURAL KILLER/T-CELL LYMPHOMA

HISTORY AND EXAMINATION

Previously known as *midline destructive granuloma* or *midline lethal granuloma*, this tumour is now known to be a lymphoma but usually presents with midface destruction.

INVESTIGATIONS

Representative biopsy from beneath necrotic tissue is required for diagnosis. Imaging shows widespread bony and soft tissue destruction.

MANAGEMENT

Treatment is with radiotherapy plus or minus chemotherapy. Long-term follow-up is required because there may be late relapses.

GRANULOMATOUS INFECTIONS OF THE NOSE

Most of these infections are rare in the developed world, and treatment should be given by an infectious diseases specialist.

TUBERCULOSIS

HISTORY AND EXAMINATION

Nasal TB is uncommon, and primary nasal TB accounts for only one-third of cases. The causative organism is usually *Mycobacterium tuberculosis*. Ulcerative and nodular (lupus vulgaris) forms are seen in the nose, with an isolated granuloma occasionally found in the paranasal sinuses.

INVESTIGATIONS

Biopsy reveals caseating epithelioid granulomas, but acid-fast bacilli may not be seen and cultures may be negative. Skin testing for TB may prove infection, and serum testing such as QuantiFERON is now available.

MANAGEMENT

Extrapulmonary TB is usually managed with combination antituberculous chemotherapy.

LEPROSY

HISTORY AND EXAMINATION

Leprosy is a chronic granulomatous condition caused by the acid-fast bacillus *Mycobacterium leprae*. It is unusual in developed countries, but there are 12–15 million cases worldwide. There are two main forms of the disease, tuberculoid leprosy, which is localized, and lepromatous leprosy, which is systemic. The nasal skin is often involved with anaesthetic plaques, and nasal mucosa may be affected in systemic cases.

INVESTIGATIONS

Diagnosis is based on clinical findings with microbiological confirmation of the bacillus on biopsy.

MANAGEMENT

Long-term dapsone remains the standard therapy.

SYPHILIS

HISTORY AND EXAMINATION

Syphilis is a sexually transmitted disease caused by the spirochaete *Treponema pallidum*. It is classified into primary, secondary, tertiary and congenital forms. Primary chancre of the nose is rare but may be seen on the skin or within the vestibule. Secondary syphilis is an infectious systemic condition, with rhinitis the most common nasal symptom. Tertiary syphilis may cause a perforation of the bony septum or present as a subcutaneous nodule (gumma) which then ulcerates. Congenital syphilis most commonly presents with 'snuffles', a purulent rhinitis with eventual excoriation of the upper lip.

INVESTIGATIONS

Syphilis is usually diagnosed with serological tests, but smears from a lesion may show the organism.

MANAGEMENT

Parenteral penicillin is the antibiotic of choice for all stages.

MUCOCUTANEOUS LEISHMANIASIS

HISTORY AND EXAMINATION

Leishmaniasis, a parasitic disease caused by *Leishmania spp.*, is endemic in more than 80 countries, with 12 million cases worldwide. It may present in cutaneous, mucocutaneous or visceral forms. The mucocutaneous form can cause swelling and erythema of the external nose with erosion of the internal nose, septum, palate and trachea, and has been reported to mimic GPA.

INVESTIGATIONS

Diagnosis is difficult, but biopsy may show granulomatous inflammation without vasculitis. Biopsy of involved skin may be more helpful than nasal mucosa.

MANAGEMENT

Treatment is usually with amphotericin or a pentivalent antimony compound.

RHINOSPORIDIOSIS

HISTORY AND EXAMINATION

Rhinosporidiosis, a chronic granulomatous infection caused by *Rhinosporidium seeberi*, is most commonly seen in India and Sri Lanka. The nasal mucosa becomes granular and polypoidal with a strawberry-like appearance.

INVESTIGATIONS

Histological examination shows the organism's spores.

MANAGEMENT

Treatment typically involves surgical excision of the lesions followed by medical therapy such as dapsone, griseofulvin, amphotericin and diaminodiphenylsulfone, but none of these preparations has proved particularly successful.

RHINOSCLEROMA

HISTORY AND EXAMINATION

Klebsiella rhinoscleromatis causes this progressive granulomatous infection of the nose and upper respiratory tract, with laryngeal involvement in up to 50 per cent of cases. There are three stages: atrophic, with crusting similar to atrophic rhinitis; granulomatous or proliferative, with nodule formation; and cicatrizing, with stenosis and adhesion formation.

INVESTIGATIONS

The diagnosis is usually made in the later stages, based on the typical histological findings of granulomatous infiltrates and Mikulicz cells.

MANAGEMENT

Prolonged antibacterial treatment with ciprofloxacin or trimethoprim-sulfamethoxazole is required, but initial surgical debridement may be helpful.

KEY LEARNING POINTS

- Systemic granulomatous conditions often present with ENT symptoms. Although they are unusual diseases, it is important to have a high index of suspicion to avoid delay in diagnosis.
- Always suspect a vasculitis if there is general malaise disproportionate to the clinical findings.
- Nasal crusting and abnormal mucosa should prompt investigation for granulomatous disease, as should recalcitrant symptoms of chronic rhinosinusitis despite appropriate management.

- There is no one diagnostic test; diagnosis is based on the clinical picture together with examination findings, imaging, serological and histological tests.

REFERENCES

1. Jennette JC, Falk RJ, Bacon PA, et al. 2012 Revised International Chapel Hill Consensus Conference Nomenclature of Vasculitides. *Arthritis and Rheumatism.* 2013; 65: 1–11.
2. Rasmussen N. Management of the ear, nose and throat manifestations of Wegener granulomatosis: an otorhinolaryngologist's perspective. *Current Opinion in Rheumatology.* 2001; 13: 3–11.
3. Sproson E, Jones N, Al-Deiri M, Lanyon P. Lessons learnt in the management of Wegener's Granulomatosis: Long-term follow-up of sixty patients. *Rhinology.* 2007; 45: 63–67.
4. Rasmussen N, Jayne DRW, Abramowicz D, et al. European therapeutic trials in ANCA-associated systemic vasculitis: disease scoring, consensus regimens and proposed clinical trials. *Clinical and Experimental Immunology.* 1995; 101 Suppl 1: 29–34.
5. Cormorand C, Pagnoux C, Khellaf M, et al. Eosinophilic granulomatosis with polyangiitis (Chrug-Strauss syndrome): clinical characteristics and long-term follow-up of the 383 patients enrolled in the French Vasculitis Study Group cohort. *Arthritis and Rheumatism.* 2013; 65: 270–281.
6. Morgenthau AS, Teirstein AS. Sarcoidosis of the upper and lower airways. *Expert Review of Respiratory Medicine.* 2011; 5: 823–33.

FURTHER READING

Fuchs HA, Tanner SB. Granulomatous disorders of the nose and paranasal sinuses. *Current Opinion in Otolaryngology and Head Neck Surgery.* 2009; 17: 23–27.

Lund VJ, Howard DJ, Wei W. *Granulomas and Conditions Simulating Neoplasia.* In *Tumours of the Nose, Paranasal Sinuses and Nasopharynx*. New York: Thieme, 2014.

Bahadur S, Thakar A. 2008. *Specific Chronic Infections.* In *Scott-Brown's Otorhinolaryngology, Head and Neck Surgery.* Eds. Gleeson M, Browning GB, Burton MJ, et al. London: Hodder Arnold, 2008: 1458–68.

6

Chronic rhinosinusitis

ROBIN YOUNGS

CHRONIC RHINOSINUSITIS

Rhinosinusitis is the term used to describe inflammation and infection within the nasal cavity and paranasal sinuses. This condition frequently coexists with nasal polyps. Chronic rhinosinusitis (CRS) is very common and accounts for a large number of visits to both primary care physicians and specialists. It is estimated that chronic rhinosinusitis affects between 5 per cent and 15 per cent of the general population in Europe and the United States.

DEFINITION

The 2012 update of the European Position Paper on Rhinosinusitis and Nasal Polyps (EPOS) defines chronic rhinosinusitis in adults as the following:

- Inflammation of the nose and paranasal sinuses characterized by two or more symptoms, one of which should be either nasal blockage/obstruction/congestion or nasal discharge (anterior/posterior nasal drip)
- +/- Facial pain/pressure
- +/- Reduction or loss of smell

and either

- Endoscopic signs
  - Nasal polyps, and/or
  - Mucopurulent discharge primarily from middle meatus and/or
  - Oedema/mucosal obstruction primarily in middle meatus and/or
- Computed tomography (CT) changes
- Mucosal changes within the osteomeatal complex and/or sinuses

for at least 12 weeks without resolution.

AETIOLOGY

The aetiology of CRS is multifactorial. The disease process depends on the complex interactions between the sinus respiratory epithelium, micro-organisms, allergy, and external factors such as environmental pollutants and tobacco smoke.

The role of micro-organisms in the aetiology of CRS is not fully understood. This is partly because the nasal cavity is home to a normal microbial population. The most common bacterial pathogen associated with CRS is *Staphylococcus aureus*. One possible explanation for the inflammation seen in CRS is the staphylococcal superantigen hypothesis, which suggests that bacterial toxins produce inflammation in the sinus mucosa. The presence of bacterial biofilms has been implicated as a factor in CRS. The aggregation of bacteria in biofilms renders them more resistant to host defences and antibiotics. Fungal infection has also been implicated in the aetiology of CRS, although this is controversial and not universally accepted.

The mucosa of the nasal cavity and paranasal sinuses is of a ciliated respiratory type. Diseases in which the function of the nasal and paranasal sinus cilia is impaired are associated with CRS. The most notable of these is cystic fibrosis, which is commonly associated with CRS and nasal polyps (Figure 6.1). Other ciliary disorders associated with CRS include primary ciliary dyskinesia and Kartegener's syndrome.

The role of nasal allergy in CRS is not completely clear. It may be that the inflammation of the nasal mucosa in allergic rhinitis predisposes to CRS, with swelling of the nasal mucosa producing obstruction of sinus ventilation and thereby infection.

Patients with immune deficiency are more likely to suffer with CRS. This includes human immunodeficiency virus (HIV)–related immune deficiency, in which opportunistic micro-organisms such as fungi, microsporidia and *Pseudomonas aeruginosa* can infect the sinuses.

Anatomical variation within the paranasal sinuses and nasal cavity such as nasal septal deviation and an enlarged cystic middle turbinate (concha bullosa) can be associated with CRS, and it is thought that these variations can cause blockage of the sinus ostia. These variations, however, are common in the general population without CRS, and it is unlikely that they can cause CRS in the absence of other aetiological factors.

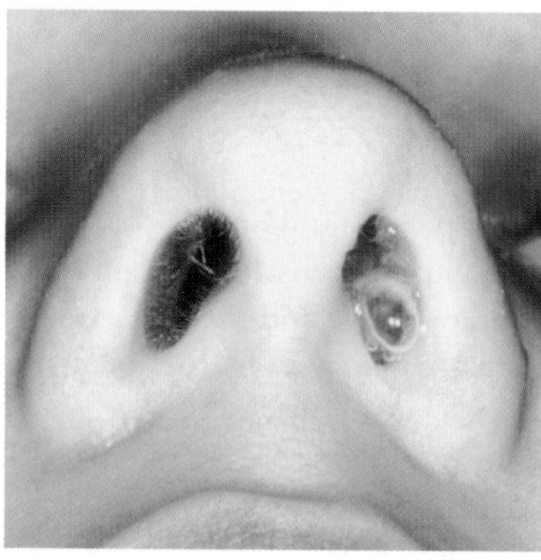

Figure 6.1 Chronic rhinosinusitis in an 11-year-old patient with cystic fibrosis.

CLINICAL PRESENTATION

Local symptoms of CRS include nasal blockage, nasal discharge, facial discomfort and reduction in sense of smell.

Nasal blockage in CRS is due to oedema of the nasal cavity mucosa. Co-existing nasal polyps can also block the nasal cavity. The blockage can be unilateral or bilateral.

Nasal discharge can be anterior, coming out of the nostrils, or posterior, where ciliary flow takes it into the pharynx. It can be unilateral or bilateral. The discharge in CRS is usually mucopurulent, having a yellow/green colouration (Figure 6.2). Many people wrongly interpret the normal physiological postnasal discharge, in which clear white mucus passes into the pharynx, as representing CRS.

Facial discomfort is not a prominent feature of CRS, although a mild dull ache, particularly in unilateral cases, can occur. Of the patients who are referred to ear, nose and throat (ENT) departments from primary care with a possible diagnosis of rhinogenic facial pain, less than 15 per cent actually have CRS. Other causes, such as migraine, cluster headaches, tension headaches and facial neuralgia, should also be considered.

A reduction (hyposmia) or loss (anosmia) of the sense of smell can occur with CRS but is much

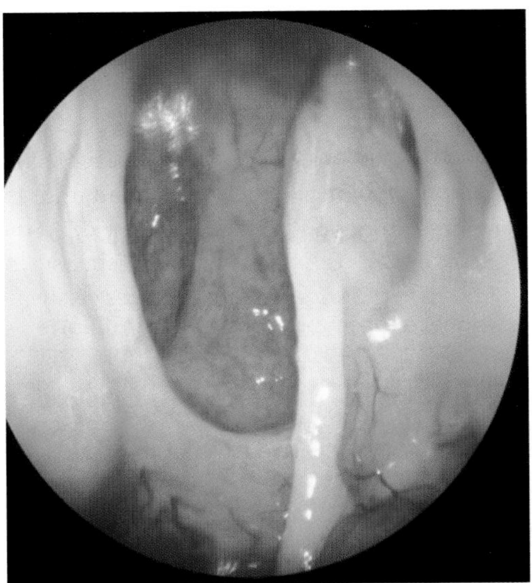

Figure 6.2 Endoscopic view of purulent post-nasal discharge in CRS.

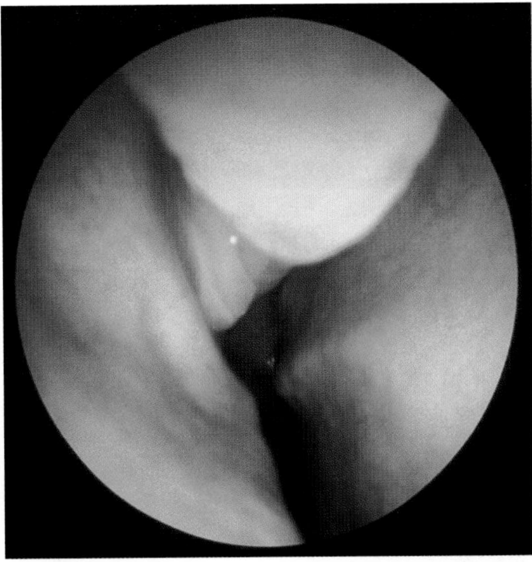

Figure 6.3 Endoscopic view of mucopurulent discharge in the middle meatus in CRS.

more common when co-existing nasal polyps are present.

CRS can also be accompanied by systemic and distant symptoms, such as malaise, pyrexia, cough, hoarse voice and sore throat (Table 6.1).

DIAGNOSIS

Most cases of CRS in primary care are diagnosed on symptoms alone. In secondary care, nasal endoscopy and CT scanning are used as additional diagnostic tools.

Table 6.1 Symptoms of chronic rhinosinusitis

Local
Nasal blockage
Nasal discharge (anterior and posterior)
Facial discomfort
Reduction in sense of smell
Distant and systemic
Cough
Sore throat
General malaise and pyrexia
Dysphonia

Nasal endoscopy

Nasal endoscopy can be undertaken in an outpatient setting. A rigid or flexible endoscope can be used, and the examination can be facilitated by the application of topical local anaesthetic and decongestant nasal spray. In CRS the presence of mucosal oedema, mucopurulent discharge and nasal polyps will be noted (Figure 6.3). In addition anatomical variation such as septal deviation or large turbinates will also be recorded. Endoscopically guided microbiological swabs can be taken if purulent discharge is seen. Anterior rhinoscopy alone, in which the nasal cavity is inspected by means of a torch or headlight, is of limited value in the diagnosis of CRS because only the anterior part of the nasal cavity can be clearly seen.

Sinus CT scanning

CT scanning is the radiological investigation of choice in CRS. Normally, however, this investigation is undertaken only when initial medical treatment has failed and surgical treatment is planned, or when complications are suspected. Most sinus CT data are collected in the axial plane and then reconstructed in the axial, coronal and sagittal

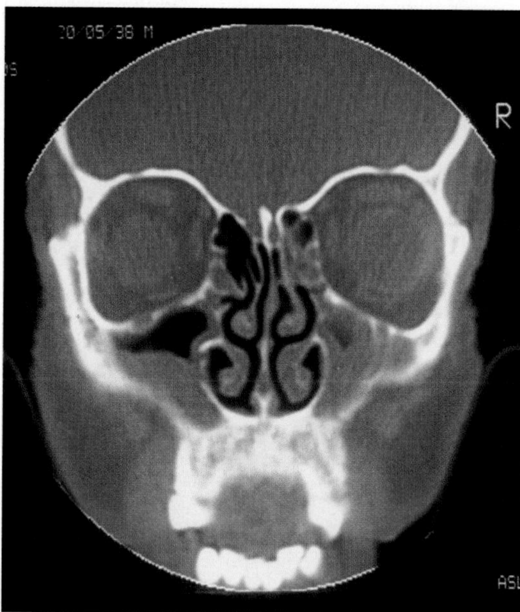

Figure 6.4 Coronal sinus CT showing sinus opacity in CRS.

planes. In CRS the usual finding on CT scanning is sinus opacity (Figure 6.4) due to swelling of the sinus mucosa and/or retained secretions. A commonly used method of quantifying CT involvement in CRS is the Lund-Mackay scoring system, in which individual sinuses are rated for opacity and then aggregated. CT scans cannot be used alone to diagnose CRS because radiological abnormalities are common in the 'normal' asymptomatic population. The diagnosis should be made by considering symptoms and endoscopic findings in addition to CT abnormalities. Plain sinus x-rays are of little value in the diagnosis of CRS. CRS can also be diagnosed with magnetic resonance imaging (MRI) scans, which have the advantage of no radiation dose. MRI scans, however, do not show the bony anatomy well and frequently demonstrate minor mucosal swelling of doubtful significance.

TREATMENT

Medical management of CRS includes corticosteroids, antibiotics and saline irrigations. In a proportion of patients, surgical treatment is also needed (Table 6.2).

Table 6.2 Treatment of chronic rhinosinusitis

Medical
Intranasal corticosteroids
Short-term antibiotics
Long-term antibiotics
Saline nasal irrigation
Surgical
Functional endoscopic sinus surgery (FESS)

Medical management of CRS

CORTICOSTEROIDS

Corticosteroids act in CRS by moderating the inflammatory processes in the disease, particularly those mediated by eosinophils. These drugs are usually administered in spray or drop form directly to the nasal mucosa. Because of their mode of action, symptomatic relief is noticed only after about 7 days, and they have to be administered daily to be effective. There is little evidence to favour one preparation over another, although those that are used once a day may have better patient compliance. Preparations in common use are beclomethasone, fluticasone and mometasone. Long-term use of intranasal corticosteroids is safe, although side effects can occur, including nasal dryness, crusting and epistaxis. In CRS without nasal polyps, systemic corticosteroids are generally not used owing to the potential for serious long-term systemic side effects.

ANTIBIOTICS

Antibiotics are an important treatment for CRS, and they can be used in short or long-term courses. Antibiotics used in short courses (less than 4 weeks) are usually prescribed for acute infective exacerbations and are broad spectrum drugs such as amoxicillin/clavulanic acid, cephalosporins, macrolides or doxycycline. There has been much interest in the use of long-term antibiotics for CRS following their initial success in patients with chronic lower respiratory conditions such as diffuse panbronchiolitis. There is evidence that long-term antibiotics may influence the inflammatory response in CRS in addition to any antimicrobial effects. Macrolide antibiotics such as clarithromycin or azithromycin have been most frequently used, although doxycycline is an alternative preparation. Long-term antibiotics in CRS should be considered when treatment with nasal steroid sprays and saline irrigation fail to control symptoms.

SALINE NASAL IRRIGATION

Saline nasal irrigation is a treatment for CRS that has seen a revival in recent years. Regular saline irrigation produces symptomatic relief possibly through washing away purulent secretions, although the mode of action is not certain. This treatment is well tolerated with minimal side effects.

Surgical management of CRS

Modern surgical management of CRS is normally by the technique of functional endoscopic sinus surgery (FESS). In this technique, endoscopes are used to remove tissue that is considered to be blocking the ostia of the paranasal sinuses. The common method is to follow the disease using an anterior to posterior dissection. In this way removal of the uncinate process provides access to the anterior ethmoidal sinuses, and partial removal of the basal lamella of the middle turbinate provides an opening into the posterior ethmoidal sinuses. The ostium of the maxillary sinus can be enlarged. Clearance of the anterior ethmoid may facilitate ventilation of the frontal sinus through the frontal recess. The optimal extent of surgery in CRS is controversial and ranges from minimal approaches with mucosal preservation to complete sinus exenteration with removal of diseased mucosa. Surgery is particularly effective where nasal obstruction is a prominent feature. Post-nasal discharge and hyposmia are much less likely to respond to surgery. A major effect of FESS surgery in CRS is to produce a larger 'sinus cavity', which is more accessible to topical corticosteroids and saline irrigation.

Endoscopic balloon dilatation of paranasal sinus ostia (balloon sinuplasty) has also been advocated as a treatment for CRS with the rationale of improving sinus ventilation. Its use, however, is controversial, and long-term clinical evaluation is awaited.

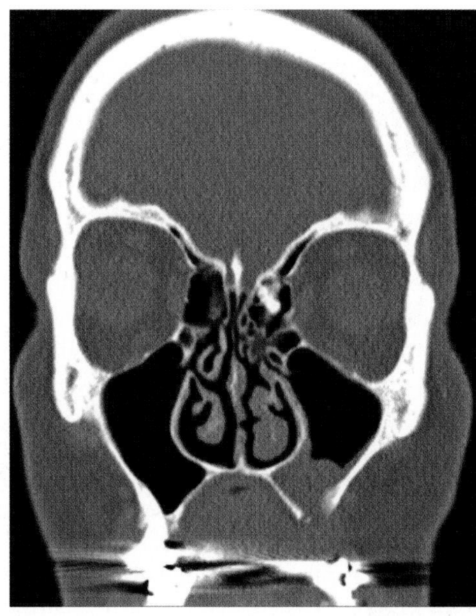

Figure 6.5 CT scan showing maxillary sinusitis secondary to chronic dental disease with an oro-antral fistula.

SINUSITIS OF DENTAL ORIGIN

Chronic sinus infections can also arise secondary to dental infection (Figure 6.5). This is by virtue of the upper molar teeth being related to the floor of the maxillary antrum. In some cases, particularly after dental extraction, an oro-antral fistula can form. Treatment is with antibiotics and appropriate dental treatment to the diseased dental root.

NASAL POLYPS

The term *polyp* when applied to the nasal cavity is purely a descriptive one, referring to the appearance of an abnormal pedunculated lesion. Nasal polyps are frequently associated with chronic rhinosinusitis. Other types of nasal polyps include antrochoanal polyps and neoplastic polyps.

NASAL POLYPS IN ASSOCIATION WITH CHRONIC RHINOSINUSITIS

This condition, which is also known as chronic rhinosinusitis with nasal polyps (CRSwNP), produces the largest group of patients with nasal polyps.

AETIOLOGY

Many of the inflammatory changes seen in CRS are also seen in patients with nasal polyposis. In particular, inflammation mediated by eosinophils and to a lesser extent neutrophils is important. There are a number of important clinical associations in patients with nasal polyps (Table 6.3). The most common association is with coexisting asthma, particularly non-atopic and late onset. In this subgroup of asthmatics, 10–15 per cent have nasal polyps. Nasal polyps are common in patients with cystic fibrosis, with about a third of these patients having nasal polyps. Cystic fibrosis should be considered in children with nasal polyps, although the diagnosis will have normally been made in early childhood. The so-called aspirin triad is the association of nasal polyps, asthma and aspirin hypersensitivity. The disease manifestation in these cases is particularly severe. Nasal polyps are also seen in allergic fungal sinusitis, a condition that is not completely understood. Allergic fungal sinusitis is associated with nasal polyps, thick eosinophilic mucus, lack of fungal invasion into tissues and type-1 hypersensitivity to fungi. The condition is also characterized by bony erosion seen on CT scanning.

CLINICAL PRESENTATION

The principal symptoms of nasal polyps are nasal obstruction and a reduction in or loss of the sense of smell. There is a large variation in disease severity. Some patients have minor symptoms or small nasal polyps that are discovered as an incidental examination finding. Other patients may have severe symptoms with complete nasal obstruction and anosmia. Nasal polyps are associated with CRS; hence, there may be additional symptoms of nasal discharge and facial discomfort.

Table 6.3 Conditions associated with nasal polyps (CRSwNP)

Asthma (non-atopic and late-onset)
Cystic fibrosis
Aspirin hypersensitivity
Allergic fungal sinusitis

DIAGNOSIS

Nasal endoscopy

In advanced cases, nasal polyps can sometimes be seen in the anterior part of the nasal cavity with the naked eye. Occasionally, on anterior rhinoscopy alone the inferior turbinate is mistaken for a nasal polyp. Nasal endoscopy is the key diagnostic tool, with nasal polyps having the appearance of pale, gelatinous pedunculated lesions (Figure 6.6). There have been numerous attempts to stage or grade nasal polyps, usually with reference to the extent of disease in relation to the middle turbinate. Most nasal polyps originate from the anterior and posterior ethmoidal sinuses. Anterior ethmoidal polyps tend to present in the middle meatus, whereas posterior polyps occupy the spheno-ethmoidal recess and the posterior nasal cavity.

CT scanning

CT scanning is undertaken in nasal polyposis when surgery is planned or complications are suspected. As in CRS, the degree of sinus opacity and any anatomical variation that may affect a surgical approach are noted. In the most severe

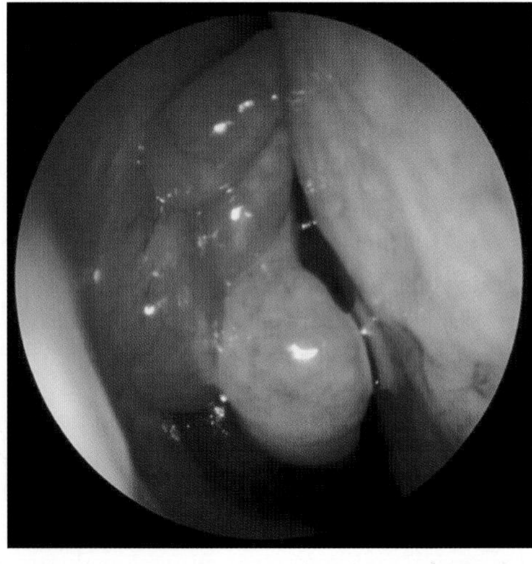

Figure 6.6 Endoscopic view of nasal polyps.

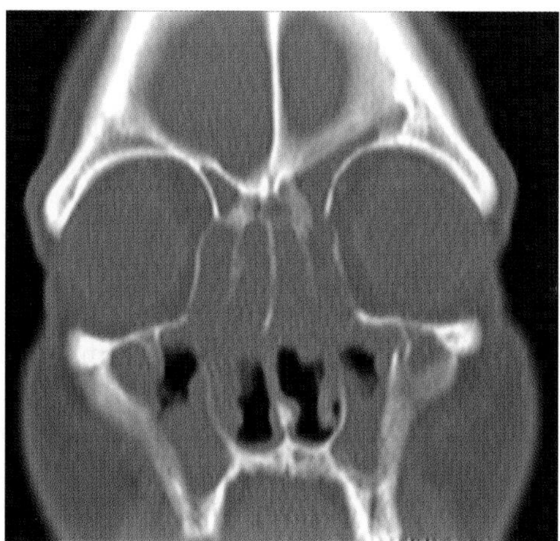

Figure 6.7 CT scan of severe nasal polyps showing widening of the ethmoidal sinuses.

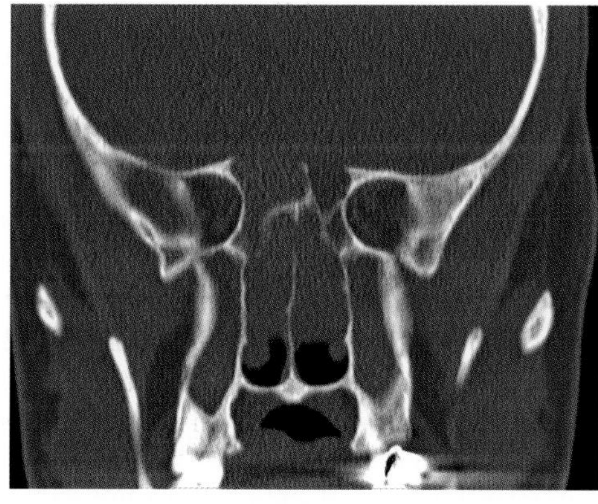

Figure 6.8 CT scan of allergic fungal sinusitis showing mixed opacity of 'fungal' mucus and bony erosion of the roof of the posterior ethmoidal sinuses.

cases of nasal polyps, there can be widening of the ethmoidal air cells with lateral displacement of the lamina papyracea, usually bilaterally. In cases where nasal polyps are seen in association with allergic fungal sinusitis, characteristic additional features are mixed density of 'fungal' mucus and bony erosion (Figures 6.7 and 6.8).

Histological examination

Histological examination of polyps removed at the time of surgery is normally undertaken. In nasal polyps associated with CRS, the notable features are an oedematous stroma with eosinophilic or neutrophilic infiltration and the absence of any features suggesting neoplasia.

TREATMENT

Because nasal polyposis is a reflection of underlying mucosal inflammation, there is no surgical cure in the majority of cases. Medications, surgery and combinations of both are used in an individualized manner depending on symptom profile, symptom severity and extent of disease.

Medical treatment

The most effective medical treatment for nasal polyposis is corticosteroids, which can be administered locally in spray or drop form, or systemically. As in CRS, commonly used corticosteroid sprays for nasal polyps are mometasone, beclomethasone and fluticasone. Nasal corticosteroid drops can be more effective than sprays in the treatment of hyposmia associated with nasal polyps. Common corticosteroid nasal drops are betamethasone and fluticasone. Care must be taken in the use of nasal corticosteroid drops because overdose can lead to significant systemic absorption and subsequent side effects. Systemic corticosteroids can be given in short courses of up to 3 weeks as initial therapy, in severe cases and as an adjunct to surgical treatment. Prednisolone is the most commonly used preparation in doses of up to 50 mg daily. When nasal polyps are associated with infection, antibiotics can be given in addition in a similar fashion as in CRS.

Surgical treatment

Surgical treatment is often indicated when nasal blockage is a prominent symptom and is best undertaken using endoscopes for visualization. Simple removal of nasal polyps is known as nasal polypectomy. As in CRS without nasal polyps, the optimal extent of surgery is controversial and ranges from polypectomy to radical sinus exenteration. Creation of a larger space in the nasal cavity to facilitate topical corticosteroid treatment after surgery is important. Patients in whom a loss of sense of smell is the prominent symptom are frequently disappointed with the outcome of surgery, because their symptoms often recur within a few months after initial transient improvement.

ANTROCHOANAL POLYPS

Antrochoanal polyps originate from the maxillary antrum and pass into the nasal cavity, where they occupy the floor and posterior part of the nasal cavity (Figures 6.9 and 6.10). They are almost always unilateral and often occur in children and young adults, presenting as unilateral nasal obstruction. The maxillary antral component is often fluid filled and cystic and passes through an abnormally large accessory maxillary ostium. In advanced cases, the polyp can pass into the nasopharynx and oropharynx.

Diagnosis is by nasal endoscopy and CT scanning. Treatment is surgical because these polyps are resistant to corticosteroid therapy. Complete removal of the nasal and antral components is required; otherwise recurrence is common. An endoscopic approach is adequate using angled endoscopes and curved instruments to access the antral portion. Histological analysis is mandatory to exclude neoplasia because inverted papilloma originating from the maxillary antrum can present in a similar way.

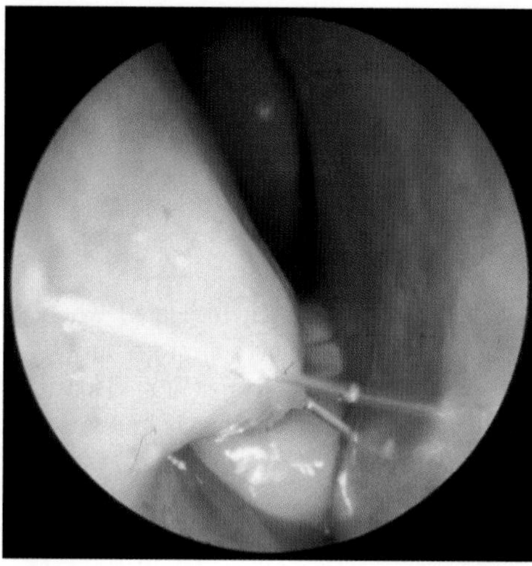

Figure 6.9 Endoscopic view of an antrochoanal polyp lying in the posterior nasal cavity.

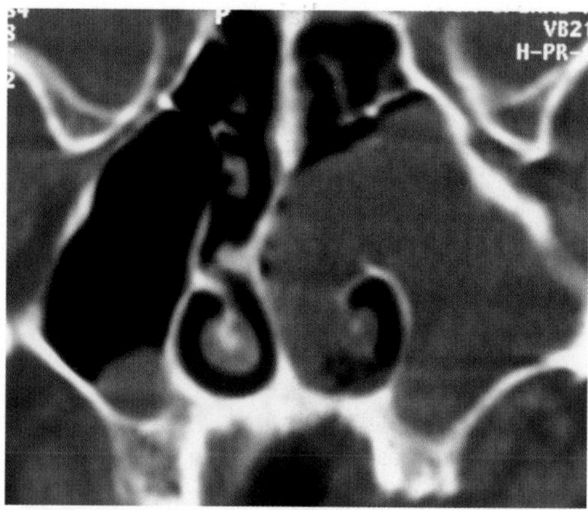

Figure 6.10 CT scan showing an antrochoanal polyp.

PARANASAL SINUS MUCOCELES

A mucocele is an epithelial-lined sac containing mucus within one of the paranasal sinuses. This is in contrast to a blocked sinus simply containing retained or infected secretions. Mucoceles can be seen in association with CRS and nasal polyps, or they can be an isolated finding. Mucoceles have the capacity to expand and erode the bone of the sinus walls. The fronto-ethmoidal region is the most common site for mucoceles, where they can present with displacement of the orbital structures and subsequent proptosis (Figure 6.11). Erosion of the posterior table of the frontal sinus can also occur with large mucoceles. Treatment is surgical

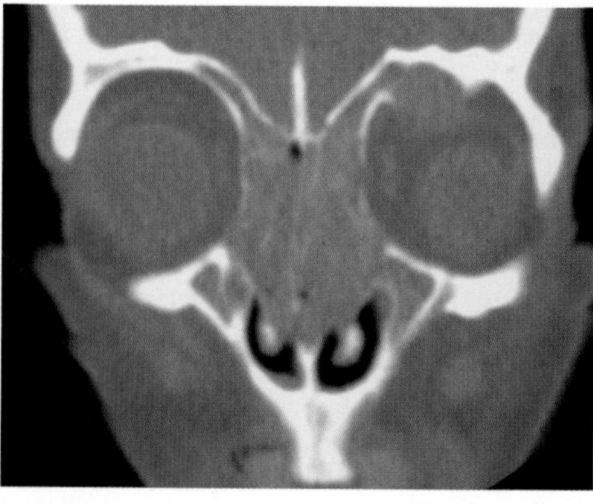

Figure 6.11 CT scan showing a left frontal mucocele with displacement of the orbit.

by endoscopic marsuplialization into the frontal recess.

KEY LEARNING POINTS

- Chronic rhinosinusitis is characterized by nasal blockage, nasal discharge and facial pain.
- Nasal endoscopy and CT scanning are key tools in diagnosis.
- Medical treatment of CRS is with antibiotics, topical corticosteroids and saline irrigation.
- Nasal polyps present with nasal blockage and decreased sense of smell.
- Treatment of nasal polyps is medical (with corticosteroids) or surgical.

FURTHER READING

Chan Y, Kuhn FA. An update on the classification, diagnosis, and treatment of rhinosinusitis. *Current Opinion in Otolaryngology and Head Neck Surgery*. 2009; 17: 204–8.

Fokkens WJ, Lund VJ, Mullol J, Bachert C, et al. European position paper on rhinosinusitis and nasal polyps 2012. *Rhinology*. 2012; 50: Suppl 23.

Ah-See KL, MacKenzie J, Ah-See KW. Management of chronic rhinosinusitis. *BMJ*. 2012; 345: 40–44.

Bhattacharyya N, Lee LN. Evaluating the diagnosis of chronic rhinosinusitis based on clinical guidelines and endoscopy. *Otolaryngology – Head and Neck Surgery*. 2010; 143: 147–51.

Wallwork B, Coman W, MacKay-Sim A, Grieff L, Cervin A. A double-blind randomized, placebo-controlled trial of macrolide in the treatment of chronic rhinosinusitis. *Laryngoscope*. 2006; 116: 189–93.

Poetker DM, Mendolia-Loffredo S, Smith TL. Outcomes of endoscopic sinus surgery for chronic rhinosinusitis associated with sinonasal polyposis. *American Journal of Rhinology*. 2007; 21: 84–8.

Kennedy D. Functional endoscopic sinus surgery. Technique. *Archives of Otolaryngology*. 1985; 111: 643–9.

Foreman A, Boase S, Psaltis A, Wormald P-J. Role of bacterial and fungal biofilms in chronic rhinosinusitis. *Current Allergy and Asthma Reports*. 2012; 12: 127–35.

7

The blocked nose

PAUL S WHITE

Nasal obstruction or nasal blockage is the sensation of reduced airflow through the nose and can be bilateral or unilateral. In normal respiration, the physiological pathway is via the nose, and the sensation of nasal obstruction occurs when this process is impaired. If this is severe, mouth breathing will also be evident. In emergency situations, and during extreme exercise, the higher ventilation requirements mean that physiological mouth breathing may have to come into play, as a necessary supplement to nasal respiration. Occasionally, athletes may become concerned about this and are best reassured that it is not unusual to have to resort to some mouth breathing during exercise. Normal physiological changes mean that nasal patency can be influenced by factors other than exercise. These include the humidity and temperature of the surrounding air and the position of the body, with the supine position being associated with more congestion when compared with being erect. The average rate of ventilation during nasal breathing at rest is approximately 6 litres per minute. During exercise, this will increase to 50–60 litres per minute, and at this level will be shared jointly as nasal and mouth breathing.

The highest velocity of flow occurs through the internal nasal valve, which is the narrowest point in the nasal airway. Consequently, disorders acting to reduce the cross-sectional area in the nasal valve will have a disproportionate effect on the reduction in nasal patency and the increase in resistance to flow. Conditions that interfere with the normal airflow pattern in the nasal valve area can also accentuate the symptom of nasal obstruction. Examples of this include deformities such as anterior septal perforation, which interfere with the laminar flow patterns necessary for the sensation of normal nasal breathing.

The sensation of normal nasal flow occurs through stimulation of flow receptors in the nasal valve area. The nose, when compared with the oral airway, is a resistant airway, and the normal perception of flow requires a background level of resistance along with the presence of a laminar airflow pattern. Nasal resistance is the difference between air pressure at the nasal vestibule and air pressure in the nasopharynx. This is normally between 8 and 20 mm H_2O, and supplementary mouth breathing begins at pressure differences above 40 mm H_2O. This explains why conditions associated with low resistance, such as 'empty nose syndrome' caused by excessive loss of turbinate tissue, are associated with the sensation of nasal obstruction, because a minimum level of resistance (normally greater than 6–8 mm H_2O) is needed for the normal perception of flow. Physiologically, the resistance of the nasal airway is necessary for the fulfillment of complex functions of the nose as a respiratory and olfactory organ.

Another factor affecting physiological airflow is the nasal cycle, during which each side of the nasal airway undergoes an alternating cycle of congestion and decongestion. In the normal state, this cycle is not noticeable, but when concurrent disorders such as rhinitis affect the nasal airway, cyclical alternating nasal obstruction may become apparent. The regulation of the nasal cycle is controlled by the influence of the parasympathetic and sympathetic nervous systems on vascularity of the erectile tissue of the inferior turbinate and septum. This, in turn, will cause a variation in the respective nasal resistance of each nasal airway. This explains the positive influence of exercise, during which increased sympathetic nervous system tone enables vasoconstriction via stimulation of nasal mucosal vascular α-adrenergic receptors. Adrenaline analogue drugs such as xylometazaline work in the same way. This demonstrates why intranasal vasoconstrictors may relieve nasal obstruction by causing mucosal decongestion.

AETIOLOGY

Otolaryngology is a specialty that covers a broad demographic; when considering possible underlying aetiologies, it is useful to keep in mind the influence of patient age, race and geographic location. Choanal atresia, if bilateral, will be evident at birth. Because neonates are obligate nasal breathers, the resultant posterior nasal airway obstruction causes a potentially life-threatening situation. Adenoid hypertrophy is generally a condition affecting young children and is rare in adults. In contrast, vasomotor rhinitis is a condition usually seen in adults and is a frequent cause of nasal obstruction and/or rhinorrhoea in the elderly. It is also commonly seen in pregnant women and patients on anti-hypertensive medication. Cross-border variations in aetiology are sometimes evident. For example, when compared with its prevalence in other European counties, perennial allergic rhinitis due to house dust mite (HDM) allergy is especially common in the United Kingdom. The nature of home environmental conditions in the United Kingdom is such that levels of the HDM allergen are high. Racial differences are another factor to consider. For example, differences in facial structure mean that septal deformities are more frequently seen in Caucasians compared with other racial groups, such as Asians and Black Africans. It follows that there are many different causes of nasal obstruction (Table 7.1), with the most common aetiologies being the various forms of rhinitis. When considering relevant causes, it is useful to consider four different subdivisions:

1. Conditions affecting the mucosa, e.g. rhinitis, polyps, sinusitis and neoplasms
2. Septal disorders including deviation and perforation
3. Nasal valve collapse
4. Nasopharyngeal disease

Many patients with nasal obstruction will have more than one disorder. Examples of this include the child who has both allergic rhinitis and adenoid hypertrophy, the atopic individual with rhinitis and nasal polyps, and the elderly patient with internal valve collapse secondary to age-related degeneration of the upper lateral cartilages who also has vasomotor rhinitis.

Certain patterns of nasal obstruction may herald the presence of underlying neoplasia or a different need for urgent treatment. Children with unilateral nose block, especially when associated with discharge, may have an underlying foreign body. Nasal polyps in children are rare and require further investigation to exclude conditions such as mucoviscidosis, encephalocoele and juvenile angiofibroma. In general, unilateral nasal obstruction, especially if associated with pain or bleeding, should be investigated as a matter of urgency.

EVALUATION AND DIAGNOSIS

The symptom of nasal obstruction is the most common complaint seen in the various disease processes that affect the nose and paranasal

Table 7.1 Different causes of nasal obstruction

Subdivision	Aetiology	Common characteristics
Mucosa/skin/lining	Common cold	Coryzal prodrome
	Seasonal allergic rhinitis	Sneezing, rhinorrhoea, itch
	Perennial allergic rhinitis	House dust mite, animal dander
	Vasomotor rhinitis	Temperature, posture, stress
	Nasal polyps	Hyposmia, post-nasal discharge
	Nasal vestibulitis	Bleeding and crusting
	Chronic infective sinusitis	Purulent discharge
	Acute sinusitis	Pain, fever, discharge
	Rhinitis medicamentosa	Increasing need for vasoconstrictors
	Inverting papilloma	Unilateral blockage gradual progression
	Atrophic rhinitis	Ozaena, crusting and blockage
	Antriochoanal polyp	Unilateral blockage, nasopharynx mass
	Sarcoid	Can mimic rhinosinusitis
	Wegener's granulomatosis	Bleeding, crusting, systemic symptoms
	Encephalocoele	Unilateral mass, may pulsate
	Olfactory neuroblastoma	Slowly progressive hyposmia
Septal	Septal dislocation	Can be familial
	Septal fracture	History of trauma or childhood trauma
	Haematoma	Sudden bilateral block after trauma
	Perforation	Crusting, whistling, epistaxis
	Bleeding polyp of the septum	Unilateral bleeding mass
Nasal valve	Weak upper laterals	Can be with narrow middle third
	Weak lower laterals	Seen more often in the elderly
	Post-rhinoplasty	Main effect on the nasal valve
	Saddle deformity	Reduced septal height affects valve
	Foreign bodies	Usually impact in the valve
Nasopharynx/ posterior	Adenoids	Mouth breathing and snoring
	Choanal atresia	Evident at birth or early childhood
	Nasopharyngeal angiofibroma	Increasing blockage +/- epistaxis
	Nasopharyngeal carcinoma	Neck mass and other symptoms
	Lymphoma	Systemic and middle ear manifestations

sinuses. It is worth noting that there may be subtle differences between subjective nasal obstruction or 'nose block' and the sensation of nasal congestion or nasal stuffiness. Some patients will use the terms *congested* or *stuffy* to describe a mid-facial or nasal discomfort; this may or may not be associated with true blockage, and only with good history taking can these relative meanings be teased out.

HISTORY

One should begin by characterizing the nature of the obstruction, taking into account duration, periodicity, nocturnal variation, seasonal effects, laterality, association with trauma, and any alleviating or provoking factors. Knowledge of the presence or absence of associated symptoms, such as hyposmia, anosmia, rhinorrhoea and post-nasal discharge, is not only useful diagnostically but also helps to create a picture of the level of quality of life impairment suffered. Chronic nasal obstruction is often associated with sleep disturbance and may be a contributing factor to snoring. Persistent hyposmia or anosmia is frequently seen with nasal polyposis and/or allergic rhinitis. It is important to enquire about allergies and any previous allergy tests, hay fever, asthma and the presence of any animals in the home. A history of cigarette smoking is relevant because it may potentiate the symptoms of allergic rhinitis, and vasomotor rhinitis is sometimes seen as a cause of nasal obstruction during smoking withdrawal. The presence of psychosomatic overlay is common in patients with rhinological conditions, and, although rare, perceptive nasal obstruction is occasionally seen in patients whose symptoms are found to have no organic basis. Such individuals should be investigated thoroughly, including formal nasal airflow testing, because results of these tests often prove to be a valuable tool in subsequent patient counseling. Although empirical medical treatment for rhinitis in this situation is worth contemplating, the temptation to perform speculative surgical interventions such as septoplasty without a clear diagnostic basis should be avoided.

The character of any nasal discharge can give clues to an infective versus an allergic origin. In children with constant chronic nasal obstruction and mouth breathing, the possibility of adenoid hypertrophy should be considered. In this case, there will usually be a history of snoring and occasionally sleep apnoea. A previous history of nasal trauma including fractured nose and epistaxis may suggest nasal obstruction resulting from traumatic septal deformity. Increasing nasal obstruction associated with epistaxis, especially when unilateral, may be suggestive of a benign or malignant neoplasm.

It is relevant to consider the previous medical history. Surgical procedures such as rhinoplasty, alar base reduction and cleft palate surgery can all have a restrictive effect on the nasal airway. Many systemic diseases have nasal manifestations including nasal obstruction. Wegener's granulomatosis is a systemic vasculitis in which nasal obstruction is associated with diffuse crusting of the nasal mucosa. Other conditions with a similar symptom profile include sarcoidosis, Churg-Strauss vasculitis and Bechet's syndrome. Chronic infections such as rhinoscleroma, tuberculosis and rhinosporidosis can cause local nasal tissue destruction such as septal perforation and consequent nasal obstruction. Cocaine abuse and habitual nose picking can cause septal crusting, septal perforation and saddle deformity, all of which have the potential to cause nasal airway impairment.

The pharmaceutical history will sometimes reveal nasal obstruction occurring as an unwanted drug side effect. Nonsteroidal anti-inflammatory drugs (NSAIDs) such as aspirin and ibuprofen in patients who have NSAID/aspirin hypersensitivity can trigger non-infective rhinitis and rhinosinusitis. Nasal obstruction associated with vasomotor rhinitis (VMR) is seen as a potential side effect of a number of drugs. These include anti-hypertensives (such as β-blockers and calcium channel blockers), sedatives, phenothiazines, antidepressants, oral contraceptives and drugs used to treat erectile dysfunction. Also, overuse of decongestant nasal sprays can cause a type of VMR called rhinitis medicamentosa.

CLINICAL EXAMINATION

A comprehensive approach to examination of the nose can be developed with practice. This should include the examination of the external nose, anterior rhinoscopy, nasendoscopy and an evaluation of flow.

Examination of the external nose should begin with careful inspection and palpation of the nasal bones and cartilages. The detail should include an evaluation of skin type, skin scars, soft-tissue envelope thickness, integrity of the alar cartilages, nasal tip support, nares shape and integrity of the nasal valve. These factors can offer useful information on the more subtle causes of nasal obstruction, such as nasal valve insufficiency. Relevant abnormalities will include saddle deformity, septal deviation and deficiency of the alar cartilages. Anterior rhinoscopy is performed with an appropriate-sized Thudichum's speculum prior to any decongestion. Specific evaluation of the turbinates, anomalies of the septum, secretions and crusting as well as the presence of any mass lesions such as polyps is noted. Determining the relevance of subtle septal deviation can be difficult, especially because most Caucasian individuals will have some degree of septal misalignment. In this regard a simple grading system for each of Cottle's areas of the septum can help to improve inter-observer agreement (Table 7.2).

Table 7.2 Grading system for classification of septal deviation for use in conjunction with each Cottle's area

Grade of deviation	
0	Central
1	Minimal
2	Deviated but less than 50 per cent
3	Deviated greater than 50 per cent
4	Mucosal contact with lateral wall
Cottle's areas	
1	Caudal
2	Nasal valve
3	High mid-septum
4	Low mid-septum
5	Posterior

Simple clinical patency tests such as the digital occlusion test, Cottle's test and the nasal vapour condensation test may be helpful. The occlusion test is achieved by occluding one nostril with a thumb, then asking the patient to sniff through the nose. The vapour condensation test can be performed with a metal tongue depressor or a Glatzel calibrated mirror (Figure 7.1) and gives a ready reckoning of relative flow.

In Cottle's manoeuvre, the cheek is pulled laterally with the index finger applying traction to the alar to increase the internal nasal valve angle. When applying Cottle's test (Figure 7.2) in patients with nasal valve collapse, the sensation of nasal flow should improve, although differentiation between internal or external valve insufficiency is not possible. In addition, other causes of obstruction, including septal deviation in the nasal valve area, will often give a positive test.

When the suspicion of nasal valve insufficiency is raised, other clinical tests can help confirm the diagnosis. Internal valve collapse caused by weakness of the upper laterals may respond to a useful diagnostic trial of *Breathe Right* strips. Similarly, nasal vestibule stents such as Francis alar dilators can have a positive effect on both valve areas.

NASENDOSCOPY

Nasendoscopy is a necessary investigation for all patients referred for a specialist investigation of nasal obstruction. This is best performed after the application of local anaesthetic and decongestant, when the effect of the vasoconstriction on the turbinate mucosa will give a useful indication of the reversibility of any rhinitic congestion. Endoscopic evaluation using a three-pass technique should encompass imaging of the inferior meatus, middle meatus, superior meatus, spheno-ethmoidal recess, olfactory cleft, septal areas and nasopharynx. Conditions causing severe obstruction of the anterior airway such as a dramatic septal deviation or a large polyp may preclude endoscopy beyond this level, but they will emphasize its clinical relevance. Any nasal masses should be evaluated for colour, consistency, vascularity and origin. Classic bilateral nasal polyps need not be biopsied unless the mucosal appearance is unusual. Biopsy performed

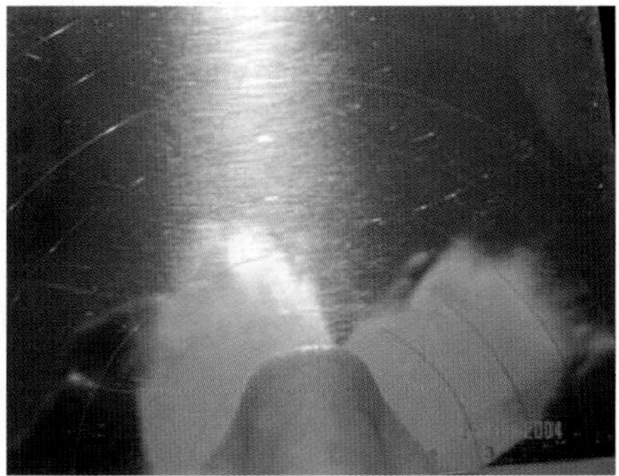

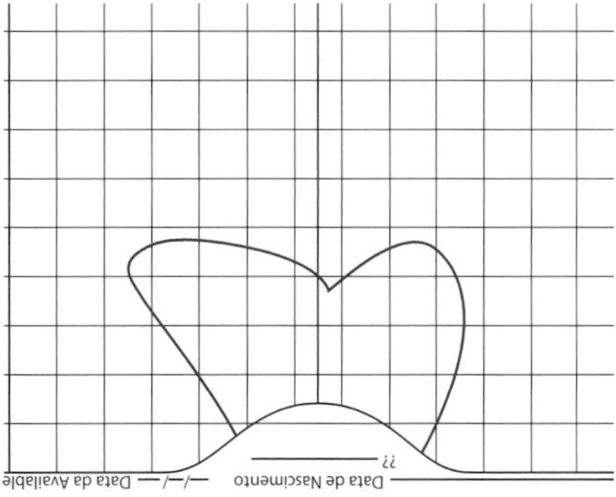

Figure 7.1 Nasal vapour condensation shadow as seen with a calibrated Glatzel mirror.

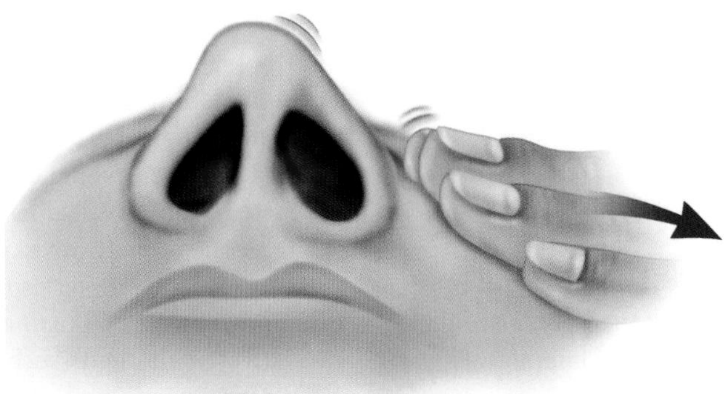

Figure 7.2 Cottle's cheek retraction test.

in a clinic situation for a unilateral mass should be considered if the risk of vascularity is low and the origin does not appear to be from the skull base area. Preparations should be made for the potential for epistaxis following biopsy. Vascular-appearing masses that raise the suspicion of a diagnosis of juvenile angiofibroma should first undergo computed tomography (CT) imaging with enhancement. If biopsy is then considered necessary, it is best performed in the operating theatre.

INVESTIGATION OF NASAL OBSTRUCTION

Nasal airway testing can offer supportive diagnostic information for conditions such as nasal valve collapse, subclinical septal deviation and perceptive nasal obstruction. These investigations can also be useful in situations where there is some diagnostic uncertainty, for which they offer supportive objective information beyond the usual subjective clinical evaluation. Although advanced functional tests such as acoustic rhinometry and rhinomanometry may not be available in all centres, PNIFR (peak nasal inspiratory flow rate) measurement is inexpensive and offers good correlation with patient symptoms.

Acoustic rhinometry (AR) is a technique in which acoustic wave pulses are directed into the internal structures of the nasal airway and the measured acoustic reflections are used to construct a static map of the nasal airway. These depict the cross-sectional area (CSA) of the nasal airway as a function of distance from the nares, which is exhibited as a characteristic waveform (Figure 7.3). Narrow points in the airway are represented as depressions or troughs in the CSA. The first depression after the nosepiece is the minimal cross-sectional area (MCA). This corresponds to the narrowing of the internal nasal valve and includes a contribution from the anterior end of the inferior turbinate. Reliability of AR can be affected by test/retest error; to achieve appropriate levels of reproducibility, it is best performed by a trained technician.

Rhinomanometry is a test of nasal flow that measures nasal resistance, the ratio between differential pressure and airflow. It offers a genuinely objective measure of the degree of impairment of nasal airflow. In contrast to AR, it is a dynamic technique; it measures flow as a function of the differential pressure as this changes during the nasal breathing cycle. It is normally represented as a sigmoid pressure-flow curve plotted with inspiration and expiration, and a different graph for the right and left nasal airway (Figure 7.4). Accordingly, patients with genuine nasal obstruction will be expected to have high resistance, which graphically is seen as a decreasing slope on the pressure-flow curve because greater negative pressures are required to generate flow. The roles of acoustic rhinometry and rhinomanometry are complementary. Rhinomanometry is a valuable objective test for substantiating complaints of nasal obstruction and quantifying nasal resistance, whereas AR is useful for confirming specific sites of airway restriction. Both are useful measures of response to treatment.

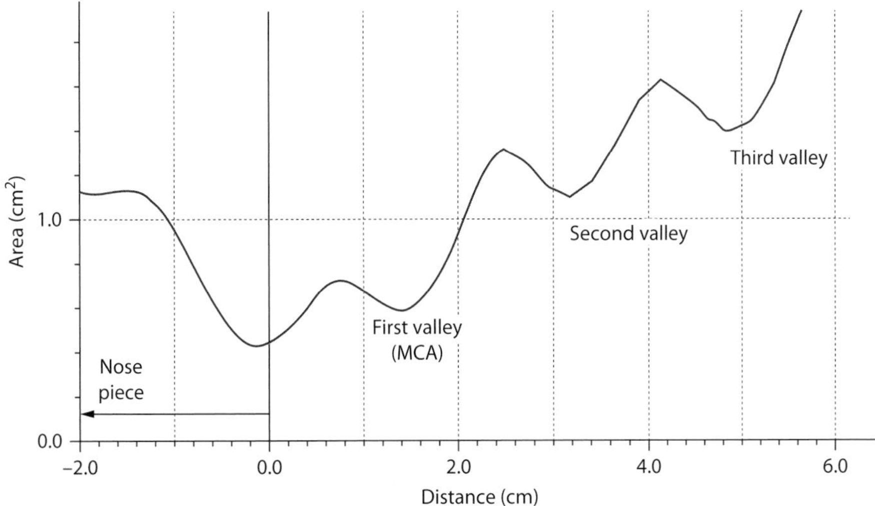

Figure 7.3. A typical acoustic rhinogram waveform showing the depressions that occur at narrow points in the nasal airway. The first depression after the nosepiece, the minimal cross-sectional area (MCA), corresponds to the narrowing of the internal nasal valve.

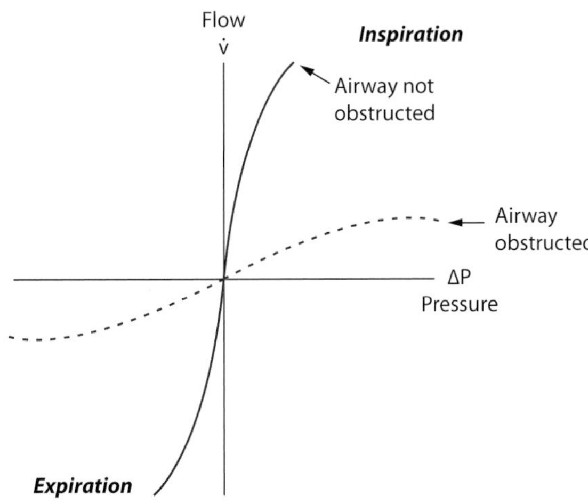

Figure 7.4 Rhinomanometry pressure-flow curve, with airflow increasing with increased transnasal pressure. With the obstructed airway, flow fails to increase, and nasal resistance is shown to be high.

Peak nasal inspiratory flow is a straightforward and inexpensive means of measuring nasal obstruction, because test results have been shown to correlate well with the severity of symptomatic nasal obstruction (Figure 7.5). The patient is required to perform a forced sniff at maximum effort via a flowmeter, with the flow peak being measured using a cursor. Peak nasal inspiratory flow appears to be the best validated technique for home monitoring of nasal obstruction in clinical trials and is quick to perform in a clinic situation. Because readings are effort dependent, they measure peak nasal inspiration, which may not necessarily mirror nasal breathing at rest. Furthermore,

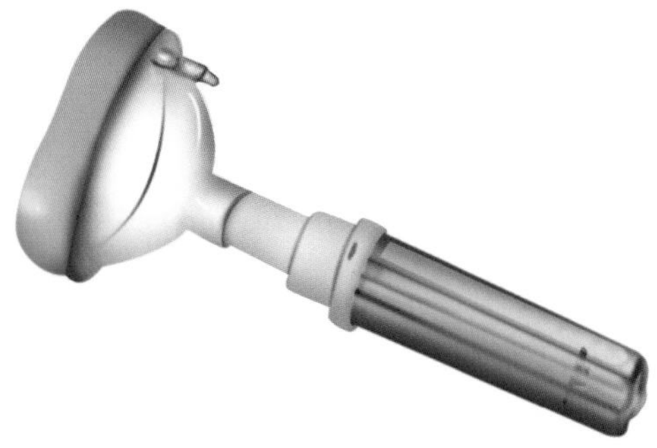

Figure 7.5 Face mask and flowmeter used for measuring peak nasal inspiratory flow (PNIF).

the level of patient cooperation required may generate false positive results in patients unable to generate the necessary inspiratory effort.

ALLERGY TESTING

Patients with rhinitis and polyps should be assessed for inhalant allergy. This can comprise skin testing and/or measurement of allergen-specific IgE by the radioallergosorbent test (RAST). The skin prick test is performed on the volar aspect of the forearm and tests a wide variety of allergens including house dust mite, various pollens and animal dander. These are compared with positive (histamine) and negative (saline) controls, the latter being important to exclude patients with dermatographia. If skin testing is inconclusive or contraindicated, then the RAST, although less sensitive than skin testing, should be performed. These investigations offer the patient useful information on the nature of any allergic conditions causing the nasal obstruction and can bring about options for behavioural change in terms of allergen avoidance. In addition, clinical knowledge of the presence of atopy can influence decisions on drug interventions.

IMAGING

Although not normally indicated in the evaluation of the more common causes of nasal obstruction such as rhinitis and septal deformity, both CT and magnetic resonance imaging (MRI) are useful for the evaluation of nasal obstruction caused by mass lesions and other conditions such as choanal atresia. In this context, CT scanning is most commonly performed as a preoperative investigation of patients undergoing endoscopic sinus surgery for chronic rhinosinusitis or nasal polyps.

TREATMENT OF NASAL OBSTRUCTION

The individual choice of treatment for nasal obstruction is determined by the relevant underlying diagnosis and by patient preference. The goal of treatment is to address all the specific problems that are causing the obstruction, which can be multifactorial. More common conditions such as chronic rhinitis will usually respond to medical treatment and, where appropriate, behavioural change such as allergen avoidance. Significant structural deformities cannot be resolved with medication and will usually require surgical management. However, if medical treatment has failed, surgeons should avoid the 'workman-like' approach of recommending nasal airway surgery on account of medical treatment failure. Instead, a comprehensive diagnostic workup should be completed to exclude conditions such as nasal valve collapse and perceptive nasal obstruction. Septoplasty, turbinate surgery and nasal valve surgery should be considered when appropriate. Care should be taken not to be overly aggressive with tissue removal when performing turbinate reduction surgery, because the normal functions of the nose require preservation of a minimum level of resistance. In other words, 'more space' does not necessarily mean better function.

KEY LEARNING POINTS

- The history is a good source of diagnostic information.
- The aetiology is often multifactorial.
- Structural causes may have complex involvement of the nasal valve.
- The nose is a resistant airway - radical surgery to create 'more space' may not equate with better function.

8

Allergic rhinitis

MARTYN L BARNES AND QUENTIN GARDINER

INTRODUCTION

Allergic rhinitis is a disease characterized by inflammatory nasal changes secondary to exposure to inhaled allergens termed *aeroallergens*. It occurs in previously exposed individuals who have gone on to express allergen-specific immunoglobulin E (IgE), which coats tissue mast cells through binding to cell surface receptors. Any later aeroallergen exposure acts through this complex to trigger mast cell activation, with release of preformed histamine granules ('degranulation') and synthesis of other inflammatory mediators.

Clinically, this results in the classic features of allergic rhinitis: mucosal irritation, nasal vascular engorgement and loss of mucosal integrity resulting in sneezing, itching and rhinorrhoea acutely and nasal obstruction with more chronic exposure.

Our greatest scientific understanding of the disease is well presented in the report of the Allergic Rhinitis and its Impact on Asthma (ARIA) workshop[1] in conjunction with the World Health Organization (WHO) and the 2008 update.[2]

EPIDEMIOLOGY

Allergic rhinitis is a common disease, affecting roughly a quarter of populations with a Western lifestyle, which in common with most forms of allergy has an increasing international prevalence. It is often associated with other allergic diseases, especially allergic asthma.

The traditional explanation for the increasing prevalence (the 'germ theory' or 'hygiene hypothesis') relates abnormal immune function to a lack of exposure to infection (mainly bacterial and viral) in childhood, resulting from modern standards of cleanliness and safety (with fewer significant wounds).

A more recent explanation is the 'worm theory'. This is a similar concept but with a greater focus on the striking changes in parasitic disease seen in modern society. Intestinal worms were uniformly widespread until the early twentieth century but in developed countries have now become a rarity. There are supporting comparative epidemiological studies and early interventional studies demonstrating that iatrogenic helminth infections lead to symptomatic improvement in some allergic and autoimmune diseases. A simplified pathophysiology is presented in Figure 8.1.

In addition to this backbone of allergic drive, other mechanisms contribute. Allergens are proteins, often with enzymatic activity and likely direct immunological effects. These effects are certainly implicated in the development of initial sensitivity.

IgE receptors are also found on basophils and low affinity varieties on the broader spectrum of leucocytes, antigen presenting cells, and platelets, allowing for a more complicated pathophysiology.

The inflammatory cascade released by mast cell degranulation includes not only histamine but also other granule contents (serine proteases, heparin) and newly synthesized eicosanoid mediators (leucotriene C4, prostaglandin D2, thromboxane and platelet-activating factor, or PAF).

The most acute effects are, however, driven by histamine released from mast cells, as is reflected in the clinical efficacy of antihistamines in most acute allergic reactions.

Although allergic rhinitis symptoms are focused on the nose, the disease is best considered systemic. We now recognize that aeroallergen sensitization affects the nose (allergic rhinitis) and the lungs (allergic asthma) together. Indeed, these diseases are increasingly considered to be a single entity, with a spectrum of respiratory allergic response, termed the *unified allergic airway*. They have a common epidemiology, pathophysiology and, in many cases, treatment approach. Treatment of allergic rhinitis can improve asthma control, reduce medication requirements and prevent hospital admissions. There is some evidence that early treatment of allergic rhinitis may prevent the later onset of asthma.

Recent exposure of the nose to an allergen may lead to asymptomatic eosinophil infiltration and a pro-inflammatory mucosal environment – a concept known as priming. Such changes are also likely to be reflected in the bone marrow, with an increased production of allergy-associated cellular and biochemical mediators that are effective

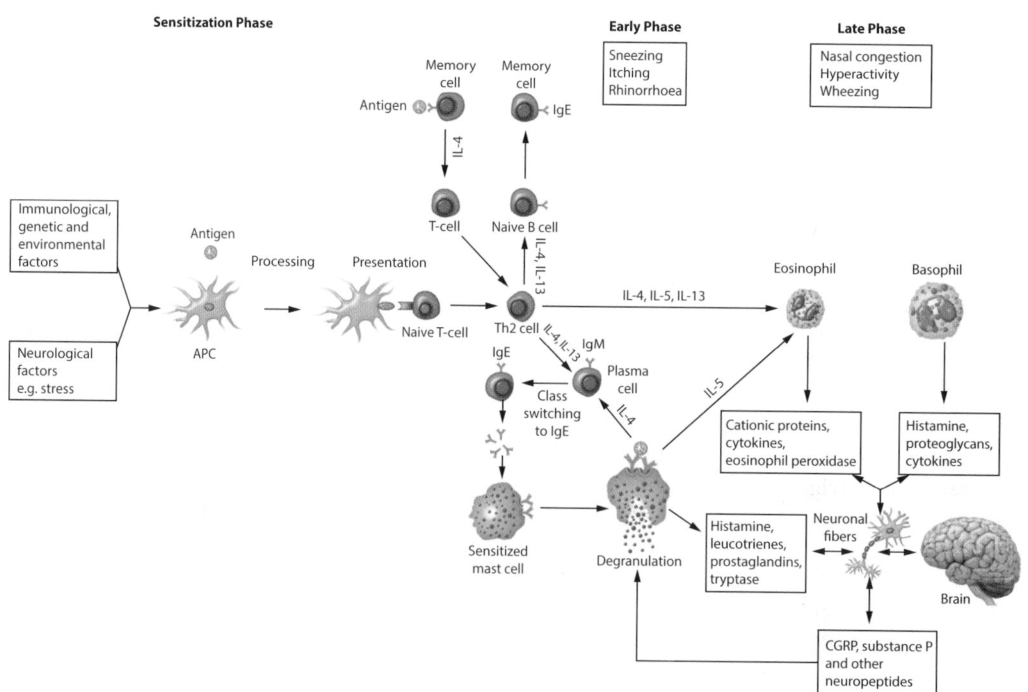

Figure 8.1 Pathophysiology of allergic rhinitis. Reproduced with permission from International Immunopharmacology.[4]

systemically. These changes further unite the clinical diseases we identify in the nose and lung and rationalize the demonstrated need to treat both together for optimal therapeutic control.

PRESENTATION, DIAGNOSIS AND DIFFERENTIAL DIAGNOSIS

Allergic rhinitis is primarily a clinical diagnosis. Pattern recognition is paramount. The disease is very common, but there are rarer important differential diagnoses to exclude. The typical presentation to an ear, nose and throat (ENT) department in the United Kingdom is of chronic persistent allergic rhinitis (predominantly young to middle-aged adults with obstructive complaints) or severe intermittent allergic rhinitis (irritant symptoms, often in association with ocular symptoms and most commonly in a recognized severely atopic child or young adult).

In primary care, and often undiagnosed and uncomplaining in the community, is a larger group of individuals with intermittent or less severe allergic rhinitis. Some will self medicate, and others dismiss their own symptoms as an upper respiratory tract infection or hay fever that they simply live with. It is all too easy to be dismissive of the significant impact of their disease (see the following section on Complications/Prognosis).

Endonasal examination is obligatory and may demonstrate the 'textbook' appearances of mucosal congestion with pale, sticky exudate. This is typical of the acute presentation, but in more chronic cases, generalized congestion and prominent engorged turbinates may be more subtle findings.

Additional pointers to the diagnosis include the association with asthma and other forms of atopy, as well as recognized triggers (e.g. the season, pets at home).

COMPLICATIONS/PROGNOSIS

Allergic rhinitis is an underestimated disease in terms of not only its prevalence but also its impact. It is easy to be dismissive of a 'snotty' nose or 'a touch of hay fever', but it should be appreciated that this disease leads to a significant impact on quality of life, affecting many domains, including sleep, work and school performance. Performance is further exacerbated by ill-informed administration of sedative antihistamines. The economic impact of this highly prevalent disease is enormous – 39 million sufferers in a 1994 study, totalling $1.2 billion in health care costs.

Children with allergic rhinitis are three times more likely to develop asthma than negative controls, and poor allergic rhinitis control leads to a higher risk of severe asthma and hospital admission.

CLASSIFICATION

The variation in clinical presentation relates primarily to two factors: whether exposure is intermittent or constant, and how severely the patient manifests the disease. On this basis, contemporary classification (after the ARIA guidelines[2]) is divided into intermittent or persistent and mild/moderate or severe allergic rhinitis (Figure 8.2). As already described, chronicity may lead to more obstructive, less irritant type symptomatic presentations.

DIFFERENTIAL DIAGNOSIS AND INVESTIGATIONS

Nasal polyposis and chronic rhinosinusitis are excluded clinically (by the mucopurulent character of rhinorrhoea, facial pressure, aspirin sensitivity and more prominent anosmia) and by endoscopy (visualization of polyps, congestion or oedema focused on the middle meatus or mucopurulent discharge). Sinonasal computed tomography (CT) scans may be helpful, although changes associated with transient infection or simple allergy may be misleading.

In patients presenting with nasal congestion, septal deviation and adenoid hypertrophy should be excluded by endoscopy, noting that adenoid hypertrophy may be associated with allergic exposure.

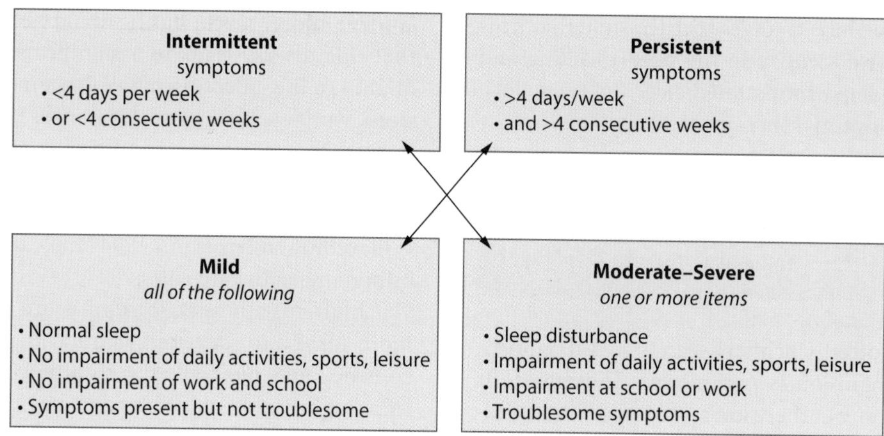

Figure 8.2 Classification of allergic rhinitis. Licensed for reproduction from the ARIA Pocket Guide for Physicians and Nurses.[5]

Turbinate congestion should be noted; it is an inflammatory marker of the condition, also seen transiently in upper respiratory tract infections.

Ultimately, diagnosis is based on the recognition of this clinical pattern, in conjunction with demonstrated exposure and proven sensitivity through radioallergosorbent test (RAST) or skin-prick tests.

In severe or atypical presentations (especially in the presence of cartilage or mucosal loss, cosmetic changes, systemic illness or refractory bleeding), exclusion of other inflammatory or neoplastic diseases is important.

Initial inflammatory markers – erythrocyte sedimentation rate, plasma viscosity, C-reactive protein and a blood eosinophil count – may be helpful screening tests. When presentation is markedly atypical, a direct assay of anti-neutrophil cytoplasmic antibodies (ANCA), serum angiotensin-converting enzyme, serum calcium levels, IgE total and fungal antigen specific titres can aid diagnosis.

Positive ANCA results with a cytoplasmic staining pattern (cANCA) suggest granulomatosis with polyangiitis (previously termed Wegener's granulomatosis). Specific auto-antibody affinity can then often be demonstrated for proteinase (PR3) and myeloperoxidase (MPO) by enzyme-linked immunosorbent assay. Positive cANCA and pANCA (perinuclear staining pattern) may also be seen in Churg-Strauss syndrome.

Elevated serum angiotensin-converting enzyme (ACE) and occasionally calcium levels may be seen in sarcoidosis. A chest X-ray may demonstrate lymphadenopathy, infiltrates, or fibrocystic changes, and in cases with identifiable mucosal changes a biopsy can be diagnostic.

Serum total IgE levels are a non-specific marker but may be markedly elevated in allergic disease, Churg-Strauss syndrome, and allergic fungal sinusitis. In the latter, skin-prick or RAST specific IgE may be demonstrated towards fungal antigens.

Neoplasia tends to present with unilateral symptomatology – nasal discharge, blockage, refractory (usually minor) bleeding or anosmia. The diagnosis may become clear on endoscopy or CT.

MEASURING ACTIVITY

The ARIA workshop recommended quantification of severity in allergic rhinitis on the basis of the impact of symptoms on daily activities, leisure, work, school or sleep (see Figure 8.2).

Direct patient questioning may be supplemented by symptom or visual analogue scores and patient reported outcome measures (PROMs). Well-established PROMs include the Rhinoconjunctivitis Quality of Life Questionnaire, the Chronic Sinusitis Survey, and the Sino-Nasal

Outcome Test 22 (SNOT-22). The latter is recommended by the Clinical Audit and Practice Advisory Group of ENT-UK.[3]

Limited objective assessments can be made of the endonasal mucosal appearance.

Formal acoustic rhinometry and rhinomanometry may have little advantage over peak nasal inspiratory flow rates, which are readily and cheaply obtained in clinic.

Systemic inflammatory markers, including blood eosinophil counts and eosinophil cationic protein (ECP) assays, are more often used in research settings, as are local inflammatory markers such as nasal lavage eosinophil counts, nasal nitric oxide levels and reactivity to nasal challenge (with, e.g. allergen, histamine or adenosine monophosphate).

MANAGEMENT

MEDICAL

Management is well guided by the recommendations of the ARIA workshop group[2] (Figure 8.3). Allergen avoidance is advocated in all cases, but there is little evidence base of efficacy – total avoidance tends to be impossible, and symptomatic disease persists, requiring pharmacotherapeutic intervention. Significant pet dander, for example, remains present in a house for several years after removal of the animal, and total avoidance of house dust mite can only really be achieved by moving the patient to an environment where it is too dry for the mite to live – e.g. the Swiss Alps. Identification of sensitization through skin-prick or RAST testing can, however, consolidate diagnosis and improve patient understanding and possibly compliance with treatment. In the case of industrial exposure or animal sensitization outside the home, avoidance may be important and effective.

In mild intermittent disease (primarily 'hay fever'), systemic antihistamines are effective, but these patients may self-medicate or be treated in primary care, rarely presenting to an ENT clinic. First-generation antihistamines should be avoided, noting their sedative effects, which exacerbate the adverse effects of the disease on school and work performance.

This leaves the mainstay of treatment in the form of topical intranasal corticosteroids, the choice of which should be based on efficacy, adverse effects and cost. Efficacy is well established for common corticosteroids, but early examples (beclometasone and especially betamethasone) have a greater systemic bioavailability and potential side effects. Cost savings may not justify these compromises.

The greatest concerns with regard to adverse effects are those of growth reduction in children, bone density loss and exacerbations of diabetes, hypertension or glaucoma. The topical nasal administration of modern corticosteroids within licensed doses rarely causes any form of measurable systemic activity; certainly less than commonly administered regimens in asthma. In patients (as commonly encountered) requiring concomitant asthma treatment, care should be taken, although nasal administration may also be effectively 'steroid sparing' for the inhaled dose. More common corticosteroid side effects are mild – nasal dryness and minor bleeding – but mucosal injury and even septal perforation have been attributed to their use.

In those with persisting symptoms despite maximal licensed dose topical corticosteroids, systemic corticosteroids can give significant benefits. However, prolonged treatments are usually inappropriate. Equally, short courses may be inadvisable, unrealistically raising expectations. Further treatments in such refractory cases tend to be best directed at specific symptomatic complaints or, where possible, immunotherapy (see later discussion).

Those with prominent rhinorrhoea may benefit from topical ipratropium nasal sprays, although these can be over-effective and lead to problems with dryness. Rhinorrhoea in the elderly may be usefully addressed in this way.

Persistent nasal obstruction or congestion may benefit from short courses of topical decongestant, noting that courses in excess of 10 days can lead to rhinitis medicamentosa (RM) and should be avoided. Concomitant intranasal corticosteroid may reduce the likelihood of RM, but the problem is very common in cases

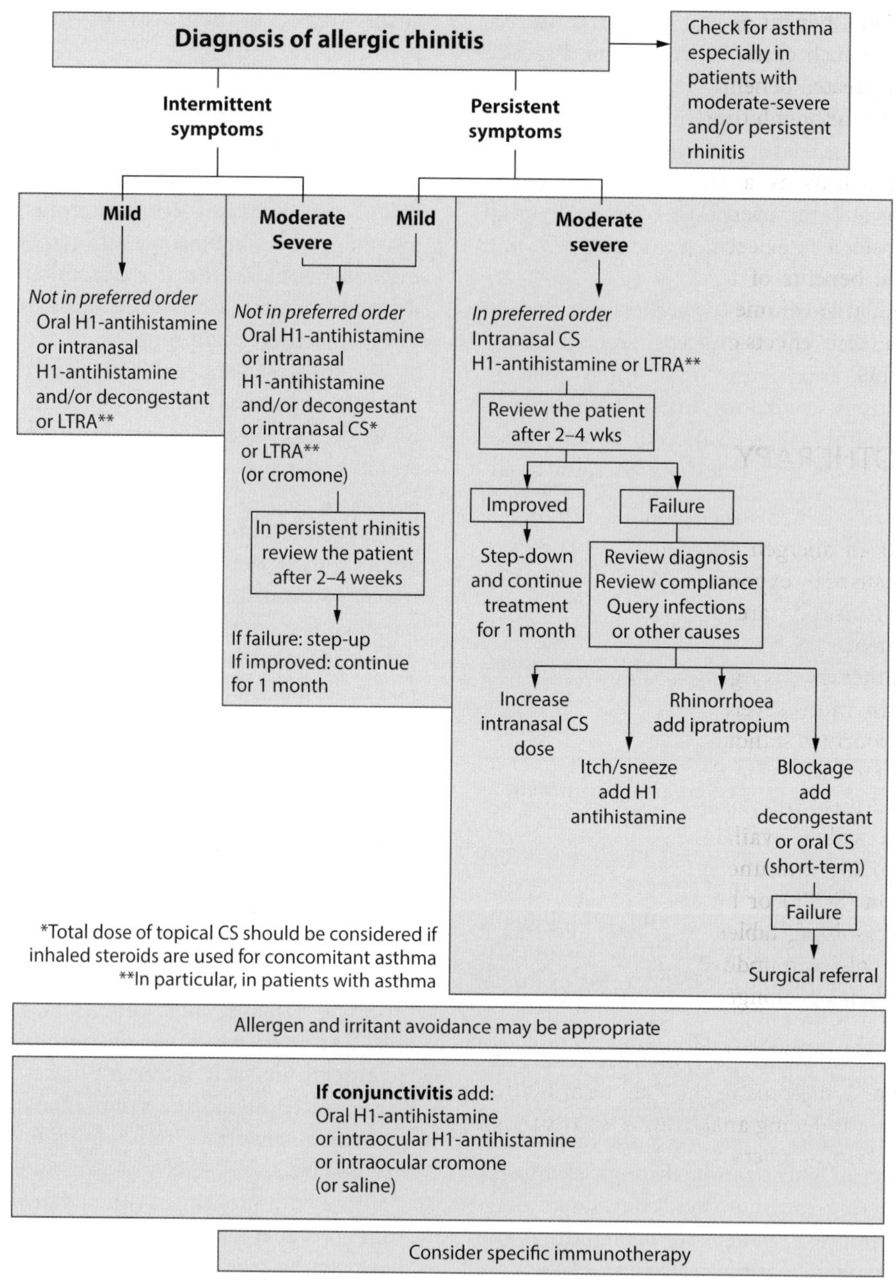

Figure 8.3 Management of allergic rhinitis. Licensed for reproduction from the ARIA Pocket Guide for Physicians and Nurses.[5]

of self-medication and should not be underestimated. Oral decongestants are much less likely to cause RM but are associated with systemic side effects, and they should be avoided in those with hypertension.

In cases of more severe allergic symptoms (often in children), acute type irritant symptoms tend to be prominent (itch, sneeze, rhinorrhoea, ocular irritation, redness and tearing). Antihistamines and leucotriene receptor antagonists may have some additional benefit as add-on to topical corticosteroids in such cases. Topical antihistamines may have a greater benefit, and cromones are a further option, although their efficacy is limited at best.

Saline douching is a recent and important addition to our therapeutic options. Although frequently used as a placebo in clinical trials, the symptomatic benefits of topical nasal saline are marked, and large-volume douches especially may exceed the clinical effects of more typical pharmaceutical agents.

IMMUNOTHERAPY

Immunotherapy is a treatment designed to induce tolerance to an allergen and therefore to reduce symptoms caused by exposure to it. *Desensitization* and *hyposensitization* are terms that refer to the same treatment.

Immunotherapy is generally reserved for patients with more severe symptoms who have responded poorly to standard medical treatment.

The common allergens (grass and tree pollen; dog, cat and dust mite; as well as bee and wasp venom) are widely available. Allergens can be presented to the immune system by subcutaneous injection (SCIT) or by the sublingual route (SLIT) as dissolving tablets or drops. Treatment generally involves an updosing phase over several weeks and then a prolonged (3-year) maintenance phase.

Immunotherapy has the potential to significantly reduce symptoms in the long term but has a small risk of inducing anaphylaxis, so treatment should be carefully supervised.

SURGERY

Finally, surgery may have a role in selected cases. Where symptomatic nasal obstruction has any structural element, surgical techniques may have a role, but it should be noted that an improved nasal airway may lead to an increased allergen delivery, so medical treatment must be maintained and optimal. Inferior turbinate reduction may be of particular benefit in chronic cases when turbinate engorgement has become irreversible.

KEY LEARNING POINTS

- Allergic rhinitis is better considered as the unified allergic airway, or even a systemic disease – with inflammatory changes in the circulation and bone marrow.
- Diagnosis is based on symptomatic presentation, exposure and demonstration of sensitization.
- The disease has a strong association with asthma and an underestimated prevalence, cost and impact on quality of life.
- There are important differential diagnoses in atypical/severe presentations.
- The mainstay of contemporary treatment is topical corticosteroids, but immunotherapy has a reemerging role, and surgery can be an adjunct.

REFERENCES

1. Bousquet J, Van Cauwenberge P, Khaltaev N. Allergic rhinitis and its impact on asthma. *Journal of Allergy and Clinical Immunology.* 2001 Nov; 108 (5 Suppl): S147–34.
2. Bousquet J, Khaltaev N, Cruz AA, Denburg J, Fokkens WJ, Togias A, et al. Allergic rhinitis and its impact on asthma (ARIA) 2008 update (in collaboration with the World Health Organization, GA(2)LEN and allergen). *Allergy.* 2008 Apr; 63 Suppl 86: 8–160.
3. Clinical outcome: Approved ENT-UK CAPAG (clinical audit and practice advisory group) patient reported outcome measures (proms). Available from: https://entuk.org/professionals/clinical_outcomes. Accessed 6 February 2013.
4. Mandhane SN, Shah JH, Thennati R. Allergic rhinitis: An update on disease, present treatments and future prospects. *International Immunopharmacology.* 2011 Nov; 11(11): 1646–62.
5. Bousquet J, Reid J, van Weel C, Baena Cagnani C, Canonica GW, Demoly P, et al. Allergic rhinitis management pocket reference 2008. *Allergy.* 2008 Aug; 63(8): 990–6.

9

Facial pain

NICK S JONES

Most patients who are referred to an ear, nose and throat (ENT) clinic with facial pain or headache have received a provisional diagnosis of sinusitis. There is an increasing awareness that non-sinugenic causes of headache and facial pain are responsible in the majority of patients. If facial pain and pressure are the primary symptoms, it is unlikely to be due to sinus disease, particularly in the absence of any nasal symptoms.

In patients with facial pain who have no objective evidence of sinus disease at nasal endoscopy, it is very unlikely that sinusitis is the cause. Most patients with pain due to sinusitis have acute bacterial sinusitis with nasal symptoms and signs and respond to antibiotic therapy. It is of note that more than 80 per cent of patients with purulent secretions visible at nasal endoscopy and chronic infective sinusitis have no facial pain,[1] and those who do normally have pain during an acute exacerbation. The majority of patients with idiopathic nasal polyposis do not have pain unless they have an acute infective episode.[2] In previous series of patients undergoing endoscopic sinus surgery, a significant proportion of patients were noted to have persisting facial pain,[1,3] making it likely that other causes were overlooked.

Headaches are common in the general population and are rarely due to sinusitis. Pain of vascular origin such as migraine, cluster headache and paroxysmal hemicrania[4] can be associated with autonomic rhinological symptoms such as nasal congestion and rhinorrhoea. This has led to confusion in arriving at a correct diagnosis.

It is important to be aware that a proportion of patients who mistakenly undergo surgery for non-sinogenic pain experience temporary relief from their symptoms, although their pain returns within a few weeks and nearly always within 9 months. It is hypothesized that the reason for a temporary or partial reduction in their pain is either the effect of cognitive dissonance or the effect of surgical trauma on the afferent fibres going to the trigeminal nucleus, which alters its threshold for spontaneous activity in the short term. In some patients surgery does not significantly affect the pain, and in a third the pain is made worse.[5]

PAIN SECONDARY TO SINUSITIS

In cases of facial pain secondary to genuine sinusitis, patients almost invariably have coexisting symptoms of nasal obstruction, hyposmia and/or a purulent nasal discharge,[2] and there are usually endoscopic signs of disease.[6] In those who fail to respond to medical treatment, endoscopic sinus surgery has been shown to alleviate facial pain in 75–83 per cent of cases.[1]

In examining the criteria for diagnosing chronic rhinosinusitis, it is important to note that the inclusion of facial pain/pressure 'on its own does not constitute a suggestive history for rhinosinusitis in the absence of another major nasal symptom or sign'.[7] The evidence that a vacuum within a blocked sinus can cause *protracted* pain is poor. Transient facial pain in patients with other symptoms and signs of rhinosinusitis can occur with pressure changes when flying, diving or skiing, but this resolves. Patients who repeatedly suffer these symptoms during a pressure change are often helped by surgery to open the ostia. It is interesting to note that patients with 'silent sinus syndrome', which is due to a blocked maxillary sinus with resorption of its contents to the extent that the orbital floor prolapses into the maxillary sinus, experience no pain.

HISTORY

Acute sinusitis usually follows an acute upper respiratory tract infection and is usually unilateral and severe and associated with pyrexia and unilateral nasal obstruction. In maxillary sinusitis, unilateral facial and dental pain are good predictors of true infection confirmed by nasal endoscopy, and the condition is helped by antral lavage if it does not respond to antibiotics. This differs from chronic sinusitis, where there is a poor correlation between the site of facial pain and evidence of sinus pathology. Chronic sinusitis is usually painless, with pain occurring only during an acute exacerbation or if there is obstruction of the sinus ostia. An increase in the severity of pain on bending forward has traditionally been thought to be diagnostic of sinusitis, but this is non-specific and it can occur in many other types of facial pain.

Here are some of the key points to ask:

1. What are the main symptoms you have now?
   This provides a starting point and is often efficient because it can help to direct further questioning.
2. Ask the patient to point to the area of his or her pain.
   The manner and the gestures used can give useful information about the emotional significance of the symptom as well as its site. If it is symmetrical across the forehead, then tension-type headache should be considered, and if it is symmetrical involving the face, then mid-facial segment pain is likely. Severe unilateral pain centred near the medial canthus may be cluster headache or paroxysmal hemicrania. A vague motion that crosses the midline asymmetrically may make it difficult to arrive at a recognized diagnostic category. Seeing the patient on later occasions, after he or she has kept a diary of symptoms, may help to clarify the clinical picture.
3. Is the pain continuous or intermittent?
   Pain described as continuous or present on a daily basis is unlikely to be sinogenic or migrainous in origin, and is more likely to represent mid-facial segment pain or be neuropathic. Intermittent pain that occurs more than twice a year is unlikely to be due to bacterial sinusitis unless there are other coexisting symptoms (nasal obstruction, mucky discharge, pyrexia) or endoscopic signs of disease. Having more than two episodes of bacterial sinusitis a year is unusual unless the patient's immunity is deficient. Pain that is unilateral and progressive can be due to infection or a tumour; although the latter is rare, this possibility must be considered and excluded.
4. Character of the pain: Is it sharp, dull, throbbing, burning, aching or pressure, and what score out of 10 would the patient give it for severity?

Pain that is vascular in origin tends to be throbbing in nature, with cluster headaches being particularly severe, and is scored 10 out of 10. Mid-facial segment pain is often described as pressure, although the term *blockage* can be used. The patient may point over the dorsum of the nose, yet there is no restriction to the nasal airway. Trigeminal neuralgia causes a stabbing pain that is initiated by a trigger point. A burning or a nagging ache describes neuropathic pain.

5. What precipitates or is associated with the pain?
   Sinogenic pain usually only occurs after an upper respiratory tract infection and is associated with the rhinological symptoms of nasal obstruction and infected secretions. *The symptoms of catarrh, postnasal drip, lethargy, dark rings under the eyes, puffy eyes, clicking and popping in the sinuses, worse pain bending forwards and tenderness when touching the cheeks are unreliable, although they have historically been said to be associated with sinusitis.* Classic migraine may have an aura, but common migraine usually does not. However, both are often associated with nausea. Cluster headaches are frequently triggered by alcohol and wake the patient. The pain of temporomandibular joint dysfunction is exacerbated by chewing, and trigeminal neuralgia is normally provoked by trigger points in the mandibular or maxillary division of the trigeminal nerve.
6. What relieves the pain?
   Patients with facial pain due to sinusitis generally respond to antibiotics. Be aware that patients with intermittent severe episodes of pain due to migraine may often say that they respond to antibiotics because when they are given them their pain stops within 72 hours of onset. However, this would have happened in any event because migraine rarely lasts more than 72 hours.
7. What effect does the pain have on daily life?
   Patients with atypical facial pain often describe their pain in dramatic terms as severe and unrelenting despite sleeping and not appearing to be in pain. There is often a mismatch between the description of their symptoms and the patients' affect. Severe crippling pain that wakes the patient, who is then incapable of doing anything during its duration because of its severity, is typical of cluster headache.
8. Has the pain progressed?
   Continuous pain for more than a year is unlikely to be vascular in origin and is more likely to be mid-facial segment pain, tension-type headache or neuropathic pain; it is unlikely to be due to sinusitis. Pain that progresses day to day warrants investigation because there is likely to be a significant underlying pathologic disorder, whether it be an infected pyocoele, pachymeningitis from vasculitis or a tumour.
9. What is the response to treatment?
   There are few investigations that are diagnostic for most types of facial pain, so a provisional diagnosis should be made, and response to treatment can then help confirm or refute the provisional diagnosis. A good response to antibiotics makes sinusitis likely. Response to indomethacin helps confirm a diagnosis of paroxysmal hemicranias. A response to four or more out of six triptan tablets, each given early in the onset of the pain, results in a diagnosis of migraine.
10. Is the history unclear?
    If the history is unclear or uncertain, ask the patient to keep a diary of symptoms, then review his or her history. This often helps define the frequency, the distribution and the severity of the symptoms.
11. Was a holistic assessment considered?
    A holistic assessment of the patient is worthwhile. Patients who have a history of myalgic encephalomyelitis, chronic fatigue or irritable bowel syndrome are over-represented in clinical groups with tension-type headache and mid-facial segment pain, although many patients with the latter do not have the former three symptoms. Some patients somatize; a history of many other symptoms and investigations without any pathological findings may raise this possibility. To effectively manage patients with facial pain, the psychological aspects of this condition must be considered, and in some patients these may be an important factor. An example is a patient with facial pain who has previously sustained a nasal injury during an assault without resolution

of the psychological insult. This is more likely to persist if there is ongoing compensation or legal issues that are outstanding.

EXAMINATION

Neurological signs are uncommon, but when they occur they often indicate significant underlying pathologic disorder due to an inflammatory disease such as vasculitis, demyelination or a skull base tumour. Rigid nasal endoscopy is helpful in confirming infective rhinosinusitis. If the findings are normal, it is unlikely that the paranasal sinuses are responsible.

INVESTIGATIONS

Beware ordering either computed tomography (CT) or magnetic resonance imaging (MRI) of the paranasal sinuses, because these have a high prevalence of an incidental finding of mucosal thickening in an asymptomatic population. Plain sinus x-rays are so insensitive and non-specific that they are deemed to be of no use in the diagnosis of chronic sinusitis. CT scans must also be treated with caution. If CT is clear, this helps exclude rhinosinusitis as a cause, but the presence of mucosal swelling or a fluid level is not necessarily the cause of any pain; these changes might well be incidental, as they are in a third of asymptomatic people. Specific investigations are warranted to confirm or refute particular diagnoses (e.g. cANCA for Wegener's granulomatosis), and a biopsy is justified for most masses or abnormal tissue. MRI should be considered for suspected trigeminal neuralgia, in the young to consider demyelinating disease or for someone who develops migraine over the age of 55.

Patients who have two or more bacterial sinus infections within 1 year should be investigated for an immune deficiency.

TREATMENT

The majority of patients with bacterial sinusitis respond to treatment with antibiotics. The common pathogens are *Streptococcus pneumoniae* and *Haemophilus influenzae* and less commonly *Staphylococcus aureus, Moraxella catarrhalis* and various streptococci. A minority have anaerobes such as bacteroides and anaerobic streptococci.

In chronic bacterial rhinosinusitis, defined by its persistence for more than 12 weeks, anaerobes and staphylococci are more prevalent, and pseudomomas is cultured in a small proportion of patients. In patients who fail to respond to medical treatment, the possibility of a fungal infection or immunodeficiency should be investigated.

It is unusual for acute sinusitis not to respond to medical treatment, but when there is progressive excruciating pain, the patient will benefit from drainage of the affected sinus. Placing a dressing soaked with a vasoconstrictor adjacent to the ostium of the affected sinus will occasionally be enough to establish drainage; otherwise, maxillary antral lavage or trephining the frontal sinus will be required. Acute frontal sinusitis is normally an isolated event and does not warrant an intranasal approach because this runs the risk of causing stenosis of the frontal recess. In acute or intermittent sinusitis, antral washouts have not been shown to add any benefit to a 10-day course of antibiotic.

TENSION-TYPE HEADACHE

Eighty per cent of the population suffers from a headache every year, and 50 per cent have at least one a month, 15 per cent one a week and 5 per cent one a day. The main quality of the pain is symmetrical pressure that may be confined to a small area just above the nasion or extend across the whole forehead. There is often an occipital component. There are often no exacerbating or relieving factors, although bending forwards can sometimes aggravate them, a symptom often incorrectly said to mean that the patient must have rhinosinusitis. There is often some hyperaesthesia of the soft tissues in the area. Patients are often taking many analgesics although they say they do little to help. Analgesic-dependent headache can complicate the picture. Withdrawal from analgesics for several weeks alone may be sufficient in this group but is rarely tolerated without starting other treatment for headache. However, this is an option. The prevalence of headache increases sharply during the second decade and then levels off until the age of 40–50, after which it reduces.

MID-FACIAL SEGMENT PAIN

Over the past decade or more, studies on facial pain have shown that there is a distinct group of patients who have a form of facial neuralgia that has all the characteristics of tension-type headache with the exception that it affects the midface; this is called mid-facial segment pain.[8] Patients describe a feeling of symmetrical pressure, although some patients may say that their nose feels blocked when they have no nasal airway obstruction. Mid-facial segment pain may be located at the nasion, under the bridge of the nose, on either side of the nose, in the peri- or retro-orbital regions, or across the cheeks. The forehead and occipital region may also be affected at the same time in about 60 per cent of patients. There are no consistent exacerbating or relieving factors. Patients often take a range of analgesics, but they have no or minimal effect apart from ibuprofen, which may help a few to a minor extent. There may be hyperaesthesia of the skin and soft tissues over the affected area. This is similar to the tender areas over the forehead and scalp seen with tension-type headache. Nasal endoscopy and CT, if done, are typically normal. (Note the reservations expressed earlier about ordering these because of the incidence of false-positive changes.) The majority of patients with this condition respond to low-dose amitriptyline but usually require up to 6 weeks of 10 mg at night and occasionally 20 mg before it works. Amitriptyline should then be continued for 6 months. In the 20 per cent of patients whose symptoms return when they stop it, amitriptyline should be restarted if the pain returns. Other antidepressants are not effective; again, this is akin to tension-type headache. If amitriptyline fails, then relief may be obtained from gabapentin or pregabalin.

MIGRAINE

Migraine is an episodic headache lasting 4–72 hours with distinguishing features. Migraine without aura (previously called common migraine) affects almost 75 per cent of migraine sufferers. It is characterized by a headache, which can be severe, and is typically unilateral, pulsating and often accompanied by nausea and photophobia that last 4–72 hours. There is no premonition. The second type, migraine with aura (previously called classic migraine), affects 25 per cent of migraine sufferers. The attacks are preceded by neurological symptoms such as visual disturbances or numbness. It is three times more common in women, and there is often a family history. Stress, diet, the premenstrual state and barometric pressure can induce attacks. Coexisting nasal obstruction and rhinorrhoea occur in many patients with facial migraine.

CLUSTER HEADACHE

Cluster headache is characterized by recurrent, unilateral attacks that typically wake the patient and are retro-orbital or centred at the medial aspect of the orbit, of great intensity and usually last up to 1 hour and rarely 3. The pain is also accompanied by ipsilateral signs of autonomic dysfunction, such as the parasympathetic signs of rhinorrhoea, lacrimation, and sympathetic signs of miosis and ptosis. Bouts may last 8–10 weeks annually and are separated by remission when the patient is pain free for 2 weeks.

PAROXYSMAL HEMICRANIA

Paroxysmal hemicrania has been described as an excruciating unilateral pain that is usually ocular and frontotemporal with short (5–45 minutes) frequent attacks (usually more than five a day). At least one of the following autonomic symptoms should be present: nasal congestion (40 per cent), rhinorrhoea (40 per cent), conjuctival injection (40 per cent), lacrimation (60 per cent) or, rarely, ptosis, eyelid oedema, heart rate changes (bradycardia, tachycardia and extrasystoles), increased local sweating, salivation and facial flushing. Attacks may occur bilaterally even though they are usually more pronounced on the symptomatic side. These last between 5 and 45 minutes on each occasion, and they recur many times a day. Remission ranges from 4 months to 3 years. Rarely do these headaches develop into the chronic form. Overall, the average age of onset is usually 30–40 years, but the spectrum ranges from 6 to 80 years. The episodic form tends to have an earlier age of onset. The condition's complete or rapid response to indomethacin is said to differentiate paroxysmal hemicrania from cluster headache.

SUNCT

Short-lasting unilateral neuralgiform headache with conjunctival injection and tearing (SUNCT) is an uncommon idiopathic headache syndrome. It is a form of primary headache marked by trigeminal pain, particularly in the orbital or periorbital area, associated with autonomic symptoms, in which conjunctival injection and tearing are the most prominent features. Attacks last 15–60 seconds and recur 5–30 times an hour. These attacks may be precipitated by chewing movements and certain foods such as citrus fruits.

ANALGESIC-DEPENDENT HEADACHE

This entity is all too often unrecognized and mismanaged. Patients with tension-type headache or mid-facial segment pain often take a great number of analgesics in spite of the fact that they have little effect. Drug-induced headache is usually described as dull, diffuse and band-like and usually starts in the early morning. The original headache (migraine or tension headache) has often been present for many years, and the regular intake of drugs often started several years earlier. Patients take on average 30 or more tablets per week, often containing several different substances. Withdrawal is problematic because patients' symptoms take several weeks to resolve. However, chronic headache disappears or decreases by more than 50 per cent in two-thirds of the patients.

TRIGEMINAL NEURALGIA

The characteristic presentation of trigeminal neuralgia – paroxysms of severe lancinating pain induced by a specific trigger point – is well recognized. In more than one-third of sufferers, the pain occurs in both the maxillary and mandibular divisions, while in one-fifth it is confined to the maxillary division. In a small number of patients (3 per cent), only the ophthalmic division is affected. Typical trigger points are the lips and naso-labial folds, but pain may also be triggered by touching the gingivae. A flush may be seen over the face, but there is no sensory disturbance in primary trigeminal neuralgia. Remissions are common, but the condition can also increase in severity. Younger patients should undergo MRI to exclude other pathology such as disseminating sclerosis, which is identified in 2 to 4 per cent of patients with trigeminal neuralgia. Tumours such as posterior fossa meningiomas or neuromas are found in 2 per cent of patients presenting with trigeminal neuralgia, reinforcing the need for imaging to exclude such disorders.

ATYPICAL FACIAL PAIN

This is very much a diagnosis of exclusion, and care must be taken in reaching this conclusion, even when the patient has received previous opinions and no pathologic disorder has been identified. The history is often vague and inconsistent, with widespread pain extending from the face into other areas of the head and neck. The pain may move from one part of the face to another between different consultations, and other symptoms, such as 'mucus moving' in the sinuses, are often described. A number of patients have such completely fixed ideas about their condition that they will not be convinced otherwise, whatever the weight of evidence to the contrary. Pain is often described in dramatic terms in conjunction with an excess of other unpleasant life events. Many of these patients have a history of other pain syndromes, and their extensive records show minimal progress despite various medications. They have often undergone previous sinus or dental surgery and may be resentful about their treatment. Many patients with atypical facial pain exhibit significant psychological disturbance or a history of depression and are unable to function normally as a result of their pain. Some project a pessimistic view of treatment, almost giving the impression that they do not wish to be rid of the pain that plays such a central role in their lives.

A comprehensive examination (including nasendoscopy) is essential, and imaging studies such as MRI are advisable to exclude pathologic disorders before the patient is labeled as having atypical pain. The management of such patients is challenging, and confrontation is nearly always counterproductive. Patients should sympathetically be made aware that psychological factors may play a role in their condition, and referral to a clinical psychologist or psychiatrist may be helpful. Drug treatment revolves around a gradual build-up to the higher analgesic and antidepressant levels of amitriptyline (75–100 mg) at night. Referral to a pain clinic is often helpful.

KEY LEARNING POINTS

- If facial pain and pressure are the primary symptoms, this is unlikely to be due to sinus disease in the absence of any nasal symptoms or signs.
- Patients with facial pain who have no objective evidence of sinus disease at nasal endoscopy are very unlikely to be helped by surgery.
- Neurological causes are responsible for a large proportion of patients with headache or facial pain.
- Pain that is unilateral and progressive can be due to infection or a tumour; although the latter is rare, this possibility must be considered.
- Facial pain described as continuous or present on a daily basis is unlikely to be sinogenic or migrainous in origin and more likely to represent mid-facial segment pain or be neuropathic.

REFERENCES

1. West B, Jones NS. Endoscopy-negative, computed tomography-negative facial pain in a nasal clinic. *Laryngoscope*. 2001; 111: 581–86.
2. Fahy C, Jones NS. Nasal polyposis and facial pain. *Clinical Otolaryngology*. 2001; 26: 510–13.
3. Tarabichi M. Characteristics of sinus-related pain. *Otolaryngology – Head and Neck Surgery*. 2000; 122: 84–87.
4. Jones NS. The classification and diagnosis of facial pain. *Hospital Medicine*. 2001; 62(10): 598–606.
5. Khan O, Majumdar S, Jones NS. Facial pain after sinus surgery and trauma. *Clinical Otolaryngology*. 2002; 27: 171–74.
6. Hughes R, Jones NS. The role of endoscopy in outpatient management. *Clinical Otolaryngology*. 1998; 23: 224–26.
7. EPOS. EAACI position paper on rhinosinusitis and nasal polyps. Working Party from the European Academy of Allergy and Clinical Immunology. 2012; Suppl 22, 1–299.
8. Jones NS. Mid-facial segment pain: implications for rhinitis and sinusitis. *Current Allergy and Asthma Reports*. 2004; 4: 187–92.

FURTHER READING

Jones NS. *Mid-facial Segment Pain: Implications for Rhinosinusitis*. In *Nonallergic Rhinitis*. Eds. Baraniuk JN, Shusterman D. New York: Marcel Dekker, 2007: 323–33.

Jones NS. *Practical Rhinology*. London: Edward Arnold, 2010: 1–184.

Woolford T, Jones NS. *Facial Pain*. In *Scott-Brown's Otorhinolaryngology, Head and Neck Surgery*. 7th ed., Volume 2. Eds. Gleeson M, Browning G, Burton MJ, et al. London: Hodder Arnold, 2008: 1718–30.

10

Nasal and facial trauma

PETER D ROSS

INTRODUCTION

Significant facial trauma can result in acute life-threatening situations, permanent disfigurement and disability. Up to 10 per cent of all emergency department visits involve injury to the face. Fortunately, the majority of this facial trauma is relatively minor, with nasal fractures making up approximately 40 per cent of all facial fractures seen. Because of the sensitive cosmetic nature of the face, as well as the major functions undertaken in the foreface, trauma to this area often involves litigation. This necessitates good note keeping and timely clinical care to ensure appropriate outcomes for the patient.

MECHANISM OF INJURY

The pattern of the injuries found in facial trauma is directly related to the mechanism of injury to the face. It ranges from simple soft tissue injuries to the life-threatening situation caused by massive tissue loss and airway compromise. Therefore, initial assessment is dictated by the mechanism of injury as well as the stage of treatment that is involved.

INITIAL ASSESSMENT

The initial assessment should focus on managing and stabilizing the potential life-threatening injuries. This is done using the structured approach of the advanced trauma life support (ATLS) primary survey, a compulsory part of all surgical training.

THE PRIMARY SURVEY

- Airway with cervical spine control
    - The potential of airway compromise may be apparent or predictable. Significant facial trauma may lead to instability of the mandible or foreface, significant airway oedema, or haemorrhage into the airway. With evaluation, early involvement of the anaesthetist will allow for appropriate

management of the airway, be this observation, intubation or a surgical airway.
  - The cervical spine must also be managed in this first part of the survey, to prevent long-term disability. It is potentially damaged in all cases of major facial trauma. In the unconscious patient, it will need to be stabilized with a collar, sandbags/head blocks, and strapping to prevent movement. Only when the patient is conscious and the cervical spine has been cleared should they be removed. In the conscious patient, the symptoms, signs and radiological findings will dictate when the cervical spine protection can be removed.
- Breathing
  - After establishing that there is an adequate airway, effective ventilation is required to optimize gas exchange – deliver oxygen and remove carbon dioxide. Thoracic trauma should be identified and addressed.
- Circulation
  - Life-threatening haemorrhage will generally be apparent and must be controlled. After establishing large-bore intravenous access, pressure should be used to prevent ongoing loss until definitive management can be undertaken. Epistaxis is managed with caution. If there is potential of a skull base fracture, care is required with packing to prevent intracranial penetration of the packing.
- Disability
  - With significant facial and head trauma, intracranial consequences may occur. Conscious level needs to be frequently assessed, as well as examination for cranial nerve or other neurological dysfunction.
- Exposure
- Adequate exposure of the patient should be undertaken to ensure that all other injuries are identified and managed.

TYPES OF FACIAL FRACTURE

When considering fractures of the midface, they can be classified as central (nasal, naso-orbito-ethmoid and maxillary) and lateral (zygomatic).

CENTRAL FACIAL FRACTURES

Nasal trauma

HISTORY AND EXAMINATION

Nasal trauma is frequently seen in assault, sports injuries and road traffic accidents. It can reflect injury to more than just the external structures of the nose. Swelling and bruising become established rapidly, making early assessment difficult. After initial presentation to the emergency department, uncomplicated cases should be reviewed at 5 to 7 days after the injury. This will allow for the swelling to improve and for adequate assessment of any deformity.

Required history

- Details of mechanism of injury, though often unreliable
- Change in function
  - Breathing
  - Sense of smell
- Change in appearance
- Change in vision
- Epistaxis
- Watery rhinorrhoea

Examination (with clear documentation)

- Condition of skin
- External deformity
  - Bony alignment
  - Septal and cartilage alignment
- Palpable fractures of the nose
- Integrity of orbital rim
- Internal
  - Septal alignment
  - Septal haematoma?
- Nasal function/air entry
- Eye movements
- Infraorbital nerve sensation

Classification of nasal deformity

1. Straight nasal bones
2. Bones deviated, displaced less than half the width of the nasal bridge
3. Bones deviated, displaced half to one full width of the nasal bridge

4. Bones deviated, displaced more than one full width of the nasal bridge
5. Bones almost in contact with cheek

Patterns of nasal fractures

Class 1: A blow to the anterior nose, causing depression or displacement of the distal portion of the nasal bone. A fracture of the cartilaginous septum, running from the dorsum towards the bony septum, may also occur (Chevallet fracture).

Class 2: Lateral trauma to the nose, resulting in lateral deviation of the bony nasal pyramid, and a horizontal or C-shaped fracture of the nasal septum.

Class 3: A high-energy injury to the nose, which leads to a complex fracture which extends into the ethmoid bone. The bony septum at the perpendicular plate of the ethmoid rotates backwards, taking the septum with it into the face. The nasal tip is also rotated upwards, giving greater show of the nostrils. There will be a saddle-type deformity, and the nose will have a 'pig-like' appearance. As a result of the disruption of the medial canthal ligament attachment, there may be telecanthus.

INVESTIGATION

No investigation is needed in simple cases of nasal fracture. However if there is concern of facial or skull fracture, plain radiographs will assist in identifying such fractures. CT scanning may be subsequently used to assess the extent of these injuries.

MANAGEMENT

Soft tissue

Wounds to the nose should be cleaned and closed at the first opportunity after the injury. Tetanus immunization status should be checked in open wounds. Swelling and bruising can be reduced with the use of ice.

The nasal bones

Timing. Once assessment is made and deformity of the bones is identified, there is a limited window of opportunity to manipulate the fracture to improve position. This is ideally 7–10 days postinjury, but can be attempted at up to 3 weeks. The longer after the injury, the more callus will have formed, and the less likely the manipulation will be successful. Fractures can also be reduced straight after the injury (within 1 hour), before the oedema has developed.

Anaesthesia. Either local or general anaesthesia is appropriate for reduction of nasal fractures. Both have been shown in studies to be suitable, with similar outcomes. The choice therefore is determined by patient choice, service design and local expertise. Local anaesthetic can be injected into the dorsum of the nose along the fracture sites, over the nasal bridge, and to the infraorbital foramen to give a field block to the nose. Additional topical local anaesthetic may be applied to nasal cavities by spray or patties soaked in the chosen preparation.

Reduction techniques. Closed digital manipulation, with or without instruments, is the main technique for reduction of nasal bone fractures. The bones should be reduced to their original position by disimpaction and realignment with appropriate lateral force. If there is infracture, or posterior displacement, a Walsham's forceps should be used to elevate the fragment. Following elevation, temporary packing under the previously depressed nasal bone may be required to maintain the position. External splinting or taping is advisable when the bones are very mobile and unstable following manipulation because they are at risk from inadvertent displacement.

Nasal septum. Management of the septum is often unsuccessful when managing acute nasal bone fractures. Digital manipulation may lead to improvement; however, the septum will usually return to its pre-intervention position. Therefore, it tends to be addressed after at least 6 months, once the swelling has resolved and healing is complete. Septoplasty or septorhinoplasty may be required for significant septal deformities.

COMPLICATIONS

Epistaxis

Traumatic epistaxis usually settles once the tissue oedema is established and vessels tamponaded. However, patients who present with severe brisk bleeding episodes, greater than 48 hours after a nasal fracture, can prove challenging and require surgical intervention. Because the bleeding is commonly from the fracture site high in the nose, anterior ethmoid artery ligation may be required.

Cerebrospinal fluid leak

A cerebrospinal fluid (CSF) leak may occur after nasal or facial trauma when the fracture involves the cribiform plate or the lateral lamella of the cribriform plate. These are the thinnest areas of the skull base, where the dura is very adherent to the bone and tears when the bone fractures. The most common presentation is unilateral watery rhinorrhoea, with a positive result for β2-transferrin (asialotransferrin) on testing the rhinorrhoea. β2-Transferrin is a product of neuraminidase activity within the central nervous system and is therefore only found within the CSF, the perilymph and the aqueous humour.

The majority of traumatic CSF leaks resolve within 7–14 days with conservative management. This includes strict bed rest and elevation of the head with avoidance of straining, retching or nose blowing. Antibiotics may mask meningitis, and discussions with the neurosurgeon are advised to check local policy. If the leak does not settle, the location should be identified with high-resolution computed tomography (CT) scanning of the skull base, with magnetic resonance imaging (MRI) if required. Endoscopic repair of the leak should be undertaken as soon as possible if conservative management is not sufficient because there is a significantly increased risk of meningitis (0.3–10 per cent per year).

Septal haematoma

This is the presence of a haematoma under the perichondrium of the septum. The blood supply to the cartilage is disrupted when the perichondrium is elevated by bilateral haematoma. This may lead to ischaemia and septal necrosis with perforation or septal collapse. Another risk is infection, which carries the risk of meningitis, brain abscess, cavernous sinus thrombosis and septal collapse. It can easily be confused with an anterior septal deformity. To differentiate, the area should be gently probed; a haematoma will be fluctuant and compressible, a deviation of the septum will not. Aspiration will also confirm the presence of blood.

Management involves draining the haematoma and securing the perichondrium back to the cartilage with quilting sutures, packing or nasal splinting. This can be achieved under local or general anaesthetic. Because the collection will often be too organized to aspirate, it is often best approached with formal incision and drainage. Owing to the high re-accumulation rate, the patient will need to be reviewed 2 to 4 days after discharge to ensure that there is not an additional collection, which would require a further procedure.

Traumatic anosmia

The olfactory nerve fibres within the nose and cribriform plate may be damaged with nasal or head injuries. This can lead to a loss of sense of smell, which is rarely recovered.

Naso-orbital-ethmoid complex fractures

DEFINITION

These are fractures involving the nose, orbits and frontals, ethmoids and skull base. They are frequently comminuted and complex.

HISTORY AND EXAMINATION

Patients who have fractures of the complex may present with loss of nasal projection, upward rotation of the nasal tip, widening of the nasal base, telecanthus, epiphora and CSF leak. The telecanthus reflects disruption to the medial canthal ligament insertion, which migrates laterally, while the epiphora is secondary to damage to the nasolacrimal system.

INVESTIGATIONS

Plain films are of little use in the assessment of these complex fractures. Three-dimensional imaging is required to adequately assess the fractures to allow reconstruction.

MANAGEMENT

Surgery is generally required to restore normal anatomy. The fractures are managed with miniplates, and the instability of the medial canthal tendon needs to be addressed with miniplates or wires. If there is evidence of damage to the nasolacrimal system, it may require lacrimal intubation or dacryocystorhinostomy.

Orbital floor fractures

HISTORY AND EXAMINATION

The orbit is a smooth, bony box in which the orbital muscles, fat, optic nerve, vessels and globe sit. For it to function normally, the orbit must be intact. Trauma to the globe or orbital bones can lead to fracture of the weak orbital floor, and this disruption to the orbit will affect the function of the contents.

The signs of an orbital floor fracture are the following:

- Enophthalmos
- Subtarsal hollowing
- Infraorbital nerve paresthesia
- Palpable step in orbital rim
- Restricted vertical movement of the eye
- Subconjunctival haemorrhage
- Diplopia
- Periorbital ecchymosis
- Surgical emphysema around orbit on nose blowing

INVESTIGATIONS

Plain radiography (occipitomental views) is used to screen for orbital floor fractures. Features to suggest fracture include the following:

- Teardrop sign. A polypoidal mass hanging from the orbital floor into the maxillary antrum, usually in the shape of a teardrop. It represents the herniation of orbital contents through the fracture, usually periorbital fat and inferior rectus muscle. It is this herniation that leads to possible entrapment of the inferior rectus and limited vertical movement of the globe.
- Opacification or an air-fluid level in the maxillary sinus. This occurs as a result of the presence of blood in the sinus from the fracture.

CT scanning is subsequently used to show in greater detail the soft tissue and bone involvement (Figure 10.1).

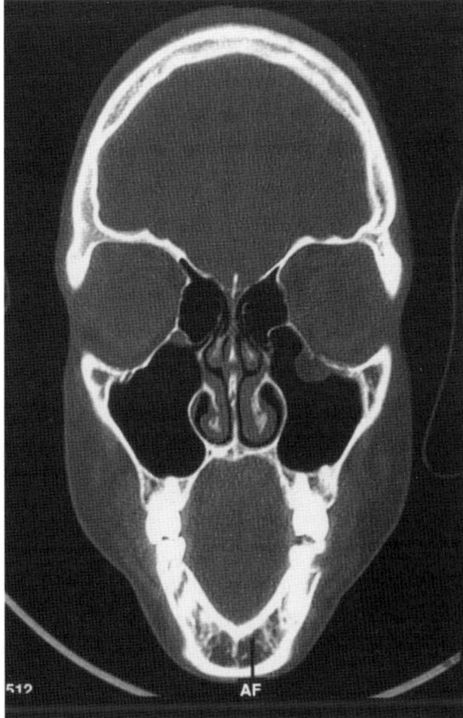

Figure 10.1 Orbital floor fracture.

MANAGEMENT

Surgical management is required when there is evidence of restriction of eye movement, diplopia, significant enophthalmos (>2 mm) or significant loss of support due to the fracture (>50% of orbital floor). The aim of surgery is to fill the defect in the orbital floor. This is done with either a graft of the patient's own bone or an implant. Those who do not require surgery will heal without significant consequence.

Maxillary fractures

HISTORY AND EXAMINATION

The maxilla is intimately related to the nose, orbits, skull base and oral cavity. Therefore the signs and symptoms of fractures in the area will be related to these sensitive functional and cosmetic areas. High energy to the face is required to fracture the maxilla; because of this, other injuries to the brain or cervical spine should be considered.

Swelling makes assessment of the underlying deformity challenging, so careful examination of the internal relations of the maxilla will point to possible fracture. Signs of maxillary fracture include the following:

- Facial oedema
- Flattening or lengthening of the face
- Periorbital ecchymosis
- Malocclusion of bite with premature contact of the molars and anteriorly open bit
- Facial emphysema
- Mobility of the mid-face
- Haematoma at junction of soft and hard palate
- Airway compromise due to posterior maxillary displacement

The Le Fort Classification of mid-face fractures provides a simplistic but helpful structure to understanding fractures in this area (Figure 10.2).

A Le Fort 1 fracture runs above the floor of the nasal cavity, through the nasal septum, maxillary sinuses and inferior parts of the pterygoid plates.

A Le Fort 2 fracture runs from the floor of the maxillary sinuses superiorly to the infraorbital margins, then extends through the zygomaticomaxillary suture. In the orbit, it passes across the lacrimal bone to the nasal bridge. The infraorbital nerve can be damaged if it is involved with this fracture.

A Le Fort 3 fracture traverses the medial wall of the orbit to the superior orbital fissure and exits across the greater wing of the sphenoid and zygomatic bone to the zygomaticofrontal suture. Posteriorly, this fracture line runs inferior to the optic foramen, across the lesser wing of the sphenoid to the pterygomaxillary fissure and sphenopalatine foramen. The zygoma arches are also broken. This fracture disconnects the facial skeleton from the cranial base.

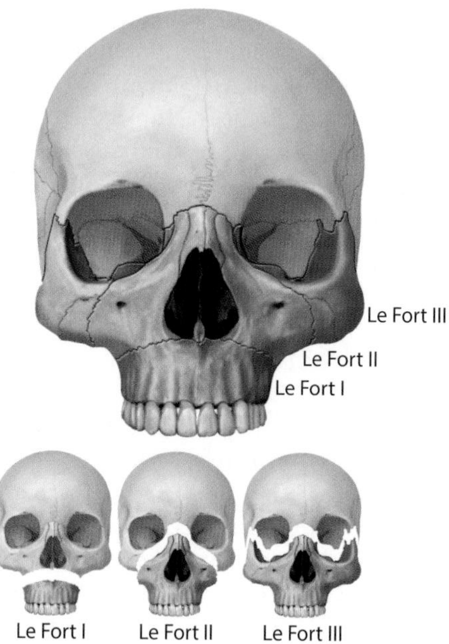

Figure 10.2 Le Fort classification.

INVESTIGATIONS

Plain radiographs may provide some information as to the likelihood of maxillary fracture and are required to assess the cervical spine. However, CT is the imaging modality of choice. It will allow for analysis of the fracture, and 3D reconstruction is used for planning of fracture treatment.

MANAGEMENT

Initial management focuses on treating the life-threatening injuries. Subsequent surgery targets fixation of unstable fracture segments and realignment of significant anatomical relationships. This is undertaken for two reasons: (1) to improve the cosmetic appearance by restoring mid-facial height and projection and (2) to realign the occlusional plate for the functional outcomes of mastication and dental occlusion.

Historically, this was done with external fixation. However, this has now been superseded by internal fixation with miniplates.

LATERAL FACIAL FRACTURES

Zygomatic complex fractures

HISTORY AND EXAMINATION

Trauma to the lateral aspect of the mid-face is common, second only to nasal fractures. The zygomatic complex has important roles in cosmesis, providing the definition of the cheeks, and in function, supporting the globe and anchoring the muscles of mastication. Patients may complain of diplopia (due to reduced eye movements), pain on mouth opening/trismus, or reduced projection of the cheek (due to zygoma depression, a late sign caused by swelling). There is usually lateral subconjunctival haemorrhage, and if the zygomaticotemporal or zygomaticobuccal branches of the infraorbital nerve are involved, there will be paraesthesia of the overlying skin. Examination should look directly at the area for bony deficiency or displacement, as well as those structures that can be indirectly involved – the eye and brain.

INVESTIGATIONS

Plain radiography (15° and 30° occipitomental views) will show most fractures. To identify fractures, it is advisable to study the following:

- The orbital outline: Look for a break in the outline or a 'teardrop' sign for orbital floor fracture.
- The sinus outline: Opacification or fluid level within the maxillary sinus suggests a fracture involving the sinus.
- The 'elephant's trunk': Follow the zygomatic line laterally and the maxillary line medially to check the zygomatic arch's integrity.
- The coronoid processes: These should be equidistant from the maxillary line bilaterally. If one is not, it suggests that a fracture is present.

CT is useful to plan when surgery is required. There is a potential role for ultrasound to identify fractures and check reduction to reduce radiation exposure through imaging.

MANAGEMENT

When there is no significant displacement of the fracture, conservative management is appropriate. Patients should be advised not to blow their nose for 2 to 3 weeks, and they should be reviewed after the swelling has resolved (approximately 10 days) to make sure there is no subsequent displacement. If there is enough displacement to lead to functional or cosmetic issues, reduction of the fracture is required. This is done with simple elevation or open reduction with internal fixation, depending on the fractures.

MANDIBULAR FRACTURES

History and examination

Mandibular fractures are seen predominantly in the young male population, with women and children being much less at risk unless involved in domestic violence (Figure 10.3).

The most commonly fractured sites are the following:

- Body (29 per cent)
- Condyle (26 per cent)
- Angle (25 per cent)
- Symphysis (17 per cent)
- Ramus (4 per cent)
- Coracoid (1 per cent)

Presentation usually reflects a significant force to the mandible as a result of sports, assault, road traffic accident or fall. Other injuries to structures such as the neck and brain should be suspected and excluded. Patients may report pain on eating, an inability to occlude their teeth properly, or missing teeth. Examination should note any abnormality in facial symmetry and shape of the mandible. Movement should be assessed as best as possible and occlusion checked. Palpation may demonstrate a step or bony crepitus. Loose and fractured teeth should be counted and assessed. If any are missing and unaccounted for, a chest x-ray should be considered to ensure that teeth have not been aspirated. Neurological status of the supplying branches of the trigeminal and facial nerve should be checked and documented (inferior alveolar and marginal mandibular nerves).

Investigation

Plain radiology is used for initial assessment of the mandible in many centres. It does not show the mandible well, with large areas of overlap, making fracture identification difficult. Panoramic radiographs, known as orthopantomograms (OPGs), are plain x-rays taken while moving the x-ray detector around the mandible to generate a flat image of the mandible. This allows for satisfactory fracture identification in all areas but the condyles. It has been shown to be almost as good as CT in fracture

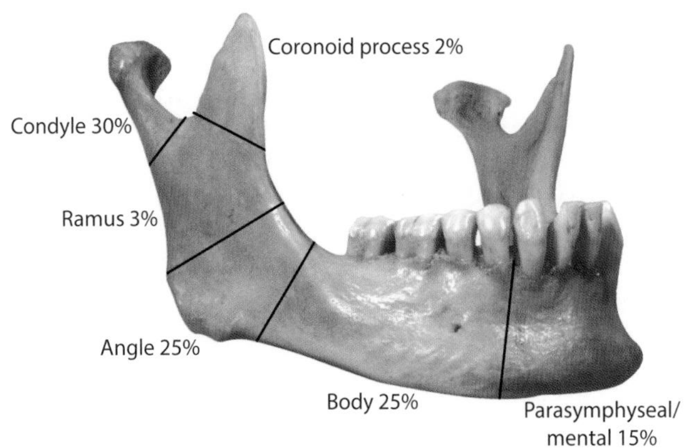

Figure 10.3 Frequency by location of nasal mandibular fracture.

identification, and the choice of CT or OPG is determined by local facilities, expertise and preference.

Management

The mandible is a highly functional part of the skeleton, and therefore fractures are painful and readily affect function. After management of the acute life-threatening injuries has taken place, reduction will be required to allow for return of function and pain control.

Antibiotics have been shown to be of benefit and should be given. The fractures should be considered open into the mouth, owing to the thin covering of mucosa and connection with dental sockets.

Reduction of the fracture can be undertaken open or closed. Because of the significant forces across the mandible resulting from the various muscles that attach, fixation will be required to maintain the reduction. This can be done by indirect or direct skeletal fixation.

Indirect fixation involves using the teeth as an anchor for an arch bar or wire. They are placed so as to support either side of the fracture intraorally and are left for 2 to 8 weeks depending on the age of the patient and the pattern of fracture. It is used in the paediatric population, because direct fixation risks damage to the unerupted teeth still lying within the mandible.

In direct fixation, the open approach is used, and wires or plates with screws are placed over the fracture site. This method has higher morbidity and complication rates than indirect fixation. It is used in complex fractures or in edentulous patients. Newer absorbable plates may increase the use of open reduction techniques.

KEY LEARNING POINTS

- Facial trauma can be life threatening.
- Mechanism of injury will point to possible fractures and other craniofacial injuries.
- Early manipulation of nasal fractures is advisable.
- Septal haematoma needs to be identified to prevent septal necrosis.
- Plain radiographs are useful in the identification of facial fractures, but CT is the main imaging modality used.
- Unsafe/unstable facial fractures or those with significant cosmetic impact will require surgical intervention.

11

Facial plastic surgery

TIM J WOOLFORD

INTRODUCTION

This chapter provides an overview of plastic surgery of the nose, ear and facial flaps. The chapter covers septorhinoplasty, nasal reconstruction, pinnaplasty, ear reconstruction, and the commonly used bilobed and rhombic flaps.

Patient assessment and selection are of key importance, and the various aspects of this are discussed. Informed consent must be taken from any patient undergoing surgery; it is particularly important in the field of facial plastic surgery, where there is a higher incidence of medico-legal action.

PATIENT SELECTION

The fundamental decision in facial plastic surgery is whether the individual patient is a candidate for surgery. It is of key importance that patients have realistic expectations and accept the limitations of surgery. This is particularly important when a rhinoplasty is being considered, and for this reason most surgeons will see patients on two occasions to discuss this operation.

Facial plastic surgery can be a very positive experience for many patients. However, this is not always the case, and a significant minority of patients should not undergo surgery. In the preoperative discussion, the surgeon must make sure that the patient does accept that a 'perfect' result is not achievable.

On occasion, patients exhibit extreme and excessive anxiety about a particular cosmetic feature, most commonly (but certainly not exclusively) their nose. This is a recognized psychological disorder known as body dysmorphic disorder. These patients often describe minor abnormalities in very dramatic terms, and their concerns have a very negative impact on their quality of life. Although they are often desperate to undergo surgery, this is almost invariably counterproductive and leads to more unhappiness. Referral to a clinical psychologist or psychiatrist with an interest in this field is the way forward. In reality many of these patients reject this option and continue to seek surgery.

NASAL PLASTIC SURGERY

SEPTORHINOPLASTY

Patients who are considering a septorhinoplasty have either cosmetic concerns alone or both cosmetic and functional concerns. On rare occasions patients have no cosmetic concerns; however, the external structural shape of their nose is affecting the nasal airway, and a septorhinoplasty will be required to improve this. In terms of definitions, *rhinoplasty* is surgery to the external structure of the nose, and *septorhinoplasty* affects both the external structure and the nasal septum. Almost all rhinoplasty procedures also involve the septum to a lesser or greater degree, and many surgeons refer to all such procedures as septorhinoplasty.

Preoperative assessment

As described earlier, patients should be offered a septorhinoplasty only if they have realistic expectations. As part of the preoperative assessment, clinical photographs must be taken. This is a medico-legal requirement but is also very helpful to discuss the aims of surgery with the patient using these photographs.

Examination

Clinical examination initially involves inspection of the external shape of the nose. Palpation is often helpful as well. The patient's skin type is particularly important in rhinoplasty, with thin skin tending to show irregularities and thicker skin reducing the definition that can be achieved. Anterior rhinoscopy is performed to examine the nasal septum and turbinates. The dynamic function of the nose should be examined, particularly any collapse of the nasal valves on inspiration. Examination of the nasal cavity and postnasal space with an endoscope is often indicated if the patient has airway obstruction or other rhinological symptoms.

Aesthetic assessment

An extensive description of analysis of the nose is beyond the scope of this chapter; however, it is important to stress that the nasal anatomy must be fully understood and the anatomical abnormality leading to the aesthetic or functional problem identified. Only then can the surgeon plan a suitable operation to address these.[1]

Key features to be examined on front view include the width and any deviation of the nasal bones. The upper lateral cartilages and septum make up the mid third of the nose, and any deviation or asymmetry should be identified. Finally, the symmetry and definition of the nasal tip is studied.

On profile view the height of the nasal dorsum is examined, as well as the presence of a dorsal hump or need for augmentation. The ideal aesthetic profile will, of course, differ between men and women. An important feature of the nose is the projection of the nasal tip. This is the distance that the nasal tip projects forwards from the face, and any over- or under-projection of the tip of the nose in relation to the nasal dorsum should be recognized. The rotation of the nasal tip is the angle between the nasal columella and the lip. Again, this differs between the male and female nose, with an ideal angle of approximately 90° in men and an increase in rotation in women to 100–110°.

Informed consent for septorhinoplasty

The preoperative discussion must include the possible complications. The complications discussed must include bleeding, bruising, infection, numbness, septal perforation and a poor outcome requiring further or revision surgery. Other possible problems such as loss of smell, skin changes and nasal obstruction are also recorded by many surgeons. Septorhinoplasty is a common cause of medico-legal action, and it is very important that these complications are not only discussed but also recorded in the case notes and consent form. Written information should also be given and this action recorded in the case notes and on the consent form.

Surgical techniques in septorhinoplasty

There are two approaches used in septorhinoplasty: the endonasal approach and the open or external approach. In endonasal septorhinoplasty, all incisions are made inside the nose. In the open approach, however, a small incision is made across the columella and the skin, and soft tissues are elevated from the underlying cartilages and bone.[2]

There are advantages and disadvantages to each approach. The type of surgery performed will depend upon both the complexity of the surgery required and the experience and training of the surgeon. In general, more complex cases such as revision or cleft nose surgery are performed via an open approach, and more straightforward primary cases are performed using an endonasal approach. There is actually great variation even amongst those who specialize in this area of surgery, with some surgeons performing the majority of cases open and others preferring an endonasal approach.

Surgery may involve reduction in the size of the nasal bones and cartilage to reduce a dorsal hump, and osteotomies and fracture of the bones are often required to narrow the nasal bridge. The lower lateral cartilages can be reduced and the shape modified with sutures to improve the shape of the nasal

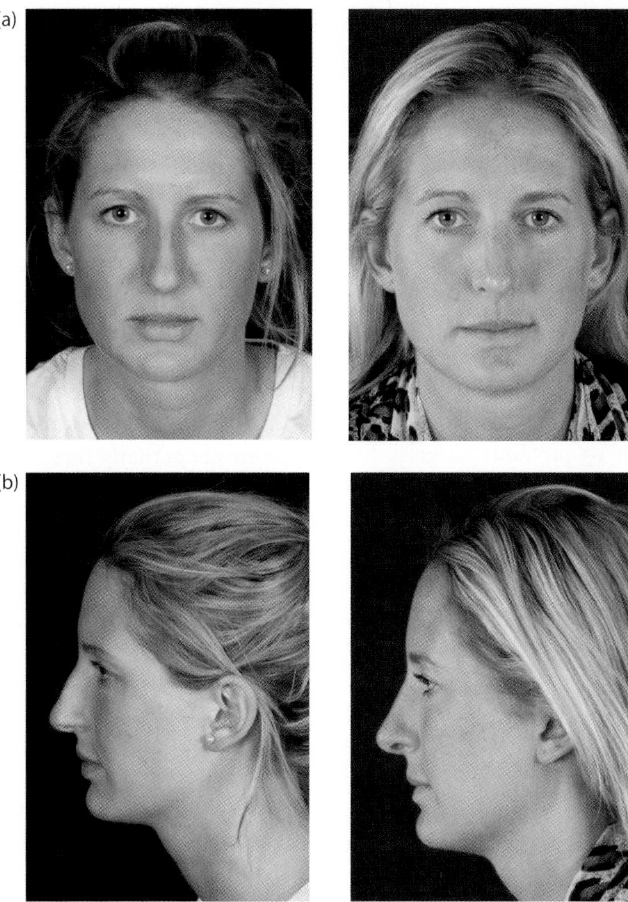

Figure 11.1 Preoperative rhinoplasty photographs on the left, with post-operative on the right, showing a patient with a deviation, a small dorsal hump and a bulbous nasal tip. *(Continued)*

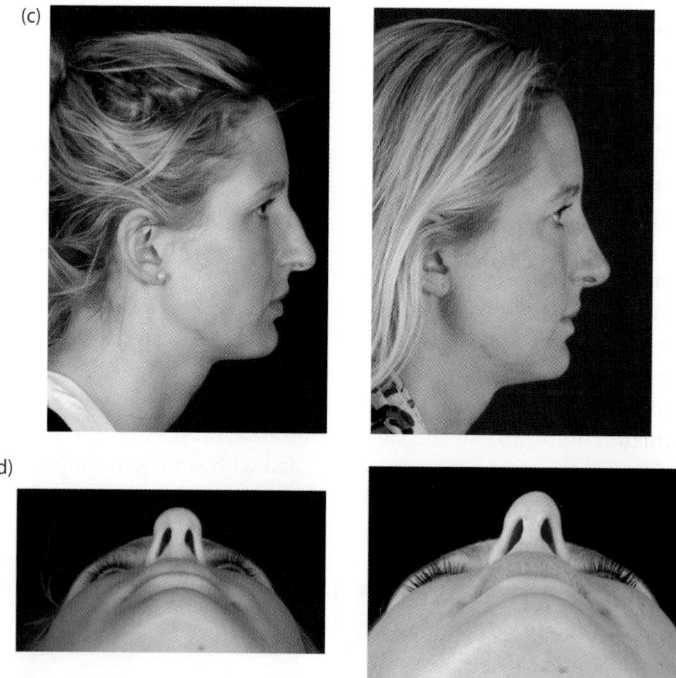

Figure 11.1 (Continued)

tip. The results of an open septorhinoplasty are shown in Figure 11.1a-d. Cartilage grafts to augment, support or straighten the nose are frequently placed during septorhinoplasty. These grafts may be harvested from the nasal septum or from the pinna if there is insufficient cartilage in the septum due to injury, infection or previous surgery. On occasion, rib cartilage is used when large or strong structural grafting is required. Synthetic grafts may be used, although these are not favoured by a number of surgeons owing to an increased risk of extrusion and infection.

The nose is protected with an external splint for a week or so. It takes a number of months for the swelling of the nose to settle before the final result can be judged, and patients must be made aware of this.

NASAL RECONSTRUCTION

A nasal reconstruction is required when a significant part of the external nose, including skin, requires reconstruction. A variety of cases require nasal reconstructive surgery, including congenital abnormalities, trauma and complications of surgery. By far the biggest group of patients requiring a nasal reconstruction are those with nasal skin cancer.

The defect of the nose may involve skin, cartilage, bone and the underlying mucosa. Defects of bone are actually rare. A defect that involves skin, cartilage and mucosa is described as being full thickness. The key principle of a nasal reconstruction is to reconstruct the nose in these three layers and replace like with like.

A mucosal defect is replaced with mucosal flaps from the nasal cavity, often the nasal septum. The defect in the cartilage is replaced using cartilage from the conchal bowl of the pinna or rarely the septum.

The approach used to reconstruct the skin defect depends on the size and location of the defect, a concept known as the 'reconstructive ladder'. Small defects may be closed primarily or be allowed to heal by secondary intention, although this is rare. Full-thickness skin grafts may be used to reconstruct certain smaller defects.

They give the best results in areas where the nasal skin is thin such as over the bony dorsum or sidewall. Where the skin is thicker, particularly over the nasal tip, full-thickness skin grafts often do not give a favourable cosmetic result. It is important to involve patients in the decision-making process at an early stage. Patients of course prefer more straightforward surgery; however, it must be explained that this may not result in a favourable long-term cosmetic result.[3]

Certain defects can be closed using local flaps; the bilobed flap is the most common example in nasal reconstruction. As seen in Figure 11.4, these flaps often cause distortion of the nasal tip and remain rather visible. A composite graft of skin and fat from the forehead is a good alternative for smaller nasal tip defects. Larger defects require a distant flap, and two varieties are most commonly used for nasal reconstruction. In the first, skin from the cheek is used to reconstruct a defect of the nasal ala or columella. This flap is called the melolabial or nasolabial flap. Larger defects affecting the nasal tip, sidewall and dorsum are usually reconstructed using a paramedian forehead flap. This so-called workhorse flap of nasal reconstruction is based on the supratrochlear artery, and the whole of the nasal skin can be replaced with this flap if required.

The melolabial and paramedian forehead flaps ideally should be interpolated, that is, they bridge normal skin. The flaps are divided at 3 to 4 weeks once the reconstructed skin has developed a blood supply. Refinement procedures to thin and contour the flaps are often required. The various stages of reconstruction of a full-thickness nasal tip defect are shown in Figure 11.2.

PLASTIC SURGERY OF THE EAR

PINNAPLASTY

The operation to correct prominent ears is called an otoplasty or pinnaplasty. Prominent ears (now rarely referred to as 'bat' ears) are a relatively common aesthetic problem affecting approximately 1 in 20 children. Children with this condition may be subject to teasing at school, although this is rare in very young children. For this reason surgery is usually performed from about 7 years of age. Although a pinnaplasty may be performed in younger children, delaying surgery until this age is preferable because the child will express a wish to undergo the surgery, has a greater understanding and can be involved in the decision process. Surgery does not need to be performed at this age, however, and may also be performed in older children or on rare occasions in adults.

The anatomical causes of a protruding ear include unfolding of the antihelix of the pinna, a deep conchal bowl and projection of the lobule. Often the cause is a combination of these factors, and a correct anatomical diagnosis must be made and surgery planned accordingly.

As in all operations the consent process is important. Children and their families must be made aware of the risks of bleeding, infection,

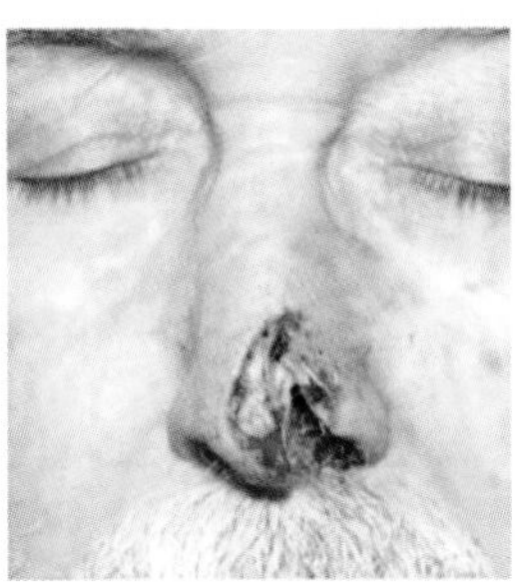
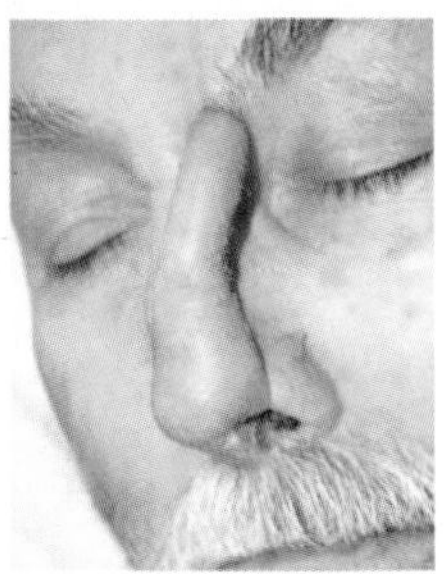
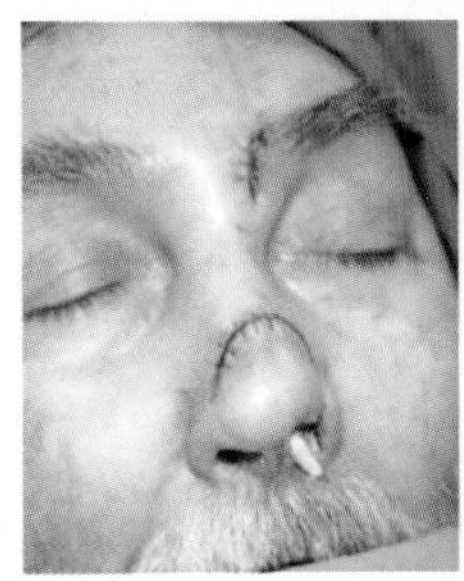
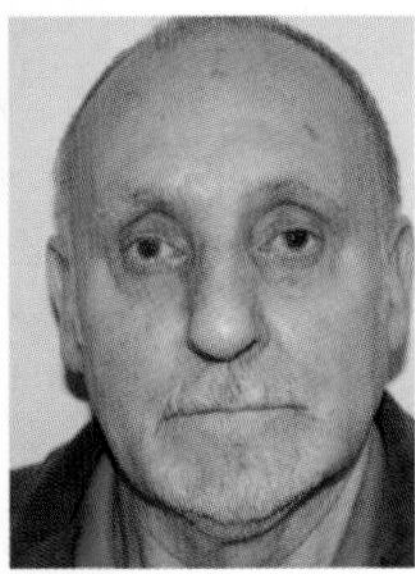

Figure 11.2 A full-thickness nasal tip defect after excision of skin cancer. The first stage of the reconstruction was a mucosal rotation flap and cartilage support, using cartilage harvested from the pinna. A paramedian forehead flap was used to reconstruct the skin defect. The final result of the reconstruction at 1 year after surgery.

excessive (keloid) scarring and numbness and that both ears may not be exactly the same. As in all cosmetic procedures, there is a possibility that further surgery will be required.

There are two main surgical techniques used to correct prominent ears: anterior scoring or suturing. In the scoring technique, changes are made to the shape of the pinna by making numerous partial-thickness incisions to weaken the cartilage and create an antihelical fold. In the suture technique, the antihelical fold is formed by sutures.[4] After formation of an antihelical fold, correction of a deep conchal bowl is often required. This is achieved either by the placement of sutures between the conchal bowl and the mastoid process or, when necessary, by excision of conchal bowl cartilage. Correction of a projecting lobule is the final step and is particularly challenging.

Post-operative advice following surgery varies between surgeons. Children generally wear a bandage for a week or so, and it is my practice to advise them to avoid contact sport for a month. Pre- and post-operative photographs of a pinnaplasty patient are shown in Figure 11.3.

EAR RECONSTRUCTION

There are a variety of different conditions that result in partial or total loss of the pinna, with the most common acquired causes being skin cancer and trauma. In the United Kingdom, the most common traumatic cause of a defect of the pinna is a human bite injury. A congenitally small or absent ear is called microtia. This condition affects approximately 1 in 8000 children, with 10 per cent of congenital cases being bilateral.

Microtia is usually associated with an absent ear canal, known as atresia, and this causes a severe conductive hearing loss. The majority of children with this condition, however, have a normally functioning cochlea and no underlying sensorineural hearing loss. In the vast majority of children with microtia, the ear abnormality is not part of a wider genetic abnormality, although this condition may be a feature of Goldenhar and Treacher Collins syndrome.

When part or all of the pinna requires reconstruction, the technique required will of course depend upon the size of the defect. Smaller defects involving only skin are reconstructed using skin grafts or local flaps. Larger defects often require more complex multistage surgery involving carved rib cartilage grafts and various soft tissue flaps and grafts. An alternative to surgical reconstruction is an implant retained prosthetic ear. These artificial ears clip onto titanium bone-anchored implants, similar to those used for bone-anchored hearing aids. These prosthetic ears are very realistic when made by a skilled prosthetist and are a good alternative to a surgical reconstruction for some patients.

The most common type of condition requiring total ear reconstruction is congenital microtia. It is important that children with microtia and their families are given a comprehensive and

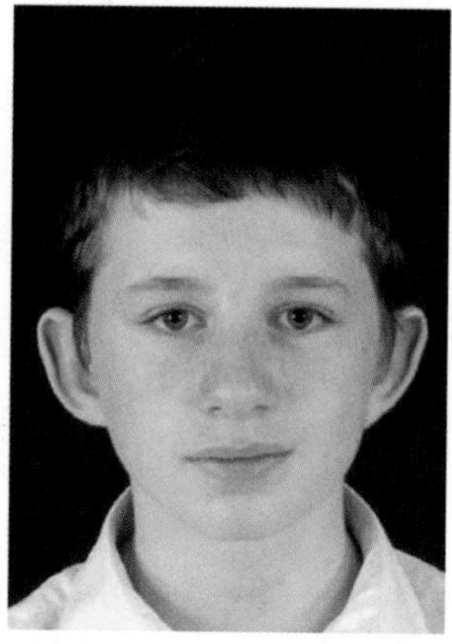
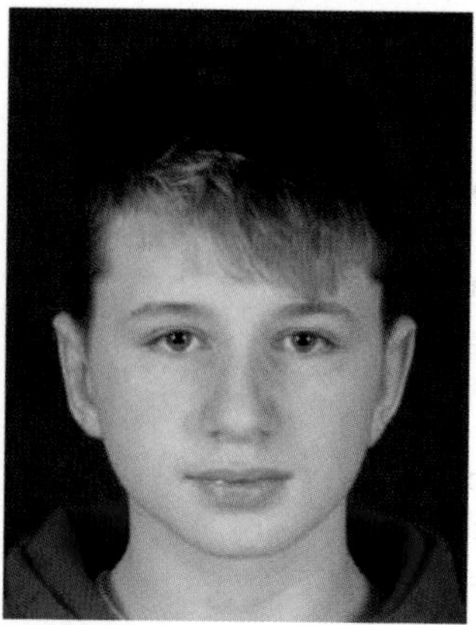

Figure 11.3 Pre- and post-operative pictures of a pinnaplasty patient.

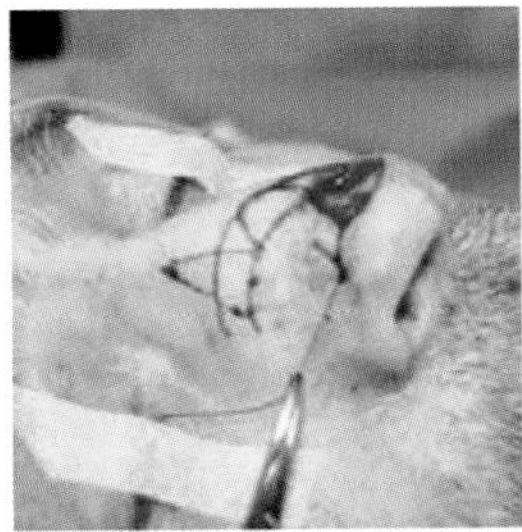
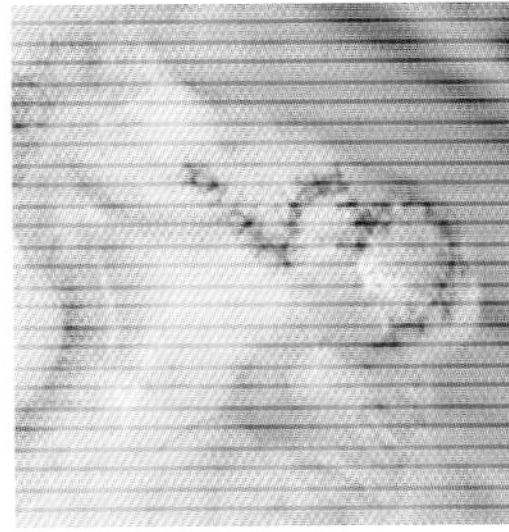
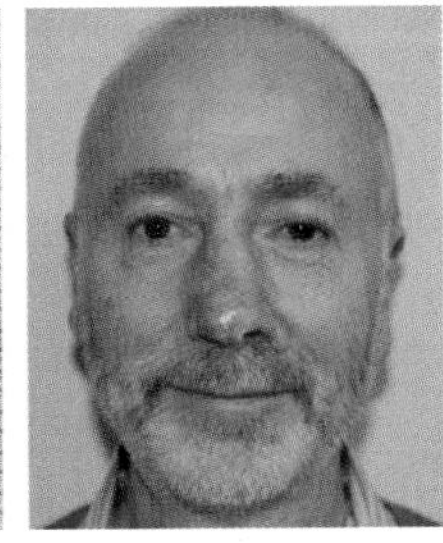

Figure 11.4 A nasal tip defect with a bilobed flap designed. The flap is rotated and sutured in place. The final result at 1 year (right). Note that there is some distortion of the nasal tip and telangiectasia of the skin, which are common with this flap.

balanced view of all aspects of their condition. This includes the management of the hearing loss and the options for reconstruction. Ear reconstruction is usually performed from the age of 8 years. At this age, children have sufficient rib to carve a new framework, and importantly they are old enough to request surgery and have an understanding of what is involved. Some children decide against surgery. That decision must be respected and no pressure placed on them to proceed.

Ear reconstruction takes two to four stages. Surgery involves carving a new ear framework from rib cartilage based on a template taken from the normal ear.[5] Any cartilage remnant is generally removed, the ear lobe transposed to the correct position and the new framework placed in a subcutaneous pocket. After a few months the framework is elevated, and the posterior surface of the new ear is covered with a skin graft.

FACIAL FLAPS

Skin defects that are too large for primary closure require either grafts or flaps for reconstruction. Where possible, local flaps are generally preferred owing to their close texture and colour match with the surrounding skin, resulting in a favourable aesthetic outcome.

In many cases a number of different flaps may be used to reconstruct a particular facial cutaneous defect. The flap selected depends on a number of factors, including the size and location of the defect. Possible distortion and functional impairment of adjacent structures by the reconstructive technique used must also be considered, for instance in defects near the eyelid or lip. Larger defects are, of course, more challenging to reconstruct, and on occasion a less aesthetically pleasing technique must be adopted to ensure that function is not compromised.

The most common facial flaps are the bilobed and the rhombic flap, and both are examples of pivotal local cutaneous flaps.

THE BILOBED FLAP

The bilobed flap is a double transposition flap that shares a single base. The flap has a number of applications on the face; however, the most common use is to reconstruct defects of the nasal tip. The flap must be designed with geometrical accuracy, and the principle is that the first lobe is the same diameter and height as the defect. The width of the second lobe is slightly less, and the height is double. Each lobe rotates through 45°. The donor site of the second lobe is closed first, the first lobe reconstructs the defect and the second lobe is trimmed to close the first lobe donor site. Finally, any standing cutaneous deformity at the base of the defect is removed. A bilobed flap is illustrated in Figure 11.4.

THE RHOMBIC FLAP

The rhombic flap is a transposition flap where a rectangle of skin is transposed to reconstruct a similar sized defect. The most common application is to reconstruct defects of the medial and lateral cheek.

The rhombic flap must be designed bearing in mind the skin laxity and proximity to other structures. A rhombic defect is created with two angles of 60° and two of 120°. An adjacent rectangle is marked parallel with the base of the rhombic defect. This rectangle is transposed to reconstruct the defect, and a standing deformity of variable size at the base of the flap is excised.

KEY LEARNING POINTS

- Assessment and patient selection are key in facial plastic surgery.
- Informed consent must be obtained and documented, with written information also given.
- In rhinoplasty the patient's skin type must be taken into consideration as it is one of the key factors to the outcome.
- Nasal reconstruction must involve reconstruction of all three layers of any defect: mucosa, cartilage and skin.
- In pinnaplasty and rhinoplasty, a diagnosis of the anatomical abnormality is required to enable the surgeon to plan the procedure required.

REFERENCES

1. Tardy ME. *Practical Surgical Anatomy.* In: *Rhinoplasty, The Art and the Science, Volume 1.* Ed. Tardy ME. Philadelphia: WB Saunders, 1997: 2–125.
2. Adamson PA. Open rhinoplasty. *Otolaryngologic Clinics of North America.* 1987; 20(4): 837–52.
3. Burget GC, Menick FJ. The sub-unit principle in nasal reconstruction. *Plastic and Reconstructive Surgery.* 1985; 76: 239.
4. Mustarde JC. The treatment of prominent ears by buried mattress sutures: A ten-year survey. *Plastic and Reconstructive Surgery.* 1967; 39: 38–86.
5. Brent B. Ear reconstruction with an expansile framework of autogenous rib cartilage. *Plastic and Reconstructive Surgery.* 1974; 53: 619.

FURTHER READING

Nolst Trinite GJ, Ed. *Rhinoplasty: A Practical Guide to Functional and Aesthetic Surgery of the Nose.* The Hague, Netherlands: Kugler Publications, 2005.

Baker SR, Naficy S, Eds. *Principles of Nasal Reconstruction.* St. Louis, Missouri: Mosby, 2002.

12

Pituitary surgery

JOHN HILL AND SEAN CARRIE

The development of the operating endoscope has made a significant change to the delivery of pituitary surgery over the past 10 years. The improved visualization of the operative field afforded by the endoscope is leading to decreased morbidity and better results. It has also necessitated the move to more joint work between neurosurgeons and otolaryngologists, which fits well with modern multidisciplinary patient management and should lead to safer advances in extended skull base surgery in the future.

Historically, development in pituitary surgery has been driven by the improvement in the optics. Sir Victor Horsley in 1906 performed the first successful transfrontal craniotomy for a pituitary tumour. Herman Schloffer first described a nasal approach in 1907, but Harvey Cushing[1] is most associated with the transseptal, transsphenoidal approach. He started his series of cases in 1909, but he abandoned this approach and reverted to a transcranial approach because he was struggling with post-operative infections and, not surprisingly, difficulty in visualizing the operative field when using only a relatively primitive headlight.

In the 1960s the operating microscope allowed the switch back to the per-nasal transseptal route.[2,3] By using an operating microscope[4] the surgeon gets excellent illumination, 3D perception and two hands free for operating. This has been the mainstay of pituitary surgery until recently.

Otolaryngologists started using rigid endoscopes for endoscopic sinus surgery in the late 1980s, and the first use in pituitary surgery was by an otolaryngologist, Roger Jankowski, in 1992. Since then the techniques have been refined.[5,6]

Pituitary tumours are relatively common in that they constitute approximately 12 per cent of all primary brain tumours. The majority are adenomas and are benign. Malignant disease in the pituitary is extremely rare.

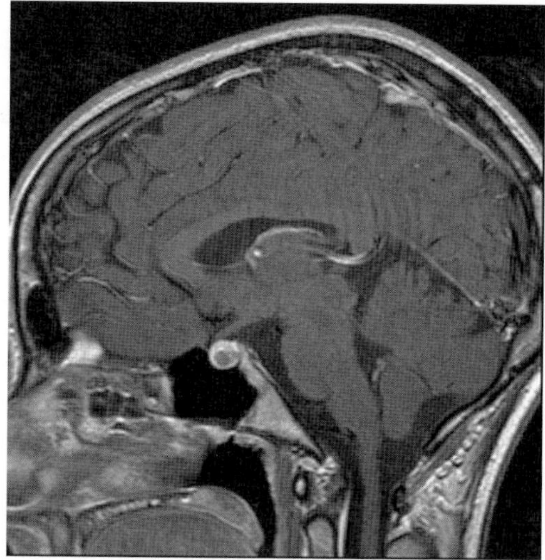

Figure 12.1 Sagittal MR view of a micro-adenoma placed centrally in a normal-sized pituitary gland.

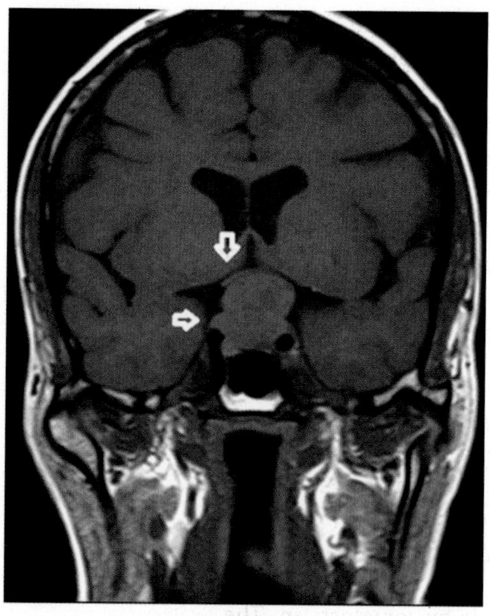

Figure 12.2 Coronal MR view showing macro-adenoma elevating the optic chiasm (down arrow) and extending over the carotid artery in the right cavernous sinus (horizontal arrow).

Adenomas are classified by both their size and their function. Tumours that are less than 1 cm in diameter are classified as micro-adenomas. Macro-adenomas are those that are greater than 1 cm in diameter. Approximately 50 per cent of adenomas are nonfunctioning and will present by virtue of their size as a space-occupying lesion. The other 50 per cent of adenomas are functioning and will therefore present by the effects that they have via excess hormone secretion (Figures 12.1 and 12.2).

PRESENTATION OF PITUITARY TUMOURS

PROLACTINOMAS

Adenomas that produce prolactin are the most common of the secreting adenomas. The adenoma produces raised levels of circulating prolactin, and in women this will have the effect of causing secondary amenorrhoea and galactorrhoea. In men the effects of raised prolactin levels are less obvious. A degree of impotence is often the only symptom, and tumours are often extensive before they are diagnosed.

Prolactin secretion from the anterior pituitary lobe is controlled by prolactin releasing hormone, which is secreted from the hypothalamus. The hormone is dopamine, and it controls prolactin secretion by inhibiting its release. This is the basis of medical treatment in that dopaminergic compounds can be used to inhibit the secretion of prolactin. Initially, bromocriptine was used, but this has been superseded by more effective agents such as cabergoline. These medications can be taken orally and lead to circulating prolactin levels returning to normal and the adenoma itself resorbing. Medical treatment is very effective and is all that is required in 95 per cent of cases. Surgical intervention or radiotherapy is only considered in patients who are unable to tolerate the side effects of medical treatment.

GROWTH HORMONE-SECRETING ADENOMAS

Adenomas that increase circulating growth hormone level lead to acromegaly. In adulthood the symptoms are due to an increase in the size of soft tissues and membranous derived bones. The classical appearance is of coarsening of the facial features with prognathism, and the hands and the feet increase in size leading to an increase in shoe and ring sizes. Patients are often lethargic and sweaty with macroglossia leading to sleep apnoea. The internal changes lead to hepato-splenomegaly, hypertension and increased risk of cardiomegaly. It is these changes that lead to a significantly reduced life expectancy in untreated patients. Growth hormone secretion is controlled by growth hormone releasing hormone, which is released from the hypothalamus. This is a positive releasing hormone. Growth hormone leads to increased production of insulin-like growth factor 1 (IGF1), and both circulating growth hormone and raised levels of IGF1 can be measured in affected patients. The effects of growth hormone are mediated in the body by somatostatin. The basis of medical treatment for acromegaly is to block the effects of somatostatin with agents such as octreotide. Medical treatment needs to be given by subcutaneous injection and remains relatively expensive. Not all tumours respond to these agents, but in those that do there will be a reduction in the clinical symptoms of acromegaly and a slight shrinkage in the size of the tumour.

Surgery remains the treatment of choice in the majority of these tumours. Transsphenoidal surgery for a micro-adenoma has a good chance of curing the patient. When the tumour is a macro-adenoma, complete clearance of the tumour is unlikely, but significant de-bulking of the tumour tissue will lead to an improvement in the symptoms and easier control with subsequent treatment, whether it be radiotherapy or somatostatin analogues.

ADRENOCORTICOTROPHIC HORMONE-SECRETING ADENOMAS

Adrenocorticotrophic hormone (ACTH)-secreting adenomas produce the clinical syndrome of Cushing's disease. The ACTH leads to an increase in circulating glucocorticoids, which gives the classical appearance of central obesity with wasting of the proximal limbs, moon face, acne, striae and fat deposition around the nape of the neck producing a buffalo hump. Cushing's disease is associated with significant morbidity and mortality. The internal effects of the raised glucocorticoid levels are hypertension, diabetes and cardiovascular complications. Untreated Cushing's disease can lead to significant mortality rates over only a few years.

There is no particularly satisfactory medical treatment for Cushing's disease. High doses of antifungal agents such as ketoconazole can restrict the effects of Cushing's disease, but these are only partially effective and have complications at the required high doses.

Adenomas that produce ACTH are usually very active and present when the adenomas are small. Surgical adenomectomy therefore is the treatment of choice. Small tumours can be difficult to locate at presentation and may not be evident on magnetic resonance (MR) scanning. Diagnosis can be helped by inferior petrosal sinus sampling, which allows ACTH levels to be assessed in both petrosal sinuses – first by confirming that the Cushing's disease is due to an adenoma in the pituitary area, and second by comparing levels between the two sides – to indicate the likely side of the lesion if it is laterally placed in the pituitary fossa. Pituitary adenomectomy is usually the simplest surgical procedure to control Cushing's disease, but the alternative surgical option is bilateral adrenalectomy. This is increasingly done endoscopically but is still a procedure with a higher morbidity than pituitary surgery and is therefore used as a second-line treatment.

OTHER SECRETING PITUITARY TUMOURS

Thyroid stimulating hormone (TSH) tumours that produce TSH, luteinizing hormone (LH) and follicle stimulating hormone (FSH) compose less than 1 per cent of pituitary tumours.

MASS EFFECT PRESENTATION

Approximately 50 per cent of adenomas will present with the hyper-secretion syndromes already mentioned, but the other 50 per cent of adenomas are nonsecreting in nature and will present by virtue of their size alone.

Increasingly, nonsecreting adenomas are being picked up incidentally on MR scans. The classical presentation of a nonsecreting tumour is that of bitemporal hemianopia, headaches or hypopituitarism.

As a tumour grows and becomes a macro-adenoma, it will extend beyond the pituitary fossa. Extension inferiorly into the clivus is usually asymptomatic. Extension laterally results in invasion of the cavernous sinus. Tumour in the cavernous sinus is also usually asymptomatic. It tends to wrap itself around the sinusoidal shape of the carotid artery or the siphon, which makes surgical removal more difficult; the III, IV, V and VI cranial nerves are placed laterally in the cavernous sinus, however, and therefore are very rarely affected by direct pressure. The immediate superior relation of the pituitary fossa is the diaphragmatica sellae. Increasing pressure on the diaphragm can lead to low-grade headaches; however, most of these tumours are slow-growing, so it is not a reliable feature. Further growth in the supra-sellar region will lead to pressure on the optic chiasm. Early compression affects the visual fields, initially producing unilateral upper quadrant anopia. With increasing pressure, this can become bilateral and take the form of the classical bitemporal hemianopia.

As the nonsecreting tumour increases in size, it will cause compression of the residual normal pituitary tissue, resulting in pan-hypopituitarism with hypothyroidism, amenorrhoea, impotence and a hypo-functioning steroid axis. Clinically, these patients present with a steady decline in energy levels, generalized ill health, hypotension and pallor.

The nonsecreting tumours cannot be treated medically, and surgical regimens are the mainstay of treatment. Surgical removal of an adenoma or decompression will relieve the pressure from the optic chiasm, which may be all the treatment that is required or may be combined with radiotherapy.

OTHER LESIONS IN THE PITUITARY FOSSA

Ninety-five per cent of lesions in the pituitary fossa are adenomas, but other disorders include Rathke's cleft cysts, craniopharyngiomas, meningiomas, chordomas and, rarely, aneurysms of the vessels of the circle of Willis. Secondary metastases from primary malignancies, typically breast adenocarcinoma, are occasionally seen.

Cystic lesions of the pituitary fossa present as space-occupying lesions with visual field defects and occasionally headache. Treatment is surgical with drainage of the cyst, but the lesions have a tendency to recur.

RADIOTHERAPY IN THE MANAGEMENT OF PITUITARY ADENOMA

Radiotherapy is widely used in the treatment of pituitary adenomas despite the fact that these are benign rather than malignant tumours. However, it is not suitable for large tumours because of the risk of damage to the adjacent optic chiasm, which is relatively radiosensitive. Radiotherapy can be an effective treatment for smaller adenomas and hyper-secretion syndromes, but it does have the disadvantage that it can take 2 to 5 years to take effect, during which the hyper-secretion syndrome will be ongoing. Normal pituitary function will also decline with time, requiring long-term endocrine monitoring and hormone replacement to support the pituitary axis. For these reasons, radiotherapy is often used as a post-operative treatment after the de-bulking of large macro-adenomas or in patients with residual raised hormone secretion levels as a result of partially successful surgical treatment. Stereotactic radio-surgery in the form of the gamma knife or cyber knife also appears to have advantages in terms of improved control of hyper-section and a decreased reduction in residual pituitary function over conventional radiotherapy.

SURGICAL ANATOMY

The normal pituitary gland is approximately 0.5 cm^3 in volume. It sits in the sella turcica in a pocket of dura, which lines the floor of the sella; a layer of dura forms the roof of the pituitary fossa (diaphragma sellae). The stalk of the pituitary pierces this diaphragm. The diaphragm separates the intracranial space from the pituitary fossa. Cerebrospinal fluid (CSF) is present intracranially but not normally in the fossa. The small defect in the diaphragm that accommodates the pituitary stalk is therefore a potential route for a CSF leak. Laterally, the pituitary tissue is adjacent to the venous sinusoids of the cavernous sinus. The internal carotid arteries ascend in a vertical portion in the inferior part of the cavernous sinuses, turn forwards at the level of the pituitary gland and then double back on themselves to perform a siphon in the carotid artery that can often be seen on either side of the pituitary fossa as it indents the posterior wall of the sphenoid sinus. Carotid arteries pass posteriorly from this bulge and then medially to the anterior clinoid processes into the anterior cranial fossa. The oculomotor (III), trochlear (IV), trigeminal (V) and abducens (VI) nerves are placed laterally in the wall of the cavernous sinus. The optic nerves pass posteromedially and superiorly from the orbital apex to indent the superior aspect of the sphenoid sinus just above the bulge formed by the carotid artery before meeting in the optic chiasm, which lies just anterior to the stalk of the pituitary gland (Figure 12.3).

The degree of pneumatization and the position of septae in the sphenoid sinus are highly variable. In the majority of cases the pituitary fossa will form a bulge in the posterior or posterosuperior region of the sphenoid and is easily identifiable with the operating endoscope. The rostrum of the sphenoid, where it is in contact with the posterior edge of the plate of the ethmoid bone forming the posterior end of the nasal septum, is in the midline. If there is a sphenoid sinus septum in contact with the anterior wall of the sphenoid sinus, it will usually contact it in the midline. The posterior attachment of intrasphenoid septae is highly variable and will often veer to one side or another and insert close to the carotid artery (as in Figure 12.5). Multiple vertically and transversely placed septae that may or may not extend from the posterior wall of the sphenoid sinuses as far as the anterior wall are often encountered. The degree of pneumatization of the sphenoid is variable, with approximately 1 per cent of sphenoids being full of cancellous bone with no aeration at all. In approximately 10 per cent of cases, the pituitary fossa is behind the posterior wall of the sphenoid with no air space below it.

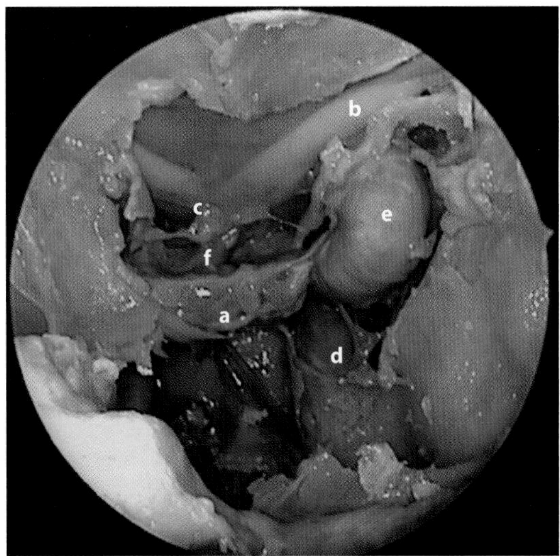

Figure 12.3 Cadaveric dissection of pituitary fossa and left cavernous sinus. The bone of the roof of the posterior wall of the sphenoid sinus and the diaphragma sellae have been removed to demonstrate the normal pituitary gland (a), optic nerve (b), optic chiasm (c), vertical portion of the carotid artery (d), carotid siphon (e) and pituitary stalk (f).

SURGICAL MANAGEMENT OF PITUITARY DISEASE

The evolution of pituitary surgery has been driven by the steady improvement in surgical equipment. Harvey Cushing is considered the father of pituitary surgery because of his introduction of the transseptal, transsphenoidal route from 1912–25, but he battled with the restricted view in the days before good artificial illumination and magnification and ultimately reverted to a transfrontal craniotomy approach. The introduction of the operating microscope in the 1960s stimulated the move away from high-morbidity transcranial approaches to surgery. Transseptal and transethmoidal techniques became the standard approach.

The endoscopic approach refines this surgery further with improved visualization of the pituitary fossa and further reductions in morbidity and improved endocrine outcomes.[7]

The main advantage of the endoscopic approach is the improved view. The operating microscope gives good visualization of the anterior pituitary wall and opening into the pituitary fossa, but the view inside the fossa is restricted by the size of the opening. The fisheye lens of the endoscope allows a better view of the contents of the fossa. For a small adenoma, the endoscope can be positioned right at the opening of the fossa. In cases where the fossa has been expanded, the endoscope is placed inside the fossa, allowing better assessment of tumour clearance laterally towards the cavernous sinuses and superiorly towards the diaphragm. In our series the average operating time is the same as for the transseptal approach (1¼–1½ hours). The patients still go home on the second post-operative day, but there is a reduction in morbidity in that there is no sublabial incision and the anterior septum is left undisturbed.

Transcranial approaches are still occasionally required for very large macro-adenomas extending into the third ventricle or anteriorly into the anterior cranial fossa.

PREOPERATIVE MANAGEMENT

The endocrinologists who need to establish whether the lesion is a nonfunctioning or a functioning adenoma assess patients initially. If the lesion is causing hypersecretion, the hormone type and baseline hormone levels are established, and then suitability for medical treatment is assessed. The residual pituitary function needs to be established because surgery on patients with a suppressed or absent steroid response is potentially hazardous. Cases considered suitable for treatment are managed by a multidisciplinary team including endocrinologists, radiologists, oncologists and pituitary surgeons (ideally both otolaryngologists and neurosurgeons). Preoperative MR scanning is mandatory because this will show the extent of the growth of the adenoma and spread into the cavernous sinus, clivus and supra-sellar regions, but computed tomography (CT) may give additional information in relation to the bony anatomy of the sphenoid sinus. If the surgical anatomy is unclear on scanning, it will be necessary to use an intraoperative surgical navigation system, which will give orientation in three planes, or an image intensifier, although this only gives support in two dimensions.

Endoscopic technique

PREPARATION

Thorough decongestion of the nasal mucosa is essential. We use topical co-phenylcaine applied to the nasal mucosa when the patient is awake 10 minutes before going through to the anaesthetic room, followed by 10 mL of Moffat's solution instilled into the nasal cavity for 10 minutes when the patient is anaesthetized in the reverse Trendelenburg position on the operating table. Further decongestion can be achieved by injecting a 1:80 000 solution of adrenaline using a dental needle or Moffat's solution on small Neuro Patties as necessary.

STEP 1: SPHENOIDOTOMY

The sphenoid sinus ostia are identified and enlarged using Stammberger sphenoidotomy punch forceps and Kerrison and Hajek punches, so that the front wall of the sphenoid is taken down to the level of the floor of the sphenoid sinus.

STEP 2: RESECTION OF POSTERIOR SEPTUM AND ROSTRUM

To achieve good access to the sphenoid sinuses, it is necessary to remove the rostrum of the sphenoid. This is performed with a Killian's type incision 1 cm anterior to the front wall of the sphenoid. Use of a ball diathermy electrode minimizes mucosal bleeding. The muco-perichondrial flap raised from the incision to the sphenoidotomy is removed with a micro-debrider. The bone of the posterior septum is carefully removed and sections preserved for potential use in closing the anterior wall of the pituitary fossa. The rostrum of the sphenoid is removed with Tilley Henkel forceps, and the muco-perichondrial flap on the side opposite to the incision is removed with the micro-debrider. There

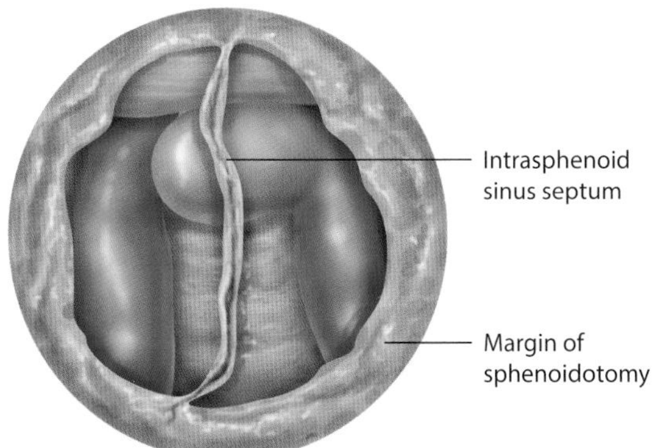

Figure 12.4 Diagram of sphenoid sinus and intrasphenoid sinus septum.

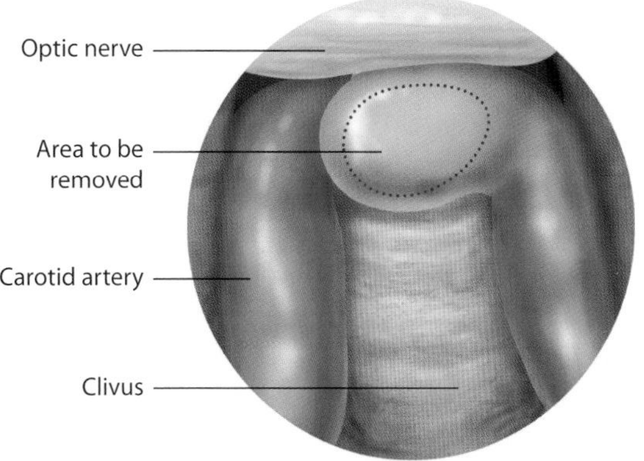

Figure 12.5 Diagram of posterior wall of sphenoid showing area of bone to be removed to open the pituitary fossa. Figures 12.4 and 12.5 reprinted with kind permission of the *Journal of Laryngology and Otology*.

should now be good access to the sphenoid sinus on both sides of the nose (Figure 12.4).

STEP 3: IDENTIFICATION OF LANDMARKS

The intrasphenoid sinus septae are highly variable but are visible on preoperative MR scans. The septae are reduced to allow access to the posterior wall of the sphenoid. In most cases it is then possible to identify the positions of the carotid arteries, the bulge of the pituitary fossa and possibly the optic nerves in the sphenoid. Careful correlation of the preoperative radiology and the observed anatomy usually allows accurate identification of the front wall of the pituitary fossa, but the use of an image intensifier or a surgical navigation system will be necessary in a small minority of cases (Figures 12.5 and 12.6).

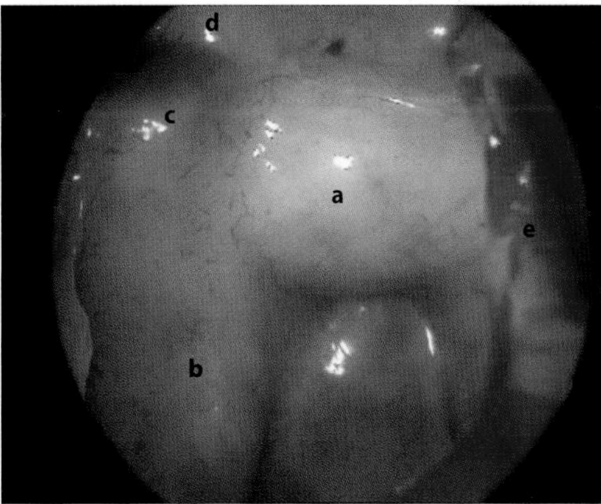

Figure 12.6 Peri-operative view of the posterior wall of the sphenoid showing the bulges over the pituitary fossa (a), the vertical portion of the right carotid artery (b), the right carotid siphon (c), the right optic nerve (d) and the intrasphenoid septum (e). The intrasphenoid septum is still in place and obscures the view of these same structures on the patient's left.

STEP 4: OPENING OF THE PITUITARY FOSSA

The bone over the front wall of the pituitary may be thin if a tumour has caused local expansion but usually will require gentle drilling in the midline. When through the bone, the opening is enlarged with a Stammberger sphenoidotomy punch or Kerrison forceps without breeching the dura. The dura is opened in the midline with a pointed diathermy needle in the form of an *X* to allow entry into the pituitary fossa (Figure 12.7).

STEP 5: ADENOMECTOMY

The pituitary fossa is explored using standard pituitary ring curettes. At this point it is useful to have a second surgeon available to manipulate a sucker through the other nostril. Gentle manipulation of the ring curettes allows a soft pituitary adenoma to be gently teased out of the fossa. A normal pituitary gland appears yellower than tumour tissue and is more adherent to the walls of the fossa. This makes it possible to perform a selective adenomectomy and leave normal tissue behind. In cases with

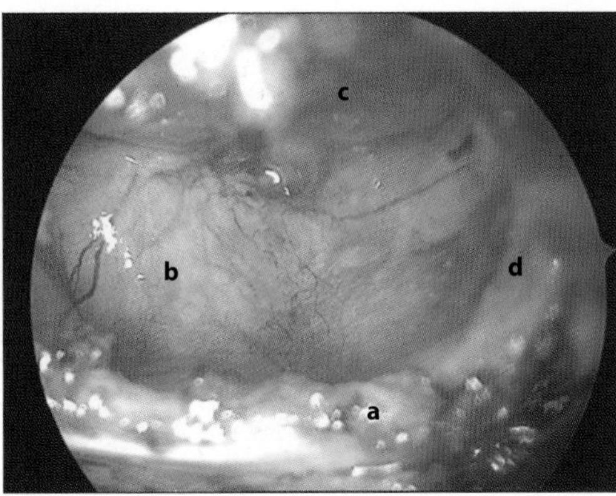

Figure 12.7 Peri-operative endoscopic view into the pituitary fossa after removal of a cystic macro-adenoma showing the inferior margin of the dural opening (a), the posterior wall of the fossa (b), the diaphragm bulging down into the fossa (c) and the lateral wall formed by the cavernous sinus (d).

an expanded pituitary fossa, it is possible to look inside the pituitary fossa by positioning the tip of the endoscope inside the fossa. Care is taken not to breach the diaphragm above the pituitary fossa. It is unusual for CSF to be encountered in the fossa. Large tumours are resected by gently removing the inferior margin of the tumour. Intracranial pressure will push supra-sellar components down into the fossa, and piecemeal resection can usually be continued without having to dissect above the confines of the pituitary fossa.

STEP 6: CLOSURE

Small balls of moistened Spongistan are placed within the fossa. The dura of the anterior pituitary wall is not repaired, but if possible the bony defect is repaired by placing a patch of bone taken from the posterior septum just inside the bony opening in the pituitary fossa wall. A flattened piece of moistened Spongistan is then placed over the opening into the pituitary fossa and the sphenoid sinus is packed with ribbon gauze. If there is no suggestion of a CSF leak, Vaseline-coated ribbon gauze will suffice and can be removed after 24 hours. If there is excessive bleeding or concern of a possible CSF leak, a BIPP (bismuth iodine paraffin paste) pack can be used because this can be left *in situ* for longer (Figure 12.7).

Equipment required

- Good-quality endoscopes with three-chip camera and monitor
- Neurosurgical pituitary instruments and standard FESS (functional endoscopic sinus surgery) instruments
- Micro-debrider
- Endoscrub +/– image intensifier
- Surgical navigation equipment

COMPLICATIONS

Bleeding

Bleeding from the pituitary fossa is usually venous in origin and comes from the small inter-cavernous connecting sinuses that run across the anterior pituitary floor or from the cavernous sinuses themselves. This bleeding is low pressure and is usually controlled by gentle tamponade of the fossa from inside with Spongistan absorbable balls. Arterial bleeding is most likely to result from damage to the spheno-palatine artery as it crosses the front wall of the sphenoid, during creation of the sphenoidotomy. Carotid artery damage is rare because the arterial wall is relatively robust, but it is associated with high mortality and morbidity. Damage can occur when extending the opening into the pituitary fossa laterally or when dissecting in the cavernous sinus. Immediate nasal packing will probably provide short-term control, but neuroradiological help and stenting is the treatment of choice.

Cerebrospinal fluid leak

Cerebrospinal fluid leak occurs in 2–5 per cent of cases in most large series. CSF is not usually present in the fossa, but it may be encountered when the pituitary fossa is opened because the adenoma has forced a breach in the diaphragm or widened the opening around the pituitary stalk. The diaphragm can also be damaged during tumour removal, particularly when a large tumour with supra-sellar extension has caused thinning of the diaphragm. Options for dealing with a leak are the use of synthetic sealants/glues/dural substitutes to repair the anterior pituitary fossa floor, autologous fat or muscle plugs to the fossa itself or reinforcement of the anterior pituitary wall with nasal muco-perichondrium, either as a free graft or in the form of a Hadad transposition flap. Small leaks may settle with a lumbar drain alone.

Infection

The concern about a persisting CSF leak is that it may lead to pneumocephalus or meningitis. Covering antibiotics are usually given for a week pre- and post-operatively, but meningitis is extremely rare.

Visual problems

Direct trauma to cranial nerves II to VI is possible but rare. A post-operative haematoma or infarction of residual adenoma can cause swelling and pressure on the chiasm or nerves III, IV and VI in the cavernous sinus.

Endocrine problems

Diabetes insipidus due to decreased secretion of anti-diuretic hormone (ADH) from the posterior lobe as a result of direct peri-operative surgical trauma occurs in 2–5 per cent of cases. Diuresis is noted 12–24 hours post-operatively. It is often self-limiting, but if it persists it is treated with DDAVP. Pituitary hypofunction will be detected by repeat endocrine assessment 6 weeks post-operatively, with the exception of a possible reduction in steroid response, which is treated prophylactically with steroid cover at the time of surgery and steroid replacement for the first 6 weeks until the function of the steroid axis can be assessed at 6 weeks.

POST-OPERATIVE MANAGEMENT

Neurological observation is recommended for the first 12–24 hours to watch for cranial nerve and intra-cranial complications.

Fluid balance charts and daily urea and electrolytes are monitored to exclude diabetes insipidus, and the patient is instructed not to blow his or her nose for 48 hours.

A regimen of steroid cover is required. This will vary with the pathology and is best done, along with the rest of the patient management, in conjunction with an endocrinologist.

Antibiotic cover is necessary for 7 days.

KEY LEARNING POINTS

- Transsphenoidal surgery has been done with the operating microscope since the 1960s but is increasingly being superseded by endoscopic techniques.
- Pituitary disease management requires a multidisciplinary team of endocrinologists, radiologists, oncologists, otolaryngologists and neurosurgeons.
- Endoscopic techniques allow better identification of the sphenoid anatomy and improved visualization inside the fossa.
- Complications include bleeding, CSF leak and pneumocephalus, diabetes insipidus and upper cranial nerve palsies.

REFERENCES

1. Cushing H. *Pituitary Body and Its Disorders.* Philadelphia: J.B. Lippincott Co., 1912.
2. Hardy J. Transsphenoidal removal of pituitary adenomas. *L'Unión Médicale du Canada.* 1962; 91: 933–45.
3. Guiot G, Thibant B. L'extirpation des adenomes hypophysaires par voie trans-sphenoidale. *Neurochirurgia.* 1959; 1: 133–49.
4. Jankowski R, Auque J, Simon C, et al. Endoscopic pituitary tumor surgery. *Laryngoscope.* 1992; 102: 198–202.
5. Cappabianca P, Alfieri A, de Divitiis E. Endoscopic endonasal transsphenoidal approach to the sella: Towards functional endoscopic pituitary surgery (FEPS). *Minimally Invasive Neurosurgery.* 1988; 41: 66–73.
6. Jho HD, Carrau RL, Ko Y. *Endoscopic Pituitary Surgery.* In: *Neurosurgical Operative Atlas.* Eds. Wilkins H, Rengachary S. Park Ridge, IL: American Association of Neurological Surgeons, 1996: 1–12.

7. Dorward NL. Endocrine outcomes in endoscopic pituitary surgery: A literature review. *Acta Neurochirurgica*. 2010; 152: 1275–79.

FURTHER READING

Cappabianca P, Alfieri A, De Divitis E, Tschabitscher M. *Atlas of Endoscopic Anatomy for Endonasal Intracranial Surgery*. New York: Springer-Verlag, 2001.

Greenspan FS, Gardner DG. *Basic and Clinical Endocrinology*. New York: Lange Medical Books/McGraw-Hill, 2001.

Tabaee A, et al. Endoscopic pituitary surgery: A systemic review and meta-analysis. *Journal of Neurosurgery*. 2009; 111: 545–54.

13

Smell and anosmia

EMMA MCNEILL AND SEAN CARRIE

INTRODUCTION

Olfaction is the sensation arising from the nasal cavity following stimulation of the olfactory epithelium by volatile compounds. A normal sense of smell plays a vital role in the enjoyment of food and detection of environmental hazards, and some occupations depend heavily on an intact sense of smell (e.g. cooks and wine tasters). Olfactory perception has a strong association with memory and emotion, owing to projections into the limbic system. Olfactory symptoms may also be the primary manifestation of serious intracranial pathology. European studies have described a 20 per cent prevalence of olfactory dysfunction, composed of approximately 14 per cent with hyposmia and 6 per cent with anosmia. Men appear to perform less well in olfactory testing, and olfactory sensitivity deteriorates with age.

PHYSIOLOGY OF OLFACTION

Olfaction is mediated via cranial nerves I (olfactory) and V (trigeminal). The olfactory nerve is responsible for the identification of odorants via specialized olfactory epithelium, and the trigeminal nerve is responsible for the perception of chemical irritants and detection of pungency. The olfactory mucosa is a 1 mm thick area of specialized neuroepithelium overlying the cribriform plate, within the olfactory cleft. The olfactory cleft is accessed by both orthonasal (via direct inspiration into the nasal cavity) and retronasal (the passage of odorant molecules via the mouth and postnasal space) airflow. Olfactory mucosa extends over the superior turbinate, below the anterior middle turbinate and onto the nasal septum, more anteriorly and inferiorly than originally thought. This is generally unrecognized but should be borne in mind when performing nasal surgery.

Odorant molecules interact with olfactory mucus before binding with the olfactory receptor cells. Olfactory receptor neurons are bipolar, with a cilia-bearing, club-shaped peripheral receptor. Their thin, unmyelinated axons become ensheathed by Schwann cells and pass through the 15–20 foramina of the cribriform plate before synapsing in the olfactory bulb. Each neuron expresses a single receptor and can combine with a range of odorant molecules before its associated axon projects to glomeruli in the olfactory bulb. It is suggested that an odorant provides an 'olfactory code' by activating a set pattern of receptors and glomeruli, which is recognized by the olfactory cortex and identified as a specific odour. Olfactory neurons generate continuously, but this ability seems to decrease with age. The ability to regenerate is thought to be related to the constant exposure of the olfactory mucosa to environmental conditions. The vomeronasal organ (Jacobson's organ) is an accessory olfactory organ found in mammals, which is thought to have a role in pheromone perception. It is thought to be situated in the anterior septum in humans, but its role as an active sensory organ appears to be open to debate.

The primary olfactory cortex is represented by the prepyriform and periamygdaloid areas of the medial aspect of the temporal lobe and is responsible for primary odour identification. The amygdala and entorhinal areas of the pyriform lobe make up the secondary olfactory cortex. These are part of the limbic system and are involved in the affective aspects of olfaction. Projections from the olfactory pathways to the thalamus, the forebrain and the limbic system are thought to mediate the associations between odour perception, memory and emotional stimuli. The olfactory pathway is mediated by cyclic adenosine monophosphate (AMP) (Figure 13.1).

PATHOPHYSIOLOGY OF OLFACTORY DISORDERS

Olfactory disorders (dysosmia) manifest in a number of ways.

1. A reduced or absent sense of smell – hyposmia or anosmia
2. A distorted sense of smell
    a. Parosmia/troposmia – distorted quality of a perceived odorant
    b. Phantosmia – perceived smell in the absence of an olfactory stimulant
    c. Cacosmia – perception of an unpleasant smell in the absence of olfactory stimulation
    d. Hyperosmia – increased olfactory acuity

Such disorders can be total, partial or specific to certain smells.

Analogies have been drawn between causes of olfactory disturbance and causes of hearing

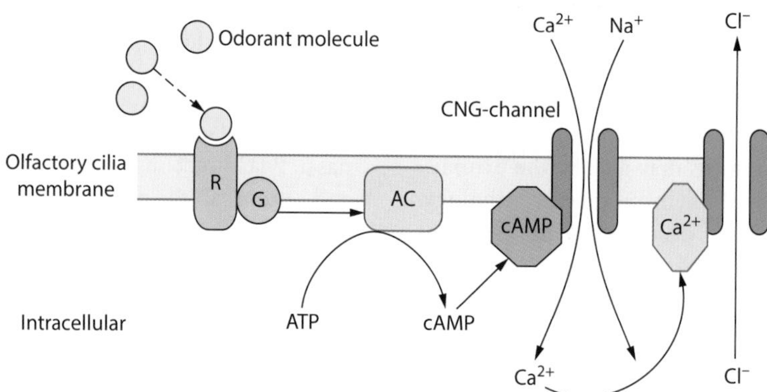

Figure 13.1 Olfactory transduction – interaction of odorant molecules with olfactory neurons. Reprinted with permission from Harish Viswanathan and ENT News.

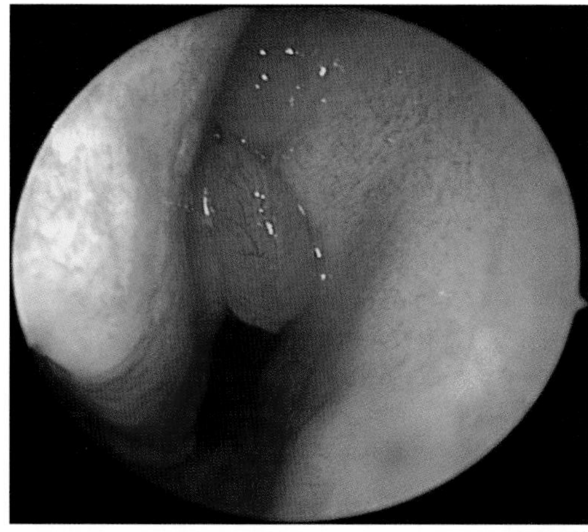

Figure 13.2 Nasal polyps causing reduced olfactory acuity.

loss. 'Conductive' disorders result from odorant molecules failing to access the olfactory mucosa, e.g. nasal polyps or rhinosinusitis (Figure 13.2). 'Sensory' losses are caused by olfactory mucosal damage, e.g. chemical exposure, viruses or neoplasms, whilst neural causes result from defects in the peripheral or central neural pathways, e.g. head injury. In individual cases olfactory loss may be a combination of both conductive and sensory losses. Twenty per cent of cases of dysosmia are idiopathic, and iatrogenic causes of hyposmia should always be considered. The most common causes of olfactory dysfunction are trauma, viral infections, nasal pathology and neurological disease. This is summarized in Table 13.1.

Studies suggest that head injuries account for up to 18 per cent of olfactory disturbances. In such cases, olfactory insult can result from damage to nasal mucosa, shearing of olfactory fibres due to cribriform plate fracture, and oedema of the olfactory tracts and bulbs. Damage to peripheral olfactory apparatus results in anosmia, whereas central olfactory damage may manifest as an inability to discriminate odours. The anterior temporal lobes and orbitofrontal poles are most vulnerable.

Table 13.1 Causes of olfactory loss

Aetiology	Percentage of patients (approximate)
Post URTI	35
Nasal/sinus disease	20
Idiopathic	20
Head injury	17
Miscellaneous	5
Congenital	3

Note: Miscellaneous causes included solvent abuse, abuse of nasal decongestants, Parkinson's disease, therapeutic radiation and cerebral infarction.

Upper respiratory tract infections (URTIs) commonly result in olfactory dysfunction. Temporary anosmia can occur following URTI, when oedema prevents odorant molecules from reaching the olfactory cleft. Viral URTI accounts for up to 20–30 per cent of identified olfactory losses, typically parainfluenza 3 virus. Viral infections may also cause reduction in olfactory receptors with replacement by respiratory epithelium, resulting in a permanent olfactory impairment. The purulent nasal secretions associated with chronic rhinosinusitis may cause a patient to complain of a persistent unpleasant smell.

Olfactory acuity deteriorates with age but is also associated with a number of neurological conditions. Disturbance of the sense of smell occurs in more than 95 per cent of patients with idiopathic Parkinson's syndrome and can precede the motor symptoms by up to 6 years. Dysosmia is also associated with Alzheimer's disease, Huntington's disease and motor neuron disease. The olfactory pathology is thought to be central in origin in these conditions.

There seems to be an association between phantosmia and various neurological conditions, including epilepsy, migraine, schizophrenia, head injury and neuroblastoma. Both central and peripheral pathology can play a role, with incorrect signalling at the level of the neurons, or the active or abnormal function within the brain. The symptoms can last from a few seconds to a number of hours, and the odours experienced may be pleasant or unpleasant.

ASSESSMENT OF OLFACTORY DISORDERS

HISTORY

A thorough clinical history should be taken. The duration, speed of onset and pattern of olfactory disturbance should be determined. The presence of associated nasal symptoms, such as nasal obstruction, discharge, postnasal drip and facial pain, suggests rhinosinusitis. The patient may be able to identify an episode of viral URTI preceding his or her symptoms. Patients often complain of taste disturbance, which has an underlying olfactory component in 80 per cent of cases.

Details of any head injury should be elicited, particularly regarding loss of consciousness, direction of impact and radiological findings. Iatrogenic causes must be considered, including medications, illicit drugs, neurosurgical intervention, radiotherapy and previous nasal surgery. Clearly, a patient with a laryngectomy or tracheostomy is likely to notice a decrease in olfactory acuity, mainly as a result of the reduction in nasal airflow, although smell can still be active via retronasal airflow. Table 13.2 summarizes details of medical conditions and prescribed medications that should be explored. A neurological history should be performed, particularly in patients with phantosmia.

Occupational history is relevant because it may reveal exposure to noxious chemicals, e.g. formaldehyde or benzene, but the impact of the olfactory disturbance on the patient may be significantly greater if the patient's occupation requires an intact sense of smell. Alcohol, nicotine and cocaine reduce olfactory sensitivity. Family history should be elicited because conditions such as primary congenital anosmia and Kallman syndrome (hypogonadotrophic hypogonadism and anosmia) may be familial. Anosmia with associated premature baldness and vascular headaches has been described with a dominant inheritance pattern.

Table 13.2 Medical causes of olfactory dysfunction

Congenital	Kallman syndrome Familial, e.g. primary congenital anosmia
Neurological	Alzheimer's disease Epilepsy Multiple sclerosis Parkinson's disease
Metabolic/endocrine	Chronic renal/liver failure Diabetes Hypo/hyperadrenalism Hypothyroidism
Trauma	Head injury
Inflammatory	Rhinosinusitis/nasal polyposis Sarcoidosis Wegener's disease
Neoplasms	Olfactory neuroblastomas Anterior skull base tumours
Degenerative	Age
Infective	Viral upper respiratory tract infection
Iatrogenic	Radiotherapy to skull base Neurosurgical procedures Sinonasal surgery Laryngectomy
Medication	Local anaesthetics, e.g. cocaine Antihypertensives, e.g. nifedipine, diltiazem Immunosuppressants, e.g. methotrexate Antidepressants, e.g. amitriptyline
Others	Psychiatric

CLINICAL EXAMINATION

Congenital disorders of smell, including isolated absence/hypoplasia of the olfactory bulbs, are associated with Kallman syndrome, primary congenital anosmia, Turner syndrome and premature baldness, and may be diagnosed on assessment of the patient's habitus. Nasendoscopy may show evidence of rhinosinusitis, turbinate hypertrophy or polyposis or may reveal no abnormality (Figure 13.2). There may be clinical evidence of previous sinonasal or neurosurgical intervention. It should be apparent if the patient has a tracheostomy or laryngectomy. Cranial nerve examination should always be included, and a patient should be examined for papilloedema if there is suspicion of a cranial space-occupying lesion. Neurological assessment should be considered in cases in which Parkinson's disease or similar motor pathologies are suspected.

INVESTIGATIONS

Radiological evaluation of olfactory dysfunction

Currently, there are no guidelines regarding the indications for imaging in olfactory disorders. Computed tomography (CT) is felt to be more appropriate for patients with sinonasal disease, particularly as an aid to surgical planning. However, magnetic resonance imaging (MRI) is the gold standard for diagnosis of olfactory apparatus abnormalities and parenchymal disease, particularly in congenital disease (Figure 13.3). Decreased volume of the olfactory bulbs is noted with increasing age. Absent olfactory bulbs are described in congenitally absent olfactory disease, and hypoplastic olfactory sulci and loss of temporal and/or frontal lobe volume have been noted in Kallmann syndrome (Figure 13.3). Phantosmias and olfactory hallucinations may have peripheral or central origins and should always be imaged. Accurate diagnosis of the site of skull fracture and associated parenchymal injuries may allow prediction of the likelihood of recovery of smell. A positive correlation has been shown between the number of plaques and olfactory function in patients with multiple sclerosis. Functional MRI is used to measure blood flow within the brain, with the theory that an area of higher activity has a higher blood flow and can be identified as a result. It is rarely used clinically, but studies have shown reduced frontal lobe blood flow in patients with schizophrenia and olfactory disorders.

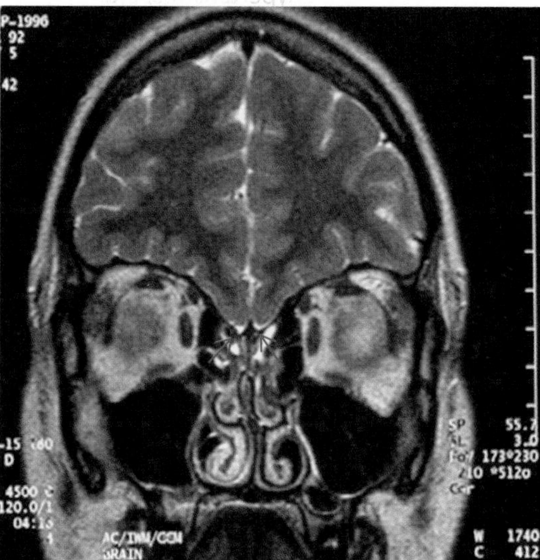

Figure 13.3 MRI scan demonstrating absent olfactory apparatus (indicated by arrows).

Olfactory testing

Three criteria have been described as necessary to maximize odour recognition in olfactory testing.

1. Odours must be familiar to the patient.
2. There should be a long-standing association between the odour and its name.
3. Help should be given to recall the name.

Reliability is improved by using both threshold testing and odour discrimination assessment. Threshold testing identifies the concentration at which an odorant is reliably perceived. A simple threshold test can be performed using butanol or phenylethylalcohol, which are used because of their minimal trigeminal stimulation effects. Varying dilutions of the olfactory stimulant (4 per cent being the lowest dilution) are presented to the patient in a random order. Patients have to make a choice between the odorant and two control samples as to which they can smell, and the lowest concentration that can be perceived is documented. This is repeated until the lowest concentration that is reliably perceived is determined. 'Forced-choice' procedures reduce response bias because patients scoring less than chance are likely to be malingering, as are those who fail to identify trigeminal nerve stimulants, such as ammonia. Formal olfactory testing allows monitoring of the progression or resolution of dysosmia, particularly following surgical or other therapeutic intervention.

The UPSIT (University of Pennsylvania Smell Identification Test) system is commonly used by clinicians in North America. This is a forced-choice supra-threshold test with 40 microencapsulated odours, acting as a 'scratch-and-sniff' test. The test indicates a level of smell function, i.e. mild to total anosmia, and has score ranking for age and gender. However, the system has not been validated on a UK population. The Cross-Cultural

Smell Identification Test (CCSIT) is a self-administered 12-item test based on UPSIT that can be carried out in 5 minutes. Sniffin' Sticks are a test of olfactory function based on felt-tip pens and assess odour threshold, discrimination and identification (Figure 13.4). The UPSIT and Sniffin' Sticks tests were developed in the United States and Germany, respectively, and some of the odorants may not be familiar to a UK population. The Combined Olfactory Test is a test designed and validated in the UK and assesses odour discrimination and threshold testing.

There is considerable variation in the reliability of olfactory tests related to length of testing. Results from different testing methods should not be compared because variations may result from differing reliabilities rather than reflecting clinical findings.

Electrophysiological methods are available to assess olfactory function. The electro-olfactogram (EOG) measures the electrical potential evoked in the olfactory mucosa when an odorant is presented in the nasal cavity and reflects the generator potential of the olfactory neurons. The technique has a role in the investigation of olfactory processing but is technically demanding and has high inter-individual response variability. The presence of olfactory event-related potentials (OERPs) is taken to indicate that the ability to smell is present; however, an olfactory stimulus of defined duration, concentration and stimulus rise time must be provided. The aim of such techniques is to provide an objective olfactory assessment, but they are rarely used beyond the realms of specialist olfactory centres.

Finally, olfactory function can be assessed using the retronasal route by placing 'taste powders' in the mouth and using forced choice questionnaires to identify the powders. Given that a truly anosmic patient would only be able to detect sweet, sour, bitter, salty and umami, the technique can be used to evaluate the authenticity of a patient's clinical perception.

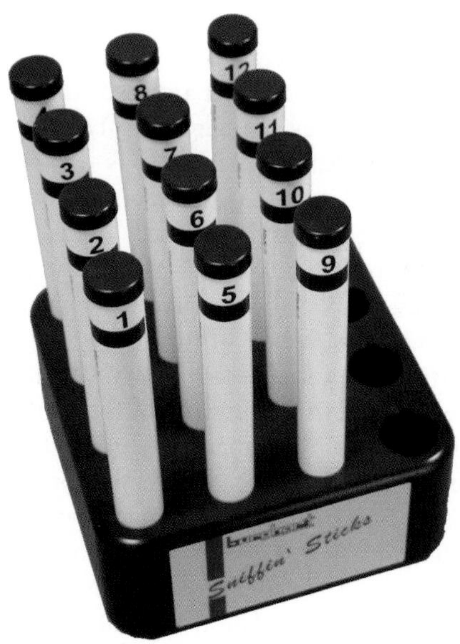

Figure 13.4 Sniffin' Sticks screening 12 olfactory test – an example of qualitative and quantitative olfactory testing. Reprinted with permission from Burghart Messtechnik GmbH.

TREATMENT OF OLFACTORY DISORDERS

PHARMACOLOGICAL THERAPY OF OLFACTORY DISORDERS

Ideally, a specific aetiological cause for the olfactory disorder would be identified during the assessment of the patient, and treatment directed towards the cause. Unfortunately, evidence for the use of specific pharmacological therapies in dysosmia is variable.

A trial of oral corticosteroids may be useful. Improvements in subjective and objective olfactory measurements have been described, particularly in anosmic patients with allergic rhinitis, chronic rhinosinusitis and nasal polyposis. The cause of improvement is unclear but is likely to be due to a reduction in mucosal oedema, even when a conductive olfactory loss may not be apparent. However, while hyposmic patients appear to improve, they may not return to normosmia, and anosmic patients show minimal improvement in olfactory scores. The recommended doses and length of treatment vary between studies. A trial of prednisolone 0.5 mg/kg for 7 days would seem reasonable. Patients should be asked to 'test' their sense of smell during the treatment period to assess for any improvement.

Corticosteroid nasal sprays have a role in the treatment of inflammatory nasal conditions but seem to be less effective in improving olfactory scores and symptoms. It is thought that their effect results from the reduction of oedema in the olfactory cleft. Their use has been shown to maintain the effects of an initial response to oral steroids or following endoscopic sinus surgery.

Antidepressants and anticonvulsants have been used in the treatment of olfactory distortions. The presence of a neurological or psychiatric disorder needs to be established as part of the patient's investigations and treated accordingly. Topical cocaine hydrochloride can temporarily disrupt olfactory neurons, but the patient should be fully informed of potential complications, including permanent anosmia or phantosmia. The effectiveness of therapies other than steroids, including zinc replacement, herbal remedies, alpha-lipoeic acid and caroverine, has been assessed, with no reliable evidence to recommend their use in anosmia or hyposmia.

The potential for neural plasticity in the olfactory system has been targeted by the use of olfactory training. Olfactory ability has been shown to improve on formal testing, at least in the short term, by structured exposure to intense odours. This 'odour gymnastics' involves smelling four different odours each morning and evening for 4 to 6 months. A single study showed positive effect in patients with anosmia secondary to URTI and head trauma, with improvements in approximately 25 per cent of patients compared to those who did not carry out training. More research is required to separate the potential for a degree of spontaneous remission from genuine therapeutic effect.

SURGICAL INTERVENTION FOR OLFACTORY DISORDERS

It seems logical that treating mucosal oedema and polyposis to improve access of odorant molecules to the olfactory apparatus would result in symptomatic improvement. However, the surgeon should always take care to avoid damage to normal olfactory mucosa during all nasal surgeries. The effectiveness of surgical intervention for hyposmia secondary to chronic rhinosinusitis has been debated. A correlation between nasal airflow and odour identification in patients with chronic rhinosinusitis has been demonstrated. A number of studies have shown improvements in subjective and objective measures of olfactory functions. The improvements may be maintained by continuing use of nasal steroids. Permanent impairment in olfactory function in patients with chronic rhinosinusitis may be due to reduction in olfactory epithelium and replacement with normal respiratory mucosa. Inflammatory changes within the olfactory mucosa may account for hyposmia, independent of airflow alteration. Recovery of smell in patients with chronic rhinosinusitis/polyposis seems to be time dependent, with prolonged disease resulting in a less satisfactory outcome.

Other surgical techniques have been described in the management of patients with olfactory distortions. These include bifrontal craniotomy with removal of the olfactory bulbs, and excision of the olfactory mucosa via an endonasal approach. Both approaches result in permanent anosmia, but the potential complications and uncertainty of outcome mean these are rare procedures.

PROGNOSIS

Post-traumatic olfactory impairment is more pronounced with less chance of recovery than in chronic rhinosinusitis or post-infection. Predictive factors may allow identification of likelihood of recovery. Factors noted to negatively influence recovery include a Glasgow Coma Scale (GCS) score of <13 at presentation, loss of consciousness >1 hour, post-traumatic amnesia and radiological abnormalities with occipital, frontal and skull base fractures. Forty per cent of such patients suffer an olfactory deficit, although this may only manifest on formal testing. Recovery of normal smell following head injury is unlikely, although recovery has been noted up to 5 years post injury.

The prognosis for recovery from URTI-induced hyposmia varies in the literature from 6 months to 3 years, although other studies describe minimal recovery. Stem cells may persist in the olfactory mucosa with the potential for regeneration.

However, in a small percentage, olfaction remains permanently distorted, particularly in women (70–80 per cent) and in those aged between 40 and 60 years. This is partly due to cumulative degeneration of the olfactory apparatus with age. With regard to endoscopic sinus surgery, approximately 10 per cent of patients have no improvement and 6 per cent have been shown to have experienced a deterioration in olfaction at 5 years post surgery. In practice, managing such patients requires the judicious use of both steroid therapy and careful surgery. Patients should be given a realistic indication of the prognosis for the recovery of smell when preparing for nasal surgery.

QUALITY-OF-LIFE ISSUES

It is very important for the evaluating clinician to appreciate the effect that an impaired sense of smell can have on a patient's quality of life. Studies have reported that almost 75 per cent of dysosmic patients have problems with cooking food, and 50 per cent report inadvertently eating spoiled food. Occupations that depend heavily on an intact sense of smell include wine tasting, cosmetic and perfume manufacturing and catering. Altered mood and difficulty in the perception of one's own body odour can also put a significant strain on a patient's daily life, and the clinician should be sensitive to this. Finally, it is vital to advise patients of the potential risks associated with reduced smell, with particular regard to detection of environmental hazards, e.g. smoke and gas.

CONCLUSIONS

Patients with olfactory disorders should undergo a comprehensive clinical assessment. CT imaging is most appropriate for planning surgery for sinonasal disease, while MRI evaluates the olfactory apparatus more accurately. Olfaction may remain permanently distorted following head injury, viral infection and chronic rhinosinusitis. However, recovery has been documented over longer periods than previously thought. Oral corticosteroids appear to be the only effective pharmacological treatment for hyposmia at this time.

KEY LEARNING POINTS

- The quality of life can be significantly reduced by olfactory disorders.
- Nasendoscopy should be a mandatory assessment to visualize the olfactory epithelium.
- Formal chemosensory testing can assist with both the diagnosis and the monitoring of olfactory disorders.
- Oral corticosteroids appear to be the only current effective pharmacological treatment for hyposmia.
- Patients should be advised of the potential risks associated with reduced smell.

FURTHER READING

Briner HR, Jones N, Simmen D. Olfaction after endoscopic sinus surgery: Long-term results. *Rhinology*. 2012; 50(2): 178–84.

Doty RL, Mishra A. Olfaction and its alteration by nasal obstruction, rhinitis, and rhinosinusitis. *Laryngoscope*. 2001; 111(3): 409–23.

Hummel T, Landis, BN, Hüttenbrink KB. Smell and taste disorders. *GMS Current Topics in Otorhinolaryngology, Head and Neck Surgery*. 2011; 10: Doc04. Epub 2012 Apr 26.

Hummel T, Rissom K, Reden J, et al. Effects of olfactory training in patients with olfactory loss. *Laryngoscope*. 2009; 119 (3): 496–9.

Leopold, DA. Distortion of olfactory perception: Diagnosis and treatment. *Chemical Senses*. 2002; 27: 611–15.

Martinez-Devesa P, Patiar S. Oral steroids for nasal polyps. *Cochrane Database of Systemic Reviews*. 2011 Jul 6; (7):CD005232. Review. 622.

McNeill EJM, Ramakrishnan Y, Carrie S. Diagnosis and management of olfactory disorders: Survey of UK-based consultants and literature review. *Journal of Laryngology and Otology*. 2007; 121(8): 713–20.

14

Tumours of the nose and sinuses

KIM W AH-SEE

INTRODUCTION

The nose and paranasal sinuses can be the site of both benign (relatively common) and malignant (rare) neoplasms.

The variety of tissue types that constitute the nose and sinuses results in a wide range of histological tumour types. Tumours can thus arise from epithelial tissue, bone, cartilage and neurological, vascular and lymphoid tissue and muscle. Tumours will be benign or malignant in their behaviour; however, some may have malignant potential, for example the inverted papilloma.

ANATOMY

The anatomy of the nose and paranasal sinuses is complex, and a detailed description is beyond the scope of this chapter. However, it is worth highlighting certain points.

This complex bony skeleton occupies the anterior portion of the skull and consists of air-containing cells varying in size from small ethmoid cells to the large maxillary antra. It is of importance surgically to be aware of the fragile nature of the bony boundaries of the ethmoid complex of sinuses with the 'paper-thin' lamina papyracea laterally between ethmoids and orbits and the perforated cribriform plate superiorly forming part of the floor of the anterior cranial fossa. The frontal sinuses are protected behind the thick frontal bone of the skull with a thinner inner plate anterior to the frontal lobes of the brain. The centrally place sphenoid sinuses are closely associated with the cavernous sinuses, optic nerves and internal carotid arteries laterally and the pituitary gland superiorly. Both the frontal and sphenoid sinuses typically are asymmetrical with bony partitions that are off-centre. The large maxillary sinuses or antra are pyramidal in shape with the apex directed laterally into the zygomatic process. The floor is closely related to the upper dentition. Superiorly lies the orbit, with the nasal cavity medially, while posteriorly the pterygoid plates are attached, creating the pterygomaxillary fissure, which leads into the pterygopalatine fossa medially and the infratemporal space laterally.

The nasal cavity is divided in two by the vertically placed septum. This structure is composed of two bones, the vomer and the perpendicular plate of the ethmoid, and one quadrilateral hyaline cartilage, which lends support and projection to the nose along with the supporting upper and lower lateral cartilages. Superiorly it is attached to the cribriform plate while inferiorly it sits in the groove of the maxillary crest. The floor of the nasal cavity is the roof of the mouth, thus the nasal cavity runs horizontally from nostril to nasopharynx – a point worth remembering when packing a nose. The lateral wall of the nose consists of the three turbinate (or conchal) bones: superior, middle and inferior. The spheno-ethmoidal recess sits postero-superior to the superior turbinate and receives drainage from the sphenoid sinuses, while the posterior ethmoids drain just under the superior turbinate. Most remaining paranasal sinuses drain into the hiatus semilunaris under the middle turbinate, while the only structure to drain under the large inferior turbinate is the naso-lacrimal duct.

The blood supply of the nose and paranasal sinuses is via the external and internal carotid artery systems, principally the maxillary artery and the ethmoid arteries. This leads to the well-known watershed on the anterior nasal septum called 'Little's area' (Keisselbach's plexus), which is the source for many nosebleeds (Figure 14.1).

The mucosal covering throughout the nose and paranasal sinuses is respiratory-type columnar ciliated epithelium, except in the roof of the nasal cavity where the neuro-epithelium of the olfactory mucosa sits.

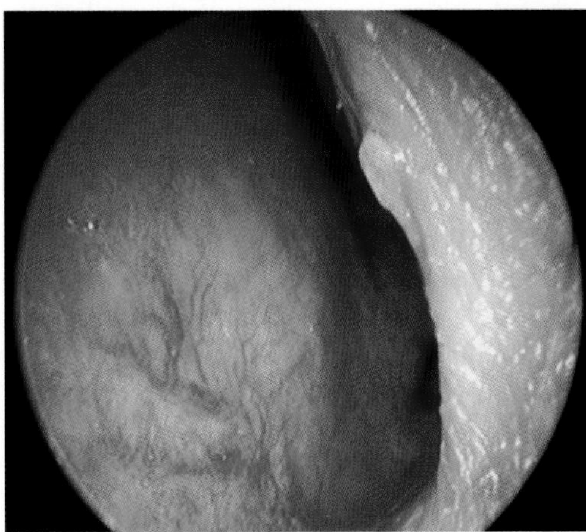

Figure 14.1 Little's area of septum.

The lymphatic drainage of the anterior nose is to the submandibular level I nodes, while the posterior nose drains to the retropharyngeal and level II neck nodes. This principle is true also for the paranasal sinuses with all anteriorly placed sinuses draining to the submandibular lymph nodes, while the posterior ethmoid and sphenoid sinuses drain to the retropharyngeal and level II nodes.

AETIOLOGY

The aetiology of many sinonasal tumours remains unknown. Certain risk factors are known for malignant disease, such as smoking and hardwood exposure in ethmoid adenocarcinoma. Other environmental pollutants may have a role in some benign conditions. Human papillomavirus (HPV) infection has been associated with inverted papillomas, in particular HPV types 6, 11, 16 and 18. HPV types 16 and 18 are most likely to be associated with malignant transformation in an inverted papilloma.

CLINICAL FEATURES

Tumours of the nose or paranasal sinuses can present with any of the commonly recognized symptoms:

- Nasal blockage
- Rhinorrhoea
- Epistaxis
- Facial pain
- Hyposmia/anosmia

Certain features, however, should make one clinically suspicious:

- Red flag symptoms
- Unilateral symptoms
- Blockage
- Bleeding/blood-stained discharge
- Cacosmia
- Proptosis
- Diplopia
- Epiphora
- Neurological symptoms

CLINICAL EXAMINATION

Follow standard steps including the following:

- Nasal endoscopy, including the postnasal space
- Orbital examination, including eye movements
- Cranial nerves, especially the trigeminal nerve
- Intraoral examination, including hard and soft palate, teeth and gingiva
- Otoscopy

Evidence of a unilateral soft tissue swelling, especially if associated with pain and/or bleeding, is a highly suspicious clinical scenario, and one should endeavour to exclude malignancy.

While the benign appearance of a 'simple allergic-type' nasal polyp is well recognized, these simple polyps can demonstrate surface changes that make immediate reassurance difficult. Similarly, 'fleshy' intranasal swellings may ultimately prove benign. Further investigations are therefore likely to be required.

TISSUE TYPES

A huge range of tissue types exist within the nose and paranasal sinuses, all of which may lead to the development of benign or malignant disease (Table 14.1).

Table 14.1 Sinonasal tissue types and tumours

Tissue type	Benign	Malignant
Epithelial	Squamous papilloma Inverted papilloma (fungiform, inverted, cylindrical)	Squamous cell carcinoma Adenocarcinoma Adenoid cystic carcinoma Muciepidermoid carcinoma Acinic cell carcinoma Malignant melanoma
Mesenchymal	Osteoma Chondroma Fibroma Juvenile nasopharyngeal angiofibroma (JNA)	Osteosarcoma Chondrosarcoma Fibrosarcoma Rhabdomyosarcoma Leiomyosarcoma Malignant fibrous histiocytoma
Neural	Schwannoma Neurofibroma Meningioma	Olfactory neuroblastoma Neuroendocrine carcinoma
Fibro-Osseus	Fibrous dysplasia Ossifying fibroma Giant cell tumour Giant cell granuloma Aneurysmal bone cyst	
Vascular	Haemangioma Haemangiopericytoma Pyogenic granuloma	Angiosarcoma Kaposi sarcoma
Lymphoreticular		Non-Hodgkins lymphoma Burkitt's lymphoma Plasmacytoma
Odontogenic		Ameloblastoma

INVESTIGATIONS

The most common type of swelling within the nose and paranasal sinuses is the simple nasal polyp. Further information on this can be found in Chapter 6 and therefore will not be discussed further here.

When faced with the clinical scenario of a tumour within the nose, clinical examination should attempt to clarify whether it is confined to the nasal cavity or has originated from within the paranasal sinuses. This may be easily confirmed on nasal endoscopy; however, more often than not, imaging will be required to establish the extent of the lesion.

Computed tomography (CT) is the imaging modality of choice because of its ability to demonstrate soft tissue while providing excellent bony definition. This is of importance when suspecting malignancy because bone erosion/destruction is a sign of malignancy, while bone distortion such as bowing of a bony wall indicates a longer-term process and is less likely to indicate malignancy (Figure 14.2).

CT scanning is complemented by magnetic resonance imaging (MRI), which gives improved soft tissue definition, for example distinguishing mucus from soft tissue, and of course does not involve radiation (Figure 14.3).

The use of plain x-rays is no longer recommended owing to their poor sensitivity and specificity.

The role of positron emission tomography–computed tomography (PET–CT) scanning in these tumours is yet to be established. Angiography may be considered for vascular tumours such as juvenile nasopharyngeal angiofibroma (JNA).

Advancing technology now permits excellent 3D reconstruction of images for treatment planning.

Haematological investigations such as a full blood count may be indicated if lymphoma is suspected.

Histological confirmation of the diagnosis will require a biopsy either under local anaesthetic or during the course of an examination under general anaesthetic. The latter is generally to be recommended because bleeding may be a problem and can be dealt with more easily in this setting. It may be considered dangerous, however, to attempt

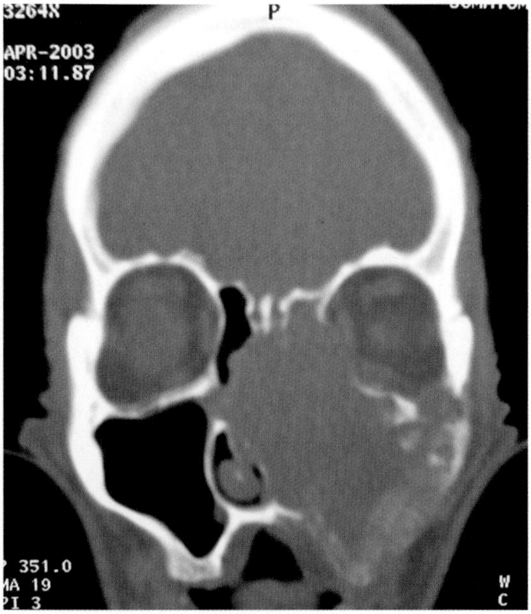

Figure 14.2 CT scan demonstrating extensive squamous carcinoma with bone destruction and involvement of orbit and soft tissue of cheek.

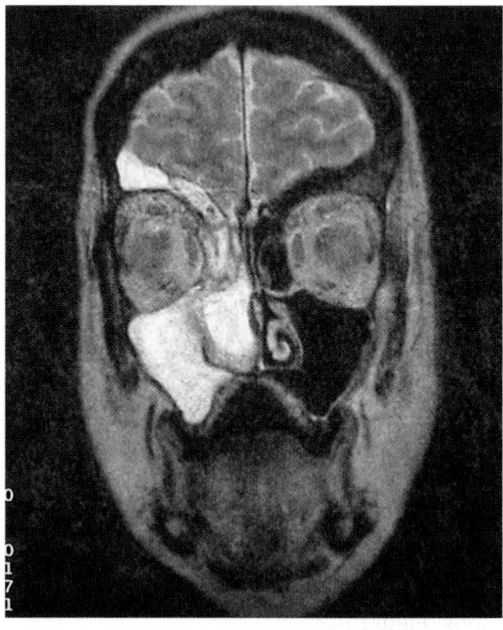

Figure 14.3 MRI of nasal tumour highlighting mucus retention in maxillary and frontal sinuses.

biopsy, and diagnosis of this condition is usually made on the basis of the clinical picture and the radiological features.

MANAGEMENT

The treatment for tumours of the nose and the paranasal sinuses will depend on the specific condition, and in particular whether it is benign or malignant. It is likely, however, that surgical intervention will be required to alleviate symptoms, the extent of which will vary from simple intranasal excision to major craniofacial resection and reconstruction.

Close multidisciplinary working is paramount under these circumstances to ensure that the correct approach is chosen because major surgical resection can be mutilating and have a significant impact on length and quality of life. Maxillofacial and plastic surgery collaboration may be required along with colleagues from restorative dentistry and prosthetics.

The use of chemotherapy and radiotherapy as adjuvant treatments should be fully discussed among the multidisciplinary team and with the patient, who should be aware of the side effects of these treatment modalities.

BENIGN TUMOURS

The nose and paranasal sinuses contain all tissue types, including epithelial, mesenchymal, vascular and neural. All tissue types can give rise to benign as well as malignant tumours.

The more common types are discussed in the following sections.

Inverted papilloma (schneiderian papilloma)

Inverted papillomas are benign tumours of the sinonasal mucosa. Their characteristic inverted mucosal surface extending into the stroma of the papilloma leads to the term *inverted* for these lesions (Figure 14.4).

They occur more frequently in men (3:1) and have an incidence of approximately 1 per 100,000 population.

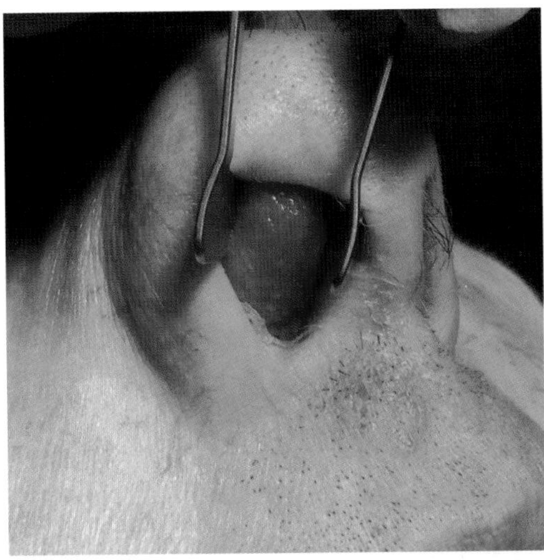

Figure 14.4 Inverted papilloma presenting at nostril.

Although benign, they behave in a locally aggressive manner, requiring wide local excision if recurrence is to be prevented. Malignant transformation can occur in up to 10 per cent of lesions but is typically reported as occurring in approximately 2 per cent. The aetiology remains unclear, and the reasons for malignant transformation similarly are unknown.

Clinical presentation is typically with unilateral nasal symptoms, especially blockage, rhinorrhoea and epistaxis. Endoscopic examination typically reveals an irregular fleshy lesion arising from the nasal mucosa. The most common site is the lateral nasal wall around the middle turbinate. Bilateral lesions are rare.

Preoperative investigations include CT scanning, which may be complemented by MRI for more detailed soft tissue definition. The extent of the disease will determine the extent of surgery (Figure 14.5).

Staging for IP was proposed by Krouse in 2001:

Stage 1. IPs confined to the nasal cavity
Stage 2. IPs involving the ethmoid sinuses, medial and superior region of maxillary sinus
Stage 3. IPs involving all paranasal sinuses, but confined to the nose and paranasal sinuses
Stage 4. IPs not confined to the nose and paranasal sinuses (i.e. orbital or intracranial extension) or with evidence of malignancy

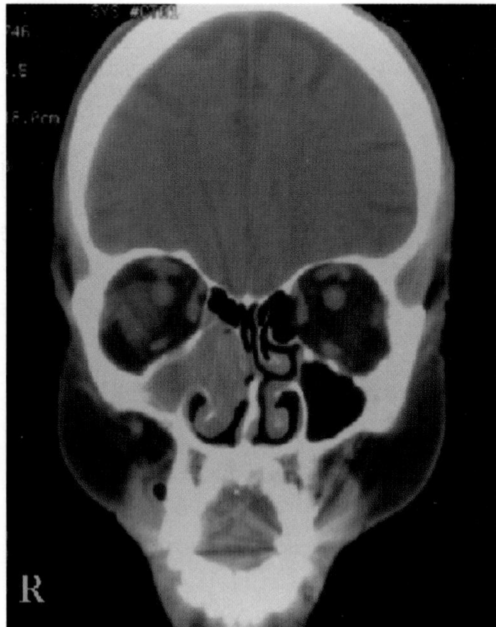

Figure 14.5 CT scan demonstrating unilateral opacification centred on the lateral nasal wall.

Table 14.2 Juvenile nasopharyngeal angiofibroma staging

I Tumour limited to nasopharynx. Bone destruction is negligible or limited to sphenopalatine foramen
II Tumour invading pterygopalatine fossa or maxillary, ethmoid or sphenoid sinus with bone destruction
IIIA Tumour invading infratemporal fossa or orbital region without intracranial involvement
IIIB Tumour invading infratemporal fossa or orbit with intracranial extradural (parasellar) involvement
IVA Intracranial intradural tumour without infiltration of cavernous sinus, pituitary fossa or optic chiasma
IVB Intracranial intradural tumour with infiltration of cavernous sinus, pituitary fossa or optic chiasma.

Staging for JNA commonly employs the system proposed by Andrews, Fisch et al.

Surgery can be either open/external approach or endoscopic. With improved technological advances the latter is gaining favour, and reports of case series around the world suggest that a low recurrence rate (11–12 per cent) can be achieved with endoscopic methods. Wide excision remains the key principle to resection of these tumours, and regular post-operative monitoring is required to detect recurrence or malignant transformation.

Juvenile nasopharyngeal angiofibroma

These are rare but locally aggressive vascular lesions that occur almost exclusively in young teenage boys. These lesions typically arise from the sphenopalatine foramen and present within the nasopharynx. Although they are benign, local extension into the skull base means that at presentation intracranial disease may be present in 10–20 per cent of cases.

Typical presentation is with progressive nasal obstruction and epistaxis in a teenage boy. Endoscopic examination of the nasopharynx is mandatory in this instance and will reveal the characteristic purple soft tissue swelling. Staging of this condition is as suggested by Fisch (Table 14.2).

Investigations include CT and MRI as well as angiography/magnetic resonance angiography (MRA). Biopsy should be avoided because the diagnosis can be made radiologically, and severe bleeding may be encountered with biopsy. The classic finding on CT scan is anterior bowing of the posterior maxillary wall, known as a Holman-Miller sign (Figure 14.6).

Surgical resection is the mainstay of treatment, and complete removal should be attempted if possible. If residual disease remains, some centres recommend radiotherapy or stereotactic radiotherapy, but evidence of their long-term benefit is currently lacking.

Preoperative embolization may be considered in an attempt to reduce tumour bulk and vascularity at surgery. If embolization is to be considered, it should take place within 24 hours of planned surgery. Angiography prior to embolization will determine the safety of proceeding with embolization because there is a risk of cerebrovascular accident if the embolizing material should pass into the cerebral circulation.

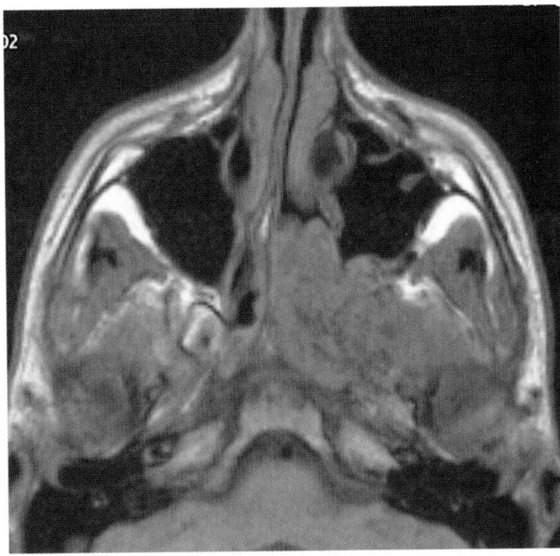

Figure 14.6 MRI demonstrating juvenile nasopharyngeal angiofibroma (JNA) distorting the posterior wall of the maxillary sinus.

As with inverted papilloma, surgical resection may be via open/external or endoscopic approaches. In general, open approaches may be favoured because they lend greater access to the field, which may be very bloody, making endoscopic techniques difficult. However, smaller tumours may be resected successfully endoscopically. A reduced risk of recurrence is reported when the basisphenoid has been drilled clean.

Open approaches may employ midfacial degloving, lateral rhinotomy or maxillary swing methods. More extensive disease will require a combined skull base approach with neurosurgery.

MALIGNANT TUMOURS

Malignant tumours of the nose and paranasal sinuses are rare, occurring in less than 1 per 100 000 population. Males over 50 years of age are the most likely candidates for this disease. Risk factors for developing sinonasal malignancy relate to inhaled carcinogens. Therefore, smoking is included, but a clear association with woodworkers has been noted as well since the late 1960s. This is especially true for adenocarcinoma of the ethmoid sinuses developing in hardwood workers. Overall 5-year survival for sinonasal malignancy is dependent on a number of factors, in particular cell type, but also the extent of disease, with involvement of the orbital apex being a poor prognostic factor.

- Squamous cell carcinoma (SCC): 5-year survival 30–50 per cent
- Adenocarcinoma: 5-year survival 45–60 per cent
- Olfactory neuroblastoma: 5-year survival of 75 per cent

Surgical management

Options:

- External approach
  - Craniofacial resection (CFR)
  - Lateral rhinotomy
  - Midfacial degloving
  - Total maxillectomy
- Endoscopic approach

Surgical resection will usually be supplemented by adjuvant chemoradiotherapy regimens. The surgical modality may consist of open external approaches or endoscopic techniques if appropriate expertise is available.

More traditional open approaches will include total maxillectomy, typically via a Weber-Ferguson incision (Figure 14.7).

Lateral rhinotomy gives excellent access for medial maxillectomy. Mid-facial degloving and maxillary swing are other options described.

For anterior skull base involvement, a craniofacial approach in collaboration with neurosurgery will often be recommended. This approach is of particular benefit for adenocarcinoma and olfactory neuroblastoma, which tend to involve the anterior skull base.

Preservation of the orbit is an area of some debate. If the tumour has breached the periorbital periosteum (periorbita) and has invaded the periorbital fat and/or extraocular muscles, the need for orbital exenteration is likely. Any attempt to preserve the orbit must be balanced against the risk of suboptimal resection.

Reconstruction after resection may be required and may also include the need for experts in

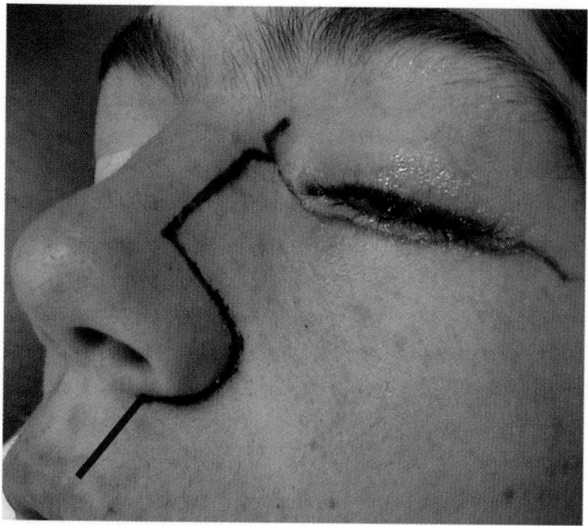

Figure 14.7 Weber-Ferguson approach. Marking out facial incision prior to maxillary swing procedure to access JNA.

prosthetics to help design obturators to fill the surgical defect following maxillectomy.

Neck node disease is relatively rare at presentation (less than 10 per cent); hence elective neck dissection for the N0 neck is probably unnecessary. Evidence of neck nodal disease will of course require treatment either as part of the primary surgical procedure or within the field of radiation.

Adjuvant therapy

Adjuvant therapy will consist of radiotherapy and/or chemotherapy. Current evidence suggests that chemotherapy (platinum-based) can improve survival by up to 10 per cent and may improve quality of life. Cisplatin acts as a sensitizer for radiotherapy and is therefore not used in isolation but in combination with radiotherapy. Clinical series report a benefit from topical 5-fluorouracil for adenocarcinoma, but this evidence is of low grade.

Radiotherapy (60–70 Gy) remains the main adjuvant treatment after surgery but is associated with complications such as wound breakdown, orbital damage (up to a third of patients), brain radionecrosis and osteoradionecrosis. These complications may be reduced with the introduction of intensity modulated radiotherapy (IMRT).

TNM (tumour, node, metastasis) staging exists for maxillary and ethmoid sinus cancers (Table 14.3).

Squamous cell carcinoma

Squamous cell carcinomas are the most common types of sinonasal cancer, with the majority arising from the lateral nasal wall or the maxillary sinus. Tumours affecting the nasal septum have a particularly poor prognosis because of the vascularity of this area and its midline position; radical surgery including total rhinectomy may be required to effect any chance of cure (Figure 14.8).

Local resection and flap reconstruction, such as a nasolabial flap, may suffice (Figures 14.9 to 14.12).

Chemoradiotherapy will complement surgical resection of sinonasal squamous cancers.

Sinonasal undifferentiated (anaplastic) carcinoma (SNUC) is a highly aggressive subset of squamous carcinomas.

Adenocarcinoma

This group of cancers constitutes about 10 per cent of sinonasal malignancy. These are related to hardwood exposure, but other carcinogens such as nickel and chrome have also been implicated. They tend to originate in the ethmoid sinuses and the region of the middle meatus; hence the need to consider craniofacial surgery, in collaboration with neurosurgery, for the more advanced tumours. Alternatively, surgical debulking via an extended maxillary antrostomy with subsequent topical 5-fluorouracil has been used with some success.

Adenoid cystic tumour

These slowly growing indolent tumours have a propensity for peri-neural invasion. This makes curative surgery difficult and late recurrence common. The overall 20-year survival is only 5 per cent; this is due to late recurrence, especially intracranially, with distant metastases to the lungs. These tumours are relatively radio-resistant, although post-operative radiotherapy may afford temporary disease control.

Table 14.3 TNM staging

TX	Primary tumour cannot be assessed.
T0	No evidence of primary tumour.
Tis	Carcinoma *in situ.*
Maxillary sinus	
T1	Tumour limited to maxillary sinus mucosa with no erosion or destruction of bone.
T2	Tumour causing bone erosion or destruction including extension into the hard palate and/or middle nasal meatus, except extension to posterior wall of maxillary sinus and pterygoid plates.
T3	Tumour invades any of the following: bone of the posterior wall of maxillary sinus, subcutaneous tissues, floor or medial wall of orbit, pterygoid fossa or ethmoid sinuses.
T4a	Moderately advanced local disease. Tumour invades anterior orbital contents, skin of cheek, pterygoid plates, infratemporal fossa, cribriform plate, or sphenoid or frontal sinuses.
T4b	Very advanced local disease. Tumour invades any of the following: orbital apex, dura, brain, middle cranial fossa, cranial nerves other than maxillary division of trigeminal nerve (V_2), nasopharynx or clivus.
Nasal cavity and ethmoid sinus	
T1	Tumour restricted to any one subsite, with or without bony invasion.
T2	Tumour invading two subsites in a single region or extending to involve an adjacent region within the nasoethmoidal complex, with or without bony invasion.
T3	Tumour extends to invade the medial wall or floor of the orbit, maxillary sinus, palate or cribriform plate.
T4a	Moderately advanced local disease. Tumour invades any of the following: anterior orbital contents, skin of nose or cheek, minimal extension to anterior cranial fossa, pterygoid plates, or sphenoid or frontal sinuses.
T4b	Very advanced local disease. Tumour invades any of the following: orbital apex, dura, brain, middle cranial fossa, cranial nerves other than (V_2), nasopharynx or clivus.
Nodal stage	
NX	Regional lymph nodes cannot be assessed.
N0	No regional lymph node metastasis.
N1	Metastasis in a single ipsilateral lymph node, ≤3 cm in greatest dimension.
N2	Metastasis in a single ipsilateral lymph node, >3 cm but ≤6 cm in greatest dimension, or metastases in multiple ipsilateral lymph nodes, ≤6 cm in greatest dimension, or in bilateral or contralateral lymph nodes, ≤6 cm in greatest dimension.
N2a	Metastasis in a single ipsilateral lymph node, >3 cm but ≤6 cm in greatest dimension.
N2b	Metastases in multiple ipsilateral lymph nodes, ≤6 cm in greatest dimension.
N2c	Metastases in bilateral or contralateral lymph nodes, ≤6 cm in greatest dimension.
N3	Metastasis in a lymph node, >6 cm in greatest dimension.
Metastatic disease	
M0	No distant metastasis.
M1	Distant metastasis.

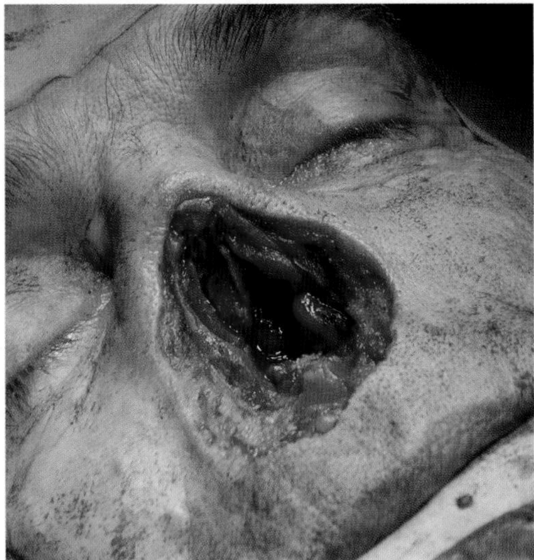

Figure 14.8 Intraoperative picture of total rhinectomy for nasal septal carcinoma.

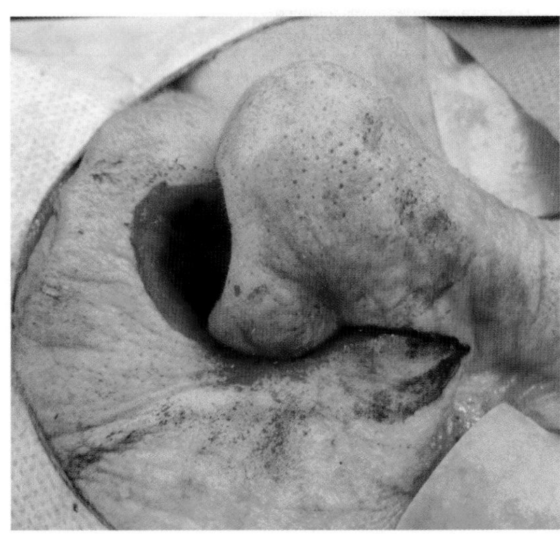

Figure 14.10 Septal squamous carcinoma undergoing wide local excision with local nasolabial flap reconstruction.

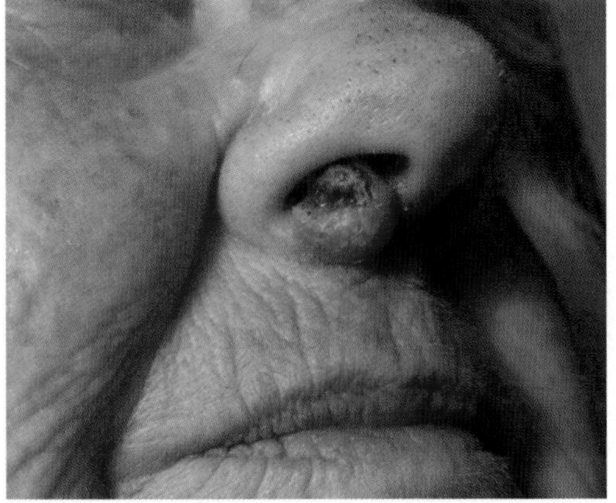

Figure 14.9 Septal squamous carcinoma undergoing wide local excision with local nasolabial flap reconstruction.

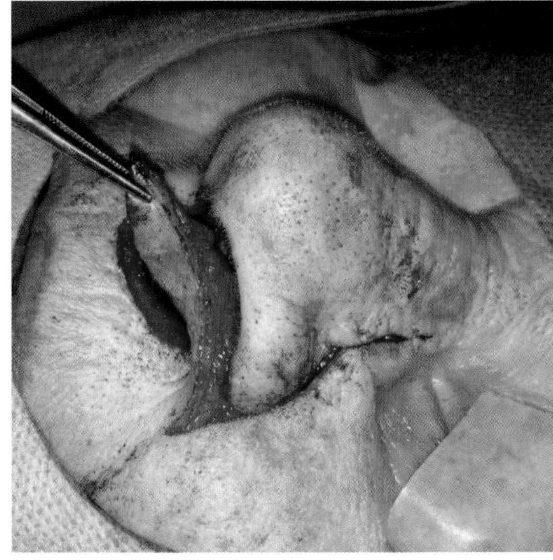

Figure 14.11 Septal squamous carcinoma undergoing wide local excision with local nasolabial flap reconstruction.

Olfactory neuroblastoma

Also known as esthesioneuroblastoma, these arise from the olfactory epithelium of the nasal cavity and hence often present late with intracranial extension. These tumours will typically require craniofacial resection and adjuvant radiotherapy.

Malignant melanoma

These are rare mucosal melanomas occurring within the nasal cavity. They can be locally aggressive with

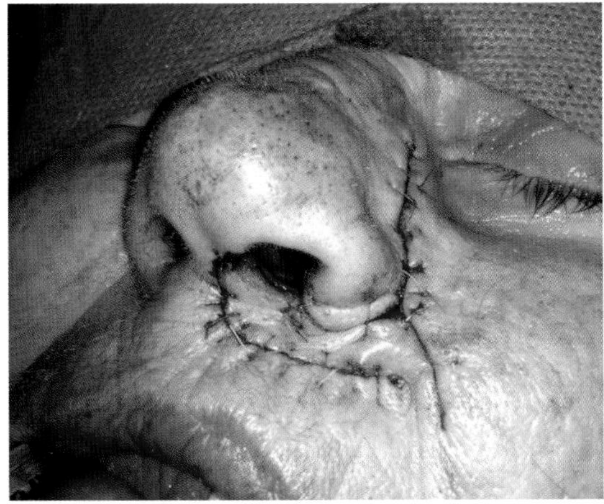

Figure 14.12 Septal squamous carcinoma undergoing wide local excision with local nasolabial flap reconstruction.

multiple distant metastases. They tend to occur in elderly females more often than males. Patients have been known to survive for years with satellite lesions that are managed with local measures such as resection or laser vapourization. Referral to a specialist melanoma service will allow consideration of chemotherapy agents in management.

Lymphoma

This form of extra-nodal lymphoma can be locally destructive and will require early histological diagnosis and CT staging to permit the appropriate choice of chemoradiotherapeutic regimens for treatment.

SUMMARY

Tumours of the nose and paranasal sinuses consist of a wide variety of lesions originating from the various tissue types found within this anatomical area. While the initial presentation may be similar for the various conditions, subsequent examination and investigations will allow a more accurate diagnosis to be made. Biopsy may be required although should be avoided with JNA.

Imaging using CT and MRI is often required, with both modalities complementing each other, CT helping with bone definition and MRI with soft tissue definition. The use of surgical navigation tools is popular in some centres, especially for complex skull base disease.

Recent advances in endoscopic techniques have allowed radical surgery to be performed, achieving excellent rates of disease clearance while reducing patient morbidity. There remains, however, a place for open approaches for cases where a wide surgical field is required.

Surgical approaches include external approaches, but improved technology has allowed endoscopic techniques to develop, which are showing promise in achieving similar cure rates while reducing morbidity.

KEY LEARNING POINTS

- Tumours of the nose and paranasal sinuses are rare.
- They present with common nasal symptoms.
- CT imaging is crucial to staging.
- Surgical advances include navigation systems and extended endoscopic techniques.
- Prognosis remains poor.

FURTHER READING

Andrews JC, Fisch U, Valavanis A, Aeppli U, Makek M. The surgical management of extensive nasopharyngeal angiofibromas with the infratemporal fossa approach. *Laryngoscope.* 1989; 99: 429–37.

Gleeson M (ed.). *Scott-Brown's Otorhinolaryngology, Head and Neck Surgery.* 7th ed. London: Hodder Arnold, 2008.

Harvey RJ, Sheahan PO, Schlosser RJ. Surgical management of benign sinonasal masses. *Otolaryngologic Clinics of North America.* 2009; 42: 353–75.

Hofmann T, et al. Endoscopic resection of juvenile angiofibromas – Long term results. *Rhinology.* 2005; 43: 282–89.

Kennedy DW, Hwang PH. *Rhinology: Diseases of the Nose and Sinuses, and Skull Base*. 1st ed. New York: Thieme, 2002.

Krouse JH. Endoscopic treatment of inverted papilloma: Safety and efficacy. *American Journal of Otolaryngology*. 2001 Mar-Apr; 22(2): 87–99.

Lund VJ, Clarke PM. *Nose and Paranasal Sinus Tumours*. In: *Head and Neck Cancer Multidisciplinary Management Guidelines*. London: ENT UK, 2011.

Robbins KT, et al. Contemporary management of sinonasal cancer. *Head and Neck*. 2011; 33: 1352–65.

Watkinson JC, Gilbert RW. *Stell & Maran's Textbook of Head and Neck Surgery and Oncology*. 5th ed. London: Hodder Arnold, 2012.

Wood JW, Casiano RR. Inverted papillomas and benign nonneoplastic lesions of the nasal cavity. *American Journal of Rhinology and Allergy*. 2012; 26, 157–63.

15

Specific chronic nasal infections

SALIL NAIR

INTRODUCTION

In the Western world chronic nasal infections have decreased in incidence. However, they continue to play a key role in nasal pathology in many developing countries. Migration from countries where these diseases are endemic means that they are encountered in the West, albeit rarely. In addition, they can occur in any immunocompromised patient, and it is important that this is recognized and managed early.

Most of these conditions fall under the umbrella of granulomatous nasal diseases and include syphilis, tuberculosis and leprosy and are discussed elsewhere. These conditions are highlighted in Table 15.1 and are challenging to manage. This chapter covers the specific chronic nasal conditions secondary to bacterial, fungal and protozoal infections.

Table 15.1 Granulomatous disease involving the nose

Infections	
Bacterial	Rhinoscleroma
Fungal	Histoplasmosis
Protozoan	Leishmaniasis
	Rhinosporidiosis
Mycobacteria	Tuberculosis (TB)
	Leprosy
	Atypical TB
Treponemal	Syphilis
Vascular	
Granulomatosis with polyangiitis (Wegener's granulomatosis)	
Churg-Strauss syndrome	
Others	
Sarcoidosis	

BACTERIAL INFECTION

RHINOSCLEROMA

In 1870, von Hebra described this condition and coined the term *rhinoscleroma*. The histological features were described by Mikulicz in 1877, and the causative agent, *Klebsiella rhinoscleromatis* (KR), was identified by Von Frisch in 1882. Rhinoscleroma is found predominantly in rural areas with poor socioeconomic conditions.[1] The disease is endemic to regions of Africa, Southeast Asia, Mexico, Central and South America, as well as Central and Eastern Europe. Rhinoscleroma does not generally affect the lymphatic system like other granulomatous diseases, such as tuberculosis and leprosy. There is no worldwide consensus on the incidence and prevalence of the disease. Untreated severe infection can lead to life-threatening airway obstruction.[2]

History and examination

Patients will most often present with a combination of persistent common nasal symptoms such as nasal obstruction, epistaxis, nasal discharge and dryness. Hoarseness may indicate laryngeal involvement. In non-endemic regions a history of travel should raise suspicion. It is important to enquire about a family history because more than 15 per cent will be positive. Young adults (third and fourth decade) appear to be at highest risk. The spread of disease is enhanced by malnutrition, poor hygiene and crowding. The transmission of the disease is via airborne spread, and humans are the only known hosts.

A complete ear, nose and throat (ENT) examination should be performed including nasal endoscopy and fibre-optic laryngoscopy. The nasal mucosa is involved in almost all cases (95–100 per cent), followed by the pharynx (18–43 per cent), paranasal sinuses, trachea and bronchi. Nasal involvement may present as septal perforation and thickening, crusting, choanal fibrosis, scarring, granulations and purulent discharge. Endoscopy may reveal polypoid masses involving the inferior turbinates or maxillary and ethmoid sinuses. Laryngo-tracheal involvement may present with oedema, ulceration, nodular lesions and vocal cord adhesions. Oropharyngeal inspection may reveal soft and hard palate granulations. The absence of the uvula, called the 'uvula sign', is highly suggestive of the disease. This is thought to occur either secondary to extensive fibrosis, causing shrinkage, or by scarring, causing fixation of the uvula in the nasopharynx. Cutaneous lesions on the face usually appear as reddish-yellow erythematous papules.

Rhinoscleroma is typically classified clinically and histologically into three stages.

1. CATARRHAL STAGE

This is also known as the atrophic stage. Patients present with nonspecific rhinitis symptoms that progress to a foul-smelling purulent nasal discharge and nasal obstruction. On examination, there is crusting and atrophy of the nasal mucosa. The thin mucosa appears 'draped' over the underlying bone. Histologically, epithelial squamous metaplasia with subepithelial infiltrate of polymorphonuclear cells and granulation tissue are seen.

2. PROLIFERATIVE STAGE

This stage is also known as the hypertrophic or granulomatous phase. Patients complain of widening of the nasal pyramid, epistaxis (secondary to granulations), anosmia and destruction of the cartilaginous nasal septum and soft palate. Other complaints include hoarseness and epiphora. On examination, bluish-red rubbery granulomatous lesions are seen. The histopathological features include mucosal infiltration by chronic inflammatory cells and the presence of Mikulicz cells and foamy histiocytes. Their presence is a hallmark sign of rhinoscleroma.

3. FIBROTIC STAGE

In the final stage, fibrosis and scarring result in increasing deformity and stenosis. Histologic examination reveals large amounts of fibrosis and scar tissue with few or no detectable Mikulicz cells or Russell bodies.

Pathophysiology

The primary infectious agent responsible is the capsulated gram-negative bacterium *Klebsiella rhinoscleromatis* (KR). However, the true mode of action is unknown. It is likely to be related to impaired cellular immunity in patients with a reversal of the CD4:CD8 ratio. It appears that following bacterial invasion, neutrophils phagocytose KR, but the bacteria escape digestion and remain viable. KR is then taken up by histiocytes, which become Mikulicz cells as their phagsomes dilate. (Figure 15.1 illustrates Mikulicz cells with foamy cytoplasm.) The Mikulicz cells are unable to kill KR, and the bacteria are eventually released back into the interstitium. Genetic susceptibility is likely to predispose to infection, because mutations affecting genes encoding complex components are known to cause susceptibility to *K. pneumoniae* infection in mice, and similar haplotypes are thought to be strong risk factors for respiratory rhinoscleroma.

Diagnosis

The diagnosis of rhinoscleroma in endemic areas is relatively straightforward and based on clinical symptoms, biopsy, culture and imaging. Where cases are sporadic, it can be more difficult to diagnose, and it must be borne in mind in the differential diagnosis of bacterial chronic rhinitis associated with granulations or atrophic nasal mucosa and the absence of lymphadenopathy.

Differential diagnoses include bacterial infections such as tuberculosis, actinomycosis and leprosy. Fungal infections include histoplasmosis and blastomycosis. Other conditions include leishmaniasis and Rosai-Dorfman disease and inflammatory conditions such as sarcoidosis, granulomatosis with polyangiitis and malignancy such as lymphomas.

Simple markers for chronic inflammation such as the erythrocyte sedimentation rate (ESR) are usually elevated.

IMAGING

Computed tomography (CT) imaging is most useful. Nasal lesions present as homogeneous non-enhancing masses with a distinct edge. If involved, the inferior aspects of the ethmoid and maxillary sinuses are most at risk. Affected turbinates may appear deformed or be completely absent.

Magnetic resonance imaging (MRI) has no distinctive features. Lesions can appear homogeneous

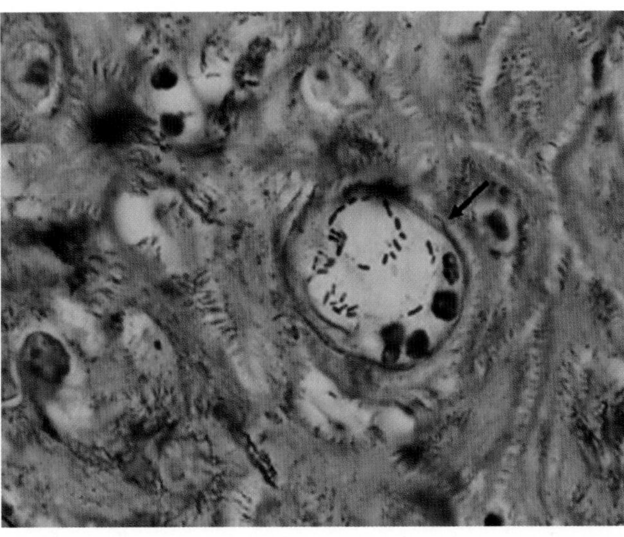

Figure 15.1 Mikulicz cells (arrow) with foamy cytoplasm and *Klebsiella rhinoscleromatis* (Warthin-Starry stain; × 1000 original magnification).[2]

and isosignal on T1 weighted images and hyposignal on T2.[3]

HISTOCHEMISTRY AND BACTERIOLOGY

These are the most useful tools in diagnosis. The laboratory should be informed of the possibility of KR. A panel of stains is best performed and includes Warthin-Starry to identify the characteristic Mikulicz cells and Russell bodies (Figure 15.2), stains for acid-fast bacilli, Gram's and periodic acid–Schiff (PAS) stains for bacteria and histiocytes, and Grocott's silver methenamine to stain fungal elements.

Blood cultures are positive for KR in about 50 per cent of cases.

Immunohistochemical stains (such as CD68) can be helpful in distinguishing the condition from other rarities.

PATHOLOGY

Biopsies are likely to yield useful information if taken from the most active sites or septum and inferior turbinate.

Management

Treatment is challenging and relapses are not uncommon because it is difficult to eradicate the disease. Treatment may involve a combination of conservative surgical debridement and long-term antibiotic treatment. There is no consensus on either the duration of treatment or the optimal antibiotic therapy. However, most studies suggest at least a 6-month course of single or combination therapy. Antibiotics that have been shown to be effective include streptomycin, doxycycline, rifampicin, second- and third-generation cephalosporins and fluoroquinolones (e.g. ciprofloxacin). Historically, tetracycline has been the treatment of choice but is contraindicated in children and pregnancy. KR is an intracellular bacterium, and rifampicin can achieve high intracellular concentrations. Similarly, ciprofloxacin has excellent anti–Gram-negative bacilli activity. A combination of ciprofloxacin and rifampicin would be a reasonable dual therapy choice. Treatment should continue until biopsy and culture results are negative.

Surgical debridement should be considered for significant airway obstruction and may help to reduce the disease load. In some advanced cases, radiotherapy may be effective in preventing disease progression.

Early diagnosis and treatment are important to eradicate the bacteria, not only to limit the fibrotic scarring sequelae but also to prevent progression

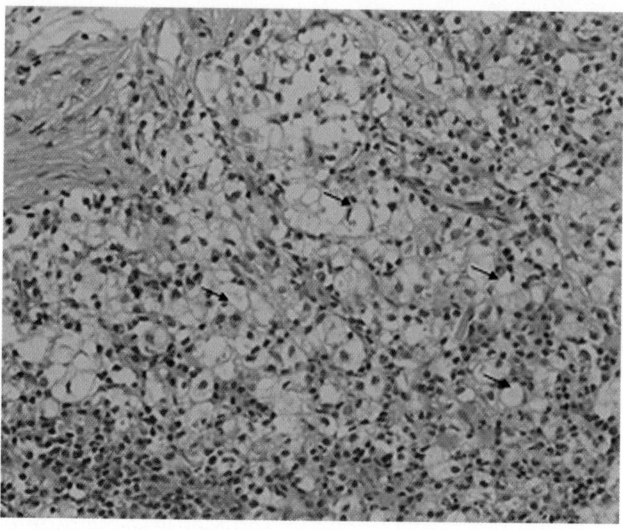

Figure 15.2 Mikulicz cells, Russell bodies (arrows) and congested and dilated vessels with a lymphoplasmacytic infiltrate (hematoxylin-eosin stain; × 400 original magnification).[2]

to the fibrotic stage, when antibiotic therapy is less effective.

PROTOZOAN INFECTIONS

RHINOSPORIDIOSIS

Rhinosporidiosis is a rare chronic granulomatous disease caused by *Rhinosporidium seeberi.* It is endemic in some areas of Asia such as South India and Sri Lanka but has been reported in the Americas, Africa and Europe as well. Once again increased migration may be responsible for the disease found in the tropics. There has been much debate about the etiological agent. Considered a fungus by most microbiologists, the microbe's taxonomy has been debated. Genetic studies have suggested that this is an aquatic protozoan parasite belonging to a novel group of fish parasites, *Mesomycetozoea*, located phylogenetically between fungi and animals.[4]

History and examination

Typically, patients present with painless nasal obstruction secondary to vascular polyps. These grow from the mucosal surfaces within the nasal cavity. The polyps are often unilateral and pedunculated. There may be a history of epistaxis or unilateral nasal discharge. Other sites affected include the conjunctiva, lips, palate, larynx and trachea. The disease has a slow course, and lesions may be present for many years before becoming symptomatic. It is reported to be more common in younger age groups, particularly in men.

On examination the friable polypoid lesion may resemble a strawberry because the surface is studded with white flecks, which are mature sporangia.[5] Nasal endoscopy can reveal tumour-like masses involving the nasal cavity, maxillary sinus and nasopharynx. Systemic disease is rare but can include multiple mucocutaneous, hepatosplenic, renal, pulmonary or bone lesions.

There may be a history of contact with stagnant water or contaminated soil, and the disease is prevalent in rural settings. The mode of transmission is thought to be via traumatized epithelium – 'transepithelial infection'.

Diagnosis

The diagnosis is established by a combination of clinical features, looking for the characteristic features of the organism in tissue biopsies and imaging. CT imaging of the nose and paranasal sinuses is useful in evaluating the extent of disease and site of origin. Differential diagnoses include antrochoanal polyps and inverted papilloma.

CULTURE

Rhinosporidium seeberi are notoriously difficult to grow in culture. Nasal smears may have a role in routine preliminary screening. By using Gridley staining, the chitinous wall appears bright purple and the endospores stain brown.

PATHOLOGY

Biopsy of the friable polypoid tissue is required. Histopathology shows sporangia with stroma infiltrated by lymphocytes, plasma cells, polymorphs and eosinophils. Giant foreign body cell reactions are seen around the sporangia. Occasionally, collapsed membranes of sporangia demonstrate liberated spores.

Management

Spontaneous regression of the disease is rare. A combination of medical and surgical treatment provides the best chance of cure. Wide local excision of the mass with the use of electrocautery to the base of the lesion is the treatment of choice.[4] This aids in haemostasis and is thought to reduce the risk of recurrence. The use of endoscopes facilitates a thorough removal under direct vision. When only limited surgical excision is feasible, post-operative medical therapy is advocated. Anti-fungal therapy has been used with varying success. More recently, encouraging results have been reported with the use of dapsone. Dapsone arrests the maturation of sporangia and promotes stromal fibrosis.[5]

LEISHMANIASIS

The protozoan Leishmania causes leishmaniasis. Approximately 12 million people worldwide suffer from this disease. Cutaneous leishmaniasis (CL) occurs in the Americas, Middle East, North Africa and Asia. CL typically presents with an ulcer usually involving the exposed parts of the body. Atypical variants include lupoid, sporotrichoid, verrucous, chancriform and erysipeloid types, amongst others. Nasal involvement is not uncommon in CL. The lupoid variety commonly affects the face.[6]

History and examination

Patients often present with a history of a slow-growing painless nodule of the nose. Lesions often progress from a papule/nodule to an infiltrated, indurated, crusted plaque. The lesion often discharges over a period of 3–4 months forming a well-circumscribed ulcer, which slowly heals over a period of 3–12 months.[7]

Examination may reveal a well demarcated, painless granulomatous nodular lesion. The lesion usually has an erythematous large raised border with numerous papules and mild scaling.

Diagnosis

Diagnosis is made based on the history of origin of the patient, whether the patient is from an endemic region and the clinical characteristics. Typically these are painless, non-itchy, slowly evolving nodules/ulcers on exposed body parts that are refractory to conventional antibiotic therapy.

HISTOLOGY AND CYTOLOGY

Slit skin smear, direct smear from the exudate or fine-needle aspiration cytology of the nodule is useful. When cytology proves inconclusive, a skin biopsy is required to make the diagnosis. Specimens are stained with Giemsa for Leishmania parasite. Histopathology reveals hyperkeratosis, parakeratosis and acanthosis within the epidermis. The dermis may show aggregates of large pink histiocytes with dot-like organisms and the presence of chronic inflammatory cells.[6]

Management

The treatment of choice is meglumine antimoniate, which is a drug belonging to a group of compounds known as pentavalent antimonials. Difficult lesions have been treated with a combination of systemic steroids and CO_2 lasers with varying results. Recent reports have suggested a possibility of some benefit with the use of cryotherapy to treat persistent nodular facial lesions.

FUNGAL INFECTIONS

HISTOPLASMOSIS

Histoplasmosis is a systemic mycosis caused by *Histoplasma capsulatum*. This potentially virulent fungus is endemic in many parts of the world. The clinical manifestations and indeed the primary site of infection are predominantly pulmonary. Mucocutaneous histoplasmosis is not rare in immunocompromised patients (e.g. those with acquired immunodeficiency syndrome [AIDS]). Nasal involvement, seen as a nasal swelling with nasal obstruction, can occur rarely in immunocompetent individuals.[8]

History and examination

One should enquire about a history of immunosuppression. This may be secondary to drugs or systemic disease. Nasal endoscopy might reveal an uncomfortable ulcerative lesion involving the septum and lateral nasal wall. Crusting and bleeding may be present. Infection is localized to mucosal lined surfaces.

Diagnosis

As with many fungal infections, a high index of suspicion in immunocompromised patients is crucial. A careful history and examination are important because these patients rarely present directly to the ENT service.

IMAGING

CT and MRI are useful in assessing the extent of disease, bony and cartilaginous erosion and soft tissue extension.

PATHOLOGY

A biopsy of the lesion is essential. Tissue should be submitted for both histological and microbiological analysis.

Histologically, there is evidence of necrosis with fibrinopurulent material. Hematoxylin and eosin staining will confirm the presence of noncaseating granulomatous inflammation. Gomori methenamine silver stains are necessary to highlight the *H. capsulatum*.

Management

First line of treatment is with itraconazole. Severe or recalcitrant disease can be treated with amphotericin B. Surgery is usually reserved for diagnostic purposes. Extensive surgical debridement, as is often required with other fungal infections such as mucormycosis, is not necessary because *H. capsulatum* is not angioinvasive.[8]

KEY LEARNING POINTS

- A good history, including a family and travel history, is important.
- Diagnosis is made based on history, examination and tissue histology.
- Imaging is not diagnostic but can help assess the extent of sinonasal involvement.

REFERENCES

1. Tan SL, Neoh CY, Tan HH. Rhinoscleroma: A case series. *Singapore Medical Journal*. 2012; 53(2): 24–27.
2. Zhong Q, Guo W, Chen X, et al. Rhinoscleroma: A retrospective study of pathologic and clinical features. *Journal of Otolaryngology Head and Neck Surgery*. 2011; 40(2): 167–74.
3. Bailhache A, Dehesdin D, Francois A, et al. Rhinoscleroma of the sinuses. *Rhinology*. 2008; 46: 338–41.
4. Das S, Kashyap B, Barua M, et al. Nasal rhinosporidiosis in humans: New interpretations and a review of the literature of this enigmatic disease. *Medical Mycology*. 2011; 49: 311–15.
5. Venkatachalam VP, Anand V, Bhooshan O. Rhinosporidiosis: Its varied presentations. *Indian Journal of Otolaryngology Head and Neck Surgery*. 2007; 59: 142–44.
6. Mlika RB, Hammami H, Sioud A, et al. Lupoid leishmaniasis of the nose responding well to cryotherapy. *Dermatology Therapy*. 2011; 24: 378–79.
7. Ul Bari A, Raza N. Lupoid cutaneous leishmaniasis: A report of 16 cases. *Indian Journal of Dermatology, Venereology and Leprosy*. 2010; 76: 85.
8. Rizzi M, Batra P, Prayson R, Citardi M. Nasal histoplasmosis. *Journal of Otolaryngology Head and Neck Surgery*. 2006; 135: 803–04.

FURTHER READING

Pignataro L, Torretta S, Capaccio P, Esposito S, Marchisio P. Unusual otolaryngological manifestations of certain systemic bacterial and fungal infections in children. *International Journal of Paediatric Otorhinolaryngology*. 2009; 73S: S33–S37.

Zargari O, Elpern DJ. Granulomatous diseases of the nose. *The International Society of Dermatology*. 2009; 48: 1275–82.

16

Snoring and OSA in adults

BHIK KOTECHA

INTRODUCTION

Most patients with obstructive sleep apnoea syndrome (OSAS) are known to snore heavily, but not all snorers have OSAS. Snorers without OSAS are termed *primary snorers*. Primary snoring and severe obstructive sleep apnoea (OSA) represent opposite extremes of sleep-related breathing disorders. The prevalence of snoring in middle-aged men is in the range of 25–50 per cent, whereas OSA affects 1–4 per cent of the adult population, with the male to female ratio being 2:1.[1] Sleep medicine is a relatively new field; the management of patients presenting with sleep disorders may require a multidisciplinary approach that could include input from a respiratory physician, otolaryngologist, neurologist, maxillofacial surgeon or a dental practitioner. Otolaryngologists are well positioned to assess and evaluate the upper airway and may be able to surgically rectify some pathological features that are causing the upper airway obstruction. The respiratory physician, on the other hand, may attract more referral from primary care practitioners of patients complaining of obvious apnoeic episodes for consideration of treatment with nocturnal ventilation.

Snoring is thought to occur as a result of a turbulent airflow through the upper airway, with the obstructive anatomical segment being anywhere from the nose to the larynx. Quite commonly, the turbulence is a result of repeated vibrations or oscillation of redundant pharyngeal mucosa. Indeed, in many cases it is thought that the obstruction can be multisegmental. Mild snoring may create a sound of about 40 dB, whereas severe snoring can be as loud as 90 dB. Needless to say, depending on how light a sleeper the partner is, there is a strong possibility that the sleep disturbance would affect both the patient and the partner. Sleep fragmentation and deprivation can result in significant daytime somnolence and thus impair the ability to function normally during the day. If the problem remains untreated and is a long-term issue, it could result in increasing chances of the patient developing other medical disorders in addition to the social issues. In OSA, as the name suggests, there are obstructive

Table 16.1 OSAS symptoms

Snoring
Apnoeic episodes
Choking sensation
Restless sleep
Nocturia/enuresis
Night sweats
Palpitations
Morning headaches
Daytime sleepiness
Impaired memory/concentration
Acid reflux
Decreased libido

episodes of breath-holding during sleep that result in oxygen deprivation. The obstruction could be purely anatomical, such as secondary to hypertrophy of the palatine tonsils or a bulky tongue. In many cases a neurogenic mechanism causes a generalized failure of dilator muscle tone of the muscles controlling upper airway patency.

Patients with OSAS can present with various symptoms (Table 16.1), which can include crescendo snoring, apnoeic episodes with gasping or choking sensation, and excessive daytime sleepiness. Untreated OSA can lead to patients having a much higher chance of developing hypertension, cardiac arrhythmias, angina, myocardial infarction, cerebral vascular accidents, type 2 diabetes and various cognitive dysfunctions.[2] If left untreated, the end sequelae would be that of cor pulmonale. It is also thought that in untreated OSA patients, there is a higher incidence of road traffic accidents because they have excessive daytime sleepiness. Thus, it would be prudent to diagnose and treat this condition in the interest of the patient's health as well as the economic health of the nation.

CLINICAL HISTORY

The clinical history should be obtained not only from the patient but also from the partner if present. In general, patients presenting to the clinic will have problems with socially intrusive snoring, and the partner may express concerns about witnessed apnoeic episodes lasting a few seconds. These patients are commonly sleep deprived and will have problems with excessive daytime sleepiness. A useful guide in gauging the severity is the Epworth Sleepiness Scale (Table 16.2). Scores of 10 or more on this scale are thought to be significant and warrant further investigations.

On direct questioning patients may admit to having morning headaches, night sweats,

Table 16.2 Epworth Sleepiness Scale

How likely are you to doze off or fall asleep in the following situations, in contrast to just feeling tired?
Please tick one box on each line using the following scale:

0 = Would never doze
1 = Slight chance of dozing
2 = Moderate chance of dozing
3 = High chance of dozing

Situation	0	1	2	3
Sitting and reading				
Watching television				
Sitting inactive in public place (e.g. theatre or meeting)				
As a passenger in a car for an hour without break				
Lying down in the afternoon when circumstances permit				
Sitting and talking to someone				
Sitting quietly after lunch without alcohol				
In a car, while stopped for a few minutes in traffic				

palpitations during sleep, impaired concentration and memory, and in general to being quite restless in their sleep. Quite commonly, patients may complain of nasal congestion in conjunction with the snoring, and further questioning in this regard is also important. Mouth breathing accentuates the problems of snoring by causing further retraction of the tongue base as well as by increasing the palatal vibrations if the patient has a lax soft palate.

An enquiry with regard to social history is also important, particularly relating to alcohol intake or consumption of tranquillizers such as diazepam because these would aggravate snoring and OSA by acting as a muscle relaxant. Other factors that are important in the history are co-existing morbidities such as hypertension, ischaemic heart disease or diabetes, because these would lower the clinician's threshold for ordering further special investigations.

CLINICAL EXAMINATION

General inspection can sometimes give a clue to the underlying root of the problem, e.g. obesity, retrognathia, fractured nose, alar collapse and clinical features of other conditions such as acromegaly or hypothyroidism. The patient's height and weight measurements are taken to calculate the body mass index (BMI). The neck circumference is also measured; it is more common to encounter problems of upper airway obstruction if this value is greater than 17.5 inches.

Oropharyngeal examination is necessary to ascertain the size of the tonsils, the position and the laxity of the soft palate and the size of the uvula. Furthermore, the lack of teeth or general dentition status should be noted because this may be an important factor in the treatment of patients with mandibular advancement devices. Friedman tongue position (Figures 16.1–16.4) assessment is sometimes a useful guide in patient selection for palatal surgery. This is performed by asking the patient to open the mouth and phonate without using a tongue depressor to see how much of the soft palate is visible. Tongue positions one and two would do better with palatal surgery than three or four.

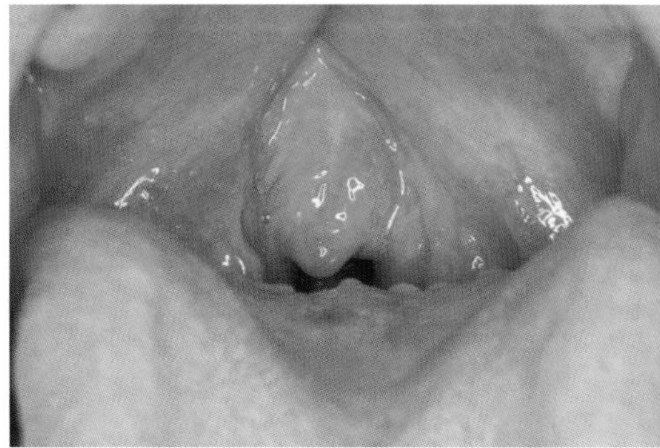

Figure 16.1 Friedman tongue position I.

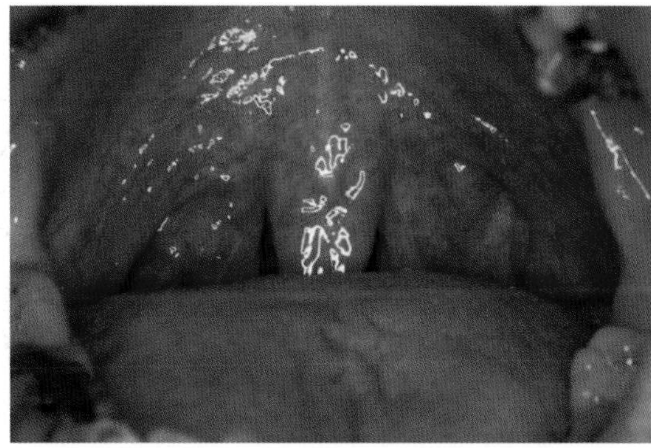

Figure 16.2 Friedman tongue position II.

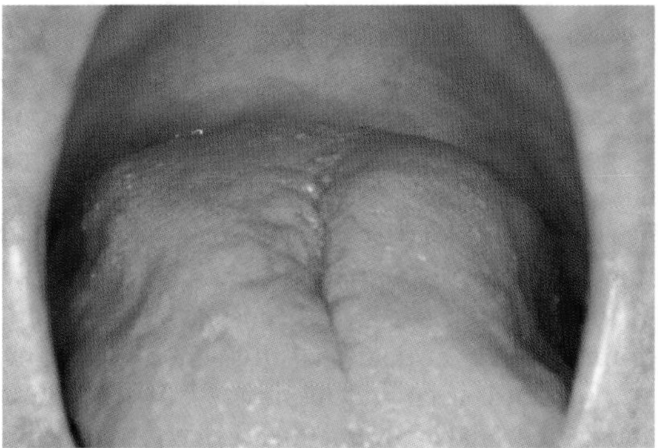

Figure 16.3 Friedman tongue position III.

Upper airway evaluation is best performed using a flexible fibre-optic nasendoscope. In the nasal cavity, special attention is given to identifying a deviated nasal septum, nasal polyposis, allergic rhinitis or sinusitis. Careful examination

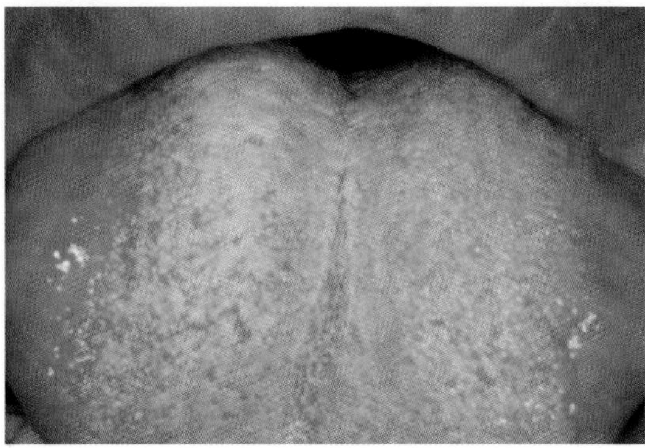

Figure 16.4 Friedman tongue position IV.

is then carried out of the postnasal space oropharynx and hypopharynx. The bulkiness of the base of tongue is noted. With the scope in position, the patient could be asked to simulate the snoring sound and to perform the Müller manoeuvre, which essentially is a reverse of the Valsalva manoeuvre. However, one must bear in mind that the dynamics of the upper airway during wakefulness may differ considerably from that during sleep because the variation in muscle tone may be significant. Hence, limited emphasis should be placed on the 'awake' assessment.

SPECIAL INVESTIGATIONS

A very basic investigation using only pulse oximetry is satisfactory as a baseline for some patients but may be inadequate in many because the specificity and sensitivity are not very good. The gold standard investigation to confirm or refute the diagnosis of OSA is a full hospital-based polysomnographic evaluation. This entails looking at a patient's nasal and respiratory airflow, chest and abdominal movements, oxygen saturation and sleep architecture. However, this may not be widely available and may be be quite expensive. A more commonly available and cost-effective way of adequately investigating these patients is an ambulatory sleep study, in which equipment could be hooked up for the patient to take home and sleep with in his or her own bed. All parameters mentioned earlier except sleep architecture can be measured with this device. The main parameters and objective values that are looked at are the apnoea/hypopnea index (AHI), the average oxygen saturation values and the oxygen desaturation index. The AHI is the number of apnoea episodes plus the number of hypopnea episodes per hour of sleep. By definition, apnoea is said to occur when there is cessation of airflow for 10 seconds or more at the nasal and oral cavity. If the tidal volume or vital capacity is diminished by more than 30 per cent, this is considered to be an episode of hypopnea. The values of AHI are used to determine the severity of OSA, with values of 5 or less being regarded as normal, between 5 and 15 representing mild OSA, values between 16 and 30 regarded as moderate and AHI of more than 30 representing severe OSA. However, these values should not be used on their own to assess severity but should be taken in conjunction with other factors such as the patient's symptoms and co-morbidities before deciding the treatment options best suited for the individual patient.

Another investigation that is useful for some of these patients is drug-induced sedation endoscopy (DISE) or sleep nasendoscopy.[3] Essentially, this is utilized in evaluating the upper airway obstruction and can identify specific anatomical obstructive sites by allowing visualization of the various parts of the pharyngeal lumen in three dimensions and in the dynamic mode. It is thought to be useful not only in deciding what kind of surgical intervention may be required but also in predicting which patients would do well with appliances such as a mandibular advancement device. However, controversy exists in the use of DISE, mainly because (1) the drug-induced sleep may not be identical to natural physiological sleep and (2) the DISE may provide only a snapshot of what may be happening in regard to the snoring and OSA. Clinical assessment of the upper airway when a patient is awake can be quite different from when a patient is asleep, because there may be considerable variation in muscle tone. Hence, DISE is the closest method we have at present to determine what may be happening to the upper airway during natural physiological sleep.[4]

Imaging with cepahalometry, computed tomography (CT) and magnetic resonance imaging (MRI) scanning can be used to evaluate the upper airway, but these would not allow a dynamic assessment and would provide information only about upper airway dimensions in the static phase. Acoustic analysis and pressure measurements have also been utilized to evaluate upper airway obstruction.

In addition to the investigations mentioned, haematological investigations such as a full blood count and thyroid function tests may prove useful in excluding other conditions causing tiredness.[5]

MANAGEMENT OF SNORING AND OSA

Treatment modalities in these patients may be used in combination and include simple lifestyle changes, medication, appliances and surgical intervention.

LIFESTYLE CHANGES

Making simple lifestyle changes such as reducing body weight are directly helpful in improving symptoms and also in managing patients in whom upper airway surgery is being considered. Reducing alcohol intake is recommended because alcohol is a muscle relaxant and aggravates upper airway obstruction by relaxing the tongue and other pharyngeal muscles. Sleeping supine also contributes in some cases by worsening tongue base obstruction; these patients may be able to avoid sleeping on their back by stitching tennis or golf balls into their nightwear. Modern technology using what is known as 'positional therapy' is at present being evaluated. This form of therapy involves a sleep position sensor that detects the position in which a patient is sleeping and gently vibrates to alter the position to non-supine, thus reducing the number of obstructive episodes.

MEDICATION

In some patients, medications such as intranasal steroids and antihistamines used for treating allergic rhinitis may prove to be useful in improving nasal symptoms by reducing nasal resistance and thus improving sleep quality. However, there is little or no evidence to demonstrate any objective improvement in OSA when this modality is used on its own. Numerous nonsteroidal sprays for the nose and oral cavity are available over the counter that claim to help with snoring, but again no clinical evidence exists to support the use of these agents. Drugs such as orlistat can be used to help patients with obesity to lose weight, and this in turn would improve their symptoms. This drug works by inhibiting pancreatic and gastric lipases and thus reduces fat absorption. There are other drugs, such as sibutramine, that may suppress appetite and therefore limit caloric intake.

APPLIANCES

Appliances or devices used in treating snoring and OSA include nasal dilators, mandibular advancement devices (MADs) and nasal continuous positive airway pressure (nCPAP) devices.

Nasal dilators

Nasal dilators are devices that dilate the nasal vestibule and improve the ability to breathe through the nose. This can be done intrinsically by using Nozovent, which is a plastic device inserted in a similar manner to Thudichum's nasal speculum to stent the inner aspect of the alar cartilage. It is particularly useful in patients with alar valve collapse. Similarly, Breathe Right could be applied externally to improve breathing. However, these devices are not effective for OSA and should be used only in patients with primary snoring presenting with nasal obstruction. If these improve the patients' symptoms subjectively, then it may be worth considering these individuals for reconstructive nasal surgery.

Mandibular advancement devices

In the past few decades, MADs have become popular in the management of snoring and OSA. There are various types available, including a monobloc type that is non-adjustable and a two-piece device that can be adjusted. They enjoy the benefit of not causing adverse effects or the pain that may result from surgical intervention, but, as with all appliances, they have to be used every night. They are difficult to use in patients who have poor dentition or who are edentulous, in patients with temporomandibular joint dysfunction or in individuals who have poorly controlled epilepsy. Essentially, MADs allow protrusion of the mandible and the hyoid bone anteriorly, and by doing increase the contraction of the genioglossus muscle as well as the retroglossal distance. In some cases, these devices may also reduce palatal vibrations. This was demonstrated in a study addressing objective evidence of MAD effectiveness whereby DISE was performed in patients with and without the device *in situ*. Long-term use can result in loosening of teeth and mild changes in occlusion. Patients with a sensitive gag reflex find an MAD difficult to tolerate, and in general compliance is in the range of 60–70 per cent.

Nasal CPAP

According to the National Institute for Health and Care Excellence (NICE) guidelines, the treatment of choice for moderate or severe OSA is nasal continuous positive airway pressure (nCPAP). To overcome the failure of dilator muscle tone in OSA patients, the nCPAP works by increasing the pressure within the pharyngeal lumen and acting like a pneumatic splint. It was first introduced in the 1980s by Sullivan; prior to this the only effective treatment for OSA was to perform a tracheostomy. This form of therapy requires a machine or a generator that is operated by electrical means and extracts air from the room, which is regenerated at a positive pressure and subsequently transmitted via tubing through the face mask or nasal pillows. The older version of nCPAP was more cumbersome and, as the name suggests, provided continuous pressure at a fixed setting. The newer models are auto-titrating and work by sensing airflow limitation or detecting an increase in impedance that may suggest airway narrowing. Thus, this autoset nCPAP kicks in only when required and is more acceptable to the majority of patients. In spite of these advances, the nCPAP treatment modality still remains relatively unpopular because it would need to be used every night; patient acceptability, adherence to treatment and compliance are somewhat poor, approximately 60 per cent. Other problems encountered by patients using nCPAP include aerophagia, nCPAP-induced rhinitis and, in some cases, claustrophobia. In patients who find nCPAP difficult to use, the upper airway should be carefully evaluated, and significant obstructive pathology – e.g. a grossly deviated nasal septum, nasal polyposis or tonsillar hypertrophy – should be surgically addressed. This would allow the CPAP pressure requirement to drop and hence facilitate easier use of this device.

SURGICAL INTERVENTION

In general, surgery could be considered in patients with simple snoring and mild OSA because in this group CPAP is unnecessary and MAD may not be desired. In patients who have moderate or severe OSA and have failed the CPAP mode of therapy or refused to accept it, surgery could be considered as an adjunctive treatment modality. Great care must be taken with the use of some premedication and analgesic agents, especially in the patient who has significant OSA, because some of these drugs may further suppress respiration. Patient selection is naturally of utmost importance, and usually patients with a higher BMI do more poorly. Site-specific targeted surgery is ideally what is required, and to this effect DISE could prove to be a useful investigation to identify the site of anatomical obstruction responsible for the symptoms. In some cases the choice to operate may be very straightforward; for example, in a slim individual with grade 3 or 4 tonsils and no other comorbidities, tonsillectomy should resolve the problem. However, in most cases there are issues with multilevel obstruction, and these patients require a more careful workup to determine what surgical intervention would be most appropriate.

Nasal surgery such as septoplasty and functional endoscopic sinus surgery can work fairly well in reducing some symptoms of simple snorers but does not suffice as a single procedure in patients with more severe problems.[6] Nasal surgery alone has been proven to be useful as an adjunctive procedure in CPAP users because it significantly reduces the pressure requirement and hence improves CPAP compliance.

Palatal surgery is probably the most common surgery performed in this group of patients. When surgery to the soft palate is being considered, patients should be divided into two categories: those who require minimally invasive intervention without changing the contours of the soft palate, and those requiring a more radical procedure to shorten and stiffen the soft palate. In the minimally invasive group, the soft palate can be scarred or stiffened by applying radiofrequency thermotherapy, by injecting sclerosing agents or by inserting pillar implants.[7] In this group, treatment is provided by using unipolar radiofrequency (Somnus) or bipolar devices (Celon) or the Coblation technique. Pillar implants are inserted interstitially within the soft palate in parallel to each other and are thought to help in patients with simple palatal snoring. In the more radical group, Fujita introduced traditional uvulopalatopharyngoplasty (UPPP), but many consider this procedure to be aggressive and radical and so use it less commonly.[8] Furthermore, UPPP is associated with high morbidity and can result in nasopharyngeal stenosis and incompetence. It can also interfere with future use of CPAP if required, but this could be overcome by using a full face mask. As a result, a number of different techniques using the laser to address the soft palate have been described with a view to reducing the amount of tissue resection. Some of these techniques are performed under local anaesthesia, but in others general anaesthetic may be necessary, especially if other procedures such as tonsillectomy are carried out simultaneously to address the multilevel problem.

Surgery to address problems in the region of the hypopharynx can be quite challenging. The simpler procedures include minimally invasive radiofrequency to the tongue and slightly more involved procedures such as midline glossectomy. Hyoid suspension also has been described to improve hypopharyngeal obstruction. This can be achieved by advancing the hyoid bone anteriorly and superiorly to hook it up to the mandible or anteriorly and inferiorly to the thyroid cartilage. More aggressive and radical, but extremely effective, is the procedure of maxilla-mandibular advancement, which can improve both retropalatal and retroglossal dimensions. Recently, transoral robotic surgery using the da Vinci system has been used to address problems associated with tongue base and/or epiglottic obstruction. Electrical stimulation using various implants and pacemaker devices has been used to stimulate the hypoglossal nerve in patients with OSA. This, however, is in an experimental stage and not widely available as yet.

CONCLUSION

Though sleep medicine is a relatively new field, patients with snoring and OSA commonly present to the otolaryngologist. There are numerous treatment modalities available to help these patients, but careful evaluation and selection, especially for those chosen for surgical intervention, is very important. Combined treatment modalities are commonly required, and thus a multidisciplinary approach to snoring and OSA is advocated.

KEY LEARNING POINTS

- Sleep-related breathing disorder is a spectrum consisting of primary snoring at one end and severe obstructive sleep apnoea at the other.
- Untreated OSA increases the incidence of ischaemic heart disease, stroke and type 2 diabetes.
- Lifestyle changes such as losing weight and decreasing alcohol intake are helpful.
- nCPAP is the treatment of choice for moderate or severe OSA.
- Surgical intervention may be useful in simple snorers and in mild OSA but may also be used in an adjunctive capacity for severe OSA to facilitate CPAP therapy.
- Multidisciplinary approach is required.

REFERENCES

1. Stradling JR, Crosby JH. Predictors and prevalence of obstructive sleep apnoea and snoring in 1001 middle-aged men. *Thorax*. 1991; 46: 85–90.

2. Marshall NS, Wong KKH, Liu PY, Cullen SRJ, Knuiman MW, Grunstein RR. Sleep apnea as an independent risk factor for all-cause mortality: The Busselton Health Study. *SLEEP*. 2008; 31(8): 1079–85.
3. Croft C, Pringle M. Sleep nasendoscopy: A technique of assessment in snoring and obstructive sleep apnoea. *Clinical Otolaryngology*. 1991; 16: 504–9.
4. Kotecha BT, Hannan AS, Khalil HMB, Georgalas C, Bailey P. Sleep nasendoscopy: A 10-year retrospective audit study. *European Archives of Otorhinoloaryngology*. 2007; 264: 1361–67.
5. Georgalas C, Garas G, Hadjihannas E, Oostra A. Assessment of obstruction level and selection of patients for obstructive sleep apnoea surgery: An evidence-based approach. *Journal of Laryngology and Otology*. 2010; 124(1): 1–9.
6. Kotecha B. The nose, snoring and obstructive sleep apnoea. *Rhinology*. 2011; 49: 259–64.
7. Farrar J, Ryan J, Oliver E, Gillespie MB. Radiofrequency ablation for the treatment of obstructive sleep apnea: A meta-analysis. *The Laryngoscope*. 2008; 118: 1878–83.
8. Verse T, Pirsig W. *Laser-Assisted Uvulopalatoplasty: A Meta-Analysis*. In: *Surgery for Snoring and Obstructive Sleep Apnoea Syndrome*. Eds. Fabiani M, Saponara M. The Hague, Netherlands: Kugler Publications, 2003: 463–74.

FURTHER READING

Friedman M. *Sleep Apnoea and Snoring: Surgical and Non-Surgical Therapy*. Philadelphia: Saunders Elsevier, 2009.

Kotecha B, Hall A. Role of surgery in adult obstructive sleep apnoea. *Sleep Medicine Reviews*. 2014; 18: 405–13.

Shneerson J. *Sleep Medicine: A Guide to Sleep and Its Disorders*. 2nd ed. Oxford: Blackwell Publishing, 2005.

SECTION II

Throat/Head and Neck

17

Anatomy of the larynx and pharynx

RICHARD M ADAMSON AND SAFINA ALI

ANATOMY OF THE LARYNX

INTRODUCTION

The larynx principally has three functions: breathing, protecting the airway during deglutition and phonation. In adults the larynx lies at the level of the C3–C6 vertebrae, being slightly higher in infants at C2–C3, descending as they grow. At puberty the larynx of the male increases in size in all dimensions. The framework of the larynx consists of a series of cartilages (nine in total), ligaments, membranes and muscles (intrinsic and extrinsic). Interiorly, it can be divided into supra-glottis, glottis and sub-glottis. The mucosal lining of the larynx is continuous above with that of the pharynx and below with that of the trachea.

EMBRYOLOGY

Laryngeal development occurs during the fourth week *in utero*. The laryngo-tracheal groove in the ventral wall of the pharynx gradually deepens, and its edges fuse to form a septum, separating it from the pharynx and the oesophagus. This tube is lined with endoderm from which the epithelium of the airway develops. The cranial end of this laryngo-tracheal tube forms the larynx and the trachea, and caudally the two main bronchi form. The laryngeal structures develop from the fourth and sixth branchial arches (Table 17.1); accordingly, the

Table 17.1

Structure	Branchial arch
Thyroid cartilage	4th arch
Arytenoids, corniculate, cricoid and tracheal cartilages	6th arch
Epiglottis	Hypobranchial eminence
All muscles except cricothyroid	4th arch
Cricothyroid muscle	6th arch

nerve supply of the larynx includes the recurrent laryngeal and superior laryngeal nerves.

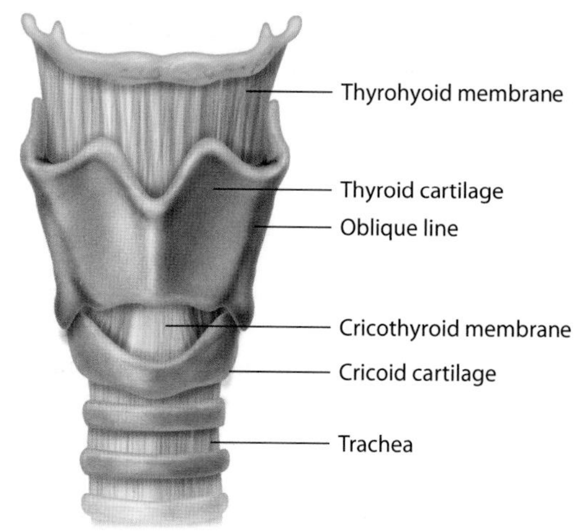

Figure 17.1 Cartilaginous framework of larynx.

LARYNGEAL FRAMEWORK

The larynx is formed by a series of cartilages, linked by ligaments and membranes that are controlled by the action of two groups of muscles (intrinsic and extrinsic).

The mucosal lining of the larynx is continuous above with that of the pharynx and below with that of the trachea.

Cartilages of the larynx

THYROID CARTILAGE

The thyroid cartilage is the largest of the laryngeal cartilages and is shield shaped. Its two laminae meet in the midline inferiorly. Superiorly, there is a palpable thyroid notch. The angle of fusion between the laminae is approximately 90° in men and 120° in women. The fused anterior borders in men form a projection that can be easily palpated, known as the Adam's apple. Posteriorly, the laminae of the thyroid cartilage diverge and form two prolongations: two slender processes known as the superior and inferior cornua. The superior cornu is long and narrow, curving upwards, backwards and medially, ending in a conical projection. The lateral thyrohyoid ligament attaches here. The inferior cornu is shorter and thicker than the superior cornua. It curves downwards and medially, and at its lower end the cricoid cartilage articulates (Figure 17.1).

The outer surface has an oblique line extending from the superior thyroid tubercle to the inferior thyroid tubercle. The superior thyroid tubercle is situated in front of the root of the superior horn, and the inferior tubercle is situated on the lower border of the thyroid lamina.

The oblique line gives attachment to the following muscles (see Figure 17.1):

- Thyrohyoid
- Sternohyoid
- Inferior constrictor

CRICOID CARTILAGE

The cricoid cartilage is shaped similar to a signet ring, with the higher segment oriented posteriorly. On the superior surface of the posterior aspect are the articular facets of the arytenoids.

ARYTENOID CARTILAGES

The arytenoids sit on the posterolateral aspects of the cricoid cartilage. The arytenoids are shaped like an inverted *T* with three processes: vocal, muscular, and apical.

EPIGLOTTIS

The epiglottis forms the anterior wall of the larynx. Its primary function is to protect the airway during deglutition.

OTHER CARTILAGES

The corniculate cartilages are cone shaped and sit directly on top of the arytenoid cartilages. The cuneiforms are found in the aryepiglottic fold. Their primary role is to provide elastic force to separate the medialized aryepiglottic folds.

Ligaments attached to the thyroid cartilage

THYROEPIGLOTTIC LIGAMENT

This is the elastic ligament connecting the stem of the epiglottis to the angle of the thyroid cartilage.

VESTIBULAR LIGAMENT/FALSE VOCAL CORD

This narrow band of fibrous tissue is attached to the angle of the thyroid cartilage just below the attachment of the root of the epiglottis.

VOCAL LIGAMENT/TRUE VOCAL CORD

The vocal ligament is responsible for production of voice. It is considered to be the thickened superior portion of the cricothyroid ligament.

Membranes

EXTRINSIC

The extrinsic membranes connect the laryngeal apparatus to the surrounding structures. The thyrohyoid membrane is a fibro-elastic structure connecting the hyoid bone to the thyroid cartilage. It is pierced laterally by the internal laryngeal nerve and artery.

The cricothryroid membrane is also a fibro-elastic structure that includes the cricothyroid ligament connecting the cricoid and thyroid cartilages. This is the structure pierced in a cricothyroidotomy during access for an emergency airway.

INTRINSIC

The intrinsic membranes connect various laryngeal cartilages and help regulate direction and degree of movement.

- Conus elasticus: Connects the thyroid, cricoid, and arytenoid cartilage to each other.
- Quadrangular membrane: Arises from the lateral epiglottis and adjacent thyroid cartilage. It attaches the corniculate cartilages and medial surfaces of arytenoids. Inferiorly, its fibres thicken and become the ventricular ligament.
- Aryepiglottic folds: These membranes and ligaments completely seal off the spaces in the laryngeal structure, thus creating a sphincter that protects the larynx and the lungs from foreign bodies.

Muscles

These can be divided into intrinsic and extrinsic muscles. The extrinsic muscles of the larynx connect the laryngeal cartilages to the hyoid bone above and the trachea below. The intrinsic muscles of the larynx interconnect the laryngeal cartilages and help in their mobility. The intrinsic muscles can be divided into three groups.

- Those that open and close the glottis (lateral and posterior cricoarytenoid muscles, transverse and oblique arytenoids)
- Those that control the tension of vocal ligaments (thyroarytenoids, vocalis and cricothyroids)
- Those that alter the shape of the inlet of the larynx (aryepiglottis and thyroepiglottis)

Interior of the larynx

The laryngeal cavity extends from the level of the third cervical vertebra to the lower border of the cricoid cartilage (C6). The whole laryngeal cavity is divided by the presence of vestibular and vocal folds into three compartments. The larynx above the vestibular fold is known as the superior vestibule. The ventricle or sinus of the larynx lies between the vestibular and vocal folds. Below the vocal folds is the subglottic space, which extends up to the level of the lower border of the cricoid cartilage (Figure 17.2).

The fissure present between the vestibular folds is known as the rima vestibularis, while the fissure between the vocal folds is known as the rima glottidis.

The laryngeal inlet is bounded superiorly by the free edge of the epiglottis and on each side by the aryepiglottic folds. Posteriorly, the inlet is bounded by the mucous membrane between the two arytenoid cartilages.

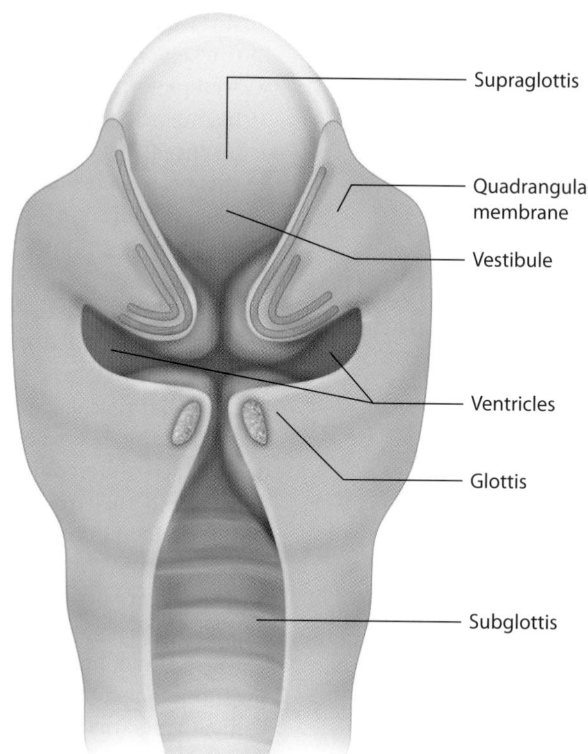

Figure 17.2 Cross-sectional view of the interior larynx.

Subsites of the larynx

The larynx is subdivided into three compartments that have relevance in the TNM staging of laryngeal cancer.

1. SUPRA-GLOTTIS

- False vocal cords
- Arytenoid cartilages
- Epiglottis
- Aryepiglottic folds

2. GLOTTIS

- True vocal cords
- Anterior commissure
- Posterior commissure

3. SUB-GLOTTIS

- Inferior aspect of the glottis to the first tracheal ring

Spaces in the larynx

The spaces adjacent to the larynx again have relevance in the spread of disease.

PRE-EPIGLOTTIC SPACE

The pre-epiglottic space is a wedge-shaped space lying in front of the epiglottis. Anteriorly, it is bounded by the thyrohyoid ligament and the hyoid bone. Laterally, it is continuous with the para-glottic space.

PARA-GLOTTIC SPACE

The para-glottic space is a potential space on either side of the glottis. It is bound by the mucosa covering the lamina of thyroid cartilage laterally, the conus elasticus and quadrangular membranes medially and the anterior reflection of the piriform fossa posteriorly.

VENTRICLE

This is the area between the vestibular and vocal folds.

RIMA GLOTTIDIS

The rima glottidis is an elongated fissure present between the two vocal folds. It is limited behind by the mucous membrane between the arytenoids.

Infant larynx

There are a few key differences in the infant larynx that have surgical relevance.

The infant larynx is funnel shaped, unlike the adult larynx, where the glottis is narrowest; the narrowest point in the infant is the sub-glottis. There is also more redundant mucosa; therefore, even a slight swelling of the mucosa produces a serious obstruction to breathing. The laryngeal cartilages in infants are more supple and hence collapse easily during forced inspiratory effort.

HISTOLOGY OF VOCAL CORDS

The vocal folds are multilayered and contain an epithelial layer, the lamina propria, and the vocalis portion of the thyroarytenoid muscle (Figure 17.3).

The epithelial layer of the vocal folds forms the outer cover and contains three different types of mucosa. The upper and lower edges of the vocal fold are composed of typical respiratory (pseudostratified ciliated columnar) epithelium. The vibrating edge of the cord is covered with non-keratinized stratified squamous epithelium.

The lamina propria is divided into three layers:

- Superficial layer (Reinke's space) containing scant amounts of loosely bound elastic and collagen fibres
- Intermediate layer containing branching elastic fibres
- Deep layer comprising mostly dense collagen fibres running parallel to the vocal cord

Together, the intermediate and deep layers of the lamina propria comprise the vocal ligament. The vocalis muscle is simply the medial fibres of the thyroarytenoid muscle.

BLOOD SUPPLY

The blood supply is derived from the laryngeal branches of the superior and inferior thyroid arteries and the crico-thryoid branch of the superior thyroid artery. The veins leaving the larynx accompany the arteries: the superior vessels drain to the internal jugular vein via the superior thyroid or facial veins, and the inferior vessels drain via the inferior thyroid vein into the brachiocephalic veins.

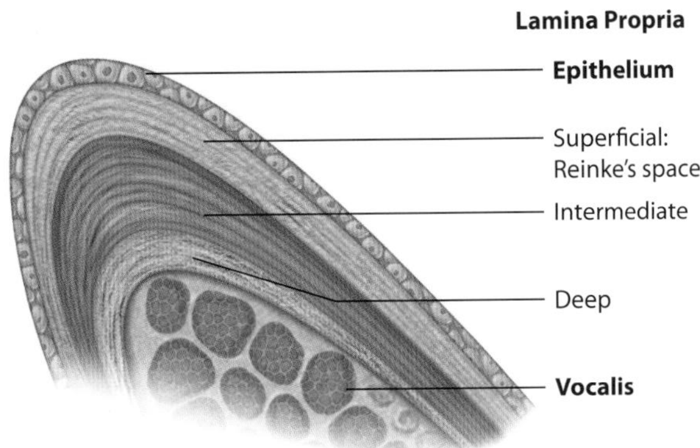

Figure 17.3 Layers of vocal cords.

LYMPHATIC DRAINAGE

The lymphatics of the larynx are separated by the vocal folds into an upper and lower group. The part of the larynx above the vocal folds is drained by vessels accompanying the superior laryngeal vein, whereas the zone below the vocal folds drains together with the inferior vein into the lower part of the deep cervical chain, often through the prelaryngeal and pretracheal nodes. The vocal folds are devoid of lymphatics.

NERVE SUPPLY

The larynx is supplied by branches of vagus nerve (superior and recurrent laryngeal nerves). The superior laryngeal nerve descends lateral to the pharynx, behind the internal carotid artery and at the level of the greater horn of hyoid bone, and divides into a small external laryngeal branch and a larger internal laryngeal nerve branch. The internal laryngeal nerve pierces the thyrohyoid membrane above the entrance of the superior laryngeal artery. The internal branch supplies general sensation, including pain, touch, and temperature, to all structures superior to the vocal folds. The external branch enters the cricothyroid muscle laterally on its deep surface. The external laryngeal nerve provides motor supply to the cricothyroid and inferior constrictor muscle.

RECURRENT LARYNGEAL NERVE

The recurrent laryngeal nerve (RLN) deserves special mention because the nerve takes different pathways on either side of the neck. The right RLN branches from the right vagus nerve in the neck, anterior to the right subclavian artery. It travels inferiorly and posterior to the subclavian artery to ascend in the neck between the trachea and the oesophagus (in the tracheoesophageal grove), behind the right common carotid artery.

The left RLN branch has a longer course because it arises from the left vagus nerve in the thorax. It loops around the arch of the aorta posterior to the liagamentum arteriosum before its ascent into the neck in the tracheoesophageal grove. The terminal portion of both RLNs passes superiorly, deep to the inferior border of the inferior pharyngeal constrictor muscle, just posterior to the cricothyroid joint.

ANATOMY OF THE PHARYNX

INTRODUCTION

The pharynx is a fibromuscular tube extending from the skull base to, and in continuity with, the oesophagus. It is divided into three parts defined by the openings on its anterior surface. These parts from superior to inferior are the nasopharynx opening into the nasal cavity, the oropharynx opening into the oral cavity and the laryngopharynx opening into the larynx. Posteriorly, the pharynx is in contact with the pre-vertebral fascia, the space between the two allowing free movement during swallowing and also a plane for infection to extend to the posterior mediastinum.

The function of the pharynx is to support breathing and swallowing, and to effectively and safely separate the two. It is made up of four curved sheets overlapping posteriorly and sitting inside each other like stacked beakers. The superior most sheet is the pharyngobasilar fascia, and below this lie superior, middle and inferior constrictor muscles.

THE NASOPHARYNX

This part of the pharynx extends from the skull base to the soft palate and communicates with the nose anteriorly through the posterior choanae. In its posterior wall is a collection of lymphoid tissue, the pharyngeal tonsil or adenoids. On the lateral wall is the opening of the auditory (eustachian) tube, which is surrounded superiorly, posteriorly and inferiorly by a prominent ridge, the torus, formed by the medial end of the cartilaginous auditory tube. Posterior to this is a slit-like space, which is the fossa of Rosenmuller.

THE OROPHARYNX

The oropharynx extends from the soft palate to the upper border of the epiglottis. It communicates anteriorly with the oral cavity. At this junction laterally lie the palatine tonsils, surrounded anteriorly and posteriorly by mucosal folds overlying the palatoglossus and the palatopharyngeus muscles, respectively.

The palatine tonsil has anterior and posterior borders and an upper and lower pole. Its medial surface is covered with pharyngeal mucosa and has up to 20 crypts. Its lateral surface is covered by a thickening in the submucosa, the tonsillar capsule, which lies on the superior constrictor muscle. The blood supply of the palatine tonsil is from the tonsillar branch of the facial artery, which pierces the superior constrictor. There are smaller contributions from branches of the lingual, the ascending pharyngeal and the ascending palatine arteries. The venous drainage is via a venous plexus that pierces the superior constrictor muscle.

THE LARYNGO-PHARYNX

This extends from the superior part of the epiglottis to the cricoid cartilage, where it becomes continuous with the oesophagus. At either side of the epiglottis the lateral glossoepiglottic folds separate it from the oropharynx. Below these folds lie the piriform fossae, which sit lateral to the quadrangular cartilage of the larynx and medial to the internal surface of the thyroid cartilage inferiorly and the thyrohyoid membrane superiorly. The piriform fossae narrow inferiorly and are connected by the post-cricoid area. This area is known clinically as the hypopharynx.

THE PHARYNGOBASILAR FASCIA

The pharyngobasilar fascia is a dense, fibrous thickening of the submucosa filling the gap between the skull base and the superior constrictor muscle. The stiffness of this fascia maintains the patency of the nasopharynx during breathing.

In the midline posteriorly running the length of the pharynx is the pharyngeal raphe. This receives fibres from all the constrictor muscles and attaches to the pharyngeal tubercle on the clivus. The attachment of the pharygobasilar fascia then passes laterally and anteriorly over the foramen lacerum to just in front of the carotid canal. It then leaves its bony attachment and is attached to the cartilaginous portion of the auditory tube before attaching to the posterior border of the medial pterygoid plate to the hamulus.

The inferior edge of the pharyngobasilar fascia is at the level of the hard palate within the superior constrictor muscle and is visible as Passavant's ridge as this muscle constricts during swallowing. Passavant's ridge allows the soft palate to more effectively close the nasopharynx during swallowing and prevent nasopharygeal regurgitation.

THE SUPERIOR CONSTRICTOR MUSCLE

The superior constrictor lies outside the pharyngobasilar fascia, sharing its attachment to the medial pterygoid plate. At the hamulus the superior constrictor attachment continues inferiorly along the pterygomandibular raphe to the mandible at the posterior end of the mylohyoid line level with the border of the last molar. Attachment to this raphe is shared by the buccinator muscle, which extends anteriorly, whilst the superior constrictor extends posteriorly.

As with the other constrictor muscles, the fibres of the superior constrictor extend around the pharynx to join in the midline at the pharyngeal raphe. Most of the superior constrictor fibres extend upwards, but the muscle is present as low as the level of the vocal cords within the middle constrictor muscle.

THE MIDDLE CONSTRICTOR MUSCLE

The middle constrictor arises from the lower third of the stylohyoid ligament. As this ligament attaches to the lesser cornu of the hyoid bone, the middle constrictor attachment extends along the superior surface of the greater cornu of the hyoid bone. The fibres again extend posteriorly to meet at the pharyngeal raphe, diverging widely. The uppermost fibres of the middle constrictor can completely enclose the superior constrictor muscle, and inferiorly fibres again extend as far as the vocal cords.

The space between the superior and middle constrictor muscles is filled by the tongue base. Passing through this space are the structures that pass from outside the pharynx to the oral cavity, the stylopharyngeus muscle and the glossopharyngeal and lingual nerves.

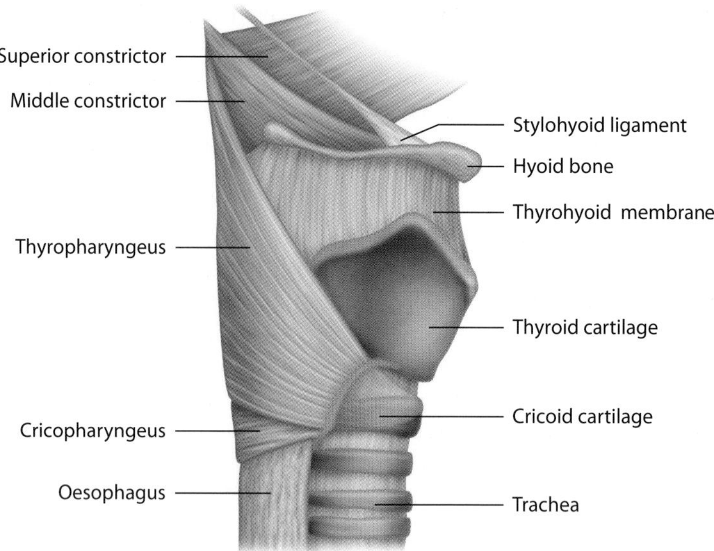

Figure 17.4 The pharyngeal constrictors from the right.

THE INFERIOR CONSTRICTOR MUSCLE

The inferior constrictor is split into two parts (Figure 17.4).

The thyropharyngeus arises from the oblique line on the thyroid lamina and inferior to this from a fibrous arch overlying the cricorthyroid muscle, ending at the inferior border of the cricoid cartilage. Its fibres diverge widely as it passes backwards enclosing the middle and superior constrictor muscles to the pharyngeal raphe. The thyropharyngeus fibres extend superiorly almost to the level of the pharyngeal tubercle. The inferior fibres travel horizontally with the superior edge of the cricopharyngeus muscle. The gap between the middle constrictor muscle and the thyropharyngeus muscle is closed by the thyrohyoid membrane. Passing through this gap are the internal branch of the superior laryngeal nerve and the superior laryngeal vessels.

Whilst the other constrictor muscles are flat sheets of muscle, the cricopharyngeus muscle is rounder and thicker and extends fully around the pharynx without joining the pharyngeal raphe. It is in continuity inferiorly with the circular muscular layer of the oesophagus and acts as a sphincter between the lowest extent of the pharynx and the upper oesophagus. This sphincter remains closed except during swallowing, which prevents air from being sucked into the oesophagus during inhalation. The cricopharyngeus muscle may be supplied by the recurrent laryngeal nerve or the external laryngeal nerve directly rather than from the pharyngeal plexus.

The area posteriorly between the superior border of the cricopharyngeus muscle and the inferior border of the thyropharyngeus muscle is known as Killian's dehiscence and is a potential weakness in the pharyngeal wall. Through this pharyngeal mucosa can herniate, causing a pharyngeal pouch.

OTHER FEATURES OF THE PHARYNX

The soft palate

The soft palate is a mobile fold of muscle and mucosa attached to the posterior edge of the hard palate and fused with the pharynx laterally. It can be raised and lowered and closes the nasopharynx during swallowing.

The soft palate is made up of an aponeurosis, which is acted on by five paired muscles. Much of the bulk of the soft palate is made up by the mucous membrane and associated minor salivary glands.

The tensor palati is a triangular muscle attaching to the scaphoid fossa on the medial pterygoid plate, the lateral edge of the auditory tube and the spine of the sphenoid. From this broad insertion the muscle comes together as a tendon at the pterygoid hamulus, where it turns at a right angle and enters the pharynx. The tendon now broadens out, forming the aponeurosis of the soft palate attached anteriorly to the crest of the palatine bone and blending in the midline. The aponeurosis is concave towards the mouth so that when the tensor palati contracts, the soft palate is flattened inferiorly. Because this muscle attaches to the auditory tube, contraction also pulls on this structure, opening it and allowing equalization of pressure between the nasopharynx and the middle ear.

The levator palati muscle is a round muscle arising at the quadrate area of the petrous bone and the adjacent medial side of the cartilaginous auditory tube. It inserts onto the nasal surface of the aponeurosis between the two heads of the palatopharyngeus. Contraction of this muscle pulls the soft palate upwards and posteriorly and again opens the auditory tube.

The palatoglossus arises from the inferior surface of the aponeurosis and passes downwards to interdigitate with the styloglossus. This muscle forms the anterior tonsillar pillar and delineates the junction between the oral cavity and the oropharynx.

The palatopharyngeus arises from two heads, one attached to the hard palate and one on the aponeurosis on either side of the levator palati muscle. The two heads fuse and head inferiorly, forming the posterior pillar of the tonsil, and insert into the posterior border of the thyroid lamina passing deep to the constrictors.

Other muscles

The salpingopharyngeus muscle is a thin muscle arising from the lower part of the cartilaginous auditory tube and passes inferiorly to blend with the palatopharyngeus muscle.

The stylopharyngeus muscle arises from the styloid process and inserts into the posterior border of the thyroid lamina. This muscle is supplied by the glossopharyngeal nerve directly and not the pharyngeal plexus.

NEUROVASCULAR SUPPLY OF THE PHARYNX

Blood is supplied by many arteries to the pharynx including the ascending pharyngeal, lingual, tonsillar, greater palatine and superior and inferior laryngeal arteries. Venous drainage is into the venous pharyngeal plexus at the back of the middle constrictor, which drains into the pterygoid plexus and the internal jugular vein.

The motor supply of the pharynx is from the pharyngeal plexus lying on the posterolateral wall of the pharynx and is made up by branches of the vagus and glossopharyngeal nerves and the cervical sympathetic trunk. Sensory supply of the nasopharynx is from the pharyngeal branch of the maxillary nerve, and the sensory supply of the oropharynx is from the glossopharyngeal nerve other than the vallecula, which is supplied by the internal branch of the superior laryngeal nerve. The rest of the pharyngeal mucosa is supplied by the internal branch of the superior laryngeal nerve and the recurrent laryngeal nerve.

KEY LEARNING POINTS

- The laryngeal structures develop from the 4th and 6th branchial arches and carry their nerve supply.
- The adult larynx is at the level of C3-C6 vertebrae.
- The subsites and spaces of the larynx are important.
- The boundaries of nasopharynx, oropharynx and hypopharynx are well defined.

18

Investigation of pharyngeal disease

NIMESH PATEL

Pharyngeal diseases are common. The challenge is to distinguish between those with benign disease and those with serious conditions without over-investigating the former.

Sore throat or pain in the throat is common. Frequently, this will be due to viral pharyngitis or tonsillitis, but unilateral symptoms should alert one to focal and possibly more serious disease. Persistence beyond a period that would be expected for common infections also warrants attention/concern (4 weeks is a sensible time point). Pain originating from the tonsil will be made worse by swallowing and may be referred to the ear because the glossopharyngeal nerve supplies both sites. Persistent pain and trismus suggest either quinsy or spread of an oropharyngeal tumour to the pterygoid muscles.

'True' dysphagia is a real difficulty in swallowing food or drink. These may come back into the mouth or 'go down' slowly. There may be an inability to swallow certain foodstuffs, for example lumps of meat. The patient may lose weight. Swallowing may progressively deteriorate. Carcinoma of the hypopharynx and oesophagus need to be excluded.

A sensation of a lump in the throat is a very frequent complaint. This may be an early symptom of cancer but is more commonly due to other things, including cricopharyngeal spasm, oesophageal dysmotility, pharyngeal pouch, laryngopharyngeal reflux and external compression from a thyroid goitre or globus pharyngeus. The last is a functional condition in which there is no true dysphagia.

Swallowing may be difficult due to pain. Painful swallowing (odynophagia) is most commonly caused by tonsillar infections but can be a symptom of cancers of the pharynx.

Regurgitation, especially of recently eaten but undigested food, suggests a pharyngeal pouch.

The speech may be altered. Large swellings of the hypopharynx or oropharynx will muffle speech, and large nasopharyngeal masses will result in hyponasality with obstruction of the choanae and pushing down of the soft palate.

Nasopharyngeal lesions can present with nasal obstruction and epistaxis. Furthermore, invasion of the skull base by a nasopharyngeal tumour can result in cranial nerve palsies presenting as diplopia, facial pain, uncoordinated swallowing, hypernasality from a paralyzed palate and dysphonia from a paralyzed vocal fold. Conductive hearing loss can result from glue ear secondary to nasopharyngeal disease.

EXAMINATION

NASOPHARYNX

Although previously examined with a nasopharyngeal mirror, the nasopharynx should be examined with a rigid nasal endoscope (or fibre-optic nasolaryngopharyngoscope). These modern instruments consistently provide an illuminated, magnified and detailed view. All areas should be assessed including the eustachian tube orifices, the fossae of Rosenmuller, the roof of the nasopharynx and the posterior nasal choanae.

OROPHARYNX

A tongue depressor should allow a good view of the tonsils, fauces, soft palate and posterior pharyngeal wall; all should be systematically examined. The tongue base and vallecula should be assessed with a laryngeal mirror with the tongue held forward or specifically examined during fibre-optic nasolaryngopharyngoscopy.

The lateral oropharynx and the base of the tongue should be palpated, because oropharyngeal tumours can arise deep within tonsillar crypts and present at the surface late.

HYPOPHARYNX

The hypopharynx may be examined with a mirror but should also be examined with a fibre-optic nasolaryngopharyngoscope. Topical local anaesthesia and/or decongestion of the nose may or may not be used. The evidence base for the use of these is not strong. However, in the very sensitive patient or the patient with a congested nose, topical decongestant and local anaesthesia should be used.

NECK

The neck should be palpated in a systematic and thorough manner (see Chapter 36). Any lumps need to be described carefully, including documentation of position, size, number, distribution and fixation. Description of fixation should include an assessment of what the lump is fixed to, because fixation does not always indicate inoperability. Position and distribution may be stated using the nomenclature of anatomical triangles of the neck or, for malignant nodes, the nomenclature of levels (see Chapter 36).

Nodal distribution can give clues to the diagnosis or the source of primary pathology. For example, posterior triangle lymph nodes are often enlarged in viral illness, including mononucleosis and toxoplasmosis. Supraclavicular lymphadenopathy can be present in gastro-intestinal, lung and breast disease.

The larynx will move on swallowing, and the laryngeal cartilages should be palpated and mobility assessed. Thyroid enlargement will present as a low neck mass that moves upon swallowing.

OTHER AREAS

The larynx must be examined during nasolaryngopharyngoscopy with clear documentation of airway patency and vocal cord paralysis. The latter can occur with hypopharyngeal tumours (due to direct laryngeal invasion or nerve involvement in the neck) or nasopharyngeal tumours (nerve involvement at the skull base).

The eardrums should be examined for evidence of otitis media and other causes of referred pain. Tuning fork tests and audiometry may be helpful.

Horner's syndrome and trismus suggest extrapharyngeal tumour spread.

INVESTIGATIONS

PLAIN RADIOGRAPHY

Plain film of the nasopharynx

This is an investigation to assess the soft tissues of the nasopharynx, in particular the size of the adenoid pad. It is rarely used now because the nasopharynx is readily examined with a nasendoscope, and even in children a paediatric nasolaryngoscope will afford an excellent view.

Plain film of the lateral soft tissues of the neck

This is a useful investigation to examine the hypopharynx especially. It is used to look for foreign bodies (beware as many are unfortunately radiolucent), free air in the soft tissues suggesting a tear in the pharynx or soft tissue swelling, as with retropharyngeal collections. If the pre-vertebral soft tissues are greater than the diameter of a vertebra, this is abnormal.

Plain postero-anterior chest x-ray

This study is useful to investigate for pulmonary metastasis or the presence of tuberculosis.

Plain mandibular film and orthopantomogram (OPG)

These studies will show invasion of the mandible in advanced tonsillar cancer; however, computed tomography (CT) and magnetic resonance imaging (MRI) are better for this. Both films are useful in planning osteotomies, and the OPG is especially useful for assessing dental health prior to radiotherapy.

CONTRAST FILMS

Barium swallow

Barium swallow will show strictures, sinuses and pharyngeal pouches. It is imperfect for mucosal lesions and examining the oropharynx. If the results are normal and clinical concern remains, a panendoscopy needs to be considered. Water-soluble contrast is used if a pharyngo-oeosophageal perforation is suspected.

Video swallow (fluoroscopy)

This is a contrast swallow taken with a greater number of frames per second (typically 30 frames per second) than the barium swallow (less than 5 frames per second). Also, the patient may be given modified consistencies of food, such as bread coated in barium, to swallow. The study can be conducted in conjunction with a speech therapist, who may ask the patient to swallow with modified techniques. Therefore, the video swallow is a technique to investigate swallowing function and can be in part a therapeutic procedure through its use in video feedback. It can be useful after laryngectomy to investigate poor voice after surgical voice rehabilitation.

SCANNING

Ultrasound scanning

Ultrasound scanning is essential for any neck lump and is usually used to guide fine-needle aspiration for cytology.

CT scanning

CT scanning is useful for assessment of pharyngeal primary pathology including malignancy. It is better than ultrasound scanning to investigate parapharyngeal space lesions, including abscesses and tumours. CT is useful in assessing invasion of the mandible by oropharyngeal cancers. It is required for staging of neck lymphadenopathy in malignancy. Also, CT of the thorax has largely replaced bronchoscopy in the hunt for second (lung) primaries in head and neck cancer. It is important in the assessment of bony invasion and intracranial spread of nasopharyngeal cancers.

MRI

MRI is better than CT for examining the oropharynx; the tongue base especially benefits from its soft tissue definition. It can, however, be readily spoiled by motion artefact. MRI is important in identifying intracranial extension of nasopharyngeal cancer. It is essential in the investigation of primary parapharyngeal tumours and parapharyngeal spread of oropharyngeal cancers.

FUNCTIONAL ENDOSCOPIC EVALUATION OF SWALLOWING (FEES)

FEES is the assessment of swallowing with a fibre-optic nasolaryngopharyngoscope in place. The patient is given foodstuffs of different consistencies to swallow with the endoscope in place just beyond the soft palate. The test especially allows observation of aspiration and failure to clear foodstuffs (stasis and soiling). Different food consistencies and swallowing techniques can be tested to see if they affect the swallow. The examination can be watched by the patient in real time and used therapeutically through video feedback.

LABORATORY INVESTIGATIONS

A full blood count and erythrocyte sedimentation rate (ESR) can be helpful. In the severely septic patient, they can be used to monitor treatment response. In the well patient with overt infection, these tests are of questionable value. A Monospot should be requested in the young patient with a sore throat and malaise. If this is negative but symptoms are those typical for glandular fever, consider testing for toxoplasma, cytomegalovirus, brucella and human immunodeficiency virus (HIV).

If Paterson–Brown-Kelly syndrome is suspected, measuring only haemoglobin is insufficient. One should also test serum iron and iron-binding capacity.

For a patient with weight loss, one should test urea, electrolytes, serum proteins and thyroid function.

The Venereal Disease Research Laboratory (VDRL) test and the *Treponema pallidum* haemagglutination (TPHA) test may be indicated, especially in regions where syphilis is prevalent or in high-risk patients.

ENDOSCOPY AND TISSUE DIAGNOSIS

PANENDOSCOPY

This is a comprehensive examination of the upper aerodigestive tract under general anaesthesia. It offers the particular advantages of a thorough, bimanual palpation.

TRANSNASAL OESOPHAGOSCOPY

This is a fibre-optic outpatient technique performed under local anaesthesia. The fine endoscope has a side channel to allow insufflation of air and biopsy forceps. The technique shows promise especially in outpatient investigation of the patient with a sensation of a lump in the throat. However, to allow adequate visualization of the hypopharynx, high-speed video must be taken and reviewed in slow motion.

Nasopharynx

This may be performed under local anaesthesia, but often lesions bleed, and local anaesthesia is difficult to achieve adequately in this area.

Under general anaesthesia, the area should be palpated. Following this, the nasopharynx may be examined with Jacques catheters to hold the soft palate out of the way and a laryngeal mirror passed through the mouth.

A better assessment may be made with a rigid nasendoscope through the decongested nose followed by biopsy. If no lesion is seen, then random (not blind) biopsy specimens should be taken from the fossae of Rosenmuller and the midline. This is important to do in the presence of unilateral glue ear.

If a juvenile angiofibroma is suspected, the mass should not be biopsied. Radiological investigations should be able to secure this diagnosis.

Oropharynx

As part of panendoscopy, the oropharyngeal tumour should be assessed both visually and, more important, by palpation. Good representative samples should be taken from the centre of the ulcer or mass, not just the edge.

Hypopharynx

Again, this should be investigated as part of panendoscopy because the oesophagogastroscope gas insufflation technique rarely allows adequate distension of the organ and a proper assessment. The upper and lower limits of a lesion need to be defined as well as fixation.

KEY LEARNING POINTS

- History and examination aid the choice of investigations.
- Barium swallow and video fluoroscopy help define the integrity of the oesophagus and the swallowing function.
- Functional endoscopic evaluation of swallowing allows assessment of swallowing in real time.
- Transnasal oesophagoscopy can be done as an office procedure.

FURTHER READING

Branstetter IV BF. *Diagnostic Imaging of the Pharynx and Esophagus*. In: *Cummings Otolaryngology – Head and Neck Surgery*. 5th ed., Vol. 2. Ed. Flint PW, et al. Philadelphia: Mosby Elsevier, 2010: 1393–1420.

19

Benign disease of the pharynx

STEPHEN R ELL

INTRODUCTION

This chapter covers laryngo-pharyngeal (silent or airway) reflux and globus syndrome (globus pharyngeus or globus pharyngis), Eagle syndrome, pemphigus and pemphigoid and Castleman disease. Many other benign conditions that affect the pharynx are covered in other chapters, including benign pharyngeal tumours, infections, dysphagia, pharyngeal pouch, snoring, obstructive sleep apnoea in both adults and children and choanal atresia.

The pharynx is divided into three parts, like a stack of three bottomless paper cups with one side missing, each of which opens anteriorly towards the nose, mouth and larynx – called, respectively, the nasopharynx, the oropharynx and the hypopharynx (laryngo-pharynx). Because the pharynx is a conduit, conditions that affect the nose and mouth tend also to affect the naso- and oropharynx; similarly, the hypopharynx may be affected by both oropharyngeal and oesophageal conditions.

LARYNGO-PHARYNGEAL (AIRWAY) REFLUX

DEFINITIONS

Reflux affecting the pharynx may be divided into two types, which may occur separately or together. First is classic gastro-oesophageal reflux disease (GORD), in which a tidal wave of stomach fluid is regurgitated up the oesophagus. Second is laryngo-pharyngeal reflux (LPR), also known as 'airway' or 'silent' reflux, in which a mist of gastric fluid drifts around the upper aerodigestive tract affecting the pharynx, larynx, lungs, eustachian tubes and middle ear. This type is the main subject of this section.

PATHOLOGY

GORD is mainly acid mediated, hence the term *acid reflux*; however, there are many other active components of gastric fluid, which include duodenal reflux at the pylorus and which may reach as high as the laryno- and oropharynx. The refluxate is cleared swiftly by peristalsis, and acid is neutralized by bicarbonate in saliva. GORD may be associated with hiatus hernias and Barrett's oesophagus.

LPR is mainly pepsin mediated, and episodes may be non-acidic as well as acidic or weakly acidic. Each droplet of mist contains not only hydrochloric acid but also proteolytic enzymes, mainly gastric pepsins, and pancreatic trypsin and chymotrypsin, bacteria and bile salts, which all affect the upper airway mucosa adversely. Droplets of mist landing on the upper airway mucosa release acid, proteolytic enzymes and bile salts, inflaming the surface. Though the acid may be partly buffered by mucus secretion, the pepsin and bile salts remain in contact with the surface mucosa.

In the stomach, pepsinogen is activated to pepsin by acidic conditions below pH 4, but pepsin remains active up to pH 6.5 and is irreversibly deactivated only above pH 8. Pepsin may bind to upper aerodigestive mucosal surfaces but can also enter cells by receptor mediated endocytosis and is held within the cells in vesicles. Gradually, it becomes less active in a neutral pH but can be reactivated by further reflux or ingested acids (vinegar, citrus fruits and some fizzy drinks), and the cells autodigest.

In addition, a reduction in gastric acid secretion, perhaps after distal gastrectomy or treatment with proton pump inhibitors (PPIs), allows an increase in gastric bacteria that can unconjugate bile acids. Free bile acids weaken the lipid components of the lipoprotein membrane of upper aerodigestive mucosa cells more than conjugated bile acids, and the overall result is mucosal inflammation. Also, pancreatic trypsin from pyloric refluxate, which is active between pH 6 and pH 10, may have a greater effect in LPR in these circumstances.

There is also an up-regulation of the cough reflex receptors, both in number and in sensitivity, to clear this gastric mist, which results in greater sensitivity to mild irritants such as heavy perfume or cigarette smoke.

HISTORY

All chambers of the pharynx are affected, and the symptoms may be understood from the protective reactions of the mucosa. The Reflux Symptom Index (RSI) is a commonly used questionnaire, completed by the patient, that is useful for diagnosis and subsequent monitoring of treatment.

The nasopharynx responds by producing excess thickened mucus, which characteristically is clear and is described by the patient as a continual post-nasal drip or catarrh. Nasal mucosal oedema may be associated with nasal blockage. Sneezing may be a feature but is unrelated to a specific allergen.

The oropharynx becomes more sensitive, and patients may describe various symptoms such as a foul taste and a tickly throat (like a hair laid over the tonsils), an inconsistent mobile foreign body sensation that may move about the oropharynx, or a feeling of a lump located high in the throat. There may also be a general soreness of the throat.

The laryngo-pharynx produces excess mucus, though mucus from above may also gather here.

There may be increased tonicity of the upper oesophageal sphincter, at the level of the crico-pharyngeus muscle, so that swallowing saliva or liquids, in particular, may fail to relax the muscles completely, giving rise to a globus sensation.

Laryngeal symptoms due to LPR are important because the laryngeal respiratory mucosa is less able to tolerate acid, proteolytic enzymes and bile acids. Patients may complain of constant throat clearing of excess mucus, choking and coughing, even cough syncope, and also wheeziness; they may have been diagnosed with late-onset asthma. They may also present with dysphonia and difficulty in swallowing ('pseudodysphagia') but do not eat more slowly or exhibit weight loss or true odynophagia.

These symptoms of airway reflux may be exacerbated by talking, singing, jogging, circuit training, lying down or bending forwards after a large meal or playing a wind instrument. Smoking or drinking alcohol, or both, increase the propensity for airway reflux in those susceptible by reducing the tone of the lower oesophageal sphincter, delaying gastric emptying and increasing gastric secretion.

PAST MEDICAL HISTORY

Laryngo-pharyngeal reflux may be a factor in conditions such as 'sinusitis' with post-nasal drip, eustachian tube dysfunction, chronic sore throats, chronic laryngitis, 'brittle' asthma, chronic obstructive pulmonary disease (COPD) and chronic cough. These may be exacerbated if not caused by LPR, and it may be difficult to know if LPR is a small or large aetiological factor. A trial of anti-reflux treatment may reveal to what degree airway reflux is contributing to these conditions. If LPR is a significant part, its treatment will help prevent disease progression and allow disease-specific treatments to be more effective. The difficulty facing the clinician is how to unravel the contribution that LPR is making to the symptoms of patients who are wholly convinced that they have another disorder.

Oropharyngeal and laryngo-pharyngeal reflux may exacerbate the chronic inflammation associated with smoking, spirits, spices and sepsis. Airway reflux affecting the larynx, the trachea and the bronchi may present as chronic laryngitis or pulmonary disease, or both. Any sinister features require investigation to exclude sinister causes.

EXAMINATION

Clinical findings may be subtle and lack specificity, reflecting diffuse inflammation. Flexible nasopharyngeal laryngoscopy may reveal greater inflammation in the post-nasal space than in the nasal cavity, lingual tonsil hypertrophy, three-point inflammation of both arytenoids and the base of the epiglottis, inter-arytenoid oedema or posterior commissure hypertrophy, and a pseudosulcus of the vocal cords associated with vocal cord oedema. Rarely, pyogenic granulomas, either unilateral or bilateral, may form on the mucosa over the vocal process of the arytenoid. These are associated with coughing and, if they are large, inspiratory stridor due to obstruction of the laryngeal inlet. Intralaryngeal mucus is thick, and there may be obliteration of the ventricles. The Reflux Finding Score (RFS) is a record of the examination findings and is a useful instrument aiding diagnosis and monitoring treatment.

Findings not specific to LPR may also be variously associated with inhaled irritants, smoking and alcohol consumption, voice abuse, viral infections and allergy.

INVESTIGATIONS

Most patients are diagnosed clinically and do not require further investigations. Specific features of the history and examination suggesting other diagnoses warrant appropriate investigation. For LPR, a trial of treatment, as a clinical trial of one, will help establish the diagnosis, or, in complicated cases, will give the clinician a measure of the contribution of LPR to the patient's symptoms.

A contrast swallow is no longer used as a routine test for pure LPR but may be of value in patients with dysphagia or odynophagia and may reveal a pharyngeal pouch, oesophageal dysmotility, strictures or Schatzki rings. Some ear, nose and throat (ENT) departments have access to transnasal oesophagoscopy (TNO), which allows more accurate assessment of the oesophagus for a hiatus hernia or Barrett's oesophagus at the first visit and appropriate onward referral to upper gastro-intestinal (GI) surgeons or gastroenterologists. Otherwise, when there is associated GORD, oesophago-gastro-duodenoscopy (OGD) may be requested.

The gold standard investigation is 24-hour, dual-channel pH monitoring, with or without impedance, with electrodes placed just above the lower sphincter and at the upper sphincter to capture both GORD and LPR. Some consider any reflux reaching the upper oesophageal sphincter as abnormal, whereas others consider four or more episodes in 24 hours abnormal. The addition of multichannel intraluminal impedance (MCII) picks up weakly acidic and non-acidic events, improving diagnostic accuracy; only 25 per cent of pharyngeal reflux episodes are acidic. These investigations, however, are invasive, are not well tolerated and may not be readily available. Monitoring of the upper airway pH to detect aerosolized reflux via a minimally invasive probe is now possible (ResTech, Respiratory Technology Corporation, San Diego, CA, USA), making an accurate pH diagnosis accessible. Pharyngeal secretions can be tested for pepsin (Peptest, RD Biomed Limited, Hull, UK) and, if detected, LPR is highly likely. Patients with cough-related LPR who test positive for *Helicobacter pylori* improve after successful *Helicobacter* eradication.

TREATMENT

There are three aspects of treatment: all patients require dietary and lifestyle advice, many require medical treatment and a few require surgery.

Dietary and lifestyle changes can be summarized in an advice sheet and should include the avoidance of fatty foods (anything fried, chips, crisps, pastry and even chocolate), the avoidance of fizzy drinks and fruit juices, and not eating between meals. Smoking and alcohol, particularly spirits and wine, should be avoided. If symptoms are worse lying down, propping up the head of the bed and lying on the left side reduces reflux, and not eating within 3 hours of lying down is beneficial. Jogging, circuit training, obesity and tight clothing exacerbate symptoms; therefore, light exercise, dieting and loose clothing are beneficial. A session with a trained speech and language therapist (SLT) improves compliance.

Medical treatment for LPR consists of liquid alginate preparations, e.g. Gaviscon Advance (Reckitt Benckiser, Hull, UK), which is effective in controlling symptoms, either alone or with a proton pump inhibitor (PPI). Alginates are non-systemic and can be used in reflux associated with pregnancy. PPIs work indirectly, reducing the activation of pepsin, since, at present, there are no drugs to oppose pepsin.

For mild symptoms, the dose for Gaviscon Advance is 5 mL three times a day after meals and 10 mL last thing at night, after which the patient should be nil by mouth until morning. For moderate symptoms, a low-dose PPI should be added, taken twice a day half an hour before meals, to block gastric secretions, since all PPIs last for 12–14 hours. For severe symptoms, the PPI dose may be doubled. H_2 antagonists are less effective but may have a role at night for those with nocturnal acid breakthrough despite higher dose PPIs. Not all patients respond to the same PPI, and it is worth trying another if the first PPI fails to help.

Treatment should continue for 2 to 3 months before its benefit is assessed. Most patients require 6 months' treatment before the PPI can be gradually reduced, to avoid acid rebound. Liquid alginates can help control rebound symptoms after the PPI has been withdrawn. Since liquid alginate coats the oesophagus and forms a raft over the stomach contents, reducing gastric mist formation, the mucosa is protected, especially during sleep. Should reflux occur, there is a greater chance of the refluxate being alginate rather than gastric secretions.

Most patients can manage their symptoms in the long term by lifestyle and dietary modification, perhaps with a liquid alginate at night, but for a restaurant meal with wine, an occasional PPI is required.

For the few who fail to respond in whom 24-hour dual-channel pH (+/- MCII) monitoring confirms LPR, laparoscopic fundoplication can be effective.

REFLUX IN CHILDREN

Reflux in children is an important part of paediatric practice, and LPR has been thought to be wholly or partly responsible for childhood sinusitis, otitis media with effusion, recurrent croup and laryngomalacia. LPR, if not recognized and treated, may make laryngeal papillomatosis worse, and airway reconstructions for subglottic stenosis do badly.

GLOBUS SYNDROME (GLOBUS PHARYNGEUS, GLOBUS PHARYNGIS)

INTRODUCTION

Patients with globus syndrome complain of a feeling of a lump in the throat (FOLIT) brought on or made worse by anxiety with no other organic cause, which makes it a diagnosis of exclusion. It can happen to anyone, even the most calm, given enough stress and is an example of somatization. It affects men and women equally over 50 years of age, though women are more likely to seek help. Women younger than 50 years of age are affected more than men. Stress from any source – family, social, education, employment, financial or psychological – is a feature of the history, but the often unvoiced fear of throat cancer heightens anxiety, exacerbating the symptoms. These issues have to be dealt with openly (but better at the end of the consultation) once rapport is established and alternative explanations given.

Globus may also be due to reduced mucosal sensation, since globus is often experienced after spraying the throat with local anaesthetic. Globus may also be a minor but significant feature of laryngo-pharyngeal reflux (LPR), oesophageal dysmotility and oesophagitis with crico-pharyngeal spasm, though strong evidence of this association is lacking.

HISTORY

Typically, the sensation of a lump is there 'all the time', though most often noticed when swallowing liquids including saliva (i.e. between meals) and less noticeable or absent when swallowing solid food. Patients may describe tightness, a pressure on the throat like 'being strangled', or the feeling of something stuck, like a 'flap of skin', 'a hair', or a 'blob of phlegm'. The sensation may move from front to back or from side to side, is better on some days and worse on others, may vary during the day, is often worse in the evening and is not progressive. There is no odynophagia. Although there is 'pseudodysphagia' – the feeling of difficulty in swallowing – there is no true dysphagia; patients do not eat more slowly than before and there is no unexplained weight loss. Symptoms of reflux may be a feature. Asking about the intensity of recent stress is important. In patients with true globus, excessive smoking or alcohol consumption is not usually a feature; however, if the 'globus' is constant, progressive and painful, especially on swallowing, and associated with a past history of carcinogen consumption, consider a sinister cause.

EXAMINATION

Look for signs of anaemia, angular cheilitis, glossitis and koilonychia. Examination of the midline neck viscera is often unremarkable; if there are any remarkable features, consider another diagnosis. Nasopharyngeal laryngoscopy (NPL), with particular attention to the pyriform fossae, is essential and may reveal signs of reflux. Palpation of the neck may reveal some tenderness of the laryngeal muscles but no lymphadenopathy. TNO is a small step for ENT surgeons, who are used to nasopharyngeal laryngoscopy, but a giant leap in the management of pharyngeal disease, especially globus and LPR. The use of a video camera to show the patient the beauty of the pharynx is greatly reassuring and obviates the need for a barium swallow.

DIFFERENTIAL DIAGNOSIS

Globus may be associated with contact between a hypertrophied tongue base, the uvula and a curled epiglottis; heterotopic gastric mucosa; thyroid enlargement; rare benign or malignant tumours of the pharynx; excessive tension; and Eagle's syndrome (long styloid process). Cervical osteophytes at C5–C6 have also been implicated. Globus may also be a feature of GORD and associated with oesophagitis and cricopharyngeal spasm.

LPR may also present as globus, though there are usually other features. It is extremely rare, but not impossible, for carcinoma to present as a globus syndrome, though there are usually other clinical features that cause alarm and warrant further investigation.

INVESTIGATIONS

A full blood count may reveal the iron deficiency anaemia of Paterson–Brown-Kelly (Plummer-Vinson) syndrome if there is also anaemia, koilonychia, glossitis and angular cheilitis. A diagnosis of classic globus requires no more investigation than a thorough ENT examination, including NPL and, if available, TNO: normal findings should reassure most patients. Further investigations of the oesophagus are warranted only if there are clinical features of an underlying cause, such as true dysphagia. If TNO is unavailable and there is a greater index of suspicion, e.g. classic globus but with a history of tobacco and alcohol consumption, referral for flexible OGD is appropriate. The post-cricoid area is difficult to visualize with endoscopy, and ENT surgeons traditionally request a barium swallow. A barium swallow is primarily a study of the oesophagus; unless requested specifically, the pharynx, especially the post-cricoid area, is poorly demonstrated, and reflux is missed in 40 per cent of cases. In globus it often shows nothing significant, exposes the patient to unnecessary radiation and excites futile interest in cervical osteophytes. If dysphagia is present, bringing the diagnosis of globus into question, then a barium swallow is indicated to exclude a pharyngeal pouch, extrinsic oesophageal compression, achalasia, stricture, hiatus hernia or carcinoma. When transnasal oesophagoscopy becomes widely available for ENT outpatients, the need for barium swallows and OGD will diminish, and alternate diagnoses may be referred to the appropriate specialist swiftly. Some ENT surgeons have access to TNO and multichannel intraluminal impedance/dual-probe pH monitoring; diagnose oesophagitis, Barrett's oesophagus and adenocarcinoma; and work closely with gastroenterologists and upper GI surgeons. Rigid oesophagoscopy under general anaesthetic to investigate globus barely justifies the risk of this procedure.

TREATMENT

A patient with classic globus syndrome may be reassured that the sensation will diminish as the stress diminishes, however, reassurance is often not enough. If transnasal oesophagoscopy is unavailable, a trial of anti-reflux treatment and lifestyle changes to treat reflux, with follow-up in 4 to 6 weeks, is reasonable, because 30 per cent of globus patients have reflux. Most ENT surgeons wait until review before considering further investigation, perhaps with OGD; if normal, the patient may be discharged to his or her general practitioner (GP).

EAGLE SYNDROME

PATHOLOGY

Eagle syndrome is a collection of symptoms due to the presence of a long styloid process or calcified stylohyoid ligament and is associated with irritation of the glossopharyngeal nerve (neural type) or compression of the extracranial internal carotid (vascular type). Rarely, benign nerve sheath tumours of the glossopharyngeal nerve may be responsible, and injury to the internal carotid may result in dissection, cerebrovascular events, or both. For perspective, about 4 per cent of people have an elongated styloid process greater than 30 mm (normal length is <25 mm), and between 4 and 10 per cent of these are symptomatic.

HISTORY

Eagle syndrome includes the elicitation of recurrent throat and ear pain on swallowing, turning the head, or extending the tongue, but it can present with a wide range of general head and neck symptoms that blur the finding of a specific diagnosis. Eagle syndrome should be considered when patients present with symptoms that could be related to head position. Symptoms usually include pain in the throat and the neck that ranges from mild discomfort or a bruised feeling to severe burning, throbbing pain, often associated headache, all of which may be worse after sleeping. The feeling of a lump in the throat and 'pseudodysphagia' may also be a feature of Eagle syndrome.

EXAMINATION

As part of a complete head and neck examination, it may be possible, after topical anaesthetic, to palpate the styloid through the tonsillar bed, and this may evoke symptoms. Some advocate injection of the tonsillar bed with local anaesthetic to confirm the diagnosis, but this carries the risk of injecting major vessels with serious consequences.

INVESTIGATION

Plain lateral and antero-posterior (AP) neck radiographs may be sufficient, though a computed tomography (CT) scan with 3D reconstruction provides optimal information.

TREATMENT

Treatment is surgical with reduction of the elongated styloid and calcified stylohyoid ligament via an external approach. Repair of the carotid artery may be required; discussion with a vascular surgeon is desirable before surgery in patients with the vascular type of Eagle syndrome. The external approach is preferred over the transpharyngeal approach because there is less risk of deep space neck infection and better visualization of the surgical field, particularly if the carotid requires attention.

PEMPHIGUS AND PEMPHIGOID

These blistering autoimmune conditions may affect the mucosa of the mouth and oropharynx before skin lesions appear and are due to cleavage within the epithelium. Think of the cleavage plane in pemphigus as superficial, i.e. within the epithelial layers, and in pemphigoid as deep, i.e. at the level of the basement membrane; then the pathology and clinical presentation will follow.

PEMPHIGUS VULGARIS

INTRODUCTION

Pemphigus vulgaris is a rare life-threatening autoimmune disorder of mucous membranes and skin, attacking the adhesion between epithelial cells. Most cases are idiopathic; however, an association with myasthenia gravis and thymoma has been reported, and a variety of drugs have been implicated in its induction, especially penicillamine, phenylbutazone, rifampin and captopril. It is also known to occur in association with a variety of internal malignancies (paraneoplastic pemphigus).

PATHOLOGY

The cleavage plane in pemphigus occurs above the basal layer of the epithelium, leaving a layer of basal cells with rounded tops, like tombstones. Above, in the intact serum-filled bulla, are a few sloughed rounded keratinocytes resembling fried eggs, with large hyperchromatic nuclei and a rim of eosinophilic cytoplasm, which are called Tzanck cells and can be seen in a smear from a fresh blister (the Tzanck test). Once ruptured, the remaining ulcer becomes slowly covered with fibrinoid necrotic debris and develops neovascularity, and mixed inflammatory cells infiltrate the underlying stroma. At the ulcer's edge, there is intraepithelial cleavage. Direct immunofluorescence of adjacent mucosa shows a lacy or chicken-wire pattern of immunoglobulin deposits around individual spinous epithelial cells that are mainly IgG, with some IgM and IgA.

CLINICAL

Pemphigus presents in patients between 50 and 70 years of age, in women more than men, and more frequently in Ashkenazi Jews. Of all cases of pemphigus, the mouth or oropharynx is the initial site in 75 per cent, and in 50 per cent it is the only site involved. Mucosal bullae are fragile, rupture swiftly and leave flat ulcers with epithelial tags along a thin red edge but no inflammatory halo. Unlike traumatic ulcers and aphthous ulcers, the base of a pemphigus ulcer is not concave, and there is significantly less pain. The bullae may be greater than 4 cm in diameter and can affect most of the oral mucosa. Blisters can be created by pressure or friction upon a normal-appearing area of mucosa (positive Nikolsky sign).

Bullae may present on any oral or oropharyngeal surface but typically arise in the buccal, palatal and gingival regions. In time skin blisters occur and remain intact much longer, becoming the major problem. Most patients have circulating autoantibodies detected by indirect immunofluorescence using serum from other affected individuals. Titres are directly proportionate to the severity of the disease.

DIFFERENTIAL DIAGNOSIS

Paraneoplastic pemphigus may occur in patients with internal malignancy, such as lymphoma, leukaemia, sarcoma and thymus tumours. Bullae may be severe, and they can resemble erythema multiforme or bullous lichen planus and be resistant to treatment. Waldenstrom's macroglobulinemia and Castleman disease have also been associated with pemphigus.

Small lesions may be mistaken for viral vesicles, e.g. herpes simplex, herpes zoster and Coxsackie viruses. The mucosal lesions of erythema multiforme may demonstrate intraepithelial or subepithelial blistering, or both, but this unique allergic response occurs in younger patients and has an abrupt onset and limited duration, separating it from pemphigus.

TREATMENT AND PROGNOSIS

Systemic corticosteroid therapy reduces or eliminates pemphigus vulgaris, although high doses (prednisone, 400 mg daily) may be needed. Oral or intravenous cyclophosphamide, azathioprine, cyclosporine and methotrexate may reduce the dose of corticosteroids required. Topical corticosteroids can be an adjunct if the bullae are confined to the mouth.

Almost 10 per cent of patients die from electrolyte loss, wound infection, or treatment complications. Patients with paraneoplastic pemphigus may be limited to supportive treatment until the underlying neoplasm is controlled.

MUCOUS MEMBRANE PEMPHIGOID

INTRODUCTION

Pharyngeal mucous membrane pemphigoid (benign mucous membrane pemphigoid or cicatricial [scar-forming] pemphigoid), is a bullous autoimmune disease attacking the subepithelial basement membrane. It affects mucosa, not only of the pharynx, but also of the mouth, larynx and eyes, where scar formation may lead to blindness.

CLINICAL FEATURES

This disease is characterized by bullous lesions of mucous membranes, presenting in patients between 40 and 60 years of age, initially with oral lesions, and is twice as common in women. Bullae develop slowly and are small and infrequent in early disease, but may eventually become large (>3 cm in diameter) and appear as clear or slightly bluish blisters without an inflammatory halo, though the mucosal region may be erythematous. A positive Nikolsky test (creation of a blister by pressure or friction) occurs in 10 per cent of patients. A ruptured blister leaves a shallow, mildly tender ulcer bed which heals in 7–10 days with scar formation.

PATHOLOGY

Lesions occur intermittently and may affect different parts of the mucosa at different times. Separation of the epithelium from the basement membrane forms a bulla; however, most are ruptured at the time of biopsy. Direct immunofluorescence shows a continuous linear apple green band along the basement membrane. More than 50 per cent of patients have circulating autoantibodies identified by indirect immunofluorescence.

DIFFERENTIAL DIAGNOSIS

Blistering of mucous membranes may also be seen in linear IgA disease, bullous lichen planus, epidermolysis bullosa (hereditary and acquired forms), bullosa haemorrhagica, erythema multiforme, bullous pemphigoid and dermatitis herpetiformis, and also with the use of lithium, vancomycin, diclofenac, and glibenclamide.

TREATMENT AND PROGNOSIS

Mucous membrane pemphigoid can often be controlled by immunosuppressive agents such as topical or systemic corticosteroids, or cyclophosphamide, but there is no cure. Blisters elsewhere in the upper aerodigestive tract are unusual, but patients with laryngeal or esophageal involvement will develop dysphagia or oesophageal webs. Ocular and skin involvement eventually occurs, and early referral to an ophthalmologist and a dermatologist is desirable.

CASTLEMAN DISEASE

Castleman disease may present in the pharynx as a parapharyngeal mass, enlarged tonsil, or neck node. It is a rare lymphoproliferative disorder and is not considered a cancer, but is associated with a higher risk of developing lymphoma. Also known as giant lymph node hyperplasia and angiofollicular lymph node hyperplasia, it may be localized (unicentric) or widespread (multicentric), which determines prognosis.

PATHOLOGY

The actual cause is unclear, though human herpes virus 8 (HHV-8) is associated with the multicentric type, but not the unicentric type. The same virus is associated with Kaposi's sarcoma, a cancer of the blood vessel walls, which is also common in people with multicentric Castleman disease. HHV-8 may cause an excess production of interleukin-6 (IL-6) within lymphatic cells, which reproduce rapidly leading to the clinical picture of Castleman disease. Those with HIV are more likely to have both Castleman disease and Kaposi's sarcoma.

Three subtypes are described on histology: hyaline vascular (80–90 per cent), plasma cell (10–20 per cent) and mixed (rare). Since there is a lack of specific clinical, biochemical, and radiological features, the diagnosis of Castleman disease is by histopathology.

CLINICAL

Most patients with unicentric Castleman disease are asymptomatic but notice an enlarged lymph node in the neck, axilla or groin. It may present with a parapharyngeal mass or an enlarged tonsil associated with unintended weight loss, cough and anaemia. The mean age at presentation is between 30 and 40 years.

Patients with multicentric Castleman disease usually develop fever, night sweats, loss of appetite, nausea and vomiting, unintended weight loss, weakness, fatigue, hepatospenomegaly, peripheral neuropathy and enlarged peripheral lymph nodes in the neck, the axilla and the groin. The mean age at presentation is between 50 and 60 years.

PROGNOSIS

Patients with unicentric Castleman disease do well once the affected lymph node is removed, though they may have an increased risk of lymphoma.

Multicentric Castleman disease is more serious and often life-threatening. Death is associated with serious infection, multiple organ failure, lymphoma or Kaposi's sarcoma. The prognosis is worse in the presence of HIV/AIDS.

KEY LEARNING POINTS

- LPR is associated with a mist of proteolytic enzymes and bile, not just hydrochloric acid.
- Globus syndrome should be a diagnosis of exclusion based on a balance of probabilities.
- Eagle syndrome may be neural or vascular and is best investigated by CT and treated surgically via an external procedure. Vascular surgical help may be needed.
- Pemphigus and pemphigoid may present in the mouth before skin lesions appear and may be paraneoplastic.
- Think of lymphoma, HIV and Kaposi's sarcoma before you think of Castleman disease.
- The RSI and RFS are useful diagnostic and monitoring instruments.

FURTHER READING

Belafsky PC, Postma GN, Koufman JA. Validity and reliability of the Reflux Symptom Index (RSI). *Journal of Voice*. 2002; 16: 274–77.

Belafsky PC, Postma GN, Koufman JA. Validity and reliability of the Reflux Finding Score (RFS). *Laryngoscope*. 2001; 111: 1313–17.

Bove MJ, Rosen C. Diagnosis and management of laryngopharyngeal reflux disease. *Current Opinion in Otolaryngology & Head and Neck Surgery*. 2006; 14: 124–27, 133–37, 143–49.

Ford CN. Evaluation and management of laryngopharyngeal reflux. *JAMA*. 2005; 294: 1534–40.

Jaume Bauza G, Tomas Barberan M, Epprecth Gonzalez P, Trobat Company F. The diagnosis and management of globus: a perspective from Spain. *Current Opinion in Otolaryngology & Head and Neck Surgery*. 2008; 16: 507–10.

Khalil HS. The diagnosis and management of globus: a perspective from the United Kingdom. *Current Opinion in Otolaryngology & Head and Neck Surgery*. 2008; 16: 516–20.

Murtagha RD, Caraccioloa JT, Fernandez G. CT findings associated with Eagle Syndrome. *American Journal of Neuroradiology*. 2001; 22: 1401–02.

Park W, Hicks DM, Khandwala F, et al. Laryngopharyngeal reflux: Prospective cohort study evaluating optimal dose of proton-pump inhibitor therapy and pre-therapy predictors of response. *Laryngoscope*. 2005; 115: 1230–38.

Rechtweg JS, Wax MK. Eagle's syndrome: A review. *American Journal of Otolaryngology*. 1998; 19: 316–21.

Remacle M. The diagnosis and management of globus: a perspective from Belgium. *Current Opinion in Otolaryngology & Head and Neck Surgery*. 2008; 16: 511–5.

Watson MG. What's new in LPR? *The Otolaryngologist*. 2011; 4(1): 21–27.

20

Infections of the pharynx

ANDREW ROBSON

SORE THROAT

Sore throat is a common condition that will be experienced by almost everyone at some stage in life. Most people do not consult their general practitioner about this, although when they do it may be as an introduction to other health-related problems.

Sore throat is not necessarily infectious in aetiology. Non-infectious causes include:

- Inhalation of dry air (mouth breathing)
- Exposure to irritants, e.g. occupational exposure, cigarette smoking
- As a sequela to endotracheal intubation and gastroscopy
- Laryngopharyngeal reflux disease
- Globus pharyngeus
- In association with functional dysphonia
- Pharyngeal and laryngeal cancer

It is important to consider non-infectious causes of sore throat in the differential diagnosis of pharyngitis so that the symptoms can be appropriately investigated and treated.

MANAGEMENT OF SORE THROAT

A careful history and examination may establish a diagnosis without recourse to special investigations. 'Red flags' should be sought (persistence, unilateral symptoms especially associated with otalgia, association with other symptoms, e.g. hoarseness and dysphagia). Symptoms associated with specific causes and their management will be discussed later in the chapter.

Causative factors, for example exposure to irritants, should be determined and avoided if possible. Patients who smoke should be advised to stop. Nasal disease and laryngopharyngeal reflux may need treating. Simple reassurance that there is no serious cause may help with some patients. Patients often 'throat clear' in a misguided attempt to relieve their symptoms, and this should be actively discouraged. Symptomatic relief of pharyngitis can be achieved by rest, drinking plenty of fluids, a soft diet and simple analgesics, for example paracetamol. Benzydamine mouthwashes may provide relief of symptoms. Antibiotics should be avoided unless specifically indicated.

INFECTIONS OF THE PHARYNX

Pharyngitis may be viral or bacterial in aetiology, with the former predominating. The most common viruses are rhinovirus, adenovirus, coxsackievirus, parainfluenza virus and coronavirus. Other important viruses include Epstein-Barr virus (EBV, causing infectious mononucleosis), human immune deficiency virus (HIV) and cytomegalovirus (CMV) (Table 20.1).

The most common bacterial pathogen is group A beta-haemolytic streptococcus (GABHS). This is a more common cause of sore throat in children (up to a third of cases) than in adults (approximately 10 per cent).

Table 20.1 Summary of rare pharyngeal infections

Infection	Presenting features	Management
Cytomegalovirus	Mononucleosis-type symptoms. Common opportunistic infection in immunocompromised patients. Pharyngitis and adenopathy less common than with EBV infection.	Supportive.
Toxoplasmosis	Protozoal infection latent in many healthy people. Mononucleosis-type symptoms. Common potentially severe opportunistic infection in immunocompromised patients. Sore throat and lymphadenopathy.	Supportive in immunocompetent patients.
Herpes simplex infection	More common in children. Vesicular stomatitis rarer in oropharynx than oral cavity. Malaise and lymphadenopathy.	Supportive. Aciclovir may be of benefit in severe infections.
Herpes zoster infection	Reactivation of latent virus in cranial nerve distribution. Transient tonsillar vesicles associated with Ramsey-Hunt syndrome. Pain on swallowing, shallow vesicles.	Supportive; may benefit from famciclovir.
Candida	Most commonly *Candida albicans*. More common in denture wearers, those undergoing antibiotic treatment, immunocompromised patients and following chemoradiotherapy. Sore burning mouth and pharynx, white patches on mucosa that can be scraped off, erythematous patches on mucosa. Acute or chronic.	Prevention. Topical and systemic antifungal treatment.
Syphilis	Rare. Primary syphilis may present with chancre (painless ulcer) on tonsil. Non-specific systemic symptoms in secondary syphilis with hyperaemic pharynx and snail track ulcers.	VDRL (Venereal Disease Research Laboratory) testing; penicillin.
Tuberculosis (TB)	Primary TB in children; focus in tonsil with cervical adenopathy. Secondary TB associated with pulmonary TB, often seen on posterior commissure, differential diagnosis of pharyngeal cancer. More common in immunocompromised patients.	Management as per pulmonary TB.

Pharyngeal infections are generally transmitted by close contact with droplet transmission, so outbreaks are often seen in people who have been in proximity with each other.

ACUTE TONSILLITIS

Acute tonsillitis remains a common condition. The incidence varies, which may reflect the pattern of referral in different parts of the world. It is predominantly a disease of children and young adults, although it may present at any age. There tend to be peaks in incidence between 5 and 7 years of age and in late teenage years, possibly due to people being exposed to new pathogens when starting school or when moving away from home.

Like all infective causes of sore throat, tonsillitis may be caused by viral or bacterial pathogens. Throat swabs are generally not helpful because the true pathogens lie in the crypts of the tonsil, and in general the management is not influenced by the result from a throat swab.

The clue to diagnosing acute tonsillitis lies in the history. Patients present with an acute onset of sore throat, malaise and fever, usually with tender cervical lymphadenopathy. They may experience referred otalgia. The symptoms are self-limiting and resolve within 5 to 7 days, after which they are symptom free. Patients with persistent, low-grade sore throat without systemic upset or lymphadenopathy do not have acute tonsillitis and will have another cause of pharyngitis that may be non-infective. On examination they will be pyrexial and often flushed. The tonsils will be red and inflamed, often with an associated exudate. There may be associated generalized pharyngitis. In the absence of a peri-tonsillar abscess (PTA, quinsy), patients will not have trismus. They are likely to have bilateral cervical lymphadenopathy, most pronounced when caused by EBV (infectious mononucleosis). When the tonsillitis is caused by GABHS or EBV, there may be associated petechial haemorrhage on the palate and, in the case of GABHS, a punctuate erythematous rash (scarlet fever rash). It is important to remember to perform a full systemic examination because the patient may be dehydrated, have coincidental disease or have hepatosplenomegaly (suggesting infectious mononucleosis) and generalized lymphadenopathy.

Some patients develop recurrent symptoms of tonsillitis leading to a significant amount of time off from school or work. It is unpredictable which group of patients will develop recurrent symptoms. Predisposing factors for sore throat, such as exposure to irritants and smoking, should be avoided.

The differential diagnosis of acute tonsillitis includes infective and non-infective pharyngitis as well as neoplasia. The presenting symptoms of neoplasia differ from acute tonsillitis with symptoms of unilateral progressive, persistent sore throat, often associated with unilateral cervical lymphadenopathy and otalgia. Neoplasia usually presents in an older age group than for those presenting with acute tonsillitis.

Tonsillitis should be treated in the same way as other causes of pharyngitis, with reassurance, rest and plenty of fluids. The role of antibiotics is controversial, with no good evidence that routine treatment with antibiotics leads to more rapid resolution of symptoms. In a patient who is clinically deteriorating, antibiotics may be prescribed. Penicilllin V is the first-line treatment in such cases. Most patients can be managed at home. The indications for hospital referral include dysphagia and the development of symptoms of respiratory obstruction. These patients will be managed with intravenous fluids and antibiotics. Ampicillin-based antibiotics should be avoided because a rash may develop if the tonsillitis is caused by EBV. The criteria for tonsillectomy are discussed later in the chapter.

Complications of acute tonsillitis

PERITONSILLAR ABSCESS

The most common complication of acute tonsillitis is PTA, or quinsy. This is a collection of pus between the tonsil capsule and the superior pharyngeal constrictor. The causative organism is usually beta-haemolytic streptococcus, although anaerobic organisms are quite common, especially in the presence of periodontal disease. PTAs are rare in children. They are almost always unilateral.

A PTA presents on a background of acute tonsillitis that instead of resolving becomes worse. Patients complain of worsening sore throat, dysphagia and drooling of saliva. The symptoms lateralize to one side, and patients may complain of referred otalgia. On examination the patient will be unwell and may be dehydrated. The patient will usually have trismus (caused by spasm of the medial pterygoid muscle due to contact with pus) as well as unilateral cervical lymphadenopathy. Intraoral examination may be difficult as a result of trismus. Presence or absence of periodontal disease should be noted. The tonsils will look relatively normal, but the tonsil on the side of the PTA will be displaced inferomedially with a swelling lateral to the tonsil involving the soft palate. Flexible nasendoscopy is usually normal.

The differential diagnosis of a PTA may include infective disorders, such as a dental abscess, or non-infective disorders. These are rare but important and will be determined by a careful history, with an absence of preceding tonsillitis and a longer history of progressive symptoms. Important differential diagnoses include lymphoma and squamous cell carcinoma, deep lobe parotid tumours and carotid artery aneurysms.

Left untreated, many PTAs resolve spontaneously by discharging into the mouth, but they may develop into a parapharyngeal abscess. Special investigations are usually unnecessary. Curative treatment is achieved by incision and drainage. This is usually performed under local anaesthesia using a 5 mL syringe and white needle, aspirating pus which is usually sent for microbiological analysis. Some ear, nose and throat (ENT) surgeons advocate incision of the abscess with a scalpel, and this is good practice in PTAs that rapidly recur. Occasionally, tonsillectomy in the acute situation will be required for persistent PTAs that fail to settle after repeated aspiration. Patients are generally admitted to hospital for intravenous fluids and antibiotics. Some may be well enough following aspiration to be discharged, having been prescribed a single dose of intravenous corticosteroid and antibiotic.

RHEUMATIC FEVER AND GLOMERULONEPHRITIS

In the United Kingdom these are rare but serious complications of pharyngitis and tonsillitis caused by GABHS but are more common in the United States and developing countries. Routine treatment of sore throat with antibiotics is not justified in the United Kingdom, to prevent the development of rheumatic fever or glomerulonephritis.

Tonsillectomy

Tonsillectomy is a long-established surgical treatment for acute tonsillitis. It will cure acute tonsillitis. It will not cure other causes of sore throat. It is a safe procedure with a complication rate of less than 5 per cent. There has been considerable debate about the indications for tonsillectomy, with different views being held by different healthcare workers. The numbers of tonsillectomies performed in the United Kingdom has fallen considerably over the past 20 years as surgeons are encouraged to follow evidence-based guidelines for tonsillectomy, partly owing to pressure from commissioners of health care to reduce the number of operations that may be perceived as unnecessary. There is little in the way of high-quality evidence that either supports or refutes tonsillectomy as an effective surgical procedure. There is some evidence from hospital activity data in England and Wales that the number of emergency admissions for complications of acute tonsillitis is increasing as the number of tonsillectomies falls.

The natural progression is for the severity and frequency of tonsillitis to decrease with time, which must be borne in mind when considering referral.

Tonsillectomy for acute tonsillitis is a *relative* indication. *Absolute* indications for tonsillectomy include diagnostic tonsillectomy for possible malignancy, as an oncological procedure for malignancy and obstructive sleep apnoea in children. Whilst many good guidelines exist, the Scottish Intercollegiate Guideline Network (SIGN) has produced some rational guidelines that have been arrived at through a consensus approach.

The following are recommended as indications for consideration of tonsillectomy for recurrent acute sore throat in both children and adults:

- Sore throats are due to acute tonsillitis.
- The episodes of sore throat are disabling and prevent normal functioning.
  - Seven or more well-documented, clinically significant, adequately treated sore throats in the preceding year or
  - Five or more such episodes in each of the preceding two years or
  - Three or more such episodes in each of the preceding three years.

When a patient is referred to an ENT clinic, the surgeon needs to take a careful history to establish the diagnosis. It is important to enquire about the effect the attacks have on normal functioning, for example the impact they have on school or ability to work. Co-existent nasal, oral or pharyngeal disease that may contribute to the severity of the tonsillitis should be treated if possible. Enquiry into the patient's general health should be made, in particular looking for any diseases that could potentially compromise the safety of the anaesthetic. Bleeding disorders are especially important to exclude, and a careful family history of bleeding disorders should be taken. If patients have a bleeding disorder or a family history, tonsillectomy is likely to be contraindicated. Young children with coexistent respiratory disorders should be referred to a dedicated paediatric unit for perioperative management. Patients should be encouraged to stop smoking prior to surgery.

Patients and/or their caregivers should be counselled about the different management options and the benefits of tonsillectomy compared to the potential for resolution with time, possible complications and temporary incapacity following surgery.

Tonsillectomy should be performed when the patient is fit, and not during or within 2 weeks of an attack of tonsillitis. It may be performed as a day-case procedure or with an overnight stay.

There is a theoretical risk that the new variant Creutzfeldt-Jakob disease (CJD) virus may accumulate within the tonsil (lymphoid tissues) with concomitant risks of transmission of the virus on incompletely sterilized surgical instruments. In England and Wales this risk has been addressed by introducing improved decontamination facilities to cope with the requirements of sterilizing this virus, which is notoriously resistant to standard techniques. The use of disposable instruments for tonsillectomy led to an unacceptably high haemorrhage rate.

TONSILLECTOMY TECHNIQUES

There are several techniques for tonsillectomy. The most common technique in use in the United Kingdom is dissection tonsillectomy using cold steel instruments with or without the use of bipolar diathermy for haemostasis. Monopolar diathermy is associated with a higher incidence of post-operative haemorrhage. The guillotine for tonsillectomy is rarely used now, while newer techniques such as Coblation tonsillectomy or use of the harmonic scalpel have their advocates. Surgeons should be appropriately trained in the use of all techniques that they use and audit their results.

The principles of dissection tonsillectomy are as follows:

- Careful liaison with the anaesthetist to manage the 'shared airway' safely
- Good exposure of the tonsils
- Traction and counter-traction of the tonsils to allow dissection in the plane between the capsule of the tonsil and superior constrictor muscle
- Haemostasis with ties and/or bipolar diathermy
- Careful removal of clots from the oro- and nasopharynx

Healing is by secondary intention. Patients are encouraged to eat and drink normally following surgery. They may complain of earache due to referred otalgia from the glossopharyngeal nerve. Effective control of post-operative nausea is important, not least so that same-day discharge can be achieved when otherwise indicated.

Post-operatively, patients may complain of increased pain, fetor and difficulty with swallowing, which is usually due to secondary infection. This can be prevented by an adequate diet but may require antibiotics.

Haemorrhage following tonsillectomy occurs in less than 5 per cent of cases. This may be *reactionary*, occurring within the first 24 of surgery, or *secondary*, occurring 5 to 10 days after surgery. Secondary haemorrhage may be due to infection. Patients should receive specialized nursing care post-operatively; haemorrhage may not initially be apparent if a patient swallows blood rather than spitting it out. Post-operative haemorrhage should be treated seriously, especially in children, in whom hypovolaemic shock is a dangerous complication of haemorrhage. Early return to theatre is advisable especially in children to prevent further complications of bleeding.

Other rarer complications include dental trauma, temporomandibular joint dislocation, pneumonia and taste and sensory disturbance, which is usually transient.

SPECIFIC INFECTIONS

Infectious mononucleosis

Infectious mononucleosis (glandular fever) is caused by infection with EBV, which is transmitted through close contact with other individuals, usually via oropharyngeal contact. Incubation can be up to 6 weeks. It is a systemic disease and may affect the spleen, liver and central nervous system as well as the pharynx. All lymphoid tissue within Waldeyer's ring may be affected (unlike in acute tonsillitis). Patients present with fatigue, malaise, sore throat and cervical lymphadenopathy, which may be massive. The tonsils and oropharynx may be covered in a membranous exudate, and petechial haemorrhage may be seen on the soft palate. The tonsils may be so enlarged (kissing tonsils) that the patient exhibits stertor, and airway obstruction is a serious complication of infectious mononucleosis. Systemic examination may reveal a short-lived maculopapular rash, splenomegaly and rarely hepatomegaly and cranial neuropathies. Upper eyelid oedema is associated with EBV infection.

The diagnosis is both clinical and based on laboratory investigations. Abnormal lymphocytes may be present in the peripheral blood film. Heterophile antibodies develop, and these are the basis for the Paul-Bunnell and Monospot tests, in which sheep and horse red blood cells, respectively, agglutinate when exposed to the antibodies. Serological evidence of IgM-specific antibodies to viral capsid antigen is the gold standard for diagnosis. Abnormal liver function tests are often seen in infectious mononucleosis.

Treatment is supportive. Secondary bacterial infection will need to be treated with antibiotics, avoiding ampicillin-based antibiotics because a rash will develop. Steroids may be useful, especially in the presence of grossly enlarged tonsils. On rare occasions acute tonsillectomy is indicated in the presence of severe unresolving airway obstruction.

Up to 20 per cent of patients who have suffered from infectious mononucleosis will develop a chronic fatigue syndrome. It is generally recommended that this can be avoided by a prolonged period of rest following infection. Contact sports should be avoided for up to 6 weeks to avoid the risk of splenic rupture.

HIV/AIDS

HIV continues to be a disease with significant morbidity worldwide, although it can be effectively treated with antiretroviral drugs. HIV infection is associated with intravenous drug abuse and sexual intercourse between men. It may be seen in children through vertical transmission from mothers. There are very few reports in the literature of HIV acquired by healthcare workers through, for example, needle-stick injury.

In the pharynx and oral cavity, HIV may present in a variety of ways. It is rare to have isolated pharyngeal symptoms in the absence of systemic disease. Pharyngeal features of HIV infection include:

1. Acute seroconversion illness. Primary HIV infection may present with severe generalized illness, which includes malaise, sore throat, mucosal ulceration, cervical lymphadenopathy and headache, associated with non–head and neck symptoms such as gastro-intestinal disturbance, arthralgia and lethargy. The symptoms are similar to those of glandular fever.
2. Opportunistic infections. The most common in the pharynx is Candida infection, often with unusual forms of Candida other than *Candida albicans*. Other infections that may be found in association with HIV include tuberculosis, cytomegalovirus, toxoplasmosis and herpes infections. Opportunistic sinonasal infection is relatively common in HIV disease.
3. Pharyngeal neoplasms. Kaposi's sarcoma in particular, non-Hodgkin's lymphoma and squamous cell carcinoma are more common in patients with HIV infection as are skin cancers of the head and neck region. All such neoplasms are diagnosed and managed in the same way as in patients without HIV, although specific treatment regimens may need to be tailored to an individual patient (for example, taking into account systemic morbidity, which may preclude aggressive chemotherapy regimens).

KEY LEARNING POINTS

- Not all cases of sore throat are infectious. Environmental and lifestyle causes (e.g. smoking) should be addressed in management.
- Acute tonsillitis is a self limiting condition diagnosed on history.
- The most common complication is a peritonsillar abscess, which requires incision and drainage to prevent further complications.
- Tonsillectomy should be offered for acute tonsillitis only when the history fulfills the appropriate criteria for tonsillectomy.

FURTHER READING

Scottish Intercollegiate Guidelines Network (SIGN). *Guideline 117; Management of sore throat and indications for tonsillectomy.* www.sign.ac.uk. April 2010.

21

Investigations of laryngeal disease

MEREDYDD HARRIES

OPTICAL

There have been huge technological advancements in endoscopic laryngeal examination over the past 15 years. The larynx can be viewed with a flexible endoscope inserted via the nose or with a rigid angled telescope via the mouth.

FLEXIBLE TRANSNASAL FIBRE-OPTIC LARYNGOSCOPY

Flexible transnasal fibre-optic laryngoscopy is now readily available in most ear, nose and throat (ENT) outpatient departments. The transnasal approach allows examination of the larynx and the vocal cords in a more physiological posture than the transoral approach. This is ideal for observation of voice problems such as muscle misuse dysphonia where the structure of the vocal cords is normal but the technique of phonation is the problem.

The newer distal chip camera systems give excellent detail, and this technique also results in less stimulation of the patients' gag reflex when transoral examination is not possible.

Wider scopes with side channels can be used for biopsies of suspicious lesions or injections to the larynx under local anaesthetic in the outpatient setting, especially if the patient may not be suitable for a general anaesthetic. Laser fibres (usually potassium titanyl phosphate, or KTP) can also be passed down these side channels for outpatient ablation of lesions such as laryngeal papillomatosis after initial histological confirmation via a biopsy.

RIGID TRANSORAL ENDOSCOPY

In 1959, British physicist Harold Hopkins developed the rigid lens system, which has since been used for rigid endoscopy throughout ENT departments. The 'Hopkins rod' telescope can be used for rigid indirect laryngoscopy. This technique gives excellent illumination and resolution higher than with most other flexible endoscopes. Combined with the newer camera and video capture systems, a clear, bright and magnified image can be obtained for a full and detailed examination of the larynx.

Both 90° and 70° endoscopes are available, and although each gives a slightly different view, which one is used often comes down to personal choice and availability.

Technique is important, including positioning of the patient and the endoscope to minimize the gag reflex.

The technique concentrates on the larynx and the vocal cords. Owing to the abnormal position of the tongue and vocal tract during vowel phonation, it is usually impossible to make any assessment of technique of phonation, which is best done with the flexible scope, as stated earlier.

STROBOSCOPY

During phonation the vocal folds vibrate between 80 and 1000 Hertz (cycles per second).

Talbot's law – named after the British scientist William Talbot – states that the retina can only register 1 image per 0.2 seconds or 5 images per second. The vibration of the free edge of the vocal fold will therefore appear as a blur if viewed with a simple white light source.

In 1878, Oertel used a shuttered light system to view the vocal folds. By adjusting the shutter speed to a rate slightly different from the rate of vibration, he was able to produce a montage of apparent slow-motion vocal fold vibrations. This is the principle of stroboscopy. It is not, however, a true representation of vibration because successive images from different cycles are taken to form a composite continuous wave (Figure 21.1).

For accurate measurements, the vibration must be periodic and symmetrical, which is usually not

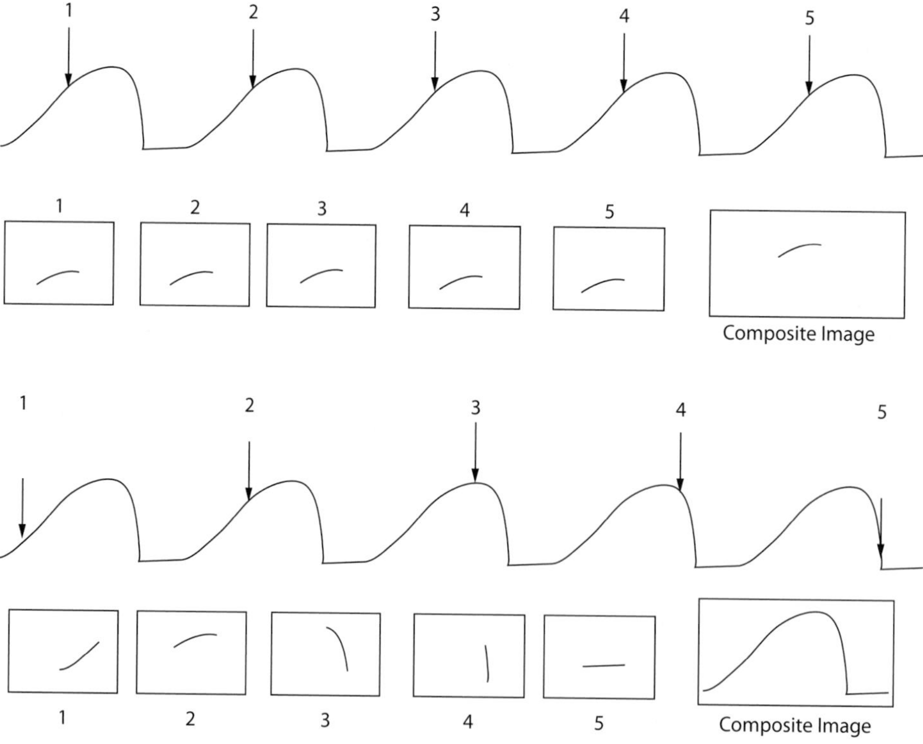

Figure 21.1 Diagrammatic representation of the principles of stroboscopy. Note that the image is a montage of different stages of vocal fold vibration rather than a true image of each vibratory cycle.

the case when a pathological disorder is present, so there are limitations to this system when applied to abnormal vibration. It remains one of the best clinical tools for examining the vocal folds during vibration and can distinguish between a pathologic disorder on the epithelium and one in the deeper layers as well as identifying segments of reduced vibration such as those caused by scarring or haemorrhage.

It can also help assess the depth of invasion of a tumour and plan for further treatment such as a laser excision biopsy of superficial lesions. Although most commonly used with the rigid endoscopes, it can now be used with the newer flexible scopes with their excellent illumination and resolution.

Stroboscopic video images provide a record of the patient's laryngeal function and allow subjective ratings of the vibratory patterns of the vocal folds. The interpretation of these images does require training, experience, knowledge of laryngeal pathophysiology and clinical judgement. The mucosal wave and vibration of the vocal folds can be altered by changing the task given to the patient and the patient's ability to comply with this task. Repeated measurements should only be done with exact replication of the examination procedure if they are to be used as evidence to support treatment regimens.

Perceptual judgements of the stroboscopic images can include:

1. Symmetry, or the degree to which the two vocal folds provide mirror images of each other
2. Periodicity, or the regularity of apparent successive cycles of vocal fold vibration
3. Amplitude, or the extent of horizontal excursion of the vocal folds
4. Presence of stiffness or adynamic (nonvibratory) segments on the vocal fold
5. Pattern of closure. This can be placed into seven categories (see Table 21.1).

Other measurements, such as plane and phase of closure, can be used, but more training is required to be competent and reliable with these.

This assessment is subjective and can be susceptible to bias, but with today's emphasis on results and the need to produce evidence, it can be a useful tool to support treatment regimens.

Table 21.1 Classification of the different patterns of closure of the vocal fold on stroboscopic examination

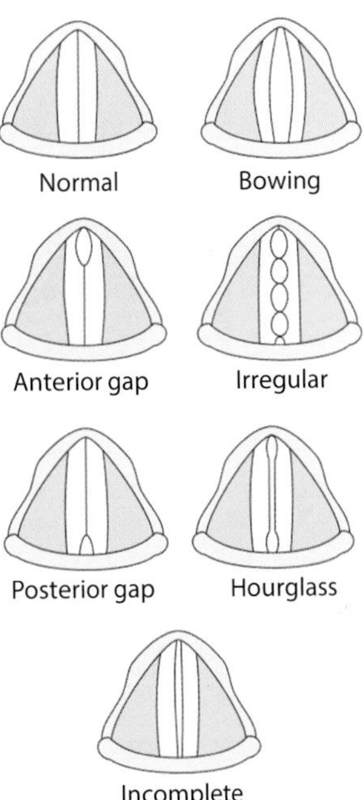

It is now recommended that all professional voice users should have access to stroboscopy during their examination in the voice clinic because of the potential added information obtained, as discussed earlier, and the limitations of white light examination.

HIGH-SPEED VIDEO IMAGING

This type of imaging of the larynx can capture the true vibratory pattern of the vocal folds, because it is capable of recording up to 8 000 frames per second. Used in the United States since the 1960s, it is not a widely available clinical tool partly because of the cost. It does allow true analysis and evaluation of the vocal cords even with disease and aperiodic vibration. One of the difficulties is in the analysis of the recording, as even a 2-second clip will take around 5 minutes to view. Which 2-second clip to use is also a matter of debate, with some clinicians using the onset of phonation and others preferring to analyze the midvoice sections. Currently, this is more of a research tool, but newer software

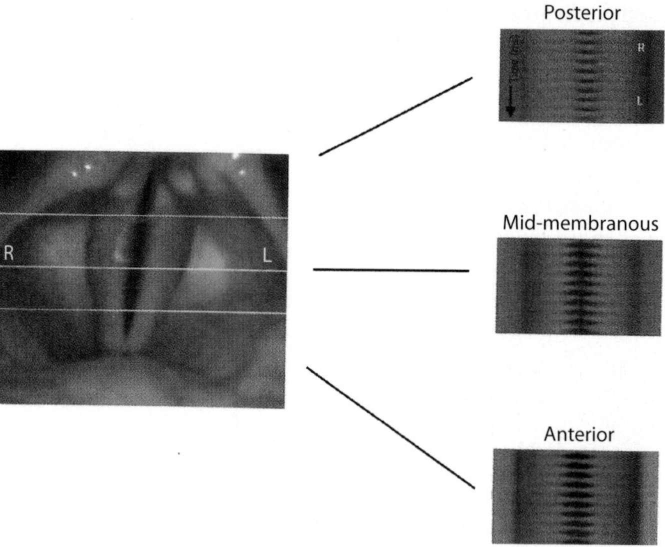

Figure 21.2 Videokymography. Photographic recording of the vibration of the vocal folds at the three different positions. A cross-sectional image of the free edge is seen on successive cycles at each position.

packages should bring this to clinical settings in the future.

VIDEOKYMOGRAPHY

Videokymography analyzes the high-speed images of oscillation at one specific horizontal position on the vocal fold. It produces a spatiotemporal image of the vibration of the medial edge of the vocal fold in that area and plots this along the vertical axis against time. Asymmetry of vibration or pathologic changes are particularly well seen with this technique, but it is not used widely in the United Kingdom.

The endoscope must be perpendicular to the fold, and for true comparison exactly the same segment must be used, which does provide some technical challenges (Figure 21.2).

NARROW BAND IMAGING

Narrow band imaging (NBI) is a technique for imaging the mucosal surfaces with selected portions of the light spectrum – usually blue (400 nm) or green (540 nm). Haemoglobin will preferentially absorb these, so that early cancers with increased vasculature give a dark signal when viewed with NBI techniques. This has proved to be useful in patients with Barrett's oesophagus. Early studies suggest that it may also have a role in early detection of laryngeal cancer and in guidance regarding the limits and location of biopsies (Figure 21.3).

Keratinization, which is common in laryngeal cancer, scatters all the visible light, and it may be better to use autofluoresence methods rather than NBI in these cases. It is a technique in its infancy, and its precise role as yet still undefined.

ELECTRICAL

LARYNGOGRAPHY

Laryngography is a quantitative assessment of laryngeal function. The electrolaryngograph consists of two electrodes placed on either side of the thyroid cartilage at the level of the vocal cords. A high-frequency current (3 MHz) is applied between the electrodes. The change in conductance correlates to the change in contact area between the

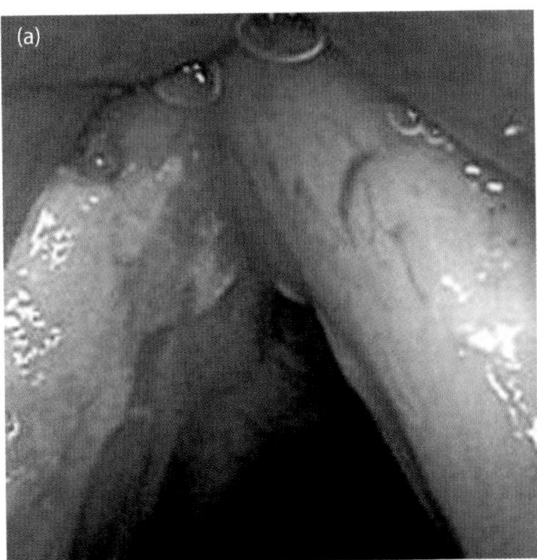

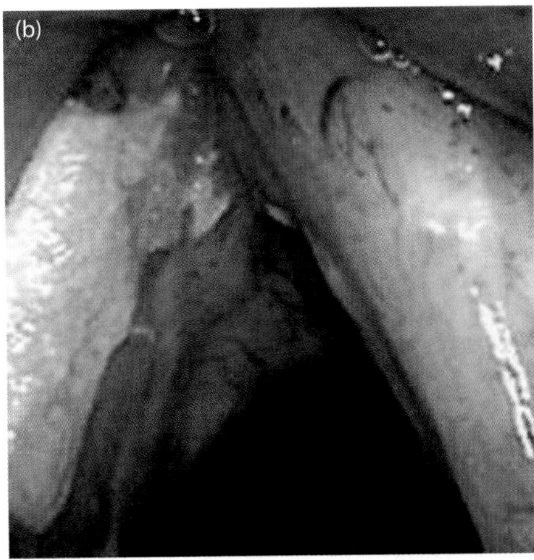

Figure 21.3 Narrow band imaging **(b)** and white light appearance **(a)** of a lesion on the anterior left vocal cord.

vocal folds during vibration. This gives an assessment of the laryngeal component of voice and is not affected by any change in the vocal tract (resonance) that is present when using a microphone to analyze the voice at the mouth.

Good contact is essential, and thick neck tissue can prevent an accurate signal.

Using sustained vowels or connected speech (read passage or spontaneous discourse) can both be useful and have their separate merits. Sustained vowels are simple components of speech and predominantly reflect vocal fold vibratory activity, whereas fluent speech may be more relevant to the patient's day-to-day experience and a listener's impression of the voice. Ideally, both should be used to give a complete quantitative assessment.

Measurements using this method include jitter (variation in frequency) and shimmer (variation in intensity), and more complex indices such as harmonics/noise ratio and percentage contact quotient can be calculated to provide measurements of laryngeal function (Figure 21.4).

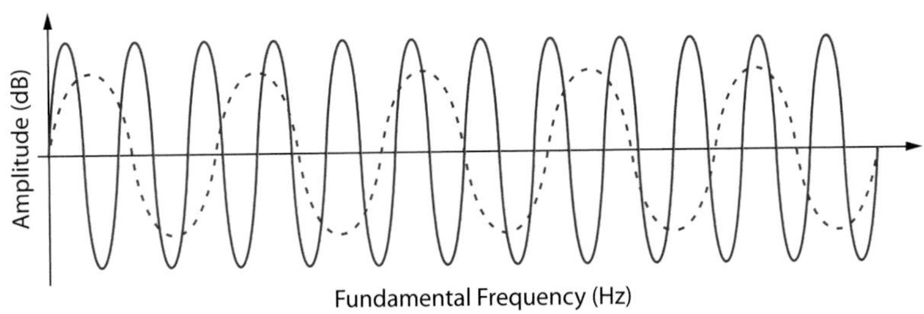

Jitter = Fundamental frequency (pitch) perturbation
Shimmer = Perturbation of amplitude (loudness)

Figure 21.4 The fundamental frequency of the laryngeal signal (dotted line) and the voice (solid line). The laryngeal signal is modified by the vocal tract to produce specific frequency harmonics and peaks, termed formants.

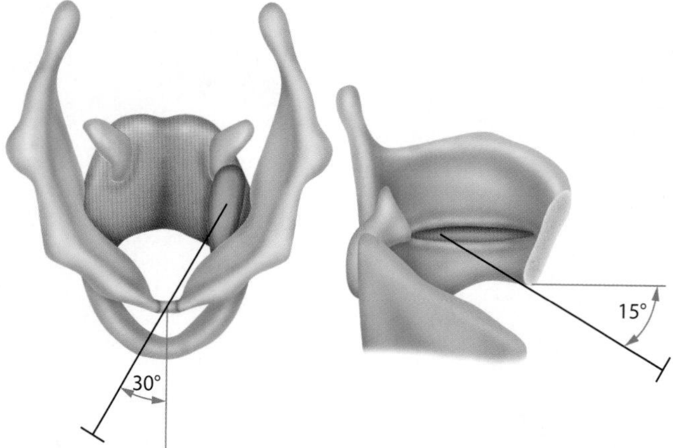

Figure 21.5 Position of needle electrode for thyroarytenoid EMG or for injection of botulinum toxin.

ELECTROMYOGRAPHY

Electromyography (EMG) measures electrical activity of muscle. This gives a visual signal of electrical activity and is usually coupled to a speaker to produce an audible output. There are three different types of electrical potential: spontaneous, insertional and volitional. Each has a specific acoustic and visual signal that can be identified by an experienced examiner, usually a neurophysiologist, and can differentiate between normal, denervated or reinnervating muscle.

Recording an EMG from laryngeal muscles can be technically challenging, and there is still lack of agreement on methodology, validity, interpretation of signal and clinical value.

Current electrodes include the monopolar and concentric needles that are inserted into the muscles in the outpatient setting, usually without need for local anaesthesia (Figure 21.5).

Many laryngologists who inject botulinum toxin will be used to this technique, but it is still recommended that a neurophysiologist be present for interpretation of the signal.

Laryngeal EMG can be used for the following:

- Differentiating laryngeal paralysis from mechanical fixation
- In cases of denervation, comparing the signal from cricothyroid muscle (innervated by the external laryngeal branch of the superior laryngeal nerve) and the thyroarytenoid muscle (innervated by the recurrent laryngeal nerve) to localize the site of the lesion and determine whether it is a high vagal (skull base) or recurrent laryngeal nerve (neck or mediastinal) problem
- Diagnosing neurological diseases such as myasthenia gravis and amyotrophic lateral sclerosis, and distinguishing between upper and lower motor neuron conditions
- Intraoperative nerve monitoring, especially in thyroid surgery
- Estimating the degree and prognosis (recovery) of paralysis/paresis

RADIOLOGICAL

ULTRASOUND

Ultrasound has limited applications in the larynx owing to the cartilaginous framework that reflects sound, thus preventing it from reaching the interior of the larynx. Using high-frequency and high-resolution probes, however, it is possible to assess the mobility of the cords, especially in paediatric patients, in whom dynamic visualization of the larynx can be difficult. It can be used to identify and assist fine needle cytology or core biopsy of possible nodes with advanced laryngeal cancer.

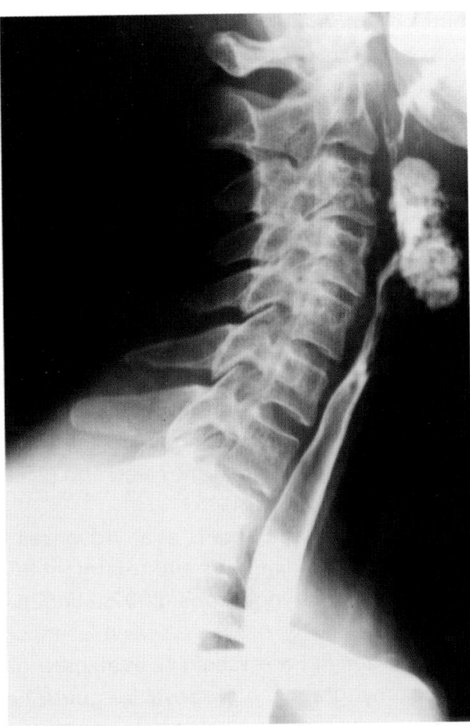

Figure 21.6 Lateral radiograph with a calcified lymph node overlying the retro-pharyngeal tissues. Note air in the oesophagus related to an impacted soft food bolus lying in the mid-oesophagus.

X-RAY

Plain radiographs, especially lateral views, can be useful in diagnosing foreign bodies, evaluating the thickness of the retropharyngeal soft tissue and identifying air in tissue planes from perforations or trauma.

Calcification in the laryngeal cartilages can mimic a foreign body and an anteroposterior (AP) and lateral view should always be obtained to exclude and identify any overlying structures such as jewelry or a calcified lymph node in the neck (Figure 21.6).

A plain chest x-ray is also useful in identifying pulmonary and mediastinal pathology in patients with left recurrent laryngeal nerve paralysis, although many units are now proceeding straight to computed tomography (CT) of the chest because of its greater accuracy.

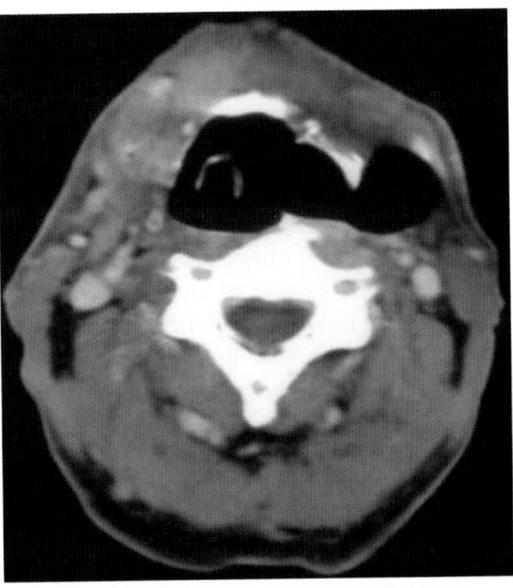

Figure 21.7 CT scan showing left laryngocoele with the sac extending through the thyrohyoid membrane. The tip of the epiglottis can be seen in the pharynx.

CT SCANNING

CT scanning is readily available, has faster image acquisition than magnetic resonance imaging (MRI) – and subsequently less motion artefact – and gives excellent detail of calcification or cortical bone (Figure 21.7).

Most agree that CT is the radiological investigation of choice for initial examination of laryngeal carcinoma to show tumour size, extent, thyroid cartilage infiltration and nodal status. It is often combined with a chest CT for tumour staging, and both procedures can be conveniently performed at the same time. CT has poorer soft tissue definition compared with MRI, does involve radiation and can be distorted by artefacts from dental restorations.

MRI SCANNING

MRI scanning does not involve ionizing radiation, gives superb soft tissue contrast and allows multiplanar images, especially in the sagittal plane. This can demonstrate the superior and inferior extent of a tumour such as in the assessment of tongue base extension of supraglottic tumours. It does take 30

KEY LEARNING POINTS

- Optical investigations – recent scientific developments have improved the visual assessment of the larynx, especially the improvements in fibre-optics in both dimensions and clarity of image. Stroboscopy should now be available in all voice clinics, and high-speed video with kymography and light of different wavelengths shows promise in improving the accuracy of laryngeal diagnosis.
- Electrical investigations – although still used mainly in audit, research and voice laboratories, both laryngography and laryngeal EMGs have been proven to have diagnostic, prognostic and quantitative roles. It is expected that these will become more commonly available, and improved standardization of technique and interpretation of results will follow.
- Radiological investigations – widely available in most units, these are invaluable in location and assessment of laryngeal pathology and its staging.

minutes or more and can be poorly tolerated by claustrophobic patients. Owing to the length of time taken, it is also prone to movement artefact and is absolutely contraindicated if there is any ferro-magnetic material in the patient such as a cardiac pacemaker or even some stapes prostheses. It is often the preferred investigation to image neck metastases and can be complementary to CT investigations.

FURTHER READING

Mehta D, Hilman R. Voice assessment: Updates on perceptual, acoustic, aerodynamic and endoscopic imaging methods. *Current Opinion in Otolaryngology, Head and Neck Surgery*. 2008; 16: 211–15.

Rosen CA, Amin MR, Sulica L, et al. Advances in office-based diagnosis and treatment in laryngology. *Laryngoscope*. 2009; 119(S2): 185–212.

Volk GF, Hagen R, Pototschnig C, et al. Laryngeal electromyography: A proposal for guidelines of the European Laryngological Society. *European Archives of Oto-Rhino-Laryngology*. 2012; 269(10): 2227–45.

Watanabe A, Fujita M. *Case Study of NBI Endoscopy: ENT for Healthcare Professionals*. Olympus Medical Systems, 2011; 2: 1–20.

22

Infections of the larynx

MICHAEL S W LEE

INTRODUCTION

The upper aerodigestive tract shares a common passage in the oropharynx. The larynx separates the airway from the digestive tract at the level of hypopharynx. It is divided into supraglottis, glottis and subglottis anatomically. The larynx serves the functions of providing a rigid framework for transmission of air on breathing, producing voice for communication and protecting the trachea and lung by preventing aspiration.

The narrowest part of the upper airway is at the glottis. Acute infection manifested as inflammation and gross oedema of the laryngeal mucosa can cause airway obstruction, which can be fatal if the condition is not recognized early. Fibre-optic nasal laryngoscopy is a very useful tool for visualization of the larynx. Some of the chronic infections of the larynx can resemble malignant neoplasm, and, therefore, direct laryngoscopy and biopsy are important in ascertaining a diagnosis.

The pattern of infection has changed over the years. Diphtheria and syphilis were common diseases more than half a century ago, but they are rare nowadays. The incidence of hospital admission for acute epiglottitis in infants has drastically been reduced following the introduction of the *Haemophilus influenzae* type b (Hib) vaccination programme decades ago.[1–3] Opportunistic infection is not uncommon in patients with acquired immunodeficiency syndrome (AIDS) and in those who are taking potent immunosuppressive medications following solid organ and bone marrow transplantation.

ACUTE LARYNGITIS

Acute infective laryngitis is the most common form of infection in the larynx. The majority of the infection is caused by viruses, including rhinovirus, adenovirus, parainfluenza virus and respiratory syncytial virus.

The presenting symptoms are sore throat, hoarse voice, fever, malaise and cervical lymphadenitis. Laryngitis is often associated with other symptoms of upper respiratory tract infection such as rhinorrhoea, nasal congestion, otalgia, hearing impairment and cough. Fibre-optic laryngoscopy reveals erythema and oedema of the true vocal cords and the mucosa of the larynx and pharynx.

The symptoms generally improve within a few days and resolve spontaneously in 1 to 2 weeks. Supportive treatment such as voice rest, water for rehydration, simple analgesia and inhalation of steam and menthol is usually adequate. Secondary bacterial laryngitis may occur and may require antibiotics if the symptoms are progressively getting worse. Patients who suffer with persistent hoarse voice and sore throat for 6 weeks warrant laryngoscopy using a fibre-optic nasendoscope to exclude any other pathologic factors. This is true particularly for smokers, who are at risk of developing laryngeal carcinoma.

LARYNGO-TRACHEOBRONCHITIS (CROUP)

Laryngo-tracheobronchitis is a subacute upper respiratory tract infection most commonly caused by parainfluenza viruses types I, II and III, accounting for 75–80 per cent of cases.[4,5] Adenovirus, respiratory syncytial virus and influenza viruses types A and B compose the remaining cases. Children between the ages of 6 months and 3 years are more commonly affected, and such cases of croup usually last for 3 to 7 days. Many cases are self-limiting, and most patients do not need admission to hospital for treatment. Croup is the most common cause of stridor in children, and approximately 5 per cent of these patients require tracheal intubation. The infection is more prevalent in autumn and winter months. The disease is uncommon in adults.

The viral infection causes inflammation and oedema in the larynx, the trachea and the bronchus. The subglottis is the most affected area. The cricoid cartilage is the only complete cartilaginous ring in the upper respiratory tract that prevents any expansion in acute inflammation. The mucosa in the subglottis has numerous mucus-secreting glands. The pseudostratifed ciliated columnar respiratory epithelium lining the subglottis is loosely adherent to the underlying perichondrium. The infection causes mucosal oedema and glandular hypersecretion. A small amount of oedema creates a great amount of reduction in subglottic airway.

The clinical features of croup are 'barking' cough, hoarse voice and low-grade fever. Barking cough is a highly predictive symptom for croup. When the patient is drooling saliva, acute epiglottis must be considered. Stridor and respiratory distress happen when the subglottic airway becomes narrowed. Usually, the symptoms are worse at night. Patients with bacterial tracheitis caused by staphylococcus and streptococcus are more systemically unwell, with high fever and leucocytosis. Non-infective causes of stridor, including subglottic stenosis due to previous prolonged intubation, foreign body, laryngomalacia, tracheomalacia, subglottic haemangioma, laryngeal web, vocal cord palsy or neoplasm, need to be excluded.[5] Flexible fibre-optic laryngoscopy can reveal subglottic inflammation and oedema as well as excluding any other pathologic changes in the larynx. An anteroposterior soft tissue x-ray of the neck, performed only if the child's airway is safe and in a stable condition, may show a symmetrical narrowing of the subglottis known as a 'steeple sign'.[4]

The treatment for croup is air humidification, nebulized adrenaline 1:1000 5 mL and systemic corticosteroids. Oral, intramuscular and inhaled steroids are shown to be effective.[6,7] The rapid onset of action of nebulized adrenaline causes mucosal vasoconstriction and reduced vascular permeability, resulting in reduction of mucosal oedema and airway obstruction within 10–30 minutes. Patients treated with nebulized adrenaline need to be reassessed 3 to 4 hours after administration in the event of regression of stridor. The anti-inflammatory action of a systemic corticosteroid may take several hours.

Tracheal intubation may be necessary in severe cases. A whole size smaller than the anticipated endotracheal tube for age and size of the child (half a size smaller for infants up to 6 months old) should be used to avoid causing intubation injury to the subglottic mucosa. The endotracheal tube should be inserted with minimal resistance. Otherwise, a smaller size of endotracheal tube is needed. A trial of extubation can be considered after 48 hours or when there is a leak of air around the endotracheal tube. Microlaryngoscopy and bronchoscopy should be considered if there is prolonged intubation as well as to rule out any other pathologies in the upper airway. The need for tracheostomy is rare unless the endotracheal tube is too small for ventilation and keeps blocking by secretion, or subglottic mucosal ulceration in the endotracheal tube area is seen during microlaryngoscopy and bronchoscopy.[4]

ACUTE EPIGLOTTITIS (SUPRAGLOTTITIS)

Acute epiglottitis is a potentially life-threatening infection due to acute inflammation and oedema of the supraglottis, in particular the epiglottis, causing laryngeal airway obstruction. Therefore, epiglottitis is also known as supraglottitis. The classic causative infectious agent is *Haemophilus influenzae* type b.[1,3] In the past, the infection predominantly affected children between 2 and 4 years old, but the incidence of acute epiglottitis in children has dramatically decreased following the introduction of the Hib vaccine.[2,3,5] The infection is now more commonly found in adults. However, acute epiglottitis can still be seen in unvaccinated children or vaccine failures. Group A *Streptococcus pneumoniae, Staphylococcus aureus, Klebsiella pneumoniae, Haemophilus parainfluenzae* and *beta-haemolytic streptococci* (groups A, B, C and F) are associated with epiglottitis in the post-vaccination era. Candida and viruses, including herpes simplex type 1, varicella-zoster and parainfluenza, can cause the infection in immunocompromised patients.

Patients often present with a short history of sore throat and fever and then rapidly deteriorate to odynophagia, dysphagia, drooling of saliva, airway obstruction and stridor within a few hours. Cervical lymphadenitis is not uncommon. In children, acute epiglottitis can be difficult to differentiate from acute laryngo-tracheobronchitis (croup). Drooling of saliva is commonly seen in children with acute epiglottis, while coughing is often a sign in croup. In adults, an acutely severe sore throat and odynophagia with no obvious sign of inflammation in the oropharynx should raise the suspicion of acute epiglottitis.

The diagnosis is made on visualization of the larynx either by using a rigid laryngoscope under general anaesthesia after securing of the airway in children or by using a fibre-optic nasendoscope in awake adults. Typically, the epiglottis looks inflamed and oedematous and is often described as having a 'red cherry' appearance. The view of the laryngeal inlet is usually obscured by the enlarged epiglottis. The rest of the supraglottis, including aryepiglottic folds, arytenoids and false vocal folds, also shows signs of inflammation and oedema. Abscess formation on the epiglottis can happen days following treatment with intravenous antibiotics.

The lateral view on radiography of the soft tissue of the neck can show a swollen epiglottis, often known as a 'thumbprint sign'. Radiography is also useful to exclude retropharyngeal abscess, which is more common in children than in adults. Patients, especially children, with suspicion of acute epiglottitis with an impending upper airway obstruction and unstable airway must not be sent to the radiology department.

The differential diagnoses of acute epiglottitis include retropharyngeal abscess, laryngotracheobronchitis, foreign body, inhalation burns, corrosive ingestion, angioedema, parapharyngeal abscess, tonsillitis, pharyngitis and laryngeal carcinoma in adults.

The immediate care of acute epiglottitis in children is different from that in adults. The child with symptoms of acute epiglottitis should be admitted to a hospital where facilities and expertise are available to manage paediatric airway emergency. The most senior otolaryngologist, paediatrician, anaesthetist and intensive care physician must be informed immediately, and at the same time the operating theatre should be organized for treating an upper airway obstruction. The child and his or her parents should be assessed and cared for in a designated area, ideally in a paediatric accident and emergency department with equipment available to deal with acute airway emergency. Nebulized adrenaline 1:1000 0.5 mL/kg can be used to relieve the airway obstruction temporarily while the child waits to go to operating theatre. Physicians should not upset the child by trying to separate the child from his or her parents or by carrying out any clinical examination or invasive procedures, such as gaining intravenous access. Attempting an examination of the child's mouth using a tongue depressor can cause distress to the child and trigger a gag reflex, turning a partially obstructed upper airway into a complete obstruction. The child and the parents should be medically escorted to the operating theatre. A rigid ventilating bronchoscope, rigid laryngoscope and tracheostomy must be prepared in advance. Surgeons and scrub nurses should be scrubbed up before starting administration of anaesthesia and be ready to intervene in the event that the anaesthetist fails to secure the upper airway by tracheal intubation. Anaesthesia should take place in the operating theatre rather than in an anaesthetic room, and gas induction technique should be used.

In contrast to children, examination of the oropharynx and larynx is safe in awake adults. The larynx should be examined using a fibre-optic nasendoscope. Medical therapy including oxygen, nebulized adrenaline 1:1000 5 mL, intravenous corticosteroids and intravenous antibiotics is commenced once the diagnosis is established. Heliox (a gaseous mixture of 79 per cent helium and 21 per cent oxygen) can also be used. Heliox has a lighter gaseous density than oxygen, allowing an easy flow of the gaseous mixture through a narrowed airway. It should be noted that an oxygen concentration greater than 21 per cent cannot be delivered via Heliox. The adrenergic effect of the nebulized adrenaline provides quick and temporary relief of the airway obstruction by causing vasoconstriction in the inflamed and oedematous mucosa. As soon as the adrenergic effect wears off, the mucosa becomes hyperaemic and oedematous (a bound effect), which can make the airway obstruction worse. A definitive airway management plan should be in place after giving nebulized adrenaline. The assessment and management of suspected acute epiglottitis in adults is illustrated in Figure 22.1.

Surgeons and anaesthetists should assess the patient jointly and agree on a strategy for securing the airway in the operating theatre. It is important to secure the airway in the quickest and safest manner. A tracheostomy with local anaesthetic performed on an awake patient is recommended when tracheal intubation is likely to fail. Tracheal intubation is performed in an anaesthetized patient when it is considered safe and highly likely to be successful in maintaining ventilation and achieving tracheal intubation. Paralyzing the patient to facilitate endotracheal intubation presents a risk of the patient's losing airway tone and becoming unable to ventilate. While preserving self-breathing in an anaesthetized patient is considered safer than paralyzing the patient, tracheal intubation is more difficult. A rigid ventilation bronchoscopy, cricothyroidotomy or emergency tracheostomy in an anaesthetized patient should be performed when tracheal intubation fails.[8] Fibre-optic intubation in an awake patient is contraindicated in acute severe upper airway obstruction. The use of sedatives, opioids and topical anaesthesia should be avoided because of the risk of precipitating complete airway obstruction.

Once the airway is secured in the operating theatre, direct laryngoscopy and pharyngoscopy are performed. Preferably a swab from the epiglottis and a blood culture should be taken for microbiology investigation before commencing intravenous antibiotics. Third-generation cephalosporin, which covers a broad spectrum of pathogens, is the first choice of antibiotic. The patient's length of stay in intensive care and in the hospital is shortened by the use of corticosteroids. Daily fibre-optic laryngoscopy in an intubated patient can be used to assess his or her progress and determine when extubation is safe, usually 48–72 hours after intubation and medical therapy.

Adult patients must be monitored closely in a high-dependency unit for rapid deterioration in airway obstruction when airway intervention is thought to be not necessary in early acute

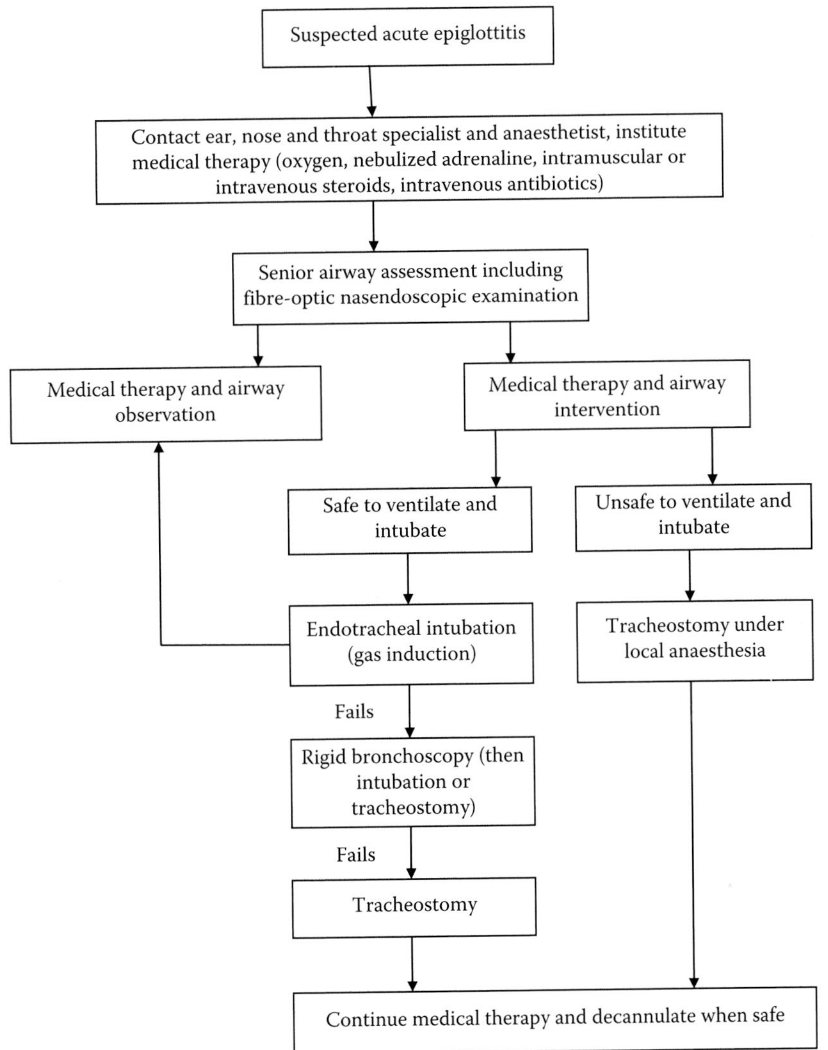

Figure 22.1 Algorithm for assessment and management of suspected acute epiglottitis. From Syed I, Odutoye T, Lee MSW, Wong P. Management of acute epiglottitis in adults. *British Journal of Hospital Medicine* (London). 2011; 72(5): M74–6.

epiglottitis. Daily fibre-optic laryngoscopy should be used to assess improvement and to detect abscess formation in the epiglottis.[9]

PERICHONDRITIS OF THE LARYNX

Infective perichondritis of the larynx is uncommon. The condition used to be associated with diphtheria, typhoid, tuberculosis, lupus and syphilis, but now it is seen in patients who have undergone radiotherapy for laryngeal carcinoma; those with trauma, including fracture of the laryngeal cartilage framework; patients with advanced-stage laryngeal carcinoma with invasion of laryngeal cartilage; and patients who are immunocompromised.

Radiation-induced chondronecrosis of the laryngeal cartilage and periochondritis can happen months or years after completion of radiotherapy for carcinoma (Figure 22.2). Residual or recurrent

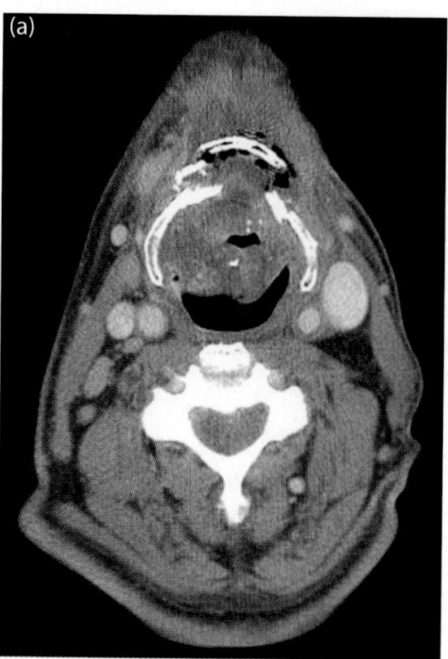

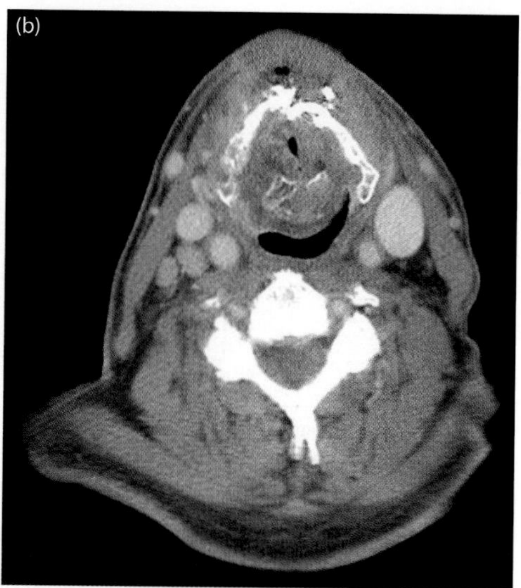

Figure 22.2 Axial CT scan with contrast shows features of radio-osteochondronecrosis in larynx. **(a)** Hyoid bone disruption with air in pre-hyoid area. **(b)** Thyroid cartilage lamina disruption with air in pre-thyroid area.

laryngeal carcinoma must be excluded if the condition happens within 2 years of radiotherapy. Patients usually present with severe sore throat, odynophagia, hoarse voice, dysphagia, aspiration pneumonia and stridor. Physical examination may show pre-laryngeal skin erythema, laryngeal tenderness and cervical lymphadenitis. Fibre-optic laryngoscopy can reveal erythema and oedema of pharyngeal and laryngeal mucosa, impaired vocal cord movement and pooling of saliva in the hypopharynx. Architectural disruption and necrosis of thyroid cartilage lamina, arytenoid cartilage and cricoid cartilage; laryngeal mucosal oedema; and emphysema can be seen on computed tomography (CT) of the larynx. Endoscopic examination of the larynx and the pharynx and laryngeal biopsy are important because coexistence of laryngeal carcinoma is possible. Intravenous antibiotics and corticosteroids are given as initial management. Tracheostomy is performed for airway obstruction. Placement of a nasogastric or gastrostomy tube endoscopically or radiologically may be necessary for enteral feeding. Total laryngectomy with primary surgical voice restoration should be considered if patients become dependent on tracheostomy and enteral feeding, i.e. have a functionless larynx, to improve their quality of life.

Perichondritis and abscess formation happen rarely in advanced-stage laryngeal carcinoma with thyroid cartilage invasion. A staging CT scan of the neck, the thorax and the liver, as well as panendoscopy and biopsy of the larynx, is needed for diagnosis and staging. The abscess should be treated with intravenous antibiotics and drainage if necessary. The definitive treatment is total laryngectomy with excision of the abscess wall, skin incision and neck dissection. It may require reconstruction of the cutaneous defect using a free or pedicle flap followed by post-operative adjuvant radiotherapy.

A laryngeal cartilage fracture can be caused by penetrative or blunt trauma (Figure 22.3). The skin or mucosal lining can be breached, exposing perichondrium and cartilage or forming a sub-perichondrial haematoma, which increases the risk of infection. Upper airway obstruction with stridor, dysphagia, odynophagia and drooling of saliva is common. A laryngeal fracture may be associated with injury to the cervical spine, the head, the pharynx and upper oesophagus, the major blood vessels and the lower cranial nerves. Skin laceration, bruising, soft tissue oedema and surgical emphysema can be found on physical examination. Fibre-optic laryngoscopy can show laceration, haematoma, erythema and oedema of

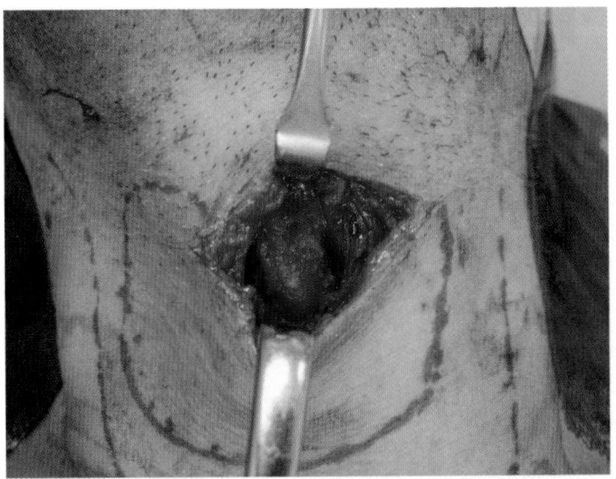

Figure 22.3 Self-inflicted penetrative neck injury with laceration of sternohyoid and thyrohyoid muscles, thyrohyoid membrane and superior part of thyroid cartilage.

the mucosa (including posterior larynx), dislocation of arytenoids, disruption of vocal cords and salivary retention in the hypopharynx. A CT scan of the neck including the larynx can show laryngeal fracture, derangement of the laryngeal structures and surgical emphysema. The patient may require tracheal intubation or tracheostomy for upper airway obstruction and insertion of a nasogastric tube for dysphagia. Intravenous antibiotics and corticosteroids are given. Open reduction and fixation of the laryngeal cartilage fracture, endoscopic reduction of the dislocated arytenoid cartilage and repositioning of the disrupted vocal cord under general anaesthesia should be performed as soon as the patient's medical condition allows.

LARYNGOPYOCELE

A saccule is located at the base of the laryngeal ventricle anteriorly, between the ventricular fold medially and the thyroarytenoid muscle and thyroid cartilage lamina laterally. The saccule is lined with pseudostratified ciliated columnar epithelium containing mucus-secreting glands. The surrounding laryngeal muscles compress the saccule and squeeze out the mucous secretion through its laryngeal opening, lubricating the true vocal cords. A laryngocele is formed when the saccule becomes dilated.[10]

The aetiology of a laryngocele can be congenital or acquired. An acquired laryngocele caused by increased endolaryngeal pressure is sometimes found in glass-blowers, musicians who play wind instruments, singers, street hawkers, pregnant woman and patients with chronic cough. Chronic inflammation, vocal cord surgery, laryngeal trauma and carcinoma arising from or involving the laryngeal ventricle can cause stenosis of the saccule neck leading to dialation and formation of a laryngocele.[10]

A laryngocele can be categorized as internal, external or mixed. An internal laryngocele is confined to the laryngeal ventricle and may extend superiorly to the glossoepiglottic vallecule. An external laryngocele extends superiorly and laterally outside the thyroid cartilage lamina and thyrohyoid membrane into the neck through an opening where the upper branch of the superior laryngeal nerve and the laryngeal blood vessels enter the larynx through the thyrohyoid membrane. When a laryngocele has both internal and external components, it is known as mixed or composite.[10]

Stasis of mucus within the laryngocele and impaired mucociliary clearance can result in bacterial infection, causing laryngopyocele. The common pathogens are *Staphylococcus aureus*, haemolytic group B *Streptococcus*, *Escherichia coli* and *Pseudomonas aeruginosa*.[10] Patients often present with sore throat, odynophagia, dysphagia, hoarse voice, breathing difficulty, painful neck mass and fever. The laryngoscopic findings include bulging of false vocal cord, aryepiglottic fold or glossoepiglottic fold. In a large mixed or external laryngopyocele, the larynx can be displaced medially with a tender neck mass and cervical lymphadenopathy (Figure 22.4). CT or magnetic resonance imaging (MRI) with contrast of the soft tissue of the neck is useful in making a diagnosis when a fluid-filled cavity is seen within the laryngeal ventricle and/or lateral to the thyrohyoid membrane and thyroid cartilage lamina. Fine-needle aspiration via the neck with or without ultrasound scan guidance can be used to obtain a pus specimen for microbiology investigations. Appropriate intravenous antibiotics should be given. Repeat fine-needle aspiration or formal surgical incision and drainage through

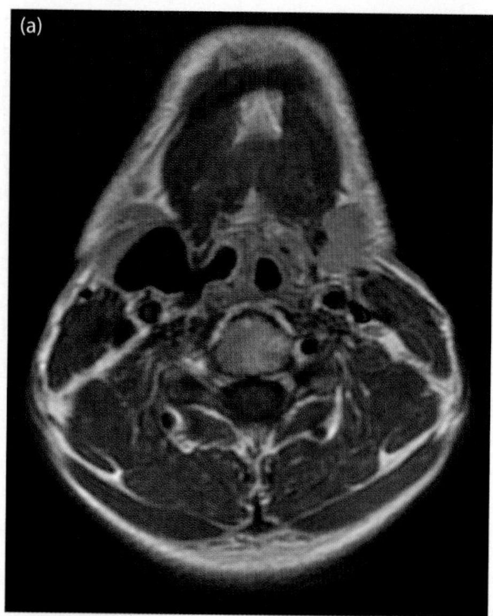

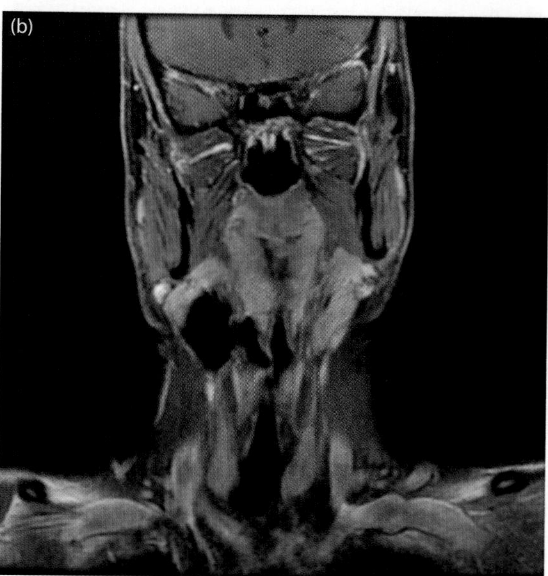

Figure 22.4 MRI of a composite laryngocele showing displacement of submandibular salivary gland and medial deviation of laryngeal airway. **(a)** Axial T1 post contrast. **(b)** Coronal T1 fat saturation post-contrast.

the neck may be necessary in a large external and mixed laryngopyocele. An internal laryngopyocele can be drained via an endolaryngeal approach. Tracheal intubation or tracheostomy should be considered in patients with acute airway obstruction.[11] Caution must be taken to avoid rupture of the internal component of a laryngopyocele during tracheal intubation. The laryngeal ventricle must be examined carefully to exclude any pathological disorders, in particular carcinoma, once the infection has settled.

Surgical excision can be planned 6 weeks after the infection is resolved (Figure 22.5). An internal laryngocele can be removed via an endolaryngeal approach using a carbon dioxide laser.[12] An external approach is used for an external or mixed laryngocele. A lateral horizontal skin crease incision is made at the level of the thyrohyoid membrane. A sub-platysmal myocutaneous flap is raised superiorly and inferiorly to expose the external laryngocele, thyrohyoid membrane and thyroid cartilage lamina. The laryngocele is dissected towards the thyrohyoid membrane. The sternothyroid and thyrohyoid muscles are retracted anteriorly and may need to be divided. After a perichondrial flap is raised, the inferior portion of the thyrohyoid membrane and the upper portion of the thyroid cartilage lamina can be removed to gain access to the laryngeal ventricle for excising the internal component of the laryngocele. The perichondrial flap is then sutured to the residual thyrohyoid membrane. The sternothyroid and thyrohyoid muscles are repaired if divided. A suction drain is sited and the wound is closed.

DIPHTHERIA

Diphtheria is a disease caused by *Corynebacterium diphtheriae*, a Gram-positive rod exotoxin producing bacillus, transmitted by direct contact or by respiratory droplets through sneezing and coughing. The disease has been almost eradicated following implementation of mass vaccination programmes in developed countries, but it is still an endemic disease in developing areas such as South America, India and Afghanistan. Outbreaks of the disease in developed countries are usually caused by patients who have visited the endemic

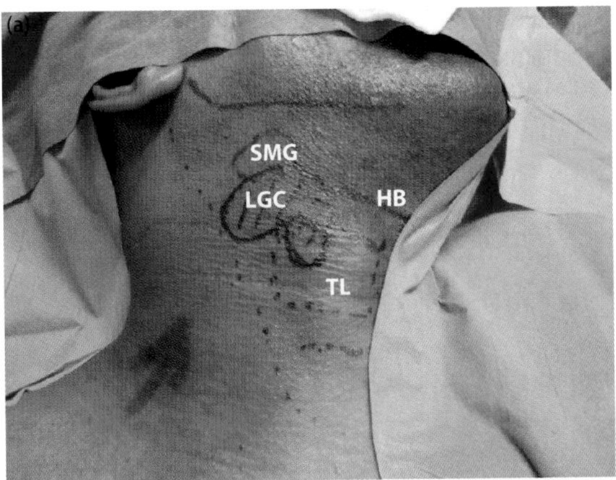

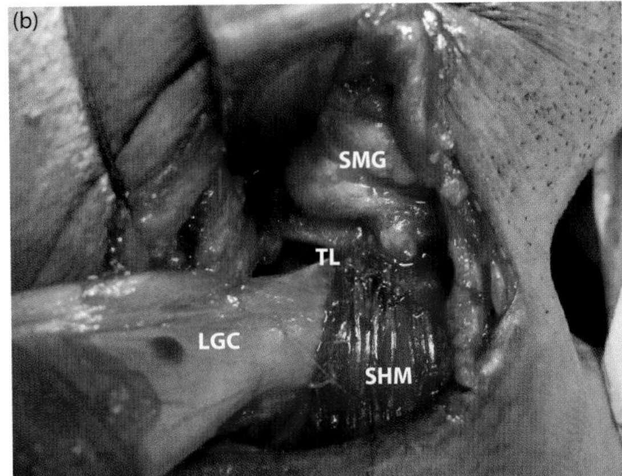

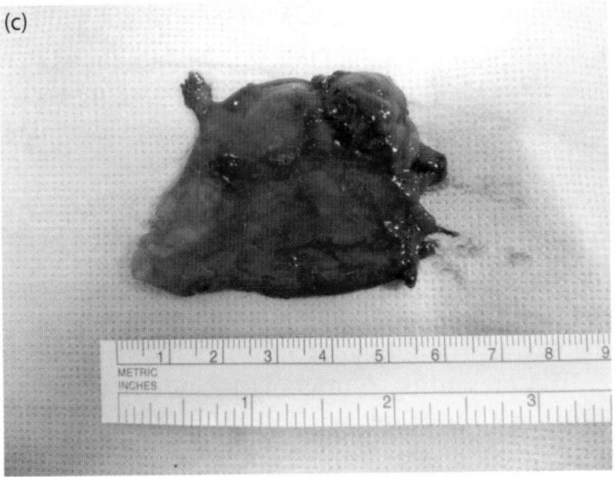

Figure 22.5 Intraoperative photographs of laryngocele excision. **(a)** Surgical planning. **(b)** Laryngocele extended out of thyrohyoid membrane lying medial and posterior to the sternohyoid muscle. **(c)** Laryngocele specimen (SMG = submandibular gland; LGC = laryngocele; HB = hyoid bone; TL = thyroid lamina; SHM = sternohyoid muscle).

areas. Non-immune children are commonly affected before the age of 5 years, but the disease affects any age group.

C. diphtheriae usually localizes in the upper respiratory tract, causing ulceration of the mucosa and an inflammatory pseudomembrane. Bleeding occurs when trying to remove the pseudomembrane from the vascularized and ulcerated mucosa underneath it. The oropharynx, including the tonsillar pillars, the palatine tonsils, the soft palate, the uvula and the posterior pharyngeal wall, is the most commonly affected area in the upper respiratory tract. The oral cavity, including the hard palate, the buccal mucosa, the upper and lower lips, and the tongue, can also be affected. The pseudomembrane can extend into the nasopharynx, the larynx, the trachea and the bronchus. In the larynx, the epiglottis is commonly involved. Primary laryngeal diphtheria is very uncommon (about 5 per cent of cases). Tracheobronchial diphtheria is thought to be caused by overspilling of the *C. diphtheriae*-containing pseudomembrane from the larynx. The potent exotoxin produced by the bacteria is absorbed into the circulation and affects other organs in the body. Myocardium and peripheral nerves are most affected. Acute cardiac failure and cardiac arrhythmia can happen weeks after resolution of the infection and may be fatal. Ninth and tenth cranial neuropathy can cause dysphagia, aspiration and nasal regurgitation. Peripheral motor neuropathy can affect the upper and lower extremities. Sensory peripheral neuropathy may result in glove-and-stocking neuropathy. The liver, the kidney, the adrenals, the spleen, the lung and the skin can also be affected by the exotoxin.[13–16]

Diphtheria is classified into four different forms according to the severity of the clinical features: the catarrah form (erythema of the pharynx without membrane), the follicular form (patches of exudates over pharynx and tonsils), the spreading form (a membrane covering tonsils and posterior pharynx) and the combined form (two anatomical sites involved).[16]

The presenting symptoms are sore throat, fever, odynophagia, dysphonia and breathing difficulty.[13,15,16] Multiple large areas of cervical lymphadenitis and neck soft tissue oedema can cause a 'bull neck' appearance. A history of diphtheria immunization should be established. The differential diagnosis includes severe streptococcal tonsillitis, glandular fever and Vincent's angina. The presence of a pseudomembrane on the pharyngeal and laryngeal mucosa, which bleeds on being peeled off, is characteristic of the exotoxin strain *C. diphtheriae* infection. The mortality rate of *C. diphtheriae* infection is about 12–25 per cent, and most patients die of acutely rapid airway obstruction.[13,15–17] A tracheostomy or tracheal intubation should be considered when patients are first hospitalized, especially when laryngeal pseudomembrane is seen on laryngoscopy.[13]

Microbiology swabs are taken from the throat and the nasopharynx, as well as from the cutaneous lesions, if any. A sample of the pseudomembrane should also be sent for microscopy and culture. The specimens are cultured on blood agar and selective tellurine media. Pathogenic strains are identified by biotyping using commercial kits. There are four biotypes of *C. diphtheriae*: *var gravis, var milis, var intermedius* and *var belfani.* Toxigenicity is detected by using the Elek immunoprecipitation test, polymerase chain reaction (PCR) or enzyme immunoassay (EIA).[18]

The treatment for diphtheria is administration of diphtheria antitoxin (20 000 to 1 000 000 units) and penicillin or macrolides (erythromycin or clarithromycin), if allergic to penicillin, and corticosteroids intravenously. Tracheostomy or endotracheal intubation is indicated in the event of airway obstruction. Close contacts and relatives of the patients should be traced and immunized.

BACTERIAL GRANULOMATOUS DISEASE

TUBERCULOSIS

Tuberculosis, infection with *Mycobacterium tuberculosis*, usually affects the lung, but laryngeal tuberculosis can present with or without pulmonary tuberculosis. The posterior part of the larynx, including the posterior true vocal cords, the arytenoid cartilage and the inter-arytenoid area, can be affected in severe pulmonary tuberculosis because of the infected mucus being brought up by mucociliary clearance to the larynx from the trachea.[19] Laryngeal tuberculosis in the absence of pulmonary tuberculosis is believed to be caused by haematogenous or lymphatic spread of the organism.[20]

The presenting symptoms include hoarseness, dysphagia, odynophagia, cough and weight loss. The glottis is the area most commonly affected, but all parts of the larynx can be involved. The laryngeal examination usually reveals mucosal ulceration or a nodular exophytic lesion, which can cause upper airway obstruction.[21] The clinical appearance of laryngeal tuberculosis can resemble a squamous cell carcinoma. It is important to obtain a biopsy from the laryngeal lesion for histopathologic analysis to exclude any malignant diseases, and for microbiological examination including culture and sensitivity.

Diagnosis is usually made on tissue and sputum microscopy and culture for acid-fast bacilli. Caseating granulomas, Langhans-type giant cells and acid-fast bacilli are often seen on histopathological examination. Rapid polymerase chain reaction testing may give false negative results and not be able to provide drug sensitivity testing. CT scan of the soft tissue of the neck is useful to assess the extent of laryngeal disease and cervical lymphadenopathy. Assessment of pulmonary involvement using chest radiography or CT is useful. Tests for patients for immune deficiency diseases such as human immunodeficiency virus (HIV) should be considered. The treatment is primarily medical, using prolonged anti-tuberculous therapy. Surgical management using a laryngeal microdebrider for de-bulking of the disease or tracheostomy is indicated in obstructive laryngeal tuberculosis. The disease can cause laryngeal stenosis and vocal cord fixation following treatment.[22]

LEPROSY

Leprosy, also known as Hansen's disease, is caused by *Mycobacterium leprae* (Hansen's bacilli), which spreads by direct contact via skin, mouth or nasal discharge. The disease is classified into five descriptive types based on whether the lesions are tuberculoid or lepromatous. The tuberculoid lesions have a marked cell-mediated immune reaction, whilst the lepromatous lesions show minimal cellular reaction.[19]

The infection affects primarily skin and peripheral nerves. Most infected patients develop acute cutaneous lesions, which heal spontaneously with fibrosis and scar formation. It can also affect the nasal mucosa, causing ulceration and nasal septal perforation. The larynx is the second most commonly affected site in the head and neck. The supraglottis, especially the epiglottis and aryepiglottic fold, is initially involved, showing features of erythematous or nodular oedema, which progresses to involve the glottis. The nodules are painless, and patients commonly present with a muffled voice rather than hoarseness. If the disease is left untreated, the nodules become enlarged and ulcerated, then heal by fibrosis, which can lead to laryngeal stenosis and upper airway obstruction, necessitating tracheostomy. Tissue biopsy is required for making a diagnosis. The histopathological exanimation shows an abundance of the acid-fast Hansen's bacilli in numerous large foam cells within a background of chronic inflammation and oedema in a lepromatous lesion, but much fewer in a tuberculous lesion, and the findings may be mistaken as other granulomatous diseases. Leprosy is treated with oral diaminodiphenylsulfone, rifampicin and clofazimine for 1 to 2 years after the organism can no longer be identified on biopsy samples of affected areas. The therapeutic period may be as long as 5 to 10 years.[20]

SYPHILIS

Syphilis, a sexually transmitted infection caused by spirochete *Treponema pallidum*, is classified as acquired or congenital. Acquired syphilis presents in primary, secondary and tertiary stages. In the primary stage, a painless ulcer or chancre presents at the contact point, usually on the genital, oral or anal mucosa, which heals within a few weeks. The secondary lesions present as widespread erythematous nodules that appear on cutaneous or mucosal surfaces when the primary lesion is resolving. The tertiary stage of syphilis appears years to decades later, when gummatous lesions involve almost any body tissue. Syphilis rarely affects the larynx, but if it does, secondary and tertiary stages of disease are more common than primary stage disease. The supraglottis, including the epiglottis and the aryepiglottic folds, is mainly affected.[20]

The presenting symptoms are hoarseness and dysphagia but rarely pain. In secondary stage syphilis, the supraglottis appears diffusely erythematous with maculopapules on the mucosa. In tertiary laryngeal syphilis, the mucosa looks diffusely nodular, and the nodules coalesce into a painless ulcer. The disease can develop laryngeal chondritis and fibrosis.[21] The laryngeal features can resemble tuberculosis and carcinoma.[19] Serological tests for syphilis, including the Venereal Disease Research Laboratory (VDRL) test, fluorescent treponemal antibody absorption (FTA-ABS) test, *Treponema pallidum* particle agglutination assay (TPPA) and *Treponema pallidum* haemagglutination assay (TPHA), are used to confirm the diagnosis. The treatment is high doses of penicillin.

ACTINOMYCOSIS

Actinomycosis is an infection caused by *Actinomyces bovis* and *Actinomyces israelii*, Gram-positive, anaerobic filamentous bacteria. It is a commensal saphrophyte of the normal mouth flora, commonly found in the tonsillar crypts and in the gingival and oral mucosa. It can become a pathogen when exposed to an anaerobic environment, such as in trauma and in devitalized tissue. The oral cavity is the most common site of infection in the head and neck. Laryngeal actinomycosis is uncommon. It can present as an indurated tissue in the cervical or submandibular area that progresses to an abscess and ruptures, developing a discharging sinus involving the paralaryngeal region. The larynx may look erythematous, oedematous and firm. Most often the diagnosis is made from histopathologic analysis when sulphur granules of *Actinomyces* organisms are seen. Microbiology culture, which requires an aerobic culture medium and may take up to 2 weeks to grow, is not always helpful. In one study, microbiology culture helped make a diagnosis of actinomycosis in only 20 per cent of cases. The treatment is several weeks of oral penicillin or tetracycline for superficial infection, or intravenous medication followed by oral for deep-seated infection.[20,23–26]

NOCARDIA

Nocardia is an infection caused by an organism of the *Actinomyces* species. The species are soil saprophytes. The mode of infection is through local cutaneous trauma or by inhalation. Farm workers who are exposed to large amounts of soil and dust are prone to contract the infection. The disease has non-specific features and resembles other infective granulomatous diseases. Aerodigestive tract involvement is common. Immunocompromised patients, including those with solid organ transplants, are at risk of contracting the infection and can present with vocal cord palsy and laryngeal abscess. The treatment is intravenous sulfisoxazole.[19,27]

SCLEROMA (RHINOSCLEROMA)

Scleroma is a chronic infection of the upper respiratory tract caused by *Klebsiella rhinoscleromatis*. The disease is more common in tropical and temperate climates and in populations with poor social circumstances.[19]

The nasal cavity is commonly affected. Scleroma can also involve the larynx, mainly the glottis and the subglottis. The disease progresses in three stages: catarrhal, granulomatous and sclerotic. In the catarrh stage, there is marked mucopurulent rhinorrhoea with nasal crusting, whilst in the granulomatous stage, small painless granulomas are noted. In the final sclerotic stage, sclerosis and scar tissue develop within the nose, the palate and the larynx and may cause upper airway obstruction.[19,21,28]

Diagnosis is confirmed by microbiology culture of the organism and by histopathology when Mikulicz cells (foamly vacuolated histiocytes) and Russell bodies (bloated plasma cells with red birefringent inclusions) are seen.[28] CT and MRI are useful in evaluating the extent of the disease.

The medical treatment is rifampicin, trimethoprim-sulfamethoxazole, ciprofloxacin or cephalosporin for 3 to 4 months. Relapse of the disease is common after treatment. Surgical procedures – including division of pharyngeal adhesions, microlaryngoscopy and removal of laryngeal granuloma, excision of nasal granulomas, tracheostomy, bronchoscopy with dilatation of subglottic and tracheal stenosis, and laryngo-tracheal reconstruction – may be required.[21,28–31]

FUNGAL GRANULOMATOUS DISEASE

CANDIDIASIS

Candidiasis is caused by *Candida albicans.* The predisposing factors include use of systemic antibiotics or systemic or inhaled corticosteroids; diabetes mellitus; alcoholism; inhalational and thermal injury; leucopenia and haematological malignancy; AIDS; use of immunosuppressive medications or systemic cytotoxic chemotherapy; and local radiotherapy to the upper aerodigestive tract, including the larynx, the pharynx, the oral cavity and the neck.[21] The oral cavity, the oropharynx and the oesophagus can also be affected by candidiasis.

Sore throat, odynophagia and dysphonia are the most common presentations. Dysphagia can happen in candidal oesophagitis. The features of candidiasis are mucosal erythema with white plaques, cheesy material and exudate. The supraglottis and glottis are commonly affected in the larynx. The appearance can mimic malignant neoplastic lesions and mucosal ulcerations. Direct laryngoscopy, microlaryngoscopy and biopsy of the lesions for histopathology may be necessary to exclude laryngeal carcinoma (Figure 22.6). Swab and tissue specimens should also be sent for microbiologic analysis for culture, special fungal stain and microscopy. Investigation and management of

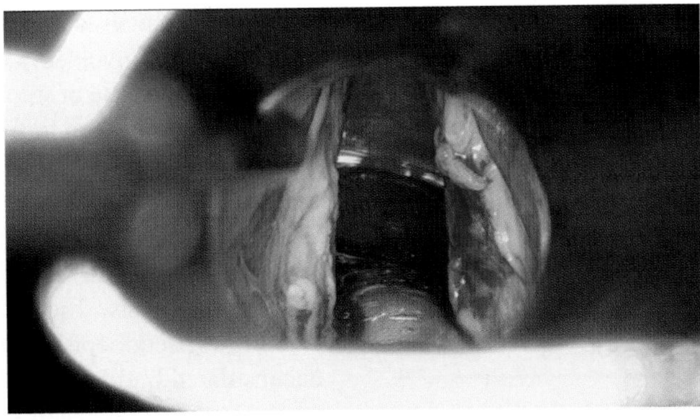

Figure 22.6 Microlaryngoscopic view of glottis showing features of candidiasis on true vocal cord bilaterally. A biopsy was taken from the right vocal cord.

any underlying medical conditions are important. Oral nystatin suspension for several weeks is often effective. Systemic antifungal agents, such as fluconazole or ketoconazole, are necessary in immunocompromised patients and in severe cases.[20,26]

ASPERGILLOSIS

Aspergillosis is an opportunistic infection, caused by *Aspergillus fumigatus* or *Aspergillus flavus*. *Aspergillus* is widespread and is transmitted by airborne spores. It usually causes saprophytic infection in the nasal cavity and the paranasal sinuses. Invasive aspergillosis occurs mainly in immunocompromised patients. Primary laryngeal aspergillosis is very rare. The infection is usually invasive and necrotizing with a very poor prognosis. The treatment is aggressive: surgical debridement of necrotic tissue until fresh viable tissue is identified, which may require total laryngectomy, and long-term intravenous amphotericin B.[26]

HISTOPLASMOSIS

Histoplasmosis is an infection caused by *Histoplasma capsulatum*. The fungus is in a dimorphic form, which lives as yeast at normal body temperature and as a mycelium in soil with high nitrogen content, usually derived from avian faeces.[20]

The mode of infection is through inhaled spores, which cause acute upper respiratory tract infection that resolves, then forms small calcification deposits in the lungs and the spleen. Occasionally, the disease may progress, developing pulmonary cavitation and indolent widespread disease in the body. Laryngeal histoplasmosis usually occurs in the disseminated form of the disease with features of mucosal ulcerations in the upper aerodigestive tract and heptosplenomegaly. The anterior larynx and epiglottis are commonly affected.[21]

Most patients with otolaryngological involvement are immunocompromised. Dysphonia, sore throat, dysphagia, fever, night sweats, lethargy and weight loss are the common symptoms on presentation.[19] Diagnosis is made with microbiology culture and microscopy with special fungal stains revealing intracellular yeast buds. Chest radiography can show multiple small calcifications in the lungs. A complement fixation test for histoplasmosis is useful in making a diagnosis. There are non-specific granulomatous features on histopathology. Intravenous amphotericin B is used for treatment.[20,26,32]

BLASTOMYCOSIS

Blastomycosis is caused by *Blastomyces dermatitidis*, a dimorphic fungus. It is usually found in damp areas with decaying wood. The infection is contracted through inhaled spores. The disease can affect multiple organs, with the lungs and the skin most commonly involved. The larynx is infrequently involved. Patients usually present with dysphonia. Laryngoscopy may reveal granular exophytic masses with mucosal ulcerations commonly involving the glottis and the false vocal cord. The clinical findings can resemble laryngeal carcinoma. The histopathologic examination shows features of acute and chronic inflammation, micro-abscesses, giant cells and pseudoepitheliomatous hyperplasia. The latter feature can be mistaken for carcinoma. Fungal culture and stains are useful in confirming the diagnosis. The treatment is long-term oral itraconazole or amphotericin B.[20,21,26,33,34]

COCCIDIOIDOMYCOSIS

Coccidioidomycosis is a fungal infection caused by *Coccidioides immitis,* a soil fungus. The disease is endemic in the southwestern United States, northern Mexico and parts of Central and South America. It is primarily a pulmonary infection via inhalation of spores. Patients with the infection are frequently asymptomatic. Extra-pulmonary or disseminated disease affecting skin, lymph nodes, bone, joints and meninges occurs in about 1–2 per cent of infected individuals. Immuncompromised patients are at risk of developing aggressive and disseminated disease. The presenting symptoms include fever, malaise, cough, dysphagia, odynophagia and dysphonia. Upper airway obstruction may occur with laryngeal involvement, requiring tracheostomy. The laryngeal examination reveals mucosal oedema, ulceration, granulation tissue and impaired vocal cord movement. Chest radiography or CT scan may show calcified granulomas in the lungs. The diagnosis is made from histopathologic analysis, with fungal stain showing typical *Coccidioides* spherules that contain endospheres. Specimens should also be taken for fungal culture. *Coccidioides* IgM and IgG antibody and complement fixation titres are useful. The treatment is systemic amphotericin B and azole antifungal agents.[26,35–37]

CRYPTOCOCCOSIS

Cryptococcosis is a fungal infection caused by *Cryptococcus neoformans* and *Cryptococcus gattii,* which are found in soil. The infection is through inhalation of spores, and it affects the lung primarily. Cryptococcosis commonly affects immunocompromised patients with AIDS, with haematological malignancy or who are on immunosuppressive drugs. Less commonly, the infection affects immunocompetent individuals. The brain and the meninges of the central nervous system are commonly involved. Laryngeal involvement is rare. Prolonged use of inhaled corticosteroid therapy may contribute to local laryngeal infection.

Persistent dysphonia is the usual presentation, and the vocal cords are most commonly affected. The exophytic laryngeal lesion may mimic carcinoma. Biopsy and fungal culture are needed to make a diagnosis. The histopathologic examination shows pseudoepitheliomatous hyperplasia and encapsulated budding yeast cells. The treatment is systemic antifungal agents such as amphotericin B and azole.[4,20,26,39–41]

HERPESVIRUS INFECTION

HERPES SIMPLEX VIRUS

Herpes simplex virus most often causes reactivation infection but may also cause primary infection. Herpes simplex laryngitis is rare and can affect immunocompetent and immunocompromised young children and adults.[42–44] It can be associated with herpes simplex gingivostomatitis and pharyngitis and, rarely, acute herpes simplex laryngo-tracheitis.

The clinical features are sore throat, odynophagia and hoarse voice. History of organ transplantation, HIV infection or immunosuppressive medication should be established. Multiple small vesicles and ulcers are seen in the oral cavity and the oropharyngeal and laryngeal mucosa. The vesicles rupture and coalesce, forming large ulcers. In the larynx, ulcers can be found in the epiglottis, the aryepiglottic folds and the vocal cords. When the epiglottis is involved, the condition can be misdiagnosed as acute bacterial epiglottitis. An ulcerative mass in the larynx can resemble carcinoma.[45] It can cause laryngeal airway obstruction, laryngeal cartilaginous framework destruction and vocal cord palsy.[46,47] The diagnosis is established on herpes simplex viral serological examination, including IgM and IgG, viral culture on tissue or vesicular fluid, and histological examination with immunohistochemistry on laryngeal biopsy specimen.

Tracheal intubation or tracheostomy is needed for upper airway obstruction. Intubation may cause worsening in laryngeal and subglottic mucosal ulceration, leading to stenosis, particularly in children.[4] Systemic antiviral therapy with acyclovir should be started without delay while waiting for confirmation of the diagnosis from the laboratory tests. Concurrent candida fungal and superimposed bacterial infection may occur and require systemic antifungal and antibiotic treatment.[45] Laryngeal incompetence is found in children following recovery from herpes simplex laryngitis, presumably due to impaired sensory neural function in the laryngeal mucosa.[4]

VARICELLA-ZOSTER VIRUS

Varicella-zoster virus infection has two distinct clinical manifestations: primary infection (chicken pox) and reactivation of latent virus in the neurons of the cranial nerve or the dorsal root ganglia (herpes zoster) associated with impaired immune response or physical stress. The virus can infect healthy individuals but is more common in recipients of solid organ, bone marrow or haematopoietic stem cell transplants and in HIV-infected patients.[49]

Herpes zoster laryngitis is rare and often associated with unilateral multiple cranial neuropathy affecting the seventh, eighth, ninth and tenth cranial nerves.[50] Symptoms of odynophagia, sore throat, hoarse voice and dysphagia are common. There may be unilateral facial palsy, otalgia, sensory neural hearing impairment, vertigo and skin rash along sensory nerve dermatomal distribution. Laryngoscopy reveals multiple mucosal ulcers or eruptions in the tongue base, the supraglottis, the glottis and the hypopharynx. A laryngeal mass may also be found. Unilateral vocal cord paralysis is not uncommon. Examination of the oropharynx and the nasopharynx may reveal mucosal eruptions and soft palatal palsy.

The clinical diagnosis of varicella-zoster virus infection can be made from characteristic unilateral vesicular lesions in a dermatonal pattern.[51] The diagnosis is confirmed by laboratory investigations including viral culture from vesicular liquid, body fluid and tissue; varicella-zoster virus IgM and IgG titre[52]; enzyme immunoassay (EIA); and polymerase chain reaction. Anti-viral agents, such as acyclovir, are given orally or intravenously in severe infection. The treatment should be started as soon as the varicella-zoster virus infection is suspected. Systemic corticosteroids can also be given.

CYTOMEGALOVIRUS

Cytomegalovirus (CMV) infection is common in patients after solid organ, bone marrow or haematopoietic stem cell transplantation and in AIDS patients because of their impaired cellular immunity. Organs involved by cytomegalovirus in those patients include liver, brain, lung, gastro-intestinal tract and eye. However, cytomegalovirus laryngitis is rare. Laryngeal examination can show mucosal inflammation, pseudomembrane with mucosal necrosis, vocal cord palsy and obstructive laryngeal mass.

The diagnosis of cytomegalovirus infection can be made with tissue pathologic analysis by identification of cytomegalic inclusion bodies and by detection of cytomegalovirus via immunohistochemistry or DNA hybridization technique. Tube cell culture and shell vial culture techniques are used to detect replicating cytomegalovirus cells in body fluids and tissue. Viral blood culture, detection of cytomegalovirus antigenemia in blood leucocytes and PCR are also used for making a diagnosis. Antiviral agents, including ganciclovir and foscarnet, are effective.[49,53]

EPSTEIN–BARR VIRUS

Epstein–Barr virus (EBV) is known to cause infectious mononucleosis, also called glandular fever, which typically presents with sore throat, fever, malaise, lymphadenopathy, tonsillar and adenoidal hyperplasia, abdominal pain and hepatitis. EBV infection in transplantation recipients is not uncommon, and it is known to be associated with post-transplantation lymphoproliferative disease (PTLD). The incidence of PTLD varies with different organs, and the rate ranges from 1–10 per cent. The larynx is rarely affected. Patients present with chronic cough, fever, dyspnoea and a supraglottic laryngeal mass, which can cause airway obstruction. The diagnosis is made on EBV IgM and IgG serology, polymerase chain reaction and tissue biopsy for histopathology with immunohistochemistry examination.

The treatment for EBV-related localized post-transplantation lymphoproliferative disease is to use acyclovir or ganciclovir and to reduce immunosuppression. Chemotherapy and/or radiation therapy may be required in extranodal, multifocal and brain disease.[49,54–56]

KEY LEARNING POINTS

- Laryngeal infections can cause airway obstruction rapidly.
- Skill is required in the management of stridor in children and adults.
- Features of laryngeal infection can resemble malignancy.
- Prevalence of infective pathogens varies in different countries.
- Infective pathogens can be different in immunocompromised patients.

REFERENCES

1. Berg S, Trollfors B, Nylén O, Hugosson S, Prellner K, Carenfelt C. Incidence, aetiology, and prognosis of acute epiglottitis in children and adults in Sweden. *Scandinavian Journal of Infectious Diseases.* 1996; 28(3): 261–64.
2. Devlin B, Golchin K, Adair R. Paediatric airway emergencies in Northern Ireland, 1990–2003. *Journal of Laryngology and Otology.* 2007; 121(7): 659–63.
3. González Valdepeña H, Wald ER, Rose E, Ungkanont K, Casselbrant ML. Epiglottitis and *Haemophilus influenzae* immunization: The Pittsburgh experience – a five-year review. *Pediatrics.* 1995; 96(3): 424–47.
4. Shine NP, Prescott C. *Acquired Disorders of the Larynx in Children.* In: *Pediatric ENT.* Eds. Graham JM, Scadding GK, Bull PD. Berlin: Springer, 2007: 197–210.
5. Sobol SE, Zapata S. Epiglottitis and croup. *Otolaryngologic Clinics of North America.* 2008; 41(3): 551–66, ix.
6. Cetinkaya F, Tüfekçi BS, Kutluk G. A comparison of nebulized budesonide and intramuscular and oral dexamethasone for treatment of croup. *International Journal of Pediatric Otorhinolaryngology.* 2004; 68(4): 453–56.
7. Rittichier KK. The role of corticosteroids in the treatment of croup. *Treatments in Respiratory Medicine.* 2004; 3(3): 139–45.
8. Syed I, Odutoye T, Lee MSW, Wong P. Management of acute epiglottitis in adults. *British Journal of Hospital Medicine (London, England: 2005).* 2011; 72(5): M74–6.
9. Bizaki AJ, Numminen J, Vasama J-P, Laranne J, Rautiainen M. Acute supraglottitis in adults in Finland: Review and analysis of 308 cases. *The Laryngoscope.* 2011; 121(10): 2107–13.
10. Cassano L, Lombardo P, Marchese-Ragona R, Pastore A, Marchese Ragona R. Laryngopyocele: Three new clinical cases and review of the literature. *European Archives of Oto-rhino-laryngology.* 2000; 257(9): 507–11.
11. Fredrickson KL, D'Angelo AJ. Internal laryngopyocele presenting as acute airway obstruction. *Ear, Nose, & Throat Journal.* 2007; 86(2): 104–06.
12. Szwarc BJ, Kashima HK. Endoscopic management of a combined laryngocele. *Annals of Otology, Rhinology, and Laryngology.* 1997; 106(7), Pt 1: 556–59.
13. Dobie RA, Tobey DN. Clinical features of diphtheria in the respiratory tract. *JAMA: The Journal of the American Medical Association.* 1979; 242(20): 2197–201.
14. Hadfield TL, McEvoy P, Polotsky Y, Tzinserling VA, Yakovlev AA. The pathology of diphtheria. *Journal of Infectious Diseases.* 2000; 181(1): S116–20.
15. Kadirova R, Kartogiu HU, Strebel PM. Clinical characteristics and management of 676 hospitalized diphtheria cases, Kyrgyz Republic, 1995. *Journal of Infectious Diseases.* 2000; 181(1): S110–15.

16. Nandi Raj, De M, Browning S, Purkayastha P, Bhattacharjee AK. Diphtheria: The patch remains. *Journal of Laryngology and Otology*. 2003; 117(10): 807–10.
17. Rakhmanova AG, Lumio J, Groundstroem K, Valova E, Nosikova E, Tanasijchuk T, Saikku J. Diphtheria outbreak in St. Petersburg: Clinical characteristics of 1860 adult patients. *Scandinavian Journal of Infectious Diseases*. 1996; 28(1): 37–40.
18. Efstratious A, Engler KK, Mazurova IK, Glushkevich T, Vuopio-Varkila J, Popovic T. Current approaches to the laboratory diagnosis of diphtheria. *Journal of Infectious Diseases*. 2000; (181)1: S138–45.
19. Swift AC. *Infective Diseases of the Head and Neck*. In: *Diseases of the Head & Neck, Nose & Throat*. Eds. Jones AS, Phillips DE, Hilgers FJM. London: Hodder, 1998: 543–61.
20. James KR. *Infections and Manifestations of Systemic Disease of the Larynx*. In: *Otolaryngology Head & Neck Surgery*. 3rd ed. Eds. Cummings CW, Fredrickson JM, Harker LA, Krause CJ, Richardson MA, Schuller DE. St. Louis: Mosby, 1998: 1979–88.
21. Altman, KW, Koufman JA. *Laryngopharyngeal Reflux and Laryngeal Infections and Manifestations of System Diseases*. In: *Ballenger's Otorhinolaryngology Head and Neck Surgery*. Centennial ed. Eds. Snow JB Jr, Wackym PA. Shelton, CT: PMPH-USA, 2008: 885–97.
22. Travis LW, Hybels RL, Newman MH. Tuberculosis of the larynx. *The Laryngoscope*. 1976; 86; 549–58.
23. Brown J. Human actinomycosis: A study of 181 subjects. *Human Pathology*. 1973; 4(319).
24. Hughes RA, Paonessa DF, Conway WR Jr. Actinomycosis of the larynx. *Annals of Otology, Rhinology, and Laryngology*. 1984; 93: 520.
25. Tsuji DH, Fukuda H, Kawasaki Y, Kawaida M, Ohira T. Actinomycosis of the larynx. *Auris, Nasus, Larynx*. 1991; 18: 79–85.
26. Vrabec DP. Fungal infections of the larynx. *Otolaryngologic Clinics of North America*. 1993; 26: 1091–144.
27. Cohen E, Blickstein D, Inbar E, Samra Z, Weinberger M. Unilateral vocal cord paralysis as a result of a *Nocardia farcinica* laryngeal abscess. *European Journal of Clinical Microbiology & Infectious Diseases*. 2000; 19(3): 224–27.
28. Zhong Q, Guo W, Chen X, et al. Rhinoscleroma: A retrospective study of pathologic and clinical features. *Journal of Otolaryngology – Head & Neck Surgery*. 2011; 40(2): 167–74.
29. Gaafar HA, Gaafar AH, Nour YA. Rhinoscleroma: An updated experience through the last 10 years. *Acta Otolaryngologica*. 2011; 131(4): 440–46.
30. Holinger PH, Gelman HK, Wolfe Jr CK. Rhinoscleroma of the lower respiratory tract. *The Laryngoscope*. 1977; 87: 1–9.
31. Soliman Z, Mobashir M, Basha WM, Askar S, Elnashar I, Said AE. Surgical management of scleromatous laryngotracheal stenosis. *Auris, Nasus, Larynx*. 2013; 40(4): 388–93.
32. Gerber ME, Rosdeutscher JD, Seiden AM, et al. Histoplasmosis: The otolaryngologist's perspective. *The Laryngoscope*. 1995; 105: 919–23.
33. Hanson JM, Spector G, El-Mofty SK. Laryngeal blastomycosis: A commonly missed diagnosis. Report of two cases and review of the literature. *Annals of Otology, Rhinology, and Laryngology*. 2000; 109(3): 281–86.
34. Reder PA, Neel HB. Blastomycosis in otolaryngology: Review of a large series. *The Laryngoscope*. 1993; 103(1), Pt 1: 53–58.
35. Allen JE, Belafsky PC. Laryngeal coccidioidomycosis with vocal fold paralysis. *Ear, Nose, & Throat Journal*. 2011; (90)5: E1–5.
36. Arnold MG, Arnold JC, Bloom DC, Brewster DF, Thiringer JK. Head and neck manifestations of disseminated coccidioidomycosis. *The Laryngoscope*. 2004; 114(4): 747–52.
37. Rosen EJ, Newlands SD, Patel J, Kalia A, Friedman NR. Reactivated laryngeal coccidioidomycosis. *Otolaryngology – Head and Neck Surgery*. 2001; 125(1): 120–21.
38. Bamba H, Tatemoto K, Inoue M, Uno T, Hisa, Y. A case of vocal cord cyst with cryptococcal infection. *Otolaryngology – Head and Neck Surgery*. 2005; 133(1): 150–52.

39. Gordon DH, Stow NW, Yapa HM, Bova R, Marriott D. Laryngeal cryptococcosis: Clinical presentation and treatment of a rare cause of hoarseness. *Otolaryngology – Head and Neck Surgery*. 2010; 142(3): S7–9.
40. Mittal N, Collignon P, Pham T, Robbie M. Cryptococcal infection of the larynx: Case report. *Journal of Laryngology and Otology*. 2013: 1–3.
41. Nadrous HF, Ryu JH, Lewis JE, Sabri AN. Cryptococcal laryngitis: Case report and review of the literature. *Annals of Otology, Rhinology, and Laryngology*. 2004; 113(2): 121–23.
42. Chauhan N, Robinson JL, Guillemaud J, El-Hakim H. Acute herpes simplex laryngotracheitis: Report of two pediatric cases and review of the literature. *International Journal of Pediatric Otorhinolaryngology*. 2007; 71(2): 341–45.
43. Sharp HR, Blaney SP, Morrison GA. Neonatal stridor in association with herpes simplex infection of the larynx. *Journal of Laryngology and Otology*. 1998; 112(12): 1192–93.
44. Yeh V, Hopp ML, Goldstein NS, Meyer RD. Herpes simplex chronic laryngitis and vocal cord lesions in a patient with acquired immunodeficiency syndrome. *Annals of Otology, Rhinology, and Laryngology*. 1994; 103(9): 726–31.
45. Sanei-Moghaddam A, Loizou P, Fish BM. An unusual presentation of herpes infection in the head and neck. *BMJ Case Reports*. 2013; Jan 31, 2013.
46. Dupuch V, Saroul N, Aumeran C, Pastourel R, Mom T, Gilain L. Bilateral vocal cord abductor paralysis associated with primary herpes simplex infection: A case report. *European Annals of Otorhinolaryngology, Head and Neck Diseases*. 2012; 129(5): 272–74.
47. Sims JR, Massoll NA, Suen JY. Herpes simplex infection of the larynx requiring laryngectomy. *American Journal of Otolaryngology*. 2013; Jan 14, 2013.
48. Zhang S, Farmer TL, Frable MA, Powers CN. Adult herpetic laryngitis with concurrent candidal infection: A case report and literature review. *Archives of Otolaryngology – Head and Neck Surgery*. 2000; 126(5): 672–74.
49. Patel R, Paya CV. Infections in solid-organ transplant recipients. *Clinical Microbiology Reviews*. 1997; 10(1): 86–124.
50. Lin YY, Kao CH, Wang CH. Varicella zoster virus infection of the pharynx and larynx with multiple cranial neuropathies. *The Laryngoscope*. 2011; 121(8): 1627–30.
51. Wu CL, Linne OC, Chiang CW. Herpes zoster laryngis with prelaryngeal skin erythema. *Annals of Otology, Rhinology, and Laryngology*. 2004; 113(2): 113–14.
52. Watelet J-B, Evrard A-S, Lawson G, Bonte K, Remacle M, Van Cauwenberge P, Vermeersch H. Herpes zoster laryngitis: Case report and serological profile. *European Archives of Oto-rhino-laryngology*. 2007; 264(5): 505–07.
53. Valla F, Lévêque N, Escuret V, Galambrun C, Mialou V, Bleyzac N, Bertrand Y. Human cytomegalovirus (HCMV) laryngitis: Atypical HCMV disease presentation in haematopoietic stem cell transplantation. *Journal of Medical Microbiology*. 2008; 57(Pt 11): 1434–35.
54. Banks C, Meier JD, Stallworth CR, White DR. Recurrent posttransplant lymphoproliferative disorder involving the larynx and trachea: Case report and review of the literature. *Annals of Otology, Rhinology, and Laryngology*. 2012; 121(5): 291–95.
55. Lee HH, Lee DS, Park JH, Lee KW, Kim SJ, Joh JW, Seo JM, Kwon GY, Choe YH, Lee SK. A case of laryngeal posttransplantation lymphoproliferative disease. *Transplantation Proceedings*. 2004; 36(8): 2305–06.
56. Rafferty MA, Devaney D, Russell J. Case report: An unusual cause of stridor in a post-liver transplant 6-year old. *International Journal of Pediatric Otorhinolaryngology*. 2000; 54(2–3): 149–51.

23

Tumours of the nasopharynx

NICHOLAS D STAFFORD

Squamous type cancers of the nasopharynx are biologically distinct from those at other sites in the upper aerodigestive tract. Their histology, clinical behaviour and treatment reflect this. They are rare in the Western world, where their incidence is approximately 1 in 100 000 of the Caucasian population. In Southeast China (where they comprise 18 per cent of all tumours) their incidence is 40 times higher. They are also common in Africa (particularly Tunisia, Sudan and parts of Kenya and Uganda).

Nasopharyngeal carcinoma (NPC) is approximately three times more common in men than in women.

With China's recent socio-economic development, there would appear to be a fall in the disease's incidence locally.

AETIOLOGY

There are three main aetiological factors that predispose to the development of NPC.

VIRAL

The link between infection with the Epstein–Barr virus (EBV) and histological types II and III of NPC is now well established. Infection of the general population with this virus is relatively common, although only a very small subgroup develop NPC. It would therefore seem likely that the effect of EBV on the development of NPC is a secondary one, with the virus impairing tumour suppression by the host defences.

What is established is that post-treatment levels of EBV DNA in the circulating blood can predict both overall survival and the likelihood of disease relapse. Indeed, in a multivariate analysis of parameters such as tumour stage and histology, the only independently significant factor predicting long-term outcome was EBV DNA status.[1]

GENETIC

The high incidence of NPC noted in Southeast China would appear to lend support to a significant genetic predisposition to the disease. The Chinese retain this predisposition even when they emigrate and settle in North America or Western Europe. However, in such situations the disease incidence decreases with each new generation.

ENVIRONMENTAL

NPC development is associated with a high dietary intake of salted fish. The content of carcinogenic nitrosamines in the fish appears to be the crucial factor. The higher the level of carcinogenic nitrosamines consumed, the higher the incidence of NPC. It has certainly been shown that dimethyl nitrosamine can induce malignant tumours in the upper respiratory tracts of rats.

ANATOMY

The nasopharynx is bounded anteriorly by the posterior choanae and the posterior edge of the nasal septum. Its lateral walls include the fossae of Rosenmuller and the eustachian tube orifices. The roof slopes posteriorly and inferiorly and becomes the posterior wall of the oropharynx at the level of Passavant's ridge, essentially at the level of the hard palate. Its transverse diameter is approximately 3 cm anteriorly, widening to 4–5 cm between the fossae. The foramen lacerum is directly related to the roof of the nasopharynx. The close proximity of the eustachian tube orifices, the orbits, the skull base and maxillae and the intracranial fossa explains the diverse range of clinical manifestations of the disease.

An extensive submucosal lymphatic plexus drains primarily into the retro-pharyngeal and upper deep cervical chain nodes and is the reason for the high incidence of nodal disease at presentation.

The main arterial supply comes from the ascending pharyngeal branch of the external carotid artery on each side. Venous drainage is largely into a diffuse pharyngeal venous plexus.

The epithelium of the nasopharynx varies from stratified squamous to ciliated columnar types, with transition zones in between. There are also countless microscopic minor salivary glands as well as follicles of lymphoid tissue; hence the heterogeneity in the histological types of malignancy that can arise locally.

HISTOPATHOLOGY

The great majority of malignancies originate from the squamous mucosa of the nasopharynx, and it is this group (NPC) that forms the focus of this chapter. Other histological types include adenocarcinomas, carcinomas of salivary gland origin, sarcomas, melanomas and solid haematological malignancies.

The World Health Organization describes three histological types of carcinoma of squamous mucosal origin:

Type 1 – squamous cell carcinoma
Type 2 – keratinizing undifferentiated carcinoma
Type 3 – non-keratinizing undifferentiated carcinoma

Whilst Type 1 tumours tend to behave in a similar way to squamous cell carcinomas at other head and neck sites, the latter two types, which are associated with EBV infection, are biologically different.

STAGING

Primary tumours are staged as follows:

T1 tumour involves the nasopharynx alone or the nasopharynx and oropharynx.

T2 tumour extends into parapharyngeal tissues but does not involve bone.
T3 tumour spreads to involve bone or paranasal sinuses.
T4 tumour involves the skull base/orbit/hypopharynx/pterygopalatine fossa.

The overall tumour staging determines the treatment protocol employed.

Stage 1 – T1N0 (N0)
Stage 2 – T1N1, T2N0 or T2N1 (all M0)
Stage 3 – T3N0, T3N1, T3N2, T1N2 or T2N2 (all M0)
Stage 4A – T4N0, T4N1, T4N2 (all M0)
Stage 4B – Any T stage N3 (all M0)
Stage 4C – Any T stage, any N stage, M1

CLINICAL PRESENTATION

LOCAL SYMPTOMS

Local symptoms include nasal obstruction, nasal speech, epistaxis and nasal regurgitation of food. Orbital extension can result in proptosis or diplopia, whilst involvement of the skull base can cause chronic headache or secondary sphenoiditis. Obstruction of the ipsilateral eustachian tube will lead to a conductive hearing loss due to a middle ear effusion. Extensive disease invading the maxilla can cause swelling of the cheek or dental symptoms.

NEUROLOGICAL SYMPTOMS

The proximity of the anterior cranial fossa, the cavernous sinuses and the skull base can result in a palsy of one or more of any of the cranial nerves. Diplopia or a jugular foramen syndrome is associated with locally advanced disease. Overall, 20–25 per cent of patients have a cranial nerve palsy at presentation; of these, involvement of the fifth or sixth nerve is evident in more than half.

METASTATIC DISEASE

Approximately 50 per cent of patients will have cervical lymphadenopathy at the time of presentation. Indeed, this may be the patient's sole presenting symptom. Nasopharyngeal cancer must be considered as a possible diagnosis in any patient presenting in this way.

The likely presence of metastases outside the head and neck seems to vary geographically. It is rare in Caucasians, except in cases where the locoregional disease is very advanced. It occurs in less than 10 per cent of cases in Southeast Asia and China, whilst bony metastases are relatively common in Africans with NPC.

NPC-ASSOCIATED SYNDROMES

Syndromes associated with NPC include:

- Hypertrophic osteoarthropathy
- Inappropriate antidiuretic hormone (ADH) secretion
- Pyrexia of unknown origin (PUO) associated with a leukaemoid peripheral blood picture (seen particularly in young Africans)

CLINICAL ASSESSMENT

A full ear, nose and throat examination should be augmented by fibre-optic examination of the nasopharynx. If an obvious mass is present, then it can be biopsied in the clinic after application of a local anaesthetic. However, this should not be done if the lesion has any of the characteristics of an angiofibroma. Cranial nerve function should be evaluated, as should the appearance of the optic discs and whether a Horner's syndrome is present.

Trismus is indicative of pterygoid muscle invasion. Palpation of the neck with fine-needle aspiration of any palpable lymph nodes is also essential.

Imaging of the head and neck is very important; accurate staging of the tumour on purely clinical grounds is close to impossible. Computed tomography (CT) scanning is useful for demonstrating bone involvement or destruction, whilst magnetic resonance imaging (MRI) is better for demonstrating the soft tissue extent of the disease and involvement of adjacent muscles and neurovascular structures. For patients with advanced (stages III and IV) disease, a positron emission tomography

(PET)–CT scan will be very helpful in excluding infraclavicular metastases.

If the neck is clinically negative but MRI suggests possible nodal disease, then ultrasound scanning can be helpful in confirming or refuting such involvement. It is also a great aid to fine-needle aspiration of nodes that are less than 1 cm in diameter.

Given the preceding discussion, the only reasons a patient may require a formal endoscopy under general anaesthesia are if the tumour cannot be biopsied with the patient awake, if there is reason to suspect a synchronous second primary or if a grommet insertion is also required. Severe trismus may make intubation prior to general anaesthesia very difficult.

TREATMENT

All patients should be reviewed by the multidisciplinary team for head and neck oncology. The cornerstone of treatment for NPC is radiotherapy. However, the past decade has elucidated the important role of chemotherapy, and there is now good evidence to demonstrate that chemo-radiation is superior to radiation alone. A recent literature review showed the clear benefit of concomitant chemo-radiation but cast doubt on the efficacy of adjuvant chemotherapy.[2] However, a comparatively large study from Hong Kong has shown that such improvement in local control is offset by an increase in treatment-related mortality when platinum and 5-fluourouracil are used in combination with radiotherapy.[3]

RADIOTHERAPY

Commonly employing lateral fields and a supplementary anterior field, radiotherapy is given to a dose of 66–70 Gy in 33–35 fractions. Late complications are common (30 per cent) with a significant mortality from the treatment itself (1.4 per cent).[4] All patients should receive a dental evaluation before starting their treatment. Chronic xerostomia is the most common long-term complaint, and this exacerbates any pre-existing dental caries. Diligent dental follow-up is important. Long-term sensorineural hearing loss and trismus, resulting from pterygoid muscle fibrosis, are also commonly seen.

More than 10 per cent of treated patients demonstrate residual local disease immediately after radiotherapy. Intracavity radiotherapy is rarely practised in the United Kingdom, but intensity modulated radiation therapy (IMRT) has been used to good effect in such cases.[5]

CHEMOTHERAPY

For stage III and IV disease the synchronous use of radiotherapy and a combination of platinum and 5-fluorouracil gives improved survival over that achieved with radiotherapy alone. However, as mentioned, this is countered by increased post-treatment morbidity and mortality.

SURGERY

Histological type I NPC is not related to EBV infection and behaves more in keeping with standard squamous cell carcinomas in the region. As such, a case can be made for a neck dissection as treatment of type I nodal disease where the cervical mass exceeds 2 cm in diameter or demonstrates necrosis on imaging.

A neck dissection is also indicated for radioresistant neck disease as proven by imaging and positive needle aspiration. Otherwise, surgery does not have an established role to play in the management of NPC. Nasopharyngectomy is practised in a few centres but has not become a widely established and accepted treatment option. This is largely due to its inability to achieve satisfactory resection margins and the close proximity of vital neurovascular structures.

TREATMENT RESULTS

Over the past three decades, more accurate staging (largely enabled by proven imaging techniques), improved radiotherapy techniques (e.g. IMRT) and more comprehensive radiotherapeutic management of the neck have combined to improve survival of patients with NPC. Overall control of the primary disease is now achievable in 66–80 per cent of patients, whilst control of the neck is approximately 12 per cent better. Overall 5-year survival figures range from 37–57 per cent and are generally better for the type II and type III types.

RETREATMENT OF RECURRENT NPC

Active treatment of recurrent NPC often results in very good medium- to long-term palliation or even cure, without unacceptable morbidity or mortality.[6] In general, patients with disease that recurs within 2 years of their first treatment do less well than those in whom the disease takes longer to recur. Retreatment characteristically involves external beam irradiation and/or intracavity irradiation, though as commented earlier, experience with the latter is limited in the United Kingdom.

Recurrence in the neck should be surgically salvaged if possible.

The patient with widespread metastatic disease can be given chemotherapy; the best results have been obtained using bleomycin, epirubicin and platinum.

KEY LEARNING POINTS

- Epstein Barr viral titres can be used to monitor disease status.
- NPC is most common in southeast China.
- Concurrent chemoradiotherapy is the mainstay of curative intent treatment.
- Re-irradiation of recurrent local disease is often effective.

REFERENCES

1. Le Q-T, Jones CD, Yau T-K, et al. A comparison study of different PCR assays in measuring circulating plasma Epstein-Barr virus DNA levels in patients with nasopharyngeal carcinoma. *Clinical Cancer Research*. 2005; 11(16): 5700–7.
2. Chan ATC, Leung SF, Ngan RFC, et al. Overall survival after concurrent cisplatin-radiotherapy compared with radiotherapy alone in locoregionally advanced nasopharyngeal carcinoma. *Journal of the National Cancer Institute*. 2005; 97(7): 536–9.
3. Lee AWM, Lau WH, Tung SY, et al. Preliminary results of a randomized study as therapeutic gain by concurrent chemotherapy for regionally advanced nasopharyngeal carcinomas: NPC-9901 Trial by the Hong Kong Nasopharyngeal Cancer Study Group. *Journal of Clinical Oncology*. 2005; 23(28): 6966–75.
4. Lee AW, Law SC, Ng SH, et al. Retrospective analysis of nasopharyngeal carcinoma treated during 1976–1985: Late complications following megavoltage irradiation. *British Journal of Radiology*. 1992; 65(778): 918–28.
5. Lee N, Xia P, Quivey JM, et al. Intensity modulated radiotherapy in the treatment of nasopharyngeal carcinoma: An update of the UCSF experience. *International Journal of Radiation Oncology, Biology, Physics*. 2002; 53(1): 12–22.
6. McLean M, Chow E, O'Sullivan B, et al. Re-irradiation for locally recurrent nasopharyngeal carcinoma. *Radiotherapy and Oncology*. 1998; 48(2): 209–11.

24

Tumours of the oropharynx

PAUL PRACY

INTRODUCTION AND EPIDEMIOLOGY

In developed countries the incidence of oropharyngeal cancer has been steadily rising over the past 10–15 years. While the 'traditional' aetiological factors, smoking and alcohol, are still of importance, the increase is due to the emergence of a new aetiological factor, human papillomavirus (HPV). HPV is spread by orogenital sex, and HPV-driven tumours tend to present in younger patients and appear to carry a better prognosis than those associated with alcohol and tobacco. More than 50 per cent of oropharyngeal tumours are HPV positive, with the most common subtype implicated being HPV-16. HPV-induced tumours are particularly radiosensitive, and the oropharynx has been an area in which there has been a shift away from radical surgery towards non-surgical interventions for primary treatment, particularly through the use of chemo-radiation.[1,2]

SURGICAL ANATOMY

The oropharynx lies below the soft palate and is delineated from the oral cavity by the anterior faucial pillars; the roof is formed by the undersurface of the soft palate and the floor is the base of the tongue. The superior limit is the level of the hard palate, and the lower limit is the hyoid bone. Within this space are contained the palatine tonsils, the anterior and posterior faucial pillars, the tongue base including the lingual tonsil, the vallecula and lingual surface of the epiglottis, the pharyngoepiglottic folds, the soft palate and the posterior pharyngeal wall anterior to the second and third cervical vertebrae.

FUNCTION

The oropharynx is a complex muscular structure of crucial importance in both swallowing and speech. The soft palate influences speech by affecting the amount of air escaping through the nose during speech and by altering the volume of resonating cavities. In coordination with these palatal movements, positioning of the tongue base further modulates sound from the vocal tract. In swallowing, the palate and tongue base work together to close the nasal passages as the food bolus is propelled through the oropharynx.

PATHOLOGY

While the most common malignant tumour of the oropharynx is oropharyngeal squamous cell carcinoma (OPSCC), the preponderance of lymphoid tissue and minor salivary glands means that lymphomas and salivary gland cancers must also be considered. The lymphomas are almost always non-Hodgkin's type, while mucoepidermoid and adenoid cystic carcinomas are the most common salivary cancers.

CLINICAL PRESENTATION

Lymph node metastases are common at presentation and may be the only sign or symptom of disease. Fifty per cent of patients have palpable lymph node metastases at presentation, and an additional 25 per cent will have occult nodal disease. Where a cervical lymph node metastasis presents with an occult primary tumour, the majority of patients will turn out to have an OPSCC. However, the individual primary sites within the oropharynx can also give rise to symptoms such as dysphagia, odynophagia, otalgia, sore throat or tongue, or change of voice (the 'hot-potato' voice).

Tonsil tumours may present as unilateral tonsillar enlargement or, most commonly, as an ulcer. Tongue base tumours will most commonly appear as ulcers but may also present as endophytic masses, which are notoriously difficult to see and are better identified by palpation. See Figures 24.1, 24.2, and 24.3.

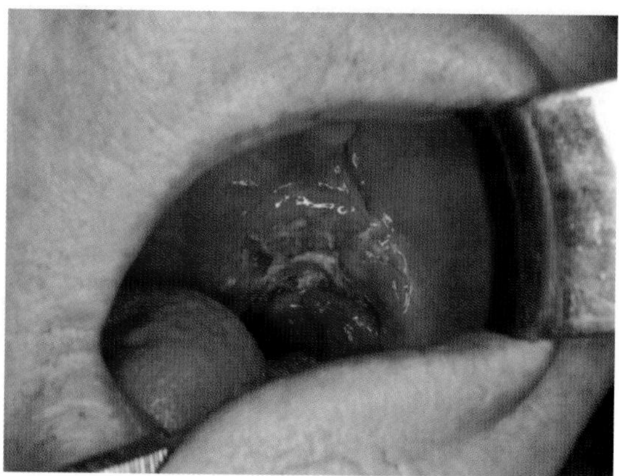

Figure 24.1 SCC of the tonsil involving the soft palate and anterior faucial pillar. Clinical photograph compliments of Mr T Martin, FRCS OMFS.

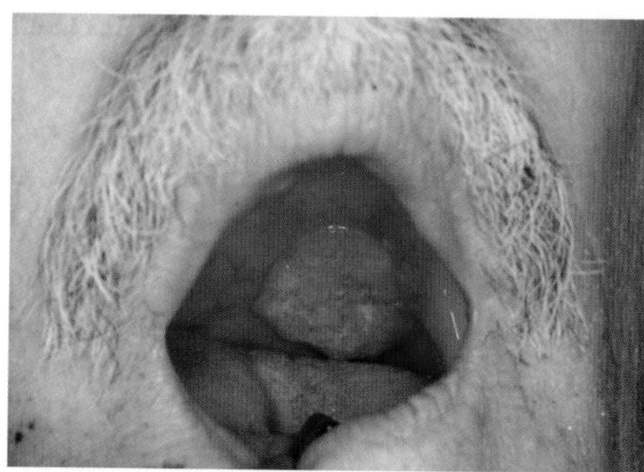

Figure 24.2 SCC of the soft palate involving the hard palate. Clinical photograph compliments of Mr T Martin, FRCS OMFS.

ASSESSMENT AND STAGING

Clinical examination must be systematic and thorough. All patients should undergo fibre-optic laryngopharyngoscopy, and an attempt should be made to palpate the tongue base (although not all patients will tolerate this).

Cross-sectional imaging is mandatory for accurate staging and treatment planning. Magnetic resonance imaging (MRI) is the best modality to assess the primary site and cervical nodes.

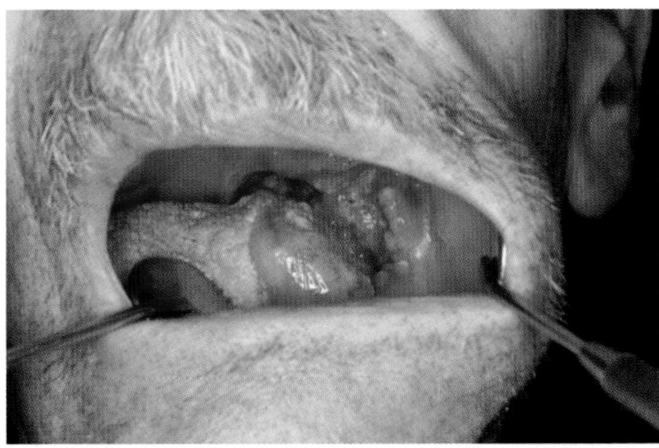

Figure 24.3 SCC of the oropharynx with involvement of the tonsil, tongue base retromolar trigone, soft palate and posterior pharyngeal wall. Clinical photograph compliments of Mr T Martin, FRCS (OMFS).

Computed tomography (CT) may be required for the evaluation of any bony involvement and offers the advantage of allowing assessment of the chest and upper abdomen at the same time.

Panendoscopy or examination under anaesthesia is not mandatory but allows better assessment for second primary tumours and additional information about the resectability of some tumours.[2]

Staging is based on the TNM classification for oropharyngeal tumours (Table 24.1).

Table 24.1 Staging of oropharyngeal tumours

TX	Primary tumour cannot be assessed
T0	No evidence of primary tumour
Tis	Carcinoma *in situ*
T1	Tumour up to 2 cm in greatest dimension
T2	Tumour larger than 2 cm but 4 cm or less in greatest dimension
T3	Tumour larger than 4 cm in greatest dimension
T4a	Tumour invades larynx, deep/extrinsic tongue muscles, medial pterygoid muscle, hard palate or mandible
T4b	Tumour invades lateral pterygoid muscle, pterygoid plates, lateral nasopharynx or skull base or encases the carotid artery

TREATMENT

The treatment of OPSCC has significantly changed over the past 20 years. Patients with early disease or who were not fit enough to undergo radical resection with reconstruction were treated with primary radiotherapy. Patients with advanced disease, who were fit enough, would be offered radical resection with reconstruction. The increased use of concomitant chemoradiotherapy through the 1990s was shown to offer better rates of survival with the presumed additional advantage of 'organ preservation'. This has resulted in a shift away from radical surgery, and chemoradiotherapy is currently regarded as the standard of care for most patients with OPSCC. However, the increased morbidity of chemo-radiation over radiotherapy has led researchers to look at alternative regimens, such as the use of intensity modulated radiotherapy (IMRT) or radiotherapy alone for the management of HPV+ve tumours. The increased use of transoral microsurgery in head and neck cancer has also seen the development of surgical techniques, often incorporating the use of robotics, for the excision of OPSCC, although the majority of patients still receive postoperative radiotherapy or chemoradiotherapy.[1–3]

EARLY TUMOURS

Early-stage tumours (T1–2 N0) can be treated with equal effect by primary surgery or radiotherapy. Cure rates of 80–90 per cent can be expected with either modality.

Surgery for early disease can be carried out using open techniques or by transoral resection. Where access is required for free flap reconstruction, it is usually necessary to perform a paramedian mandibulotomy or a lingual release and drop down of the oral cavity into the neck, while maintaining the integrity of the mandible. Small tongue base tumours can be approached via transhyoid lateral pharyngotomy. Small defects can be left to granulate or be closed primarily, while larger defects should be reconstructed with a radial forearm free flap or anterolateral thigh flap for very large defects. The use of pedicled flaps should be reserved for patients who are not fit enough to undergo microvascular free tissue reconstruction because the functional results are not as good. At the moment there is insufficient evidence to support the routine use of transoral techniques with or without the robot, because almost all of these patients receive post-operative adjunctive treatment with chemo-radiation or radiotherapy.[4,5]

The incidence of occult nodal metastases in patients with T1 and T2 tumours is 10–30 per cent, so the neck must be included in any treatment plan. Both surgery, using a selective neck dissection, and radiotherapy are effective. Where the primary tumour lies close to the midline, there is a significant risk of contralateral spread, so both sides of the neck should be included in the treatment plan.

ADVANCED TUMOURS

The management of T3/T4 N+ OPSCC is most commonly by the use of chemo-radiation. However, there remain some questions about the toxicity of this line of treatment, and the increased incidence of HPV-driven tumours (which have a better prognosis regardless of treatment modality) makes this a fertile area for research.

Surgery for advanced tumours results in a significant loss of tissue and a consequent deterioration in function. However, in the best hands, free flap reconstruction can achieve excellent functional results. Primary resection should be considered only where there is a realistic chance of achieving adequate margins, which avoids the need for post-operative chemotherapy in addition to radiotherapy.

Management of the neck is of paramount importance because the rates of nodal metastases in patients with T3/T4 tumours are in excess of 50 per cent.[3–5]

KEY LEARNING POINTS

- Increasing incidence is due to the emergence of HPV as an aetiological factor.
- HPV-related tumours have a better prognosis.
- There is a trend towards nonsurgical treatment, although this has to some extent been balanced by the development of transoral laser surgery (TLS) and transoral robotic surgery (TORS).
- Meticulous clinical and radiological assessment is crucial and will usually require both CT and MR imaging.
- High rates of nodal metastasis must be considered in the treatment plan.

REFERENCES

1. Ang KK, Harris J, Wheeler R, et al. Human papillomavirus and survival of patients with oropharyngeal cancer. *New England Journal of Medicine*. 2010; 363: 24–35.
2. Robson AK, Paleri V. Evidence based management of oropharyngeal cancer. *Clinical Otolaryngology*. 2010; 35: 273–76.
3. Parsons JT, Mendenhall WM, Stringer SP, et al. Squamous cell carcinoma of the oropharynx: Surgery, radiation therapy or both? *Cancer*. 2002; 94: 2967–80.
4. Allal AS, Nicoucar K, Mach D, Dulgueroy P. Quality of life in patients with oropharynx carcinomas: Assessment after accelerated radiotherapy with or without chemotherapy versus surgery and post operative radiotherapy. *Head and Neck*. 2003; 25: 833–40.
5. Skoner JM, Anderson PE, Cohen JI, et al. Swallowing function and tracheostomy dependence after combined modality treatment including free tissue transfer for advanced stage oropharyngeal cancer. *Laryngoscope*. 2003; 113: 1294–98.

FURTHER READING

Bernier J, Domenge C, Ozsahin M, et al. European Organization for Research and Treatment of Cancer trial 22931. Postoperative irradiation with or without concomitant chemotherapy for locally advanced head and neck cancer. *New England Journal of Medicine*. 2004; 350: 1945–52.

Bonner JA, Harari PM, Giralt J, et al. Radiotherapyplus cetuximab for squamous cell carcinoma of the head and neck. *New England Journal of Medicine*. 2006; 354: 567–78.

25

Tumours of the hypopharynx

JEAN-PIERRE JEANNON

ANATOMY

The hypopharynx is a funnel-shaped structure that includes the sub-sites of the piriform fossa or sinus (laterally), the posterior pharyngeal wall (posteriorly) and the post-cricoid oesophagus (inferiorly). The piriform fossa extends from the pharyngo-epiglottic fold to the upper end of the oesophagus. It is bound laterally by the thyroid cartilage and medially by the hypopharyngeal surface of the ary-epiglottic fold and the arytenoids and cricoid cartilage. The posterior pharyngeal wall extends from the superior level of the hyoid bone (or floor of the vallecula) to the level of the inferior border of the cricoid cartilage and from the apex of one piriform sinus to the other.

The post-cricoid area extends from the level of the arytenoid cartilages and connecting folds to the inferior border of the cricoid cartilage, thus forming the anterior wall of the hypopharynx. It is part of the upper aero-digestive tract, where the airway and the swallowing tubes separate, and is seen at the level of the fourth to the sixth cervical vertebrae. The nerve supply comes from the recurrent laryngeal nerve, a branch of the vagus (tenth cranial nerve).

AETIOLOGY/EPIDEMIOLOGY

The common causative agents that play an important role in all head and neck cancer also have a role in hypopharyngeal cancer. This type of cancer is also associated with poor socio-economic status. The incidence of this condition appears to be falling, and it is one of the rarest of head and neck cancers.

Smoking is the most important factor, followed by heavy alcohol consumption. The combined effect of these two factors greatly increases the risk of cancer at this site. Human papillomavirus (HPV) is thought to play less of a role at this site than at the oropharynx.

Carcinoma of the post-cricoid oesophagus is a distinct disease and is also associated with the Plummer–Vinson (Paterson–Brown–Kelly) syndrome. This syndrome is a rare collection of symptoms of dysphagia, iron deficiency anaemia, koilonychia, glossitis, angular stomatitis and post-cricoid web. Hypopharyngeal cancer can also be associated with a pharyngeal pouch, which is a benign diverticulum of the pharynx. Chronic inflammation associated with stasis of food contents in the pouch has been postulated as a cause of cancer, which occurs in 1 per cent of pouches.

There is a geographical variation in this cancer as it is more commonly seen in Eastern Europe than in Western Europe and has the highest incidence in Southeast Asia and South America.

CLINICAL PRESENTATION

SYMPTOMS

Hypopharyngeal cancer often presents in a late or advanced stage, which explains the poor prognosis associated with this type of cancer. The reasons for this are complex, but one explanation is that it can present with a myriad of symptoms. This cancer can only be diagnosed by a specialist who has the skills to perform a laryngoscopy.

The red flag symptoms that warrant an urgent referral are included in Table 25.1. A high index of suspicion should exist if the patient is a smoker or heavy drinker of alcohol.

Dysphagia, which is usually progressive from solids to liquids, is a common symptom initially; it is intermittent but eventually becomes persistent. Dysphonia or hoarseness can result from hypopharyngeal cancer; this is due to tumour invading the larynx. Unilateral otalgia may be the first sign of hypopharyngeal cancer and develops as a result of referred pain from invasion of a branch of the glossopharyngeal or vagus nerves, which give off branches to the ear. If unilateral otalgia exists and ear examination is normal, hypopharyngeal cancer should be suspected.

Table 25.1 Symptoms of hypopharyngeal cancer

Dysphagia
Dysphonia
Unilateral otalgia
Lymphadenopathy
Sore throat
Odynophagia
Stridor
Cough

Sore throat that persists for more than 2 weeks should alert the clinician to the possibility of throat cancer. Pain on swallowing is termed *odynophagia* and is a sinister symptom. Although the most common cause of sore throat is infection, if the patient shows no sign or symptom of sepsis, then malignancy should be considered.

Chronic cough that persists can be a first sign of cancer because the tumour may irritate the larynx and activate the cough reflex. This cough is usually non-productive. It may also be associated with swallowing and indicate aspiration with loss of the protective reflexes of the larynx.

Lymphadenopathy due to metastatic cervical lymph node involvement often presents in hypopharyngeal cancer (Figure 25.1). The lymphatic drainage from this site is rich, and this occurs even in early-stage cancer. The first echelon nodes that are affected are the upper (level 2), middle (level 3) and lower (level 4) deep cervical lymph nodes of the neck. Large hypopharyngeal cancer left undetected may obstruct the laryngeal/tracheal airway and result in stridor. Stridor is a high-pitched sound of an obstructed airway and is a medical emergency.

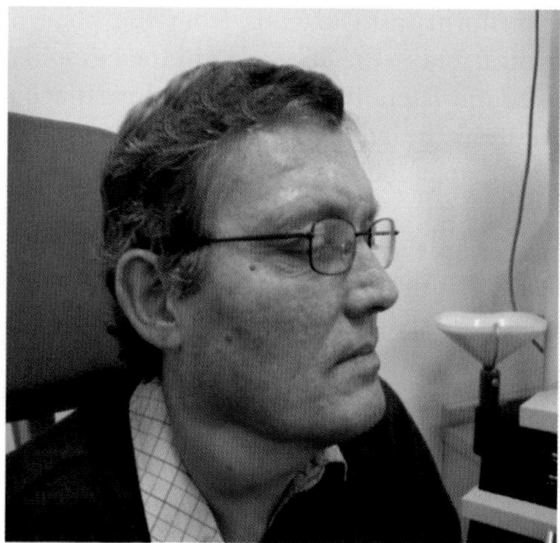

Figure 25.1 Patient with upper cervical lymphadenopathy due to metastatic involvement of lymph nodes from a hypopharyngeal cancer.

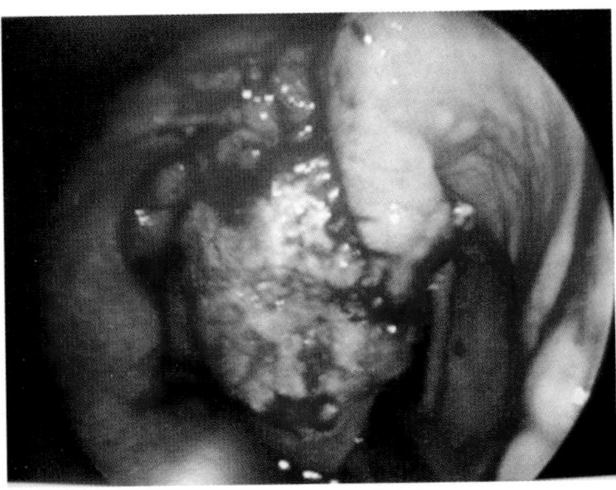

Figure 25.2 Endoscopic appearance of a hypopharyngeal cancer. Note the ulcerating tumour on the left aryepiglottic fold.

Late signs of cancer can also be present in hypopharyngeal cancer, such as weight loss and malnutrition, which result from the adverse effects of the cancer on feeding.

SIGNS

Hypopharyngeal cancer is usually diagnosed following clinical evaluation with a fibre-optic laryngoscopic examination performed in the clinic. The tumour is usually visible as an ulcerative mass in the hypopharynx (Figure 25.2). Tumours can also be exophytic and appear as a polypoidal mass at this site. Pooling of blood or saliva in the piriform fossa may indicate a tumour hidden in the hypopharynx.

An immobile or fixed vocal cord may result from hypopharyngeal cancer. This may be due to the tumour mass impairing movement of the vocal cord or recurrent laryngeal nerve invasion.

STAGING

Clinical staging of hypopharyngeal cancer is a mandatory part of the assessment of the patient, and the Union for International Cancer Control/American Joint Committee on Cancer (UICC/AJCC) TNM (tumour, node, metastasis) staging system is used (Table 25.2).

Table 25.2 TNM staging for hypopharyngeal cancer

T1	Tumour <2 cm and limited to one sub-site of hypopharynx
T2	Tumour >2 cm but <4 cm, or invades more than one sub-site of hypopharynx or an adjacent site
T3	Tumour >4 cm or with fixation of hemi-larynx
T4a	Tumour invades thyroid/cricoid cartilage, hyoid bone, thyroid gland, oesophagus, or central compartment soft tissue
T4b	Tumour invades pre-vertebral fascia, encases carotid artery, or involves mediastinal structures
N1	Metastasis in a single ipsilateral lymph node ≤3 cm
N2a	Metastasis in a single ipsilateral lymph node >3 cm but <6 cm
N2b	Metastasis in multiple ipsilateral lymph nodes <6 cm
N2c	Metastasis in bilateral or contralateral lymph nodes <6 cm
N3	Metastasis in a lymph node >6 cm

Early-stage tumours include T1 and T2 tumours; advanced tumours are T3 and T4 cases. The N staging is the same as for other head and neck sub-sites. More than 50 per cent of patients with node-negative hypopharyngeal cancer have occult or microscopic lymph node involvement; hence the primary site and the neck always have to be considered for treatment.

CLINICAL INVESTIGATION

Histological confirmation in the form of an incisional biopsy is necessary to diagnose hypopharyngeal cancer. This involves panendoscopy and biopsy. Panendoscopy involves formal assessment of the larynx, the pharynx, the upper oesophagus and the trachea under general anaesthesia.

Consideration of the safety of the airway is mandatory in managing patients undergoing panendoscopy for head and neck cancer. After the biopsy, swelling and bleeding can result, which may obstruct the airway; therefore, this complication should always be considered a possibility. Good communication between the ear, nose and throat (ENT) surgeon and the anaesthetist is necessary to plan for this possible complication, and tracheostomy may be needed to secure the airway surgically.

The biopsy specimen is sent to an expert pathologist for assessment and grading. The most common type of cancer is squamous cell carcinoma, which accounts for almost 95 per cent of tumours in this site. Rarely, other histological types may exist, such as adenocarcinoma or lymphoma.

IMAGING

Cross-sectional imaging in the form of a computed tomography (CT) scan is necessary to stage hypopharyngeal cancer. This modality of imaging allows assessment of the size of the tumour and its upper and lower extent (Figure 25.3). Invasion of local structures and spread to lymph nodes can also be determined. CT scanning also allows for detection of distant metastasis to the lungs, which may occur in this type of cancer.

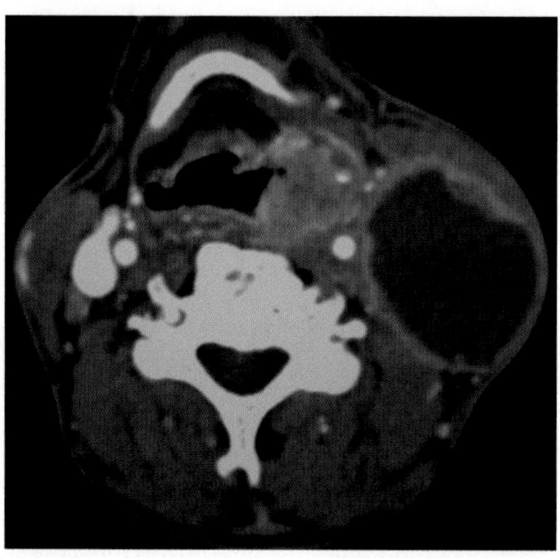

Figure 25.3 CT scan of a patient with a left-sided carcinoma of the piriform fossa. Note the tumour to the left of the larynx and a large necrotic cervical metastasis.

Other imaging modalities may be involved in staging, such as magnetic resonance imaging (MRI) or positron emission tomography (PET) scanning.

Evaluation of the overall health status of the patient is an important part of the investigation. Assessment of cardiovascular fitness, co-morbidities, nutritional state and dental hygiene is necessary for all head and neck cancer patients.

TREATMENT

Treatment of hypopharyngeal cancer follows the same principles of all cancers and can be divided into curative or palliative intention. Determining which treatment is adopted depends upon the following factors: stage, patient's co-morbidity and patient's wishes.

In general, early-stage tumours receive single-modality treatment, whilst advanced require combined-modality treatment.

Because all head and neck cancers have the tendency to adversely affect speech, swallowing and cosmetic appearance, treatments should be designed to treat the cancer effectively without adding to the patient's morbidity. All patients diagnosed with head and neck cancer are discussed in the multidisciplinary team meeting (MDT) prior to definitive treatment. Here the patient's clinical status, staging, histopathology and imaging are discussed by a panel of experts who determine the best treatment according to evidence-based practice.

The primary tumour needs to be treated along with the lymphatic basin fed by the hypopharynx, which includes levels 2 to 4 (upper to lower deep cervical chain).

Nutritional support during treatment is usually necessary. This may be in the form of oral food supplements in mild cases following radiotherapy but often requires enteral feeding via a nasogastric tube or gastrostomy feeding tube. External beam radiotherapy treatment (EBRT) is used as curative treatment for early-stage hypopharyngeal cancer. The usual dose is 65 Gray (Gy) given to the hypopharynx and neck in divided dosages called fractions.

Radiotherapy involves targeting ionizing radiation to the tumour to activate apoptosis or programmed cell death. EBRT is usually given daily over a 6-week period on an outpatient basis. Because the patient needs to lie immobilized on the treatment table to maximize accurate targeting of treatment, he or she wears an immobilization shell, which prevents movement artefact. Radiotherapy can cause acute and late toxicities. Acute toxic reaction can affect the skin in the form of erythema mimicking a burn. Mucositis is inflammation of the mucous membranes, which can affect speech and swallowing. Late toxicity can result in fibrosis and scarring of the pharynx and larynx, which can result in dysphagia.

For advanced-stage hypopharyngeal cancer, chemotherapy is added to EBRT, which is termed *chemo-radiation*. The combination of chemotherapy with EBRT increases the effectiveness of treatment but adds to the toxicity and side effects. The most common chemotherapy agent used is cisplatinum. Chemotherapy can cause neutropenia, ototoxicity, renal damage, nausea, vomiting and alopecia.

PET scanning can be employed at 3 months following completion of radiotherapy treatment to evaluate disease control. If recurrence of cancer is detected, surgery may be appropriate.

Surgery tends to be reserved for the most advanced types of hypopharyngeal cancer (stage T4) or for recurrent disease. The operation required is total laryngo-pharyngectomy; the aim is to remove all of the tumour and restore swallowing function. This is a complex, major surgical operation, which can only be performed on a patient who is fit enough for a long procedure with general anaesthetic. It involves removal of the larynx, the thyroid gland and part or all of the pharynx. The patient will therefore have a permanent tracheostomy after this surgery.

To restore swallowing function after this surgery, the pharynx must be reconstructed. If only part of the pharynx (partial pharyngectomy) is resected (Figure 25.4), then a patch repair of the pharynx is adopted. This is usually in the form of a myocutaneous flap harvested from the arm (radial forearm free flap), leg (anterolateral thigh free flap) or chest wall (pectoralis major pedicled flap).

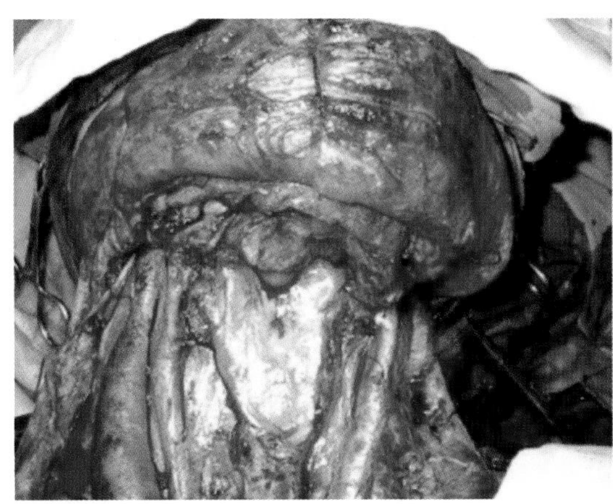

Figure 25.4 Total laryngectomy with partial pharyngectomy with neck dissection for advanced hypopharyngeal cancer. The pharynx can be reconstructed with a patch repair.

If a total pharyngectomy has been performed, then a circumferential defect has been created and needs to be restored. Reconstruction of the pharynx can be achieved using several techniques, including a jejunal free flap (Figure 25.5), anterolateral thigh free flap or a gastric transposition pedicled flap. Speech can be restored by creating a surgical tracheoesophageal fistula (TOF) as is seen after laryngectomy (Figure 25.6). A selective neck dissection, levels 2 to 4, is necessary at the time of surgery for lymph node negative (N0) patients and a modified radical neck dissection for node positive patients. Post-operative radiotherapy is usually adopted in all cases and is indicated for close or involved margins and lymph node metastases.

Major complications can occur following pharyngo-laryngectomy. These may be general (related to a prolonged head and neck operation) and specific. The main specific complications include pharyno-cutaneous fistula and hypocalcaemia. A pharyno-cutaneous fistula results when saliva or food leaks from the pharynx into the neck and onto the skin. If mild, this initially can be managed conservatively by prolonged tube feeding. In severe cases, further reconstructive surgery is needed to repair the pharynx. Hypocalcaemia can result as a result of resection of the parathyroid glands with

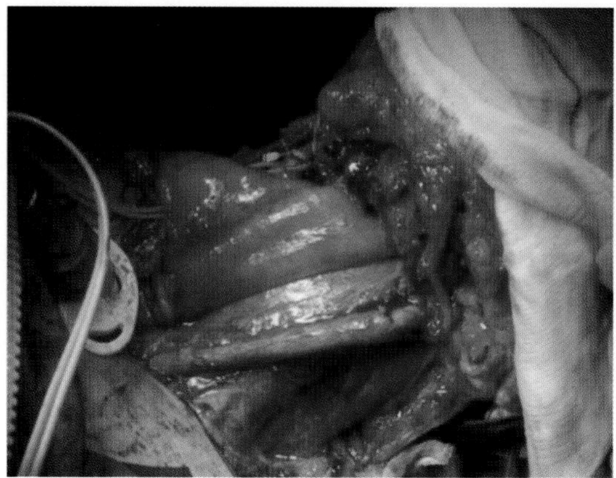

Figure 25.5 Total laryngo-pharyngectomy with neck dissection. The segmental pharyngeal defect has been reconstructed with a microvascular free-jejunal flap.

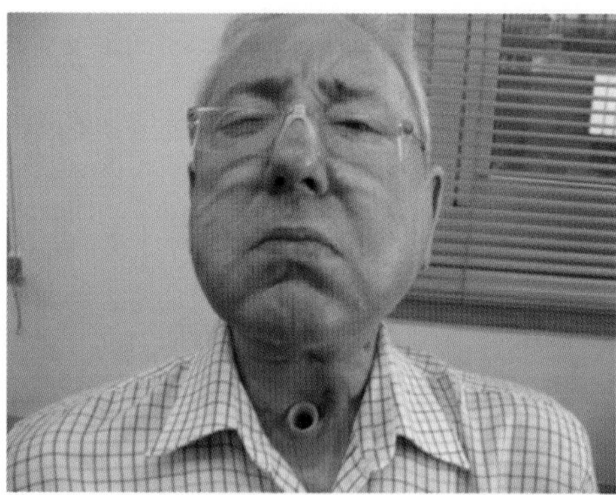

Figure 25.6 Post-operative picture of a patient who has undergone total pharyngo-laryngectomy and free jejunal transfer reconstruction. Note the permanent tracheostomy stoma and the laryngectomy tube in situ.

the tumour; calcium and parathyroid hormone may be necessary to correct this.

SURVIVAL AND PROGNOSIS

Hypopharyngeal cancer has the worst overall survival rate for any sub-site cancer in the head and neck. This is due to the advanced stage and late presentation but also to the high frequency of distant metastases. Early-stage hypopharyngeal cancer (T1 and T2) has a 5-year survival rate of between 50 per cent and 40 per cent, whereas advanced stage (T3 and T4) has a survival rate of between 30 per cent and 20 per cent. Therefore, palliative and supportive care are often necessary in managing this aggressive cancer.

KEY LEARNING POINTS

- Smoking and alcohol consumption are important factors in hypopharyngeal cancer. HPV is thought to play less of a role in the hypopharynx than in the oropharynx.
- Red flag symptoms for hypopharyngeal cancer include dysphagia, dysphonia, otalgia, odynophagia and stridor.
- On fiberoptic laryngoscopy the tumour is either an ulcerated or an exophytic mass.
- TNM staging and imaging help in the appropriate management of hypopharyngeal cancer. Nutritional support is important.
- Radiation and chemo-radiation are the mainstay of treatment. Surgery is reserved for the most advanced cases or for recurrent disease.
- Hypopharyngeal cancer has the worst overall survival rate for any subsite in the head and neck

26

Tumours of the oral cavity

PHILIP MCLOUGHLIN

ANATOMY

The oral cavity commences at the vermillion of the lips and extends posteriorly to the oropharynx. The oral cavity contains the anterior two-thirds of the tongue, the floor of the mouth, and the maxillary and mandibular alveolus, which may contain teeth, and as such there are differing relationships of mucosal coverage. The upper and lower alveolar mucosa is connected by the buccal mucosa, which lines the cheeks, and completing the oral maxillary structures is the hard palate. The surface of the oral cavity is lined with stratified squamous epithelium. This epithelium can be intimately related to the underlying bone, such as the attached mucosa of the gums or the midline of the hard palate. Other areas of the oral cavity have a more prominent sub-mucosal element containing fibrous tissue and minor salivary glands, such as the buccal mucosa and the retromolar soft tissues. The oral cavity is unique in the human body in that its integument is breeched by calcified structures, the teeth, and the presence or absence of teeth can have a bearing on the progression and spread of pathologic disorders close to the jaw.

The oral tongue comprises its anterior two-thirds, extending posterior to the V-shaped demarcation of the sulcus terminalis. Structurally, the tongue is skeletal muscle enveloped on its upper surface by gustatory epithelium and on its undersurface by non-keratinizing simple squamous epithelium. The intrinsic musculature of the tongue is responsible for changes in shape occurring during the functions of eating and speaking, but the positional changes of the tongue are largely the responsibility of the extrinsic muscles, which attach the organ to the mandible, the hyoid bone and the pharynx.

BENIGN TUMOURS OF THE ORAL CAVITY

Benign tumours of the oral cavity may originate from any of the individual structural elements. Almost all will present as a slowly growing, well-defined nodular mass, which may be sessile or pedunculated. Benign oral cavity tumours are relatively common and will occur in approximately 1 per cent of the population throughout life. The following are those most often encountered.

SQUAMOUS CELL PAPILLOMA

A papilloma is a benign epithelium neoplasm commonly occurring in the oral cavity. Papillomas may occur as single or multiple sessile warty lesions, seldom measuring more than a few millimetres. While a viral aetiology has been implicated, a true papilloma is a benign tumour, the closest differential being a viral wart. Histologically, both a papilloma and a viral wart show finger-like projections of squamous epithelium above the level of the surrounding mucosa. In most cases mild hyperkeratosis can be seen. Epithelial dysplasia is not a feature of papilloma. The distinction between squamous cell papilloma and a viral wart is largely clinical. While neither lesion enlarges to a great extent, a viral wart will involute and the telltale signs of lesions on the tips of the fingers may be present, particularly in children. Papillomas occur throughout the oral cavity. Simple excision is all that is required, and recurrence and malignant change are rare.

FOCAL EPITHELIAL HYPERPLASIA

Focal epithelial hyperplasia, also called Heck's disease, is a benign disorder of the oral mucosa. The condition is characterized by multiple papillomatous lesions, possibly caused by a virus of the Papova group. When first reported, the condition was thought to be confined to children. However, focal epithelial hyperplasia occurs worldwide and is certainly not limited to youth. The lesions measure several millimetres, have a papillomatous or fibroma-like appearance, are usually asymptomatic and can occur anywhere in the oral cavity. The tongue, however, is the usual site. With multiple lesions of this nature, clinical diagnosis is usually adequate, but biopsy will confirm. Although no specific treatment is required, cryotherapy may be useful in symptomatic cases.

FIBROMA

The true fibroma is a soft tissue neoplasm of the oral cavity, often pedunculated and covered with normal mucous membrane. The buccal mucosa is the most common site. Far more commonly, lesions referred to as fibroma are not true neoplasms but merely overgrowths caused by chronic irritation, such that the terms *fibro epithelial polyp* or *fibrous hyperplasia* are preferred for this type of lesion. More than 3 per cent of the population will experience an oral fibrous growth at some time. True fibromas rarely occur before the fourth decade and have an equal sex prevalence. Lesions that become large or symptomatic may require simple conservative excision. Once excised, recurrences are exceptional.

GRANULAR CELL MYOBLASTOMA

This is a curious benign tumour whose origin has been debated for some time. While originally thought to represent a benign neoplasm of muscle, currently a neurogenic origin seems to be more likely. Moreover, there is opinion that this lesion is not a true neoplasm but a benign proliferation of peripheral neurogenic elements, which would account for its self-limiting nature, as once reaching a critical size the lesion shows degenerative features. Granular cell myoblastoma has no preference for sex or age, although the favoured anatomical sight is the oral tongue. Presentation is a firm submucosal nodule, which may grow up to a few centimetres in diameter (Figure 26.1). Overlying mucosa is usually of normal appearance, although ulceration may occur if the size of the lesion makes it prone to trauma. There is a congenital form known as epulis of the newborn in which a histologically similar lesion occurs on the alveolar

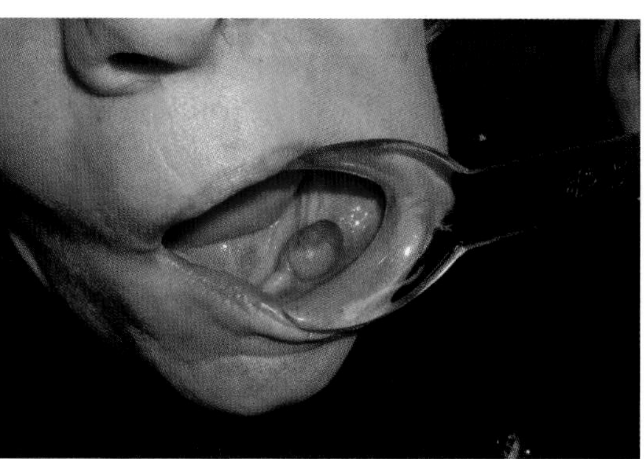

Figure 26.1 Well-demarcated benign tumour in the mouth. This is a granular cell tumour.

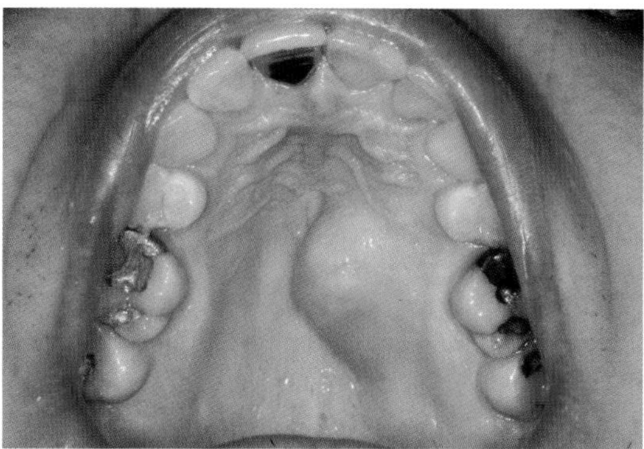

Figure 26.2 A smooth, solitary palatal lump. Biopsy showed this to be a benign salivary gland tumour, but many at this site will be malignant.

ridge of the newborn. Histology shows a circumscribed, poorly encapsulated mass; cytologically benign granular cells predominate. Management of the granular cell tumour is conservative surgical removal. Recurrence is rare.

NEUROFIBROMA

Oral neurofibroma is the most common benign nerve sheath tumour. These tumours are asymptomatic, occurring as solitary lesions more often than is appreciated. Multiple lesions are seen in von Recklinghausen's disease, where the tongue is often involved primarily. Neurofibroma in the tongue may enlarge to result in unilateral macroglossia and a significant functional disturbance. Neurofibromas occurring in von Recklinghausen's disease have approximately a 10 per cent risk of malignant change.

BENIGN TUMOURS OF MINOR SALIVARY GLANDS

There is an abundance of minor salivary glands contained within the submucosa of the oral cavity. The typical appearance of a benign salivary gland tumour, by far the most common of which is the pleomorphic adenoma, is a rounded mass occurring in the palate, the buccal mucosa or the floor of the mouth, covered by overlying mucosa of normal appearance. While benign salivary gland tumours may occur anywhere on the buccal mucosa, the typical appearance on the palate is where the submucosa is thickest – that is, in the mid-portion of the palatal vault between the midline raphe and the maxillary alveolus (Figure 26.2). A firmly enlarging tumour at this site should arouse clinical suspicion and management along appropriate lines. The distribution of histological types of tumour arising in minor salivary glands differs from that of tumours arising in the larger major salivary glands. Approximately 50 per cent of minor salivary tumours turn out to be malignant. Therefore, even when the presenting lesion is clinically benign, a biopsy is mandatory to rule out the malignant counterpart. Of those that are benign, the majority are pleomorphic salivary adenomas, although myoepitheliomas, basal adenomas and cystadenomas are occasionally found. Local surgical excision is usually curative, and recurrence is uncommon.

MISCELLANEOUS BENIGN ORAL TUMOURS

Benign tumours occasionally arise from the abundance of tissue types lining the oral cavity. True lipomas, leiomyomas and schwannomas are all occasionally found. Most, however, are incidental histopathological findings of excised, and typically benign, oral lesions.

MALIGNANT TUMOURS OF THE ORAL CAVITY

ORAL SQUAMOUS CELL CARCINOMA

Mucosal squamous cell carcinoma (SCC) is by far the most common malignant disease occurring in the oral cavity. Malignant tumours of the oral cavity affect, in order of frequency, the anterior two-thirds of the tongue, the floor of mouth, the buccal mucosa, the retromolar region, the hard palate and the gingivae. The overwhelming majority of malignant tumours are squamous cell carcinomas. Non-squamous cell carcinomas are predominantly of salivary gland origin.

Aetiology

SCC of the oral cavity may develop *de novo* or from a pre-malignant dysplastic lesion that may appear clinically as leucoplakia (white patch) or erythroplakia (speckled red-and-white patch). In both cases chronic exposure to carcinogens in tobacco or alcohol or local trauma are thought to be important. However, carcinogenesis is a multistep process involving over-expression of oncogenes and inactivation of tumour suppressor genes. The p53 tumour suppressor gene has been identified as being important in oral cavity carcinomas in patients who are smokers. The presence of human papillomavirus (HPV) expressing the p16 oncoprotein in oral cavity carcinoma in non-smokers is of significance, because it is known that such cancers tend to occur in younger patients and have a better prognosis.

The spectrum of oral cavity SCC histological subtypes contains tumours with variable prognosis, such as the verrucous carcinoma, which carries a good prognosis, and the basaloid variety of squamous carcinoma, where the prognosis is considerably less favourable.

Oral SCC may be classified according to grade depending on several histopathological features such as degree of keratinization, nuclear pleomorphism, cellular atypia and mitotic activity. This has led to the classification of well, moderate or poorly differentiated carcinomas. This is useful as a snapshot of any individual carcinoma because well-differentiated tumours tend to have a better outcome than poorly differentiated tumours. However, tumour grade is of limited prognostic value because there is considerable heterogeneity within any individual cancer.

Other pathological features have been shown to be of prognostic importance, including tumour thickness, extra-capsular spread of nodal metastasis and pattern of invasion. Oral tongue SCC of greater than 4 mm tumour thickness represents a significantly increased risk of cervical node metastatic involvement. Extra-capsular spread (ECS) of cervical lymph node metastasis is associated with a poorer prognosis; indeed, the presence of ECS is consistently associated with increased risk of loco-regional recurrence, distant spread and reduced survival. The pattern of invasion in oral SCC may help in determining prognosis. Those cancers that have a non-cohesive and invasive advancing front or that spread in a perineural or lymphovascular fashion appear to be associated with an increased risk of loco-regional relapse after treatment.

Epidemiology

Although cancers of the head and neck region account for only 5 per cent of all cancers reported annually, 30 per cent of these cancers occur in the oral cavity. In the United Kingdom, this number is approximately 2600 each year. However, in the United States, there are approximately 30 000 new diagnoses of oral or oropharyngeal cancer made every year, with an estimated 7500 deaths. In India and Sri Lanka, oral cavity and oropharyngeal cancers comprise 40 per cent of the total number of cancers reported.[1] This large incidence has traditionally been attributed to the chewing of betel quid (which is wrapped around tobacco material); however, this is now being superseded by a more Western method of tobacco usage. Oral cavity cancer occurs almost twice as often in men as in women, although this does vary with site, and the relative increase in females seen over the past 30 years still continues. Although traditionally mouth cancer occurs most commonly in the sixth and seventh decades of life, the incidence is increasing in younger adults, particularly of HPV-related malignancies.

Clinical presentation

The majority of SCCs of the oral cavity present as ulcers or mass lesions (Figure 26.3). Although lesions may be subtle and appear as flat white patches or, more usually, red-and-white patches, a non-healing ulcer is the most common presentation (Figure 26.4). It is considered that a non-healing ulcer in the oral cavity of 3 weeks' duration or longer should undergo a biopsy to confirm or deny its malignant nature. It is interesting that the gutter that represents the floor of the mouth, demarcated by the lateral border of tongue, the reflection of the lingual sulcus and the lingual gingivae, accounts for only 30 per cent of the surface area of the oral cavity, yet 70 per cent of oral cavity malignancies occur in this region.

At a later stage, advanced tumours may present with invasion of neighbouring structures. Infiltration of the mandibular bone may cause loosening of the teeth. Deep invasion of the lateral tongue involving neurological structures causes pain often referred to the ear, and the patient presents with otalgia. Cancers in the retro-molar area may spread posteriorly to involve the pterygoid musculature, leading to severe limitation of mouth opening. Tumours presenting in such a fashion generally carry a poor prognosis. Approximately 5 per cent of cases of oral SCC will present with lymph node metastasis, and a firm upper neck mass may be the presenting feature.

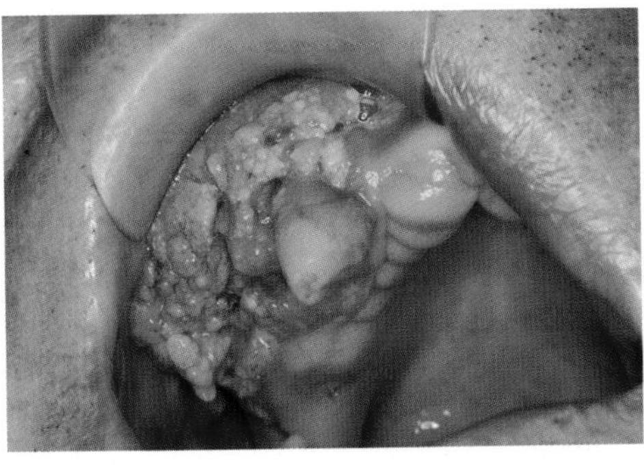

Figure 26.3 A large florid squamous cell carcinoma. The maxillary bone has been invaded.

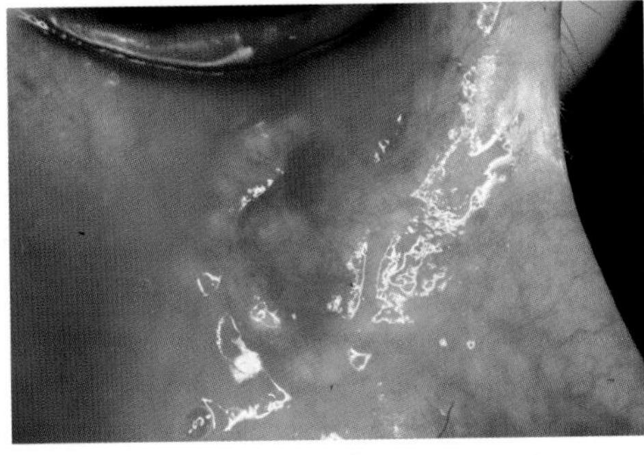

Figure 26.4 A typically ulcerated squamous cell carcinoma of the buccal mucosa.

Clinical examination

Clinical examination is probably still the most important part of diagnosis, and indeed surveillance after treatment, in oral cavity cancer. A systematic approach is important for diagnosis and treatment planning.

Surgical biopsy

A diagnosis of oral SCC should always be confirmed histologically. Biopsy within the oral cavity can usually be performed with local anaesthesia. The biopsy should be incisional and no attempt should be made to remove small lesions in total at the first attempt. The biopsy should be taken from an accessible area of the tumour close to the edge, or at the edge of the lesion. These sites give the best histological sample. A biopsy of the necrotic centre of the tumour should be resisted because histologic results may be confusing owing to the necrotic nature of the sample. Once a diagnosis is made, the patient should be considered by a multidisciplinary team, taking all relevant factors into account before reaching a treatment plan, through consensus with the patient and caregivers. Treatment intention – curative or palliative – should be clearly recorded at the outset.

Imaging

The choice of imaging for oral cavity cancers is individual and based on the site and size of the presenting tumour; often it is a multidisciplinary team decision. The team needs to know the extent of the primary tumour itself and any spread into adjacent structures. It is also important to determine whether there is any local spread into the cervical lymph

Table 26.1 T stage

T stage	Tumour maximum surface diameter
Tx	Primary tumour cannot be assessed
T0	No primary tumour
Tis	Primary lesion contains *in situ* cancer only
T1	<2 cm
T2	>2 cm <4 cm
T3	>4 cm
T4	Tumour invades deep/extrinsic muscles of tongue, pterygoid muscles, hard palate or mandible

nodes. Spread to the cervical lymph nodes increases directly with the stage of the primary tumour. With small (T1) primary SCC, it can be below 2 per cent, and in easily accessible sites such as the anterior tongue; therefore, imaging may not be necessary. As larger tumours are encountered, the incidence of lymph node metastasis increases to 30 per cent for T2 tumours, and this may rise to more than 50 per cent for T3 and T4.[2] The clinical size of the primary tumour is therefore of utmost importance. The classification is summarized in Table 26.1.

Imaging is centred on the magnetic resonance imaging (MRI) scan, which gives a good overall indication of tumour size and an excellent view of nodal metastatic spread. Computed tomography (CT) scans for oral squamous cancer are usually reserved for the assessment of bony invasion, particularly where a mandibular resection is being considered.

CERVICAL NODAL METASTASIS

Clinical examination remains the most important method of detecting lymph node metastasis. An examination of the neck should be an integral part of the clinical examination of any patient suspected of having oral SCC. Metastases occur most commonly in the upper deep cervical and submandibular nodes on the same side as the primary tumour. The more anterior the primary tumour, the more likely the involvement of submandibular nodes. The mid-deep or jugulo-omohyoid nodes are frequently affected; however, involvement of the lower deep cervical nodes is rare.

Table 26.2 N stage

N stage	Nodal status
Nx	Regional nodes cannot be assessed
N0	No regional lymph node metastasis
N1	Metastasis in a single ipsilateral node 3 cm or smaller
N2	Metastasis in a single ipsilateral node >3 cm, or in multiple ipsilateral nodes, or in bilateral or contralateral nodes, all 6 cm or smaller
N3	Metastasis in a lymph node >6 cm

Table 26.3 M stage

M stage	Distant metastasis
MX	Distant metastasis cannot be assessed
M0	No distant metastasis
M1	Distant metastasis

Contralateral nodal metastases are also infrequent and present in only about 6 per cent of cases. A simplified staging of nodal metastatic disease is given in Table 26.2.

Pre-treatment staging

Distant metastatic disease is rarely found at presentation in cases of oral cancer, although chest CT is becoming an accepted pre-treatment staging tool (Table 26.3).

At the end of clinical investigation, an overall pre-treatment staging can be determined as indicated (Table 26.4). The overall staging is directly related to known survival rates and may be useful information for the multidisciplinary team, especially when the decision is being made concerning treatments, some of which may carry significant morbidity.[3]

TREATMENT OF ORAL CANCER

SURGERY

Patient factors such as fitness for anaesthesia, the size and accessibility of the tumour and patient

Table 26.4 Overall disease stage versus survival

Stage group	TNM stage	Average 5-year survival
0	Tis	
I	T1 N0 M0	90 per cent
II	T2 N0 M0	80 per cent
III (up to)	T3 N1 M0	50 per cent
IV (greater than)	T3 N1 M0	25 per cent

choice should be considered. While there is a broad banner of surgery available for treating malignant disease, for oral cavity cancer, conventional surgical resection of accessible tumours and appropriate management of the cervical nodes are the mainstay of initial treatment, where patient factors are favourable. Intuitive surgery for cancer of the oral cavity involves resection of the tumour within an appropriate safe margin, considered to be at least 5 mm and preferably 1 cm, followed by appropriate reconstruction of the resected tissue to facilitate maintenance of function.

The size and location of the primary tumour may require the use of adjuncts such as temporary tracheostomy as well as access procedures to split the lip or even the mandible. Most tumours in the anterior aspect of the oral cavity can be accessed by the trans-oral route, avoiding scars around the mouth. However, as tumours increase in size and become more posterior, it may be necessary to perform a lip split and even mandibulotomy to effect complete tumour resection.

Reconstruction of the oral mucosa is generally performed using radial forearm free flaps or anterolateral thigh free flaps. The former is a good source to replace mucosal lining, while the latter provides useful bulk in large tongue resections. The once-popular reconstructive technique using pedicled flaps, such as the pectoralis major, is now less frequently employed, because of the superior results achieved by the use of microvascular transfers.

When the primary tumour has invaded bone, two patterns of spread may occur. Where teeth are present, the tumour spread tends to be superficial and horizontal such that a rim resection of the mandible or the maxilla, with the soft tissue overlying (a composite resection), is sufficient to ensure complete tumour ablation. In the patient who is edentulous, the nature of tumour spread within the underlying bone adopts a more vertical nature, requiring a full-thickness resection. Following such resections involving the maxilla, the maxillary sinus is entered and the patient usually requires a dental obturator to prevent oral escape of air and fluids. Full-thickness resections of the mandible can pose a significant reconstructive challenge where the surgeon has to replace soft tissue of the oral mucosa as well as the mandibular bony structure. Modern microvascular transfers using the fibula flap and the deep circumflex iliac artery (DCIA) flap or vascularized hip graft have proven significant advances in this area of reconstructive surgery.

MANAGEMENT OF CERVICAL NODES

A patient staged with a T1 tumour with a N0 neck will not usually require nodal dissection, although the patient will be closely followed in case nodal disease should present at a later date. All patients with cancers T2 and above and everyone with nodal metastasis at presentation will undergo some form of neck dissection. The current trend is to dissect levels I–IV in any patient with an N0 neck and primary staged greater than T2. In patients presenting for treatment with a node-positive neck, either a functional dissection of the nodal levels involved – at least to include levels I–IV – is performed, or occasionally a full traditional radical neck dissection involving levels I–V is used. A radical neck dissection may be modified to preserve the sternocleidomastoid muscle, accessory nerve and internal jugular vein, or any combination of these structures.

RADIOTHERAPY AND CHEMOTHERAPY

Primary radiotherapy is a very viable option for small primary tumours of the oral cavity and will be the treatment of choice in patients unfit for surgery. Similarly, primary radiotherapy will also be used in patients with very advanced unresectable disease, where a lower dose, or a so-called hypo-fractionated regimen, is given as a palliative measure in an attempt to control symptoms where curative treatment will clearly not succeed.

The current trend is to use neoadjuvant chemotherapy, which are pulses of chemotherapy given within a course of radiotherapy, because it is known to enhance the tumour's response to the ionizing radiation. Post-operative radiotherapy is used where histopathological examination following surgical resection indicates sub-optimal prognostic features. Such features include close resection margins; undiagnosed spread into adjacent tissues, which will up-stage a tumour to T4; and involvement of multiple cervical lymph nodes or cervical lymph nodes where metastatic spread has breached the lymph node capsule, the previously mentioned extra-capsular extension. In these cases a course of radiotherapy or chemoradiotherapy will be prescribed.

There is no evidence to indicate the usefulness of chemotherapy as a primary modality of treatment for oral cancer, although it may be used primarily as a palliative tool in certain instances of otherwise untreatable disease. In these cases photodynamic therapy (PDT) is currently being developed to provide additional symptomatic benefit.

SPECIFIC COMPLICATIONS OF TREATMENT

Complications of surgery

Surgical complications may occur in as many as 60 per cent of patients having treatment for oral cancer. Risk factors such as old age, poor performance status, medical co-morbidities, large aggressive tumours and complex surgery show correspondingly higher complication rates. Major surgery for oral cancer has a reported mortality of up to 4 per cent. More commonly, complications are less dramatic and of a more chronic nature.

While airway problems do occur in major oral cancer surgery, these can be largely prevented by the use of temporary tracheostomy. The immediate impact on swallowing and nutrition can be countered with the use of nasogastric feeding or even the insertion of a gastrostomy tube. Occasionally, gastrostomy tubes will be required for an extended period of time, and sometimes after the most major resections a gastrostomy tube can be a permanent feature. Wound infections following oral cancer surgery are not uncommon. The oral cavity–skin integument is a clean contaminated area, where infection rates of up to 20 per cent may be encountered. Consequent failure of wound healing and fistulation may occur in intraoral and neck wounds as a result, despite the use of antibiotic prophylaxis and local treatment.

Injuries to the facial and mandibular nerves lead to impaired lip function and sensation and are not uncommon sequelae of major surgery of this nature, particularly mandibular resection. The advances enjoyed by the development of microvascular transfers in terms of improved oral function, speech and swallowing have been significant in recent years. The failure of such flaps due to inadequate blood supply is small, in the region of less than 5 per cent. Similarly uncommon is failure of healing and subsequent orocutaneous fistulation. Donor site morbidity is minimal, although the DCIA vascularized hip graft is well known for causing reduced mobility, sometimes of a prolonged nature.

Complications of chemotherapy and radiotherapy

Although chemotherapy is seldom used alone in the treatment of oral cancer, the immediate complications of nausea and vomiting are now well controlled with antiemetics such as ondansetron. The most potent complications of radiotherapy in the treatment of mouth cancer are xerostomia, a chronic dry mouth that is very difficult for patients to manage, and the effects of radiotherapy on bone, most significantly the development of osteoradionecrosis (Figure 26.5).[4] Improvements in radiotherapy techniques, especially the development of intensity modulated radiation therapy (IMRT), have reported reduced complications following treatment. IMRT is able to avoid irradiation of salivary glands, with a reduced incidence of xerostomia and reportedly very low rates of osteoradionecrosis. Although the latter complication responds in some way to hyperbaric oxygen treatment, and a medical regimen involving tocopherol and pentoxifylline, chronic pain and bone destruction

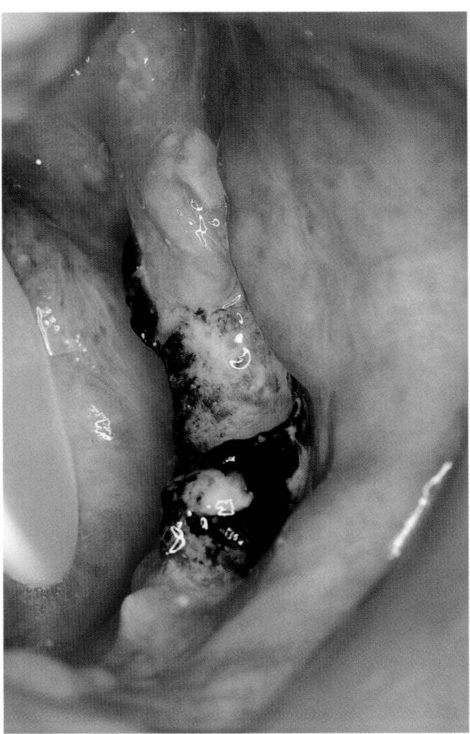

Figure 26.5 Mucosal atrophy with exposed mandibular bone in osteoradionecrosis.

can sometimes necessitate secondary mandibular resection and reconstruction with a vascularized bone graft.

SURVIVAL

The overall 5-year survival of oral SCC, irrespective of stage, at the end of the past century was of the order of 50 per cent. This incidence had not changed in the preceding three decades. New studies indicate that current overall survival of oral SCC approaches 70 per cent, irrespective of stage. This may represent improved methods of diagnosis and greater awareness within the general population that cancer does indeed occur within the oral cavity. There is certainly evidence for better use of surgery combined with adjuvant chemoradiotherpy, although full-scale randomized controlled trials are currently lacking. At present, palliative treatment of incurable disease is centred on symptom control. While most of this care is medical and supportive and is delivered by the dedicated palliative care team, there may be a role for adjuncts such as photodynamic therapy (PDT) in the future.

MALIGNANT TUMOURS OF THE MINOR SALIVARY GLANDS

While salivary gland tumours have been considered elsewhere in this book (see Chapter 28), it is worth highlighting a few salient points regarding salivary gland tumours as they pertain to the oral cavity. In the submucosa throughout the mouth, there is an abundance of minor salivary glands, which are by no means immune to forming the full range of tumours that are found in the major salivary glands themselves. The usual presentation of malignant minor salivary gland tumours is a solitary lump, although occasionally florid ulceration may be present, particularly with tumours presenting late. These solitary lumps are often found in the palate, typically at the hard/soft palate junction on either side of the midline, or in the buccal mucosa. An important feature to acknowledge with minor salivary gland tumours is that as previously mentioned, depending on the site, the reported incidence of malignancy lies between 50 and 70 per cent. For this reason primary excision should be resisted, and the suspected minor salivary gland tumour will be managed with an incisional biopsy in the first instance. Once a definitive histological diagnosis is obtained, appropriate staging can be undertaken and appropriate resection and reconstruction planned for a malignant tumour.

HAEMATOLYMPHOID TUMOURS

Haematolymphoid tumours are included in the World Health Organization (WHO) classification of oral tumours and are therefore mentioned here for completeness. Both Hodgkin's and non-Hodgkin's lymphomas may present in the oral cavity. All sites of the oral cavity may be involved, and clinical presentation is diverse. A lymphoma in the mouth may present as a solitary lump or a chronic ulcer, but lymphomatous change occurring in areas of erythroplakia and leucoplakia have been reported.

KEY LEARNING POINTS

- Tumours of the oral cavity are common and usually benign.
- Mouth cancer usually presents as a chronic ulcer.
- Squamous cell carcinoma is by far the most common mouth cancer.
- Site and size of tumour are important in prognosis.
- Surgery is the usual primary modality of treatment of oral cancer.
- Complications of radiotherapy to the jaws may be significant.
- Minor salivary gland tumours have a high incidence of malignancy.

REFERENCES

1. Langdon JD, Henk JM, eds. *Malignant Tumours of the Mouth, Jaws and Salivary Glands*. 2nd ed. London: Edward Arnold, 1995.
2. Shah JP, Johnson NW, Batsakis JG, eds. *Oral Cancer*. 1st ed. London: Martin Dunitz, 2003.
3. Scully C. Cancers of the oral mucosa. 2012. emedicine.medscape.com/article /1075729.
4. Hutchison I. Complications of radiotherapy in the head and neck: An orofacial surgeon's view. *Current Radiation Oncology*. 1996; 2:144–77.

27

Tumours of the larynx

KENNETH MACKENZIE

INTRODUCTION

The most common malignant tumour of the larynx is squamous cell carcinoma (SCC), with an incidence of 6.2 per 100 000 males and 1.3 per 100 000 females in the United Kingdom. It is rare in patients under the age of 40. The main co-aetiological factors are tobacco smoking and drinking alcohol, with a strong association with the lower socio-economic groups.

Within the larynx there are three main sub-sites, the glottis, the supraglottis and the subglottis, which comprise the vocal cords, the area above the vocal cords and the area below the vocal cords, respectively. The most frequently affected sub-site is the glottis; the next most frequent is the supraglottis; and the least is the subglottis. Smoking is the highest risk factor in glottic cancer, with alcohol playing a greater role in supraglottic tumours.

Considerable importance is attached to early diagnosis of SCC because comprehensive treatment in its early stages is associated with a very good prognosis.

PRESENTATION

The cardinal symptom associated with tumours in the larynx is hoarseness. This occurs initially because of the change in the contour of the vocal cords, and as the tumour extends and more mucosal surfaces are involved, the hoarseness will increase. If the volume of the tumour increases further and more sub-sites are involved, for example the glottis and the supraglottis, then the hoarseness and its severity will increase. The hoarseness is persistent, and although it may fluctuate, the voice does not return to normal. With increasing tumour volume, the vocal cord mobility may be reduced, with a subsequent breathy component to the voice. As turbulence of the air through the larynx increases, stridor will ensue, with marked noisy breathing most evident in inspiration. Associated with these symptoms may be referred pain to the ear. As the tumour extends beyond the larynx, there may be associated aspiration because of vocal cord immobility. So when swallowing, the patient may complain of choking attacks. Ultimately, as other structures are involved and dysphagia increases, the patient may not be able to maintain dietary intake and may experience weight loss and increasing airway compromise. Although the majority of tumours of the larynx present with hoarseness, supraglottic lesions may present as cervical lymph node metastases.

DIAGNOSIS

CLINICAL EXAMINATION

The key investigation in a patient presenting with hoarseness, particularly a smoker, is examination of the larynx by fibre-optic nasolaryngoscopy when the patient is awake. This is carried out using a fibre-optic nasolaryngoscope per nasal approach along the floor of the nose, having anaesthetized the nose initially using co-phenylcaine or topical lignocaine spray. In many patients who have repeat examinations, topical anaesthesia is not necessary because they are very compliant if a good examination technique is adopted. From this examination it is possible to assess the proximal aerodigestive tract in its 'natural' position, looking at the tongue base, the vallecula and then the laryngeal surface of the epiglottis. Thereafter, the intralaryngeal structures are examined in detail from the supraglottis to the glottis, with it being possible to visualize certain aspects of the subglottis. The remainder of the other hypopharyngeal structures, such as the posterior pharyngeal wall and the pyriform fossa, are also examined at this time. From this examination it is possible to visualize the main bulk, or epicentre, of the tumour, the vocal cord mobility and the residual airway. It is also possible to assess the symmetry or otherwise of the pyriform fossae. It is strongly advised that this examination be conducted as a routine prior to any endolaryngeal procedure being conducted for diagnostic and staging purposes. This allows definitive assessment of vocal cord mobility to be made and also gives an update of the status of the airway prior to anaesthesia administration.

Other visualization techniques, such as videostroboscopy, can be used to examine the detail of the vocal cords. Such techniques are considered by some to be of importance when contemplating endoscopic or partial laryngeal surgery.

IMAGING

When a laryngeal malignancy is suspected, imaging ideally should be carried out prior to endoscopic examination under general anaesthesia. The principal reason for this is that the endolaryngeal procedure and subsequent biopsies will disrupt the tumour and laryngeal architecture either by direct tumour removal or subsequent peri-tumour inflammation. The main imaging modality used for evaluation and staging purposes is computed tomography (CT) scanning. The key elements of tumour staging are assessment of the index primary, i.e. the tumour within the larynx, cervical lymph node status, and the presence or otherwise of metastatic disease, most commonly affecting the lung.

The presence of pulmonary disease significantly affects the treatment philosophy. For example, if there is metastatic disease, then it may change the recommended treatment to a palliative intent, whilst single synchronous primary pulmonary resection may change the treatment intent to curative if the single synchronous primary within the larynx is also early disease. For these reasons all patients with suspected laryngeal cancer should have CT scans of their neck and chest.

With regard to the larynx, the principal role of fine-cut CT scanning is to assess the extent of the tumour. This is in particular relation to the presence of tumour invasion to the subglottis or invasion into the paraglottic and pre-epiglottic spaces. The pivotal result is the involvement or otherwise of the thyroid cartilages with extension into the laryngeal soft tissues. Suspected involvement of these laryngeal cartilages is the key element in the recommendation of treatment modalities.

A CT scan will highlight any suspected lymphadenopathy. To confirm or refute this involvement, ultrasound scanning can be carried out with the associated sampling either by fine-needle aspiration cytology or by core biopsy.

The standard imaging using CT scanning can be supplemented if there is any doubt or concern about the involvement of the thyroid cartilages or extension of the tumour into the tongue base.

This is achieved by magnetic resonance imaging (MRI) scanning, which has a higher sensitivity but less specificity for laryngeal cartilage invasion. Combining these imaging modalities will provide accurate staging when taken in conjunction with the subsequent endoscopic examination under general anaesthesia. At this initial stage it is occasionally necessary to ensure that there are no distant metastases or other malignancies. For example, in a situation where a patient may have a pre-existent, but treated, malignancy prior to considering radical treatment of the head and neck cancer, it is necessary to determine if malignancy is present. In this situation positron emission tomography (PET)-CT scanning is advocated.

When assessing the imaging of a laryngeal tumour, the following should be considered:

1. Sub-site or sub-sites involved
2. Extension of the tumour into paraglottic and pre-epiglottic spaces
3. Laryngeal cartilage invasion
4. Inferior extent of the subglottis, particularly around the cricothyroid membrane
5. Extension into the hypopharynx, including the pyriform fossae and post-cricoid region
6. Tongue base
7. All lymph node levels, including levels I to VI
8. Examination by microlaryngoscopy

EXAMINATION BY MICROLARYNGOSCOPY

The aim of this procedure is to confirm the sub-site of origin of the tumour, describe the extent of the tumour by determination of the surface area of the tumour and the sub-sites involved, and obtain a tissue sample for histological diagnosis.

Following fibre-optic nasolaryngoscopy immediately pre-operatively, the most appropriate way of establishing and maintaining an airway is discussed with the anaesthetist.

In general, the anaesthetist can insert a small endotracheal tube, such as a microlaryngeal tube, with minimal trauma into the larynx and trachea; this allows the detailed examination.

In advanced malignancy, however, there may be a large obstructive lesion within the larynx and trachea that needs de-bulking prior to continuing the general anaesthesia. In this situation the tumour can be de-bulked using the CO_2 laser in conjunction with supraglottic jet ventilation or microdebrider de-bulking of the tumour with a microlaryngeal tube in place.

To establish general anaesthesia and safe ventilation of the patient, the larynx and surrounding structures are examined in detail. Each sub-site mentioned in the imaging section is examined in detail, starting with the tongue base and continuing to the vallecula, the laryngeal surface of the epiglottis, the lateral pharyngeal wall, the posterior pharyngeal wall with extension into the post-cricoid region, the cervical oesophagus, both pyriform fossae and the larynx, with specific attention being paid to the supraglottis, the glottis and the subglottis.

After the epicentre of the tumour has been identified, the surrounding area can be examined in detail with the 0°, 30° and 70° Hopkins rods in conjunction with a system to digitally record the extent of the tumour. Not only does this allow a clearly documented record for the patient, but it also provides information on the tumour extent for discussion by the multidisciplinary head and neck cancer team.

Biopsies are taken from all of the representative sub-sites using cupped biopsy forceps. Haemostasis is secured using 1:1000 adrenaline on surgical patties.

MANAGEMENT OF LARYNGEAL CANCER

Following the completion of the diagnostic investigations, the tumour is staged according to the TNM classification (Table 27.1). The recommended treatment strategy is dependent upon the clinical staging at the time of presentation; the clinical characteristics of the patient, such as the age and co-morbidities; and finally the wishes of the patient, relatives and caregivers.

After consideration of each of these treatment strategies independently and collectively, the decision is made whether the treatment will be with a curative or a palliative intent. Given the staging and

Table 27.1 TNM classification of laryngeal cancer

Supraglottis	
T1	Tumour limited to one subsite of supraglottis with normal vocal cord mobility.
T2	Tumour invades mucosa of more than one adjacent subsite of supraglottis or glottis or region outside the supraglottis (e.g. mucosa of base of tongue, vallecula, medial wall of piriform sinus) without fixation of the larynx.
T3	Tumour limited to larynx with vocal cord fixation and/or invades any of the following: postcricoid area, pre-epiglottic space or paraglottic space and/or includes minor thyroid cartilage erosion (e.g. inner cortex).
T4	
T4a	Tumour invades through the thyroid cartilage and/or invades tissues beyond the larynx, e.g. trachea, soft tissues of neck including deep/extrinsic muscle of tongue (genioglossus, hyoglossus, palatoglossus and styloglossus), strap muscles, thyroid or oesophagus.
T4b	Tumour invades prevertebral space or mediastinal structures or encases carotid artery.
Glottis	
T1	Tumour limited to the vocal cord(s) (may involve anterior or posterior commissure) with normal mobility. T1a Tumour limited to one vocal cord. T1b Tumour involves both vocal cords.
T2	T2a Tumour extends to supraglottis and/or subglottis with normal vocal cord mobility. T2b Tumour extends to supraglottis and/or subglottis and/or includes impaired vocal cord mobility.
T3	Tumour limited to larynx with vocal cord fixation and/or invades paraglottic space, and/or includes minor thyroid cartilage erosion (e.g. inner cortex).
T4	
T4a	Tumour invades through the thyroid cartilage or invades tissues beyond the larynx (e.g. trachea, soft tissues of neck including deep/extrinsic muscle of tongue (genioglossus, hyoglossus, palatoglossus and styloglossus), strap muscles, thyroid or oesophagus.
T4b	Tumour invades prevertebral space or mediastinal structures or encases carotid artery.
Subglottis	
T1	Tumour limited to subglottis.
T2	Tumour extends to vocal cord(s) with normal or impaired mobility.
T3	Tumour limited to larynx with vocal cord fixation.
T4	
T4a	Tumour invades through cricoid or thyroid cartilage and/or invades tissues beyond the larynx e.g. trachea, soft tissues of neck including deep/extrinsic muscle of tongue (genioglossus, hyoglossus, palatoglossus and styloglossus), strap muscles, thyroid or oesophagus.
T4b	Tumour invades prevertebral space or mediastinal structures or encases carotid artery.

treatment modalities at the time of presentation of laryngeal cancer patients, the vast majority are treated with curative intent.

The treatment options are considered as follows and are broadly divided into two main groups, early and advanced laryngeal cancer.

EARLY LARYNGEAL CANCER

Early laryngeal cancer is defined as a T1 or T2 lesion that affects any of the sub-sites within the larynx and with no cervical lymphadenopathy (N0) nor evidence of metastatic disease (M0).

The aim of treatment is to eradicate the disease whilst maintaining function, principally voice and swallowing. The choice of treatment is between radiotherapy or transoral endolaryngeal surgery, with each having extremely good cure rates. These can be up to 100 per cent for T1 lesions and 89 per cent for T2 lesions for endoscopic resection and similar rates for radiotherapy.[1,2,3]

There are relative advantages and disadvantages for each treatment modality. Transoral resection of the laryngeal tumour using the CO_2 laser allows the patient to be treated on a single occasion with minimal absence from work, allows confirmation of removal of the tumour histologically, and avoids the pharyngeal sequelae of radiotherapy with the final advantage of further surgery or radiotherapy as a salvage option should there be disease recurrence. The disadvantages are that it may not be appropriate in all cases as a result of difficulty in accessing the larynx comprehensively to allow tumour resection, and it tends to need repeated microlaryngeal procedures to ensure disease-free status. In addition, because it may affect the voice quality, it tends not to be used in T1B lesions where excision will involve both vocal cords across the anterior commissure. Subsequent scarring with possible webbing, even with the use of topical application of mitomycin, can result in poor voice outcomes.

In supraglottic lesions, if they are node negative, either transoral endoscopic resection or radiotherapy can be used. However, if there are suspicious or confirmed lymph node metastases, then the index site has to be radiated, as do the lymph node groups. The alternative is a selective neck dissection in conjunction with the endoscopic resection. In the latter case, it may be necessary to give adjuvant radiotherapy if there is significant involved lymph node volume or extra-capsular spread is present.

Radiotherapy tends to be used in those patients where the excision will affect the contralateral vocal cord significantly, where there is a relatively large-volume T2 lesion or the access is not sufficient to allow security in achieving a margin on excision, or in those patients where repeated endolaryngeal procedures under general anaesthesia would not be acceptable.

With the popularization of endolaryngeal surgery, the role of open partial laryngeal surgery tends now to be restricted to a few rare clinical situations, such as a patient with poor access who has refused radiotherapy or in low-volume recurrence following radical radiotherapy.[4]

ADVANCED LARYNGEAL CANCER

Advanced laryngeal cancer can be defined as T3/T4 tumour with cervical lymph node negative or node-positive disease. The key treatment option is organ preservation strategy, in the form of radiotherapy or chemoradiotherapy, or total laryngectomy. Much less commonly used techniques are transoral CO_2 laser surgery or near-total laryngectomy. In advanced laryngeal cancer, the risk of lymph node metastasis is high and can be up to 60 per cent if the supraglottis is involved. For the N1 neck, if the treatment of the primary is by surgery, then an ipsilateral selective neck dissection clearing levels II–IV is carried out followed by chemoradiotherapy where appropriate. If chemoradiotherapy is to be used as the treatment of the index primary, then in N1 disease it is also used to treat the identified lymph node metastases and the surrounding lymph node basins, which may be subject to metastatic microscopic spread of the tumour. Close monitoring both clinically and radiologically is essential thereafter to identify the persistence of the disease or recurrence.

Advanced lymph node disease, N2 and N3, again will need treatment that is dependent on the recommended treatment for the index primary. Curative-intent N3 disease generally requires clearance of the neck, possibly with a modified or radical neck dissection; N2 disease is treated with surgical clearance of large-volume disease; and lower-volume N2 disease is able to be treated by chemoradiotherapy when this is to be used for the treatment of the index tumour.

Since the early 2000s, the organ preservation strategy using radiotherapy plus or minus chemotherapy has become popular. The basis of this strategy is that it was demonstrated that it is possible to achieve the same survival outcomes for advanced laryngeal malignancy using chemoradiotherapy with salvage laryngectomy as required when compared with primary total laryngectomy.[5]

The key element in decision-making regarding which strategy is to be recommended is the presence or absence of laryngeal cartilage invasion. CT, and subsequent MRI scanning if CT is equivocal, is used to make this differentiation. The sensitivity and specificity of these combined investigations is in excess of 90 per cent. It is difficult to be certain of thyroid cartilage invasion because of the differential ossification and subsequent appearances on imaging of the thyroid cartilages. Essentially, if there is thyroid cartilage invasion, then chemoradiotherapy is not considered suitable as a curative option because it would not eradicate the disease; therefore, a total laryngectomy is recommended.

Conversely, if this is not the case, then chemoradiotherapy can be deployed with a curative intent depending on the other factors in decision-making. These factors may include the patient's lifestyle and social support network. For example, the patient may want to preserve the larynx because of his or her occupation as a lecturer or teacher. Conversely, the patient may wish to 'clear the disease'. Ultimately, it is the patient's preference, in conjunction with relatives' and caregivers' opinions, that will result in the final treatment strategy.

The standard chemoradiotherapy regimen uses concomitant or concurrent chemoradiotherapy with cisplatin and 5-fluorouracil (5-FU) in conjunction with radiotherapy schedules. The dose for those who receive radiotherapy is determined by the clinical oncological planning services and is delivered over a period of approximately 6 weeks in appropriate fractions as determined by the head and neck oncological team. Both during and following these combined treatments, it is necessary to monitor patients closely and support them well with regard to the following: their nutrition, because radiotherapy affects their per-oral dietary intake; the pain that they may experience due to the mucositis produced by the treatment regimen; the airway in advanced disease, which may be impaired because of the tumour volume; impaired vocal cord mobility; or the effect of peri-tumour oedema. Thereafter the patient is monitored on a regular basis every 4 to 6 weeks for at least the first year to 18 months, 8 weeks thereafter for the next year, and so on, with a view to identifying and treating recurrence should it arise.

Total laryngectomy clearly involves resection of the larynx with possible partial pharyngectomy and lymph node resection. Approximately 1 week post-laryngectomy, feeding is commenced if pharyngeal repair is intact. Thereafter, nutrition is generally well maintained through the neopharynx.

Following pathological assessment of the total laryngectomy specimen with partial pharyngectomy and neck dissection as indicated, a decision can be made in regard to adjuvant radiotherapy. The key indications for adjuvant radiotherapy are excision margins that are regarded as being close to or involved in the laryngeal resection specimen, or evidence of extra-capsular spread in the neck dissection. It should be noted, however, that such adjuvant therapy may affect the functional outcomes of both voice production and swallowing, and should be considered carefully when advising the patient.

Voice rehabilitation takes place using a tracheo-oesophageal voice prosthesis inserted into a tracheo-oesophageal fistula. This voice prosthesis allows air that is exhaled to be shunted through the voice prosthesis by occlusion of the stoma, with the air gathering in the neopharynx and the patient phonating thereafter. This is carried out as a primary puncture, i.e. there is a creation of the tracheo-oesophageal fistula between the posterior wall of the trachea and the cervical oesophagus at the time of laryngectomy. To allow such a voice to take place, a healed stoma is necessary because this needs to be occluded during the phonation process, and an appropriate tracheo-oesophageal valve has to be *in situ*. Some believe in the strategy of placing a tracheo-oesophageal voice prosthesis at the time of the laryngectomy. Others feel that if they wait until 3 or 4 weeks post-operatively, inserting a valve as a simple outpatient procedure gives a better measure of valve dimensions and better timing for valve use at that stage. Irrespective of which timing is used, audible sustainable speech is generally achieved in approximately 90 per cent of patients who have had a total laryngectomy.

The overall quality of life and functional outcomes following laryngectomy are very reasonable because the patients tend to be pain free, able to swallow, and able to phonate through their tracheo-esophageal voice prosthesis, but there is the clear downside of having a permanent tracheo-stoma. The best functional results after laryngectomy occur if it is carried out as a primary procedure without any adjuvant radiotherapy or as a salvage procedure following chemoradiotherapy.[6]

The complications of chemoradiotherapy are principally those that relate to the alteration in the end organ function, namely dysphonia, difficulty with communication, difficulty in swallowing and maintaining nutrition, pain and potential airway compromise necessitating tracheostomy. The principal post-surgical complication of total laryngectomy is pharyngo-cutaneous fistula formation with a prolonged stay in the hospital or the need for subsequent surgery in the form of reconstruction to seal the fistula. In the case of laryngectomy, there is an increased incidence of fistula formation in patients in whom the total laryngectomy was carried out as part of a salvage procedure as opposed to those in whom primary laryngectomy has been performed.

KEY LEARNING POINTS

- Cardinal presenting symptom is hoarseness.
- Key finding of imaging is tumour involvement of the laryngeal cartilages.
- Early laryngeal cancer treatment is endolaryngeal surgery if possible.
- Advanced laryngeal cancer treatment is radiotherapy + or - chemotherapy if no, or minimal, laryngeal cartilage involvement.
- If there is laryngeal cartilage involvement, treatment is total laryngectomy.

REFERENCES

1. Bradley PJ, MacKenzie K, Wight R, Pracy P, Paleri V. Consensus statement on management in the UK: Transoral laser assisted microsurgical resection of early glottic cancer. *Clinical Otolaryngology*. 2009; 34: 367–73.
2. Ambrosch P, Kron M, Steiner W. Carbondioxide laser microsurgery for early supraglottic carcinoma. *Annals of Otology, Rhinology and Laryngology*. 1998; 107: 680–8.
3. Dey P, Arnold DF, Wilson J, Wight R, MacKenzie K, Kelly C. Radiotherapy versus open surgery versus endolaryngeal surgery (with or without laser) for early laryngeal squamous cell cancer. *Cochrane Database of Systematic Reviews*. 2002; 2.
4. Roland NJ, Paleri V (Eds). *Head and Neck Cancer: Multidisciplinary Guidelines, 4th edition*. London: British Association of Otorhinolaryngology – Head and Neck Surgery, 2011.
5. Forastiere AA, Goepfert H, Maor M. et al. Concurrent chemotherapy and radiotherapy for organ preservation in advanced laryngeal cancer. *New England Journal of Medicine*. 2003; 349: 2091–98.
6. Robertson S, Yeo J, Dunnet C, Young D, MacKenzie K. Voice, swallowing and quality of life following total laryngectomy – Results of the West of Scotland Laryngectomy audit. *Head and Neck* (America). 2010; doi 10 1002.

28

Salivary gland disease

PATRICK J BRADLEY

INTRODUCTION

Adult salivary gland diseases and disorders occur so frequently in patients' everyday lives that they are sometimes regarded as familiar matters not requiring any detailed knowledge. When symptoms originating from the salivary glands develop, they can interfere with patients' quality of life, resulting in absences from school and work, as well as hindering leisure activities.

The management of salivary diseases and disorders requires a comprehensive understanding of embryology and anatomy; production and regulatory mechanisms of salivary production; clinical pathologies, local and systemic, that can affect the salivary glands; multiple techniques available for their investigation (analysis, imaging and biopsy); modern methods for managing ducal and parenchymal diseases; and appropriate management of salivary gland neoplasms – benign and malignant.

Thus, the investigation and management of patients with symptoms of salivary origin should be within a clinical environment of a multidisciplinary group of clinicians who have an interest in salivary gland diseases and disorders and should include surgeons, dentists, oral medicine experts, dental hygienists, radiologists, pathologists and physicians.

EMBRYOLOGY AND ANATOMY

Humans have three pairs of major salivary glands – parotid, submandibular and sublingual – and some 600–1000 minor salivary glands, which are dispersed sub-mucosally throughout the head and neck region. Each major gland develops from within the oral cavity (endoderm) and matures through a series of stages. The early stages are reliant on epithelial and mesenchymal interactions, with the basement membrane playing an important role in controlling the ductal branching morphogenesis. The final gland represents a coordinated network of acini, ducts, blood vessels, myoepithelial cells and nerves, each playing a vital role in a functioning organ.

The parotid glands are the largest of the major salivary glands. Each is a compound tubule-acinar, mepocrine, exocrine gland and is composed entirely of serous output – producing acini. Each gland is triangular shaped with the apex directed inferiorly. On average, the gland is 6 cm in length, with a maximum width of 3.3 cm. In approximately 20 per cent of the population, a smaller accessory lobe arises from the upper border of the parotid duct. The parotid duct (Stensen's duct) comes off the substance of the gland anteriorly and travels parallel to the zygoma, on the surface of the masseter muscle, and pierces the buccinator muscle to enter the oral cavity opposite the second upper molar tooth. The gland is divided into a superficial or lateral lobe, which accounts for more than 80 per cent of the glandular tissue and lies on the masseter muscle. The deep lobe, so called because it lies beneath/deep to the facial nerve and its divisions/branches, encircles the ramus of the mandible and is located in proximity to the pterygoid muscles within the parapharyngeal space. Each gland is surrounded by a fibrous capsule. The superficial layer is attached to the mandible and the temporal bone, and the deep layer covers the muscles in the parotid bed. There are many lymph nodes located within the subcutaneous tissues overlying the parotid gland, forming the pre-auricular nodes, and another lymph node group within the substance of the gland. Most of the nodes within the gland are located lateral to the facial nerve.

Each submandibular gland consists of a large, superficial lobe lying within the digastric triangle below the ramus of the mandible, and a smaller deep lobe lying within the floor of the mouth posteriorly. The two lobes are continuous with one another around the posterior border of the mylohyoid muscle. The two lobes are not true lobes, because embryologically the gland – a mixed seromucinous saliva output – is a single epithelial outpouching. The superficial lobe is partially enclosed within the two layers of the deep cervical fascia. The submandibular duct (Warthin duct) is about 5 cm long in the adult. As the duct passes forward, it passes between the sublingual gland and the genioglossus muscle to open into the floor of the mouth at the side of the lingual frenulum. The duct also runs between the lingual and hypoglossal nerves on the hyoglossus muscle.

The sublingual gland develops early (at 4 to 6 weeks of development) from a number of small epithelial thickenings in the floor of the mouth. Each thickening forms its own canal; many of these open directly onto the mucosa, and others drain into the submandibular duct. The sublingual gland is almond or 'tadpole' shaped; the oval-shaped 'head' lies in the anterior floor of the mouth, and the wedge-shaped 'tail' runs posteriorly, towards the submandibular gland. These glands are predominantly mucus-secreting saliva and are unencapsulated. Numerous minor salivary glands are widely distributed throughout the submucosa of the head and neck. The majority are located in the oral cavity and oropharynx.

SALIVA AND ITS FUNCTIONS

The majority of saliva is secreted by the major salivary glands, with the smaller glands contributing less than 10 per cent either at rest or when stimulated. The rate of salivary secretion ranges from barely perceptual during sleep to a high of 4 mL min^{-1} on maximal stimulation. In healthy, non-medicated adults, unstimulated and chewing-stimulated whole-saliva flow rates on average range from 0.3 to 1.5 mL min^{-1}, respectively. The true volume of saliva flow per day is unknown because there is considerable variation both in flow rates among individuals and for the normal volume of mixed saliva. *Hyposalivation* is a term based on objective measures of saliva secretion, when the flow rates are significantly lower than the generally accepted 'normal values' – flow rates of unstimulated saliva less than 0.1 mL min^{-1}, and those of chewing-stimulated whole saliva of 0.5–0.7 mL min^{-1}. Saliva consists of two components that re-secrete by independent mechanisms: (1) a fluid component that includes ions, produced mainly in response to parasympathetic stimulation, and (2) a protein component released mainly in response to

Table 28.1 Functions of saliva

Mechanical cleansing of food and bacteria
Lubrication of oral surfaces
Protection of teeth and oral-oesophageal mucosa
Antimicrobial activity
Dissolution of taste compounds
Facilitation of speech, mastication and swallowing
Formation of food bolus conducive for swallowing
Initial digestion of starch and lipids
Oesophageal clearance and gastric acid buffering

sympathetic stimulation. Many other factors affect saliva composition: flow rate, diurnal variation, age, drugs, salivary cells capable of contributing to saliva (serous- or mucus-acinar cells and lining cells of the ducts), hormones, diet, and so forth. Saliva has many functions (Table 28.1).

CLINICAL PRESENTATION

Symptoms of salivary gland diseases and disorders are limited in number and generally are non-specific. Patients usually complain of swelling, pain, dry mouth, foul taste and excessive salivation. While many tests are available – e.g. sialometry, sialochemistry, microbiology, serology, other blood tests – in general, after a detailed history and a thorough physical examination, the majority of patients will be given a diagnosis that will allow for the commencement of treatment or an explanation as to a likely cause and effect. In uncommon cases, further investigation may be needed. Diseases can be classified into acute, recurrent or chronic; ductal or parenchymal; localized or diffuse parenchymal; affecting a single gland or multiple glands; and neoplastic or non-neoplastic.

An acute swelling of one or more salivary glands – major and minor – may result from duct obstruction, inflammation or a neoplasm and can result in a partial or diffuse gland enlargement. An acute swelling episode of the submandibular or parotid gland (diffuse gland) accompanied by pain and related to salivary stimuli is suggestive of duct obstruction, most likely a stone. A partial swelling of a major salivary gland, most easily palpated by the patient and the clinician, can be a major diagnostic challenge. The majority of salivary lumps present slowly (months to years) and with little or no pain. The differential diagnosis rests between non-neoplastic disease; lymph nodes, cysts, abscess, and auto-immune sialadenitis; and neoplastic disease, benign or malignant. The malignant disease could be primary salivary cancer or secondary cancer from a local or distant source (Figures 28.1 and 28.2).

Pain has been reported in 3–5 per cent of patients with a benign parotid tumour, and 10–30 per cent of patients with a parotid cancer. Similarly, pain as

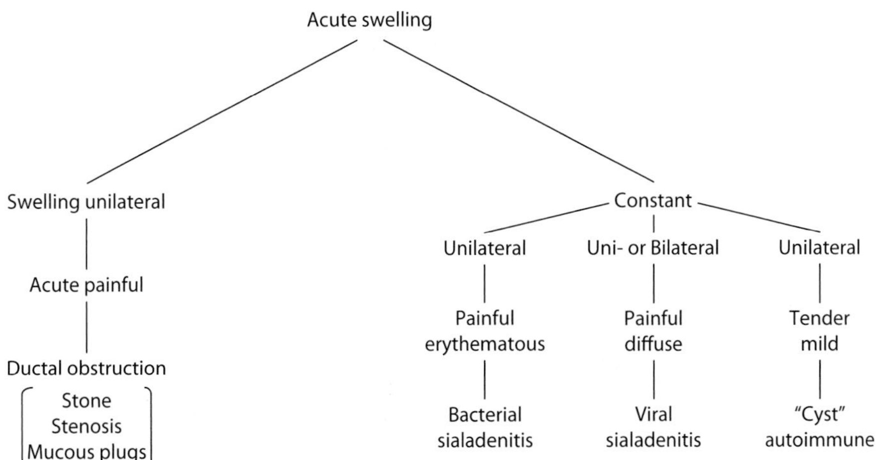

Figure 28.1 Diagnostic algorithm for acute swelling of major salivary glands.

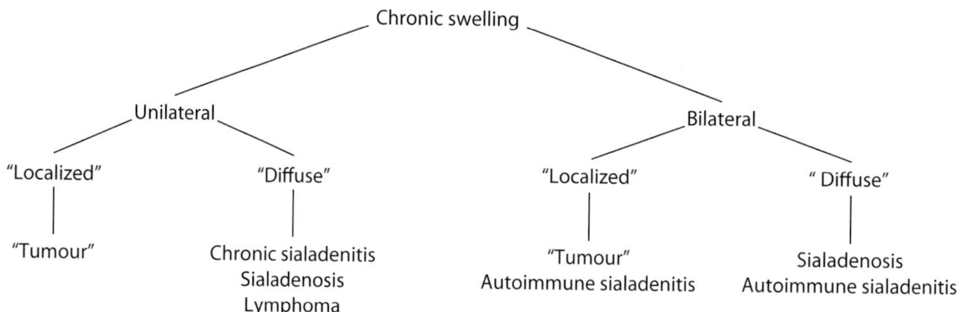

Figure 28.2 Diagnostic algorithm for chronic swelling.

a symptom is reported in patients with a submandibular benign tumour and in up to 50 per cent of patients with a malignant submandibular tumour. Thus pain as a symptom is more commonly associated with a salivary malignancy but is not of itself diagnostic of malignancy.

A history of systemic disease and of medications (naproxen, valproic acid, some antihypertensives) must be carefully assessed. Salivary gland dysfunction resulting in diffuse gland swelling may be associated with diabetes mellitus, cirrhosis, hormonal imbalance, bulimia, anorexia, chronic alcoholism, and other causes. This results in a fatty infiltration of the major salivary gland, most commonly the parotid, and may be unilateral. This condition is best diagnosed by performing magnetic resonance imaging (MRI). A middle-aged patient with a history of rheumatoid arthritis or another connective tissue disease may have Sjögren's syndrome. Lymphoma may masquerade as a local or diffuse swelling and should be considered in the differential diagnosis of the elderly.

Xerostomia and 'dry mouth syndrome' should not be confused within the clinical environment. Xerostomia may occur without the signs of hyposalivation (in mouth breathers, xerostomia as a symptom is caused by dehydration of the mucosa), and in turn hypo-salivation may occur without the symptoms of xerostomia. Altered salivary composition may occur when the salivary flow has been unaffected. Salivary gland dysfunction can be a manifestation of various systemic disorders, or it can be a result of local functional or morphological pathology. Temporary causes of salivary dysfunction include depression, local infections or the side effects of prescribed medications. Medications notorious for causing dry mouth syndrome include antidepressants, anti-anxiety agents, antihypertensive agents, diuretics and antihistamines. They are common causes of both hyposecretion and xerostomia. Another common cause is radiotherapy, which is initially of acute onset, but the effects may persist for years after treatment.

Increased secretion of saliva is called hypersecretion, ptyalism, sialorrhoea or hypersialia. The term *sialorrhoea* should be restricted to the symptom complex consisting of involuntary flow of saliva from the mouth; this is also known as drooling. The symptom of excessive salivation is very uncommon, because usually the saliva is swallowed. 'False ptyalism' is more common and is either delusional (the patient is alarmed by a sudden awareness of excessive saliva) or due to a faulty neuromuscular control, which leads to drooling despite normal salivary flow (e.g. in patients suffering from stroke, Parkinsonism, or cerebral palsy). Occasionally, hypersalivation may be associated with heavy metal poisoning (lead, mercury, arsenic) or iodine toxicity, may be temporary following the initiation of some medications (reserpine, clozapine, pilocarpine and isoproterenol) and may even follow a change of dentures.

DIAGNOSTIC INVESTIGATION

Some patients will provide only a vague complaint, such as pain, local discomfort, or a swelling, with

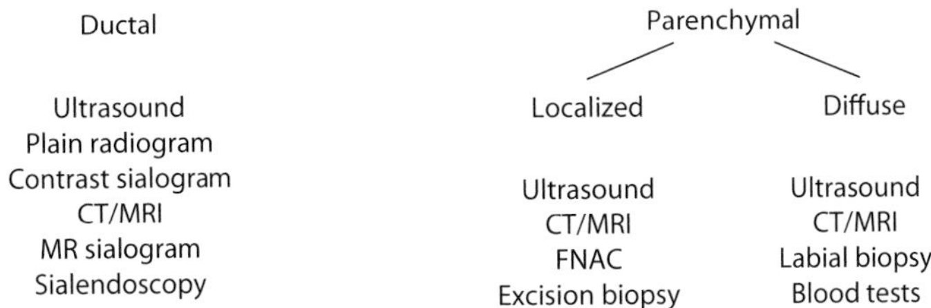

Figure 28.3 Investigation of salivary gland diseases/disorders.

little by way of any revealing physical signs. In such patients it may be necessary to follow a structured investigation process, more to exclude a serious diagnosis and to provide reassurance. When investigating salivary gland diseases and/or disorders, one should consider the major glandular functions as ductal, parenchymal or both (Figure 28.3).

When sialadenitis is suspected, an underlying ductal disease should first be considered. Investigations should be delayed until the acute episode has settled. Because the majority of cases are associated with calculi, other causes may be due to ductal stenosis or mucus plugs. Salivary stones are located in the submandibular gland system in 60 per cent of cases and in the parotid gland in 40 per cent. Because the majority of salivary stones are composed of calcium carbonate and calcium phosphate and are thus radio-opaque, they will show up on a plain radiograph. Other stones are not radio-opaque; some may be multiple; and there may be a stricture present. In these situations, other modes of imaging including magnetic resonance (MR) sialogram will demonstrate the site of the ductal narrowing. However, the use of sialoendoscopy is indicated when the cause of salivary swellings is unclear, including swellings associated with stones, strictures, inflammation or tumours and other processes that might cause obstruction of the duct. Sialendoscopy is a technique for inspecting the salivary ductal system with a fibre-optic system, which allows for manipulation of instruments to remove, dilate and biopsy lesions within the salivary duct system.[1]

The investigation of diffuse parenchymal salivary disease, either uniglandular or multiglandular, must include imaging of the head and neck, including chest x-ray, fine-needle aspiration cytology (FNAC) and consideration of performing a labial or a sub-lingual gland biopsy.[2] Before performing a salivary gland biopsy, consultation with the pathologist may help in achieving an accurate diagnosis.

DUCTAL DISEASES

SIALOLITHIASIS, DUCTAL STENOSIS, SALIVARY PLUGS

The diameter of the main duct in the submandibular gland is approximately 3–4 mm, and the parotid duct is >2 mm in a normal gland. The salivary gland ductal system branches, without systematization, and has a decreasing diameter from the main duct to the terminal duct. It is not possible to enter the third- or fourth-level branches with the current sialendoscopes.[1]

Salivary gland calculus accounts for more than 50 per cent of major salivary gland disease, with 5.9 cases per 100 000 people each year in the United Kingdom and a prevalence of 0.45 per cent. The condition most frequently affects men aged 30–60 years, with the submandibular gland affected in 80–90 per cent of cases. Small salivary stones can be removed endoscopically, employing a scope and a retrieval basket, when they are less than 3 mm in the parotid duct and less than 4 mm in the submandibular duct. Stones of a larger size or stones located within the gland itself can be removed using a combined approach with the sialendscope and an external approach, creating a ductotomy and delivering the stone, then repairing the ductal opening using a vein graft, ensuring the creation of a widening plasty of the duct at the level of impaction to minimize the possibility of duct stenosis. In the past, salivary gland excision surgery was performed for the removal of salivary stones on the assumption that the gland itself was diseased beyond repair. Clinicopathological studies have shown (1) that submandibular glands excised because of sialolithiasis did not demonstrate any correlation between the degree of gland alteration and the number of infectious episodes; (2) there is no correlation between the degree of gland alteration and the duration of evolution; and (3) despite appropriate indications for submandibular excision, close to 50 per cent of the removed glands were histopathologically normal or close to normal. Excisional gland surgery should be the exception rather than the rule for sialoadenitis, which has been associated with significant morbidity.

PARENCHYMAL DISEASE

INFECTION

Sialadenitis or infection of the salivary glands is an acute and/or chronic condition that presents as a swelling of the gland, with or without pain, and with or without systemic upset, which affects the major and minor glands. The most common pathogens identified are viruses and bacteria. The most frequent scenario is that of an adult presenting with a swelling of the parotid or submandibular gland, with a diagnosis of obstructive sialadenitis associated with sialolithiasis.[3]

Although mumps is the most common virus causing sialadenitis in children, other viruses can also cause acute diffuse gland obstruction in adults (15 per cent of adults, usually the elderly). Other more common viruses may mimic 'clinical mumps', such as influenza, parainfluenza viruses (types I and 3), coxsackieviruses A and B, echovirus and lymphangitis choriomeningitis virus. Bacterial sialadenitis may also present in an acute manner with a tender painful swelling, with the parotid gland being more frequently affected than the submandibular gland.

The parotid gland may also be involved with human immunodeficiency virus (HIV), which manifests as parotid gland enlargement due to lymphoepithelial cysts and may be an infection of the peri-parotid lymph nodes rather than the glandular parenchyma itself. Some of the salivary neoplastic diseases, including some of the malignant diseases, may also present with a 'cystic-type lesion'.

There exists a non-specific bacterial sialadenitis, which is considered to be due to a retrograde contamination from the oral cavity. Penicillin-resistant, coagulase-positive *Staphylococcus* is commonly encountered but is often mixed flora containing *Streptococcus pneumoniae* and beta-haemolytic *Streptococcus*, *Escherichia coli* and *Pseudomonas aeruginosa* as well as anaerobic bacteria. Specific bacteria have also been reported to infect salivary glands. These infections include bartonellosis (cat scratch disease), tuberculosis, actinomycosis and sarcoidosis.

AUTOIMMUNE DISORDERS

The fact that autoimmune diseases can affect salivary glands is well known, but reliance on the clinical symptoms and signs in making such a diagnosis is unsatisfactory and inaccurate. Only since 2002, with the publication of the American–European consensus criteria (AECC) for Sjögren's syndrome (SS), has gained wide acceptance, which is one of the major autoimmune diseases that affects the salivary glands.[4] The evidence of autoimmunity required for diagnosis includes autoantibodies to Sjögren's syndrome (autoantibody A [SSA or anti-Ro] or autoantibody B [SSB or anti-La]) or a positive biopsy of the minor salivary glands. The disease is found in all age groups but usually in patients between the ages of 40 and 60 years, and it is rarely seen in children and adolescents. There is often an interval of several years from the start of symptoms to confirmation of the diagnosis. An estimated prevalence of SS is 1–4 per 100 000 population, with a large female predominance (9:1 female:male). Secondary SS is defined as the occurrence of signs and symptoms of SS in conjunction with other autoimmune systemic diseases, such as rheumatoid arthritis and systemic lupus erythematosus. The most common primary disease is rheumatoid arthritis, with a prevalence of secondary SS of 10–30 per cent. The hallmark of SS is sicca syndrome of the eyes and the mouth. SS affects the parotid and submandibular glands, manifesting initially with intermittent swelling. Objective evidence of salivary gland involvement is defined by a positive result for at least one of the following diagnostic tests: (1) unstimulated whole salivary flow (>1.5 mL in 15 minutes), (2) parotid sialography showing the presence of diffuse sialectasias (punctuate, cavitary or destructive pattern) without evidence of obstruction in the major ducts, and (3) salivary scintigraphy showing delayed uptake, reduced concentration, and/or delayed excretion of tracer. Reduced exocrine function or sicca symptoms may be caused by a variety of conditions and may also be age related. The most definitive test is a biopsy of the minor salivary glands from inside the lower lip, which should demonstrate a focus as defined as an accumulation of at least 50 inflammatory cells (lymphocytes) per 4 mm^2 of glandular tissue. Treatment includes support of symptoms, reduction of mouth dryness, prevention of corneal dryness and minimization of fungal infections.

There is an increased risk (16-fold) of SS patients developing non-Hodgkin's lymphoma of the mucosa-associated lymphoid tissue (MALT) type. This is a solid tumour that originates from the B cells of the marginal zone of the MALT. It presents as a persistent enlarged or nodular parotid or submandibular gland with regional or generalized lymphadenopathy, pulmonary infiltrates, hepatomegaly, vasculitis and monoclonal gammopathy. Treatment should include surgery and radiotherapy. The overall 5-year survival rate is more than 80 per cent.

Another autoimmune disease that affects the salivary glands is graft-versus-host disease (GVHD). This is a complication of allogeneic bone marrow transplantation in which functional immune cells in the transplanted marrow recognize the recipient as 'foreign' and mount an immunological attack. Kuttner's tumour and Mikulicz disease have recently been described as similar and are thought to be IgG_4-related systemic diseases. The serum immunoglobulin G_4 (IgG_4) concentration is elevated, and IgG_4 expressing plasmacytes infiltrates the salivary glands.[5]

NEOPLASMS

BENIGN

In the United Kingdom the annual incidence of benign salivary gland neoplasms ranges from 6.2 to 7.2 per 100 000 people. The majority of salivary gland neoplasms are benign (65–70 per cent), and nearly 80 per cent are found within the parotid gland.[6] Histological analysis of benign salivary neoplasms, most recently classified by the World Health Organization (WHO) in 2005, has identified some 10 entities. However, the vast majority (80–85 per cent) are diagnosed as pleomorphic adenoma and adenolymphoma (Warthin's tumour), either by FNAC or after excision. Other benign non-epithelial lesions may present as slow-growing masses in the parotid or submandibular gland areas and include haemangioma, lymphangioma and lipomas. Before considering surgical excision, it is important that a firm diagnosis be made, because surgery may result in an angry and unhappy patient. Other lesions need to be considered in the differential diagnosis, such as lymph node disease, salivary cysts, inflammatory lesions and granulomatous lesions, many of which do not necessarily need excision surgery.

MALIGNANT

Primary malignant salivary gland neoplasms are considered rare, with an age-standardized incidence between 0.6 and 1.4 per 100 000 in Europe. In England, about 450 new cases of salivary gland malignancy are diagnosed every year, with the incidence increasing by 37 per cent between 1990 and 2006. Malignant salivary glands have been classified into 24 differing types of carcinoma.[6–8] The majority are histological variants of adenocarcinoma. The most common types (88 per cent) diagnosed include adenoid cystic carcinoma, mucoepidermoid carcinoma, acinic cell carcinoma, adenocarcinoma not otherwise specified (NOS) and polymorphous low-grade adenocarcinoma.[9] The less common cancer histopathology types are identified in the parotid and minor salivary glands. In the evaluation of patients considered to have a salivary gland malignancy, it is important to consider metastatic disease, most commonly skin cancers (squamous cell carcinoma and malignant melanoma) or the possibility that the tumour mass is a lymphoma process; or, uncommonly, a distant metastasis from a distant cancer site – lung, breast or genito-urinary system. The proportion of malignant tumours increases as the gland size decreases, with malignancy accounting for 10 per cent of parotid gland cancers, 33 per cent of submandibular gland cancers and 67 per cent of minor salivary gland cancers. A diagnosis of a benign salivary gland neoplasm of the sublingual gland is exceedingly rare.

MANAGEMENT OF SALIVARY GLAND NEOPLASM

Surgical excision is the treatment of choice for both benign and malignant salivary gland neoplasms, with an appropriate margin, ensuring that the capsule of the tumour is not breached or the tumour contents spilt into the wound.[10] Any cranial nerves in proximity should be identified and preserved. While a working diagnosis can be made preoperatively on an FNAC, complete excision ensures that a definitive diagnosis can be made and the clinical team can prognosticate the likely clinical course of the disease.[11] Most tumours are likely to continue to grow, causing a cosmetic deformity because of position or interfering with local function if located in a minor salivary gland. There is reported to be a risk of malignant degeneration/transformation associated with the salivary pleomorphic adenoma of about 8 per cent, which is thought to increase the longer the tumour remains untreated. Malignant salivary gland tumours are many, but prognosis is associated with the presence of nerve weakness or paralysis, size of the tumour, presence of cervical adenopathy, histological grade of disease, ability to ensure complete excision and whether or not post-operative radiotherapy has been applied to the tumour bed.

COMPLICATIONS AND MORBIDITY AFTER SALIVARY GLAND SURGERY

The possible early (immediate ≥4 weeks) and late (after hospital discharge) complications and morbidity are listed in Table 28.2. The most serious complication of major parotid surgery is facial or hypoglossal nerve paralysis, which might be partial or complete.[12] Temporary facial nerve paresis, which can last for weeks or months, has been reported in 29 per cent of patients; the rate of permanent palsy can be as high as 6–8 per cent. The marginal mandibular branch of the facial nerve is the branch most likely to be traumatized during surgery on the parotid and submandibular glands. Other complications are related to local effects on wound healing, wound draining and local skin numbness. Frey's syndrome (gustatory hyperhydrosis) is a nuisance in some 5–10 per cent of patients. This symptom can be treated using botulinum toxin local injections periodically. Recurrence of disease – tumour (benign or malignant) and infective – is the most frustrating event for patients and tends to manifest within 5 years of initial surgery.[13] Further surgery, when possible, presents the best likelihood of cure but carries increased risk of local complications and further recurrence of the disease originally treated.

Table 28.2 Early and late complications of salivary gland surgery

Early (immediate ≥4 weeks)	Late (after hospital discharge)
Nerve palsy	Hyperaesthesia of local skin
Facial, lingual, hypoglossal	Cosmetic deformity: divot defect
Greater auricular nerve	Hypertrophic scar
Haemorrhage/haematoma	Frey's syndrome
Seroma	First-bite syndrome
Infection	Recurrent disease – tumour/infection
Skin-flap necrosis	
Trismus	
Fistula/sialocoele	

KEY LEARNING POINTS

- Symptoms of salivary gland diseases and disorders are limited in number and are generally non-specific.
- Pain as a dominant symptom may be associated with inflammation and neoplasms but is not itself diagnostic of malignancy.
- Primary salivary gland neoplasms (benign and malignant) most often present as a 'discrete mass', not involving the whole of the salivary gland.
- 'Diffuse' major salivary gland swellings, unilateral or bilateral, are associated with systemic disease or medication; however, on occasion lymphoma may present similarly and should always be considered in a differential diagnosis.
- Xerostomia may occur without any signs of hypo-salivation; however, medications are the most frequent identifiable cause of the patient with the 'dry mouth syndrome'.
- Sialadenitis most commonly presents in adults, associated with salivary ductal stenosis with salivary stones, duct stenosis or mucus plug.
- A diagnosis of primary Sjögren's syndrome must demonstrate autoantibodies A or B or a positive biopsy of salivary gland tissue demonstrating lymphocytic infiltration.
- Patients with Sjögren's syndrome are associated with an increased risk (16-fold) of developing non-Hodgkin's lymphoma of a major salivary gland (MALT type).
- Primary salivary gland neoplasms require a confirmatory needle biopsy before proceeding to treatment, which is usually surgery but may be different if proven malignant.
- Recurrence of primary salivary gland neoplasms tends to manifest within 5 years of surgery, but some types of salivary malignant neoplasms recurrences have been reported 15 years or more after initial surgery.

REFERENCES

1. Rahmati R, Gillespie B, Eisele DW. Is sialendoscopy an effective treatment for obstructive salivary gland disease? *Laryngoscope.* 2013; 123: 1828–9.
2. Nanda KDS, Metha A, Nanda J. Fine-needle aspiration cytology: A reliable tool in the diagnosis of salivary gland lesions. *Journal of Oral Pathology & Medicine.* 2012; 41: 106–12.
3 Chung MK, Jeong H-S, Ko M-H, et al. Pediatric sialadenitis: What is the difference from adult sialadenitis? *International Journal of Pediatric Orolaryngology.* 2007; 71: 787–91.
4. Vitali C, Bombardieri S, Johnsson R, et al. Classification criteria for Sjogren's syndrome: A revised version of the European Criteria proposed by the American-European consensus group. *Annals of Rheumatology Diseases.* 2002; 61: 554–8.
5. Batti RM, Stelow EB. IgG4-related disease of the head and neck. *Advances in Anatomic Pathology.* 2013; 20: 10–16.
6. Bradley PJ, McGurk M. Incidence of salivary gland neoplasms in a defined UK population. *British Journal of Oral and Maxillofacial Surgery.* 2013; 51: 399–403.
7. van der Poorten V, Bradley PJ, Takes RP, et al. Diagnosis and management of parotid carcinoma with special focus on recent advances on molecular biology. *Head & Neck.* 2012; 13: 58–70.
8. Munir N, Bradley PJ. Diagnosis and management of neoplastic lesions of the submandibular triangle. *Oral Oncology.* 2008; 44(3): 251–60.
9. van der Poorten V, Hunt J, Bradley PJ, et al. Recent trends in the management of minor salivary carcinoma. *Head & Neck.* 2014; 36: 444–55.
10. Bradley PJ. Consent to treatment and major salivary gland surgery. *ENT News.* 2001; 10(4): 55–9.
11. Isa AY, Hilmi OJ. An evidence based approach to the management of salivary masses. *Clinical Otolaryngology.* 2009; 34(5): 470–3.

12. Marshall AH, Quraishi SM, Bradley PJ. Patients' perspective on the short and long-term outcomes following surgery for benign parotid neoplasms. *Journal of Laryngology & Otology*. 2009; 119: 1140–6.
13. Gillespie MB, Albergotti WG, Eisele DW. Recurrent salivary gland cancer. *Current Treatment Opinions in Oncology*. 2012; 13: 58–70.

FURTHER READING

Bradley PJ, Guntinas-Lichius O. *Salivary Gland Disorders and Diseases: Diagnosis and Management*. Stuttgart, Germany: Thieme, 2011.

29

Thyroid disease

OMAR J HILMI

EMBRYOLOGY

The embryology of the thyroid has been covered elsewhere.

ANATOMY

The thyroid gland is a butterfly-shaped organ that surrounds the anterolateral aspect of the trachea in the root of the neck. It has three parts: a right and a left lobe joined by the isthmus in the midline. It has a discrete blood supply from the superior and inferior thyroid arteries and venous drainage via the superior, middle and inferior thyroid veins. Lying within the pre-tracheal fascia, posterior to the strap muscles (sternohyoid and sternothyroid), it has attachments at facial condensations (Berry's ligament) fixing it to the larynx and trachea just anterior to the cricoarytenoid region on each side. Its surgically important relationships are with the right and left recurrent laryngeal nerves and to the parathyroid glands (Figure 29.1).

PHYSIOLOGY

The thyroid is an endocrine gland that produces a variety of hormones and proteins.

The thyroid epithelial cells, or thyrocytes, which are arranged in a follicular pattern (see Figure 29.1), produce the hormones triiodothyronine (T_3) and tetraiodothyronine (T_4) under the control of the pituitary thyroid-stimulating hormone (TSH),

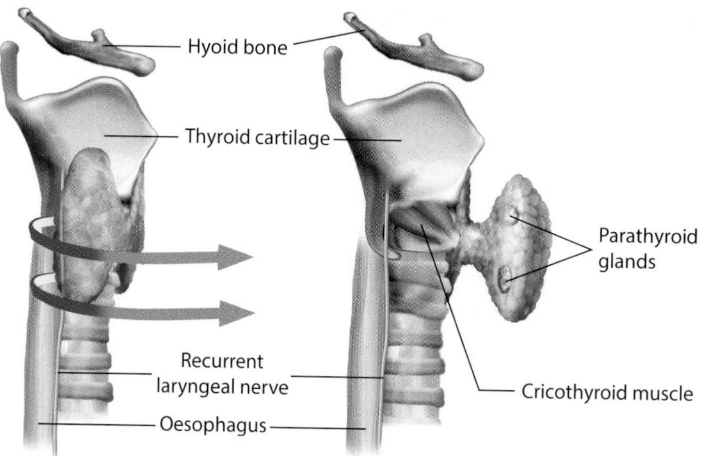

Figure 29.1 Thyroid in the neck.

which is itself controlled by thyrotropin-releasing hormone (TRH) (see Figure 29.2). T_3 and T_4 act on the body to increase metabolism, affect growth and development and increase the sensitivity to catecholamines. In addition to the metabolically active hormones, the thyrocytes also produce the protein thyroglobulin, which is stored as colloid in the follicles.

The parafollicular or C cells produce calcitonin, which acts to reduce the circulating blood levels of calcium.

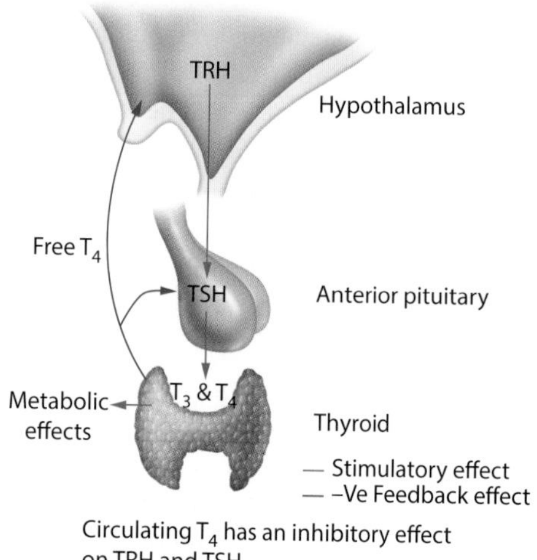

Figure 29.2 Hormone feedback diagram, T_3 and T_4.

PATHOLOGY

Diseases of the thyroid typically present with hyperthyroidism or hypothyroidism, or as a mass in the neck.

HYPERTHYROIDISM

Overproduction of T_3 and/or T_4 manifests clinically with tachycardia, diarrhoea, increased appetite, weight loss, anxiety, hyperkinesis, insomnia and heat intolerance.

HYPOTHYROIDISM

Lack of thyroid hormones presents with weight gain, lethargy, cold intolerance, coarse skin and hair loss. In adults, the conditions that affect the thyroid gland can be classified as inflammatory and autoimmune, hyperplastic and metabolic abnormalities, cysts and neoplasms (Table 29.1).

THYROID MASSES

Presentation

From a surgical perspective, thyroid masses are the most common presentation of thyroid disease.

Table 29.1 Inflammatory and autoimmune conditions

	Pathophysiology	Blood tests	Clinical presentation
Graves' disease	Thyroid hyperplasia in response to high levels of circulating antibodies to the TSH receptors in the thyroid gland (thyroid receptor antibodies [TRAB] or long-acting thyroid stimulator [LATS])	TSH — suppressed $T_3/_4$ — elevated TRAB — elevated	Diffuse goitre with clinical signs of hyperthyroidism with or without proptosis (thyroid ophthalmopathy)
Hashimoto's thyroiditis	Diffuse lymphocytic infiltration of the thyroid gland leads to progressive destruction of the gland	TSH —suppressed/ normal/elevated $T_3/_4$ Thyroid peroxidase — elevated	Diffuse thyroid enlargement with or without pain; patient may be hyper/euthyroid in the initial stages but gradually becomes hypothyroid
De Quervain's thyroiditis	Subacute granulomatous thyroiditis; normally self-limiting	TSH —elevated/ suppressed/normal $T_3/_4$ — variable depending on stage of inflammation	Diffuse painful goitre with initial hyperthyroidism, leading to hypothyroidism, ultimately becoming euthyroid
Hyperplastic/metabolic disorders			
Physiological goiter	Diffuse thyroid enlargement often comes on during pregnancy/puberty	All normal	Mild diffuse goitre
Simple/ multinodular goitre	Benign enlargement often with nodularity of the gland	All normal	Diffuse enlargement of gland may have multiple nodules on scanning/ clinical assessment
Endemic goitre	Diffuse enlargement of thyroid due to iodine deficiency, notably Sudan, Nepal, etc.	TSH may be elevated	Diffuse, massive enlargement of gland shows some nodularity
Thyroid cysts	Cystic degeneration of thyroid follicle	Normal	Thyroid mass, normally asymptomatic Occasionally can present with compressive symptoms secondary to a bleed into the cyst with rapid enlargement

(Continued)

Table 29.1 (Continued) Inflammatory and autoimmune conditions

	Pathophysiology	Blood tests	Clinical presentation
Neoplasms of the thyroid			
Papillary thyroid cancer (PTC)	Malignant growth of papillary cells	Normal or slightly elevated TSH	Mass in thyroid/neck; may have metastasis on presentation
Follicular thyroid cancer (FTC)	Malignant growth of thyroid epithelial cells	Normal or slightly elevated TSH	Mass in thyroid, rarely presents with metastatic disease
Medullary thyroid cancer (MTC)	Malignancy of parafollicular C cells; 25 per cent have genetic causality; part of MEN 2 (medullary thyroid cancer, phaeochromocytoma and primary hyper-parathyroidism)	Calcitonin elevated Carcinoembryonic antigen — elevated RET proto-oncogene — positive in 25 per cent	Mass in thyroid/neck
Anaplastic/ undifferentiated thyroid cancer	Poorly differentiated malignancy of thyroid origin; high rates of lymphovascular invasion and spread	Normal	Mass with rapid enlargement; often presents with airway compromise/dysphagia in thyroid/neck
Thyroid lymphoma	Development of lymphoma nodules within the thyroid, classically on a background of Hashimoto's thyroiditis	Normal	Mass in thyroid/neck; rapid enlargement; often presents with airway compromise/ dysphagia

This can be because of the obvious presence of a mass or compressive symptoms related to pressure on the trachea (causing breathing issues) or the oesophagus (causing swallowing problems); rarely, a retrosternal thyroid can present with superior vena cava obstruction.

The important consideration when assessing these patients is whether the mass is part of a generalized process affecting the gland or a malignant tumour. Historically, this differentiation was based largely on clinical examination. A solitary thyroid nodule was assessed as if it were potentially malignant, whereas a diffuse enlargement was more likely to be benign. Whilst the assessment technology has changed with the advent of cross-sectional imaging and ultrasound assessment, the terminology has not. Therefore, a solitary thyroid nodule may represent:

1. A clinically identified nodule
2. A radiological suspicious nodule in a more diffuse process such as a multinodular goitre
3. An incidentally found suspicious nodule in a patient scanned for other reasons

Imaging

Ultrasound is now central in the assessment of these patients. With ultrasound, it is possible to describe position, shape, size, margins, content, echogenic pattern and, whenever possible, the vascular pattern of the nodule. In addition, it can help to identify whether the nodule at risk is malignant; can stratify the nodule with a risk score based on the ultrasound findings; and, if necessary, can guide the fine-needle aspiration (FNA) biopsy. For patients with a suggestion of retrosternal extension, computed tomography (CT) is also required to define the full extent of the disease. Scintigraphy is rarely used in the assessment of thyroid masses unless the patient is thyrotoxic and clarification is required as to whether the mass is a 'hot nodule', in which case hemithyroidectomy may be curative.

Investigation

The key investigation in the assessment of any suspicious thyroid mass is fine-needle aspiration cytology (FNAC), which gives excellent assessment of nodules in which papillary thyroid cancer is present. It is of less utility in diagnosing follicular thyroid cancer because the differentiation between a benign adenoma and a carcinoma is not cytological but is based on the presence of peri-vascular or peri-capsular invasion. This requires histological assessment of the entire nodule. In surgical terms, this means a diagnostic hemithyroidectomy or isthmusectomy (Figure 29.3).

FNAC is best performed by a dedicated cytologist and/or ultrasound guidance to reduce sampling error. The optimal results are likely to be achieved by a dedicated cytologist under ultrasound guidance. Without the ability to target the sampling, the value of FNAC is reduced. In the United Kingdom, the results of the cytological examination are categorized according to the THY classification of thyroid cytology, but elsewhere the Bethesda System for Reporting Thyroid Cytology is becoming popular. The systems are similar. The THY system gives assessment categories and management strategies based on the result (Table 29.2).

THYROID CANCER

The incidence of thyroid cancer has been increasing for many years. In 1986, the overall incidence of thyroid cancer in Scotland was 1.9 cases per 100 000, but it is more common in women (2.6/100 000) than in men (1.3/100 000). By 2008, the overall incidence had risen to 3.4 cases per 100 000, with the incidence for women being 4.6 and for men being 2.1 per 100 000. This increase has been noted throughout Europe and America, although the cause for this is not clear. Thyroid cancer generally has a good prognosis, and despite this rise in incidence, the mortality rate has remained unchanged at 0.4 per 100 000. Known risk factors for thyroid cancer are radiation exposure, family history and pre-existing thyroid disease.

More than 90 per cent of thyroid cancers are differentiated thyroid cancer (DTC). Of these, there are two main histological types: papillary, which accounts for around 80 per cent of thyroid malignancies, and follicular, which involves another 10–15 per cent. Medullary thyroid cancer makes up an additional 3–5 per cent, with lymphoma and anaplastic thyroid carcinoma at 1–3 per cent.

STAGING OF THYROID CANCER

As in other cancers, the TNM system is the most commonly used. The tumour is classified according to size, and loco-regional nodal disease is assessed with ultrasound and/or CT. The presence of metastasis can be assessed by CT of the chest or chest x-ray, although this is an area of debate. Staging is then further defined according to tumour type and patient age (Table 29.3).

MANAGEMENT OF THYROID CANCER

Unlike in other head and neck cancers, in the majority of cases papillary and follicular thyroid cancer cells retain the typical characteristics of thyroid cells. These features can be used to optimize treatment.

1. They respond to TSH stimulation. Therefore, TSH suppression with hormone replacement can potentially reduce the growth rate of any residual thyroid cells.
2. They take up iodine. I-131 can be used for diagnostic purposes to assess both the completeness of the excision and the presence of metastatic disease (iodine uptake) or the destruction of residual thyroid tissue and metastatic disease with high-dose radioiodine (iodine ablation). The use of radioiodine also requires any residual thyrocytes to be metabolically active. This means having high circulating TSH levels, which is achieved by withholding hormone replacement. If T_4 is used, it must be continued

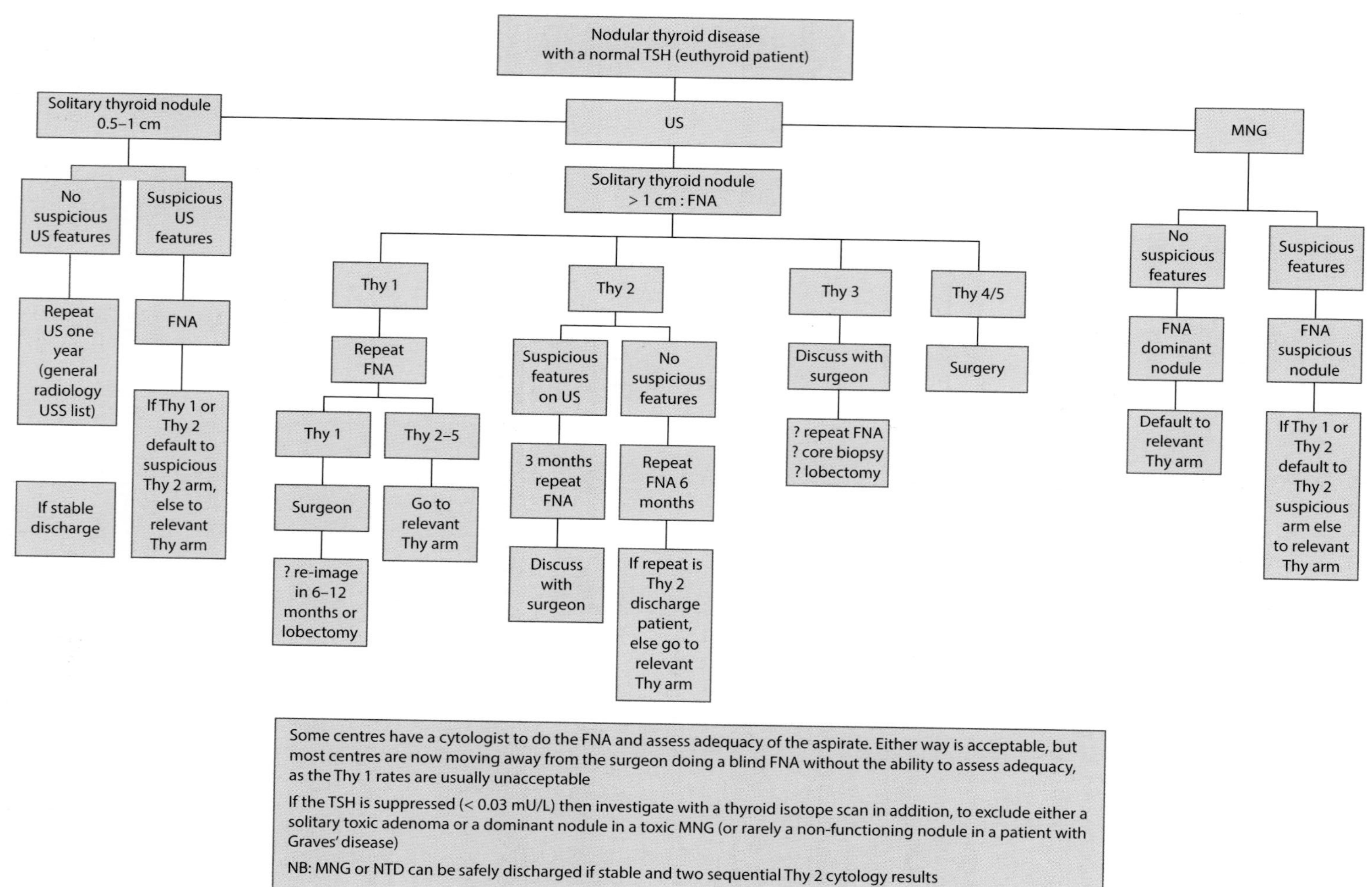

Figure 29.3 Thyroid nodule decision tree. US, ultrasound; USS, ultrasound scan.

Table 29.2 Management of thyroid nodules according to the THY cytology classification

Diagnostic category	Actions	Risk of malignancy
THY1: non-diagnostic (lack of cellularity)	Repeat fine-needle aspiration with ultrasound guidance; consider surgery if several results are nondiagnostic, especially if the nodule is solid	0–10 per cent
THY1c: clearly identified as cyst	If the cyst has been aspirated completely with no residual mass, a repeat ultrasound scan alone may be sufficient, with fine-needle aspiration only if the cyst recurs	0–10 per cent
THY2: non-neoplastic	Repeat fine-needle aspiration in 3 to 6 months	0–3 per cent
THY3: follicular lesion	Most patients should be treated by surgical removal of the lobe containing the nodule; these cases should be discussed in the MDT meeting if a therapeutic procedure is being considered; completion thyroidectomy may be necessary if the histology proves malignant	15–30 per cent
THY3a: atypical cytological findings are worrying but do not fit in the THY2 or THY4 categories	These cases should be discussed in the MDT to decide on the appropriate course of action; most will go on to a diagnostic lobectomy	5–15 per cent
THY4: suspicious but non-diagnostic	Surgical intervention is usually indicated for suspected cancer; where THY4 assessment has been given because of the absence of material for immunocytochemistry (medullary carcinoma) or flow cytometry (lymphoma), the aspirate should be repeated	60–75 per cent
THY5: suspicious for papillary carcinoma or Hürthle cell neoplasm	The diagnosis should be discussed at the MDT meeting where further management should be agreed upon; surgical intervention is indicated for DTC and MTC depending on tumour size, clinical stage and other risk factors; appropriate further investigation, radiotherapy and/or chemotherapy is indicated for anaplastic thyroid carcinoma, lymphoma or metastatic tumour	97–100 per cent

DTC — differentiated thyroid cancer; MDT— multidisciplinary team; MTC — metastatic thyroid cancer. Adapted from the British Thyroid Association.

for about 6 weeks, but in the case of T_3 supplementation, a 2-week washout period is normally enough.

3. They produce thyroglobulin. Blood levels of thyroglobulin can be used as a tumour marker to assess both response to treatment and rising potential of recurrent disease. This needs to include an assessment of thyroglobuin antibodies as well; if present, they will give a false, low result. In this situation, however, the thyroglobulin antibody level itself can act as a tumour marker.

These strategies are effective only in patients who have undergone total thyroidectomy. In clinical practice, this means that most patients undergo total thyroidectomy and post-operative radioiodine ablation.

If the tumour is a small (<10 mm) papillary or follicular carcinoma, then hemithyroidectomy alone may be satisfactory.

Medullary thyroid cancer is a malignancy of the parafollicular C cells. This is part of MEN2 (medullary thyroid cancer and phaeochromocytoma); it is subcategorized as 2a in the presence of parathyroid

Table 29.3 TNM system

Prognostic scoring systems for thyroid cancer

Staging

The 7th edition of the TNM classification is recommended

Classification according to tumour, nodes and metastases

Primary tumour

pT1 Intrathyroidal tumour, ≤2 cm in greatest dimension
pT2 Intrathyroidal tumour, >2–4 cm in greatest dimension
PT3 Intrathyroidal tumour, >4 cm in greatest dimension
pT4 Tumour of any size, extending beyond thyroid capsule
pTX Primary tumour cannot be assessed

All anaplastic carcinomas are considered stage IV:

pT4a Intrathyroidal anaplastic carcinoma
pT4b Anaplastic carcinoma with gross extrathyroidal extension

Regional lymph nodes (cervical or upper mediastinal)

N0 No nodes involved
N1 Regional nodes involved
If possible, subdivide
N1a Ipsilateral cervical nodes
N1b Bilateral, midline or contralateral cervical nodes or mediastinal nodes
NX Nodes cannot be assessed

Distant metastases

M0 No distant metastases
M1 Distant metastases
MX Distant metastases cannot be assessed

Based on these three categories, the cancer is assigned a Stage of 1, 2, 3 or 4.

Papillary or follicular carcinoma staging

	Under 45 years	**45 years and older**
Stage I	Any T, any N, M0	pT1, N0, M0
Stage II	Any T, any N, M1	pT2, N0, M0,
Stage III		pT3, N0, M0
Stage IV		pT4, N0, M0, Any pT, N1, M0, Any pT, any N, M1

Medullary cancer has a different staging. Undifferentiated or anaplastic carcinomas: All are stage IV.
Adapted from Edge SB, Byrd DR, Compton CC, Fritz AG, Greene FL, Trotti A, et al. *AJCC Cancer Staging Manual*, 7th ed. New York: Springer-Verlag; 2010.

hyperplasia and as 2b if associated with mucocutaneous neuromas.

Twenty-five per cent of patients have a mutation in the RET proto-oncogene. All patients with this diagnosis should be referred for genetic testing and counseling.

Whilst medullary cancer cells do not take up iodine, they produce calcitonin; this can be used as a diagnostic blood test and also for post-operative monitoring.

Patients with medullary thyroid cancer do not respond to radioiodine. Therefore, the minimum operation is total thyroidectomy with neck dissection and a low threshold for external beam radiotherapy.

MANAGING THE NECK IN THYROID CANCER

Neck dissection in papillary thyroid cancer

The presence of metastatic neck disease mandates a therapeutic neck dissection of the involved nodal groups to optimize the post-operative adjuvant treatments. The role of a staging central compartment clearance, in the absence of known disease, is controversial. It is known that papillary thyroid cancer metastasizes early to lymph nodes in levels 6 and 7 and that pre-operative imaging of this area is difficult. Therefore, it is justified that in greater than 20 per cent of cases, such a clearance will be therapeutic. In the node-negative cases, it may reduce the need for post-operative radioiodine.

Neck dissection in follicular thyroid cancer

Most follicular cancer is diagnosed after diagnostic hemithyroidectomy. For small lesions that are low risk on the basis of the pathology and staging scans (ultrasound, CT or both), this may be all that is needed; most, however, require completion surgery (removal of the contralateral lobe of the thyroid) and adjuvant treatment as dictated by formal staging. The presence of metastatic neck disease mandates therapeutic neck dissection of the involved levels to optimize the post-operative adjuvant treatments. Unlike in papillary thyroid cancer, there is no established benefit in doing a staging neck dissection because lymph node metastases are not frequently found.

Neck dissection in medullary thyroid cancer

Central compartment neck dissection with total thyroidecotomy is the minimum treatment for medullary thyroid cancer, and many would also do a lateral neck dissection (levels 2a, 3, 4 and 5b) on the ipsilateral side. The presence of disease in the lateral neck mandates a comprehensive dissection on that side.

SURGERY FOR ANAPLASTIC THYROID CANCER

This poorly differentiated malignancy is characterized by rapid growth, local invasion and distant metastasis. It responds poorly to chemotherapy or radiotherapy and is normally inoperable by the time of diagnosis. Median survival time from diagnosis is 4–6 months.

Historically, the only surgery advocated was biopsy or tracheotomy for airway obstruction, with or without isthmusectomy. If there is no involvement of the great vessels, then surgery in the form of total thyroidectomy and neck dissection can be performed, but this is unlikely to be curative and is aimed at reducing the chance of airway or swallowing problems.

SURGERY IN THE THYROTOXIC PATIENT

With the advent of medical treatments of thyrotoxicosis and the excellent results of radioiodine in the long-term control of thyrotoxicosis, surgical management of this condition is becoming increasingly rare. Normally, those patients who cannot be rendered euthyroid by other means present for surgery.

Surgically, these patients are a challenge, because the metabolically active gland has an increased blood supply, and global enlargement makes the surgery more complex and at higher risk of complications than do other indications for thyroid surgery. Logo's iodine can be used pre-operatively for 1–2 weeks at a dose of 0.1-0.3 mL TDS to try to render the patient euthyroid rapidly, but this carries the potential risk of initiating a thyroid crisis if surgery is delayed. Historically, subtotal thyroidectomies, preserving part of the superior pole to reduce the chance of developing hypothyroidism, were performed, but with improvements in the use and monitoring of thyroxine treatment, total or near-total thyroidectomy is the standard.

From the anaesthetic point of view, the toxic patient is prone to cardiac arrhythmias; with peri-operative manipulation of the gland, this can be exacerbated. β-blockers can be used to regulate this either pre- or peri-operatively. Post-operatively, toxic patients are at increased risk of developing hypocalcaemia as a result of hypoparathyroidism but also due to hungry bone syndrome. In this condition, post-operative reversal of phytotoxic osteodystrophy causes increased uptake of calcium in the presence of normal or high circulating levels of parathyroid hormone (PTH). Treatment is with calcium and vitamin D supplementation once recognized. Some surgeons advocate pre-operative treatment if the patient is at risk, as predicted by an elevated alkaline phosphatase level pre-operatively, with calcium and alafacalcidol. Failure to correct or recognize this serious complication can cause cardiac arrhythmias and seizure activity. Emergency treatment of symptomatic hypocalcaemia is with calcium glucuronate given intravenously. These patients should have cardiac monitoring during the infusion.

COMPLICATIONS OF THYROID SURGERY

In addition to the usual complications of surgery encountered in any sub-site of the neck, the relationship of the thyroid to the airway, the recurrent laryngeal nerves and the parathyroid glands causes specific risks.

BLEEDING

Airway obstruction secondary to a post-operative bleed is a potentially life-threatening complication. Traditionally, drains were routinely used, but their use is no longer universal, and bleeds can occur even in their presence. If there are signs of a haematoma, careful consideration should be made of returning to the operating theatre for evacuation. Most surgeons would return to the theater if faced with a haematoma, and definitely if there were signs of airway obstruction.

RECURRENT LARYNGEAL NERVE PALSY

Permanent recurrent laryngeal nerve palsy is rare after thyroid surgery (1–4 per cent of cases), but because of its implications it is imperative for all patients to be aware of it as a potential problem. Temporary weakness is probably quite common but is rarely looked for specifically. Bilateral vocal cord palsies can cause airway obstruction, and because of this patients undergoing total thyroidectomy are sometimes counselled about the possibility of tracheostomy. All patients undergoing thyroid surgery for malignancy, undergoing revision surgery or with a history of voice change should have a pre-operative vocal cord assessment, and it is good practice to do so in all cases.

HYPOCALCAEMIA

Low calcium levels post–thyroid surgery can be due to hungry bone syndrome (see earlier discussion), but hypoparathyroidism secondary to either removal or devascularization of the parathyroid glands is the most common cause. This is a very low risk for patients who have undergone hemithyroidectomy but is a potential problem in those who have undergone either total or completion surgery. Calcium levels should be monitored post-operatively and treatment commenced as appropriate.

KEY LEARNING POINTS

- The key assessment for a suspicious thyroid mass is the FNAC.
- All patients undergoing thyroid surgery for malignancy, undergoing revision surgery or with a history of voice change should have a pre-operative vocal cord assessment.
- Hypocalcaemia is a serious post-operative complication in patients who have undergone completion or total thyroidectomy.

FURTHER READING

Mehanna HM, Morton RP, Watkinson J, Shaha A. Clinical review: Investigating the thyroid nodule. *British Medical Journal.* 2009; 338: b733.

30

Benign diseases of the oral cavity

GRAHAM R OGDEN

INTRODUCTION

This chapter will consider the diseases affecting the teeth, the gingiva (gums) and the oral mucosa, since tumours of the mouth and the salivary glands and facial pain are covered in other chapters. However, where relevant, these latter topics will be briefly mentioned, since the oral cavity is often neglected within medical training.

Patients can present to the ear, nose and throat (ENT) surgeon with a variety of oral problems. Such a manifestation may mimic a more serious disease; therefore, it is important to exclude the more common conditions, not least to avoid unwanted investigations or unnecessary surgery.

CONDITIONS AFFECTING THE HARD TISSUES

TEETH

Dental caries ('tooth decay') describes decalcification of tooth enamel due to acids released from plaque bacteria following their metabolism of carbohydrates (Figure 30.1). (Fluoride in water and toothpaste aid remineralization.)

There are a number of risk factors, which include genetics, saliva flow, bacteria and diet. Saliva helps protect the teeth. Decreased saliva flow (caused by Sjögren's syndrome or certain drugs, for example diuretics, or previous radiotherapy to the major

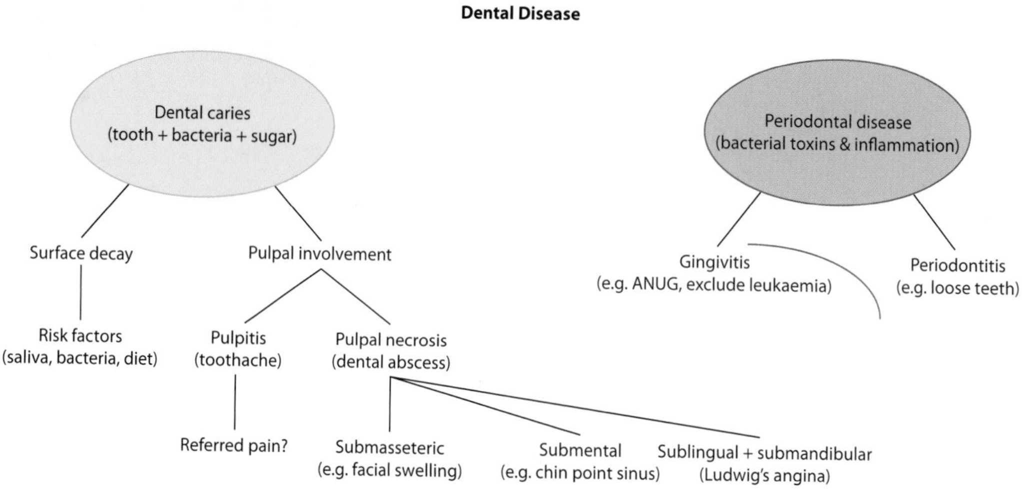

Figure 30.1 Description of the most common dental diseases.

salivary glands) may also predispose an individual to dental caries (Figure 30.2). The main acid-producing bacteria are mutans streptococci and lactobacilli.

Subsequent cavitation into dentine can cause pain ('toothache') due to pulpitis (inflammation of the dental pulp). This may lead to pulpal necrosis and the development of a dental abscess.

The importance of pulpitis to the ENT surgeon is twofold. It can cause vague pain that is difficult to localize, and it may lead to referred pain elsewhere in the mouth. (Maxillary sinusitis can also result in pain referred to the teeth.) Pulpitis may be detected by applying a cold stimulus to the tooth (e.g. ethylchloride-soaked cotton pledget), eliciting pain, which does not immediately recede once the stimulus is removed.

If the tooth becomes non-vital, a negative response to cold stimulus is found. If an abscess occurs, this can track through the fascial plains, for example to the submandibular 'space', giving rise to a unilateral swelling under the body of the mandible (Figure 30.3). A submasseteric abscess can cause trismus (inability to open the mouth) and swelling, for example unilateral fat face. A bilateral swelling involving both sublingual and submandibular 'spaces' (also known as Ludwig's

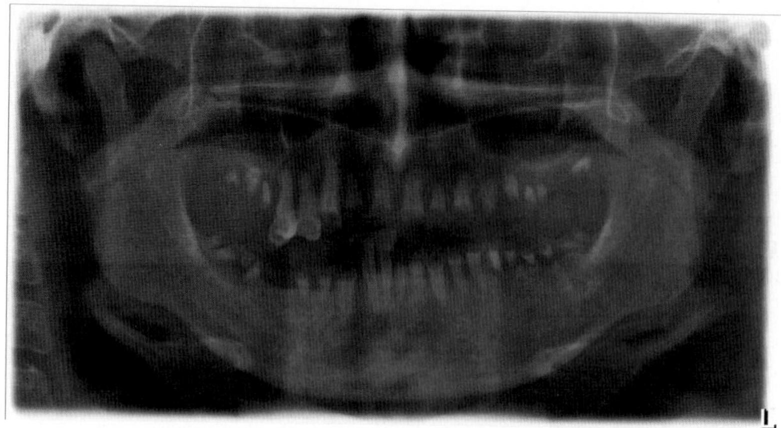

Figure 30.2 Panoramic radiograph to illustrate gross caries affecting the dentition.

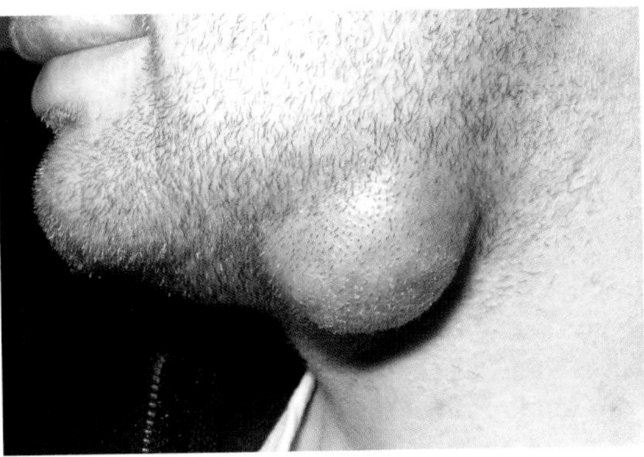

Figure 30.3 A large fluctuant dental abscess 'pointing' externally and ready for incision and drainage.

angina) is a life-threatening condition. In addition to marked trismus and a raised temperature, a patient with this condition may find it difficult to swallow or even breathe. Because of the trismus, some authorities avoid using a general anaesthetic (owing to risk of failure to intubate following use of a muscle relaxant) and prefer a local anaesthetic instead. Bilateral drains are inserted, with the incision made from the neck into the mouth through both sublingual and submandibular 'spaces'.

Such infection is painful when enclosed in bone, although temporary relief can arise when it spreads into the soft tissues. Some teeth are associated with particular swellings, for example maxillary canine around the eye, maxillary lateral incisor in the anterior palate, and mandibular molar in the face. When the swelling is fluctuant (i.e. pus is present; see Figure 30.3), it should be incised and drained, with the offending tooth either root treated or extracted. If is not, the infection may create a sinus (either intraorally or extraorally). The author has seen a sinus be mistaken for a basal cell carcinoma (Figure 30.4) that subsequently 'recurred' after excision; hence, the importance of ruling out simple dental disease. In that instance, trauma had resulted in the tooth becoming non-vital. Radiographic investigation using a panoramic radiograph gives a good general view, with gross caries seen as darkening of the white enamel (due to loss of calcification). There may also be loss of bone at the apex of the tooth, particularly when abscessed. Pain on chewing is suggestive of this. Advice to patients to reduce caries risk should

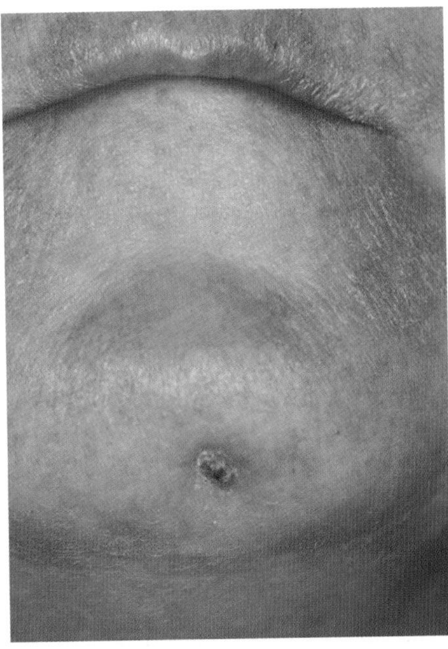

Figure 30.4 Sinus from non-infected tooth at chin point mimicking a basal cell carcinoma.

include good oral hygiene, dietary guidance, and use of fluoride therapy (toothpaste or mouthwash).

OTHER DENTAL ANOMALIES

Tetracycline antibiotics should not be prescribed to children younger than the age of 12 years because they may lead to staining of the teeth (they fluoresce under ultraviolet light).

Dental erosion is the loss of tooth enamel due to gastric acid reflux (or due to exogenous factors, e.g. fizzy drinks). It typically leads to cupping of the cusps or loss of enamel around an amalgam filling. This may be an early sign of bulimia nervosa (associated with depression, loss of self-esteem, misuse of alcohol and self-harm).

Other causes of tooth discolouration include exogenous factors (e.g. chlorhexidine mouthwash, tobacco, bacteria) or endogenous factors (trauma to pulp, fluorosis, certain drugs).

PERIODONTAL DISEASE

Gingivitis, the mildest form of periodontal disease, causes the gums to be red and swollen and bleed

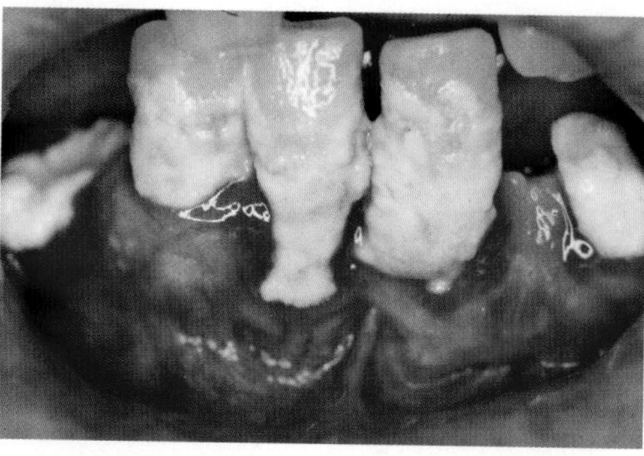

Figure 30.5 Gingivitis due to gross deposits of dental plaque.

easily. It is associated with the presence of plaque bacteria (Figure 30.5). Rarely, it can be a feature of leukaemia, although a combination of other associated features such as lymphadenopathy, bleeding, petechiae, oral ulceration, fungal infections and herpes infection is usually present too. When leukaemia is suspected, a blood film, white cell count and platelet count should be obtained. Acute necrotizing ulcerative gingivitis (ANUG; necrosis and ulceration of the gingiva) is a particular example in which halitosis, pain, gingival bleeding and systemic involvement can be confused with symptoms of leukaemia.

Untreated gingivitis can spread to periodontal disease. Toxins produced by the plaque bacteria stimulate an inflammatory response that in turn leads to damage to the periodontal ligament (tooth support) and surrounding bone (known as 'pocketing'). As the disease progresses the teeth can become loose and mobile. Multiple teeth are usually involved, and where a single tooth is found, malignant disease should be excluded. Recently, there has been much interest in the link between periodontal disease and systemic illness. Originally thought to be due to the bacteria, periodontal disease is now thought to be due to the associated inflammatory response. The main links have been to diabetes (reduced ability to control blood sugar levels and also increased periodontal disease) and cardiovascular disease (increased risk of heart disease). In these cases, referral to a dental surgeon is advised.

BONE

Sometimes a patient will present to a physician worried about a swelling that she only just noticed, which proves to be a developmental benign exostosis (torus). Common sites include the midline of the palate (palatine torus) and the lingual aspect of the mandible (usually bilateral, lingual to the premolars and unequal in size). Smooth or nodular, with an ulcerated surface if traumatized (e.g. by a toothbrush), the subsequent pain and ulceration can draw the swelling to the attention of the patient for the first time. Subsequent review will reveal no increase in size and healing of the area of ulceration (Figure 30.6).

As mentioned, the panoramic radiograph provides a general screening of the jaw bones. Common anomalies may include impacted teeth (e.g. maxillary canines, supernumerary [extra] teeth), odontomes (malformed dental tissue), cysts (e.g. dentigerous cysts or odontogenic keratocysts), benign conditions (e.g. fibrous dysplasia) and malignant disease. A cyst has a well-delineated, corticated white margin on a radiograph that may be uni- or multilocular. Those associated with the crown of a tooth are termed *dentigerous cysts* (Figure 30.7). Malignant disease is associated with resorption of adjacent tooth roots and a moth-eaten appearance to the regular corticated margin. Benign radiolucent conditions of the bone include ameloblastoma (a locally invasive tumour) and fibrous dysplasia (if polystotic, exclude Albright

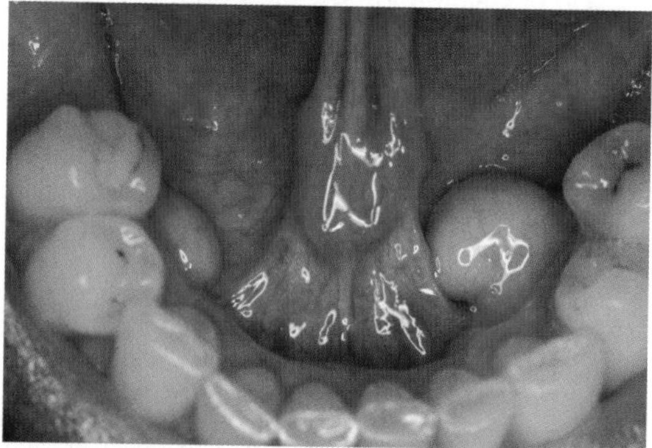

Figure 30.6 An example of tori lingual to the premolars, often bilateral and of unequal size.

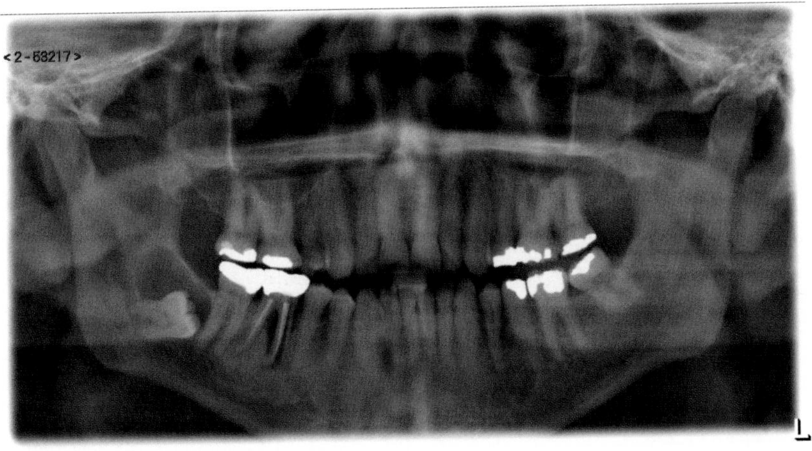

Figure 30.7 A dentigerous cyst in association with an impacted unerupted third molar.

syndrome, associated with skin pigmentation and endocrine disorders, e.g. precocious puberty in girls).

TEMPOROMANDIBULAR JOINT SYNDROME

Synonyms of temporomandibular joint (TMJ) syndrome include myofascial pain dysfunction, facial arthromyalgia and TMJ pain dysfunction syndrome. It affects approximately 10 per cent of the population at some point and commonly presents as clicking of the jaw, sometimes progressing to limitation and locking with pain in the jaw and surrounding musculature. It is most often seen in young females and associated with stress (e.g. exams) or trauma. Incoordination of the two heads of the lateral pterygoid (which is also attached to the TMJ meniscus) can lead to no displacement of the meniscus, anterior displacement with reduction (a click is heard as the meniscus snaps back into position) or anterior displacement of the meniscus with no reduction (it gets stuck and causes 'locking' of the jaw).

TMJ syndrome is not usually associated with any long-term damage and is usually self correcting, although many patients can present to their ENT surgeon complaining of pain around the ear; hence the importance of excluding the condition. There is no swelling associated with this condition. Therefore, if there is swelling, it is due to another cause. Positive findings include tenderness of the muscles of mastication (e.g. on palpating the masseteric muscle) and deviation of the jaw on opening and/or closing. Jaw exercises in the form of preventing forward posturing and encouraging opening and closing in a straight line are usually sufficient as long as the patient persists ('retraining the sprained muscle'). Referral to a dentist to exclude a dental cause, such as a high restoration (e.g. filling or crown), is advised. Note that this condition can be part of the spectrum associated with fibromyalgia, which also includes chronic headaches, sleep disorder, dizziness, other joint stiffness, dysmenorrhea, and back pain. Beware also of psychological issues such as somatization.

A panoramic radiograph is not usually indicated, although magnetic resonance imaging (MRI) can be useful to identify displacement of the meniscus (Figure 30.8).

Often there is spontaneous remission. The patient should be reassured that the 'clicking' sound is quite common and not usually associated with damage to the joint.

Initial management includes jaw exercises and analgesics. Many clinicians prescribe a bite guard, although its efficacy is disputed. Patients who fail to adhere to this regimen (or do not improve with it) can often benefit from a 6-month course

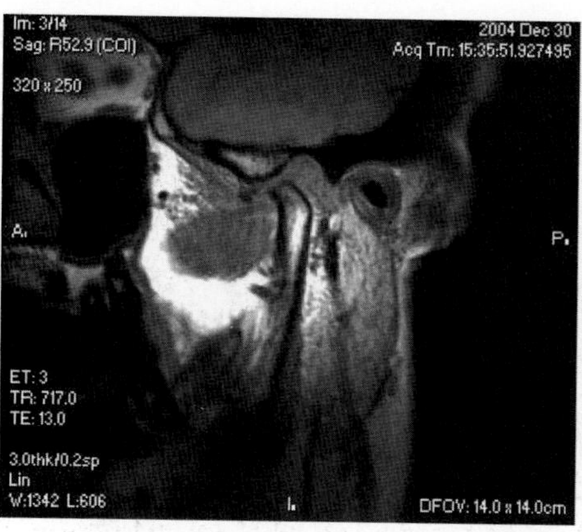

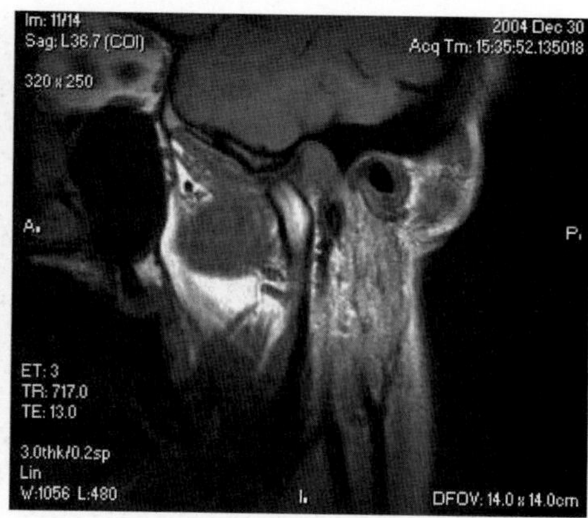

Figure 30.8 MRI scans of left (meniscal displacement) and right (healthy) temporomandibular joints. Notice the 'bow tie' appearance of the normal positioned meniscus (dark) and the anteriorly displaced, heaped up meniscus on the left.

of Prothiaden. It is prudent to exclude conditions that may have a similar presentation, including giant cell arteritis and trigeminal neuralgia. If symptoms do not improve or there is persistent pain within the joint, arthroscopy may be helpful both as a diagnostic tool and as a treatment. If MRI reveals a damaged meniscus, then repair or removal may be indicated. Another option, rarely required, is condylotomy, which reduces pressure on the meniscus, allowing it to move more freely and alleviating the pain.

DISLOCATION OF THE TMJ

Dislocation is seen when the head of the mandibular condyle leaves the glenoid fossa and cannot return. The patient will present with an elongated facial height and an inability to occlude the teeth. This can be difficult to detect if the patient is edentulous. The patient feels the strain on the stretched masseter and medial pterygoid muscles, often accompanied by pain and anxiety. Some patients are more prone to dislocation owing to laxity of the jaw joint, whilst in others it can be due to drugs, for example phenothiazines, which are associated with involuntary muscle spasm. In others dislocation arises merely on opening the mouth too wide. In the long term, if it occurs frequently, the head of the condyle can be removed (condylectomy) or the articular eminence removed (eminectomy) or enhanced (e.g. bone graft or Dautrey procedure).

In the short term, the head of the condyles must be reinserted as soon as possible. Sometimes sedation with midazolam is required. The physician should get the patient to sit next to a wall, so the patient can exert pressure against the wall with the back of his head. At the same time (with the fingers away from the occlusal surface, and on the external oblique ridge), the physician should press downwards and backwards (first one side and then the next). The condyles should slip back into position. The physician should caution the patient not to open widely for the rest of the day, particularly if the patient has received IV sedation. A barrel bondage from the chin to the head can remind the patient not to open. If this proves impossible, the use of a general anaesthetic and some bite blocks may be necessary. On the panoramic radiograph, the condyle heads are out of the glenoid fossa and there is an anterior open bite.

CLEFT LIP AND PALATE

The incidence of this condition in the United Kingdom is 1 in 700 live births. Its aetiology includes environmental, genetic (e.g. gene *IRF6*) and maternal factors (smoking; alcohol use; poor nutrition, e.g. lack of folic acid; or use of certain drugs, e.g. methotrexate). Cleft lip is unilateral in 90 per cent of cases. Cleft lip and palate occur more frequently in males, and cleft palate alone is more frequently associated with other syndromes

Table 30.1 Proportion of cleft types

Unilateral cleft lip and palate	30–35 per cent
Unilateral cleft lip	20–25 per cent
Unilateral cleft palate	20–25 per cent
Bilateral cleft lip and palate	10 per cent

(Table 30.1). It can have profound effects on speech, hearing, appearance and psychology, with long-lasting adverse effects on health and social integration. Such cases are treated in multidisciplinary teams (Figure 30.9).

A typical care plan involves counselling for the patient's parents, and hearing tests and feeding assessment for the patient from birth to 6 weeks. At 3 months of age, surgical repair of the lip is performed. Between 6 and 12 months, surgical repair of the cleft palate is performed. Speech assessment is conducted at 18 months, 3 years and 5 years. When the patient is between 8 and 11 years old, bone grafts to the cleft in the maxillary alveolus may be required, with involvement of an orthodontist, because the teeth can often be misplaced or missing. Any corrective surgery is delayed until the jaw growth is complete, after age 18. Key stages of development are recorded in the United Kingdom at ages 5, 10, 15 and 20 years to assess the effects of treatment. It is important that children receive specialist care in association with a paediatric dentist.

Cleft lip can either be a small gap or indentation (partial or incomplete cleft) or continue into the nose (complete cleft). It can be unilateral (90 per cent of cases) or bilateral and is due to a failure of fusion of the maxillary and medial nasal processes that form the primary palate. Repair at 3 months of age usually also involves the underlying muscle.

Cleft palate can be complete (soft and hard palate) or incomplete (a hole in the palate). This occurs where there is failure in formation of the secondary palate (formed from the palatine process and nasal septum). The resulting opening between the mouth and nose leads to velo-pharyngeal insufficiency, which also changes the voice (leading to speech articulation errors) and compensatory misarticulations (e.g. glottal stops and nasal fricatives).

A submucous cleft palate is one in which there is a triad of bifid uvula, a furrow along the midline of the soft palate and a notch in the back of the hard palate.

Cleft lip repair (the Millard procedure) involves a *Z*-shaped scar, which helps to restore the lips' 'cupid' bow. For a palatal cleft, a temporary obturator may be required to aid feeding.

CONDITIONS AFFECTING THE SOFT TISSUES

RED PATCHES

Inflammatory lesions

Most red patches (Table 30.2) are inflammatory, although erythroplakia (a red dysplastic lesion with an 80 per cent risk of cancer) may be present as a carcinoma *in situ* or early carcinoma,

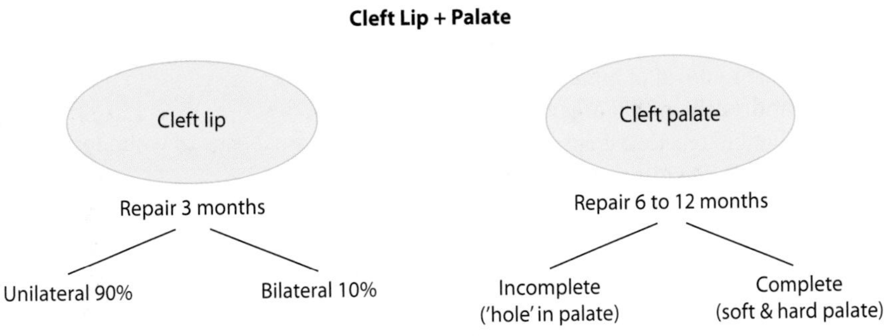

Figure 30.9 Description of the main features associated with cleft lip and palate.

Table 30.2 Causes of red lesions

Inflammatory, e.g. candida, radiation mucositis, lichen planus
Purpura, e.g. trauma, platelet disorder
Reactive, e.g. pyogenic granuloma
Neoplastic
Vascular, e.g. haemangioma

especially in a heavy drinker or smoker, and should be biopsied. Of the inflammatory lesions, most are due to infection (e.g. antibiotic sore mouth due to acute candida infection), chronic candida underneath a maxillary denture (creating a red palate) or median rhomboid glossitis (on the midline of the dorsal tongue). A past history of radiotherapy for malignant disease to the oral cavity can give rise to radiation mucositis and/or reduced salivary flow, predisposing the individual to candida infections. Viral infections include herpes simplex, either primary herpetic gingivostomatitis with raised temperature and sore inflamed gingiva, or secondary 'reactive' herpes such as a lip 'cold' sore.

Reactive lesions

Erosive lesions can be due to a burn, for example from aspirin, and skin disorders such as lichen planus, pemphigus vulgaris or erythema multiforme.

Lichen planus may arise with or without skin lesions. Its cause is unknown, although similar lesions (known as lichenoid reactions) are sometimes found in association with amalgam fillings, drugs (e.g. antihypertensives or hypoglycaemic agents) and graft-versus-host disease (in bone marrow transplant patients). The erosive or atrophic form is considered to be a potentially malignant condition and can be painful (Figure 30.10). Management may include removal of amalgam restoration (if unilateral and solely in that area), use of alternative drugs (if lichenoid reaction is suspected), topical oral steroids and chlorhexidine mouth rinse.

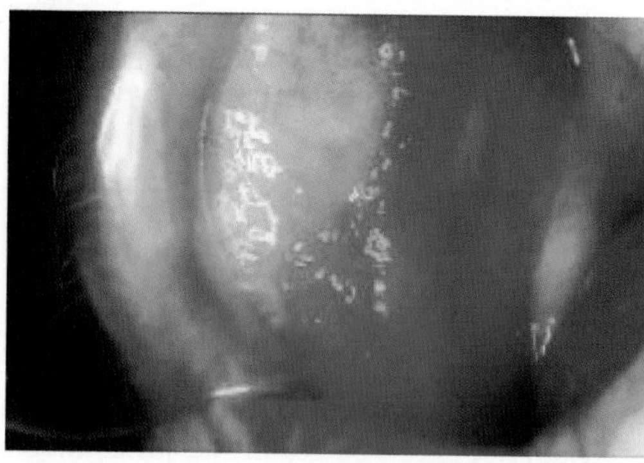

Figure 30.10 Erosive lichen planus affecting the buccal mucosa. Note the clear division between adjacent normal pink mucosa.

Other red conditions

Pyogenic granuloma is typically a red painless lesion that grows rapidly, bleeds easily and can be mistaken for a malignant tumour. It often arises at the gingival margin and is sometimes seen in pregnancy as an overreaction to plaque bacteria. Excision is curative (and histopathology is confirmatory).

Purpura can be present as petechiae, ecchymosis due to trauma, or blood platelet disorders (e.g. leukaemia).

Vascular anomalies include haemangioma (developmental but may become more obvious with age) and neoplasia.

WHITE LESIONS

The appearance of white lesions (Table 30.3) can be due to an increase in the prickle cell layer (acanthosis) or increased surface keratinization. If the lesion is due to trauma, it is usually focal and has no malignant risk. Smoker's keratosis, however, especially affecting the floor of the mouth, carries an increased risk for malignant change. *Leucoplakia*, the term given to a white patch that cannot be rubbed off and has no obvious aetiology, has a malignant risk of less than 5 per cent (compare this to erythroplakia, discussed earlier in this

Table 30.3 Causes of white lesions

Congenital, e.g. white sponge naevus, leukaemia
Infection, e.g. candida, Epstein-Barr virus, human papillomavirus
Inflammatory, e.g. lichen planus
Neoplastic, e.g. leucoplakia, carcinoma
Other, e.g. aspirin burn, trauma, furry tongue

chapter). However, squamous cell carcinoma can present as a white patch or a red-and-white patch (so-called speckled leucoplakia). Close monitoring is required, and susceptible patients should avoid alcohol and tobacco use.

Infection

Candidiasis can arise as either 'thrush' (acute pseudomembranous candidiasis), where the surface can be wiped away to reveal a red membrane, or candida leucoplakia. Thrush can arise when the normal oral flora is disturbed. Factors that can lead to this condition include xerostomia, smoking, corticosteroids, and broad-spectrum antibiotics. Investigations include fasting glucose test, full blood count, vitamin B_{12} and serum ferritin. In addition to prescribed antifungal agents, smoking cessation and adequate hydration may be required. Where candida leucoplakia is suspected, biopsy should be obtained and candida confirmed by periodic acid–Schiff (PAS) staining.

Other infections that can present as a white area include Koplik spots in measles, Epstein–Barr virus in hairy leucoplakia and warts (human papillomavirus, or HPV).

Inflammatory lesions

Lichen planus is the most common inflammatory lesion and can present in reticular (striations), papular or plaque-like form.

Congenital

White sponge naevus is typically bilateral and painless with a wrinkled appearance affecting the buccal mucosa. Leucoedema describes the faint white line seen at the occlusal level. Fordyce spots are caused by ectopic sebaceous glands and usually affect the buccal mucosa or inner lip

Other

Furry tongue (accumulation of dead epithelial cells, bacteria and food debris) is a coating often seen in otherwise healthy adults who may have poor oral hygiene or who are fasting (Figure 30.11). Scraping the tongue with a firm toothbrush usually removes the coating. Trauma (frictional keratosis) can cause whitening and can arise from a sharp tooth, poor-fitting denture or cheek biting. It has no malignant potential. Chemical burns, for example from aspirin, can cause sloughing of the epithelium and hence result in a white appearance.

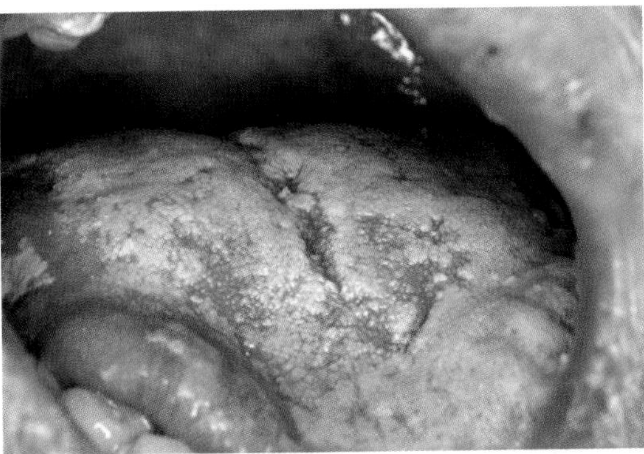

Figure 30.11 Deposits of dead cells and bacteria resulting in 'furry' tongue.

PIGMENTED LESIONS

Single pigmented lesions are probably best excised to exclude malignant melanoma (Table 30.4).

Black hairy tongue

This condition is due to elongation of the filiform papillae, which become darker, possibly owing to chromogenic bacteria. Brushing the tongue with a toothbrush and using a sodium bicarbonate mouth rinse usually eliminate the condition. A darkening

Table 30.4 Causes of pigmented lesions

Amalgam tattoo
Black hairy tongue
Drugs
Kaposi's sarcoma
Malignant melanoma
Melanotic macule
Naevus
Pregnancy
Racial pigmentation
Syndromes, e.g. Peutz-Jeghers, Addison's disease

of the dorsal surface of the tongue can also be due to smoking or chewing tobacco, eating or drinking certain foods (e.g. coffee) or using drugs (iron salts) and mouthwashes (chlorohexidine).

Other causes

Other causes of pigmented lesions include the following:

- Racial pigmentation – usually symmetrical
- Amalgam tattoo – the most common cause of a single 'lesion'; doesn't change shape or size, and if large enough will be radiodense on radiograph
- Melanotic macule – asymptomatic smooth single brown collection of melanin-containing cells usually seen near the lip and palate in Caucasians; can increase in size
- Naevi – blue-black papular lesions formed from increased melanin-containing cells; unlike the macule, they are often raised but do not change rapidly in size and are often seen in the palate
- Kaposi's sarcoma – a purple-violet lesion caused by human herpesvirus 8, seen in HIV or immunocompromised patients; intraorally may be raised and found on the palate or gingiva
- Malignant melanoma – rare and usually palatal, may arise in a previous pigmented naevus; signs of malignancy include rapid increase in size, pain, ulceration, swelling, satellite spots and regional lymphadenopathy; although usually dark, can be amelonotic

Additional causes of increased oral pigmentation include smoking tobacco (smoker's melanosis), antimalarial therapy, pregnancy and some oral contraceptives. Other rare causes include Addison's disease (hypoadrenalism), in which there is excessive production of adrenocorticotropic hormone (ACTH), which has activities similar to melanin-stimulating hormone; and Peutz-Jeghers syndrome, circumoral pigmentation associated with polyps in the small intestine (Figure 30.12).

ULCERATION

When a single ulcer has persisted for more than 3 weeks with no obvious cause, biopsy is indicated – particularly if the ulcer is not painful (and associated with tobacco and alcohol habits). Baseline tests for multiple ulcers include full blood count and iron studies.

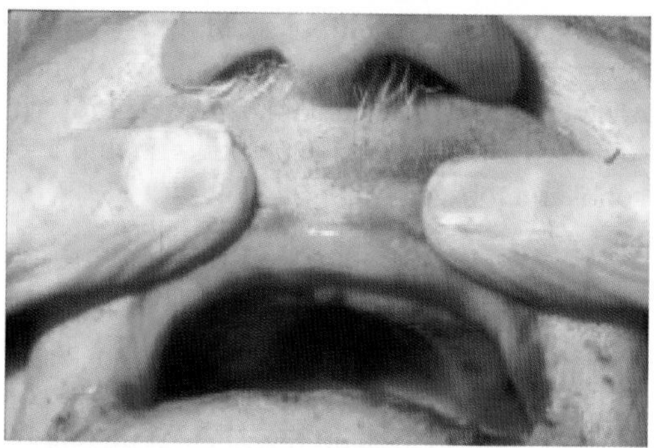

Figure 30.12 Circumoral pigmentation associated with a case of Peutz-Jeghers syndrome.

Local causes

Trauma resulting in ulceration can arise from a sharp tooth or an appliance (e.g. denture, orthodontic device) or may even be self-inflicted (Table 30.5, Figure 30.13). Ulceration of the frenulum under the upper lip may be a marker for non-accidental injury (child abuse). Chronic trauma often results in an ulcer surrounded by a white halo.

Drugs

Cytotoxics, nonsteroidal anti-inflammatory drugs and nicorandil are some examples of drugs that can cause ulcers.

Table 30.5 Causes of ulceration

Drugs
Local cause, e.g. trauma
Malignant disease
Recurrent apthae
Systemic conditions
• Blood disorders
• Gastro-intestinal disease
• Mucocutaneous disease

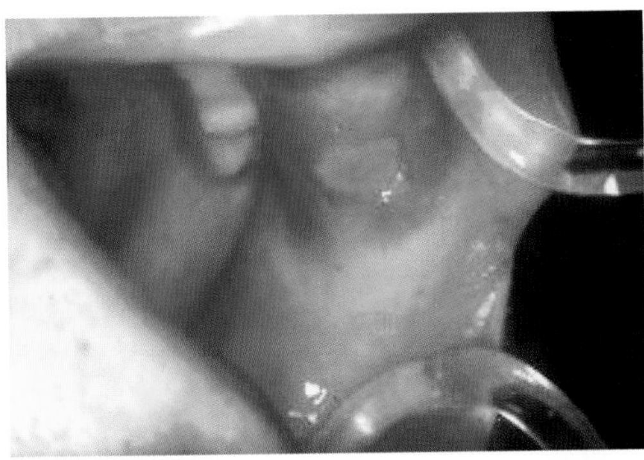

Figure 30.13 A traumatic (painful) ulcer in the buccal sulcus of an edentulous patient.

Recurrent apthae

Recurrent apthae can be classified as minor (80 per cent), major (15 per cent) or herpetiform (5 per cent). They affect at least 10 per cent of the population.

Minor apthae affect the non-keratinized sites (e.g. buccal mucosa) in younger people, are less than 5 mm in diameter, and may last for up to 2 weeks. They are painful, but often no underlying cause can be found.

Major apthae can arise anywhere in the mouth, are at least 1 cm in diameter and tend to last for more than 2 weeks, sometimes with scarring and drooling.

Herpetiform ulcers start as vesicles that form minute areas of very painful ulceration that can coalesce to create irregular areas of ulceration.

Recurrent apthae are diagnosed on clinical presentation, are usually self-limiting and occur in otherwise healthy individuals. Blood investigations are usually normal. Symptomatic relief can be obtained with benzydamine and/or chlorohexidine mouth rinses, although topical steroids may also be required. Some patients' symptoms improve when using a sodium lauryl sulphate-free toothpaste and/or avoiding fizzy drinks that contain benzoic acid as a preservative.

Systemic disease

Blood disorders that can cause oral ulceration include anaemia and haematinic deficiencies. Infections include viral (e.g. herpes simplex; hand, foot and mouth disease), bacterial (syphilis, tuberculosis), and fungal disease (angular cheilitis). Skin conditions include lichen planus, erythema multiforme and pemphigus. Gastro-intestinal diseases with oral ulceration include coeliac disease (serology for anti-endomysial antibody), ulcerative colitis and Crohn's disease. Oral manifestations of Crohn's include cobblestone buccal mucosa, gingival and labial swelling, and mucosal tags.

SOFT TISSUE SWELLINGS WITHIN THE MOUTH

Pyogenic granuloma dental abscesses and salivary gland problems (e.g. mucocele, ranula) are covered elsewhere in this book. Malignant disease can present as a swelling in the palate (e.g. lymphoma or carcinoma from maxillary antrum). Other soft tissue swellings are discussed in the following sections (Table 30.6).

Fibro-epithelial polyp

A fibro-epithelial polyp may be sessile or predunculated. Arising as a result of trauma, its surface is smooth, and it is usually seen on the buccal mucosa at the occlusal level (Figure 30.14).

Papilloma

A papilloma is an intraoral wart due to HPV.

Fibrous hyperplasia

Trauma from a poorly fitting denture flange can give rise to denture-induced hyperplasia, usually

Table 30.6 Causes of swelling

Causes of swelling
Dental abscess
Fibro-epithelial polyp
Gingival hyperplasia, e.g. drugs, pregnancy
Hyperplasia
Malignant disease, e.g. lymphoma, cancer
Pyogenic granuloma
Salivary gland problem, e.g. mucocele, ranula
Unerupted canine

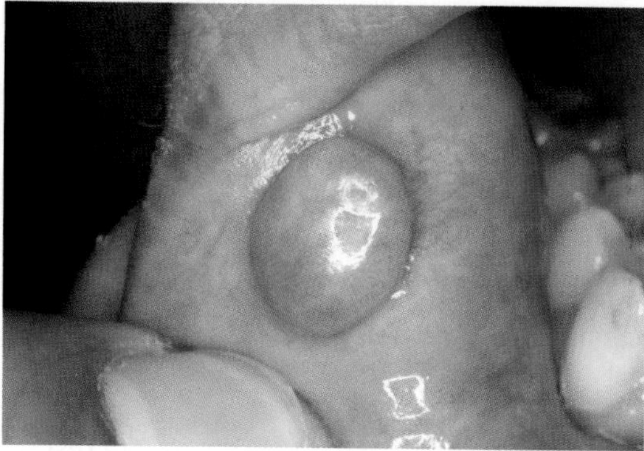

Figure 30.14 A fibro-epithelial polyp affecting the buccal mucosa. Note the overlying pink healthy mucosa.

in the anterior maxilla or mandible region, or a 'leaf' fibroma (under the maxillary denture).

Gingival hyperplasia

Gingival hyperplasia can be due to drugs (e.g. phenytoin, cyclosporins, nifedipine) or hereditary (gingivofibromatosis). It also can arise in pregnancy, either as generalized gingivitis or as discrete gingival epulis.

Burning mouth syndrome

Burning mouth syndrome (BMS) is defined as a burning sensation in the absence of any obvious organic cause. It is most frequently seen in middle-aged to older females. In approximately 20 per cent of cases, anxiety, depression or cancer phobia can be identified. It is important to exclude other conditions that can present with similar symptoms, such as geographic tongue (Figure 30.15), lichen planus, candida infection, glossitis (due to haematinic deficiency or hypothyroidism) and diabetes. Parafunctional habits such as bruxism and tongue thrusting also should be excluded.

BMS is a chronic condition that usually affects the tongue. It may be associated with dry mouth and drugs such as angiotensin-converting enzyme (ACE) inhibitors. Although patients complain of a burning sensation, they rarely take analgesics, possibly because they have tried them and found they make little difference. Management includes

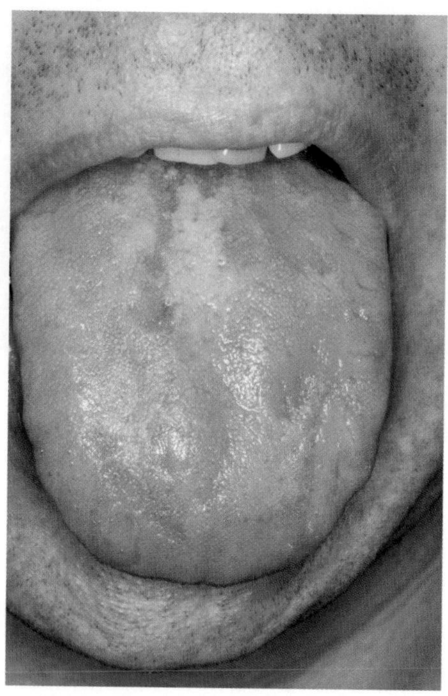

Figure 30.15 Erythema migrans (geographic tongue) affecting the dorsal surface of the tongue.

providing the patient with information, such as the fact that it is a common condition, is not infectious and so on. Screening for deficiency states (thyroxine levels, saliva, iron, B_{12}, folate levels), diabetes and denture problems is also important. Cognitive behavioural therapy may be helpful (with an empathetic approach, linking symptoms to psychological/psychosomatic problems) together with the use of antidepressants 'to treat the symptoms, not the depression' for a period of 6 months.

CONCLUSION

This chapter has been written for the ENT trainee as the patient might present with a specific problem. There are only a limited number of ways in which the oral mucosa can react, hence the subdivision of the latter section into colour change (red, white, pigmented), ulceration and swelling.

KEY LEARNING POINTS

- A dental cause for pain in the orofacial region should always be considered and, if necessary, excluded.
- All patients should be encouraged to register with a dentist.
- Teeth do not need to appear obviously decayed to cause pain.
- Maxillary sinusitis can be caused by an abscessed tooth.
- Most swellings and white patches in the mouth are benign; however, red (or red/white) lesions (especially in smokers and/or heavy drinkers) can be an early sign of cancer.
- A discrete swelling in the lower lip is likely to be a mucocoele, but in the upper lip it is more likely to be a salivary gland tumour.

FURTHER READING

Cawson RA, Odell EW. *Cawson's Essentials of Oral Pathology and Oral Medicine*. 7th ed. Edinburgh: Churchill Livingstone, 2002.

Pedlar J, Frame JW, eds. *Oral and Maxillofacial Surgery: An Objective-Based Textbook*. 2nd ed. Edinburgh: Churchill Livingstone, 2007.

Scully C. *Oral and Maxillofacial Medicine: The Basis of Diagnosis and Treatment*. London: Wright Elsevier Science, 2004.

31

Neck space infections

MUHAMMAD SHAKEEL AND S MUSHEER HUSSAIN

Neck infections can be broadly divided into superficial and deep infections (Figure 31.1). Superficial neck infections typically involve the skin and subcutaneous tissue, including the superficial fascia. These are further divided into non-necrotizing and necrotizing infections. Deep infections involve the deeper neck tissues, which are surrounded by multiple layers of fascia with potential spaces between them. It is important to have a clear idea of the deep cervical fascia and associated deep neck spaces to have a better understanding of deep neck infections and abscesses.

ANATOMY

The neck is surrounded by superficial and deep cervical fascia. The superficial fascia is a thin layer of connective tissue that lies deep to the dermis and encloses the platysma. The space deep to this layer does not constitute part of the deep neck space system and contains cutaneous nerves, superficial veins and superficial lymph nodes. The deep cervical fascia supports the muscles, the vessels and the viscera of the neck. It is condensed to form three well-defined fibrous layers and the carotid sheath. These are described as follows:[1]

- Superficial layer: Also known as the investing layer of the deep cervical fascia. This is a thick layer, arising from the spinous processes and ligamentum nuchae and encircling the neck. It splits to enclose the trapezius, the inferior belly of omohyoid and the sternocleidomastoid muscles.
- Middle layer: This is a thin layer found in the anterior neck and has two divisions: the muscular division surrounding the infrahyoid muscles and the visceral division surrounding the pharynx, oesophagus, larynx, trachea, thyroid and parathyroid glands.
- Deep layer: This is a thick layer that passes like a septum across the neck behind the pharynx and the oesophagus and in front of the prevertebral muscles and the vertebral column. It has two divisions. The prevertebral division adheres to the anterior aspect of the vertebral

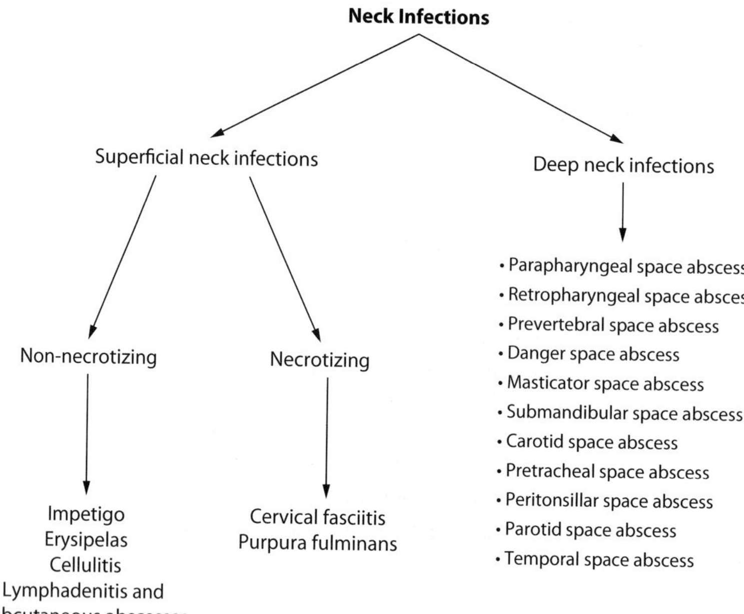

Figure 31.1 Flow chart of neck infections.

body and extends laterally to the transverse processes of the vertebrae. The alar division lies between the prevertebral division and the visceral division of the middle layer of the deep cervical fascia. Lateral extension of this deep layer on the anterior and medial scalene and levator scapulae muscles forms the fascial floor of the posterior triangle.

- Carotid sheath: This is a local condensation of all the above-mentioned three layers of the deep cervical fascia that surrounds the common and internal carotid arteries, the internal jugular vein, the vagus nerve and the deep cervical lymph nodes.

There are 11 deep neck spaces[2] that communicate with each other and are briefly described in Table 31.1.

SUPERFICIAL NECK INFECTIONS

Common examples of non-necrotizing infections include impetigo, erysipelas, cellulitis, lymphadenitis and subcutaneous abscesses in all age groups. It is important to differentiate these from skin rashes and reactions[3] (Figures 31.2 to 31.5).

Impetigo is a common, superficial bacterial skin infection primarily caused by *Staphylococcus aureus*, and it is most frequently encountered in children. The lesions are mostly located in the head and neck region. There is good evidence that topical mupirocin and topical fusidic acid are equally as effective as oral treatment, if not more effective. However, oral antibiotics may be required in patients with extensive impetigo.[4]

Erysipelas and cellulitis are the most common skin and soft tissue infections requiring in-hospital treatment. Erysipelas is a superficial skin infection that does not involve the subcutaneous tissue. It has a typically raised, well-demarcated and localized rash and is usually caused by *Streptococci*. Spreading cellulitis, on the other hand, involves both dermis and the subcutaneous tissue and is commonly due to *Staphylococci*. Community-associated methicillin-resistant *Staphylococcus aureus* is a growing problem. In diabetics and patients with suppressed immunity, a deep-seated

Table 31.1 Description of deep neck spaces[2]

Number	Deep neck space	Description
1	Parapharyngeal space	Resembles an inverted pyramid and extends between the skull base and the lesser cornua of the hyoid bone. Divided into pre-styloid and post-styloid compartments and connects posteromedially with the retropharyngeal space and inferiorly with the submandibular space. Laterally, connects with the masticator space. The carotid sheath courses through this space into the chest.
2	Retropharyngeal space	Lies between the visceral division of the middle layer of the deep cervical fascia and the alar division of the deep layer of deep cervical fascia posteriorly. Extends from the skull base to the tracheal bifurcation around T2, where the visceral and alar divisions fuse. Laterally, communicates with the parapharyngeal space. Primarily contains retropharyngeal lymphatics.
3	Prevertebral space	Located anterior to the vertebral bodies and posterior to the prevertebral division of the deep layer of the deep cervical fascia. Extends from the skull base to the coccyx.
4	Danger space	Located immediately posterior to the retropharyngeal space and immediately anterior to the prevertebral space, between the alar and prevertebral divisions of the deep layer of the deep cervical fascia. Extends from the skull base to the posterior mediastinum and diaphragm.
5	Masticator space	Situated lateral to the medial pterygoid fascia and medial to the masseter muscle. Lies inferiorly to the temporal space and is anterolateral to the parapharyngeal space.
6	Submandibular space	Bounded inferiorly by the superficial layer of the deep cervical fascia extending from the hyoid to the mandible, laterally by the body of the mandible, and superiorly by the mucosa of the floor of the mouth. Submandibular space infections may spread to the parapharyngeal space or retropharyngeal space.
7	Carotid space	Potential space within the carotid sheath.
8	Pretracheal space	Enclosed by the visceral division of the middle layer of the deep cervical fascia and lies immediately anterior to the trachea. Extends from the thyroid cartilage to the superior mediastinum.
9	Peritonsillar space	Bounded by the tonsil medially and the superior constrictor laterally. The anterior and posterior tonsillar pillars form the remaining borders of this space.
10	Parotid space	Enclosed by the superficial layer of the deep cervical fascia. This is an incomplete enclosure because the superomedial aspect of the gland is not covered. This discontinuity allows communication between the parapharyngeal space and the parotid space.
11	Temporal space	It lies between the temporalis fascia and the periosteum of the temporal bone. The temporalis muscle effectively divides the space into a deep and superficial compartment.

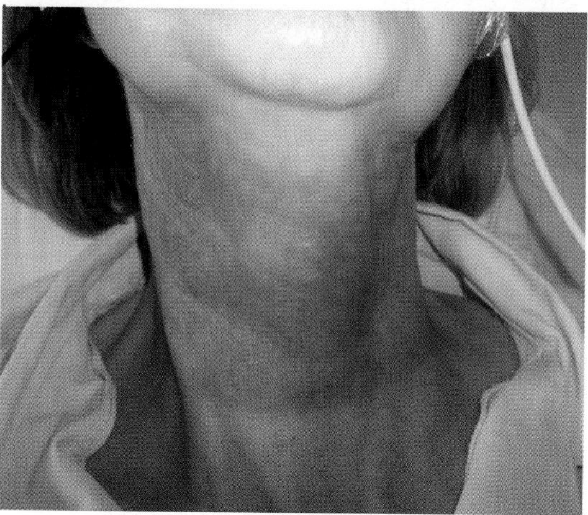

Figure 31.2 Skin reaction to radiotherapy.

infection should always be kept in the differential diagnosis of a superficial skin infection.[5,6,7]

Non-tuberculous cervico-facial lymphadenitis is a relatively common condition, particularly in children. The treatment options are varied and include a wait-and-see policy, medical therapy and surgery.

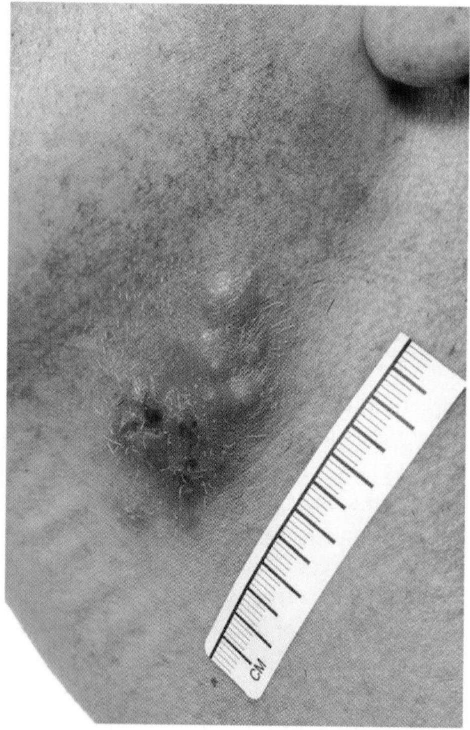

Figure 31.3 Superficial neck infection.

NECROTIZING SUPERFICIAL NECK INFECTIONS

These include necrotizing fasciitis and purpura fulminans. Both conditions have a high morbidity and mortality rate if not diagnosed and treated early.

Cervical necrotizing fasciitis is a rare and rapidly progressive infection of the superficial fascia characterized by necrosis of the subcutaneous tissue. It can lead to necrotizing mediastinitis and progressive sepsis with toxic shock syndrome. Historically, group A β-haemolytic streptococcus has been identified as a major cause of this infection. However, scientists have found that the pathogenesis of necrotizing fasciitis is polymicrobial. Diagnosis should be made as soon as possible by looking at the skin inflammatory changes, and magnetic resonance imaging (MRI) may be carried out to detect the presence of air within the tissues. Percutaneous aspiration of the soft tissue collection followed by prompt Gram staining should be conducted. Intravenous antibiotic therapy and early surgical fasciotomy and debridement are required to treat this life-threatening skin infection. Hyperbaric oxygen therapy complemented by intravenous polyspecific immunoglobulin are useful adjunctive therapies.[8,9]

Purpura fulminans is a rare syndrome of intravascular thrombosis and haemorrhagic infarction of the skin; it is rapidly progressive and accompanied by vascular collapse.[10] Clinically, it presents as septic shock. The newest revolutionary advancement in the treatment of neonatal purpura fulminans is the use of activated protein C.[8]

DEEP NECK INFECTIONS

Deep neck infections (DNIs) involve the neck structures surrounded by multiple layers of the deep cervical fascia (Figures 31.8 to 31.13). DNIs can result from the following processes: potential lymphatic spread of infection from oral cavity, face

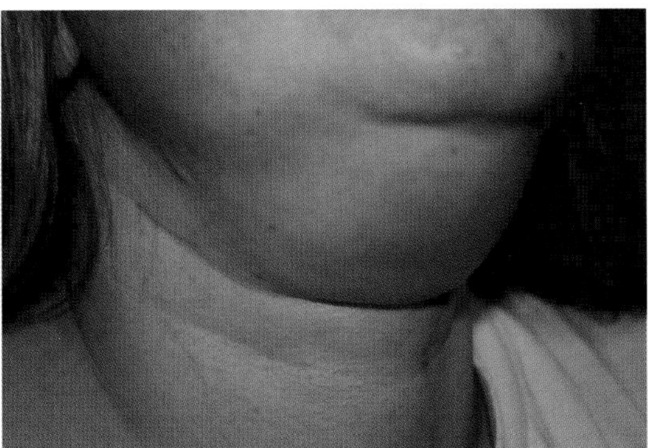

Figure 31.4 Superficial neck infection in the submental region.

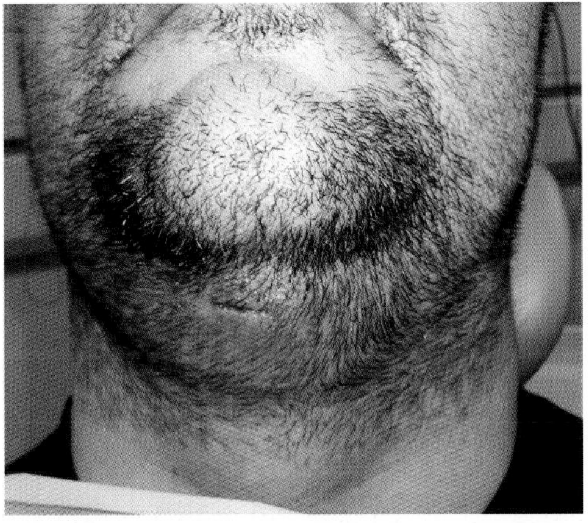

Figure 31.5 Incision and drainage of the submental abscess.

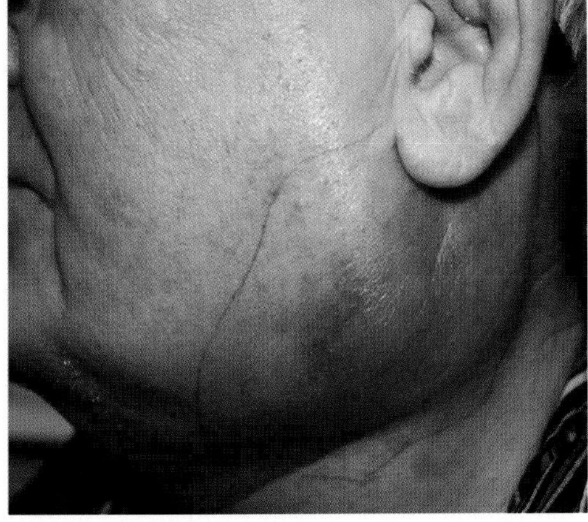

Figure 31.6 Wound infection with surrounding cellulitis.

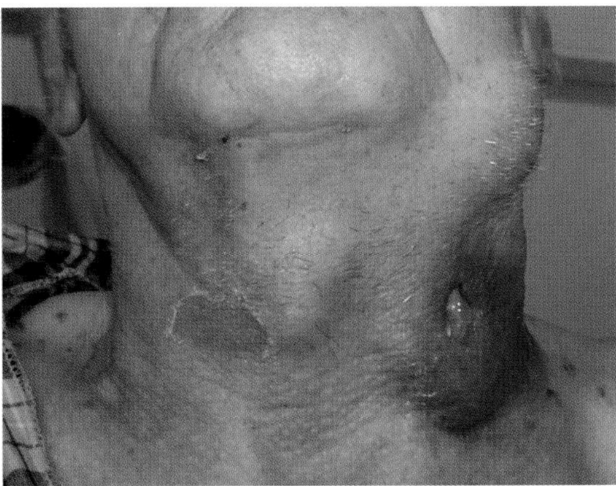

Figure 31.7 Superficial neck abscesses.

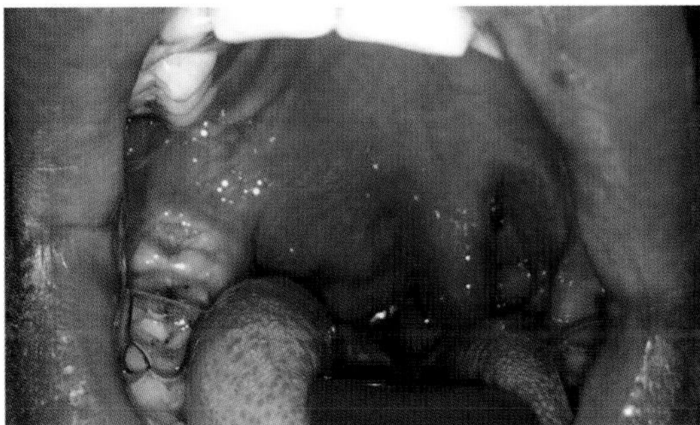

Figure 31.8 Right parapharyngeal space abscess pushing the right tonsil medially.

and superficial neck compartment to deep neck spaces; cervical lymphadenopathy, which may lead to suppuration and localized abscess formation; and penetrating trauma, which can introduce the infection to the deeper neck compartment.[2] The infection spreads along the fascial planes, and the resultant pus can expand the potential spaces between the different layers of the deep cervical fascia. The signs and symptoms of DNIs develop because of the mass effect of the inflamed tissues or abscess cavity on the surrounding structures and because of the direct involvement of the surrounding structures in the infectious process. DNIs can happen in any age group but are historically associated with patients with poor oral hygiene and lack of dental care. Depending upon the anatomical location, DNIs can be named as listed in Table 31.2.

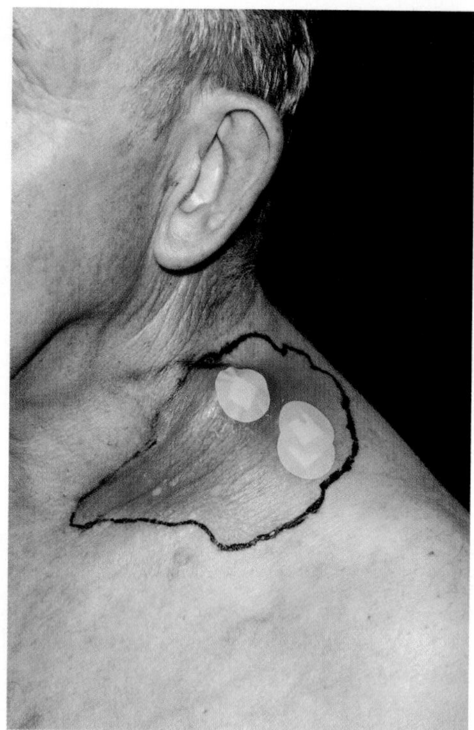

Figure 31.9 Head and neck malignancy presenting as neck abscess.

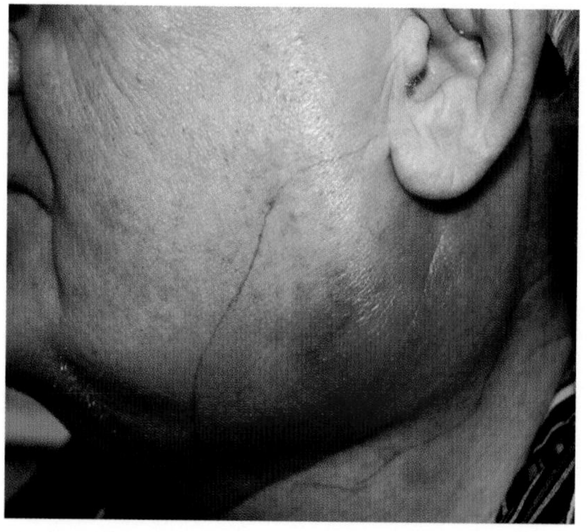

Figure 31.10 Parotid space abscess.

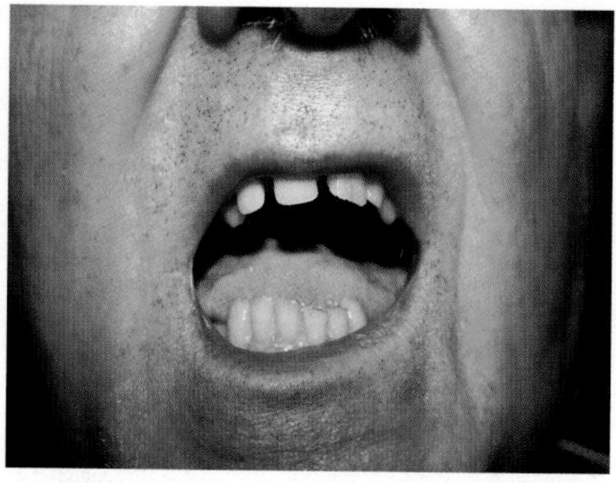

Figure 31.11 Trismus caused by parotid space abscess.

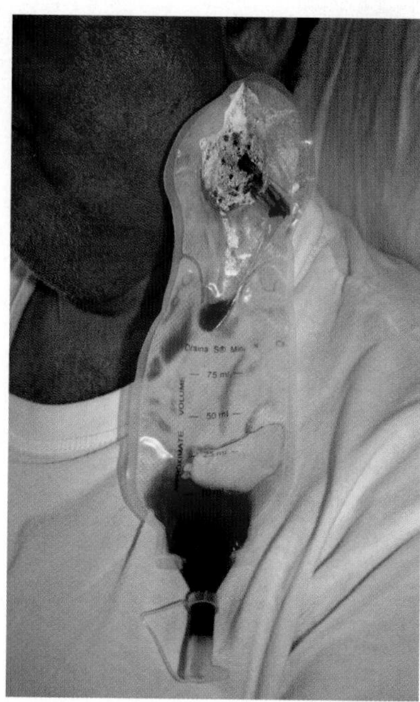

Figure 31.12 Parotid space abscess – incision and drainage.

CLINICAL PRESENTATION

A high index of suspicion is required for early diagnosis of DNIs because the patient may have only minimal symptoms and signs. However, some patients may present in distress and with

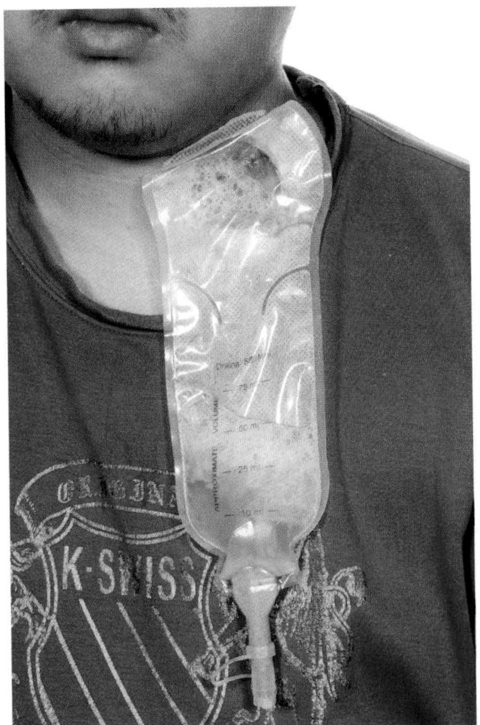

Figure 31.13 Complication after incision and drainage of deep neck abscess.

life-threatening signs. Patients may or may not have pyrexia, malaise, dehydration, sore throat, odynophagia, dysphagia, referred otalgia, drooling, respiratory distress, stridor, tismus, hoarseness, neck swelling, painful neck movements and torticollis. The predisposing factors for mediastinal extension in DNIs are older age, involvement of two or more spaces and the presence of cardiovascular and pulmonary comorbidities.[11]

AETIOLOGY

Today, tonsillitis remains the most common aetiology of deep neck space infections in children, whereas odontogenic origin is the most common aetiology of DNIs in adults.[2] Sometimes, the source of DNIs is not found, but taking a detailed patient history may help to establish the most likely aetiology (Table 31.3). Patients with a history of intravenous drug abuse and with human immunodeficiency virus (HIV) are at risk of developing tubercular deep neck space infection and abscess.

EXAMINATION

Deep neck infections are difficult to palpate and externally visualize because of normal soft tissues covering the deeper neck spaces. However, Ludwig's angina is a rapidly progressing cellulitis involving the submandibular neck space. It is characterized by induration of the submental region and floor of the mouth. It is a clinical diagnosis, and close airway monitoring is essential because upward and backward tongue elevation can result in a compromised airway.

Peritonsillar abscess (PTA) often presents with sore throat, dysphagia, peritonsillar bulge, uvular deviation, trismus and a muffled voice. The diagnosis of PTA can be made based on history and physical examination. The situation may be complicated if the patient is an uncooperative child.

Clinical evaluation may underestimate the extent of DNI in patients, which may lead to conservative treatment with worse prognosis.[12]

On clinical examination, patients with DNIs may exhibit signs mentioned in Table 31.2.

INVESTIGATIONS

Because of the complex anatomy of the neck and deep-seated nature of DNIs, precise localization on clinical grounds is challenging, and investigations are helpful in this situation. Patients should undergo laboratory tests to confirm raised markers of infection, and blood cultures are required in septic patients. The radiological assessment is carried out in consultation with radiologists. The options include a lateral neck radiograph, ultrasound scan and computed tomography (CT). It is

Table 31.2 Deep neck infections/abscesses[2]

Number	Name	Predictive descriptors on history and examination
1	Parapharyngeal space abscess	Anterior compartment infection/abscess causes • Marked trismus; odynophagia and dysphagia • Induration at the angle of mandible • Medial displacement of the lateral pharyngeal wall and tonsil Posterior compartment infection/abscess causes • Medial displacement of the posterior pillar of the tonsil and posterior pharyngeal wall • Thrombosis of internal jugular vein
2	Retropharyngeal space abscess	May present with airway occlusion at the pharynx level. Anterior displacement of one or both sides of the posterior pharyngeal wall. Torticollis and reduced neck movement. Asymmetry of neck and lymphadenopathy. Much more common in children under 5 years of age. Occasionally caused by chronic conditions such as tuberculosis
3	Prevertebral space abscess	Torticollis and reduced neck movement. Most common aetiology is iatrogenic trauma – instrumentation. Can cause vertebral osteomyelitis and spinal instability.
4	Danger space abscess	Extension of abscess from above mentioned three spaces. It can lead to mediastinitis, empyema and sepsis.
5	Masticator space abscess	Trismus. Originates from third mandibular molar infection. May spread to the parapharyngeal, parotid or temporal space.
6	Submandibular space abscess	Ludwig's angina refers to cellulitis or abscess in this space and may present with pain, trismus, drooling, odynophagia, dysphagia, neck swelling and worsening airway caused by displacement of tongue. Develops secondary to oral trauma, submaxillary or sublingual sialadenitis, or dental abscess of mandibular teeth. May spread to the parapharyngeal space or retropharyngeal space.
7	Carotid space abscess	Vocal cord paralysis Horner syndrome
8	Pretracheal space abscess	Dysphagia, odynophagia, pain, fever, hoarseness and airway obstruction. Mostly caused by perforation of the anterior oesophageal wall by endoscopic instrumentation, foreign bodies, or trauma. Can involve the superior mediastinum.
9	Peritonsillar space abscess	Trismus, throat pain, referred otalgia, odynophagia, drooling, a 'hot potato' voice and fever. There is uvular deviation, palatal asymmetry and displacement of the tonsil medially. It may spread to the parapharyngeal space. It is the most common deep neck space abscess and represents a sequela of tonsillar infections.
10	Parotid space abscess	Pain, oedema and erythema in the region of the parotid. Trismus is a later finding. Risk factors include dehydration, elderly patients with poor oral hygiene who develop salivary duct obstruction. Can spread to parapharyngeal space.
11	Temporal space abscess	Pain and trismus with or without deviation of the mandible.

Table 31.3 Aetiology of deep neck space infections/abscess[2]

1	Pharyngitis
2	Tonsillitis
3	Peritonsillar abscess
4	Odontogenic infection
5	Salivary gland infection
6	Penetrating oropharyngeal injury
7	Iatrogenic perforation of oesophagus
8	Fish bone ingestion
9	Foreign body inhalation
10	Suppurative lymph node
11	Infection in branchial cleft anomalies
12	Thyroglossal duct abscess
13	Thyroiditis
14	Mastoiditis
15	Laryngopyocele
16	Intravenous drug abuse
17	Malignant necrotic lymph node

important to note that a normal radiograph does not rule out DNIs in children.[13] A CT scan with contrast is regarded as the gold standard investigation. The presence of air indicates abscess in all cases. A CT scan can be helpful in differentiating the retropharyngeal adenitis from abscess, thereby guiding the clinician to avoid unnecessary surgical intervention.[14,15] However, a central necrotic cervical metastatic lymph node may sometimes mimic a simple pyogenic deep neck abscess on both clinical pictures and CT images. A routine biopsy of the tissue should be performed during surgical drainage.[16] The MRI scan can yield better soft tissue delineation. Arteriography is chosen if major neck vasculature is suspected to be involved in the infectious process.

The ultrasound scan not only helps in diagnosing the DNIs, but it can also be very useful for guided fine-needle aspiration for microscopy, culture and sensitivities.[17] The bacteriology of the deep neck space abscess is polymicrobial, mostly reflecting the oral flora; aerobic as well as anaerobic organisms are isolated, and both Gram positive and Gram negative organisms are cultured. In one study, children younger than 16 months and with lateral neck abscesses were at a significantly increased risk of having a *Staphylococcus aureus* infection, the majority being *methicillin-resistant Staphylococcus aureus* (MRSA).[18]

MANAGEMENT

With advancements in laboratory testing, radiological investigations and broad-spectrum antibiotics, the overall morbidity and mortality of DNIs have improved.[19]

Some patients with DNIs can present in a moribund condition with impending airway compromise. Securing the airway must take priority for such patients. They should be kept in the resuscitation section of the accident and emergency department until the airway management team can safely transfer them to a theatre to secure the airway. The anaesthetist should always be part of the team looking after these patients in a calm and controlled fashion. Orotracheal and nasotracheal intubation in patients with DNIs may be difficult because of trismus, swollen pharyngeal walls and oedema of the supraglottis impairing the vocal cords' visualization, deviation of the larynx, external tracheal compression, restricted neck movement because of paraspinal muscle spasm, and laboured breathing.[2] In such situations oropharyngeal instrumentation should be avoided because it can aggravate the pharyngeal swelling. Ideally, when diagnostic flexible pharyngolaryngoscopy is carried out, it should be as atraumatic as possible and the procedure video recorded so that the anaesthetist can have a better assessment of the airway without having to repeat the laryngoscopy. In compromised airway scenarios, it is perhaps a better option to carry out tracheostomy under local anaesthetic, and equipment should be made available for cricothyroidotomy and crash tracheostomy along with good suction facility.

Stable patients suspected to have DNIs should ideally be nursed in a close monitoring area of the ward with facilities available for prompt intervention should a need arise. These patients need adequate analgesia, fluid resuscitation, and parenteral broad-spectrum antibiotics, which should be reviewed soon after the culture and sensitivity results are available. The choice of empiric therapy should be based on local protocols, taking into account the most likely source of DNIs. The duration of medical therapy depends upon the patient's progress. If the patient continues to improve and no abscess is located on initial investigations, then parenteral antibiotics can be switched to oral ones.

A trial of high-dose intravenous antibiotics in stable children with close observation is warranted as first-line treatment, especially for small deep space neck infections.[20,21] However, if medical therapy fails, timely surgical intervention in the form of incision and drainage is essential to prevent any adverse outcome. The decision to initiate surgical drainage depends on the patient's clinical status and the accessibility of the abscess. Most deep neck space abscesses are drained transcervically, but retropharyngeal abscess is preferably drained transorally. Quinsy-tonsillectomy remains controversial but is an option. In patients unfit for general anaesthesia, needle drainage under ultrasound and/or CT guidance is a viable option but requires a motivated, experienced radiologist.

The incidence of life-threatening complications, including airway obstruction, sepsis, pneumonia and death, is significantly higher in patients with extension of DNIs into the mediastinum. Also, life-threatening complications can occur because of a delay in diagnosis or inadequate treatment (Table 31.4).

Table 31.4 Complications of deep neck infections/abscesses[2]

1	External compression of trachea
2	Rupture of DNIs into the trachea
3	Internal jugular vein thrombosis
4	Carotid artery erosion
5	Mediastinitis/empyemea
6	Cranial nerve dysfunction
7	Brain and pulmonary abscesses
8	Osteomyelitis of the spine, mandible or skull base
9	Grisel syndrome (i.e. inflammatory torticollis causing cervical vertebral subluxation)
10	Septic shock

KEY LEARNING POINTS

- Neck infections can be divided into superficial and deep depending on the anatomical region involved.
- The superficial and deep cervical fascial layers divide the neck into potential spaces, which expand by pus when infection spreads along the fascial planes.
- The symptoms and signs of deep neck infections develop because of the mass effect of the inflamed tissues or abscess cavity on the surrounding structures.
- Clinically patients may have only minimal symptoms and signs, but some may be distressed with a compromised airway.
- CT scan with contrast is regarded as the gold standard investigation. The presence of air indicates abscess in all cases.
- The bacteriology of deep neck space abscesses is polymicrobial, mostly reflecting the oral flora. Aerobic as well as anaerobic organisms are isolated.
- The incidence of life-threatening complications is significantly higher in patients with extension of deep neck infection into the mediastinum.

REFERENCES

1. Snell RR. *Clinical Anatomy: An Illustrated Review with Questions and Explanations.* 4th ed. Philadelphia: Lippincott Williams & Wilkins, 2004: 208–13.
2. Murray AD. Deep neck infections. Available from: http://emedicine.medscape.com/article/837048-overview.
3. Ely JW, Seabury Stone M. The generalized rash: Part I. Differential diagnosis. *American Family Physician.* 2010; 81(6): 726–34.
4. Koning S, van der Sande R, Verhagen AP, van Suijlekom-Smit LW, Morris AD, Butler CC, Berger M, van der Wouden JC. Interventions for impetigo. *Cochrane Database of Systematic Reviews.* 2012; 1:CD003261. doi: 10.1002/14651858.CD003261.pub3.

5. Blum CL, Menzinger S, Genné D. Cellulitis: Clinical manifestations and management. *Revue Médicale Suisse*. 2013; 9(401):1812–15.
6. Kilburn SA, Featherstone P, Higgins B, Brindle R. Interventions for cellulitis and erysipelas. *Cochrane Database of Systematic Reviews*. 2010; (6): CD004299. doi: 10.1002/14651858.CD004299.pub2.
7. Mistry RD. Skin and soft tissue infections. *Pediatric Clinics of North America*. 2013; 60(5):1063–82. doi: 10.1016/j.pcl.2013.06.011. Epub 2013 Jul 30.
8. Edlich RF, Winters KL, Woodard CR, Britt LD, Long WB 3rd. Massive soft tissue infections: Necrotizing fasciitis and purpura fulminans. *Journal of Long-Term Effects of Medical Implants*. 2005; 15(1): 57–65.
9. Sarna T, Sengupta T, Miloro M, Kolokythas A. Cervical necrotizing fasciitis with descending mediastinitis: Literature review and case report. *Journal of Oral and Maxillofacial Surgery*. 2012; 70(6): 1342–50. doi: 10.1016/j.joms.2011.05.007. Epub 2011 Aug 6.
10. Har-El G, Nash M, Chin NW, Meltzer CJ, Weiss MH. Purpura fulminans of the head and neck. *Otolaryngology – Head and Neck Surgery*. 1990; 103(4): 660–63.
11. Kang SK, Lee S, Oh HK, Kang MW, Na MH, Yu JH, Koo BS, Lim SP. Clinical features of deep neck infections and predisposing factors for mediastinal extension. *Korean Journal of Thoracic Cardiovascular Surgery*. 2012; 45(3): 171–76. doi: 10.5090/kjtcs.2012.45.3.171. Epub 2012 Jun 7.
12. Crespo AN, Chone CT, Fonseca AS, Montenegro MC, Pereira R, Milani JA. Clinical versus computed tomography evaluation in the diagnosis and management of deep neck infection. *Sao Paulo Medical Journal*. 2004; 122(6): 259–63. Epub 2005 Feb 2.
13. Uzomefuna V, Glynn F, Mackle T, Russell J. Atypical locations of retropharyngeal abscess: Beware of the normal lateral soft tissue neck X-ray. *International Journal of Pediatric Otorhinolaryngology*. 2010; 74(12): 1445–48. doi: 10.1016/j.ijporl.2010.09.008. Epub 2010 Oct 15.
14. Freling N, Roele E, Schaefer-Prokop C, Fokkens W. Prediction of deep neck abscesses by contrast-enhanced computerized tomography in 76 clinically suspect consecutive patients. *Laryngoscope*. 2009; 119(9): 1745–52. doi: 10.1002/lary.20606.
15. Shefelbine SE, Mancuso AA, Gajewski BJ, Ojiri H, Stringer S, Sedwick JD. Pediatric retropharyngeal lymphadenitis: Differentiation from retropharyngeal abscess and treatment implications. *Otolaryngology – Head and Neck Surgery*. 2007; 136(2): 182–88.
16. Chuang SY, Lin HT, Wen YS, Hsu FJ. Pitfalls of CT for deep neck abscess imaging assessment: A retrospective review of 162 cases. *B-ENT*. 2013; 9(1):45–52.
17. Nisha VA, JP, NS, AGG, Devi BKY, Reddy SS, NR. The role of colour Doppler ultrasonography in the diagnosis of fascial space infections – A cross sectional study. *Journal of Clinical and Diagnostic Research*. 2013; 7(5): 962–67. doi: 10.7860/JCDR/2013/5617.2990. Epub 2013 Mar 21.
18. Duggal P, Naseril, Sobol SE. The increased risk of community-acquired methicillin-resistant Staphylococcus aureus neck abscesses in young children. *Laryngoscope*. 2011; 121(1): 51–55. doi: 10.1002/lary.21214.
19. Osborn TM, Assael LA, Bell RB. Deep space neck infection: Principles of surgical management. *Oral and Maxillofacial Surgery Clinics of North America*. 2008; 20(3): 353–65. doi: 10.1016/j.coms.2008.04.002.
20. Wong DK, Brown C, Mills N, Spielmann P, Neeff M. To drain or not to drain – Management of pediatric deep neck abscesses: A case-control study. *International Journal of Pediatric Otorhinolaryngology*. 2012; 76(12): 1810–83. doi: 10.1016/j.ijporl.2012.09.006. Epub 2012 Oct 22.
21. Carbone PN, Capra GG, Brigger MT. Antibiotic therapy for pediatric deep neck abscesses: A systematic review. *International Journal of Pediatric Otorhinolaryngology*. 2012; 76(11): 1647–53. doi: 10.1016/j.ijporl.2012.07.038. Epub 2012 Aug 23.

32

Disorders of voice

SAMIT MAJUMDAR

"The human voice is the organ of the soul."

Henry Wadsworth Longfellow

The first cry of a baby heralds his arrival on this earth. Human voice with its meaningful distinctions bestows Homo sapiens with a unique evolutionary advantage over all other species. The larynx forms an integral part of the airway (Figure 32.1) and serves to protect the lung by its phylogenetic function as a sphincter. It also functions as a pressure valve system helping in various other human needs, such as straining. Voice is generated at the glottis, resonated, articulated and amplified in the supraglottic vocal tract to produce meaningful speech sounds, which are a rare attribute of Homo sapiens. Distal migration of the laryngeal complex through evolution has been observed among various species, and the 1:1 ratio of the parts of the tongue being present in the oral cavity and oropharynx help in the production of human speech. In primates the tongue is predominantly present in the oral cavity, which prevents them from developing sophisticated speech sounds. Phonation is a relatively recent event in evolutionary terms; it has, to some extent, compromised both the breathing and the protective functions of the larynx because of its anatomical contiguity with the hypopharynx and sharing of a common wall.

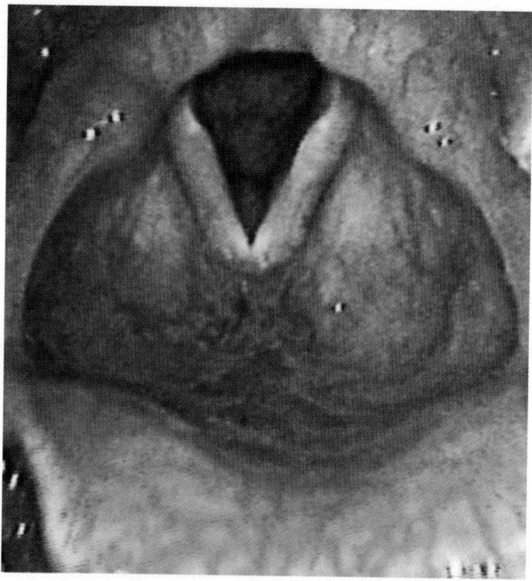

Figure 32.1 Abducted vocal folds during respiration.

DEVELOPMENT

Around 3 weeks of intrauterine life, the epiglottis shows signs of development from the embryo's hypobranchial eminence. The laryngo-tracheal groove appears as a vertical slit on the floor of the primitive foregut. The laryngo-tracheal diverticulum develops from this groove and rapidly gets separated from the foregut by the formation of the tracheoesophageal septum. The ventral portion develops into the larynx and the lower respiratory tracts. Muscles of the larynx are derived from the mesoderm of the fourth and fifth branchial arches. True and false vocal cords are developed by the tenth week of gestation.

ANATOMY AND PHYSIOLOGY

The human larynx is composed of three single and three paired cartilages held together with ligaments, membranes and intrinsic muscles of the larynx. This unique arrangement allows movements and variations of shape and volume of the supraglottic vocal tract. This is essential for regulation of the acoustic characteristics of human voice. The thyroid, cricoid and paired arytenoid cartilages are the most important structures of the larynx in relation to the vocal function. Thyroid cartilage is formed from two rectangular laminae fused at the midline. The angle between these two laminae is 90° in males and 120° in females, resulting in variation of the anteroposterior length of the laryngeal cavity. Vocal folds are, therefore, longer in males (17.5 mm–25 mm). Female vocal fold length is approximately 12.5 mm–17.5 mm. The cuneiform and corniculate cartilages are found within the aryepiglottic fold. They are believed to stiffen these folds and allow closer apposition with the epiglottis during the pharyngeal phase of deglutition, to protect the airway from the risk of aspiration. The cricoid cartilage is the only complete ring at the beginning of the lower airway. It is a signet-shaped ring with a steep superior anteromedial inclined plane that allows arytenoid gliding. The crico-arytenoid joint allows rotational and mediolateral movements. The inferior cornu of the thyroid forms a synovial joint with the articulating facet on the posterolateral aspect of the cricoid ring. This joint allows rotatory movement around a transverse axis and anteroposterior sliding. The cricothyroid membrane connects the upper border of the cricoid with the lower border of the thyroid cartilage. Contraction of the cricothyroid membrane lengthens the vocal fold. The quadrangular membrane is an elastic membrane that extends from the arytenoid to the lateral parts of the epiglottis. The superior free edge of this mast-shaped membrane is called the aryepiglottic fold; the inferior border forms the vestibular ligament. Mucosal lining draped over this ligament produces the false cord or ventricular fold. The thyrohyoid membrane connects the superior margin of the thyroid cartilage with the inferior border of the hyoid bone like a drape. The conus elasticus is a triangular-shaped fibro-elastic membrane. The base of this membrane is fixed on the superior border of the cricoid cartilage, and the apex is attached anterosuperiorly to the medial part of the inferior border of the thyroid cartilage. Medially, it blends into the vocal fold and forms the vocal ligament. Laryngeal ventricles are small spaces bound within the vertical limits of the vocal and ventricular folds and small sinus (cul-de-sac) lateral to them. These spaces are lined with mucosa with thyroarytenoid muscles on their lateral wall.

In neonates the laryngeal opening is at the level of the soft palate, thus making them obligate nasal breathers. The progressive descent of the larynx aids in the development of speech. Laryngeal descent continues until adulthood. The low larynx adds to the lengthening of the supraglottic vocal tract with its ability to change its shape and volume to produce complex and varied voice sounds.

INTRINSIC MUSCLES OF THE LARYNX

Abductor

The posterior crico-arytenoid (PCA) muscle, in essence, with the help of contraction of its horizontal part, provides most of the abduction movement of the vocal fold. Abduction of the vocal fold is necessary for the passage of airflow during inspiration and expiration. The contraction of the vertical belly of the PCA increases the length and tension of the vocal fold.

Adductors

The adductor muscles include the lateral crico-arytenoid (LCA), inter-arytenoid (IA) and thyro-arytenoid (TA). Vocal folds need to be in the adducted position, allowing intimate contact of the contralateral mucosal surfaces to initiate the rise in subglottic pressure in part of the vibratory cycle of phonation.

Tensor

The cricothyroid muscle with movement of the cricothyroid joint can change the length of the vocal folds. The vertical belly of the PCA also contributes to tensing.

EXTRINSIC MUSCLES OF THE LARYNX

The thyrohyoid, sternohyoid, sternothyroid, geniohyoid, mylohyoid, digastric and stylopharyngeus are involved in stabilization of the laryngeal position and change of the shape of the supraglottic vocal tract by variation of this.

NEUROANATOMY

The lower motor neurons from the nucleus ambiguus in the brain stem supply the larynx travelling to the neck as the vagus nerve and then as its branches to the destination. The superior laryngeal nerve (SLN) carries the general sensation from the mucosa of the glottic and supraglottic larynx. The SLN provides the motor supply to the cricothyroid (CT) muscle. The recurrent laryngeal nerve (RLN) arises from the vagus nerve in the mediastinum on the left side and loops round the aortic arch to return to the neck. On the right side the RLN loops round the subclavian artery in the neck. The PCA, IA, LCA and TA all have their motor supply from the ipsilateral RLN. All intrinsic muscles of the larynx are supplied by the RLN from the ipsilateral side except the CT muscle. The IA, being an unpaired entity on the midline, receives its motor supply from the both RLNs of the ipsilateral and contralateral side.

VOICE PRODUCTION

The fundamental frequency of sound is generated when the vocal folds are adducted into apposition on the midline (Figure 32.2) causing temporary increase in subglottic air pressure until it is able to overcome the resistance of the mucosal fold in close contact and push them apart to move a small blast of air in the supraglottic. Mucosal folds recoil to their original position owing to their inherent elasticity. This is aided by rapid passage of a laminar stream of air that causes a drop in lateral pressure (Bernoulli effect). This sustained cycle of separation and apposition of the vocal folds that chops the flow of expired air from the lung creates and sustains the fundamental sound generated at the level of the glottis. The sound waves generated through this combined muscular and aerodynamic phenomena are subsequently resonated, articulated and amplified in the supraglottic vocal tract (SGVT). The frequency of vibrations varies among adult males (100–120 Hz), adult females (180–220 Hz) and children (250–300 Hz). At puberty, in boys, the bulk of the TA muscle increases significantly under the action of testosterone. Absence of this hormone is demonstrated in the castrato type of operatic voice in history. Increase in the bulk of the vocal fold brings about the lowering of the fundamental frequency, adding more bass to the voice. In girls the vocal pitch drops as well, thus adding more maturity to the voice of a woman. Loudness of the voice increases with any increase in the amplitude of vibration, while the pitch of the voice increases with an increase in the frequency of vocal fold vibrations. The length, mass, tension and volume of the vocal folds will determine the fundamental physical characteristics of the voice. The resonance of the voice is determined by the resonating chambers of the SGVT and their natural resonance frequency. The fundamental frequency of voice (F_0) passing through the vocal tract generates multiple harmonics and gathers resonance while getting articulated. Resonance is described as formants in relation to phonetics of spoken sounds. These are distinguishing acoustic signatures that help to identify vowel sounds in speech. The first two formants (f_1 is the lowest formant frequency; f_2 is the frequency just above the first formant) determine the quality of the vowel sounds and their auditory recognition. Formant frequencies also characterize the singing voice. The first formant is characterized predominantly by the opening of the jaw, the second formant by the shape and position of the tongue and the third formant frequency is dependent on the position of the tip of the tongue.

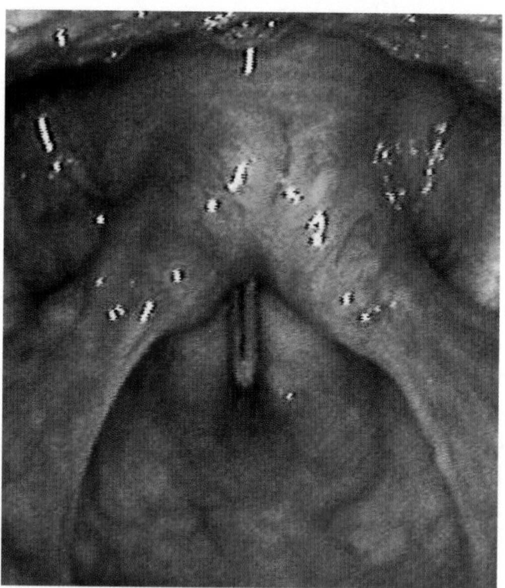

Figure 32.2 Adducted vocal folds during vocalization.

VOCAL FOLDS

The vocal fold is a trilaminar musculomembranous structure that extends from the vocal process of the arytenoid cartilage to the anterior commissure, where it meets its counterpart and is anchored into the lamina of the thyroid cartilage by the ligament of Broyle. Vocal folds are made up of five distinct layers; the rigidity of the tissue increases with its depth. The anterior two-thirds of the vocal fold contributes mainly to phonatory function, while the posterior one-third contributes to respiratory function.

SURFACE MUCOSA

The mucosal lining is approximately 0.05 to 0.1 mm in thickness and is composed of non-keratinizing squamous epithelium. This layer of tissue can tolerate a minimal degree of stretching. A transition layer between the surface mucosa and the lamina propria is described as the basement membrane zone. It has two subdivisions: lamina lucida and lamina densa. These layers are held together by collagen IV and fibronectin. Anchoring fibres, composed of collagen VII, bind the lamina densa to the superficial layer of lamina propria (SLLP). There is a significantly high concentration of these fibres in the middle third of the vocal folds, thus providing increased integrity and tensile strength to this layer.

LAMINA PROPRIA

The lamina propria is composed of three histologically and somewhat functionally distinct layers of tissues. It is made up of extracellular matrix (ECM). Collagen, elastin, fibronectin, fibromodulin, decorin and hyaluronic acid variably constitute the body of the ECM.

Superficial layer of lamina propria

The SLLP is a very thin (0.5 mm) elastin-rich layer with sparse collagen fibres embedded in mucopolysaccharide and mucoprotein matrix. The SLLP also contains macrophages, decorin, fibronectin and myofibrils with high healing potential. This layer is also described as Reinke's space. This is a highly deformable, isotropic and resilient layer with innate structural integrity to support the generation of mucosal waves.

Intermediate layer of lamina propria

The intermediate layer of lamina propria (ILLP) is characterized by the highest concentration of strongly hydrophilic glycose amino glycan (GAG) molecules. There is also an abundance of elastin fibres along with the presence of fibronectin and fibromodulin. A predominance of elastin fibre at the anterior and posterior parts of the vocal ligament may have a function in dissipation of any tension.

Deep layer of lamina propria

This layer is predominantly made of longitudinally arranged collagen fibres. There is also fibroblast, elastin, hyaluronic acid and fibronectin in the ECM.

MUSCULAR LAYER

Fibres of the vocalis muscle form the body of the vocal fold and add bulk and rigidity to it. The fibres nearest to the vocal ligament are densely innervated of slow-twitch type while the fibres at the muscularis part are of fast-twitch type in function.

DISORDERS OF VOICE

Disorders of voice can be due to physical and/or functional abnormality of the glottic and supraglottic structures or pathologies affecting movements of the vocal folds. Human voice has a significant emotional overlay; hence it may be predisposed to various psychopathologies with or without organic pathology.

LARYNGITIS

This is a common short-lasting acute inflammation of the laryngeal mucosa of multifactorial aetiology. Upper respiratory tract infections, viral infections, physical and chemical injury (coughing, voice misuse, smoking, alcohol abuse) and sometimes bacterial infection can cause laryngitis. Most patients will recover spontaneously. Voice rest, rehydration and inhalation of steam (without any additive) are effective in resolution of acute laryngitis, when toxic causes are avoided. When symptoms continue beyond 3 weeks, it is then considered to be chronic laryngitis. Laryngopharyngeal reflux, smoking, heavy alcohol ingestion, severe snoring and inhalers for asthma (if not administered correctly with precautions) may frequently predispose individuals to recurrent and chronic laryngitis. Dietary and lifestyle strategies are most effective in the management of this category of laryngitis, along with voice therapy.

Some rare systemic diseases (Wegener's granuloma, sarcoidosis, rheumatoid arthritis) may be associated with chronic inflammation of the laryngeal mucosa and present with hoarse voice and/or variable intensity of respiratory distress.

MUCOSAL INFLAMMATORY PATHOLOGY (EXUDATIVE PATHOLOGY)

Cysts

Cysts are usually associated with laryngitis, vocal trauma or laryngopharyngeal reflux. The two distinct varieties are epidermoid cysts, which are pearly in appearance and found buried in submucosa, and greyish-yellow ductal mucus retention cysts, which are often found under the free edge of the focal fold in its middle third. In a large study of benign laryngeal lesions, cysts were found in 13.6 per cent of cases. Histologically, epidermoid cysts show keratinized stratified squamous epithelium, while retention cysts show columnar epithelium (Figure 32.3).

Polyps

Polyps are pedunculated or sessile lesions, often unilateral, that arise from the free edge of the

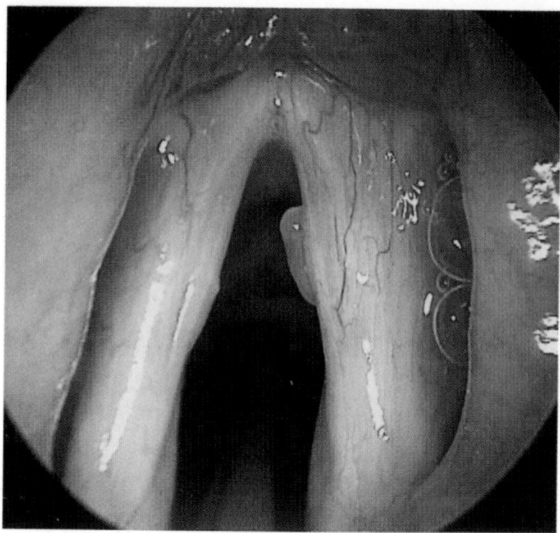

Figure 32.3 Mucus retention cyst.

vocal fold. They are associated with inflammatory changes with exudative materials being present in the lamina propria. Multiple areas of extravagated blood with surrounding endothelial cells are frequent histopathological findings in vocal polyps. Physical trauma (voice abuse, chronic cough), chemical trauma (laryngopharyngeal reflux, smoking and alcohol), infection and inflammations, and allergy have all been implicated in the aetiology of vocal polyps (Figure 32.4).

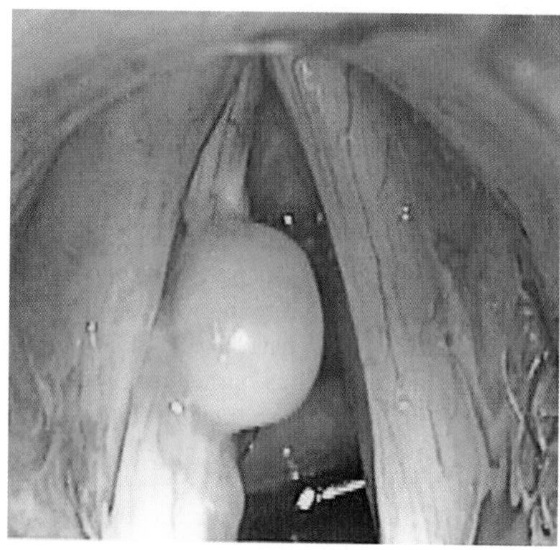

Figure 32.4 Inflammatory polyp.

Polypoid degenerations (Reinke's oedema)

Inflammatory oedema of the SLLP causing significant distension is a characteristic finding in this category. Reinke's oedema is often bilateral at presentation but can be a unilateral finding. Although it is most commonly found in smokers, polyploidy degeneration of the vocal fold can also be found in presence of severe laryngopharyngeal reflux. Increased bulk of the vocal cord causes masculinization of the voice, producing predominantly bass notes like the thicker cords in the guitar. Lateral cordotomy (mucosa-sparing approach) with the removal of viscous fluid from Reinke's space is effective in restoring voice function. If the precipitating noxious agent (smoking in most cases) for oedema is not removed, recurrence is almost inevitable.

Laryngeal granulomas

Laryngeal granulomas are characterized by continual damage of tissue creating a state of frustrated healing process.

Arytenoid granuloma, foreign body granuloma and intubation granuloma are a few examples of laryngeal granulomas. Arytenoid granuloma is often associated with a hard vocal attack at the onset of phonation. This can also be found in presence of severe laryngopharyngeal reflux. Some authorities believe that this particular type of granuloma is more common in passive-aggressive, narcissistic individuals with poor levels of tolerance to stressful situations.

Only a minority of cases of mucosal trauma during intubation result in granuloma formation, indicating possible types of cellular reactions to trauma and characteristic healing patterns of healing in some individuals.

Vocal fold nodules

Vocal fold nodules are manifestations of repetitive trauma due to misuse of the voice with overactive intrinsic muscle action. These nodules are a frequent cause of hoarseness in children who are naturally excitable and vocal. When seen in singers, the condition is called 'singer's nodules'. Failure to warm up the voice, overuse, incorrect methods of singing and amateur voice are often associated with vocal cord nodules, although this pathology also affects famous singers and performers. Nodules often start as a soft inflammatory swelling due to oedema over an area of microscopic haemorrhage (pronodules). A mature nodule is composed of fibroblasts and collagen fibres contained within the vocal fold epithelium and the superficial layer of the lamina propria. Vocal cord nodules do not have any deeper connection with the underlying tissue.

FUNCTIONAL VOICE DISORDERS

Dysphonia in this group is characterized by hyperfunction of the vocal apparatus, often in presence of normal laryngeal anatomy. Abnormal overactivity of intrinsic and extrinsic groups of muscles is often an underlying feature. Structural abnormalities and pathologies, where present, cannot match up to the abnormality of the vocal function. Patients with functional voice disorders make up nearly half of the patient traffic to the specialist voice clinic.

Muscle tension dysphonia

Muscle tension dysphonia (MTD) is the most common type of functional voice disorder. It was originally described in patients with significant vocal demand living in stressful situations. Increased and sustained tension of the laryngeal muscles leads to abnormal laryngeal movement during phonation with consequent dysphonia. The primary form is seen predominantly in females (up to 40 per cent in a voice clinic population). MTD is diagnosed in absence of any organic pathology of the vocal fold, or psychiatric or neurological pathology. Secondary MTD has an established association with underlying organic pathology. It still remains undecided whether MTD is the cause or the effect in the secondary variety. Anterior-posterior and/or lateral constriction of the supraglottis is often noted during endoscopy. Endoscopic observations that are useful ways of describing clinical findings and for communication with the voice therapist are: pitch, loudness, breathiness, timbre, prosody, fluency and intelligibility. MTD has been conveniently classified into four types, although the endoscopic findings are not always very distinct.

MTD Type 1: Hypertonic state of the posterior crico-arytenoid muscle causing posterior open chink and laryngeal isometric contraction

MTD Type 2: Supraglottic contraction with adducted ventricular folds

MTD Type 3: Anterior-posterior contraction with approximation of the epiglottis with the arytenoids; posterior migration or placement of the tongue base

MTD Type 4: Extreme anterior-posterior contraction; supraglottic squeeze. Difficult to view the entire larynx with the flexible endoscope positioned in the mid-oropharyngeal level.

The underlying factors predisposing and/or perpetuating MTD can be psychological conditions, misuse/abuse of the voice, organic pathology (local/systemic) or changes (aging) where vocal compensation is needed. Respiratory infections associated with prolonged frequent coughing, deafness, chronic snoring and laryngopharyngeal reflux (LPR) may also predispose an individual to MTD.

Recurrent respiratory papillomatosis

Prevalence of recurrent respiratory papillomatosis (RRP) in adults is 1.8/100 000 and twice as much in children in the United States. When the larynx is affected, dysphonia can be a common presentation. Human papilloma virus (HPV) types 6 and 11 are the frequently identified pathogens. These subtypes also cause genital warts. Endoscopic removal of papillomas with a microdebrider is the preferred surgical option. Recalcitrant cases need concomitant local treatment with Mitomycin or cidofovir or α-interferon. Photodynamic therapy and pulsed dye laser and photodynamic therapy have been reported to be effective. Introduction of the HPV vaccination and its availability to this group of patient holds promise.

Sulcus vocalis

This condition is characterized by the presence of a furrow/sulcus or a depression at the free edge of the vocal fold with consequent abnormality of vocal fold vibration and glottic insufficiency. It has been classified into three types depending on the depth of the sulcus and its shape. Type I is superficial and is not associated with any voice abnormality. Types IIa and IIb cause moderate and severe dysphonia, respectively. The aetiology of sulcus vocalis remains controversial, but acquired origins seem to have more support with evidence. Patients from the Indian subcontinent seem to have a higher predilection for sulcus vocalis. The presence of bilateral sulci can give a very breathy character to one's voice owing to significant air escape during vocalization as the free edges of the vocal folds cannot come in close contact during full adduction.

NEURAL PATHOLOGY (MOVEMENT DISORDERS)

VOCAL FOLD PARALYSIS

Vocal fold paralysis in association of cerebrovascular accidents predominantly presents with other neurological deficits. Wallenberg syndrome (lateral medullary infarct) is a rare neurological pathology that presents with vocal fold paralysis. The most common occurrence of unilateral vocal fold palsy is of the idiopathic type where the underlying cause cannot be identified. Iatrogenic trauma, when recognized intraoperatively, should be considered for anastomosis at the same setting. Bilateral vocal fold palsy will frequently require tracheostomy to secure the airway.

IDIOPATHIC VOCAL FOLD PARALYSIS

Twenty to forty per cent of patients with idiopathic vocal fold paralysis show spontaneous recovery. It might take up to 12 months to show signs of recovery; some patients get partial recovery with an acceptable quality of voice. Possible underlying viral aetiology (herpes zoster, Epstein–Barr virus and cytomegalovirus) has been reported by some authors as causal with the suggestions of the role of anti-inflammatory medications such as steroids (as in the treatment of facial palsy). Computed tomography (CT) or magnetic resonance imaging (MRI) scan of the brainstem to the arch of the aorta will help exclude any mitotic disease involving the vagus nerve or its RLN branch. Voice therapy is very useful and helps with the compensation from the contralateral cord in adductor paralysis. Patients with abductor paralysis often require surgical interventions such as medialization laryngoplasty, thyroplasty and so forth.

SPASMODIC DYSPHONIA

Spasmodic dysphonia (SD) is a neuropathology of focal dystonia affecting muscle groups of the larynx supplied by the RLN. The central pathology is thought to be at the basal ganglia of the midbrain and its connections. The incidence is 1 in 50 000–100 000. Adductor spasmodic dysphonia (ADSD) is the most common variety and is characterized by strained and strangulated voice. Symptoms of ADSD are more intensified during voiced reading (reading the Rainbow Passage). Abductors spasmodic dysphonia (ABSD) constitutes approximately 15 per cent of laryngeal dystonia. Combined varieties of SDs are very rare. SD may present with generalized dystonia. Public speaking, speaking to a stranger and telephone conversations are known to trigger symptoms of SD.

PARKINSON'S DISEASE

Parkinson's disease is characterized by vocal tremor with difficulty holding a conversation for long (bradykinesia of small muscles). Social isolation due to dysphonia is a common subjective finding (on the VH-10 questionnaire) in this group. Parkinson's disease affects all aspects of voice production from the generation of subglottic air pressure to the articulation and amplification of voice. The prosody and timbre of voice are also affected. Lee Silverman voice treatment (LSVT), which helps to increase the loudness of the voice, is found to be effective in this group of patients.

JOINT PATHOLOGY

Cricothyroid joint and crico-arytenoid joint involvement by trauma or systemic disease may present with the symptom of dysphonia. Intubation trauma can dislocate the crico-arytenoid joint causing immobility of the vocal fold and resultant marked hoarse voice. Timeous closed reduction is the most effective treatment in this situation.

Arthritis of the crico-arytenoid joint in rheumatoid arthritis, relapsing polychondritis and systemic lupus erythematosus has been reported; this can present with dysphonia of varying severity.

DIAGNOSIS

Anyone with dysphonia of 12 weeks' duration or more must have an endoscopic examination of the larynx to exclude mitotic pathology. High-risk patients should have this done expediently. Every patient presenting with dysphonia needs careful attention with a perceptive approach of care from a multidisciplinary team. *What matters to the patient* is the key and central theme upon which all curative and supportive efforts should be concentrated. The pace of patients' movements, at the specialist voice clinic, needs to be intuitively balanced to fulfill the needs of the patients and of the professionals. All patients attending our voice clinic complete a Voice Handicap Index-10 (VHI-10) before each consultation. Patients' own perception of the problem and its psychological and social effects are important aspects that one should always be mindful of. We find it very useful to understand *what matters to the patient*; it helps us tailor the necessary care to each individual patient with maximum sensitivity. A detailed, voice-specific history (onset, duration, constancy, precipitating and aggravating factors, hydration and fluid intake, smoking, alcohol intake, diet, voice use/demand) should be taken. The fundamental necessity to understand various psychosocial and biological aspects of the voice pathology in every patient cannot be over emphasized. Each patient is also scored using the GRBAS scale (grade, roughness, breathiness, asthenia and strain; 0 normal, 1 mild, 2 moderate, 3 severe) on the perceptual quality of their voice by two clinicians. The roughness and breathiness scores have shown very good inter-observer reliability. However, the other two parameters, asthenia (weakness) and strain, are slightly less reliable, as reported in current literature. The GRBAS scale is an excellent and easy-to-use perceptual scoring system. Other characteristics, such as loudness, fluency, intelligibility, prosody and tremor, should be recorded separately.

Measures of fundamental frequency (pitch perturbation) and amplitude perturbations are very useful in the determination of basic quality of voice. Jitter represents a variation of F_0 (fundamental frequency), and therefore pitch of the voice measured over a fixed period of time. Shimmer is a measure of amplitude (or loudness) variation over a defined timeline. A comprehensive history frequently leads to a provisional diagnosis even before any endoscopic examination is carried out. Careful listening to the patient's voice, once she or he is relaxed in the clinic, gives a good awareness of the acoustic qualities of the voice for perceptual grading. Certain dietary contents can directly or indirectly predispose the vocal tract to mucosal damage; smoking and heavy ingestion of alcoholic beverages, especially spirits, are notorious for their ability to damage the mucosa and the microenvironment of the upper aerodigestive tract. Some systemic diseases, for example pulmonary malignancy (left lung), parkinsonism, Wegener's disease, sarcoidosis, myasthenia gravis, stroke, multiple sclerosis, muscular dystrophy and generalized muscular dystonia, can manifest as disorders of voice.

Complete clinical examination of the patient's head and neck is carried out with special attention to the oral cavity, oropharynx, nose, neck muscles and the laryngeal cartilages and joints. All patients have endoscopic examination of their upper aerodigestive tract with a high-definition *chip on the tip* flexible endoscope, without local anaesthetic (if possible), after they have a careful explanation of the reasons for the procedure and what it entails. Acoustic recording of the voice is done in each patient during endoscopic examination. All structures of the larynx are carefully checked. Laryngeal function is assessed with videolaryngostroboscopy/videokymography (VLS/VKG) with voice commands and during periods of rest and movement. VLS/VKG is used to visualize and assess vocal fold mucosal movement, periodicity and symmetry of opening and closing events. Rigid endoscopy (through the oral cavity) is only used when the nasendoscope is not tolerated or cannot be negotiated owing to abnormal intranasal anatomy. The necessary prerequisites for rigid endoscopy distort the supraglottic vocal tract and laryngeal position by forced extrusion and holding down of the tongue by the endoscopist or patient. Complex physical assessment of various voice

Table 32.1 Specialist voice assessment

VHI-10: Subjective rating by patients
Perceptual assessment: Audible, Comprehensible/Intelligible, Fluent, Prosodic/Rhythmic, Tremor, Rhinophonia
GRBAS (Global Score, Roughness, Breathiness, Asthenia, Strain; normal 0, mild 1, moderate 2, severe 3)
Acoustic recording:
Short-term perturbation of fundamental frequency,
Short- or medium-term amplitude perturbation and voiceless segments
Noise vs. harmonics ratio
Long-term frequency and amplitude variation
Reading: Paragraph from standard text, i.e. the rainbow passage.
Aerodynamic assessments: MPT (Maximum Phonation Time of sound /a: /; male 25-35 sec; female 15-25 sec)
Endoscopic visualization
Videolaryngostroboscopy (VLS) / videostrobokymography (VKG)
Electroglottograph (EGG)
Electomyogram (EMG)
Voice analysis
Voice range profile
Voice strain test

parameters such as voice analysis, voice range profile, voice strain test, electroglottography and electromyography is done, as required, in patients with complex pathology and high vocal demand (Table 32.1).

MANAGEMENT

All patients with dysphonia should have his or her vocal pathology and psychosocial needs dealt with adequately. Most of the inflammatory pathology will resolve well with strict vocal hygiene measures (Table 32.2), voice therapy with diet and lifestyle advice. Phonosurgery is necessary in some cases. One should have a very cautious approach to surgery of vocal fold pathology, especially on its anterior two-thirds and its free border. Ideally, all patients should be dealt with in a specialist voice clinic setting where possible. Patients requiring surgical interventions should receive pre- and post-operative voice therapy. Vocal fold nodules should be treated with voice therapy and practice of strict vocal hygiene measures by the patient. Surgery is not the first line of treatment here, although it may be necessary in some very refractory cases. Partial vocal fold insufficiency is associated with breathy voice where the close apposition of these structures is prevented by the presence of cysts, polyps, granulomas or nodules. Unilateral vocal fold palsy unresponsive to conventional medical treatment will benefit from endoscopic medialization of the cord with injectable materials. This can be done as a day case/office procedure. Type I (medialization) thyroplasty will give such patients permanent improvement of voice quality.

Muscle tension dysphonia needs voice therapy and good patient compliance with the vocal hygiene measures. Severe cases of MTD can be difficult to differentiate from adductor spasmodic dysphonia. ADSD responds to electromyography (EMG)–guided botulinum toxin injection to the thyroarytenoid muscle, although the duration of the paralytic effect on the muscle is temporary. Voice therapy with behavioural and psychological interventions may be effective in some patients. Selective neural resection should be left as the last resort.

Table 32.2 Take care of your voice

Do not shout if at all possible.
Use voice support (microphone) if lecturing or instructing (i.e. physical instructor).
Drink up to 2 litres of still water every day.
Use steam inhalation.
Avoid using throat lozenges.
Avoid alcoholic beverages, especially spirits.
Reduce intake of tea and coffee.
Do not smoke and avoid passive smoking.
Warm up regularly and adequately before singing.
Amateur singers should consider taking singing lessons.
Rest well, sleep well and avoid physical exertion.
Identify stressful situations and develop coping strategies.
Strictly rest your voice in presence of dysphonia.
If hearing impaired, have hearing function checked and/or rehabilitated.
Sip ice cold water to stop frequent throat clearing and irritable, nonproductive dry cough.
Seek treatment for snoring when it is present.
If diagnosed with laryngopharyngeal reflux, reduce intake of dairy products; acidic, spicy or fried food; and fizzy drinks.

KEY LEARNING POINTS

- Voice disorders should be managed in voice clinics by multidisciplinary teams.
- Dietary and lifestyle strategies are very helpful in prevention of mucosal inflammatory pathologies.
- Voice problems are common in the late stage of Parkinson's disease.
- MTD can sometimes mimic the symptoms of SD.

FURTHER READING

Andrus JG, Shapshay SM. Contemporary management of laryngeal papilloma in adults and children. *Otolaryngology Clinics of North America*. 2006; 39: 135–58.

Baken RJ, Orlikoff R. *Clinical Measurement of Speech and Voice*. San Diego, CA: Singular Thomson Learning, 2000.

Bandi V, Munnur U, Braman SS. Airway problems in patients with rheumatologic disorders. *Critical Care Clinics*. 2002; 18: 749–65.

Bless DM. Measurement of vocal function. *Otolaryngology Clinics of North America*. 1991; 24(5): 1023–33.

Fairbanks G. *Voice and Articulation Drillbook*. 2nd ed. New York: Harper & Row, 1960.

Gallaghera TQ, Derkay CS. Recurrent respiratory papillomatosis: Update 2008. *Current Opinion in Otolaryngology & Head and Neck Surgery*. 2008; 16: 536–42.

Garcia Martins RH, Defaveri J, Aparecida Custodio Domingues J. Vocal polyps: Clinical, morphological, and immunohistochemical aspects. *Journal of Voice*. 2011; 25: 98–106.

Giovanni A, Chanteret C, Lagier A. Sulcus vocalis: A review. *European Archives of Otorhinolaryngology*. 2007; 264: 337–44.

Hantzakos A, Remacle M, Dikkers FG, et al. Exudative lesions of Reinke's space: A terminology proposal. *European Archives of Otorhinolaryngology*. 2009; 266: 869–78.

Harris T, Harris S, Rubin JS, Howard DM. *The Voice Clinic Handbook*. London: Whurr Publisher Limited, 1998.

Hirano M. *The Clinical Evaluation of Voice*. Vienna: Springer, 1981.

Hirano M, Bless DM. *Videostroboscopic Examination of the Larynx*. San Diego, CA: Singular Publishing, 1993.

Ho Chung J, Tae K, Seop Lee Y, et al. The significance of laryngopharyngeal reflux in benign vocal mucosal lesions. *Otolaryngology – Head and Neck Surgery*. 2009; 141: 369–73.

Houtte EV, Lierde KV, Claeys S. Pathophysiology and treatment of muscle tension dysphonia: A review of the current knowledge. *Journal of Voice*. 2011; 25: 202–06.

Koufman JA, Blalock PD. Classification and approach to patients with functional voice disorders. *Rhinology & Laryngology*. 1982: 91(4): 372–77.

Koufman JA, Blalock PD. Functional voice disorders. *Otolaryngology Clinics of North America*. 1991; 24(5): 1059–73.

Lieberman P. The evolution of human speech: Its anatomical and neural bases. *Current Anthropology*. 2007; 48(1): 39–66.

Mendelsohn AH, Berke GS. Surgery or botulinum toxin for adductor spasmodic dysphonia: A comparative study. *Annals of Otology. Rhinology & Laryngology*. 2012; 21(4): 231–38.

Sataloff RT. *Voice Science*. San Diego, CA: Plural Publishing Inc., 2012.

Schwartz SR, Cohen SM, Dailey SH, et al. Clinical practice guideline: Hoarseness (Dysphonia). *Otolaryngology – Head and Neck Surgery*. 2009; 141: S1–S31.

Silverman EP, Garvan C, Shrivastav R, et al. Combined modality treatment of adductor spasmodic dysphonia. *Journal of Voice*. 2012; 26 (1): 77–86.

Tisch SHD, Brake HM, Law M, et al. Spasmodic dysphonia: Clinical features and effects of botulinum toxin therapy in 169 patients – an Australian experience. *Journal of Clinical Neuroscience*. 2003; 10(4): 434–38.

Yun Y-S, Kim M-B, Son Y-K. The effect of vocal hygiene education for patients with vocal polyp. *Otolaryngology – Head and Neck Surgery*. 2007; 137: 569–75.

33

Vocal cord paralysis

CONRAD TIMON AND EMMA C CASHMAN

Vocal cord paralysis is commonly encountered in otolaryngology practice and is often a manifestation of disease and not a diagnosis in and of itself. True vocal cord paralysis refers to immobility of the 'true' vocal cord resulting from disruption of motor innervations to the laryngeal musculature.[1] This may be secondary to injury to either the vagus or the recurrent laryngeal nerve (RLN). As a broad entity, vocal cord paralysis has dissonant etiologies, including neurological, iatrogenic and neoplastic pathologies. A thorough knowledge of the vagus nerve, laryngeal musculature and framework is therefore vital to understanding vocal cord palsies and their clinical significance.

ANATOMY

An understanding of the anatomy of the larynx, and in particular of the relevant muscles producing abduction and adduction and their nerve supply, is fundamental to ascertaining the potential causes of vocal cord paralysis. The resting position of the cords provides an important clue as to the likely site of neural disruption. The intrinsic muscles of the larynx, with the exception of the cricothyroid muscle (the sole abductor of the vocal cords, which is supplied by the external branch of the superior laryngeal nerve [SLN]), are supplied by the RLN. The internal branch of the SLN provides the main sensory innervation to the supraglottic and glottic regions of the larynx, with some sensory contribution also to the posterior sub-glottis. The SLN is the second major branch of the vagus nerve. It branches away from the vagus at the level of the inferior cervical ganglion, coursing deep to the internal carotid artery before emerging in an anteromedial direction towards the larynx. The SLN divides into internal and external branches before supplying the larynx. In addition to supplying all of the intrinsic muscles of the larynx, with the exception of the cricothyroid, the RLN also contributes sensory branches to the glottis, sub-glottis and proximal trachea. The left RLN has a longer route than the right and branches from the vagus nerve to loop beneath the arch of the aorta, posterior to the ligamentum arteriosum, before ascending between the trachea and esophagus to reach the neck. On the other hand, the right branch of the RLN loops around the right subclavian artery.

As previously mentioned, the final resting position of the cords provides an indication as to the specific site of disruption of the nerve supply to the vocal cord. In the case of unilateral vocal cord paralysis (ULVCP), it is important to establish whether the paralysis is secondary to a RLN injury or results from disruption to the vagus nerve. The characteristic paramedian vocal cord position results from disruption below the level of the SLN. The vocal cord adopts a paramedian position due to unopposed action of the cricothyroid muscle. Paralysis of the left vocal cord is more commonly observed than right vocal cord paralysis owing to the longer and more tortuous course of the left RLN within the mediatsinum.[2]

AETIOLOGY OF VOCAL CORD PARALYSIS

UNILATERAL VOCAL CORD PARALYSIS

Unilateral vocal cord paralysis (ULVCP) is more commonly encountered than bilateral cord paralysis and represents about 75 per cent of cases.[3] ULVCP results from dysfunction of the brainstem nuclei, the vagus nerve, or the RLN supplying the involved side of the larynx. The most common cause of ULVCP remains controversial. Most recent studies cite non-laryngeal malignancy as the most common cause of ULVCP, with surgical injury reported as the second most common contributing factor.[4] Table 33.1 summarizes the main causes of vocal cord paralysis in adults.

While RLN or SLN damage was once largely limited to thyroid surgery, the types of surgery that may potentially cause ULVCP have greatly expanded and include a variety of skull base procedures, and several cervical and thoracic procedures (see Table 33.2). Idiopathic causes are next in frequency and have been the subject of debate for several decades.[5] Several recent studies have addressed the possibility of nerve injury by infectious agents, and a review of the literature

Table 33.1 Aetiology of adult vocal cord paralysis

ULVCP	
• Malignancy	25 per cent
• Iatrogenic surgical trauma	25 per cent
• Idiopathic	20 per cent
• Non-surgical trauma	11 per cent
• Intubation	7 per cent
• Neurological disorders	7 per cent
BLVCP	
• Iatrogenic	44 per cent
• Malignancy	17 per cent
• Neurological	12 per cent
• Intubation	15 per cent
• Idiopathic	12 per cent

Table 33.2 Surgical procedures associated with vocal cord paralysis

Cervical surgery
• Thyroidectomy/parathyroidectomy
• Carotid endartectomy
• Anterior approach to the cervical spine
• Repair Zenker's diverticulum
• Cricopharyngeal myotomy
Thoracic procedures
• Thoracic aneurysm repair
• Pneumonectomy
• Aortic valve repair
• Coronary artery bypass grafting
• Esophageal or tracheal surgery
• Mediastinoscopy
• Ligation of patent ductus arteriosus
Others
• Skull base or brainstem surgery
• Endotracheal intubation

reveals cases attributed to a host of infectious agents, including Lyme disease, herpes zoster, Epstein–Barr virus, herpes simplex and cytomegalovirus in the immunocompromised patient.[6] The reported outcomes in the literature for idiopathic ULVCP vary widely.[7] Larger series, however, suggest a spontaneous recovery rate of about 20–40 per cent in patients with idiopathic vocal cord paralysis, with average recovery ranging between 1 and 9 months after the onset of paralysis.[7]

BILATERAL VOCAL CORD PARALYSIS

Bilateral vocal cord paralysis (BLVCP) is a broad term that denotes reduced or absent movement of both vocal cords resulting from the impaired function of the vagus nerve or its distal branch, the RLN. There is little controversy in the literature with respect to the most common causes of BLVCP in the adult setting. Most studies cite iatrogenic surgical damage as the most common precipitating cause of BLVCP, with thyroidectomy reported as the procedure that is most likely to result in BLVCP.[8] Larger series indicate that surgical injury accounts for 44 per cent of cases of BLVCP, malignancies 17 per cent, endotracheal intubation 15 per cent, neurological disease 12 per cent and idiopathic causes account for a further 12 per cent of cases.[9]

While uncommon, mechanical disruption of the laryngeal framework, such as the crico-arytenoid joint, represents an important differential diagnosis of vocal cord paralysis. Crico-arytenoid joint fixation may arise secondary to inflammatory disease, most commonly rheumatoid arthritis or due to endotracheal intubation, external trauma or penetrating injuries. Symptoms suggestive of crico-arytenoid joint fixation include vocal fatigue, pain on phonating and loss of voice control, but ultimately symptoms will depend on the position of the immobile vocal cord. While differentiating crico-arytenoid joint dislocation from vocal cord paralysis on the basis of the clinical history may prove challenging, several findings on fibre-optic scope are suggestive of crico-arytenoid dislocation, including disparity in height of the vocal cords, arytenoid oedema or an anteriorly overhanging arytenoid. Laryngeal electromyography, discussed later in this chapter, also aids in differentiating ULVCP from crico-arytenoid joint pathology.

Table 33.3 Thyroplasty types

- Type I: Medialization of vocal cord
- Type II: Lateralization of vocal cord
- Type III: Shortening or relaxation of vocal cord
- Type IV: Elongation or tensioning of the vocal cord

Most authors recommend early treatment of crico-arytenoid fixation with some surgeons advocating arytenoidectomy via an endoscopic approach or external approach via laryngofissure.[10] However, arytenoidectomy has not been widely accepted owing to the risk of aspiration and poor airway protection associated with the procedure. Vocal cord medialization, via a type 1 thyroplasty as described by Isshiki (see Table 33.3), remains the treatment of choice for patients presenting at a later stage with crico-arytenoid fixation.[11]

It is important to note that sometimes weakness or a paradoxical motion of the vocal cords may mimic a true vocal cord paralysis. Such patients can present with a wide variety of symptoms, such as hoarseness, cough, dyspnea, stridor and reflux. During paradoxical motion of the cords, the vocal folds approximate together during inspiration as opposed to abducting normally. The exact pathogenesis of paradoxical vocal cord motion remains indeterminate, but both organic (e.g. gastro-oesophageal reflux disease, irritant induced) and non-organic (anxiety, stress) causes have been described.[12] In treating these patients the cause of the paradoxical motion of the vocal cords should first be elicited and organic causes ruled out. Heliox may be used for management in the acute phase and a multidisciplinary approach (e.g. speech therapy, psychological support) is required for long-term management of these patients.[13]

PRESENTATION

A wide variety of symptoms may be observed in vocal cord paralysis, including dysphonia or hoarseness, vocal fatigue, aphonia, shortness of breath and swallowing difficulties. Classically, patients with ULVCP present with weak, breathy, low-pitched dysphonia, and it is typically the dysphonia or hoarseness that prompts the patient to seek medical help in the first instance. Occasionally, dysphonia may be high-pitched in quality as a result of a compensatory lengthening of the vocal cords in an effort to achieve better glottic closure. Patients with ULVCP may report dysphagia, often to liquids, particularly if the ULVCP is due to the presence of a high vagal lesion, which results in impairment of both the RLN and SLN. The latter may result in significant pharyngeal hypoaesthesia and an increased risk of aspiration. To compensate for glottic incompetence, significant muscle tension may be observed in the laryngeal framework, and patients with ULVCP often describe pain or discomfort after vocalization, which may be attributable to excessive muscle tension.

The clinical presentation of BLVCP differs considerably to that observed in patients presenting with a unilateral paralysis. In contrast to ULVCP, voice quality is not usually the chief concern in patients with BLVCP. Voice quality is often only mildly affected, as the paralyzed cords tend to assume their natural position during phonation. Classically, patients with BLVCP present with symptoms of airway compromise that range from being mild to, more commonly, dyspnea and stridor. Signs suggestive of neurological involvement may also be present, such as vocal fatigue and tremor, weak or breathy voice, altered resonance or acquired dysarthria.

EVALUATION

An inventory of the patient's vocal requirements, both work-related and social, should be central to the clinical history as this will influence the type of treatment that a patient will opt for, e.g. a professional voice user may opt for a temporizing vocal augmentation in an effort to expedite his or her return to work (see Table 33.3). Any history of recent surgery should be established, with particular emphasis on any recent thyroid, cervical or thoracic procedures (see Table 33.2). Physical examination should include a complete head and neck examination with particular emphasis on the cranial nerves. Evaluation of the gag reflex and palatal elevation should also be undertaken, as a high vagal injury will cause palatal deviation to the intact side. Direct visual examination of the larynx with fibre-optic laryngoscopy provides valuable information with respect to possible aetiology of the vocal cord paralysis. Evidence of asymmetry, vocal fold bowing, the presence of any lesions and the exact position of the vocal cords should be noted: cadaveric (lateral), paramedian, median or vertical. Paralysis of the RLN results in the cords adopting a paramedian position, whereas in cases involving both the RLN and SLN the vocal cords will adopt the so-called cadaveric or lateral position. Maximal adduction and abduction can be assessed with the 'ee-sniff' manoeuvre.[14]

Commonly in cases of ULVCP there may be a temporal relation between the onset of hoarseness and a surgical injury, and in such instances further investigations may not be deemed necessary. However, where there is no identifiable aetiology, it is imperative that all patients should undergo a computed tomography (CT) (with contrast) or magnetic resonance imaging (MRI) scan from the skull base to the level of the diaphragm to rule out an extra-laryngeal neoplasia. From a neurological standpoint, the most common cause of ULVCP is a cerebral vascular accident, usually involving the brainstem. The vast majority of such patients, however, will present with additional cranial nerve involvement and associated neurological signs (e.g. paraplegia, dysphasia, aspiration), and in such cases an MRI of brain should be requested.

Video-stroboscopy is commonly deployed in the clinic setting to assess the structure and movement of the vocal cords. It is an important tool in the workup of vocal cord paralysis enabling the detection of subtle mucosal motion abnormalities. Valuable information regarding vocal fold height differences and vocal process status during phonation can be obtained with the use of video-stroboscopy. It may demonstrate, for example, increased amplitude of vibrations owing to the atrophic nature of a denervated vocalis muscle.[15]

LARYNGEAL ELECTROMYOGRAPHY

While direct visual examination can confirm the presence of vocal cord immobility or dysmobility, it cannot determine if the underling pathology represents a paralysis or paresis. By definition, paralysis (a complete loss of movement) and paresis (which denotes slight or partial paralysis) are neurological entities, and thus can only be adequately assessed with neurophysiological testing. Laryngeal electromyography (LEMG) is an important tool in accessing the neural integrity of the larynx. It provides valuable information with respect to prognosis and can affect treatment decisions and operative planning.[16] In addition, its therapeutic role in guiding the placement of botulinum toxin in cases of spasmodic dysphonia is well described.[17]

The optimal time to perform LEMG is between 1 and 6 months after the onset of ULVCP, with several recent studies suggesting that LEMG outside this time frame may yield inaccurate results.[18] If paresis is detected on LEMG, voice therapy that is specially targeted at strengthening laryngeal musculature may be beneficial. LEMG aids in determining the type and timing of surgical intervention; if there is evidence on LEMG of progressive degeneration (evidenced by the presence of positive sharp waveforms and fibrillations on LEMG), surgery may be delayed until degeneration is complete. Similarly, if regeneration is detected (characterized by the presence of polyphasic potentials on LEMG), surgery may be postponed until maximal nerve function is obtained.

MANAGEMENT OF VOCAL CORD PARALYSIS: CONSERVATIVE/ NON-SURGICAL

Patient characteristics such as age, occupation and patient preference will ultimately guide the management plan. Once an underlying neoplastic process has been definitively ruled out, expectant treatment may be indicated. As the majority of cases of ULVCP will compensate within a 6- to 18-month period, classical teaching favours a 9- to 12-month observation period before surgical options are considered.[7]

Voice therapy is widely recommended prior to restorative surgery and will aid in establishing the severity of the paralysis and evaluate the impact of vocal fold paralysis on the patient's phonation, articulation, respiration and swallowing. Speech therapy provides an important stand-alone and adjuvant treatment in the management of vocal cord paralysis, focusing on optimizing the efficiency of voice production, minimizing compensations that are counterproductive (e.g. increased effort during speech, extraneous muscle activity in head neck and shoulders during speech) and educating patients about their underlying voice disorder.

In patients with ULVCP who are deemed suitable for surgical intervention, medialization of the displaced, immobile vocal cord can be achieved in three main ways: injection augmentation, medialization laryngoplasty and selective reinnervation.

SURGICAL OPTIONS

Injection augmentation

Over the past two decades, vocal cord injection has emerged as a valuable treatment modality for vocal cord paralysis. The primary aim of injection augmentation is to implant a substance that can fill a space and restore the normal characteristics of vocal cord movement and thereby improve phonation and glottic competence. Injection augmentation confers the advantage of immediate results, is generally well tolerated by patients and may be performed in the office setting.[19]

Materials for injection augmentation are generally classified as temporary or permanent/long lasting, and the overall aim of the injected material is to match the biomechanical and viscoelastic properties of the tissue of the lamina propria of the vocal cord.[20] In the past decade, the number of available injectables for augmentation has greatly expanded, with newer materials seeking to eliminate the foreign body and inflammatory reactions observed with the use of alloplastic implants such as silicone, paraffin and, historically, Teflon.[21]

Bio-implants (e.g. autologous collagen, fat and fascia) may be incorporated into the host tissue and are associated with a lower risk of a foreign body reaction, but their main limitation has proven to be their unpredictable durability. This trend is observed with the use of autologous fat for small-to-medium glottic gaps.[22] Fat has the advantage of being readily available, and its biomechanical properties closely mirror those of the vocal fold itself. However, one of its drawbacks is the loss of a variable amount of the injected material in the first few weeks following injection.[22] This usually necessitates over-injection of the vocal cord in the initial setting. In a few reported cases, this has resulted in excess fat persisting post-injection, with resulting post-operative dysphonia.[23] Again, though rare, patients may experience airway compromise as over-injection may induce a variable amount of oedema and under-medialization is reported in a number of cases, resulting in persistent dysphonia.[24]

On the other hand, alloplastic materials are not prone to resorption and permit more permanent medialization. In addition to the aforementioned foreign body reaction, there is a risk of migration of the injected materials with such compounds.[25] Thus, as a general rule, alloplastic materials should be injected quite deeply into the thyroarytenoid muscle and paraglottic space. Various sites of preferred implantation have been described for bioimplants, and these have been shown to produce effective results when injected at levels varying from the superficial lamina propria to deep in the thryoarytenoid muscle. However, if injected too superficially, these agents can cause stiffness of the vocal cord. Newer available agents for injection augmentation include calcium hydroxlapatite, known by its trade name Radiesse Voice.[26] Results of a recent multi-institutional trial demonstrated excellent results at 12-month follow-up and showed that persistent medialization after calcium hydroxylapatite injection may be present up to 2 years or more, with an average follow-up duration of 18 months.[26]

While vocal fold augmentation is considered to be less precise than framework surgery, it does confer the advantage of a more minimally invasive approach that can be undertaken in a clinic-based setting.[19] As a general rule, injection augmentation is best deployed for treatment of mild-to-moderate glottic insufficiency (>1 to 3 mm glottic gaps).[27] With a glottic gap of greater than 3 mm, the insufficiency becomes more difficult to correct with injection augmentation and, in such cases of large posterior glottic gaps, arytenoid adduction in conjunction with medialization thyroplasty will usually yield better results.

Medialization laryngoplasty

The central aim of medialization laryngoplasty or type I thyroplasty (see Table 33.4) is to improve glottic closure by modifying the position of the vocal cords. The most common indication for laryngeal framework surgery is uncompensated or unrecovered ULVCP, with most surgeons advocating deferring surgical intervention for at least 6–12 months, to allow for spontaneous recovery.[7] Laryngeal framework surgery was first described by Payr as early as 1915; however, the procedure did not gain widespread acceptance until the late 1970s when Isshiki described his thyroplasty technique.[11] Isshiki's approach involved displacing and stabilizing a small, rectangular cartilaginous window in the thyroid lamina, at the level of the vocal cord, pushing the soft tissue medially and using Silastic instead of cartilage as the implant material.[11] Several materials in addition to Isshiki et al.'s original Silastic block, including titanium,

Table 33.4 Factors influencing treatment decisions

Aetiology of nerve injury	• Neurotemesis/axontemesis (i.e. nerve cut) favours early treatment • Neuropraxia (i.e. nerve stretched) favours conservative treatment
Clinical aspiration	• Favours early intervention
Vocal requirements of patient	• Professional voice user: Early intervention • Limited voice users: Observation
LEMG findings	• Good prognosis: Observation or temporary injection • Poor prognosis: Early ML or permanent filler

Gore-Tex and hydroxylapatite, have been described with favourable results.[28]

Medialization laryngoplasty has the advantage of being performed under local anaesthetic, allowing the patient to phonate during the procedure. Thus the degree of medialization can be determined immediately by the quality of the patient's voice. This allows for more graduated adjustments in the degree of medialization of the cords. Furthermore, while injected materials have a tendency to spread throughout the tissue in an unpredictable manner, thyroplasty can medialize a specific, targeted area.[29] The main complications reported with medialization laryngoplasty include airway compromise and implant extrusion, and in a recent study Young et al. cite a revision rate of 6 per cent.[30] A key factor necessitating revision is the presence of a persistent posterior glottic gap (indicating a lack of vocal process contact on phonation) in cases where an arytenoid adduction was not performed in conjunction with the primary surgery. Arytenoid adduction aims to reposition or displace the vocal process medially and should be considered as an adjunctive procedure in patients with evidence of impaired vocal process contact or disparity in vocal cord height on videostroboscopy.

Laryngeal reinnervation

Selective laryngeal reinnervation was originally described by Tucker in 1977 and has been predominately used in cases of unilateral paralysis of the RLN.[31] The most popular reinnervation technique involves neurorrhaphy of the ansa cervicalis to the RLN stump, with hypoglossal to the RLN anastomosis also described.[31] Laryngeal reinnervation holds several potential advantages over the techniques previously described. First, it has the potential to restore a normal or near normal voice quality without affecting vocal cord pliability, with Tucker and several other authors reporting satisfactory results.[31,32] An added advantage to selective reinnervation is that it preserves the possibility of other laryngoplasty techniques, should further intervention be necessary in the future. However, some results with selective laryngeal reinnervation have been disappointing, and limitations such as the need for a general anaesthetic, a delay in time to voice restoration (usually about 2 to 6 months before benefits are realized) and the requirement of both an intact donor and recipient nerve have prohibited its widespread use.[33]

MANAGEMENT OF BLVCP

While voice is the predominant issue in cases of ULVCP, airway is the primary concern in cases of BLVCP. Tracheotomy may be required in cases of significant airway compromise arising from BLVCP. Surgical interventions including tracheotomy, vocal cord lateralization, tissue removal and direct muscle reinnervation provide the mainstay of treatment for BLVCP. The principal procedures deployed for treatment of BLVCP are vocal cord lateralization and removal of vocal cord or arytenoid tissue.

While there was significant initial enthusiasm for lateralization, its technical difficulty has restricted its widespread use. Vocal cord lateralization aims to surgically widen the glottic opening by excising a wedge of thyroarytenoid muscle. The resulting surgical defect is then closed and the vocal cords displaced laterally by passing a suture across the cord with two needles inserted through the skin, gaining entry to the larynx above and below the level of the vocal cord. The suture is subsequently tightened to place the vocal cords in the desired position, and the suture is then secured to the surface of the skin. The sutures are removed at approximately 2 weeks post-operatively, at which time the vocal cord should be fixed in the desired position. Most authors report favourable outcomes with the advantage of reversibility. However, pain on swallowing and aspiration are recognized early complications, and patients may require additional procedures to maintain their airway.[34]

Removal of vocal cord or arytenoid tissue is an effective, albeit permanent, method of widening glottic diameter and improving the airway. Arytenoidectomy is currently the gold standard for the management of BLVCP and involves the removal of some or all of the arytenoid cartilage. Concerns with regards to aspiration observed with complete removal of the arytenoid have led to more conservative removal.[35] Arytenoidectomy can be performed endoscopically, by microsurgical or laser technique, or externally with a lateral neck approach. Outcome for arytenoidectomy is related to the amount of tissue removed and the success of healing of the residual surgical defect. The use of the CO_2 laser with the operating microscope has allowed a more conservative approach to arytenoidectomy, greater reproducibility of results and greater facility in performing the procedure in a narrower operative field.[36] The CO_2 laser permits ablation of a segment of cartilage with greater precision instead of removing the entire arytenoid, as described by earlier approaches. Partial cordectomy is the procedure of choice in our institution and involves laser excision of part of the vocal process and a C-shaped wedge from the posterior area of one vocal cord. While this technique yields excellent reproducibility of results, it is best reserved for cases where airway restriction is mild or modest.[37] If satisfactory results are not obtained, the procedure can be repeated or a cordectomy performed on the contralateral side.

VOCAL CORD PARALYSIS IN CHILDREN

Vocal cord paralysis accounts for 10 per cent of congenital laryngeal anomalies in children and is the second most common cause of stridor in the neonate.[38] Some authors observe a slight predominance of ULVCP in children, whereas others report a higher frequency of BLVCP in the paediatric setting.[38,39] BLVCP usually manifests in the neonatal period and, in addition to stridor and airway difficulty, is associated with a breathy cry, feeding difficulties and aspiration. The principal causes of neonatal BLVCP are neurological, birth trauma (especially with forceps, breach, or vertex delivery) and idiopathic. Arnold-Chiari malformation is the classical neurological cause of BLVCP and is caused by herniating contents of the posterior fossa exhibiting direct pressure on the vagus nerve as it exits the skull base.[40] An MRI scan is diagnostic once the airway has been secured. In all cases of BLVCP, airway compromise is the pre-eminent concern, and some children will ultimately require tracheostomy.

While the true incidence of ULVCP in the paediatric setting is unknown, ULVCP is more commonly observed in infants and older children. The aetiology differs from that observed in adults with iatrogenic causes accounting for most cases.[41] Cardiothoracic surgery to correct patent ductus arteriosus is reported as the most common iatrogenic precipitant, followed by traumatic and neurological causes and more rarely inflammatory and neoplastic processes.[42,43] Spontaneous recovery of vocal cord paralysis has been shown to occur in a significant number of cases. Rosin et al. observed a 16 per cent recovery in bilateral cases and 63 per cent of unilateral cases in the paediatric setting.[44] Given the chance of spontaneous recovery, particularly of ULVCP, many authors advocate conservative management in the initial setting.[7]

CONCLUSION

The aetiology of vocal cord paralysis is varied, and it is imperative that otolaryngologists are well versed in laryngeal anatomy and the disparate etiologies that may contribute to unilateral or bilateral vocal cord paralysis. The approach to ULVCP is usually conservative, with voice quality and the exclusion of malignant pathology the foremost concern, whereas in cases of BLVCP the airway will be the preeminent issue. It is important to remember that vocal cord paralysis should be considered as a physical finding and not a diagnosis in and of itself. The timing of surgical intervention, if any, will ultimately depend on patient circumstances, recovery potential and the severity of symptoms.

KEY LEARNING POINTS

- Vocal cord palsy is a manifestation of disease and not a diagnosis.
- Unilateral vocal cord palsy is more common than bilateral vocal cord palsy.
- Surgical procedures associated with vocal cord palsy include cervical and thoracic skull base surgery and endotracheal intubation.
- Bilateral vocal cord palsy may present with airway compromise. Patients with unilateral vocal cord palsy should have CT and MRI from skull base to the diaphragm.

REFERENCES

1. Tucker HM. *Anatomy of the Larynx*. In: *The Larynx*. New York: Thieme Medical Publishers, 1993.
2. Miller RH, Rosenfield DB. Hoarseness and vocal cord paralysis. In: *Head and Neck Surgery – Otolaryngology*. Philadelphia: J. B. Lippincott, 1993.
3. Terris DJ, Arnstein DP, Nguyen HH. Contemporary evaluation of unilateral vocal cord paralysis. *Otolaryngology – Head and Neck Surgery*. 1992 Jul; 107(1): 84-90.
4. Willatt DW, Stell PM. Vocal cord paralysis. In: *Otolaryngology*. Philadelphia: W.B. Saunders, 1991.
5. Maisel RH, Ogura J. Evaluation of vocal cord paralysis. *Laryngoscope*. 1974; 84: 302–16.
6. Flowers RH, Kernodle DS. Vagal mononeuritis caused by herpes simplex virus: association with unilateral vocal cord paralysis. *American Journal of Medicine*. 1990; 88: 686–88.
7. Sulica L. The natural history of idiopathic unilateral vocal cord paralysis: Evidence and problems. *Laryngoscope*. 2008 Jul; 118(7): 1303–7.
8. Chen HC, Jen YM, Wang CH, et al. Etiology of vocal cord paralysis. ORL *Journal for Oto-rhino-laryngology and Its Related Specialties*. 2007: 69(3): 167–71.
9. Hillel AD, Benninger M, Blitzer A, et al. Evaluation and management of bilateral vocal cord immobility. *Otolaryngology – Head and Neck Surgery*. 1999; 120: 760–65.
10. Sataloff RT, Bough ID, Spiegel JR. Arytenoid dislocation: Diagnosis and treatment. *Laryngoscope*. 1994; 104: 1353–61.
11. Isshiki N, Morita H, Okamura H, et al. Thyroplasty as a new phonosurgical technique. *Acta Otolaryngologica*. 1974 Nov-Dec; 78(5–6): 451–57.
12. Kellman RM, Leopold DA. Paradoxical vocal cord motion: An important cause of stridor. *Laryngoscope*. 1982 Jan; 92(1): 58–60.
13. Altman KW, Mirza N, Ruiz C. Paradoxical vocal fold motion: Presentation and treatment options. *Journal of Voice*. 2000 Mar; 14(1): 99–103.
14. Koufman JA. Approach to the patient with a voice disorder. *Otolaryngologic Clinics of North America*. 1991 Oct; 24(5): 989–98.
15. Sercarz JA, Berke GS, Ming Y. Videostroboscopy of human vocal fold paralysis. *Annals of Otology, Rhinology and Laryngology*. 1992 Jul; 101(7): 567–77.
16. Koufman JA, Postma GN, Whang SC, et al. Diagnostic laryngeal electromyography: The Wake Forest experience: 1995–1999. *Otolaryngology – Head and Neck Surgery*. 1992; 124: 603–6.
17. Eskander A, Fung K, Mc Bride S, et al. Current practices in the management of adductor spasmodic dysphonia. *Otolaryngology – Head and Neck Surgery*. 2010 Oct; 39(5): 622–30.
18. Koufman JA, Walker FO. Laryngeal electromyography in clinical practice: Indications, techniques, and interpretation. *Phonoscope*. 1998; 1: 57–70.
19. Simpson CB, Amin MR. Office-based procedures for the voice. *Ear, Nose and Throat Journal*. 2004; 83(Suppl2): 10–12.
20. Mallur PS, Rosen CA. Vocal fold injection: Review of indications, techniques and materials for augmentation. *Clinical and Experimental Otorhinolaryngology*. 2010 Dec; 3(4): 177–82.
21. Kasperbauer JL, Slavit DH, Maragos NE. Teflon granulomas and overinjection of Teflon: A therapeutic challenge for the otorhinolaryngologist. *Annals of Otology, Rhinology and Laryngology*. 1993 Oct; 102(10): 748–51.
22. Hartl DM, Hans S, Crevier-Buchman L, et al. Long-term acoustic comparison of thyroplasty versus autologous fat injection. *Annals of Otology, Rhinology and Laryngology*. 2009 Dec; 118(12): 827–32.
23. Sanderson JD, Simpson CB. Laryngeal complications after lipoinjection for vocal fold augmentation. *Laryngoscope*. 2009 Aug; 119(8): 1652–57.
24. Friedman AD, Burns JA, Heaton JT, et al. Early versus late injection medialization for unilateral vocal cord paralysis. *Laryngoscope*. 2010 Oct; 120: 2042–46.

25. Benninger MS, Gillen JB, Altman JS. Changing etiology of vocal fold immobility. *Laryngoscope*. 1998 Sept; 108: 1346–50.
26. Carroll TL, Rosen CA. Long-term results of calcium hydroxylapatite for vocal fold augmentation. *Laryngoscope*. 2011 Feb; 121(2): 313–19.
27. Dursun G, Boynukalin S, Ozgursoy OB. Long-term results of different treatment modalities for glottic insufficiency. *American Journal of Otolaryngology*. 2008 Jan–Feb; 29(1): 7–12.
28. Ustundag E, Boyaci Z, Keskin G. Soft tissue response of the larynx to silicone, Gore-tex, and irradiated cartilage implants. *Laryngoscope*. 2005 Jun; 115(6): 1009–14.
29. Bielamowicz S. Perspectives on medialization laryngoplasty. *Otolaryngology Clinics of North America*. 2004 Feb; 37(1): 139–60.
30. Young VN, Zullo TG, Rosen CA. Analysis of laryngeal framework surgery: 10-year follow-up to a national survey. *Laryngoscope*. 2010 Aug; 120(8): 1602–8.
31. Tucker HM. Selective reinnervation of paralyzed musculature in the head and neck: Functioning autotransplantation of the canine larynx. *Laryngoscope*. 1978 Jan; 88(1 Pt 1): 162–71.
32. El-Kashlan HK, Carroll WR, Hogikyan ND. Selective cricothyroid muscle reinnervation by muscle-nerve-muscle neurotization. *Archives of Otolaryngology – Head & Neck Surgery*. 2001 Oct; 127(10): 1211–15.
33. Young VN, Rosen CA. Arytenoid and posterior vocal fold surgery for bilateral vocal fold immobility. *Current Opinion in Otolaryngology & Head and Neck Surgery*. 2011 Dec; 19(6): 422–27.
34. Gupta AK, Mann SB, Nagarkar N. Surgical management of bilateral immobile vocal folds and long-term follow-up. *Journal of Laryngology and Otology*. 1997 May; 111(5): 474–77.
35. Eckel HE, Thumfart M, Wassermann K. Cordectomy versus arytenoidectomy in the management of bilateral vocal cord paralysis. *Annals of Otology, Rhinology and Laryngology*. 1994 Nov; 103 (11): 852–57.
36. Szmeja Z, Wojtowicz JG. Laser arytenoidectomy in the treatment of bilateral vocal cord paralysis. *European Archives if Otorhinolaryngology*. 1999; 256(8): 388–9.
37. Manolopoulos L, Stavroulaki, Yiotakis J. CO2 and KTP-532 laser cordectomy for bilateral vocal cord paralysis. *Journal of Laryngology and Otology*. 1999 Jul; 113(7): 637–41.
38. Daya H, Hosni A, Bejar-Solar I, et al. Pediatric vocal fold paralysis. *Archives of Otolaryngology – Head & Neck Surgery*. 2000; 126: 21–25.
39. Gentile RD, Miller RH, Woodson GE. Vocal cord paralysis in children 1 year of age and younger. *Annals of Otology, Rhinology and Laryngology*. 1986; 95: 622–25.
40. Murty GE, Shinkwin C, Gibbin KP. Bilateral vocal fold paralysis in infants: Tracheostomy or not? *Journal of Laryngology and Otology*. 1994; 108: 329–31.
41. Zbar RIS, Smith RJH. Vocal cord paralysis in infants twelve months of age and younger. *Otolaryngology – Head & Neck Surgery*. 1996; 114: 18–21.
42. Cohen SR, Geller KA, Birns JW, et al. Laryngeal paralysis in children: A long-term perspective study. *Annals of Otology, Rhinology and Laryngology*. 1982; 91: 417–24.
43. Wolfe RR, Boucek M, Schaeffer MS, et al. *Cardiovascular Disease*. In: *Current Pediatric Diagnosis and Treatment*. 12th ed. New Jersey: Lange Medical Books, 1995; 544–607.
44. Roisin DF, Handler SD, Potsic WP. Vocal cord paralysis in children. *Laryngoscope*. 1990; 100: 1174–79.

34

Laryngo-tracheal trauma

ANDREW HARRIS AND SANJAI SOOD

Injury to the larynx and trachea are rare but serious, life-threatening events. It is estimated that less than 1 per cent of trauma seen in the emergency department includes an upper airway injury.[1] A high index of suspicion is essential to identify laryngo-tracheal injury. Therefore, it is essential for the otolaryngologist to have a clear understanding of the assessment and management of upper airway injury as the condition is unlikely to be seen often by a single practitioner. This chapter aims to give the reader an overview of the mechanisms and sequalae of injury to the larynx and trachea, as well as the management options from a practical perspective.

Laryngeal and tracheal trauma can be both internal as well as external. Both pose a highly challenging situation to the clinician with possible life-threatening sequelae, along with possible long-term morbidity from poor voice or dependency on tracheostomy. It is beyond the remit of this chapter to discuss other injuries to the neck. However, one must appreciate in cases of laryngeal or tracheal injury that coexisting injuries to the pharynx, oesophagus, upper chest, thyroid gland, salivary gland, nerves and large vessels are common and must be considered during the assessment of these patients.

CLASSIFICATION

There are several ways to classify trauma to the larynx and trachea:

1. Anatomical – supraglottis/glottis/subglottis
2. Mechanism – blunt or penetrating injury
3. Zonal division – Roon and Christiansen originally described this in 1979,[2] details of which are given in Table 34.1.

Injury to the trachea and larynx falls into zones 1 and 2, respectively. The descriptive use of zones allows clinicians to understand which anatomical structures and hence which clinical problems may occur with trauma to each of the areas. It must be appreciated that trauma can extend beyond a single zone, especially in penetrative injuries.

Table 34.1 Zonal division of cervical trauma

Zone	Anatomical boundaries
1	Extends from clavicle to cricoid cartilage
2	Extends from cricoid cartilage to angle of mandible
3	Extends from angle of mandible to base of skull

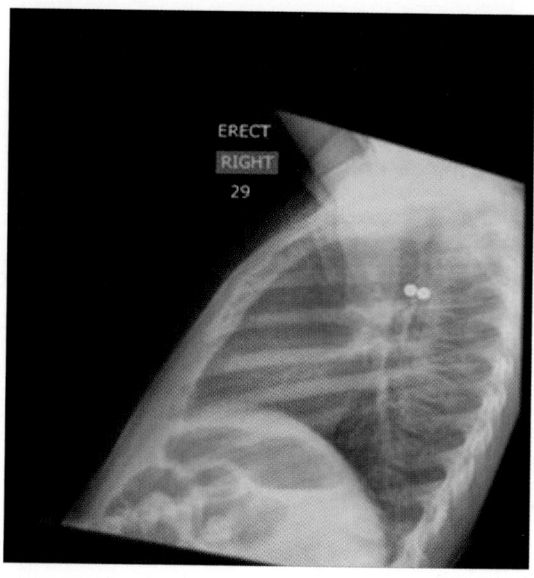

Figure 34.1 Lateral chest x-ray illustrating a foreign body that has eroded the posterior tracheal wall. A lateral chest x-ray is mandatory when assessing foreign bodies. Figure courtesy of Professor Henry Pau.

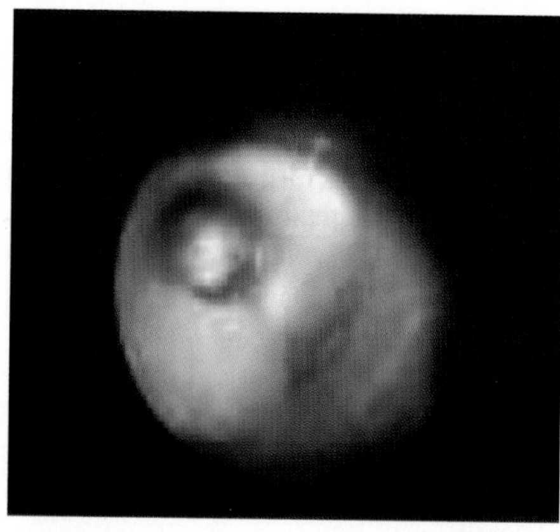

Figure 34.2 Bronchoscopy view of the foreign body seen on the chest x-ray in Figure 34.1. Figure courtesy of Professor Henry Pau.

AETIOLOGY

The incidence of trachea and larynx injury is greater in men than in women. This is in part due to a greater participation of men in contact sports. The introduction of seat belt laws and improved vehicle safety features such as airbags has led to a decrease in incidence from road traffic accidents.

The mortality from blunt trauma is considered to be higher than that from penetrating trauma. However, it is impossible to obtain accurate figures due to a significant number of deaths occurring as a result of multiple injuries at the site of the trauma. The mechanisms of trauma are outlined below:

1. Penetrating injury: for example, knife injury, gunshot wound, wires. Such injuries have a higher risk of associated oesophageal injuries.
2. Blunt injury: for example, road traffic accident, blow to the neck (contact sports) or strangulation. Blunt injuries may be further classed into low-velocity or high-velocity. It is important to appreciate that even in the absence of any external signs, internal laryngeal injury may still have occurred.
3. Internal injury: inhalation of foreign bodies (Figures 34.1 and 34.2) or caustic substances, which is usually seen in young children who accidently swallow chemical agents (e.g. weedkiller). These chemicals cause burns to the upper airway, producing oedema, mucosal haemorrhage and ultimately tissue loss. This chapter will focus on external trauma, but the principles of management of the airway remain the same for inhalation injuries to the larynx.

PATHOPHYSIOLOGY

Laryngeal fractures are relatively rare as the larynx is a mobile and elastic organ, and it is also protected by the mandible and sternum. During blunt

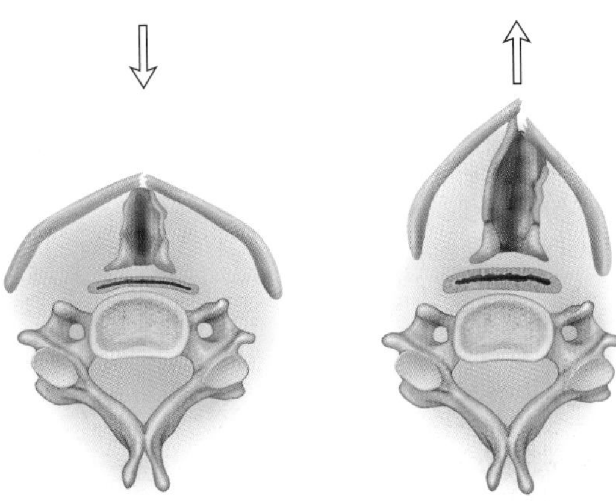

Figure 34.3 Two phases of blunt trauma to the larynx in the younger patient. Initially, the larynx is compressed against the vertebral column and is fractured along the prominence. The larynx then springs back into position. However, the vocal cords are detached at their anterior ends.

trauma, depending on the force of injury, the larynx is compressed against the cervical spine and then springs forward (Figure 34.3). This is especially true in younger patients (less than 40 years of age) as older patients generally have a calcified larynx, which is more likely to break or 'shatter' when force is applied (Figure 34.4).[3]

Blunt trauma may cause haemorrhage into the mucosa and deeper structures along with possible laceration and avulsion of tissue. This will lead to further swelling, bleeding and possible tissue fragments emerging into the laryngeal lumen. A simple way to understand blunt airway emergencies is to consider the larynx as a box. Trauma causes swelling, which will occur inside the box, thus reducing the airway. High-velocity blunt trauma can fracture the laryngeal skeleton as described above (Figures 34.3 and 34.4). In extreme force the tendon of the anterior commissure is ruptured along with the attachment petiole of the epiglottis (as would be the case in a thyroid prominence fracture, Figure 34.3). In such cases the vocal cords roll back on themselves and the epiglottis may fall back into the airway.[4] In severe cases the larynx can be sheared from the trachea at the level of the cricoid[5] (Figure 34.5).

It is imperative to note that with trauma to the larynx and trachea, other structures may be injured, e.g. in approximately 8 per cent of moderate to severe laryngeal injuries, the cervical spine

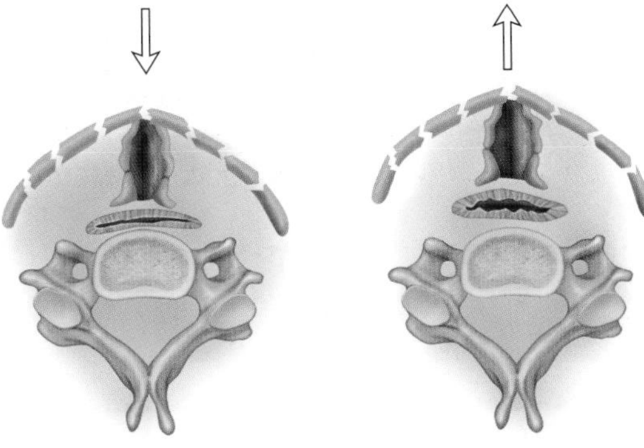

Figure 34.4 Blunt trauma to the larynx in older patients where the thyroid cartilage has ossified. The initial impact shatters the larynx, which cannot recoil. The neck is flattened and the airway is reduced.

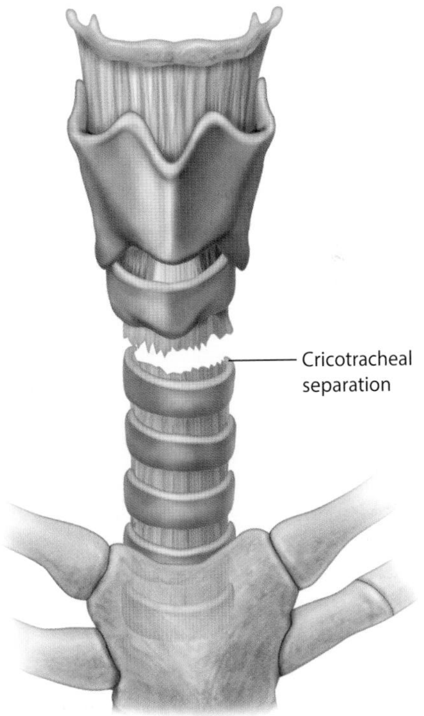

Figure 34.5 Shearing of the cricoid cartilage from the trachea.

is fractured.[6] Oesophageal injuries can also occur readily with laryngo-tracheal trauma, so other symptoms such as dysphagia and odynophagia may also be present. This is an important issue as laryngo-tracheal injuries may be underdiagnosed in the presence of multiple traumas where other presenting injuries may overshadow that of the upper airway, which can lead to serious consequences for the patient.

HISTORY AND EXAMINATION

There are three main symptoms to trauma of the upper airway: dysphonia, dyspnoea and stridor. The force and mechanism of trauma will dictate the injuries; this may be purely oedema, which typically reaches its maximal peak around 12 hours after the injury. These patients may have mild dysphonia and possibly neck pain (secondary to the trauma) as their only presenting symptoms. Coughing can also occur owing to damage to the internal larynx and secretions such as blood. Bleeding into the upper airway can also cause haemoptysis. Pain in the region should also alert the clinician to a possible laryngeal fracture.

Signs of upper airway trauma are bruising, tenderness, surgical emphysema, deformed contour of the laryngeal framework and granulations over injured cartilage.[7] Tables 34.2 and 34.3 summarize the symptoms and signs of laryngo-tracheal trauma.

The first part of the examination should be to carefully assess the airway. Several factors may in isolation or together lead to airway compromise. Bleeding into the laryngeal lumen may occur, along with fragments (such as cartilage) protruding into the lumen, and oedema. Blood in the larynx also causes spasm of the vocal cords, which further compromises the laryngeal lumen. Oedema develops over time (minutes to hours), so symptoms on first presentation may not indicate how perilous the airway may become.

Table 34.2 Symptoms of laryngo-tracheal trauma

Dysphonia
Dyspnoea
Stridor
Pain
Coughing

Table 34.3 Signs of laryngo-tracheal trauma

Bruising
Tenderness
Surgical emphysema
Abnormal contour of larynx
Granulations over cartilage

It is essential to perform a full examination of the neck. If it is deemed safe (see later discussion), then the airway should be inspected using flexible transnasal laryngoscopy, which should be done by an experienced otolaryngologist. Figures 34.6 and 34.7 depict normal and abnormal views on transnasal laryngoscopy. As these patients often have multiple injuries, it is essential to include examination of other viscera in the neck. Usually, the emergency medicine physicians will have performed a comprehensive trauma screen examination, but it is important for the otolaryngologist

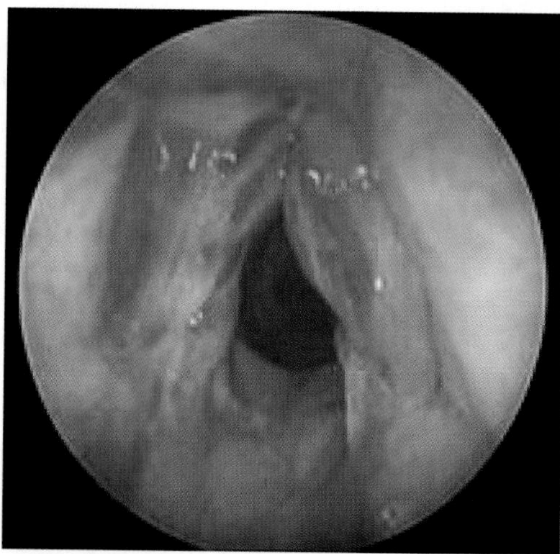

Figure 34.6 A normal larynx as viewed on flexible nasendoscopy. It can be appreciated that any blood, cartilage, oedema or disruption such as arytenoid dislocation will narrow this lumen, producing symptoms such as stridor, dyspnea and altered voice.

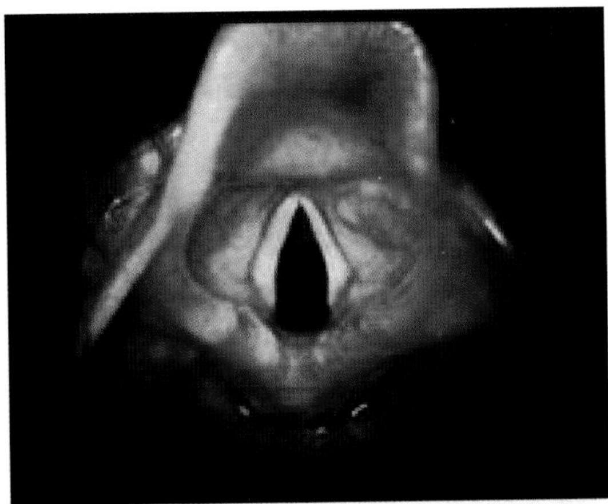

Figure 34.7 The vocal cords are oedematous and swollen with bleeding into Reinke's space.

to ensure that this has been done and note any associated injuries. Surgical emphysema is a cardinal sign of airway breach and must be investigated carefully.

AIRWAY AND GENERAL MANAGEMENT

The priority is to ensure that the patient has a safe and secure airway. A senior otolaryngologist and anaesthetist together should manage the airway. Initial management options include the following:

1. Observation in a hospital for a minimum period of 24 hours. In cases with minimal oedema on laryngeal examination, a course of intravenous steroids with observation on a high-dependency ward is a reasonable course of management. Such patients would generally be classed as group I in Schaefer's classification (see Table 34.4).
2. Surgical tracheostomy under local anaesthetic. This is considered by many to be 'the gold standard' in terms of securing an airway.
3. Endotracheal intubation. This should be done under direct supervision by an experienced anaesthetist. 'Blind intubation' is not recommended as it may lead to more damage to the laryngeal structure and if unsuccessful may lead to a very compromised airway. Use of cricoid pressure to help view at intubation is contraindicated to an already disrupted larynx.

Tracheostomy under local anaesthetic has some advantages. First, patients who are conscious will try to maintain their own airway, but if given sedative medication they may not, which then poses a risk of losing the airway in cases of failed attempts to intubate. A second advantage is the fact that whilst flexible laryngoscopy has been performed, the state of injuries may be difficult to assess with

Table 34.4 Schaefer's classification of acute upper airway injury and the management

Group	Symptoms	Signs	Management
Grade I	Minor airway symptoms	Minimal haematoma, small lacerations, no detectable fractures	Observe, humidified oxygen, possible steroids
Grade II	Airway compromise	Oedema, haematoma, minor mucosal disruption, no cartilage exposure	Direct laryngoscopy with oesophagoscopy, possible tracheostomy, possible steroids
Grade III	Airway compromise	Oedema, mucosal tears, exposed cartilage, vocal cord immobility	Tracheostomy, direct laryngoscopy with oesophagoscopy, exploration and repair, no stent necessary
Grade IV	Airway compromise	Massive oedema, significant mucosal tears, exposed cartilage, vocal cord immobility	Tracheostomy, direct laryngoscopy with oesophagoscopy, exploration and repair. Stent needed.

blood, oedema and the patient coughing. In these cases intubation may worsen the anatomical injuries along with worsening the situation if it fails. As a general principle patients with mild to moderate injuries should be transferred to the operating theatre where an experienced anaesthetist should try to intubate the patient in the presence of an otolaryngologist prepared to perform an emergency tracheostomy should intubation fail. In the case of a high-velocity injury (severe trauma) where the larynx has been split or shattered, there is a definite argument for tracheostomy under local anaesthetic being the first line management of the airway. In patients where there is any doubt to the state of the airway and symptoms are increasing in severity, a secure airway via intubation is a priority with a low threshold for tracheostomy.

Once the airway is secure, high-resolution computer tomography (CT) scanning should be undertaken along with possible pharyngo-laryngoscopy if anomalies are detected (Figure 34.8).

Once the airway has been secured and any scans have been undertaken, the patient can and should then undergo suspension micro-laryngoscopy and rigid pharyngo-oesophagoscopy to assess the extent of injuries. This must be done by an experienced otolaryngologist. Penetrating injuries (stabbings) to the larynx (giving an airway breach) will produce

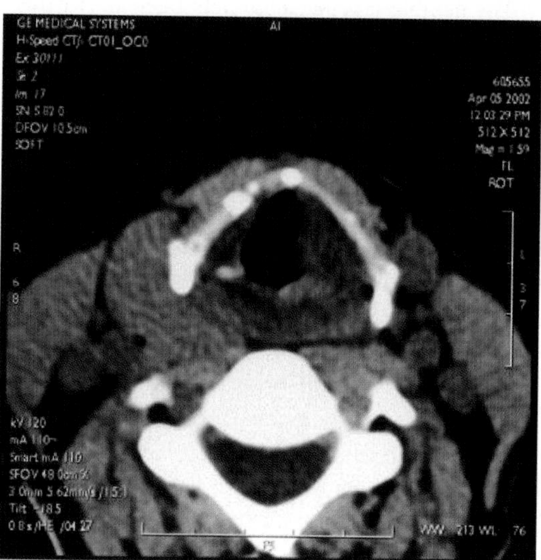

Figure 34.8 CT scan (axial view) demonstrating granuloma formation over the left vocal cord.

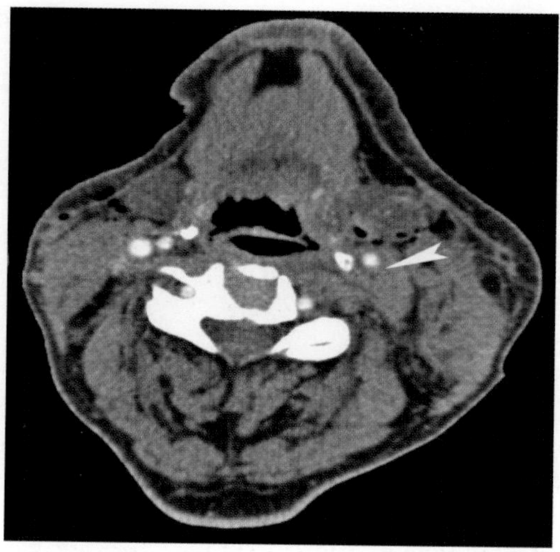

Figure 34.9 CT scan (axial view) demonstrating air bubbles in the neck. Surgical emphysema was evident on clinical examination.

the finding of crepitus (surgical emphysema) on neck examination (Figure 34.9).

Penetrating injuries will generally be diverted by the thyroid cartilage to either the thyrohyoid membrane above or the cricothyroid membrane below, as the blade usually 'slides' on the thyroid cartilage.[7] In cases of penetrating trauma, neck exploration is mandatory and the risk of intubation is less. Hence patients with these injuries are more readily intubated and taken to theatre where exploration and direct closure of tracheal and laryngeal injuries are performed. It is also important to examine the exit wound of the injury.

PRINCIPLES OF MANAGEMENT OF LARYNGEAL FRACTURES

Hyoid bone fracture occurs in strangulating injuries or blunt force injuries such as in karate. In itself a hyoid fracture warrants no treatment. These patients usually have exquisite pain on swallowing, and an internal inspection of the larynx should be performed to delineate other injuries. A bursa may form at the site of the break. This will cause malunion and may need excision, although this would be at a later stage as an elective procedure.[7]

High-velocity blunt injuries may lead to thyroid cartilage fracture. This should be treated by open reduction and fixation with (mini) plates or wire if needed. Any associated soft tissue injuries to the larynx should be repaired if possible (including mucosal tears), and, if necessary, vocal cords that have lost attachment anteriorly to the thyroid cartilage should be re-suspended. It is important to cover exposed cartilage with mucosa or perichondrium to minimize granulation tissue formation and long-term scarring.

Non-displaced laryngeal fractures may be treated expectantly. Any degree of displacement should be reduced and fixed; otherwise, impaired function will ensue. In cases where webbing is likely, adhesions forming between two areas on either side of the laryngeal lumen, a stent can be sutured into position with a covering tracheostomy. The stent should be removed in theatre typically after 10 to 14, days and the patient can often be decannulated (tracheostomy removed) at the same time. These injuries need to be corrected as soon as possible (ideally within 48 hours); otherwise, long-term sequalae are more likely.[8] Table 34.4 summarizes the management of laryngeal trauma as per Schaefer's classification.[9]

LONG-TERM COMPLICATIONS

Any trauma can lead to haematoma formation, and further organization can lead to fibrosis, scarring and webbing. Patients with laryngeal trauma can have long-term problems with phonation and breathing, ultimately needing tracheostomy. Inability to protect the airway (aspiration) may also mean long-term tracheostomy. These patients may have a narrower airway, either owing to structural damage or vocal cord palsy as a result of trauma to the recurrent laryngeal nerve. Another important potential complication is subglottic stenosis, which may form as a result of the initial trauma or as a consequence of medical intervention such as a 'high' tracheostomy (through the cricoid cartilage or first tracheal ring) or a prolonged period of intubation. Management of subglottic stenosis is challenging and should be done in specialized centres. The details are beyond the remit of this chapter but in principle range from serial dilations to resection of the stenotic segment with appropriate reconstruction.

SUMMARY

Trauma to the larynx and trachea is rare. However, such injuries need to be treated with great respect and experienced airway practitioners sought as soon as feasibly possible. These patients may have little to no airway signs at the site of trauma, and other coexisting injuries, such as overt bleeding from a chest injury, may occupy the minds of the treating team. It may not be apparent an upper airway injury has occurred until symptoms from laryngeal oedema develop some hours later or the patient fails extubation after successful surgery on another anatomical site. In contrast, other patients may have marked symptoms, such as stridor at the trauma scene, and will require swift, decisive and often courageous attempts by non-airway specialists to secure the airway as a matter of urgency. Once the airway is secured and anatomical injury has been assessed and dealt with, these patients can still have lifelong morbidity in a personal, social and employment setting from necessitating long-term tracheostomy or voice disorders.

The acute dangers and potential great morbidity from such injuries necessitate a team approach by experienced practitioners with a good understanding of the diagnosis and treatment of laryngotracheal injury. Early treatment comprises securing the airway and giving consideration to the voice. Early appropriate intervention is generally recommended to minimize long-term adverse sequelae including laryngeal scarring and subglottic stenosis.

KEY LEARNING POINTS

- The incidence of tracheal and laryngeal trauma is greater in men than in women.
- Laryngeal fractures are rare as the larynx is mobile and an elastic organ.
- Blunt trauma may compress the larynx against the cervical spine.

- Priority is to ensure that the patient has a safe and secure airway.
- 'Blind intubation' is to be avoided as it may lead to more damage to the laryngeal structures and if unsuccessful may lead to a very compromised airway.
- Schaefer's classification of upper airway injury helps in management.

REFERENCES

1. Gussack GS, Jurkovich GJ, Luterman A. Laryngotracheal trauma: A protocol approach to a rare injury. *Laryngoscope.* 1986; 96: 660–65.
2. Roon AJ, Christensen N. Evaluation and treatment of penetrating cervical injuries. *Journal of Trauma.* 1979; 19: 391–97.
3. Hussain, SM. *Laryngotracheal Trauma.* In *Logan Turner's Diseases of the Ear, Nose and Throat.* Boca Raton, FL: CRC Press, 1987.
4. Maran AGD. *Trauma and Stenosis of the Larynx.* In: *Scott-Brown's Otolaryngology.* 6th ed., Volume 5. Oxford: Butterworth Heinemann, 1997: 5/8/1–5/8/11.
5. Wu MH, Tsai YF, Lin MY, Hsu IL, Fong Y. Complete laryngotracheal disruption caused by blunt injury. *Annals of Thoracic Surgery.* 2004; 77: 1211–15.
6. Jewitt BS, Shockley WW, Rutledge R. External laryngeal trauma analysis of 392 patients. *Archives of Otolaryngology – Head and Neck Surgery.* 1999; 125: 877–80.
7. Pitkin L. *Laryngeal Trauma and Stenosis.* In: *Scott-Brown's Otorhinolaryngology, Head and Neck Surgery.* 7th ed., Volume 2. London: Hodder, 2008: 2271–85.
8. Bent JP, Silver JR, Porubsky ES. Acute laryngeal trauma: A review of 77 patients. *Otolaryngology and Head and Neck Surgery.* 1993; 109: 441–49.
9. Schaefer SD. Primary management of laryngeal trauma. *Annals of Otology, Rhinology and Laryngology.* 1982; 91: 399–402.

35

Tracheostomy

JOHN DEMPSTER

A tracheotomy is the creation of an opening into the trachea. A tracheostomy implies that this opening has a connection to an opening in the skin, i.e. the formation of a stoma. Historically, the procedure appears to have been depicted on Egyptian tablets in approximately 3600 BC. The early operations were associated with a very high mortality and became an established technique only in the nineteenth century when a large number were performed on patients suffering from diphtheria.

The overall literature on the procedure is extensive, and a significant percentage deal either with a paediatric population or with percutaneous procedures. This chapter will discuss tracheostomies that can be temporary and reversed/closed if required and will deal with the technique as it applies to an adult population. The chapter will not discuss the permanent, non-reversible tracheostomy that is performed as part of a laryngectomy.

This chapter should be read in conjunction with Chapter 59 on paediatric tracheostomy.

ANATOMY

The important anatomical structures in the neck should be palpated prior to the procedure. These include the lamina of the thyroid cartilage, usually easily identified in the central compartment of the neck by an obvious notch on its superior border. Inferior to the thyroid lamina is the crico-thyroid membrane and, in turn, the cricoid cartilage. This is a complete ring of cartilage and forms a prominent band. The trachea is attached to its inferior border and is a cartilaginous/membranous tube extending into the mediastinum and bifurcating at the carina. Posteriorly, the tracheal wall is membranous with the anterolateral walls being incomplete cartilagenous rings.

INDICATIONS FOR TRACHEOSTOMY

The list of potential conditions that may necessitate a tracheostomy is wide and differs between adult and paediatric populations. Today, the majority of tracheostomies in adults are performed electively, and this probably accounts for in excess of 85 per cent of cases. The literature suggests that the most common indication is patients in an intensive care setting who are undergoing prolonged mechanical ventilation. The list of underlying illnesses that would lead to that is extensive and includes – amongst other conditions – critical illness due to surgery and its complications, and head injury. The exact timing of such surgery is also debated but should be considered if ventilation continues for more that 14 days. Tracheostomy allows for pulmonary toilet by tracheal suctioning, should reduce the risk of aspiration and may facilitate the weaning of these patients from mechanical respiratory support. These elective tracheostomies may be of the conventional surgical type, but increasing numbers of percutaneous tracheostomies performed by either intensive care physicians or anaesthetists are undertaken.

Elective tracheostomy may also be performed as a planned event during major head and neck surgery to allow protection of the airway from bleeding and/or post-operative oedema and to eliminate endotracheal tubes from the operative field. Rarely, but effectively, it will solve significant sleep apnoea.

An emergency tracheostomy is therefore relatively uncommon. The most likely cause is upper airway obstruction, where a tracheostomy will bypass the obstruction and restore the patient's breathing. The list of pathologies that can obstruct the airway is large and includes anaphylaxis/angioneurotic oedema, infective pathology such as deep neck space infections or acute epiglottitis, neoplasia such as advanced laryngeal cancer, subglottic stenosis, and glottic stenosis due to bilateral vocal cord palsy and trauma (i.e. to the laryngeal framework or major facial injuries). An emergency tracheostomy will almost certainly be an open surgical operation performed by an ear, nose and throat (ENT) surgeon and is the default in a life-threatening situation. However, depending on the cause and severity of the upper airway obstruction, alternative interventions such as a percutaneous tracheostomy, a crico-thyroidotomy or intubation should be considered.

PROCEDURE FOR TRACHEOSTOMY

The procedure is much easier and less stressful for both patient and surgeon if done under a general anaesthetic. However, if there are contraindications to this, local anaesthesia (lignocaine 1 per cent with adrenaline 1:80 000) can be used and is injected into the skin and subcutaneous tissues overlying the trachea in the neck. Unless the situation is exceptional, it should be performed in an operating theatre on an operating table with appropriate theatre lights and supporting staff. One or preferably two assistants are required. The patient should be supine with the neck extended as much as is feasible. It is worthwhile marking on the skin the important landmarks in the neck, i.e. the laryngeal framework, the cricoid cartilage and the trachea. These can be quite difficult to feel in an obese neck and in females who have less prominent thyroid cartilage. The incision can be midline and vertical from the cricoid cartilage down to the supra-sternal notch (Figure 35.1), or horizontal midway between these two landmarks. There is no evidence that a vertical scar will lead to a poorer cosmetic outcome than a horizontal one. Should a horizontal incision be made, superior and inferior skin flaps must be elevated; this is not necessary in a vertical approach.

The trachea is a midline structure and the dissection should then proceed in the midline by identifying the midline raphe and separating the strap muscles (sternohyoid and sternothyroid), which are then retracted laterally along with the anterior jugular veins. Deep to the strap muscles within the investing fascia will be the thyroid isthmus. This typically crosses the second and third tracheal rings but is variable in size. As it lies directly on top

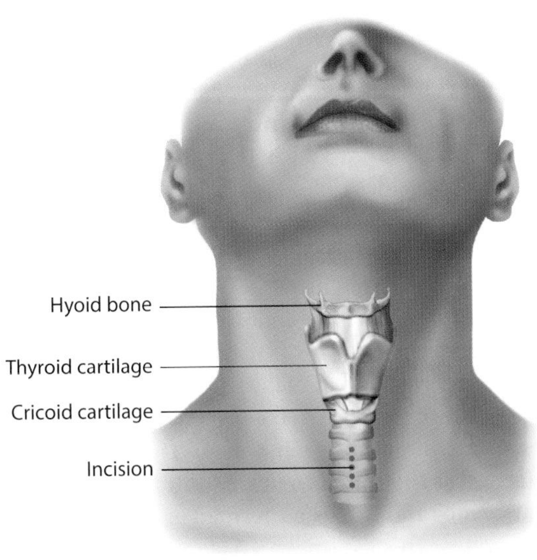

Figure 35.1 Diagram of site of vertical skin incision.

of the preferred site for the tracheotomy, it should be divided. Failure to do so leaves the potential for the isthmus to fall over and occlude the tracheotomy during early tube changes. The isthmus can be divided using diathermy or alternatively can be clamped, divided and the cut edges oversewn or transfixed. Once divided and any bleeding controlled, the lobes of the gland can be retracted laterally and the trachea will be exposed. If the trachea is low in the neck, it can be very useful to insert a cricoid hook under the inferior aspect of the cricoid and elevate the trachea into the operative site.

Various options then exist for the tracheal opening, but the important principle is to avoid the first tracheal ring. Should the cricoid cartilage or first tracheal ring be damaged, a late complication of subglottic stenosis can occur. In an adult, the cartilage of the tracheal rings can be calcified, and therefore a vertical cut, as is the preferred option in paediatric practice, is not viable. Similarly, a horizontal cut between tracheal rings is unlikely to give safe and satisfactory access. A circle or square of the anterior tracheal wall centred on the second and third tracheal rings is probably the most common opening. This can, however, leave considerable dead space between the skin opening and the tracheal opening, which can be of concern particularly in obese necks. This can be overcome by approximating the edges of the tracheal opening to the skin opening with sutures, as is common in paediatric practice. An alternative method, however, is to utilize a Bjork flap (Figure 35.2). This entails fashioning an inferiorly based *U*-shaped flap of anterior tracheal wall, again typically centred over the second and third tracheal rings. The free edge of the flap can be everted and sutured to the skin on the inferior aspect of the stoma. This eliminates dead space between the skin and

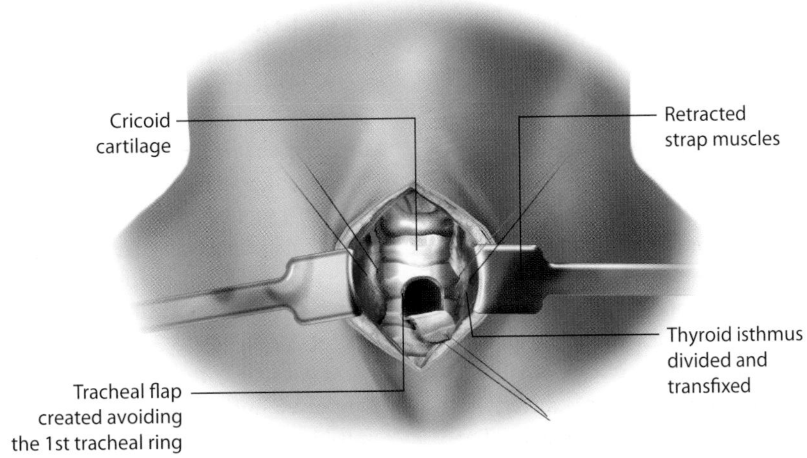

Figure 35.2 Diagram of creation of Bjork flap.

trachea and makes tube insertion and subsequent tube change more straightforward. It should help to eliminate incorrect positioning of the tube in, for example, the pre-tracheal tissues.

At the end of the operation, careful check for haemostasis should be performed, paying particular attention to the anterior jugular veins and the divided thyroid isthmus. The wound should be loosely closed with sutures around the tube, thereby lessening the risk of surgical emphysema. The tube can be secured in place either with ties around the neck or sutured to the skin. The latter may be better practice in the immediate post-operative period where the risk of tube displacement must be minimized. In either case, the tube should be secured with the neck flexed. The wound can be covered with a tracheostomy site dressing, but this is best avoided in the immediate post-operative period, allowing early detection of any bleeding.

PERCUTANEOUS TRACHEOSTOMY

First popularized in the 1980s, percutaneous tracheostomy is based on the placement of a guidewire into the tracheal lumen. This method has advantages and disadvantages over a conventional tracheostomy. It tends to be the domain of intensive care physicians and is a bedside procedure, thereby avoiding the transfer of a potentially unstable patient to the operating theatre. There is no need to have a full operating team, and it is reported in skilled hands to take approximately 15 minutes.

There are several types of percutaneous procedures, but all are reportedly safer if done under continuous fibre-optic guidance with a flexible bronchoscope. In addition, there is evidence that ultrasound control can reduce complications and is advisable if there are concerns regarding possible anatomical abnormalities in the neck. This is particularly relevant if there is vascular pulsation at the site of the proposed procedure. Once percutaneous placement of the guidewire has been performed, ideally between the second and third tracheal rings, several techniques are available. The initial Ciaglia approach utilized multiple dilators to create an opening of sufficient size, but increasingly a revised procedure using a single tapered dilator is favoured and is the most popular technique. Griggs describes the use of dilatational forceps, and the use of a screw-like device to create the opening has been reported. Upon completion of the procedure, correct tube placement should be confirmed by either endoscopic visualization or capnography.

In general, percutaneous tracheostomy is not a procedure for an emergency situation. There is, however, literature from major trauma centres where it is the initial preferred intervention in an emergency and can be performed in approximately 5 minutes. This assumes a great deal of experience and expertise. The conventional contraindications include, other than an emergency situation, awkward anatomy such as difficulty identifying the trachea or a bulky thyroid, an underlying bleeding diatheses, a short neck or obesity. Abnormal vascular pulsations should raise concern, and there are reports of accidental major vessel damage typically to the innominate vein. Any vascular pulsation over the operative area should lead to an ultrasound or, perhaps more appropriately, a change of plan to surgical tracheostomy. It is contraindicated in paediatric practice and relatively contraindicated if there has been previous tracheal/neck surgery or radiotherapy. However, with increasing use and increasing experience and skill, these all become more relative. The procedure will be unsuccessful in approximately 2 per cent of cases and require conversion to a surgical tracheostomy. The complications are outlined in Table 35.1, the list being broadly the same as for an open surgical procedure, although percutaneous tracheostomy may have a lower incidence of wound infection. Recent meta-analysis would suggest that the varying techniques of percutaneous insertion also have similar rates of success and complications. Significant early complications can occur in up to 3 per cent of patients, with a reported late complication rate of 0.7 per cent. It should be noted that intraoperative complications can be severe, indeed fatal, owing to inadvertent vascular injury, for example.

Table 35.1 Complications of surgical tracheostomy

Immediate/operative	Within first 2 weeks	Delayed
Haemorrhage	Tube obstruction	Tracheo-cutaneous fistula
Air embolism	Tube displacement	Subglottic stenosis
Pneumo-thorax	Chest or wound infection	Tracheal stenosis (narrowing >50 per cent of tracheal lumen)
Damage to recurrent laryngeal nerves, cricoid cartilage		Tracheo-malacia
Loss of airway		Trachea-innominate artery fistula

CRICO-THYROID AIRWAY PROCEDURE

As is the case with tracheostomy, crico-thyroidotomy can be an open surgical procedure or performed utilizing a Seldinger-type approach. A conventional surgical crico-thyroidotomy involves inserting a tracheostomy tube into the airway through the crico-thyroid membrane. The membrane is palpable in most necks between the inferior aspect of the thyroid lamina and the upper border of the cricoid cartilage. It is generally faster and simpler than a tracheostomy as the membrane is nearer the skin and there should be no major vessels in the area. As with tracheostomy, local anaesthetic can be used for the procedure. The neck is fully extended, the membrane palpated and a horizontal incision made through the skin and the subcutaneous tissues. This is deepened until the airway is opened horizontally. Tracheal dilators will then be needed to open up the space, allowing further division of the soft tissues to widen access and then allow insertion of a suitable tube.

The Seldinger approach involves the correct placement of a curved small-bore crico-thyroid cannula though the crico-thyroid membrane into the airway under local anaesthesia. The cannulae have a diameter of 13 Fr (inner diameter 2 mm) and when correctly placed in the airway enable the patient to be ventilated with a high-pressure oxygen injector for up to approximately 15 minutes. This gives vital time to secure a more adequate airway. This in itself may entail a conventional tracheostomy, but a Seldinger technique utilizing the cannula to insert a larger bore tube can be undertaken swiftly. Kits containing all the required equipment for both a Seldinger-type crico-thyroidotomy (Figure 35.3) and a surgical crico-thyroidotomy are commercially available.

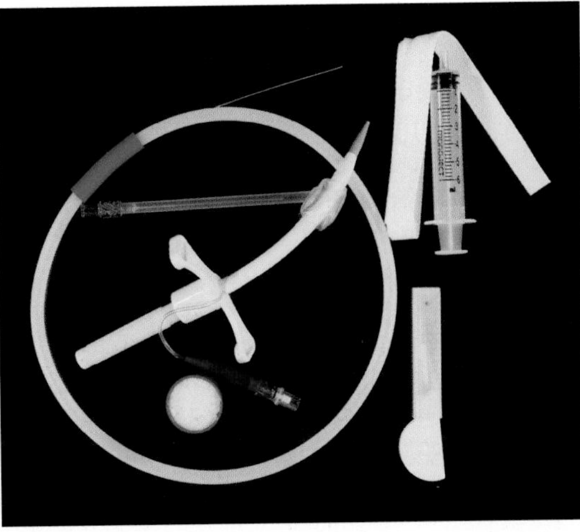

Figure 35.3 Seldinger kit for crico-thyroidotomy.

POST-OPERATIVE CARE AND TRACHEOSTOMY TUBES

Various types of tracheostomy tube are available. They vary in terms of materials (typically silicone or silver), diameters, the presence or absence of a cuff, the presence or absence of a fenestration and whether there is an inner cannula. There are tubes of standard length, longer tubes and tubes with an adjustable flange.

The tube inserted at the time of surgery will be cuffed and non-fenestrated. The patient will be at risk of blood and secretions entering the trachea and the airway will need protection. Additionally, the patient may require ventilation. The typical tube to be inserted in an adult male should have an inner diameter of at least 9 mm, and in an adult female at least 8 mm. It is standard practice to insert a tube that has an inner cannula, as it is safer, and the initial tube should not be removed until the tract from skin to trachea has stabilized, typically in 5 to 7 days. It is important to allow sufficient time for the tracheocutaneous tract to mature and thereby reduce potential complications associated with changing the tube. The most significant of these is incorrect positioning of the tube such that it is no longer in the trachea. It is good practice for the first tube change to be carried out by the surgical team that performed the procedure and for the eventual position to be checked by inserting a flexible laryngoscope down the tube. The changing of the tube over a guidewire as in a Seldinger approach may also facilitate the process.

When the tube is changed, the distal airway may no longer need protection from secretions or blood and the patient may no longer require ventilation. If these conditions exist, a cuffless fenestrated tube may enable the patient to communicate. At all times a tube with an inner cannula should be used. This is of slightly narrower calibre than the outer tube and is marginally longer. It can be removed and cleaned, obviating the need for any unnecessary removal of the outer tube.

It is vital in the early days to avoid accidental de-cannulation. This potentially disastrous event can be reduced by sound surgical technique and tube fixation, along with careful and experienced nursing skill. Post-operative care includes careful monitoring of the airway, regular inspection of the tube to ensure there is no displacement, and regular removal and cleaning of the inner tube to prevent occlusion in conjunction with regular humidification. Secretions, particularly in the early post-operative period, will require removal by gentle suction. Suctioning should be performed using a low vacuum pressure; the suction catheter should be inserted into a non-fenestrated inner cannula and then slowly withdrawn while applying suction. The cuff of the tube should be checked again on a regular basis. It is good practice to have bed head signs displaying essential information such as date of surgery, type of tracheal opening fashioned and size and type of tube inserted. Guidelines also outline the list of recommended bedside equipment, including emergency airway equipment that should be available, in addition to discussing how to assess tracheostomy patency and manage problems that may arise. Clinical consensus statements and guidelines for tracheostomy care are available.

COMPLICATIONS

Complications are an inherent part of any surgical procedure and should be considered prior to finalizing the decision to operate. The complications that can arise – typically classified as operative, early post-operative and late post-operative – are listed in Table 35.1. Typically, a 3–4 per cent figure for operative complications is quoted, and this is likely to be similar regardless of whether a surgical or percutaneous procedure is undertaken. Literature would suggest that the risk of bleeding, major operative complications and long-term complications is similar in the two groups. The most common complication is bleeding, and this is usually of a minor nature.

KEY LEARNING POINTS

- The majority of tracheostomy operations are performed electively, and an increasing proportion of these will be performed percutaneously.
- The main area of debate in an open surgical approach surrounds the type of opening made in the anterior tracheal wall and the use of skin maturation sutures.
- Intensive nursing care during the first 7 post-operative days is of paramount importance.
- ENT surgeons should have a wide knowledge of different techniques and equipment available for accessing the airway in an emergency.

FURTHER READING

Cosgrove JF, Carrie S. Indication for and management of tracheostomies. *Surgery*. 2012; 30(5): 238–43.

McGrath BA, Bates L, Atkinson D, Moore JA. Multidisciplinary guidelines for the management of tracheostomy and laryngectomy airway emergencies. *Anaesthesia*. 2012; 67: 1025–41.

National Tracheostomy Safety Project. www.tracheostomy.org.uk.

36

Neck masses

VINIDH PALERI AND HISHAM MEHANNA

INTRODUCTION

Evaluation of a patient with a neck swelling requires a careful and systematic clinical approach with sound understanding of the anatomical structures of the neck and appreciation of the pathology, which is the focus of this chapter. Neck lumps may be benign or malignant and can be the presenting symptom of loco-regional and/or systemic diseases across all age groups. A comprehensive history and assessment of the characteristics of the neck swelling, including a thorough examination of the upper aerodigestive tract followed by appropriate investigations (cytology/haematology/radiology), will provide the diagnosis in more than 95 per cent of cases. With the above structured approach, open surgical excision of neck masses should almost always be part of the planned treatment rather than a diagnostic step. Treatment of neck lumps, especially if malignant, depends on the underlying disease process, and a detailed discussion is thus outside the scope of this work.

HISTORY

The key points in the history that will help reach a diagnosis are the age of the patient, duration and location of the neck mass. A comprehensive history should explore risk factors and associated symptoms. Dysphonia, sore throat, dysphagia, odynophagia, referred otalgia and nasal obstruction may suggest a neoplasm of the upper aerodigestive tract. Weight loss, anorexia, malaise and night sweats ('B' symptoms) may suggest lymphoma or tuberculosis. Past medical history of exposure to tuberculosis, surgery, irradiation (risk factor for malignancy), occupational/sexual history (e.g. risk factors for human immunodeficiency virus [HIV] infection), foreign travel and contact with pets (e.g. cat scratch disease) are also relevant.

EXAMINATION

The neck masses should be assessed and recorded in a systematic fashion with emphasis on the number, size, site, shape and consistency. Figure 36.1 suggests one such system. It is convenient to use the neck nodal level system to describe the location of lymph node disease in the neck. Level I contains the submental and submandibular nodes. Levels II to IV contain lymph nodes along the jugular chain (upper, middle and lower). Level V contains the lymph nodes located in the occipital and subclavian triangles. The pre- and paratracheal and precricoid (Delphian) nodes are found within level VI (Figure 36.2).

Inspection of the scalp, skin over the face and neck is necessary to look for potential sources of pathology. Otolaryngologists are best placed to evaluate neck masses as clinical examination is incomplete unless the entire mucosa of the upper aerodigestive tract is examined (see Chapters 2 and 18 on investigation of nasal and pharyngeal diseases). This includes endoscopic assessment of the nasal cavity, nasopharynx, oropharynx, larynx and hypopharynx. Where facilities exist, a transnasal oesophagoscopy will allow examination of the oesophagus down to the cardia. The examination should conclude with a general physical examination to include the chest, axillae and breasts in women.

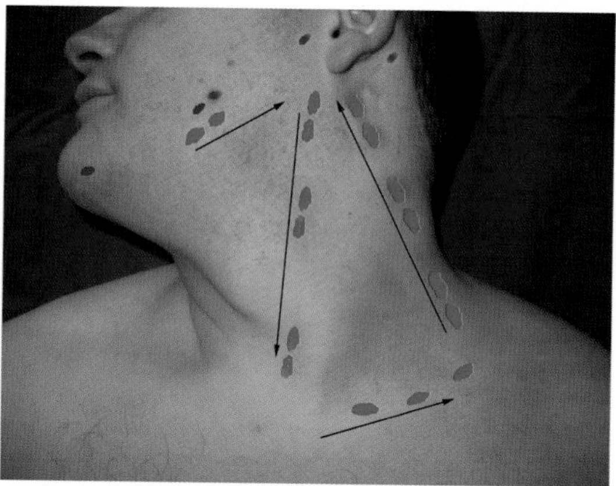

Figure 36.1 A suggested method to systematically examine the lymph nodal chains in the neck. The red dots indicate the groups of the deep cervical nodal chains, and the blue dots indicate the superficial groups. Note that the neck is turned away to the opposite side for ease of description. In real life, turning and tilting the head to the same side as the side of the neck being examined will relax the sternomastoid muscle and enable easier palpation.

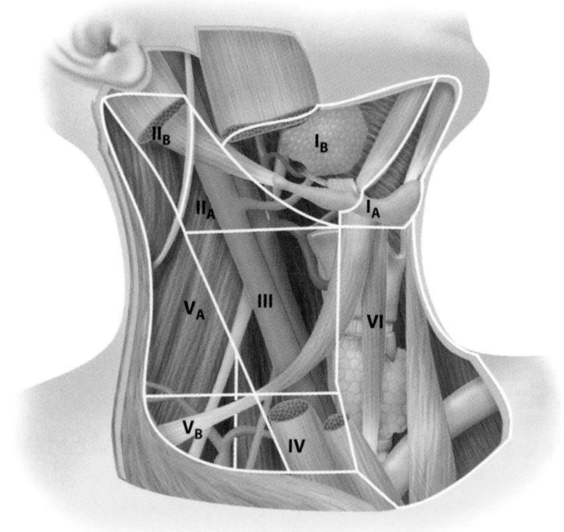

Figure 36.2 Neck levels classification system as proposed by the American Head and Neck Society and the American Association of Otolaryngology – Head and Neck Surgery.

Important signs that should raise concern include matted nodes (often felt in lymphoma), nodes that feel hard or rounded (usually indicating malignancy) and ulceration or masses in the upper aerodigestive tract (which can indicate a primary cancer).

INVESTIGATIONS

In the majority of patients with neck lumps, an ultrasound and a needle biopsy are the first-line investigations. However, these should be tailored to each individual case based on the clinical findings. For instance, if an inflammatory mass is suspected, especially in a young patient, haematological investigations including blood counts, inflammatory markers, viral titres, serology for *Brucella spp.* and *Toxoplasma spp.* and liver function tests may be indicated. An ultrasound scan may help identify an abscess. Also, a clinical trial of antibiotics and observation not exceeding 2 weeks may be instituted with close follow-up. However, a suspected neoplastic mass will need imaging and cytology as the initial diagnostic studies.

ULTRASOUND IMAGING

Ultrasound (US) is a useful modality in the evaluation of all lumps, especially of thyroid and salivary origin, with the added ability to precisely target tissue for fine-needle cytology. Currently available higher resolution probes can study the architecture of the lump and identify features that have high predictive values for benign or malignant diagnoses. It is relatively inexpensive, quick, non-invasive, and does not use ionizing radiation, but is operator dependent.

COMPUTERIZED TOMOGRAPHY

Computerized tomography (CT) is useful in identifying the presence of clinically undetectable lesions (e.g. deep-seated masses in parapharyngeal and retropharyngeal spaces) and in delineating the extent, vascularity and relationship of neck lumps to adjacent structures. It is used routinely for the staging of head and neck tumours and also in the investigation of a patient with an unknown primary presenting with metastatic neck disease.

MAGNETIC RESONANCE IMAGING

Magnetic resonance imaging (MRI) has uses that are similar to CT, but it also provides very good soft tissue contrast and is the preferred modality where soft tissue detail is important, for instance the oropharynx and parotid gland. MR angiograms are an excellent modality for vascular delineation and obviate the need for contrast injection. There is also the inherent advantage of no radiation exposure, and some of the newer MRI protocols (e.g. diffusion weighted MRI) are being tested for use in identifying recurrent or persistent cancer after treatment.

POSITRON EMISSION TOMOGRAPHY

Positron emission tomography (PET) is a functional imaging technique that depicts tissue metabolic activity and uses short-lived radioisotopes that contain protons that decay emitting positrons. PET is rarely used as a sole imaging modality, but hybrid PET-CT or PET-MRI is especially useful in assessing patients presenting with metastatic neck disease with an unknown primary (Figure 36.3) and following treatment for head and neck cancer, where differentiation between post-treatment fibrosis and residual/recurrent tumour can be difficult.

FINE-NEEDLE ASPIRATION CYTOLOGY

Fine-needle aspiration cytology (FNAC) is currently regarded as the key diagnostic modality for neck lumps and can be done with or without US guidance. Unless the mass is suspected to be of vascular origin (e.g. paraganglioma) or the diagnosis is very apparent (e.g. lipoma), an FNAC is integral to the diagnostic pathway. Although it is an easy procedure to learn, rigorous attention to detail and familiarity with the cytological processing at one's own institution are important to achieve consistently high yield rates. In addition to direct smears, needle rinses can be very useful for additional tests (immunostaining, microbiological investigations, flow cytometry or molecular testing) that can help make the diagnosis. For instance, finding p16 positivity on immunohistochemistry or high-risk human papilloma virus (HPV) on *in situ* hybridization of a needle rinse can point towards an oropharyngeal origin for a metastatic node. If the initial attempt is non-diagnostic, subsequent FNAC done under US guidance increases diagnostic rates by 10–15 per cent.

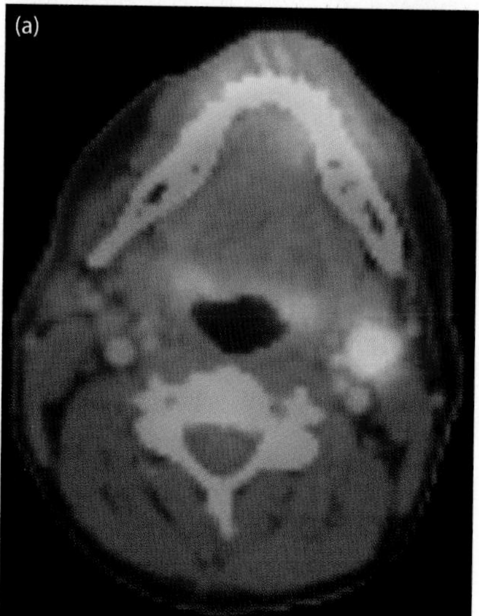

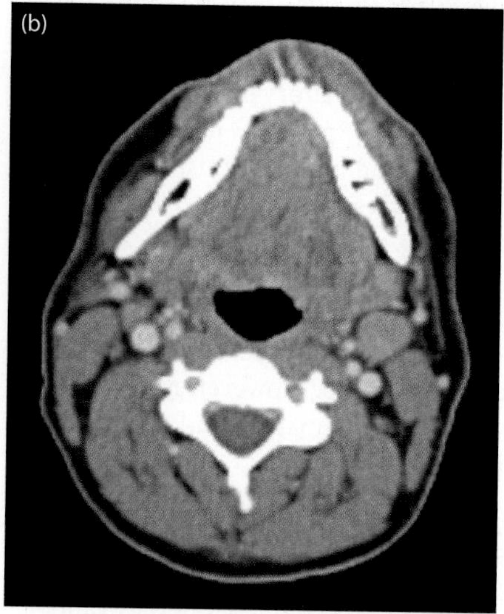

Figures 36.3 Computed tomography (CT)–positron emission tomography scan **(a)** showing high-risk human papillomavirus–positive primary cancers in both tonsils with a right-sided metastatic node. Note that the CT scan of the same patient at approximately the same level is not suggestive of tonsillar cancer **(b)**.

CORE BIOPSY

Core biopsy (CB) is a valuable adjunct to the diagnostic process when FNAC is unsuccessful. Although there had been earlier fears of seeding the CB needle tract, these are largely unfounded. CBs are especially valuable to characterize salivary gland malignancies (the heterogeneity of salivary tumours makes FNAC diagnosis difficult) and lymphomas.

OPEN BIOPSY

Open biopsy (OB) may be necessary if both FNAC and CB are unhelpful, imaging modalities suggest a malignant process but the primary is unknown or when the overwhelming diagnosis is a lymphoma. This is best undertaken by surgeons who will plan the incision to accommodate a future neck dissection if necessary. Wherever possible, an incision biopsy should be avoided in favour of excising a whole node.

APPROACH TO DIFFERENTIAL DIAGNOSIS

A basic understanding of the neck anatomy and the various disease processes is essential to direct investigations and arrive at a working diagnosis without compromising the patient's clinical outcome. There are more than 150 lymph nodes on each side of the neck, and thus lymphadenopathy is the most common neck mass seen in clinical practice and also in any part of the neck. Apart from lymph nodes, a mental checklist of the normal anatomical structures underlying the site of the palpable neck lump from which it may have originated will help with the differential. A lump high in level II of the neck is likely to be a lymph node, parotid tail mass or branchial cyst, but when it is pulsatile, consideration should be given to a carotid body tumour. A useful differential can be arrived at by considering the age of the patient (<15 years old, 15–35 or >35 years old), considering the location of the lump (central or lateral,

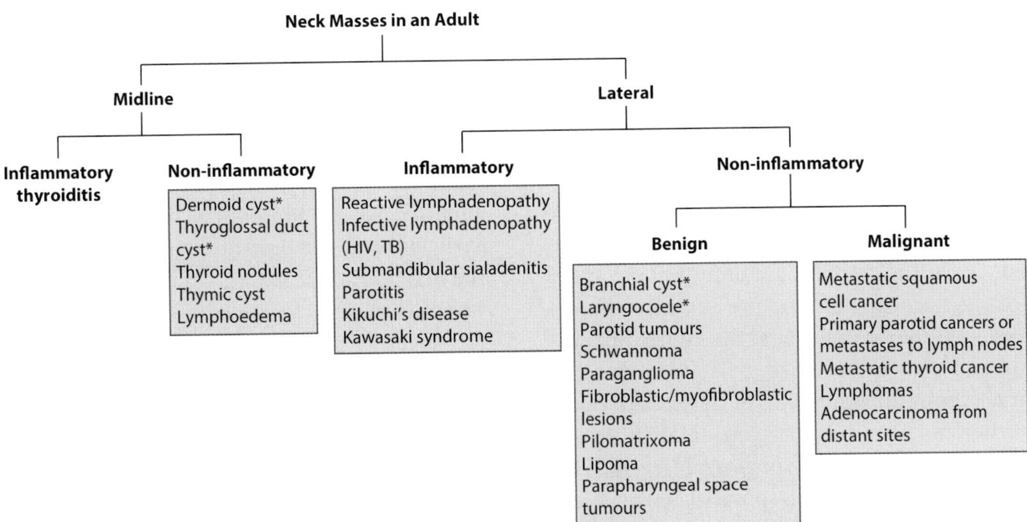

Figure 36.4 Flow chart showing the differential diagnostic options for neck masses in adults.

and if central, whether it moves with swallowing) and identifying if the lump is inflammatory or not (Figure 36.4).

In children and young adults (under the age of 35), 90 per cent of non-thyroid masses are benign, and of these up to 55 per cent may be congenital, with inflammatory swellings in second place. However, one should consider lymphoma as an uncommon but extremely important diagnosis in these patients. In adults, a lateral neck lump, even if cystic, should be considered to be malignant unless proven otherwise. The 'Rule of 80' is a useful aide memoire: 80 per cent of cervical lymphadenopathy in adults are neoplastic and of these 80 per cent are metastatic from primary cancers elsewhere in the body, while 20 per cent are of primary lymphoid origin; in the metastatic group, 80 per cent arise from primary sites above the clavicle and 20 per cent from chest and abdominal cancers. Care should be taken to ensure that the results of investigations are concordant with the clinical diagnosis. If the FNAC from a clinically malignant lump shows no signs of atypia or malignancy, it is likely to be a sampling error and additional workup is necessary. It is not uncommon to see adults with lateral cervical lymphadenopathy where a comprehensive otolaryngologic examination shows no primary site and cytology does not suggest a diagnosis. In these instances, further imaging (including PET-CT or PET-MRI) should be done to try to identify a primary site. This should be followed by CB or a carefully planned OB to confirm the diagnosis, in addition to an endoscopic assessment that includes scan-directed biopsy of putative primary sites, tonsillectomy (at least on the ipsilateral side) and tongue base biopsies. These investigations are best done in consultation with surgeons who manage these diseases on a regular basis.

APPROACH TO TREATMENT PLANNING

In the presence of benign pathology, the only treatment available is surgical excision, but patient wishes and expectations are paramount. There may be little to gain from excising a 1 cm colloid nodule of the thyroid lobe in an otherwise asymptomatic young patient, only to leave him or her with a weak voice from superior laryngeal nerve injury.

However, there is a strong argument for removing all salivary lumps given the heterogeneity in the pathology, the high incidence of false negatives and the possibility of malignant transformation with time. Thus, treatment is best tailored to the disease process at hand. In all cases, the consequences and complications of surgery and other treatments should be discussed at length with the patient. Given the complex anatomy, almost every part of the neck has a structure (usually neural) that is susceptible to injury and can cause unpleasant side effects. The following list identifies the motor nerves in different parts of the neck or operations they can be at risk in: marginal mandibular (level I), lingual (level I), hypoglossal (levels I and II), vagus (levels II–IV, VI), spinal accessory (levels II and V), facial (parotidectomy) and recurrent laryngeal (thyroidectomy). Where feasible, the surgeon should communicate his or her own personal data on complication risks.

Treatment for head and neck cancer is a rapidly evolving field, and treatment planning is best undertaken in a multidisciplinary setting where appropriate expertise is available. High-level evidence does not exist across all aspects of cancer treatment, and thus national guidelines or local protocols are often used to guide treatment. Relying on a positive FNAC alone to plan treatment in patients with head and neck cancer is a strategy beset with hazard, given the reported 3–10 per cent false positive rates. One should always try to ensure that a definitive biopsy is available before proceeding to definitive treatment.

COMMON NECK LUMPS: CLINICAL FEATURES AND MANAGEMENT

MIDLINE MASSES

Thyroglossal duct cyst

Following the descent of the thyroid gland from its origin between the first and second pouches, it remains connected to the foramen caecum in the tongue by the thyroglossal duct, which usually obliterates between gestational weeks 7 to 10. Failure of the thyroglossal duct to obliterate presents later as a midline neck lump. Although the vast majority of thyroglossal duct cysts (TDCs) present in children, these lumps are not uncommon in young adults. When they present later in life, rare malignant transformation to one of the differentiated thyroid carcinomas has been reported. In the early embryo, the base of the tongue is adjacent to the pericardial sac and thus TDCs can be seen anywhere from the tongue base to the mediastinum. However, 75 per cent occur in the vicinity of the hyoid bone, usually in the midline or slightly off to the left side. The diagnosis can be made clinically by the finding of a lump that moves on swallowing *and* on tongue protrusion (the latter differentiates it from a thyroid gland lump) (Figure 36.5a). Rupture of the cyst following an infection can lead to fistula formation (Figure 36.5b).

Management should include US imaging of the lump, with or without FNAC, to confirm the presence of a normal thyroid gland. Treatment involves surgical excision as described by Walter Sistrunk in 1920. As the thyroglossal duct can have a varying, unpredictable relationship with the hyoid bone (anterior, posterior or even within the hyoid bone), complete removal of the duct remnant is not possible unless the central portion of the body of the hyoid is removed. Recurrence rates can be reduced to fewer than 5 per cent by a well-performed Sistrunk procedure.

Thyroid nodules

Thyroid lumps are common in adults, with about 5 per cent of the adult population having a palpable nodule. This contributes to a significant proportion of the diagnostic and surgical workload. Thyroid lumps can occur across all age groups, and present as a midline neck lump that moves on swallowing (Figure 36.6). Almost 95 per cent of nodules are benign, but the presence of some clinical features should raise suspicion of cancer (Table 36.1). Malignancy risk increases with increasing age (>45 years), but thyroid masses in patients younger than 10 years should also be viewed with suspicion. US and FNAC are the only investigations necessary for the vast majority of these lumps. CT or MRI can be reserved for those patients who have retrosternal goitres or those who present with overtly

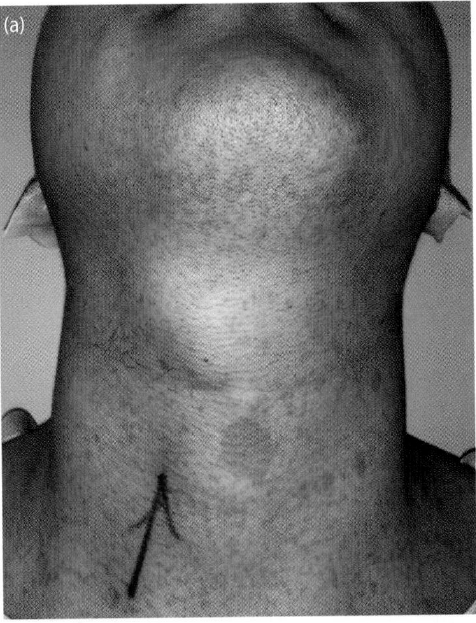

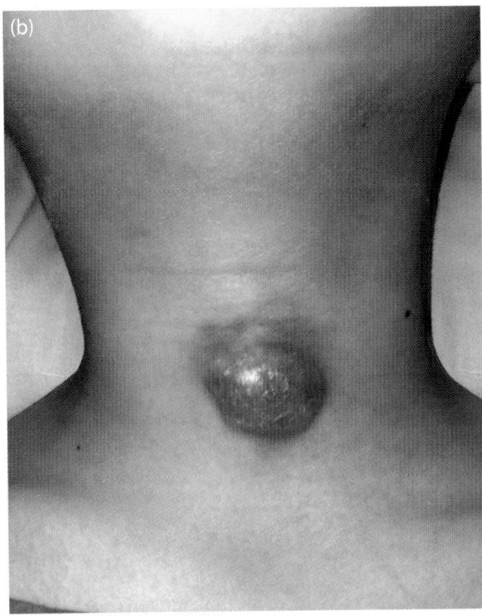

Figure 36.5 **(a)** Thyroglossal duct cyst. Note the high location of the mass around the hyoid level compared to the relatively lower location of a thyroid mass. **(b)** Infected thyroglossal duct cyst.

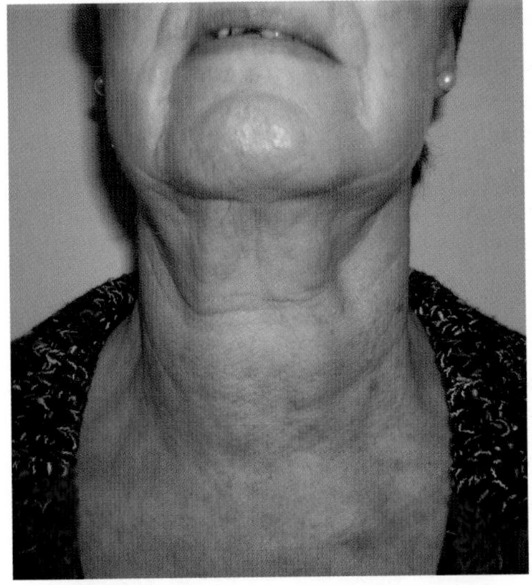

Figure 36.6 Thyroid mass. This patient had a diffusely enlarged hard mass that presented with vocal cord palsy, confirmed following investigations to be a papillary carcinoma.

malignant masses, and it is crucial to identify the extent and invasion into adjacent structures.

Treatment recommendations for thyroid masses can be based on the interpretation of FNAC findings as shown in Table 36.2. These are based on the American Thyroid Association and the British Thyroid Association guidelines.

Table 36.1 Red flag features that raise suspicion of cancer in a thyroid nodule

Family history of thyroid cancer
History of previous irradiation or exposure to high environmental radiation
Child with a thyroid nodule
Unexplained hoarseness or stridor associated with goitre
Painless thyroid mass enlarging rapidly over a period of a few weeks
Palpable cervical lymphadenopathy
Insidious or persistent pain lasting for several weeks

Reproduced with permission from Mehanna et al. 2009 BMJ doi: 10.1136/bmj.b733.

Radiation-associated lymphoedema

Radiation therapy (RT), with or without chemotherapy, is a key treatment modality in the

Table 36.2 Management algorithm for thyroid nodules based on the Thy classification

FNAC Thy classification	Interpretation	Suggested management
Thy 1	Non-diagnostic aspirate	Repeat FNAC with US guidance. Consider surgery if repeatedly non-diagnostic, especially if the nodule is solid.
Thy 1 cyst	Cystic aspirate containing colloid and histiocytes only in the absence of epithelial cells	If the cyst has been aspirated completely with no residual mass, a repeat US alone may be sufficient, with FNAC only if the cyst recurs. Consider surgery if several results are non-diagnostic.
Thy 2	Non-neoplastic	Repeat FNAC in 3–6 months.
Thy 3f	Follicular lesion, suspected follicular neoplasm	Proceed to lobectomy.
Thy 3a	Cytological findings are worrying but do not fit in the Thy 2	Discuss at a multidisciplinary forum to decide appropriate course of action.
Thy 4	Suspicious but non-diagnostic of papillary, medullary, anaplastic carcinoma or lymphoma	Discuss at a multidisciplinary forum. Proceed to surgery (lobectomy or total thyroidectomy) as appropriate.
Thy 5	Diagnostic of malignancy	Discuss at a multidisciplinary forum. Proceed to surgical intervention for differentiated thyroid cancer and medullary thyroid cancer as indicated. Other cancers should be treated appropriately.

Note that the American Thyroid Association uses different nomenclature for the various categories.

management of head and neck cancer. Following RT, the lymphatic drainage of the neck is significantly affected, and the tissue fluid tends to accumulate in the submental space, where loose areolar tissue and lack of gravity-assisted drainage enhances the process. Clinical presentation is that of ill-defined soft swelling that is not painful or inflamed and can persist for years after treatment (Figure 36.7).

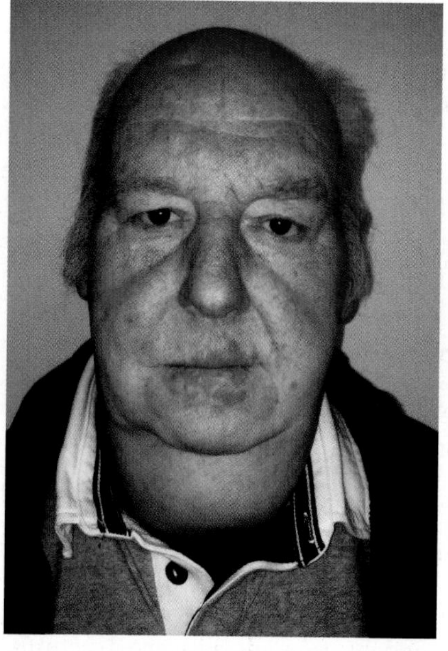

Figure 36.7 Post-radiation lymphoedema seen as an ill-defined swelling in the submental region.

LATERAL MASSES

Malignant lymphadenopathy

Metastatic disease to the neck as a cause of neck mass should be excluded in every patient over the age of 35 who presents with a neck lump (Figure 36.8). Metastatic lumps are often firm to hard but can be cystic (see the following discussion of cysts). When metastatic disease is suspected, every effort should be made to identify

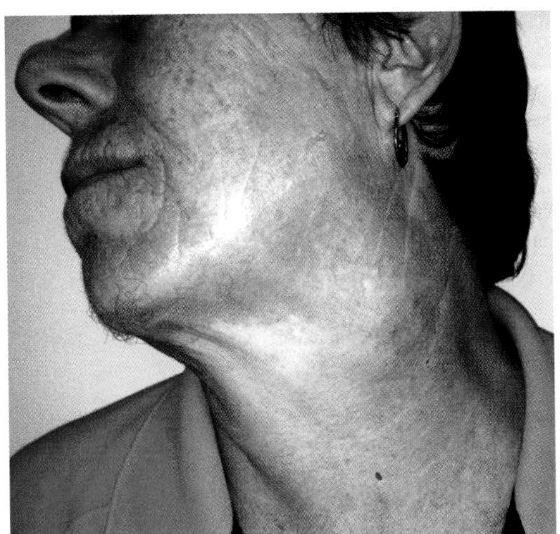

Figure 36.8 Metastatic lymphadenopathy in levels II and III in a woman with a primary site in the oropharynx.

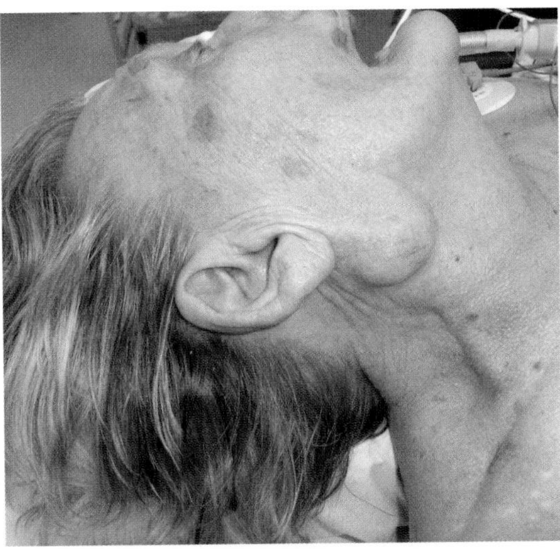

Figure 36.9 Parotid tail mass in a 72-year-old woman that was confirmed to be an adenocarcinoma arising from the parotid.

the histological nature and site of the primary cancer. Thus cross-sectional imaging and usually FNAC or CB will be needed as part of the investigative repertoire. Confirmation of the diagnosis by OB of the primary site is highly recommended. Squamous cell cancers usually arise from primary sites in the head and neck aerodigestive tract, and the distribution of the lymphadenopathy follows certain well-defined patterns based on the site of the primary. If the tissue diagnosis suggests adenocarcinoma, the primary site is more likely to be infra-clavicular. Tumour markers and further histological characterization may be needed to identify the site of origin for metastatic adenocarcinomas.

Parotid lumps

The parotid gland accounts for the majority of lumps arising from salivary glands, of which 80 per cent are benign and present solely as a lump in the parotid region. Lumps arising from the parotid gland cause the ear lobule to be pushed out, whereas skin-associated lumps (cysts and skin tumours) and lymphadenopathy in the same region do not. Features suggestive of malignancy include pain, skin fixity, facial nerve weakness and associated lymphadenopathy. As for other lumps, diagnosis is achieved by considering the constellation of clinical findings and imaging. Despite the heterogeneity seen in salivary neoplasms, FNAC has high specificity in ruling out malignancy and is thus useful. Tumours of the deep lobe of parotid can present with a barely visible and palpable lump, but will have a substantial deep-seated component that may not be detected except on intra-oral examination (where the lateral pharyngeal wall can be pushed medially) or imaging investigations (Figure 36.9).

Branchial cysts

These are squamous-lined cysts that are hypothesized to be caused by epithelial inclusions within lymph nodes that occur during the development of the neck from the pharyngeal arches. They present in the upper neck of the young adult (Figure 36.10). The clinical picture, US imaging and FNAC findings will help clinch the diagnosis. Cystic masses in patients, especially males, over the age of 35 can be metastatic from an oropharyngeal or thyroid malignancy, and thus extreme care should be taken before making a diagnosis of branchial cyst in this population. Branchial cysts are usually treated by surgical excision.

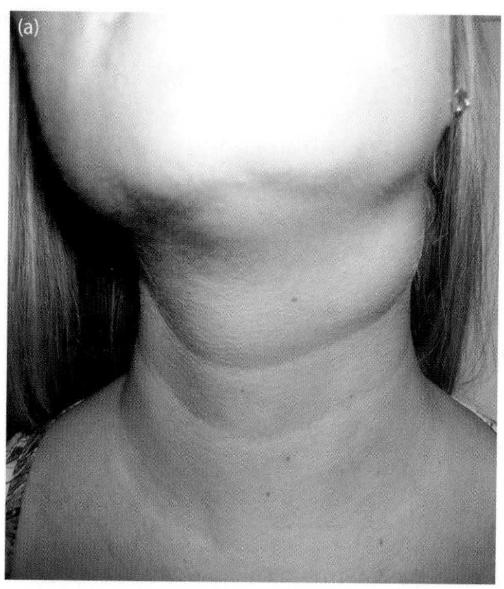

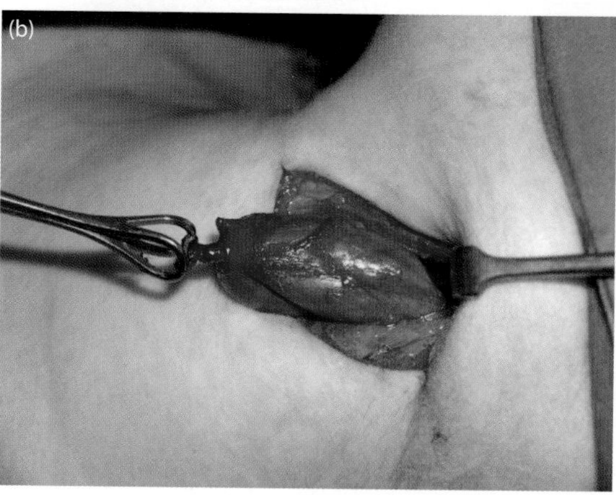

Figure 36.10 Preoperative **(a)** and intraoperative **(b)** pictures of a branchial cyst in the neck of a woman aged 22. Note the location in the anterior triangle, usually in the jugulo-digastric region.

External laryngocele

The laryngeal saccule is a blind pouch that arises from the roof of the ventricle anteriorly. When the saccules enlarge, they extend into the pre-epiglottic and paraglottic spaces and exit the laryngeal compartment through the thyrohyoid membrane, presenting as a neck lump. Frequently, the lump is air filled and is visible only on straining. If fluid filled, the lump can be persistently visible to one side in the region of the thyrohyoid membrane, difficult to separate from the larynx and moves on swallowing. Rarely, they can be associated with laryngeal carcinomas, and thus need full workup as for a laryngeal malignancy. Treatment involves excision of the lump through a thyrotomy approach and repairing the mucosal defect (Figure 36.11).

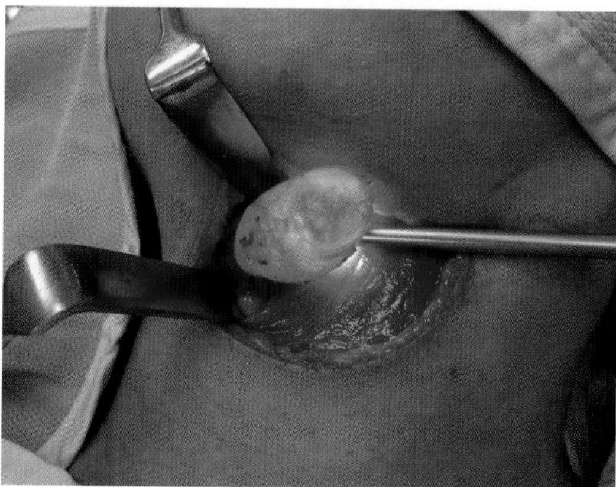

Figure 36.11 Operative picture showing a brilliantly transilluminating air-filled laryngocele. Excision was performed by tracking the laryngocele through the thyrohyoid membrane.

KEY LEARNING POINTS

- A careful and systematic clinical approach with appropriate investigations should achieve a diagnosis in over 95% of neck lumps.
- A good knowledge of neck anatomy helps in the differential diagnosis.
- Fine needle cytology, core biopsy and radiological imaging are integral in achieving a diagnosis.
- Open surgical biopsy of a neck lump should be the last option in the diagnostic algorithm.

- The most common neck mass seen in clinical practice is an enlarged lymph node.
- Neck lumps in people over 35 years should be considered malignant unless proven otherwise.
- Treatment planning for malignant diseases of the neck must be undertaken in a multidisciplinary setting where appropriate expertise is available.

FURTHER READING

Cooper DS, Doherty GM, Haugen BR, Kloos RT, Lee SL, Mandel SJ, Mazzaferri EL, McIver B, Pacini F, Schlumberger M, Sherman SI, Steward DL, Tuttle RM. Revised American Thyroid Association management guidelines for patients with thyroid nodules and differentiated thyroid cancer. *Thyroid*. 2009; 19: 1167–214.

Gleeson MJ, Browning GG, Burton MJ, Clarke R, Hibbert J, Jones NS, Lund V, Luxon L, Watkinson J (eds.). *Scott-Brown's Otorhinolaryngology: Head and Neck Surgery*. 7th ed. London: CRC Press, 2008.

Mehanna HM, Jain A, Morton RP, Watkinson J, Shaha A. Investigating the thyroid nodule. *BMJ*. 2009 Mar 13; 338: b733. doi: 10.1136/bmj.b733.

Mehanna H, McQueen A, Robinson M, Paleri V. Salivary gland swellings. *BMJ*. 2012 Oct 23; 345:e6794. doi: 10.1136/bmj.e6794.

Perros P, Boelaert K, Colley S, et al. British Thyroid Association. Guidelines for the management of thyroid cancer. *Clinical Endocrinology (Oxford)*. 2014; Jul(81 Suppl 1): 1–122. doi: 10.1111/cen.12515.

Roland NJ, Paleri V (eds.). *Head and Neck Cancer: Multidisciplinary Management Guidelines*. 4th ed. London: ENT UK, 2011.

37

Dysphagia

CHARLES E B GIDDINGS AND FRANCIS M VAZ

DEFINITIONS

Dysphagia can be defined as a disorder of swallowing either solids or liquids. Dysphagia is thought to influence up to 20 per cent of people older than 50, greater numbers of patients admitted to hospitals and even greater numbers admitted to nursing homes. Impairment of swallowing decreases quality of life and can cause significant morbidity and mortality. Dysphagia may arise from the oral cavity, oropharynx, hypopharynx or along the length of the oesophagus. It is not to be confused with other associated symptoms such as odynophagia (pain on swallowing) or globus sensation (a sensation in the throat, commonly of a 'lump'). Dysphonia is a disorder of voice, dysarthria a disorder of speech and dysphasia one of language. It is important to understand these definitions to tease out a collection of frequently overlapping presenting symptoms, of which dysphagia is commonly the most important to the patient.

ANATOMY

The oral cavity is defined as the area from the lips to the junction of the hard and soft palate and includes the teeth and the anterior two-thirds of the tongue. Beyond that it becomes the oropharynx containing the posterior third of the tongue, the tonsils and the soft palate. The hypopharynx is directly below the oropharynx and is the widened start of the upper cervical oesophagus that is just posterior to the larynx. Food has to pass through all of these areas; therefore, pathology in any area or combination of areas can result in dysphagia.

Thirty-two teeth are housed in the oral cavity along with the tongue and ductal orifices to the major salivary glands – parotid, submandibular and sublingual. The epithelium is of the stratified squamous type and houses a rich supply of minor salivary glands. The sensory innervation of the oral cavity is from the mandibular and maxillary branches of the trigeminal nerve, with special sense (taste) to the tongue via contributions of the chorda tympani to the lingual nerve. The motor supply to the muscles of the tongue is via the hypoglossal nerve, and the muscles of mastication are supplied via the mandibular branch of the trigeminal.

The oropharynx and hypopharynx are a fibromuscular tube in continuity with the nasopharynx where the tube attaches to the skull base. The tube is formed from three overlapping constrictor muscles with contributions from the stylopharyngeus and palatopharyngeus. The nerve supply to the musculature of the pharynx is via the pharyngeal plexus with fibres from the vagus and glossopharyngeal nerves and a small contribution from sympathetics. The plexus is centred on the posterolateral wall of the pharynx. The sensory innervation is via the glossopharyngeal nerve to the pharyngeal mucosa and posterior third of the tongue, with some contribution from the internal branch of the superior laryngeal nerves inferiorly.

The oesophagus is variable in length and, starting from the lower border of the cricoid cartilage, is approximately 25 cm long, passing through the diaphragm to join the stomach. Along its journey through the mediastinum, it is crossed by the great vessels and left main bronchus, with an upper cricopharyngeal sphincter and a lower sphincter at the gastro-oesophageal junction. The blood supply to the oesophagus is segmental, superiorly supplied by the inferior thyroid arteries, below that by the aorta and bronchial arteries and inferiorly by the left gastric artery. The recurrent laryngeal nerves supply the uppermost part of the oesophagus. Inferiorly, the innervation is via two plexuses contributed to by the greater splanchnic nerves, sympathetic fibres and the parasympathetic vagus nerves: the submucosal plexus of Meissener and the myenteric plexus of Auerbach, found between the two muscular layers. The oesophagus is composed of four layers. The mucosa is non-keratinizing stratified squamous epithelium which becomes columnar at the gastro-oesophagal junction. Deep to the mucosa is the submucosa and a muscular tube composed of two layers; a circular and an outer longitudinal muscular layer wraps the mucosa and submucosa.

PHYSIOLOGY OF SWALLOWING

A normal swallow is a complex coordination of voluntary and involuntary movements that results in the propulsion of a food bolus to the stomach within 20 seconds. Swallowing can be divided into three phases: oral, pharyngeal and oesophageal, each with its distinct neuromuscular mechanism. In the voluntary oral (or preparatory) phase, intact dentition and saliva production allow formation of a food bolus coordinated by movements of the tongue and the muscles of mastication via cranial nerves V, VII and XII. The tongue elevates, pressing the bolus against the soft palate and propelling it backwards until it passes through the palatoglossal arch, initiating the involuntary pharyngeal phase of swallowing. This reflex is triggered by receptors on the tongue, palatoglossal and palatopharyngeal arches (afferent limb via IX and efferent limb via the pharyngeal plexus); it is the fastest phase of swallowing, lasting less than a second, but is the most complex.

The first action in this second phase of swallowing is raising and tensing of the soft palate to close off the nasopharynx and prevent nasal regurgitation. This occurs in conjunction with contraction of the superior constrictor, known clinically as Passavant's ridge. The base of the tongue pushes onto a raised pharyngeal muscular tube as the larynx and hyoid bone rise and closure of the laryngeal inlet occurs. The reflex closure of the larynx is stimulated by the superior laryngeal nerve and is airway protective with rapid adduction of the vocal folds, false cords and arytenoids. The pharyngeal constrictors direct the bolus to the piriform sinuses and posterior pharyngeal wall, and the cricopharyngeus opens to allow passage of the bolus into the upper oesophagus. The third or oesophageal stage of swallowing is involuntary and slower, with the peristaltic wave pushing the bolus to the stomach.

Investigations for pharyngeal disease are covered in Chapter 18, but the core investigations comprise a contrast swallow, functional endoscopic evaluation of swallow, videofluoroscopy, manometry and cross-sectional imaging.

CLINICAL IMPORTANCE OF DYSPHAGIA

Immediate clinical consequences of severe dysphagia include dehydration; in less severe cases, malnutrition and a catabolic state will occur with time. Eating and drinking is of critical importance for patients, as demonstrated by significant psychosocial outcomes and a large reduction in quality of life scores in dysphagic patients. Frequently, dysphagia is complicated by aspiration of food contents requiring cessation of oral feeding; short-term alternatives of nasogastric feeding tubes or long-term feeding options such as gastrostomy tubes are not popular with patients.

INVESTIGATIONS AND MANAGEMENT

Investigation and management of dysphagia must be done via a multidisciplinary team approach with allied health professionals including speech and language therapists and dieticians. This allows early identification of at-risk patients, reduces the risks associated with dysphagia, aspiration and refeeding, and keeps patients swallowing longer with physical therapies and rehabilitation. Congenital, infectious and neoplastic causes of dysphagia are covered in greater detail elsewhere, so they will not be discussed further here.

AETIOLOGY

The causes of dysphagia are multiple and best classified according to a surgical sieve (Table 37.1).

Table 37.1 Causes of dysphagia

Congenital	
Congenital	Choanal atresia, cleft lip and palate, laryngo-malacia, laryngeal clefts, tracheoesophageal fistula, unilateral vocal fold paralysis and vascular rings
Acquired	
Infections	Acute bacterial infections (tonsillitis, quinsy, infectious mononucleosis, supraglottitis, epiglottitis, tuberculosis, abscesses of neck spaces), candidiasis, herpes
Trauma	Blunt and penetrating trauma, burns and caustic strictures, head injury and cranial nerve injury
Inflammatory	Acid-related disorders, Plummer–Vinson syndrome and sarcoid
Autoimmune	Scleroderma/CREST, systemic lupus erythematosus, dermatomyositis, pemphigoid, Sjögren's, rheumatoid arthritis, Crohn's and Behcet's
Neoplastic	Benign and malignant tumours of the oral cavity, pharynx, larynx and oesophagus; lymphomas, thyroid enlargement and skull base tumours
Neurological	Stroke, Parkinson's, recurrent laryngeal nerve injury, multiple sclerosis, myasthenia gravis and motor neurone disease
Motility disorders	Age-related motility disorders, achalasia and nutcracker oesophagus
Iatrogenic	Tracheostomy, surgery and chemoradiotherapy
Mechanical	Stricture, pharyngeal pouch and foreign body

TRAUMATIC

History and examination

Following resuscitation and primary survey, a more detailed history of a traumatic injury should include when and what mechanism of injury occurred, especially in a penetrating injury to the neck. Any history of head or cervical spine trauma, unexplained oropharyngeal bleeding, dysphonia and neck swelling should be included. Examination should include visualization of the upper aerodigestive tract and systematic testing of cranial nerves. Ingestion of caustic substances requires identification of the substance to allow appropriate systemic management in addition to managing the local oral, pharyngeal and oesophageal injury. Careful examination for entry and exit wounds, surgical emphysema and blood-stained secretions should be undertaken, and may suggest a penetrated viscus.

Investigations

In addition to a trauma series, tailored cross-sectional imaging of the head, skull base, neck and chest with oral contrast may reveal a mucosal breach or cause for a cranial nerve injury. In penetrating injuries, computed tomography arteriography (CTA) can exclude a vascular injury. Should the severity of injury not allow this, a separate contrast swallow at a later date will be helpful.

Management

Primary resuscitation of the patient is of paramount importance; thereafter, exclusion of a head or cervical spine injury is mandatory. Synchronous assessment of the airway should be considered, as disruption of swallowing may be an early sign of impending airway compromise. If a perforated viscus is suspected without a vascular injury, then cessation of oral intake, rigid endoscopy when practicable and insertion of a nasogastric tube will inform management. Isolated penetrating injury to the pharyngeal or oesophageal mucosa will heal quickly but should be covered with antibiotics. Caustic injuries frequently affect the distal oesophagus, and after healing, any stricture formation is treated with dilatation.

REFLUX DISEASE

History and examination

Reflux of acid, pepsin and bile may give a classical history of indigestion, retrosternal discomfort or burning, regurgitation, persistent cough, intermittent dysphonia and in severe cases even chest pain. Steroids and anti-inflammatory preparations should be enquired about as they may exacerbate symptoms. Examination can be normal, but there may be signs of oedema and erythema, particularly in the posterior larynx.

Investigations

Patients presenting with a classical history and examination suggestive of reflux, and without suspicious features, may be started on an empirical trial of either proton pump inhibitors (PPIs) or histamine (H2) antagonists.

Management

Failure of symptomatic improvement despite empirical treatment requires further investigation with an oesophago-gastroscopy to visualize the lower thoracic oesophagus and to exclude hiatus herniation. Oesophagitis and metaplastic change (Barrett's oesophagus) has an association with the development of adenocarcinoma. pH studies over a period of 24 hours may be helpful in establishing the diagnosis, and manometry can inform on oesophageal and sphincteric function. Lifestyle and dietary changes, including smoking cessation, are essential in conjunction with a stepwise management of barrier alginates and PPIs. For cases refractory to these measures, surgery may be appropriate, including fundoplication of the stomach.

PATERSON-BROWN-KELLY (UK) OR PLUMMER–VINSON (USA) SYNDROME

History and examination

This syndrome describes the association of dysphagia, upper oesophageal webs and iron deficiency anaemia. An intermittent history of dysphagia to solids with some aspiration may be found, typically in middle-aged females, although the incidence is declining. Signs and symptoms of iron deficiency anaemia may also be present, including lethargy, glossitis, angular chelitis, koilonychia and pallor.

Investigations

A full blood count and iron studies (serum iron and total iron binding capacity) will identify iron deficiency anaemia, and a contrast swallow will outline the appearance of the upper oesophagus (Figure 37.1). Direct or flexible oesophagoscopy may be performed and will aid in excluding the rarely associated post-cricoid carcinoma but may not demonstrate an abnormality.

Management

Correction of iron deficiency anaemia may resolve any symptoms and the web; for those in whom it does not, then oesophagoscopy and dilatation may be successful.

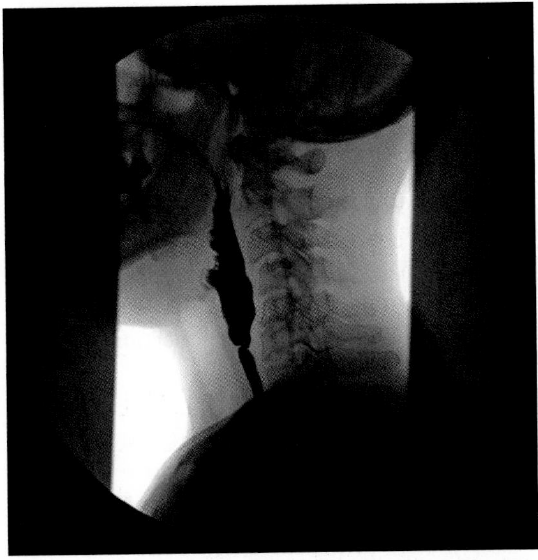

Figure 37.1 A contrast swallow demonstrating an anterior web in Plummer–Vinson syndrome.

SCLERODERMA/CREST

History and examination

This group of autoimmune connective tissue diseases is characterized by progressive fibrosis of the skin, chronic inflammation with collagen deposition in affected organs and vascular alteration. Scleroderma may be divided into two forms: limited systemic sclerosis, also known as CREST (calcinosis, Raynaud's phenomenon, oesophageal dysfunction, sclerodactyly and telangiectasias); and diffuse systemic sclerosis, affecting the skin as well as major organ systems including kidneys, heart, lungs and oesophagus.

Tightening and induration of the skin may be seen with Raynaud's phenomenon (recurrent vasospasm with colour change in fingers and toes), especially in the hands. Dysphagia with reflux and aspiration may manifest with progressive dyspnoea. Signs of heart failure and chronic renal impairment may be present in addition to musculoskeletal involvement.

Investigations

Blood tests include an autoimmune profile and erythrocyte sedimentation rate (ESR). Imaging of those organs suspected of involvement is also performed. Functional endoscopic evaluation of swallowing and videofluoroscopy will aid in dysphagia management.

Management

In combination with a rheumatologist to aid in the treatment of the underlying condition, immunosuppressants are prescribed and affected organs are managed. Management of the dysfunctional swallow is done in combination with speech and language therapists using rehabilitation and compensatory strategies.

NEUROLOGICAL

History and examination

Acute neurological injury such as a cerebrovascular accident may involve one or more cranial nerves influencing the oral and pharyngeal phases of swallowing. Typically, there are other focal neurological deficits, and the prognosis is one of gradual improvement with rehabilitation.

Chronic neurological diseases may have a more indolent presentation with progressive symptoms and reduction in function of swallowing, speech, and voice and increasing aspiration in combination with systemic neurological problems. Signs may include dysphonia, dysarthria, tongue wasting, difficulty managing secretions, cranial nerve paralysis and limb weakness.

Investigations

Investigations and mitigation of the underlying neurological condition in conjunction with neurologists are key. Endoscopic assessment of swallowing and videofluoroscopy will inform decisions on the safety of oral feeding.

Management

Regular re-evaluation of swallowing with speech and language therapy and dietician involvement is essential for keeping this group of patients swallowing safely. After acute injury, exercises are helpful in the rehabilitation of swallowing; in conditions with progressive dysfunction, compensatory strategies such as posturing and supraglottic swallowing may allow oral feeding to continue. Altering food consistencies is also helpful in preventing aspiration, as thicker consistencies are considered easier to manage. Patients with a high risk of aspiration may need to cease oral feeding and have a gastrostomy tube inserted as a palliative measure.

ACHALASIA

History and examination

Oesophageal motility disorders include uncoordinated spontaneous and non-peristaltic 'tertiary contractions' (Figure 37.2) and 'nutcracker oesophagus'. Achalasia is an oesophageal motility disorder characterized by aperistalsis in the body of the oesophagus and failure of relaxation of the lower oesophageal sphincter caused by impairment of the myenteric plexus of Auerbach's inhibitory neurones in the distal oesophagus. An elderly patient may present with a long history of intermittent dysphagia with occasional aspiration and regurgitation; younger patients may experience retrosternal pain from dysmotility and spasm.

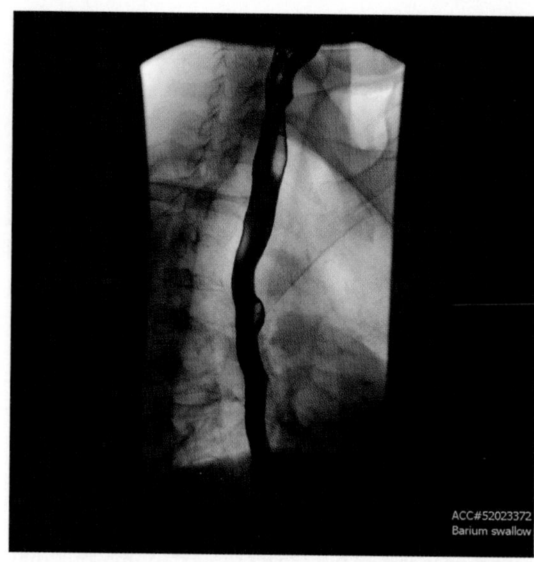

Figure 37.2 A contrast swallow demonstrating tertiary contractions.

Investigations

Contrast swallow tests may initially be normal until oesophageal dilatation and elongation occur in the later stages, revealing the classical findings of contrast retention with a tapering distal gastro-oesophageal segment into a closed sphincter, also described as a 'bird's beak' (Figure 37.3). Oesophageal manometry is the standard for the diagnosis of achalasia, and gastro-oesophagoscopy is also performed to exclude an underlying malignancy. Very rarely, similar appearances may also be found in Chaga's disease (infection with the protozoan *Trypanosoma cruzi*).

Management

Gastroenterology expertise aids in the management of achalasia. Calcium channel blockers, Botox injections into the lower oesophageal sphincter and sphincter dilatation or myotomy are the mainstay of management.

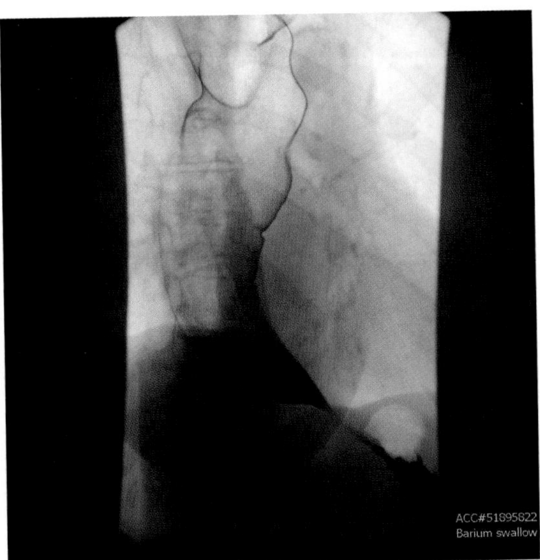

Figure 37.3 A contrast swallow demonstrating achalasia.

IATROGENIC

History and examination

A thorough history must be taken, including previous conditions, treatments including surgery and radiotherapy and current medications. Disruption of swallowing may occur as a complication of a wide range of treatments delivered via multiple specialties. Surgery to the head and neck, including posterior fossa neurosurgery, surgery to the spine and oncological surgery to the mouth, base of tongue, hypopharynx and oesophagus, may cause damage to the pharyngeal plexus, cranial nerves or muscles involved in deglutition. Drug-induced dysphagia may occur by influencing oesophageal motility or by direct mucosal injury. Radiotherapy given with or without chemotherapy agents in the oncological management of head and neck cancers is a well-recognized cause of acute and chronic dysphagia. Chemoradiotherapy is often delivered under the premise of 'organ preservation', for example in cancer of the larynx that would otherwise be treated surgically with a laryngectomy. Comparable survival rates can be achieved, but toxicity following chemoradiotherapy may give worse long-term functional outcomes and consequently reduced quality of life.

Investigations

Bedside assessment of swallowing, contrast swallow, videofluoroscopy and endoscopic evaluation of swallowing form the mainstay of investigations.

Management

Early involvement of speech and language therapists is essential to diagnose and manage the acute and chronic manifestations of treatment. During treatment, aggressive therapy and rehabilitation may reduce the need for long-term gastrostomy tube feeding. Surgery in the form of dilatations of strictures of the pharynx and oesophagus may help with mechanical causes.

PHARYNGEAL POUCH

History and examination

A pharyngeal pouch, also known as Zenker's diverticulum, is a propulsion outpouching of the hypopharynx (epithelium and lamina propria only). It develops between a weakness in the inferior constrictors (oblique fibres of thyropharyngeus and the cricopharyngeus muscle's transverse fibres). This area, also known as Killian's dehiscence, is an established weakened area that allows herniation, more commonly on the left. It has also been proposed that the cricopharyngeal sphincter may have a higher than normal resting tone. Frequently, it is elderly patients who present with regurgitation of undigested food, recurrent chest infections secondary to aspiration and halitosis in addition to dysphagia. There may be no physical signs but occasionally borborygmi may be elicited by palpation of the neck as the pouch is emptied into the pharynx.

Investigations

A contrast swallow will delineate the size and position of the diverticulum, with an opening into the cervical oesophagus usually placed high and anteriorly. It is for this reason that endoscopy must be performed with care as the endoscope will naturally pass into the pouch, not the oesophagus.

Management

Management decisions are based around the symptoms and effects on quality of life; a small pouch with minimal symptoms may require no intervention. A pouch causing symptoms or recurrent chest infections may require endoscopic division. This is performed under general anaesthetic with a split pharyngoscope (Figure 37.4) whose arms are positioned with one in the pouch and the other in the cervical oesophagus. Division of the interpositioned pharyngeal bar will not only divide the mucosa but will also divide the fibres of cricopharyngeus. Patients in whom sufficient endoscopic access cannot be achieved may require an external approach, when the pouch is excised and the defect repaired. In addition, a cricopharyngeal myotomy is performed to reduce the chance of recurrence. The excised pouch should be sent for histology as there have been reports of carcinoma occurring within the pouch.

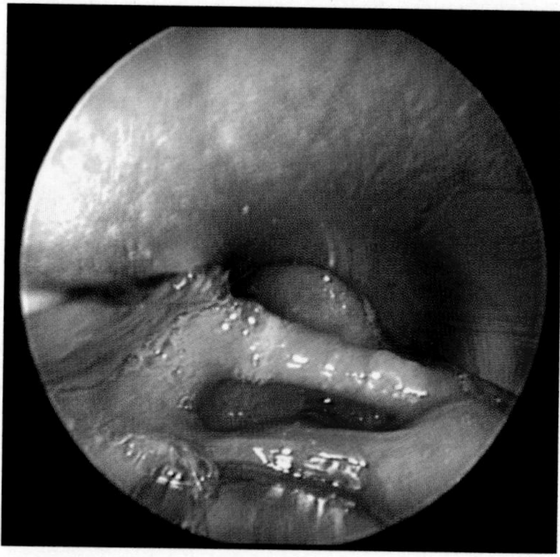

Figure 37.4 Endoscopic appearances of a pharyngeal pouch.

KEY LEARNING POINTS

- Dysphagia has a significant impact on quality of life.
- Swallowing has a complex mechanism and occurs in three phases.
- Malignancy must be excluded in progressive dysphagia.
- A multispecialty approach is essential, with speech and language therapists and dieticians.

FURTHER READING

Cook IJ. Oropharyngeal dysphagia. *Gastroenterology Clinics of North America*. 2009; 38(3): 411–31.

Domsic R. Gastrointestinal manifestations of systemic sclerosis. *Digestive Diseases and Sciences*. 2008; 53(5): 1163–74.

Richter JE. Oesophgeal motility disorders. *Lancet*. 2001; 358(9284): 823–8.

Schindler JS. Swallowing disorders in the elderly. *Laryngoscope*. 2002; 112(4): 589–602.

38

The parathyroid

MUHAMMAD SHAHED QUARISHI

INTRODUCTION

The parathyroid gland was the last major gland to be identified in the human body. Richard Owen wrote about the parathyroid glands in 1862 in the 'Transactions of the Zoological Society'.

Primary hyperparathyroidism (pHPT) is the most common cause of hypercalcaemia in the outpatient population and second only to malignancy in the inpatient population. It is usually characterized by elevated serum calcium with an unsuppressed parathyroid hormone (PTH) level. The incidence of pHPT is estimated to be between 5 and 50 per 10 000 and is more common in patients over 45 years of age, with a male-to-female ratio of 1:3. The incidence of pHPT is increasing owing to early detection since the advent of multichannel serum auto analyzers identifying hypercalcemia in asymptomatic patients.

There are two types of pHPT. One is sporadic (95 per cent), of which 80 per cent are solitary adenomas, 15–20 per cent due to glandular hyperplasia and 1 per cent carcinoma. Hereditary (5 per cent) are those associated with multiple endocrine neoplasia (MEN) Type 1. Parathyroid surgery is becoming more popular and gradually establishing itself as the acceptable definitive treatment for pHPT.[1]

EMBRYOLOGY AND SURGICAL ANATOMY

There are four parathyroid glands in total. The parathyroid gland is about 5–7 mm in size, soft, mobile and has an average weight of 30–40 μg. It is oval in shape, and the colour is variable from light yellow in older people to reddish-brown in younger patients, depending upon fat content and proportion of oxyphil cells. Parathyroid glands are placed as a superior and inferior pair on the posterolateral aspect of each thyroid lobe, with the upper pair being more constant in position. Parathyroid glands are derived from the endoderm of the third and fourth pharyngeal pouches. The developing parathyroid cells may be arrested at any point during their migration from the neck to the mediastinum. Supernumerary fifth glands have been reported in 5 per cent of cases and are often found in thymic tissue. The nerve supply is from fibres from the superior and middle cervical sympathetic ganglion or from the perivascular plexus of the thyroid gland. The venous drainage of the gland is from the superior and middle thyroid veins, which drain the upper and central parts of the thyroid and parathyroid glands.

The inferior glands develop along with the thymus from the third branchial pouch and have their blood supply from the inferior thyroid artery. In 50 per cent of cases the inferior glands are found around 1 cm inferior, lateral or posterior to the lower pole of the thyroid lobe. They are on a ventral plane in relation to the recurrent laryngeal nerve, caudal to the inferior thyroid artery, where they cross the recurrent laryngeal nerve. In 25 per cent of cases the inferior parathyroid gland may be found within the thyrothymic horn. In the remaining 25 per cent of cases their position is very variable, located some distance lateral to the thyroid (12 per cent) or adjacent to the trachea. Less often they may be situated ectopically in the mediastinal thymus below the suprasternal notch, near the carotid sheath, sometimes as high as the carotid bifurcation, and rarely the inferior gland may be intrathyroidal (0.5–4 per cent).

The superior parathyroid gland is dorsal (deeper) to the recurrent laryngeal nerve in the coronal plane and is quite often symmetrical in position and shape. In 80 per cent of cases the superior parathyroid gland is found adjacent to the cricothyroid junction, posterolateral to the upper half of the thyroid lobe and approximately 1 cm cephalic to the junction of the recurrent laryngeal nerve and the inferior thyroid artery. The main blood supply is from the inferior thyroid artery, while in 35–40 per cent of cases it may also be from the superior thyroid artery. In 3 per cent of cases the superior parathyroid glands may be found in a retropharyngeal, retrolaryngeal or retroesophageal position. In rare cases (1 per cent) they may be positioned above the superior pole of the thyroid or in the posterior mediastinum.

HISTOPATHOLOGY

Parathyroid glands have a thin connective tissue capsule with multiple septa that divide them into lobules. The stroma consists of islands of secretory cells interspersed with fat cells and a rich sinusoidal capillary network. There are two cell types: 'chief or principal cells' and 'oxyphil' cells. Chief cells are the predominant cell type in children and synthesize PTH. The oxyphil cells are larger and their number increases with age. In elderly patients there is a decrease in the number of chief cells with 60–70 per cent of the mass being occupied by fat cells. The adenomatous portion of the parathyroid may consist predominantly of chief cells with a suppressed rim of 'normal' parathyroid tissue differentiating it from a hyperplastic gland. Chief cell hyperplasia causes 15 per cent of all pHPT cases, and in 20 per cent of cases it is familial and may be related to MEN syndrome.

PHYSIOLOGY

In pHPT the excess PTH is uninfluenced by other biochemical factors and is produced by either neoplastic or hyperplastic parathyroid parenchymal cells. In secondary HPT chronic stimulation of the parathyroid gland leads to parathyroid cell proliferation and usually reverts to normal once the stimulus is removed. In chronic renal failure, low calcium and a high phosphate burden causes parathyroid proliferation. There is also reduced responsiveness of calcium receptors to PTH secretion owing to metabolic acidosis during renal failure. Prolonged use of lithium and vitamin D deficiency are related to secondary HPT. In chronic renal failure, after prolonged stimulus the hyperplastic gland may become autonomous and may not revert to its normal state after the stimulus has been removed. This results in 'tertiary' hyperparathyroidism.

Familial HPT is associated with MEN1, MEN2, neonatal severe hyperparathyroidism, hyperparathyroidism-jaw tumour syndrome, familial isolated hyperparathyroidism and autosomal dominant mild hyperparathyroidism. The penetrance of the MEN1 gene is high (95 per cent), and along with multigland HPT is associated with pituitary tumours and pancreatic and gut carcinoids. MEN2 has a mild hypercalcaemic picture and may require no treatment or removal of enlarged glands. They are both linked to medullary thyroid carcinoma and pheochromocytoma.

CLINICAL ASSESSMENT

Patients presenting to surgeons are typically referred by endocrinologists and have biochemically confirmed pHPT. The majority of patients with pHPT are asymptomatic (80 per cent), and their hypercalcaemia is picked up incidentally on biochemical screening for other reasons. These patients are then further evaluated with PTH-assay, 24-hour urinary collection for calcium level and creatinine clearance/glomerular filtration rate (GFR). A raised PTH-assay, hypercalcaemia and hypercalciuria confirm the diagnosis of pHPT.

Few patients today would present with the classical rhyme of 'bones, stones, abdominal groans and psychic moans' described in the 1930s, which possibly implied late presentation. Most symptomatic patients have non-specific complaints such as fatigue, lethargy, depression, loss of concentration and joint and bone pain. The neurocognitive symptoms can mimic dementia in the elderly population.

Table 38.1 Causes of hypercalcaemia

- Hyperparathyroidism: primary/secondary/tertiary
- Malignancy: breast, lung, PTH-secreting tumours, parathyroid carcinoma
- Drugs: thiazide diuretics, Vitamins A and D, calcium, aluminum, lithium
- Granulomatous lesions: sarcoidosis, tuberculosis, histoplasmosis
- Excess calcium intake: milk alkali syndrome
- Prolonged immobilization
- Familial: MEN syndromes, familial hypocaliuric hypocalcaemia
- Endocrine disorders: thyrotoxicosis, Addison's disease

Gastro-intestinal symptoms may include abdominal pain, chronic constipation, peptic ulceration and pancreatitis. Recent studies report the incidence of nephrolithiasis (20 per cent) and hypercalciuria (40 per cent) of all patients with pHPT.

It is important to ask about risk factors for hyperparathyroidism (lithium therapy, neck irradiation) and investigate other causes of hypercalcaemia (Table 38.1). In young patients with pHPT, family history of MEN should be investigated. MEN patients tend to have multiple gland disease and are managed differently from those with solitary adenomas. In some cases, pHPT is associated with metabolic and potential cardiovascular manifestations, including diabetes, hypertension and left ventricular hypertrophy.

MANAGEMENT OPTIONS

PRIMARY HYPERPARATHYROIDISM

The treatment modality for pHPT may range from watchful waiting to surgical intervention. The symptomatic patient should be offered surgery for a curative outcome. The asymptomatic patients may be managed conservatively with adequate hydration, avoidance of thiazide diuretics and control of calcium and parathormone levels by treating with bisphosphonates.

Table 38.2 Guidelines for parathyroid surgery in asymptomatic pHPT[3]

Serum calcium (>upper limit of normal)	0.25 mmol/L
24-hour urine for calcium	Not indicated in the absence of renal stones/nephrolithiasis*
Creatinine clearance	<60 mL/min
Bone mineral density	T-score <–2.5 at any site and/or previous fracture
Age	<50 years
Patients for whom effective medical surveillance/ follow-up is not possible.	

* Some centres consider 24-hour urinary calcium >400 mg as an indication.

Since 2004, calcimimetic drugs have been used to control serum PTH levels, mostly in secondary parathyroidism. They work by mimicking calcium at the parathyroid receptors.

Over 10 years, nearly 1 in 4 asymptomatic patients may require surgery owing to deterioration of symptoms. If a conservative management option is chosen, annual calcium, PTH, bone mineral density and renal functions should be assessed. The indications for surgery in asymptomatic patients are given in Table 38.2.

FAMILIAL HYPERPARATHYROIDISM

MEN1

Hyperparathyroidism associated with MEN1 may be associated with up to 20 per cent of failed parathyroid surgery owing to its aggressive form of parathyroid gland hyperplasia. In patients with osteoporosis or Zollinger–Ellison syndrome, surgery is required as a priority. Subtotal parathyroidectomy with bilateral thymectomy is the usual practice, leaving 20–30 mg of the smallest parathyroid gland marked with a non-absorbable suture. Total parathyroidectomy and forearm auto transplantation of 30–60 mg of the smallest gland is recommended in patients with significant four-gland enlargement.

MEN2A

Parathyroid disease in MEN2A patients is usually mild. The majority of patients are asymptomatic, and few have nephrolithiasis or hypercalcaemia. Patients with MEN2A undergo total thyroidectomy for medullary carcinoma, and only enlarged parathyroids identified at the time are removed to prevent permanent hypoparathyroidism.

SECONDARY AND TERTIARY HYPERPARATHYROIDISM

Parathyroid surgery for these patients is usually decided by renal physicians after failure of medical treatment. The main indications for surgical intervention are to control symptoms such as pruritus, muscle weakness, bone pain, fracture risk, mood swings and/or to correct the biochemical parameters. Total parathyroidectomy with autotransplantation is recommended for patients with marked four-gland enlargement. To avoid permanent hypothyroidism some surgeons prefer subtotal parathyroidectomy, leaving a parathyroid remnant with a vascular pedicle, often half of the most normal-looking gland.

PREOPERATIVE LOCALIZATION INVESTIGATIONS

Preoperative localization investigations are highly recommended to determine the best surgical approach to achieve cure with minimal risk of complications in patients diagnosed with HPT. The commonly used non-invasive studies for patients with single gland adenomas are ultrasonography and sestamibi scans for anatomical and functional details, respectively. In localizing ectopic glands, computed tomography (CT) or magnetic resonance imaging (MRI) are helpful tools. Invasive procedures such as image-guided fine-needle aspiration (FNA) with PTH assay and selective venous PTH sampling are best used for revision surgery.[2]

SESTAMIBI SCINTIGRAPHY

Technetium-99m methoxyisobutylisonitrile (sestamibi) is the radioisotope used in this metabolic scan. Sestamibi is a monovalent lipophilic cation that diffuses through cell membranes and accumulates almost exclusively within mitochondria. Parathyroid tissue has a high metabolic rate with high mitochondrial activity, which explains its high uptake of sestamibi. Normal thyroid tissue has a lower mitochondrial content, and therefore sestamibi washes out faster than it does from parathyroid adenoma tissue. Parathyroid adenoma with >20 per cent oxyphil cell content is more likely to be associated with a positive sestamibi (MIBI) scan compared to parathyroid adenomas formed mainly of chief cells.

The MIBI scan is good at detecting solitary adenoma (Figure 38.1) and has a sensitivity of around 85 per cent and positive predictive value (PPV) of between 91 and 96 per cent. The sensitivity and PPV decrease in the presence of thyroid nodules. One way of trying to improve the localization accuracy of scintigraphy is to employ dual-phase imaging with double tracer (99m-Sestamibi and Iodine-123) subtraction. This exploits the radiotracer washout characteristics of parathyroid adenomas (the washout of tracer is quicker in thyroid tissue compared to parathyroid tissue). Parathyroid images are taken 20 minutes (early-phase) and 2 hours (late-phase) after administration of sestamibi. Additional imaging of the thyroid is also performed after Iodine-123 administration. The image of the thyroid is then subtracted from the early-phase and late-phase parathyroid image. This further improves the visualization of the abnormal parathyroid adenoma. The dual-phase double-tracer subtraction technique has been reported to improve sensitivity compared to the dual-phase single-tracer technique.

ULTRASOUND SCAN

In experienced hands, preferably a dedicated radiologist, high-frequency ultrasound scan (USS) has an overall sensitivity of 89 per cent and PPV of 98 per cent for localizing solitary adenomas.

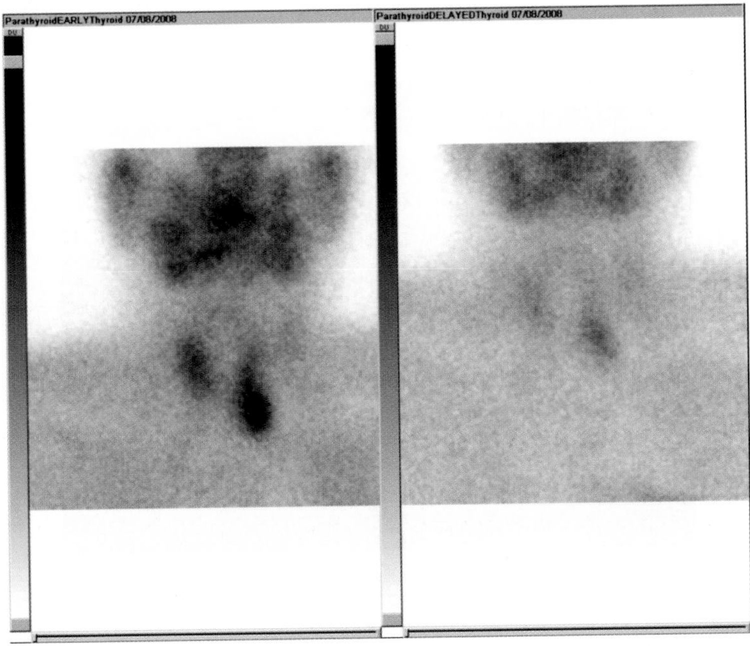

Figure 38.1 Sestamibi dual-phase scan with left lower parathyroid adenoma.

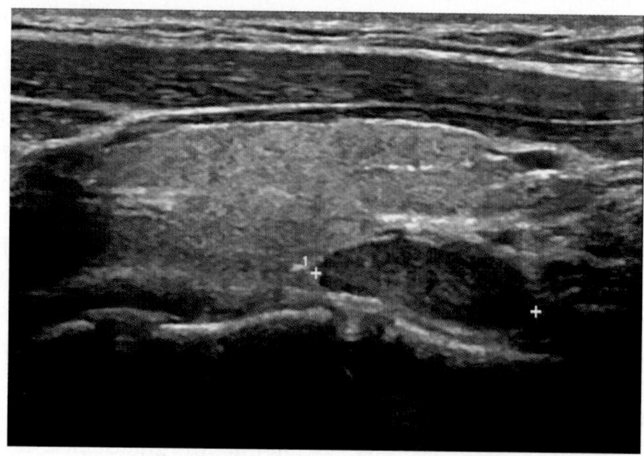

Figure 38.2 Ultrasound scan showing a solitary parathyroid adenoma.

The abnormal gland is identified by its appropriate anatomical location; enlarged, oval or triangular shape and homogeneously hypoechoic texture (Figure 38.2). Colour flow Doppler (CFD) also demonstrates peripheral blood flow of the abnormal parathyroid gland (Figure 38.3) in contrast to a vascular pedicle in a lymph node. USS provides the anatomic relationships between the enlarged gland and surrounding structures to guide surgery. The disadvantages of USS is that it may not pick up deep-seated adenomas or retrotracheal, retroesophageal, superior mediastinal or other ectopic parathyroid tissue and is dependent on the skill of the sonographer. Its sensitivity may decrease in the presence of thyroid nodules.

USS OR MIBI, OR BOTH

Though USS is cheaper and avoids exposure to ionizing radiation when compared to MIBI, opinion

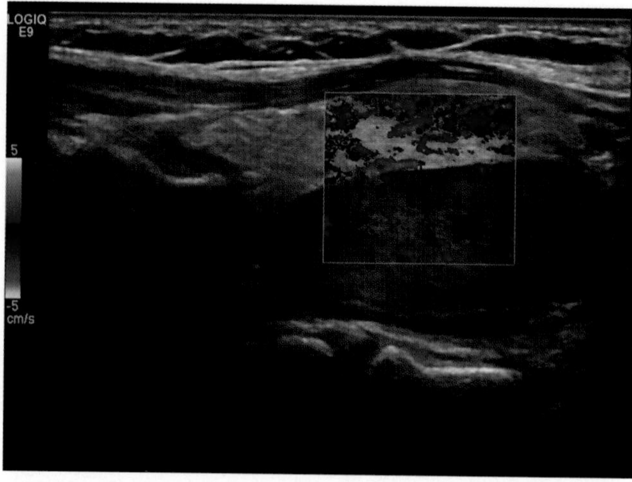

Figure 38.3 Doppler ultrasound scan showing periphery blood flow around the solitary large parathyroid adenoma as identified.

varies as to which is more helpful and should be the first localization investigation. The common practice is to have both USS and MIBI scans to help localize solitary adenomas.

Parathyroidectomy in cases with concordant USS and MIBI scans have been reported to have up to a 95–99 per cent success rate defined by normocalcaemia.

CT, MRI AND PET

CT scans and MRI scans play a small role in parathyroid imaging. They are less sensitive compared to MIBI or USS. In high-resolution CT scans at 2.5–3 mm slices with contrast enhancement and the novel four-dimensional CT (4D-CT), the sensitivity for localizing parathyroid adenomas ranges from 46 to 87 per cent. MRI scans may be able to help localize ectopic or mediastinal glands (up to 71–88 per cent sensitivity).

Fluorodeoxyglucose (FDG)-PET scans have very good sensitivity (86 per cent) and acceptable specificity (78 per cent) for solitary adenomas. They may be useful in negative or equivocal MIBI and USS localization scans or before revision surgery.

FINE-NEEDLE ASPIRATION

FNA performed under US or CT scan guidance to test for PTH assay is generally recommended in revision surgery. Cytology is less sensitive as follicular thyroid neoplastic cells may mimic parathyroid tissue.

VENOUS SAMPLING

This is a more invasive procedure and used only when imaging studies have been negative. It may be used in a re-operative situation or in patients who have had negative imaging. Selective venous sampling has a high overall sensitivity (93–95 per cent) in both a primary operation setting and a re-operative situation. This can help regionalize (neck/mediastinum) and lateralize (right/left) the abnormal parathyroid gland.

INTRAOPERATIVE LOCALIZATION TECHNIQUES

The four known modalities in intraoperative localization techniques include the use of intraoperative PTH monitoring (IOPTH), radio-guided parathyroidectomy (RGP), frozen section and methylene blue injections. These can be employed in various situations to improve surgical outcomes.

INTRAOPERATIVE PTH MONITORING

IOPTH is the most common intraoperative localization technique. It can be performed from a central or peripheral site but should be consistent for any whole procedure. It is recommended that IOPTH is used in discordant preoperative localization studies and in reoperative parathyroidectomy. IOPTH may be helpful in deciding intraoperatively if a biochemical cure has been achieved following surgery for pHPT. Cure is defined as greater than or equal to 50 per cent decay from the highest (pre-incision or pre-excision) value within 10 minutes of removing the hyperfunctioning gland(s).

RADIO-GUIDED PARATHYROIDECTOMY

RGP is intraoperative localization of parathyroid tissue with a gamma probe after preoperative MIBI administration. The dose and timing of MIBI administration varies, and there is no published MIBI protocol that is more superior. This intraoperative adjunct should be used only when there is a positive MIBI scan and is contraindicated in pregnancy or MIBI allergy/sensitivity.

The use of RGP is a useful adjunct during minimal access parathyroidectomy but could potentially prolong surgery. RGP is currently considered as an alternative technique to other intraoperative adjuncts such as IOPTH and frozen section. Its main benefit is in localizing and confirming ectopic glands and in revision surgery.

FROZEN SECTION

Frozen section (FS) is very reliable in differentiating between parathyroid and non-parathyroid tissue (e.g. lymph node, thyroid tissue) with a high degree of accuracy and has a turnaround time of 20 minutes. Differentiating between adenomas and multigland hyperplasia is often difficult.

METHYLENE BLUE

Methylene blue (MB) selectively stains parathyroid tissue and can therefore facilitate surgery. This is administered preoperatively via intravenous infusion of MB 5 mg/kg body weight, diluted in 100 mL normal saline, infused about 60 minutes prior to surgery or just before induction of general anaesthesia. Its use may be limited owing to the fact that it may interfere with pulse oximetry and recent reports of toxic encephalopathy.

SURGICAL APPROACHES TO pHPT

The traditional bilateral neck exploration (BNE) is the gold standard and benchmark for other surgical approaches. In approximately 95 per cent of cases using BNE, normocalcaemia has been achieved post-operatively. The choice of undertaking a targeted approach via a minimally invasive parathyroidectomy (MIP) or an open approach depends on the skill of the surgeon and patient factors. MIP under local anaesthesia or general anaesthesia is the recommended choice for single gland adenomas, while BNE is useful in multigland disease, recurrent/residual disease or unhelpful preoperative localization imaging.

Over the last 20 years, MIP has gained popularity, with improved localization imaging techniques being the main factor. It has less morbidity, reduced cost and shorter operating time with comparable success rates. The surgical techniques/access for MIP are summarized in Table 38.3. Current available evidence would favour open mini-incision MIP, which is less complicated and carries less risk to the recurrent laryngeal nerve when compared to video-assisted or endoscopic MIP.

Table 38.3 Surgical techniques/access for minimally invasive parathyroidectomy (MIP)

Surgical access for MIP	Technique
Open mini-incision MIP (OMIP)	Small horizontal cervical skin incision (approximately ≤2.5 cm) on neck as positioned as per image localization.
Video-assisted MIP (VAP)	Rigid endoscope without gas insufflation. Magnified view with optimal lighting.
Endoscopic MIP (EP)	Rigid endoscope with gas insufflation. Access via midline between the strap muscles or lateral access via the para-carotid gutter. Magnified view with optimal lighting.

After a skin crease incision is made (Figure 38.4), superior and inferior subplatysmal flaps are elevated and retracted with self-retaining Joules retractors. The medial edge of the sternomastoid muscle is separated from the strap muscles and laterally retracted. The carotid sheath, including the internal jugular vein, is identified and retracted laterally with a right-angled retractor. The surgical assistant then rotates the ipsilateral thyroid lobe with a retractor and thus exposes the posterolateral edge of the thyroid lobe. Depending on the preoperative localization of the parathyroid adenoma, it is identified (Figure 38.5) and gently dissected out with a combination of blunt dissection using a blunt artery clip, moist swab and meticulous haemostasis with a bipolar diathermy. Post-excision intraoperative PTH, FS or both may be done according to local practice. Usually, no drain is required, and after a two-layer closure some subcutaneous local anaesthesia is infiltrated around the incision. Nerve monitoring is used by some if general anaesthesia is being administered, while others use it only for selected cases such as revision surgery or if the suspected adenoma is more deeply placed. Single-gland exploration is performed as a

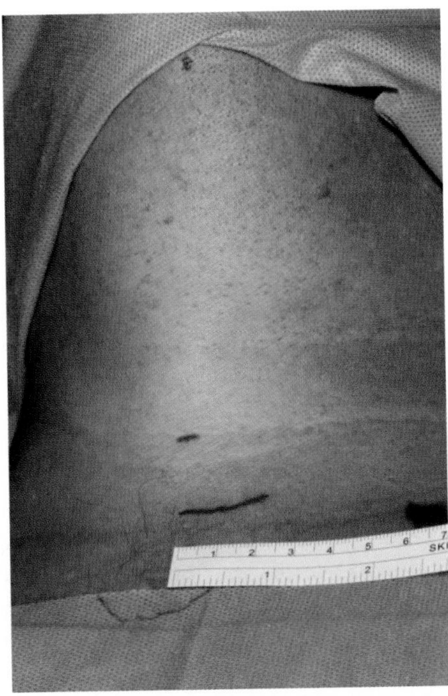

Figure 38.4 Small horizontal cervical skin crease incision for open minimally invasive parathyroidectomy (OMIP).

day-case procedure unless patient factors do not allow it.

Following successful parathyroidectomy, patients rapidly return to normocalcaemia with resolution of hypercalcaemic symptoms. Bone density has also been shown to improve over time with a significant decreased risk of bone fracture in both symptomatic and asymptomatic patients.

In the traditional four-gland exploration, ideally all four glands are exposed via bilateral dissection by either an open or endoscopic technique, and the macroscopically abnormal gland is excised. The gland may then be sent for FS tissue analysis, and IOPTH is performed to confirm biochemical cure. If negative, then additional glands may be dissected out.

The main indications for four-gland exploration as the initial procedure are:

- Secondary or tertiary hyperparathyroidism with renal failure
- Suspected MEN syndromes
- As extension of single-gland surgery when PTH levels do not fall
- Negative imaging localization studies
- Surgeon preference

LOCAL ANAESTHESIA CONSIDERATIONS

In minimally invasive surgery, local and regional block anaesthesia with or without intravenous sedation can also be considered. The local anaesthetic techniques described include local infiltration, superficial cervical block and deep cervical block.

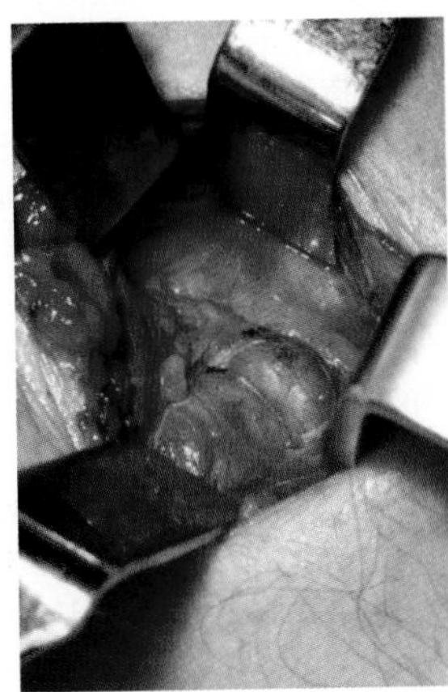

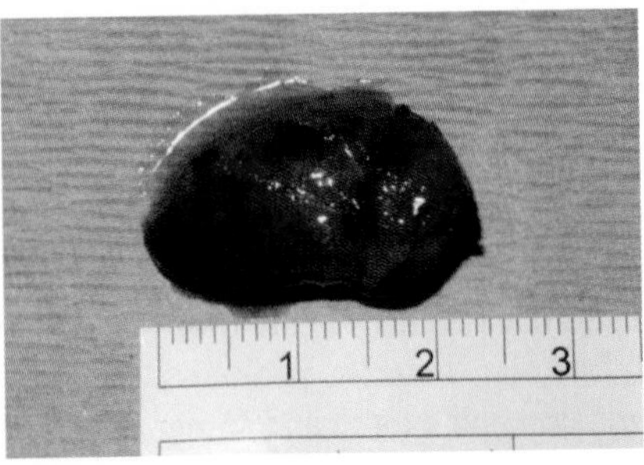

Figure 38.5 Inferior parathyroid adenoma exposed at the lower pole of the left thyroid lobe and excised gland.

Local anaesthesia can be used for older patients with severe co-morbidities where general anaesthesia is contraindicated or carries too high a risk and has a shorter recovery time with fewer symptoms like pain or nausea. Good patient selection with positive localization scans; thin, long neck; non-ectopic parathyroid glands and a cooperative patient are helpful for local anaesthetic procedures.

FAILED INITIAL EXPLORATION, PERSISTENT AND RECURRENT HYPERPARATHYROIDISM, AND RE-EXPLORATION

Surgical treatment for sporadic pHPT in experienced hands carries a success rate of more than 95 per cent with morbidity lower than 1 per cent. If the HPT is diagnosed 6 months after initial surgery, it is classified as a recurrent disease.

The most common cause of persistent sporadic pHPT has been shown to be inadequate neck exploration in up to 80 per cent of cases. This is followed by failure to locate or remove an ectopic adenoma located at various sites in the neck, superior or middle mediastinum (25 per cent), supernumerary parathyroid glands (5 per cent) and MGD (10–15 per cent).

Re-exploration should be performed preferably in a tertiary referral centre, adopting a systematic approach. Normocalcaemia after re-operative surgery in expert centres is achieved in 84–98 per cent of patients.

PARATHYROID CARCINOMA

Carcinoma of the parathyroid is a rare condition occurring in 0.5–5 per cent of patients with pHPT. It tends to occur in the fifth to sixth decade and has an equal sex incidence. It usually has a rapid onset with severe hypercalcaemia, muscle weakness, fatigue, polyuria, depression and nausea and sometimes presents with a neck mass or vocal cord palsy. Parathyroid cancer typically runs an indolent, albeit tenacious, course because the tumour has a rather low malignant potential. It locally invades the thyroid gland, muscles, recurrent laryngeal nerve, trachea or oesophagus. Serum calcium is usually very high (≥3.75 mmol/L) and the PTH may be 5 to 50 times the normal level.

Medical management is primarily geared towards management of the hypercalcemia that is often quite severe. Resistance to long-term control is usually the cause of death.

If surgery is performed, *en bloc* removal is the procedure of choice (hemithyroidectomy, paratracheal nodes and fat, thymic tissue ± modified/radical neck dissection in gross nodal involvement).

Post-operatively, there is a risk of decrease in calcium levels owing to 'hungry-bone syndrome', and patients should be monitored closely. There is an approximately 50 per cent postsurgical recurrence (2 to 5 years), with hypercalcemia preceding physical evidence of recurrence, locoregional in two-thirds of cases. The morbidity and mortality primarily result from the metabolic consequences of the disease and not directly from malignant growth. A 49 per cent 10-year survival rate has been reported in the US database of 286 patients.[4]

KEY LEARNING POINTS

- Parathyroid neoplasias are the most common cause of hypercalcaemia.
- Parathyroid tumours are benign in more than 99 per cent of cases, and more than 80 per cent are single-gland adenomas.
- Parathyroid tumours are more common in females and in the over-45 age group.
- More than 80 per cent of patients are asymptomatic on presentation but may have complications of hypercalcaemia as indications for surgery.
- Minimal access single-gland exploration is the procedure of choice for the majority of pHPT cases.
- Secondary hyperparathyroidism is usually due to chronic renal failure and may require subtotal/total parathyroidectomy.
- Parathyroid carcinoma is a rare occurrence.

REFERENCES

1. Ferris RL. *Chapter 66: Parathyroidectomy for Sporadic Primary Hyperparathyroidism.* In: *Operative Otolaryngology, Head and Neck Surgery.* Vol 1, 2nd ed. Ed. Myers EN. Philadelphia: Saunders Elsevier; 2008: 559–64.
2. Mihai R, Simon D, Hellman P. Imaging for primary hyperparathyroidism – An evidence-based analysis. *Langenbeck's Archives of Surgery.* 2009; 394: 765–84.
3. Bilezikian JP, Khan AA, Potts JT Jr. Guidelines for the management of asymptomatic primary hyperparathyroidism: Summary statement from the Third International Workshop. *Journal of Clinical Endocrinology and Metabolism.* 2009; 94(2): 335–39.
4. Hundahl SA, Fleming ID, Fremgen AM, et al. Two hundred eighty-six cases of parathyroid carcinoma treated in the U.S. between 1985–1995: A National Cancer Data Base Report. The American College of Surgeons Commission on Cancer and the American Cancer Society. *Cancer.* 1999; 86(3): 538–44.

FURTHER READING

Grant CS, Thompson G, Farley D, van Heerden J. Primary hyperparathyroidism surgical management since the introduction of minimally invasive parathyroidectomy. *Archives of Surgery.* 2005; 140: 472–79.

Harrison BJ, Triponez F. Intraoperative adjuncts in surgery for primary hyperparathyroidism. *Langenbeck's Archives of Surgery.* 2009; 394: 799–809.

SECTION III

Ear

39

Anatomy and physiology

LIAM M FLOOD

This chapter provides an introduction to applied anatomy and physiology of the ear that is strictly of clinical relevance. See the references at the end of this chapter for several excellent textbooks covering these topics in great detail.

TEMPORAL BONE

Osteology is a popular traditional examination topic and opens many temporal bone courses. Some anatomists argue as to the four parts of the temporal bone, but they are best thought of as two that ossify in cartilage and two in membrane. The former comprise the styloid process and the petromastoid, the latter the squamous temporal bone and tympanic 'ring' (a misnomer for what it is actually – a curved plate, like a gutter).

The first challenge is to orientate the bone and confidently identify it as right or left.

The lateral surface is notable for:

- The bony external auditory canal, with the tympanic ring forming the floor as an incomplete semi-cylinder. Note the sutures, the petrotympanic and tympanomastoid.
- The squamous temporal bone and especially the temporal line, a landmark for the level of the middle cranial fossa dura when exploring. The overlying muscle, the temporalis, is of less importance to ear, nose and throat (ENT) physicians than the covering layer of fascia, which is ideal graft material.
- The mastoid process, which develops in infancy to progressively cover what is initially a very exposed stylomastoid foramen and facial nerve. MacEwan's triangle, with its spine of

Henlé, is the surface landmark for the antrum, when starting to drill into a mastoid.

The posterior surface shows (Figure 39.1):

- The internal auditory canal (IAC), divided into upper and lower segments by the transverse crest, but one has to gaze deep in to see it. The upper segment is again divided by a small vertical partition. That, not the horizontal division, is called Bill's bar. Anything nerve-like that is anterior to it is the facial nerve, and posterior to it is the superior vestibular nerve, where vestibular schwannomas arise.
- The cochlear aqueduct. Directly below the IAC and passing in a similar plane is this much smaller canal, allowing communication between the cerebrospinal fluid (CSF) and cochlear perilymph (although there is great scepticism as to its patency in adults).
- Venous markings. It is worth recognizing the inferior and superior petrosal sinuses, as they can challenge the neurosurgical approach to the IAC. The grooves of the transverse and sigmoid sinuses and jugular foramen are more obvious. Their clinical relevance is in septic thrombosis secondary to chronic suppurative otitis media (CSOM) or the cranial neuropathies associated with glomus jugulare tumours (Figure 39.2).
- The cranial opening of the vestibular aqueduct. Here lies the elusive endolymphatic sac, just awaiting 'decompression'.

The superior surface shows:

- The groove of the middle meningeal artery, actually on the medial surface of the squamous bone and exposed to trauma.
- The arcuate eminence, a dome that is an inconsistent landmark for the superior semicircular canal.
- Various nerves escaping from the roof of the middle ear. The most important is the hiatus for the greater superficial petrosal nerve. Following this back is a way of finding the geniculate ganglion and facial nerve from the middle fossa. This nerve is destined to stimulate lacrimation, hence the dry eye of Bell's palsy.

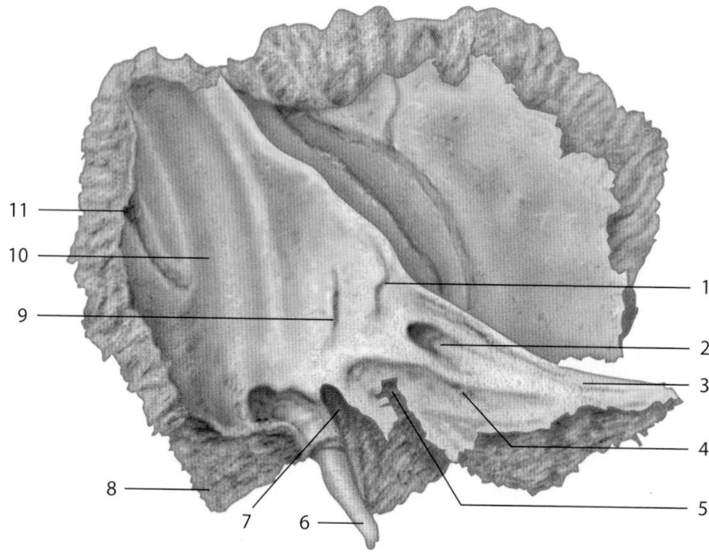

Figure 39.1 Posterior aspect of left temporal bone. 1, Fossa subarcuata; 2, internal acoustic meatus; 3, groove for superior petrosal sinus; 4, groove for inferior petrosal sinus; 5, canaliculus cochleae (cranial opening of perilymphatic aqueduct); 6, styloid process; 7, fossa jugularis (jugular bulb); 8, mastoid process; 9, cranial opening of aqueduct of vestibule; 10, groove for transverse sinus; 11, mastoid foramen (for mastoid emissary vein).

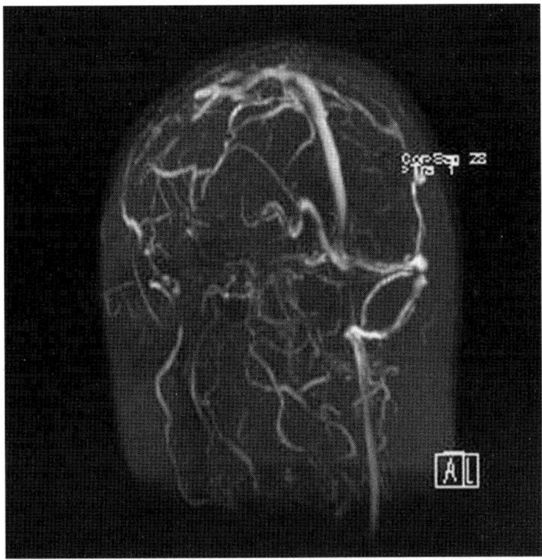

Figure 39.2 Magnetic resonance venography demonstrating flow through the upper midline (sagittal) sinus and through the lateral and sigmoid sinuses and internal jugular, on the right side of the image. Thrombosis has prevented any flow on the corresponding opposite side.

- The roof of the petrous apex is probably the only feature of interest in what is a relatively 'silent' area, beyond the IAC. It is marked by a depression, which makes up the floor of Dorello's canal. Its relevance is the proximity of the trigeminal and abducens nerve roots and the rare Gradenigo syndrome. In those with highly pneumatized temporal bones, mastoid sepsis can extend to the petrous apex causing retro-orbital pain and diplopia (due to a lateral rectus palsy) with a discharging ear.

The inferior surface looks particularly daunting. Structures worth noting include:

- The digastric groove. This is an anteroposterior dent in the undersurface of the mastoid giving attachment to the posterior belly of the digastric. Follow it forward to the stylomastoid foramen, where the facial nerve exits the skull base. In mastoid drilling, its reversed inner surface, now the digastric ridge (not groove), is a similarly useful landmark for the exit point of the descending facial nerve.
- The great vessels, especially the carotid in front and internal jugular vein behind, passing from the posterior cranial fossa into the neck.
- The bony eustachian tube. If the physician looks closely, he or she can see a canal within a canal; the tendon for the tensor tympani passes this way also, all worryingly close to the carotid canal.

EXTERNAL EAR

Most obvious is the auricle or pinna. This is composed of skin-covered yellow elastic cartilage but for the lobule, which is purely fatty areolar tissue. The relative safety of piercing the lobe, avoiding cartilage, is obvious to clinicians. The tragus is anterior to the external meatus, a source of cartilage or perichondrium in tympanoplasty. Above it is the one gap in the cartilage that allows the endaural incision. The antihelix is, of course, the fold that can be lacking and augmented in pinnaplasty correction of bat ears.

The external canal in adults is about 2.5 cm long. With the oblique lie of the tympanic membrane, the anterior canal is longer, passing into the acute tympanomeatal sulcus. The outer one-third of the canal is cartilage and the medial two-thirds bony, but the two do meet at an angle; hence the need for traction on the pinna to straighten the canal at otoscopy. Only the outer third has wax glands and hair follicles, but defects in the floor, the fissures of Santorini, are notorious routes of infection from necrotizing otitis externa spreading to the parotid and skull base. Deeper in the bony canal are two longitudinal sutures, a challenge to any surgeon in raising an intact tympanomeatal flap. The tympanomastoid and, especially, a well-developed petrotympanic suture line can only be exposed by sharp dissection, if flaps are not to tear.

The innervation of the pinna and the external ear canal has some clinical relevance. Cranial nerves V, VII, IX and X; the great auricular (C2 and 3); and the lesser occipital (C2) all contribute. Hence the vesicles seen in Ramsay Hunt syndrome, the cough on stimulating the ear, the earache of tonsil cancer and the occasional numb pinna after parotidectomy.

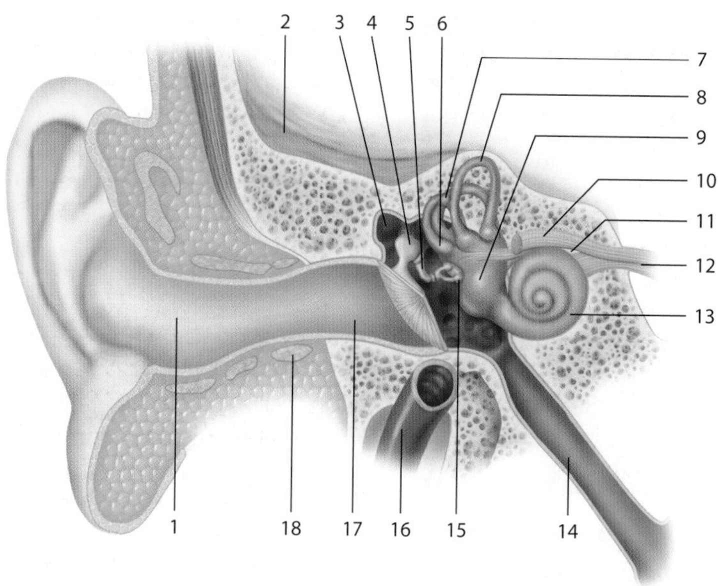

Figure 39.3 Vertical coronal diagrammatic section through right ear. (After Brödel.) 1, External meatus, cartilaginous part; 2, middle cranial fossa; 3, attic; 4, malleus; 5, incus; 6, position of lateral semicircular canal; 7, position of posterior semicircular canal; 8, superior semicircular canal; 9, vestibule; 10, facial nerve; 11, vestibular nerve; 12, cochlear nerve; 13, cochlea; 14, eustachian tube; 15, stapes; 16, internal carotid artery; 17, bony part of external meatus; 18, cartilage.

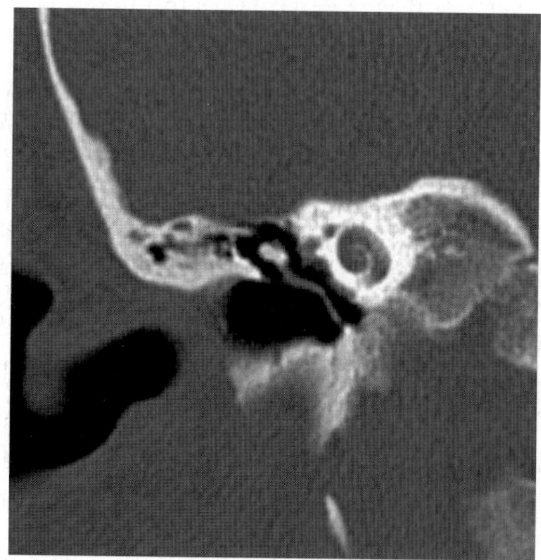

Figure 39.4 Coronal computed tomographic scan. Compare with diagram of ear anatomy in Figure 39.3.

The blood supply comes from the superficial temporal and post-auricular arteries, whilst the deep meatus is supplied by a deep auricular branch of the maxillary artery. What is clinically important is how rich this supply is. Thus a pinna can survive a combined endaural and post-aural incision, with only a worryingly narrow pedicle remaining inferiorly (Figures 39.3 and 39.4).

TYMPANIC MEMBRANE

This is a conical-shaped membrane separating the external and middle ear. Its diameter is approximately 1 cm and its area 85 mm^2, of which only 55 mm^2 is physiologically effective. The otoscopic lateral view shows few features in health. The pearly grey membrane of the pars tensa will show a light reflex unless inflamed but is generally too opaque to allow clear view of the ossicles, other than the handle of the malleus. This runs almost vertically from the lateral process superiorly, down the manubrium to the umbo, in the centre of the drumhead. Retraction of the drum can produce a foreshortened appearance to the handle. A few blood vessels will pass vertically, parallel to and immediately posterior to the handle in health. The joint between the incus and the stapes lies deep to the posterosuperior segment but is rarely evident unless the drum is thinned or retracted onto it. If it is visible, confirming its integrity is fundamental to evaluation of conductive losses. In the same quadrant, the chorda tympani nerve passes from posteriorly, lateral to the long process of the incus and medial to the neck of the malleus. It is at risk of trauma in elevating the membrane for any middle ear exploration, and taste disturbance in the ipsilateral tongue may result.

The membrane itself is said to show the elasticity of rubber and is made up of three layers. Superficially is keratinizing squamous epithelium, a curious finding in an area not expected to experience wear and tear. A failure of migration of this keratin is the basis of diseases such as keratosis obturans or cholesteatoma. The middle layer, the lamina propria, shows radiating and circular fibres. Atrophic loss of this layer weakens the drumhead and allows retraction pockets and adhesions. Conversely, hyaline degeneration and calcification produce the characteristic white plaques of tympanosclerosis. The inner layer is the expected mucous epithelium of the middle ear. The tympanic fibrocartilaginous annulus encircles the membrane edge and sits in the corresponding bony sulcus. Elevating and separating these is the basis of raising a tympanomeatal flap.

Superiorly, the middle layer is deficient (but not absent), forming the pars flaccida, easily overlooked by the novice otoscopist but the origin of many a cholesteatoma. Above the level of its superior bony margin, but deeply in the attic, lies the bulk of the ossicular chain, the heads of the malleus and the incus. Unless there is significant bony marginal erosion of the outer attic wall or scutum, these are invisible to the examiner.

MIDDLE EAR CLEFT

This is a complex, air-filled structure running posteriorly, from the bony eustachian tube through the tympanic cavity (what most call 'the middle ear') and the aditus, a small connection with the mastoid antrum (itself a single large cavity), and then connected to a variable number of mastoid air cells. Indeed, air cells can extend well beyond the mastoid to the petrous apex or into the root of the zygoma, with obvious implications in disease. The cavity is lined with a modified respiratory mucosa that undergoes a transition passing posteriorly. In health, only the most anterior and inferior portions show typical mucociliary epithelium with goblet cells. The majority show a flat, squamous but non-keratinizing lining. Chronic middle ear sepsis profoundly alters this distribution.

The relationships of the cleft are best considered for their clinical relevance. Superiorly lies the temporal lobe in the middle cranial fossa, separated from the upper middle ear, the 'epitympanum' or attic, by a thin plate of bone, the tegmen. Deficiency can lead to dural/cerebral herniation and even CSF rhinorrhoea (leakage down the eustachian tube). The dura frequently dips even lower laterally, over the external canal, tending to drive the unguarded surgeon progressively lower in drilling and towards the descending facial nerve.

Inferiorly, equally thin bone, which can indeed be dehiscent, protects the bulb of the internal jugular vein from the myringotome, passing deep to the vestibular system. More anteriorly, the carotid passes anteromedially, deep to the cochlea. The anterior wall is pierced by the eustachian tube and the canal for the tensor tympani, and laterally lies the tympanic membrane and outer attic wall.

The posterior wall shows landmarks of greater surgical relevance. The aditus leads into the antrum, but most importantly guides one to that essential surgical landmark, the prominence of the lateral semicircular canal, immediately medial to the short process of the incus. The pyramidal eminence lies on the posterior wall below the aditus and is there to allow the stapedius tendon to insert into the stapes neck. It is, however, also a landmark dividing two vertical grooves, fundamental to the evolution of mastoid surgery. The stapedius muscle is innervated by the facial nerve, and so the trunk, in its descending portion just deep to the pyramid, forms a vertical ridge. Anything lateral to that and deep to the drum margin, the bony annulus, is the facial

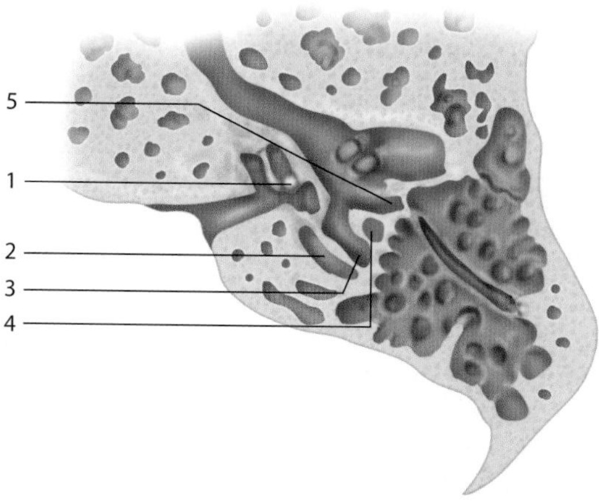

Figure 39.5 Axial section of temporal bone showing: 1, basal turn of cochlea; 2, posterior semicircular canal; 3, sinus tympani; 4, facial canal and pyramid/stapedius tendon; 5, facial recess.

recess. Disease here was traditionally accessed by a 'canal wall down' technique, to take away the bony annulus and leave an open cavity. The later intact canal wall approach uses a 'posterior tympanotomy', a transmastoid approach directly into the facial recess, between the facial and chorda tympani nerves. Unfortunately, there is a second groove deep to the pyramid and facial nerve, the sinus tympani, of varying depth and relatively inaccessible (Figure 39.5).

The medial wall is what the exploring surgeon encounters and what separates the middle from the inner ear. To allow sound passage, it is pierced by the oval and round windows. The first accommodates the stapes footplate, the latter, below it, is less obvious. The true round window membrane lies oblique to the view at tympanotomy, within a deep round window niche. Mucosal folds within this cavity are easily mistaken for the membrane itself, especially by the credulous, when seeking a perilymph fistula. Anterior to both windows is a distinct convex bulge, created by the basal turn of the cochlea, the promontory. The smooth surface may show superficially the nerves of the tympanic plexus or Jacobson's nerve. Tympanic neurectomy here has long been an option in attempts to reduce salivation stimulation, for example in Frey's syndrome (Figure 39.6).

Familiarity with the course of the facial nerve here is indispensable. A consistent landmark for the geniculate ganglion is the processus cochleariformis, especially as it is relatively resistant to erosion. (*Cochleariform* means 'hooked' and has nothing to do with the hearing part of the inner ear.) The tensor tympani, having travelled up the eustachian tube, here gives off its tendon, which turns laterally to insert into the neck of the malleus. All books agree on its value in finding the entry point of the facial nerve; few accurately describe how the two relate. The geniculate ganglion is immediately superior to this bony process. Lying in a bony tunnel, it must be slightly more medial than the processus cochlearformis. Do not confuse this with medial to; it is just above. The facial nerve then passes in the horizontal or fallopian canal, which rarely lacks some dehiscence, especially above the oval window. Passing posteriorly and slightly downwards, it courses superior to the stapes footplate, hopefully not so dehiscent as to challenge footplate surgery. It will now pass inferior to the lateral semicircular canal, towards its second turn or genu. Erosion of the lateral canal by disease is commonly associated with facial nerve exposure (and resulting paralysis) at just this point. Just as the lateral semicircular canal is curving back into the labyrinth, at its posterior end, the facial nerve takes that right angle turn into its descending portion. Clinicians have seen its branch then pass to the stapedius. Approximately 5 mm from its exit point, the stylomastoid foramen, it also gives off the chorda tympani, which passes all the way back up to the tympanic membrane.

OSSICLES

The malleus is attached to the tympanic membrane by its handle and umbo; it has well-developed anterior and posterior ligaments and various suspensory folds, all of which stabilize it. Its head lies in the attic but is often removed in surgery of CSOM by division at its neck. The stapes is secured by the stapedius tendon and the annular ligament, which, unless obliterated by oto- or tympanosclerosis, allows it to still vibrate in the margins of the oval window. It is the smallest bone in the body; its weight is that of an adult mosquito at 2.5 mg, and it

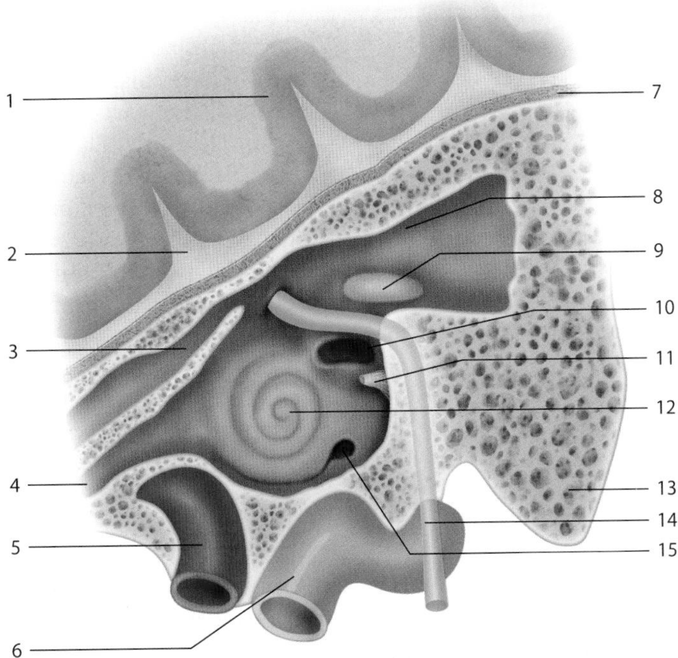

Figure 39.6 Relations of the left tympanic cavity and the facial nerve. 1, Cerebral cortex; 2, subarachnoid space; 3, canal for tensor tympani; 4, eustachian tube; 5, internal carotid artery; 6, jugular bulb; 7, dura mater; 8, aditus; 9, lateral semicircular canal; 10, oval window; 11, pyramid; 12, promontory; 13, mastoid process; 14, facial nerve; 15, round window.

is remarkably like a true stirrup with its footplate, two crura and head. The incus is less stable, almost floating between its two companions. It articulates with the malleus head via a synovial joint and with the stapes via its long process, and its posterior short process provides further ligament support. Skull trauma causing conductive loss usually indicates incus dislocation, however. The tenuous blood supply to the incudo-stapedial joint (ISJ; those tiny vessels have far to go to pass up the crura and down the long process to its tip, the lenticular process) is easily compromised by chronic sepsis, and ISJ erosion is common. The heads of the ossicles are surrounded by eponymous folds and spaces (such as the notch of Rivinius, the pouch of von Troeltsch and Prussak's space), but quoting them is less important than recognizing that cholesteatoma may either stay lateral to the ossicles or pass medially, with major implications for surgical prognosis.

EUSTACHIAN TUBE

The eustachian tube passes from the nasopharynx to the tympanic cavity, upwards, backwards and laterally (as it must, to run from a midline structure to the lateral temporal bone). It is 36 mm long in the adult, with the child's tube being shorter, wider, more horizontal and less efficient. It is the reverse of the external ear canal, being one-third bony and two-thirds cartilaginous. This reflects its role as a dynamic, moving and complex structure, not a simple conduit. In cross section proximally, it is described as a cartilaginous shepherd's crook, an inverted *J* or a fishhook. Its lateral cartilage-free margin is membranous. It is normally closed but opens owing to the contractions of the tensor and levator palati, unless of course there is a congenital abnormality, as in cleft palate. Distally, the bony tube is separated from the medially lying internal carotid canal by what may, at most, be a thin bony partition. Attempts at dilatation and intubation of the canal have raised the spectre of breaching this, with unfortunate consequences.

INNER EAR

The physiology of the inner ear is of greater clinical import to most surgeons than its structure, as few will venture there. There is a bony labyrinth containing a floating membranous labyrinth, following its every twist and turn. The bony labyrinth has an endosteal lining, and in erosive disease (e.g. cholesteatoma) a fistula is usually walled off by this delicate membrane, so, hopefully, perilymph will not pour out if one lifts the matrix (Figure 39.7).

Anteriorly is the cochlea with its two-and-one-half spiral turns. The vestibule is the connection between this and the posterior and slightly higher vestibular apparatus with its three semicircular canals. The vestibule is the site of sound entry through the oval window, with the round window membrane also piercing its lateral wall. The medial wall of the vestibule allows nerves to pass from the internal auditory canal but also, with the cochlear aqueduct, allows CSF and perilymph to communicate. The vestibule contains the saccule

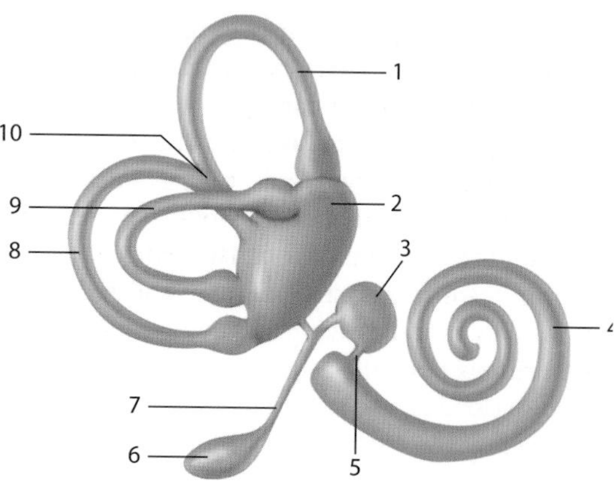

Figure 39.7 Membranous labyrinth (right side, lateral view). 1, Superior semicircular canal; 2, utricle; 3, saccule; 4, cochlea; 5, ductus reuniens; 6, endolymphatic sac; 7, endolymphatic duct; 8, posterior semicircular canal; 9, lateral semicircular canal; 10, crus commune.

and the utricle, with the former immediately deep to the stapes footplate and at risk in stapedotomy. The remaining vestibular apparatus comprises the three semicircular canals, each with its 'ampullated end', the part that contains the sensory end organ, anteriorly. Each canal then passes in its own orientation (superior, posterior and lateral or horizontal) in a large arc to pass back to the vestibule once more. As the superior and inferior canal meet, just before regaining the vestibule, there are only five orifices into the cavity. The ampullated end of the inferior canal is deep to the descending facial nerve, with obvious risks in osseous labyrinthectomy. The arc of the posterior canal is at risk in approaches to the endolymphatic sac, whilst the horizontal canal is important as a surgical landmark for the facial nerve. The endolymphatic sac at the end of its duct acts as a site of surgery for Ménière's disease.

COCHLEA

The ascending spiral takes its two-and-one-half turns around the central bony modiolus. The stairway in the middle allows nerves to ascend. Getting stimulating electrodes close to these in cochlear implantation led to the design of the modiolus hugger. A projecting bony plate follows off this central pillar in the spiral canal, winding back down again. Now the nerves can pass to the membranous labyrinth and things get complicated. Essentially, three soft tissue tubes are joined together. The upper is the scala vestibuli, so called because it runs from the vestibule, where the stapes footplate is located. The lowermost is the scala tympani, its name reflecting that it is heading back down to the round window membrane (or 'tympanum'). Both contain perilymph, essentially modified CSF; they meet at the apex of the spiral, the helicotrema, allowing sound transmission from one to the other. Then comes the scala media, the mysterious third space that contains endolymph, far more like intra- than extra-cellular fluid. Dilatation of this space, 'endolymphatic hydrops', is suggested as the basis for Ménière's disease, and consequent membrane rupture, allowing endolymph and perilymph to meet, has profound otoneurological consequences. At its simplest, the scala media is almost an isosceles triangle in cross section, its floor the basilar membrane, which vibrates on sound stimulation. The hypotenuse is Reissner's membrane, and the vertical limb is the stria vascularis, thought to be essential in homeostasis of endolymph (whether removal or production remains controversial). Within the scala media lies the whole *raison d'être*, the organ of Corti, with the hair and supporting cells, the tectorial membrane and the cortliymph, all to be considered under physiology (Figure 39.8).

The blood supply of the vestibule, the labyrinthine artery, is of clinical relevance, as it is tenuous. Derived from the basilar or anterior inferior cerebellar artery, it is an end artery. The lack of any potential for collateral circulation means that disturbance causes profound ischaemia, a likely mechanism for much sudden sensorineural hearing loss or vertigo. Because it is derived from the internal carotid circulation, the ultimate model of homeostasis and self-regulation to ensure constancy of blood supply to the brain, the potential for any claimed cochlear 'vasodilators' must be questioned.

Clinically, it is sufficient to know of the cochlear nerve and the superior and vestibular nerves. The superior vestibular nerve supplies the utricle, the ampullated ends of the superior and lateral semicircular canals and the anterior macule of the

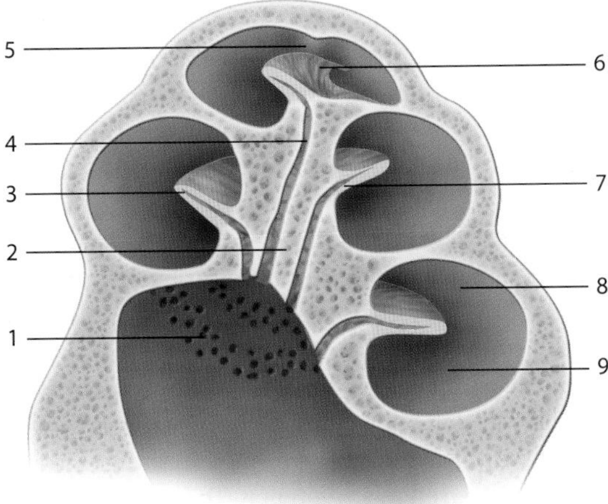

Figure 39.8 Diagram of cochlea. 1, Tractus spiralis foraminosa; 2, modiolus; 3, osseous spiral lamina; 4, central canal; 5, apex (contains helicotrema); 6, hamulus; 7, spiral canal of modiolus; 8, scala vestibuli; 9, scala tympani.

saccule. It is therefore the nerve tested by caloric irrigation. The inferior vestibular is the nerve of the posterior semicircular canal and saccule and is probably best known for its role in benign positional vertigo.

PHYSIOLOGY OF HEARING

Hearing is the perception of sound vibrations in our gaseous, fluid atmosphere, so is usually achieved by air conduction. Waves of alternate condensation and rarefaction may be conveying essential environmental information, such as beware that predator or truck, ensuring the sophisticated communication of speech or allowing the pleasure of music. Quantum physics insists that the sound of the tree falling in the forest actually needs an observer for it to even exist. Certainly, the characteristics of sound, such as pitch (frequency) and loudness (intensity), are subjective impressions of the listener.

EXTERNAL EAR

The pinna and its postauricular muscles seem almost redundant in humans, but the external ear retains some role in sound localization. The pinna here is most effective for higher frequencies and in distinguishing between sounds coming from in front or behind. Middle frequency localization depends more on the 'shadow effect' of the skull and, for lower frequencies, the phase difference between the two ears predominates. More importantly, the external ear canal acts as a resonator, maximally at 3–4 kHz. This is therefore the frequency for which the auditory system is most sensitive; hence the characteristic loss of noise-induced deafness.

MIDDLE EAR

The middle ear transformer mechanism is designed to overcome an 'impedance mismatch'. Sound does not easily pass from air into liquid, such as the perilymph that is seen in the cochlea. Impedance, the reluctance of the system to conduct sound onwards, is determined by the mass, the stiffness and the resistance of friction in the system. That air-fluid interface is a potential barrier.

The drum and ossicles provide a mechanical advantage, not strictly amplification, worth more than 30 dB of hearing. This is due to:

- A cone-shaped tympanic membrane
- A large drum connecting to a small footplate
- That connection through a lever system
- A baffle effect

Loudspeaker designers quickly learned the advantages of the cone acoustically. The drum is most free to vibrate when pressures to either side (external and middle ear) are equal; hence the importance of the connection to the outside world through the eustachian tube. A well-developed mastoid cell system may provide a useful air reservoir to dampen minor pressure changes. Gas exchange across mastoid mucosa has also been suggested, as has a role for the pars flaccida in protecting the inner ear from sudden atmospheric pressure changes.

The tympanic membrane is connected ultimately to a much smaller footplate. A true areal ratio of 20:1 is, in practice, more like 14:1 functionally, as discussed earlier. Direct contact between them, a columella, works perfectly well in birds and in many tympanoplasties. An artificial strut – a total ossicular replacement prosthesis (TORP) – can connect the drumhead to the footplate. A retraction of the drum onto the stapes head can produce a natural type III effect and, in both situations, audiograms with 10 dB of normal can result.

However, the ossicular lever effect, the differing lengths of the malleus handle and the long process of the incus, gives a further mechanical advantage, calculated at 1.3:1. The worst conductive losses come not from large perforations but from an intact drum with a break in the ossicular chain. Now the drum is acting as a 'baffle', preventing sound entry.

Curiously the 'baffle', in health, actually conveys an additional benefit. Inner ear liquids are (by definition) incompressible. If every inward excursion of the footplate is to efficiently create vibration, it is best that somewhere else there is a compensatory outward movement, here of the round window membrane. Therefore, ideally, the ossicles focus all sound onto the oval window and keep it well away from the round window membrane. Simultaneous pressure onto both produces no vibration. Therefore, the membrane is buried well inside a bony niche, it lies oblique to the direction of sound and the intact drum is a barrier to its exposure to sound.

The transmitting power of the ossicular chain is influenced by two intra-tympanic muscles and what may be protective reflexes. Both stapedius and tensor tympani stiffen the ossicular chain on contraction, stimulated by loud noise or a startle response. Any protective role is disputed because until very recently mankind rarely experienced, in nature, noises of 80–90 dB intensity (as required here) except in thunderstorms. Even then, the latency suggests that any damage is already done. Sustained contractions do attenuate or mask low-frequency background noise and may improve speech discrimination, but this 'cocktail party effect' seems even less applicable to all but our most immediate ancestors' lifestyle.

COCHLEA

The potential of the cochlea is truly remarkable, whether for its frequency or sound intensity range of hearing. Although tested clinically only up to 8 kHz in audiometry, the upper limit of hearing is well above 16 kHz in healthy youth, with an overall 10-octave range. For intensity, the 'dynamic range', the difference between the threshold at which sound is just perceived and the level when it becomes painful, represents a 10-million-fold increase in energy. Even 130 dB of sound, a highly damaging level, produces pressure variations of only 0.2 per cent of atmospheric pressure. At threshold levels, drum vibration is at molecular dimensions.

Because of this huge range of sound intensities perceived, a log scale is necessary. The decibel is, at its simplest, the ratio of two sounds: the measured sound compared to a reference. The reference happens to be 10–12 watts/m^2, which is the threshold of the 'average' (20-year-old) human at 1 kHz. What is far more important to remember, clinically, is that the scale is not linear; it is logarithmic. An apparently modest 20 dB hearing gain from surgery seems more impressive when considered as a tenfold increase in amplitude. Also, beware studies that quote a 'mean' of a series of results expressed in dB; that simply cannot be done.

This auditory miracle is achieved through vibrations first in liquid and ultimately stimulating nerve endings, the hair cells. Think of sound as passing in via the scala vestibuli (passing from the footplate) and back out via the scala tympani (as one might see in that round window reflex noted in surgery). The vibrations distort the basilar membrane, on which sit the rows of resonating hair cells. They are themselves tipped with even smaller 'hairs' or stereocilia, embedded in the tectorial membrane. The resulting shearing force or angulation causes depolarization, and off goes the auditory signal (Figure 39.9).

Although this might seem simple, it turns out that there are three times more nerves going to the cochlea (efferent) than away from it (afferent), which is a bit odd for a seemingly passive sensory organ. There is a single row of inner hair cells behaving as expected, but no fewer than three rows of outer hair cells, away from that central spiral, with a totally different mechanical function. These are contractile, and they stiffen the basilar membrane locally. Interaction between inner and outer hair cells leads to fine-tuning and precise frequency perception. The basilar membrane is displaced by a travelling wave. It is less stiff at its apex, so that area will respond more to low-frequency vibration, whilst the basal turn is naturally high frequency sensitive. The outer hair cells are unique to mammals, but, unfortunately, are particularly fragile and easily damaged by noise or toxins. Their positive feedback system allows the truly sensory inner hair cell to be remarkably selective in identifying its own 'chosen' frequency for response. A hair cell destined to passively respond to a range from 1000 to 2000 cycles per second of vibration in the basilar membrane can now detect far less intense sounds at, for example, 1050–1070 cycles per second, while ignoring all other frequencies – all because its neighbouring outer hair cells stiffened that very area of the basilar membrane. Loss of this remarkable system results in recruitment, the narrowed dynamic range. For a quiet noise, fine-tuning is lost, and no sound is perceived by any hair cells anywhere. Increase the stimulus and the patient remarks, 'I still cannot hear you'. Suddenly, the threshold for a large range of now far

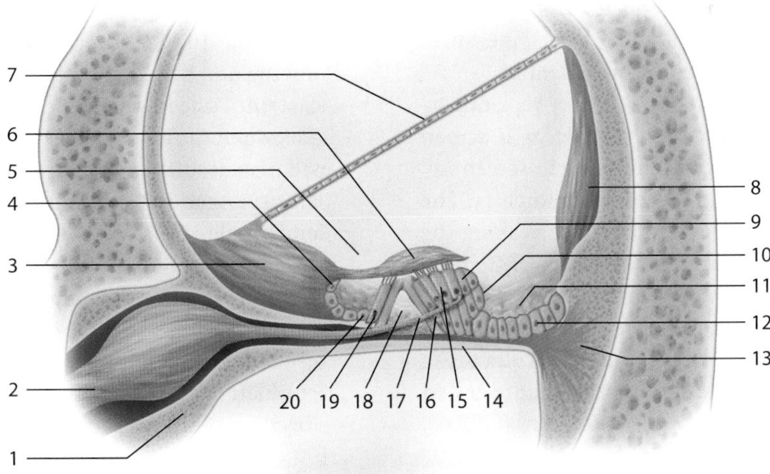

Figure 39.9 Scala media with organ of Conti. 1, Osseous spiral lamina; 2, spiral ganglion; 3, spiral limbus; 4, vestibular lip of spiral limbus; 5, inner sulcus; 6, tectorial membrane; 7, Reissner's membrane; 8, stria vascularis; 9, space of Nuel; 10, cells of Hensen; 11, outer sulcus; 12, cells of Claudius; 13, spiral ligament; 14, basilar membrane; 15, outer hair cells; 16, outer pillar of tunnel of Corti; 17, nerve fibres; 18, tunnel of Corti; 19, inner hair cells; 20, tympanic lip of spiral limbus.

less selective hair cells is reached and all respond suddenly, and the patient remarks, 'that is too loud'. The challenge for hearing aids is obvious.

Hair cell vibration produces the sound of the otoacoustic emission, the basis of much screening audiology. Their electrical activity, the cochlear microphonic, or the action potential of the resulting nerve impulse, is studied in electrocochleography. The frequency specificity associated with ascent up the cochlea is exploited in cochlear implantation. Multichannel electrodes will selectively stimulate different regions to allow frequency information. Single-channel stimulation is limited by the frequency of nerve response imposed by the refractory period, which implies maximal neural response of 200 impulses per second, not too helpful for speech. Slightly higher frequencies can still be encoded by adjacent nerves transmitting out of phase.

HIGHER AUDITORY PATHWAYS

Whilst essential for central processing of sound, especially speech, detailed knowledge of the pathways is unnecessary. The drive to earliest diagnosis of congenital hearing loss stems from the recognition that without early auditory stimulation, higher pathways do not, and will never, develop. Certainly by 5 years of age and ideally by 2 years, measures such as cochlear implantation are essential.

The auditory brain stem response, replaced by magnetic resonance imaging (MRI) as a screen for acoustic neuroma, is still of value in screening, site of lesion testing and objective audiometry. The five wave forms, I–V, correspond to sites along the anatomical pathway surely of interest solely to neuroanatomists. The popular mnemonic is ECOLI (Eighth nerve, Cochlear nucleus, superior Olivary complex, Lateral lemniscus, Inferior colliculus). The highest centres, in the brain itself, are tested in cortical electrical response audiometry (CERA).

VESTIBULAR SYSTEM

Surely the least understood part of the ear, the vestibular system's importance becomes obvious when bilaterally destroyed by ototoxic drugs such as systemic streptomycin. The patient is rendered severely ataxic with bobbing eye movements on walking termed *oscillopsia*. Balance requires a combined input of information from the eyes (e.g. viewing the horizon), proprioception (more weight on one leg than the other perhaps) and what the inner ear is telling him or her. Walking on uneven ground in the dark requires a reliable vestibular input as the only functioning of these systems. Flying in fog, a pilot must conversely totally ignore all vestibular warnings and rely on instruments, because direction of gravity, acceleration and linear velocity are all easily confused (Figure 39.10).

The vestibular apparatus comprises:

- Three semicircular canals for each inner ear. These are orientated at right angles to each other, and each is opposed to its partner in the opposite ear. The two 'horizontal' canals are angled at 30° to the true horizontal plane (hence the ideal position to establish convection currents in caloric irrigation) and work together to provide information in regard to lateral head turning. Asymmetry results in each superior canal on one side being opposed by the posterior canal on the opposite side. Endolymph inertia on head turning will cause endolymph to move through the corresponding canal. (In practice, it is the walls that are moving and the endolymph is staying still, at least until one finally gets off the fairground ride, when the reverse does truly apply.) This will displace the cupula on the crista, the sensory organ in the ampullated end of that semicircular canal. This does have a resting baseline rate of discharge, but that increases with flow towards the ampulla and reduces with flow away. The most obvious consequence results from the vestibulo-ocular reflex (VOR). Stimulation and increased discharge cause a slow drift of the eyes to the opposite side but a fast central compensation to try to maintain vision. Traditionally nystagmus is described by the fast phase direction, even though that is the result of optic fixation, not the vestibular input. To the observer, it is the most dramatic component and most easily seen. Irritative vestibular lesions (e.g. the fistula test) are also mimicked

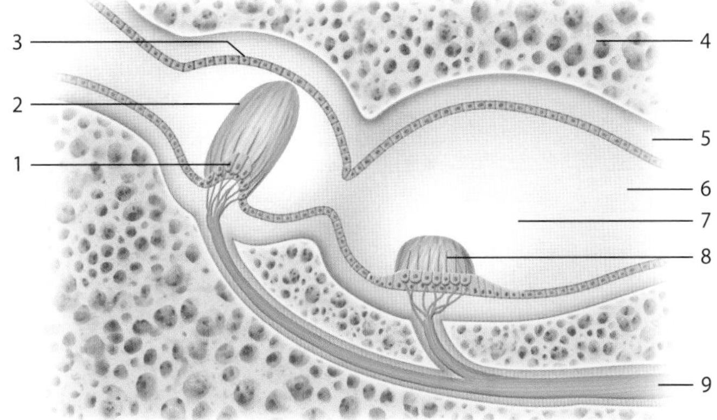

Figure 39.10 Schematic diagram of semicircular canal and utricle. 1, Hair cells; 2, crista; 3, ampulla; 4, temporal bone; 5, perilymph; 6, endolymph; 7, utricle; 8, otolith organ; 9, nerve fibres.

by caloric irrigation, with warm water producing convection currents in the endolymph. This simple explanation was totally spoiled by Skylab experiments showing that orbiting astronauts could still show caloric-induced nystagmus in zero (strictly micro) gravity - 'no gravity, no dense liquids sink' phenomenon (Figure 39.11).

- The utricle and saccule. These lie in the vestibule, the former orientated in the plane of the horizontal canal, the latter in the vertical plane. The receptor organs are the maculae. As in the cochlea, hair cells are embedded in a roof of a gel layer now containing calcium carbonate crystals. Denser than endolymph, these are the notorious otoliths of cupulo- or canalolithiasis.

Vestibular reflexes are responsible for:

- Maintenance of posture to compensate for gravity even at rest (via the maculae and not the semicircular canals). Einstein reminded us that gravity is just another way of describing acceleration.
- Maintenance of equilibrium and a stable visual field during movement (via the otoliths for linear acceleration and canals for angular acceleration).
- Maintenance of muscle tone. Information about head position creates head-righting

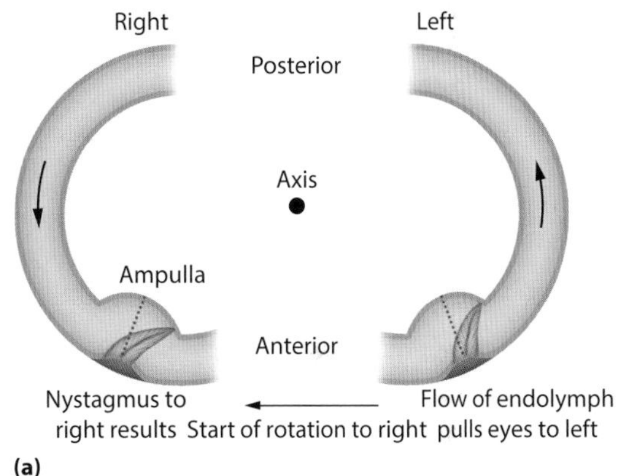

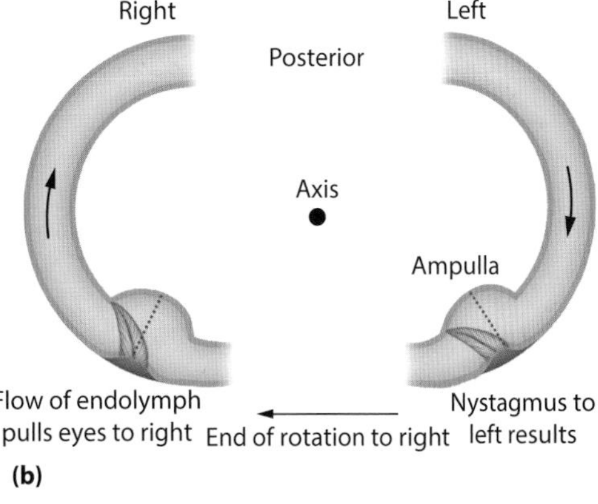

Figure 39.11 Diagram of movement of endolymph in rotation tests. **(a)** Beginning of clockwise rotation; **(b)** end of clockwise rotation.

reflexes, as seen in vestibular evoked myogenic potentials associated with sternomastoid contractions.

CONCLUSION

A single chapter can act only as an introduction to the complexity of the workings of the ear, concentrating on what is most clinically relevant. The books listed at the end of this chapter are recommended for further study.

KEY LEARNING POINTS

- Familiarity with temporal bone anatomy and surgical landmarks is fundamental to otologic practice, and advances in imaging and monitoring cannot substitute.
- The middle ear transformer mechanism conveys a mechanical advantage to sound transmission to overcome an impedance mismatch.
- Successful tympanoplasty must reproduce the areal ratio and lever action of the tympanic membrane/ossicular complex in order to reverse conductive loss.
- Cochlear hair cells are not the passive receptors once imagined, but show a remarkable ability for self tuning. Dysfunction results in recruitment and reduced speech discrimination.
- The vestibular apparatus is just one component in the maintenance of balance but does provide essential sensation of movement and of orientation in a gravitational field.

FURTHER READING

Alberti P. *The Anatomy and Physiology of the Ear and Hearing*. www.who.int/occupational_health/publications/noise2.pdf.

Flint PW, Haughey BH, Lund VJ, et al. *Cummings Otolaryngology – Head and Neck Surgery*. 5th ed. Philadelphia: Mosby, 2010.

Gleeson M, ed. *Scott Brown's Otorhinolaryngology, Head and Neck Surgery*. 7th ed. London: Hodder Arnold, 2008.

Merchant SN, Nadol JB. *Schuknecht's Pathology of the Ear*. 3rd ed. Shelton, CT: PMPH-USA, 2010.

Snow JB, Wackym PA. *Ballenger's Otorhinolaryngology Head and Neck Surgery*. 17th ed. Shelton, CT: PMPH-USA, 2009.

40

Tests for hearing

DESMOND A NUNEZ AND LI QI

INTRODUCTION

The purpose of this chapter is to introduce common hearing tests for adults and children. Bedside, behavioural and electrophysiological hearing tests are discussed. The most commonly used bedside hearing tests are the voice and tuning fork tests. Bedside hearing tests provide a basic hearing screen. Pure tone audiometry and speech tests are behavioural tests. Pure tone audiometry quantitatively measures behavioural hearing thresholds. The speech recognition threshold (SRT) and word recognition score (WRS) are the most commonly used speech test parameters. A strong correlation exists between SRT and pure tone average thresholds. WRS may provide diagnostic information of the site of lesion. Tympanometry, ototacoustic emission (OAE) and auditory brain stem response (ABR) tests are electrophysiological hearing tests. Tympanometry is used to assess middle-ear function in adults and children. OAE tests are used to evaluate outer hair function and have been used for monitoring ototoxicity and noise-induced hearing loss. ABR tests are clinically used to assess retro-cochlear pathology or estimate infants' hearing thresholds. OAE and ABR tests are widely used in newborn hearing screening programmes. Visual reinforcement audiometry (VRA) and play audiometry are used to evaluate behavioural hearing thresholds for toddlers and young children. In summary, there are a variety of hearing tests. To make an accurate diagnosis, different hearing tests should be utilized. The effects of age, motivation and cognitive function on hearing always need to be considered.

CLINICAL TESTS OF HEARING

The assessment of a patient's hearing begins at the start of the clinical encounter. If you are seeing the patient in an outpatient setting and need to call him or her from a waiting area or when going through your initial introduction, note if you need to raise your voice or repeat what you have said more than usual to be understood. Is the patient wearing a hearing aid? Make it a part of your routine to converse with the patient whilst undertaking the otoscopic examination or other parts of the consultation where the patient is unable to see your lips as you speak. Vary the intensity of your spoken voice during the consultation to get an idea of the patient's hearing threshold.

A clinical voice test is a more structured assessment of hearing that can be performed easily in almost any clinical setting with a high level of reliability in adult patients.[1] This test assesses each ear independently by masking the contralateral ear. The masking noise is produced by the examiner's index finger gently massaging the tragus against the conchal bowl of the patient's non-test ear as shown (Figure 40.1).

The sound produced distracts the non-test ear during the evaluation. Place your other hand over the patient's eyes to remove visual cues. Instruct the patient to repeat the words you say. Bi-syllabic words with equal stress on both syllables are the most suitable test stimuli. Starting the test speaking at a volume that you have determined to be audible to the patient based on his response to your 'free field' assessment of his hearing earlier in the consultation will allow you to quickly determine if the patient followed your instructions.

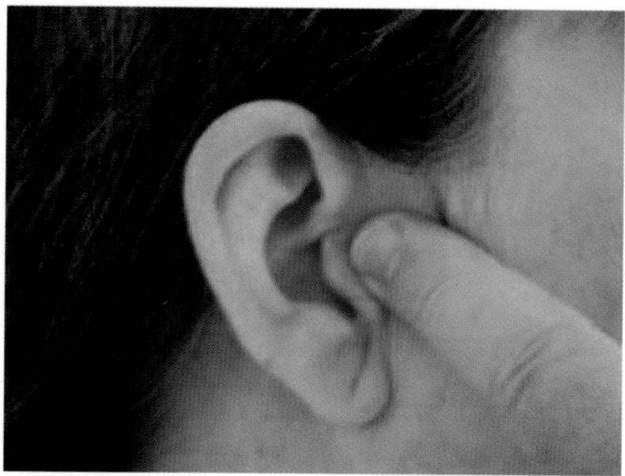

Figure 40.1 Tragal massage to mask the non-test ear in a clinical voice test.

Continue testing by presenting your voice first at ear level (6 cm) then at arm's length (60 cm) from the patient's test ear. Speak at varying intensities to cover the range of whisper, conversational and loud voice as necessary to discover the patient's threshold. Note the level at which the patient repeats some but not all the syllables. A normal hearing individual will be able to hear a whispered voice presented at 20 cm from the test ear in the normal examination room. If there is a hearing impairment, further evaluation with tuning forks will help characterize the hearing loss.

Hearing losses can be categorized by the site of the pathological lesion into conductive and sensorineural. Conductive losses refer to conditions in the outer or middle ear that impede the transfer of sound energy to the inner ear. These can include the mundane, such as impacted cerumen in the outer ear, to more esoteric conditions, such as otosclerosis that reduces the mobility of the ossicular chain. Sensorineural hearing loss refers to conditions of the inner ear and the neural pathway from the ear to the auditory cortex. The causes vary from primary disorders of the cochlea, such as noise-induced hearing loss (leading to outer hair cell damage), to a vestibular schwannoma reducing auditory nerve function.

TUNING FORK TESTS

Tuning fork tests are utilized to make the distinction between these two major categories of hearing loss. The Rinne and Weber tests are the most widely used. These tests are most reliably performed with low-frequency tuning forks, and whilst there is debate about the merits of the 512 Hz over the 256 Hz, it is agreed that higher frequency tuning forks of 1024 Hz or greater are not appropriate. A typical tuning fork is illustrated (Figure 40.2).

The Rinne test compares the perceived intensity of sound delivered via two routes, air versus bone, and is the clinical correlate of the pure tone audiogram comparing air with bone conduction thresholds. In the classical tests the examiner strikes the tines of the tuning fork and places the base plate upon the patient's mastoid process, maintaining contact by stabilizing the patient's head with the opposite hand. Ask the patient to report when the stimulus is no longer audible. The natural tendency is for the patient to withdraw from the cold tuning

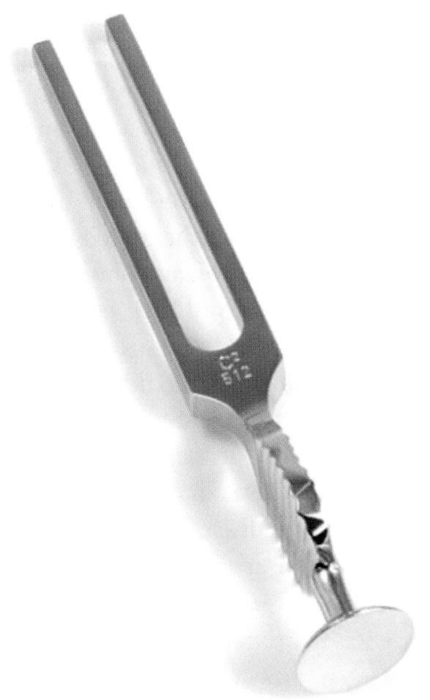

Figure 40.2 A tuning fork used in the Weber or Rinne test.

fork, thus reducing the contact between the same and the mastoid, and the subsequent transfer of the sound stimulus (see Figure 40.3).

Once the tuning fork vibrations decay to a point that the transferred sound stimulus is below the patient's bone conduction auditory threshold and the patient reports that it can no longer be heard, the tuning fork is removed from the mastoid process

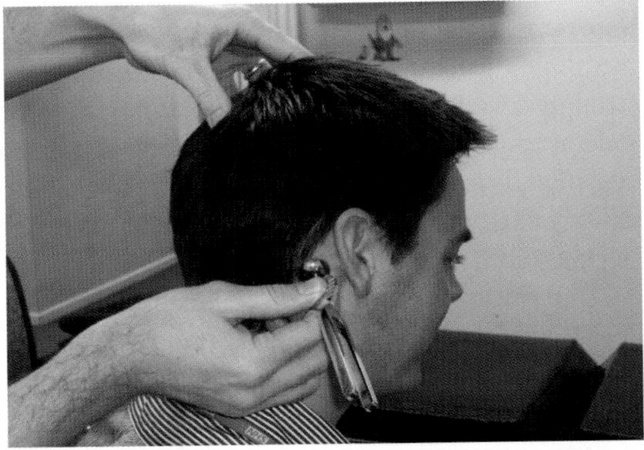

Figure 40.3 The tuning fork placed on the mastoid process during the Rinne test whilst the examiner's other hand stabilizes the patient's head.

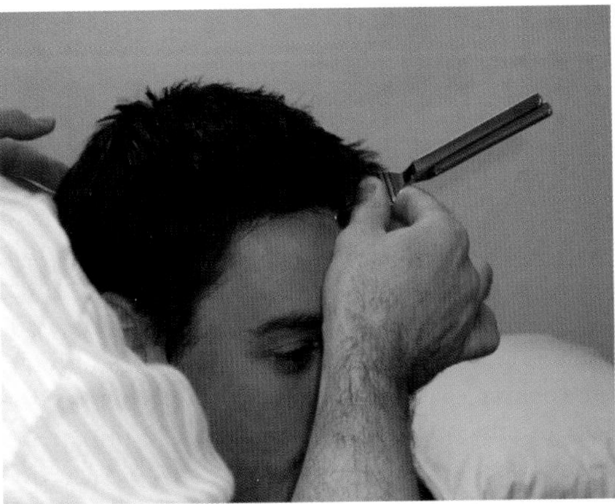

Figure 40.4 The Weber test being performed.

and the tines presented at ear level. The patient is asked if it is audible. Those with normal hearing or with a sensorineural hearing loss will report that the second sound signal is audible, whilst those with a conductive hearing loss will not. A bone conduction stimulus is more audible than an air conduction stimulus in a patient with a conductive hearing loss.

The examiner places the vibrating tuning fork onto the centre of the patient's forehead in the Weber test as shown in Figure 40.4 and asks the patient to describe where the sound is localized. Is it central, or does the sound appear to emanate from one side of the head or ear? Remember to stabilize the patient's head. In a patient with a unilateral conductive hearing loss, the Weber response lateralizes to the ear with the hearing loss. In a patient with a sensorineural loss, the Weber response lateralizes to the opposite ear.

PURE TONE AUDIOMETRY

Pure tone audiometry is the most clinically used hearing test. The purpose of pure tone audiometry is to quantitatively measure behavioural hearing thresholds. Pure tone audiometry is ideally performed in a sound-treated or soundproofed booth using a calibrated audiometer. The hearing thresholds obtained over standardized frequencies are displayed graphically in the audiogram. The thresholds for sound delivered by air conduction and bone conduction are determined. Air-conduction sounds assess the entire auditory pathway using insert earphones or headphones. Bone-conduction sounds estimate the sensory-neural hearing reserve using a bone vibrator placed on the mastoid to stimulate the cochlear directly. Masking noise is sometimes needed to obtain ear-specific hearing thresholds. Although bone-conduction tests bypass the outer and middle ear, changes in the outer or middle ear may affect bone-conduction thresholds owing to changes in the inertial responses of the outer and middle ear. One example is the poor bone-conduction thresholds usually observed around 2000 Hz in patients with a conductive hearing loss as in otosclerosis that is abolished by a successful stapedotomy and known as Carhart's notch.

American Speech-Language-Hearing Association,[2] American Academy of Otolaryngology – Head and Neck (AAO-HNS)[3] and the British Society of Audiology[4] recommend that in air-conduction pure tone testing, hearing thresholds should be measured at octave frequencies 250, 500, 1000, 2000, 4000 and 8000 Hz. If there is a 20 dB or more difference in hearing thresholds between two adjacent octaves, inter-octaves (750, 1500, 3000 and 6000 Hz) should be tested. The AAO-HNS Committee on Hearing and Equilibration guidelines on the evaluation of a conductive hearing loss recommend that 3000 Hz thresholds be either measured or estimated.[3] Bone-conduction thresholds are typically measured at octave frequencies up to 4000 Hz.[2,4]

A comparison of hearing thresholds obtained in response to air-conduction and bone-conduction tests provides information about the degree, type and configuration of a hearing loss. The audiogram of a patient with a classical conductive hearing loss shows bone-conduction thresholds within normal limits and air-conduction thresholds elevated above normal levels (see Figure 40.5). In a pure conductive hearing loss case, the air-conduction thresholds usually do not exceed 70 dB HL. In a pure sensory-neural hearing loss case, both bone-conduction and air-conduction thresholds are elevated and the air-bone gap (difference between air-conduction and bone-conduction thresholds) is equal or less than 10 dB. It should be noted that that up to 14 per cent of people tested can have at least one air–bone gap of 15 dB or more at a particular frequency.[5] In addition, a vibro-tactile response will likely be reported by a patient at 250 and 500 Hz for bone-conduction stimuli presented between 40 and 60 dB HL. Therefore, a false air–bone gap may occur in persons with sensorineural hearing loss at these frequencies. Any thresholds considered to be vibro-tactile should be labelled in an audiogram. A mixed hearing loss is diagnosed when both air-conduction and bone-conduction thresholds are elevated and thresholds are greater for air-conduction stimuli. Figure 40.5 shows a left ear pure-tone audiogram: (a) left ear conductive hearing loss, (b) left ear sensory-neural hearing loss (SNHL), (c) left ear mixed hearing loss.

Pure tone audiometry is the most widely used test in audiology. Results of pure tone audiometry are often considered the 'gold standard'.

SPEECH TESTS

The SRT and WRS are the most commonly used speech test parameters.

The test stimulus in speech test is presented as either recorded speech or the audiologist reading from a word list. The signal is presented either through earphones or free field through speakers in a soundproofed room. The speech signal consists of phonetically balanced bi-syllabic words presented at varying amplitudes when measuring the SRT. The SRT is the lowest amplitude level at which an individual can repeat 50 per cent of the presented spondaic words (such as *iceberg*, *cowboy*, *pancake*). The SRT reflects hearing disability rather than impairment. The latter is measured by the pure tone thresholds. Impairment and disability are, however, strongly correlated, and as a rule of thumb, the pure tone average is within 5 to 10 dB of the SRT. The lack of agreement between SRT and pure tone audiometry can be an indicator of a non-organic hearing loss or unreliable pure tone audiogram.

The WRS is recorded in response to typically 25–50 monosyllabic words (such as *carve* and *sun*) presented at 30 dB SL or higher; thus it is supra-threshold response. The number of words the subject can recognize is reported as a percentage of the total number of stimulus words. The WRS reflects the hearing ability of the individual in response to normal conversational or louder speech. WRS

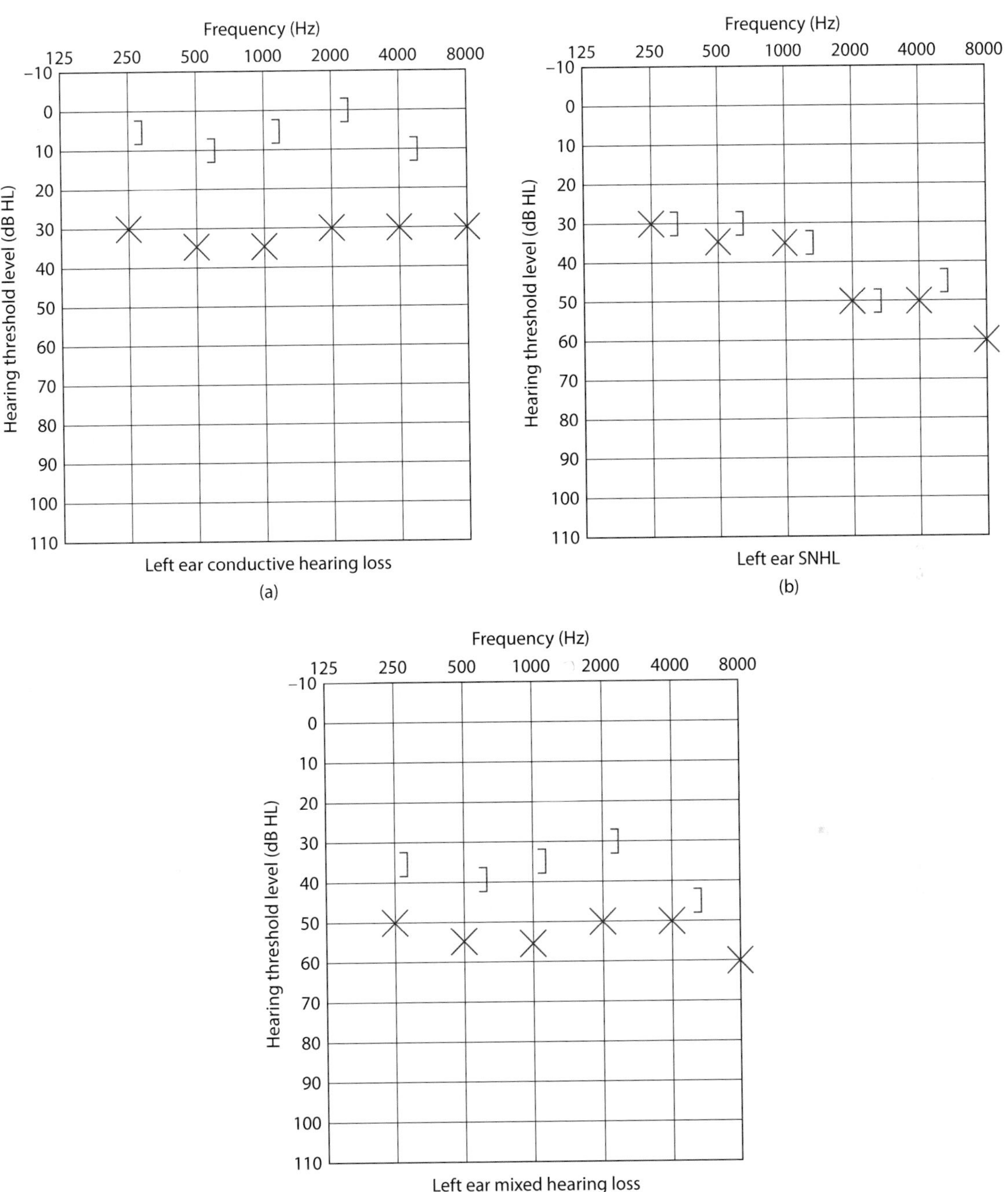

Figure 40.5 Pure tone audiogram illustrating a left ear conductive hearing loss **(a)**, a sensory-neural hearing loss **(b)** and a mixed hearing loss **(c)**. X = left ear air-conduction threshold;] = left ear masked bone-conduction threshold.

results are categorized into excellent (90–100 per cent), good (78–88 per cent), fair (66–76 per cent), poor (54–64 per cent) and very poor (<52 per cent).

WRS can help to categorize the nature of a patient's hearing loss. Patients with conductive hearing losses usually show improved recognition scores when the speech signal intensity is increased. Patients with sensory-neural hearing losses usually do not improve their recognition scores with increasing intensity because increasing loudness produces distortion of the speech signal. Patients with retro-cochlear pathology may show a reduction of recognition scores with increasing intensity, a phenomenon described as the 'rollover' effect. Rollover refers to the distortion in word recognition that occurs at high volumes, reflective of a lesion in the eighth nerve.

The SRT and WRS are measures of hearing disability in quiet, which is at variance with the real-world setting where disability and handicap are experienced in background noise. There is also increasing evidence that the cochlear processes speech information presented in background noise differently to speech presented in quiet, leading to the expansion of hearing in noise test protocols.

TYMPANOMETRY

Tympanometry is a fast and simple hearing test routinely used in clinics for the evaluation of middle-ear function. Tympanometry measures the acoustic admittance of the middle ear in the presence of a range of static pressures. In clinical tympanometry measurement, a handheld probe is inserted into the ear canal and forms a leak-free seal from the probe tip to the eardrum. Then a low-frequency tone is delivered into the ear canal while the pressure is varied within the sealed canal. The sound pressure reflected back from the tympanic membrane (TM) is measured at the probe tip location. This measurement result is then displayed in graph form, called the tympanogram.

Jerger and Liden first classified the tympanogram shapes into three patterns, as shown in Figure 40.6. The patterns are:

- Type A: Normal admittance. Peak admittance near atmospheric pressure (0 daPa)
  - Type Ad: A subcategory of Type A; hypermobile admittance (high admittance)
  - Type As: A subcategory of Type A; hypomobile admittance (low admittance)
- Type B: Rounded or flat tympanogram with no measurable peak
- Type C: Abnormal negative middle-ear pressure

OTOACOUSTIC EMISSION TEST

Otoacoustic emissions (OAEs) are low-level sounds that are generated in the outer hair cells and travel

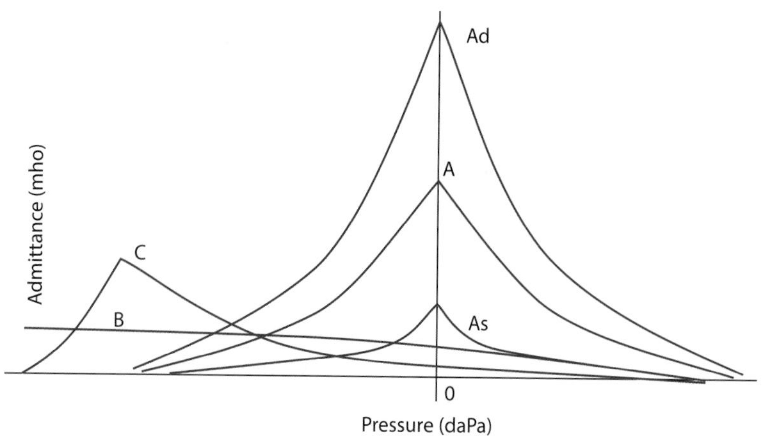

Figure 40.6 Jerger-Liden classification of three types of tympanograms.

back through the middle ear into the ear canal, where they can be recorded by a miniature microphone. Transient evoked OAEs (TEOAEs) and distortion product OAEs (DPOAEs) are two widely measured OAEs.

TEOAEs are elicited by transient stimuli such as clicks or tone bursts; DPOAEs are elicited by two continuous tones at moderate intensity levels, e.g. 55 and 65 dB SPL. TEOAEs are typically recorded from 500–4000 Hz, and DPOAEs can be recorded from 1000–8000 Hz. TEOAEs are reported to be more sensitive for hearing loss at 500 and 1000 Hz, while DPOAEs have better clinical performance for hearing loss at 4000 Hz.[6]

TEOAEs and DPOAEs are fast, easy to obtain, non-invasive tests. OAE tests typically are not affected by the patient's attention, cognitive levels or motivation. Therefore, OAE tests are widely used in the audiological assessment of children and difficult-to-manage adults, such as persons with non-organic hearing loss or learning disabilities.

OAE tests play an important role in monitoring ototoxicity and noise-induced hearing loss (NIHL) because OAEs can detect outer hair cell dysfunction earlier than a pure tone audiogram can. Typically, DPOAEs are used for monitoring ototoxicity and NIHL because (1) DPOAEs test higher frequencies than TEOAEs, and therefore can detect changes in the cochlear frequency spectrum first affected by these pathologies; (2) DPOAEs measurements can be obtained in the presence of more hearing loss than TEOAEs; (3) DPOAEs can provide some indication of degree and configuration of the hearing loss.[7]

OAE test results are affected by the patient's middle-ear status, the ambient noise level and the patient's internal noise level (e.g. breathing or movements), amongst other factors. Therefore, the results of OAE tests should be interpreted in conjunction with those of other tests (pure tone audiometry, tympanometry, and so forth).

AUDITORY BRAIN STEM RESPONSE

The auditory brain stem response (ABR), also called brain stem evoked response (BSER), is an electrophysiological measurement. It plays an important role in the assessment of the function of the auditory nerve and the integrity of auditory pathways in the lower brain stem.

ABR testing was widely used to assess the presence of retro-cochlear pathology and to objectively determine the hearing threshold. This section focuses on using ABR testing for the assessment of retrocochlear pathology. The use of ABR testing for hearing threshold determination is covered in the section on newborn hearing screening.

ABR tests typically require four electrodes placed on the vertex, forehead and on each ear lobe or mastoid, respectively. Insert earphones or headphones are used to deliver broadband click stimuli. The elicited auditory evoked responses are recorded by the skin surface electrodes.

The elicited responses consist of a series of positive waves (with respect to the vertex), which are labeled with sequential Roman numerals I–V, as shown in Figure 40.7. These waveforms normally

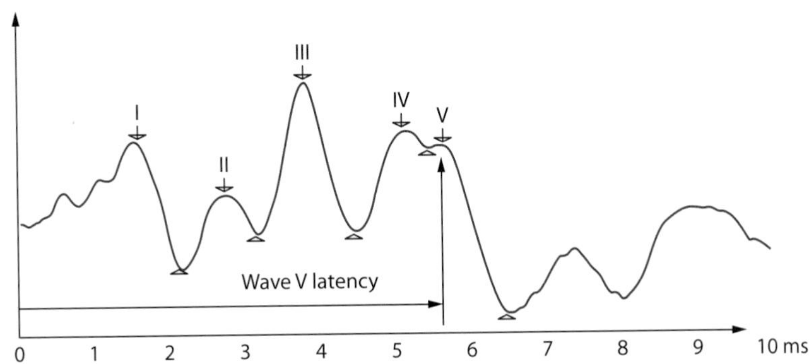

Figure 40.7 Auditory brain stem response wave V latency measurement.

occur approximately within a 15-millisecond time period from the onset of the stimulus.

Retro-cochlear pathology, e.g. acoustic schwannomas, can lead to a delay of the ABR peak latencies. Peak latency is a measure of the time between the onset of the stimuli and the occurrence of a peak in the ABR. A measurement of wave V peak latency is shown in Figure 40.7. The most clinically used ABR criteria are absolute wave V latency, wave I–V inter-peak interval difference and inter-aural wave V latency difference. Although generalized normative data is available for ABR, it is recommended that each audiological facility develop its own set of standardized norms for its ABR equipment.

Studies have shown that ABR testing has a high sensitivity (approximately 90 per cent) for detecting large tumours; however, many small tumours (less than 1 cm) may be missed. Physicians increasingly recommend magnetic resonance imaging (MRI) in high-risk patients instead of ABR results, or if ABR results are within normal limits, because MRI is a more sensitive and specific test for an acoustic neuroma. ABR waves are usually absent when a patient has a severe or profound hearing loss. A conductive hearing loss also attenuates cochlear stimulation, and increases ABR wave latencies.

NEWBORN HEARING SCREENING

TWO-STAGE SCREENING

Children whose hearing loss is identified and corrected within 6 months of birth are likely to develop better language skills than children whose hearing loss is detected later. It is recommended that all infants be screened for hearing loss by 1 month of age; all infants who do not pass the hearing screening need to complete a diagnostic hearing evaluation by 3 months of age, and all children identified with permanent hearing loss need to receive appropriate intervention by 6 months of age.[8] This plan is also called the 1-3-6 plan.

A two-stage hearing screening process has been widely used by newborn hearing screening programmes. Typically, well babies are screened with the automatic otoacoustic emission (AOAE) test, and if they pass the AOAE test, they will be classified as normal hearing. Children who do not pass the initial AOAE test will be screened with the automatic auditory brain stem response (AABR) tests. For high-risk babies, such as neonatal intensive care unit (NICU) babies, both AOAE and AABR tests are used for initial hearing screening.

Both AOAE and AABR tests can be administered by trained staff such as audiologists' assistants or nurses. It typically takes up to 5 minutes for the AABR to assess one ear, while it takes the AOAE approximately 2 minutes for one ear. However, AABR has an advantage in that it can detect auditory neuropathy spectrum disorder (ANSD), whereas AOAE can not.

The outcome of the AOAE or AABR is a 'pass' or a 'refer' result. A 'refer' result means that the child needs to have a diagnostic audiologic assessment to determine the true hearing status.

DIAGNOSTIC HEARING TESTS FOR YOUNG INFANTS AND TODDLERS

Infants who do not pass hearing screening need to complete a diagnostic audiological assessment. Infants under about 6 months of age often can be assessed by frequency-specific ABR with insert earphone and/or bone vibrator in natural sleep. Infants older than 6 months or difficult-to-manage children (e.g. children with autism spectrum disorder or Down's syndrome) are likely to require sedation. To date, frequency-specific ABR is considered the 'gold standard' for evaluating hearing thresholds in young infants and difficult-to-manage children.

Infants with normal hearing typically show a wave V at 35 dB normalized hearing level (nHL) for 500 Hz, 30 dB nHL for 1000 and 2000 Hz, and 25 dB nHL for 4000 Hz for air-conduction ABR; and 20 dB nHL for 500 Hz and 30 dB nHL for 2000 Hz for bone-conduction ABR. Studies of 1000 and 4000 Hz bone-conduction ABR for infants are sparse. Therefore, 1000 and 4000 Hz bone-conduction ABR normative data have not been established. Table 40.1 shows the air-conduction and bone-conduction ABR normal thresholds criteria in infants and young children. It should be noted that thresholds obtained from frequency-specific

Table 40.1 Air-conduction and bone-conduction tone-ABR thresholds criteria (in dB nHL) in infants and young children with normal hearing.

	Air-conduction ABR (dB nHL)	Bone-conduction ABR (dB nHL)
500 Hz	35	20
1000 Hz	30	Not available
2000 Hz	30	30
4000 Hz	25	Not available

From Seewald R, Tharpe AM, eds. *Comprehensive Handbook of Pediatric Audiology*. San Diego, CA: Plural Publishing, 2011.

ABR (dB nHL) are not directly equivalent to the thresholds obtained from behavioural tests (dB HL). The thresholds estimated from the frequency-specific ABR (dB nHL) are typically higher when compared to behavioural thresholds (dB HL). Correction factors between dB nHL and dB HL have been established.[9]

When we interpret frequency-specific ABR threshold results for infants, we *do not* assess whether a wave V latency is 'normal' or 'prolonged'. Instead, the results should be interpreted as 'Wave V present', 'Wave V absent' or 'Could not be interpreted owing to insufficient replication and/or noisy data'.

VISUAL REINFORCEMENT AUDIOMETRY AND PLAY AUDIOMETRY

Infants between 6 months and 2 years of age usually can be behaviourally assessed by visual reinforcement audiometry (VRA). The child is trained to turn his or her head towards a sound source. If a correct response is performed, the child is 'rewarded' through a visual reinforcement. For toddlers, conditioned play audiometry can be applied. The child is trained to perform an activity each time a sound is heard. The activity may involve putting a block in a box or putting a plastic toy into a water tank. VRA or conditioned play audiometry can be performed with insert earphones or headphones. Results obtained on sound field testing do not provide ear-specific information, although it might be useful for initial conditioning or demonstration purposes.

KEY LEARNING POINTS

- Pure tone audiometry quantitatively measure behavioural hearing thresholds.
- A comparison of hearing thresholds obtained in response to air-conduction and bone-conduction stimuli provides information about the degree, type and configuration of a hearing loss.
- Pure tone results are affected by factors such as patients' attention, motivation and cognitive function.
- A strong correlation exists between SRT and pure tone average thresholds.
- WRS may provide diagnostic information of the site of lesion.
- Tympanometry is routinely used for the evaluation of middle-ear function.
- Tympanogram shapes are classified into three patterns.
- TEOAEs are more sensitive for identification of hearing loss at 500 and 1000 Hz.
- DPOAEs are more sensitive for identification of hearing loss at 4000 Hz.
- DPOAEs are used for monitoring ototoxicity and NIHL.
- ABR testing is used to assess retrocochlear pathology.
- The most widely used ABR test criteria are the wave V latencies, inter-aural wave V latencies and wave I-V inter-peak inter-aural latencies differences.
- The ABR is not sensitive enough to detect small vestibular schwannomas.
- The 1-3-6 plan is a newborn hearing screening management plan.
- AOAE and AABR tests are used in newborn hearing screening.
- For infants 6 months of age or younger, 1000 Hz tympanometry is used to assess middle-ear function.
- Frequency-specific ABR is considered the 'gold standard'.

- *Do not* assess wave V latency for infants.
- VRA and play audiometry are behavioural tests for older infants and toddlers.

REFERENCES

1. Bagai A, Thavendiranathan P, Detsky AS. Does this patient have hearing impairment? *JAMA*. 2006; 295(4): 416–28.
2. American Speech-Language-Hearing Association. Guidelines for manual pure-tone threshold audiometry. 2005. Available from: www.asha.org/policy.
3. Committee on Hearing and Equilibrium guidelines for the evaluation of results of treatment of conductive hearing loss. American Academy of Otolaryngology – Head and Neck Surgery. *Otolaryngology – Head and Neck Surgery*. 1995; 113: 186–67.
4. British Society of Audiology. Recommended Procedure Pure-tone air-conduction and bone-conduction threshold audiometry with and without masking. 2011. Available from: http://www.thebsa.org.uk/docs/Guidelines/.
5. Schlauch RS, Carney E. A multinomial model for identifying significant pure-tone threshold shifts. *Journal of Speech, Language and Hearing Research*. 2007; 50(6): 1391–403.
6. Gorga MP, Neely ST, Bergman B, Beauchaine KL, Kaminski JR, Peters J, et al. Otoacoustic emissions from normal-hearing and hearing-impaired subjects: Distortion product responses. *Journal of the Acoustical Society of America*. 1993; 93(4, Pt 1): 2050–60.
7. American Academy of Audiology's Position Statement and Practice Guidelines on Ototoxicity Monitoring. 2010. Available from: http://www.audiology.org.
8. Joint Committee on Infant Hearing; American Academy of Audiology, American Academy of Pediatrics, American Speech-Language-Hearing Association, Year 2000 position statement: Principles and guidelines for early hearing detection and intervention programs. *Pediatrics*. 2000; 106: 798–817.
9. Foxe JJ, Stapells DR., Normal infant and adult auditory brainstem responses to bone-conducted tones. *Audiology*. 1993; 32(2): 95–109.

FURTHER READING

Henry KS, Heinz MG. Diminished temporal coding with sensorineural hearing loss emerges in background noise. *Nature Neuroscience*. 2012; 15(10): 1362–64.

Katz J, Medwetsky L, Burkard R, Hood L, eds. *Handbook of Clinical Audiology*. 6th ed. Philadelphia: Lippincott Williams & Wilkins, 2010.

Seewald R, Tharpe AM, eds. *Comprehensive Handbook of Pediatric Audiology*. San Diego, CA: Plural Publishing, 2011.

41

Tests for balance

PETER A REA AND JASWINDER S SANDHU

INTRODUCTION

Human balance involves the integration of information arising from the vestibular, visual and proprioceptive sensory inputs at the level of the brain stem and midbrain with modulation from higher centres. As a result, any lesion affecting the structure or function of the sensory inputs, the central nervous system structures or the effector pathways is likely to result in a balance disorder. The history and examination may therefore need to be wide-ranging and may need to be complemented by carefully targeted investigations in some, but certainly not all, patients. The assessment of the balance patient begins with a comprehensive history starting with the time frame (episodic versus continuous), symptoms (carefully define what the patient means by 'dizziness') and onset of the complaint, but then extending to a review of the cardiovascular, neurological and musculoskeletal systems if required.

Eliciting a history in a concise manner from 'dizzy' patients can be challenging as the complaints are often vague, and it is not uncommon for an anxiety overlay to be present. However, a clear history is crucial in helping to decide which additional tests are likely to help with the diagnosis. The tests available can be broadly subdivided into two categories: the bedside evaluation, which can be considered to be part of the physical examination, and laboratory testing, which requires specialist equipment and expertise.

PHYSICAL EXAMINATION

AURAL EXAMINATION

Examine the external auditory meatus and the tympanic membrane to exclude peripheral causes of imbalance such as perforation, infection, otitis media, cholesteatoma and otosclerosis (Schwartze sign). Glue ear is a common cause of clumsiness in children. It is also clinically useful to observe for nystagmus whilst applying positive and negative pressure to the tragus (Hennebert's sign), during Valsalva or with a loud noise (Tullio's phenomenon).[1] Positive responses are found in patients with perilymph fistula, hypermobile stapes, superior-canal dehiscence and occasionally in Ménière's disease.

ASSESSMENT OF HEARING

Rinne and Weber tuning fork tests distinguish conductive from sensorineural hearing loss. However, in most balance patients a pure-tone audiogram and tympanometry are needed as aberrations in these tests can help identify certain pathologies. Examples include the low-frequency sloping sensorineural hearing loss associated with Ménière's disease, the characteristic improved bone-conduction thresholds, air–bone gap and type A tympanogram seen in superior canal dehiscence syndrome, or a unilateral sensorineural hearing loss seen in labyrinthitis or rarely an acoustic neuroma.

ENT AND MEDICAL EXAMINATION

A complete ear, nose and throat (ENT), cardiovascular and neurological examination is essential to exclude non-otological causes of imbalance. This will be guided by the patient's symptoms but may include lying and standing blood pressure looking for a postural drop, reflexes, muscle tone, plantar responses, peripheral sensation (looking for a peripheral neuropathy), speech and fundoscopy (looking for papilloedema).

ASSESSMENT OF STANCE AND GAIT

It is important to assess posture and gait as the patient enters the consultation room, noting any aids that the patient may use. However, a formal assessment is also required.

Romberg's test

The patient is asked to first stand with the feet together, eyes open and arms folded across the chest for 30 seconds and then closed for 30 seconds. The test is described as a positive test if the patient is stable with eyes open but there is increased body sway with the eyes closed. This is usually ascribed to a reduced proprioceptive input; however, an acute vestibular deficit also results in a positive test. A sharpened Romberg's test can also be used whereby the patient stands heel-to-toe. This variant is sensitive to the same pathologies as the normal Romberg's test but also can detect chronic vestibular deficits. A 'wooden soldier' fall straight backwards is often non-organic. Romberg's is a relatively non-specific test.

Unterberger's test

The patient is asked to march on the spot 50 times with the arms outstretched and eyes closed. In the absence of auditory cues and musculoskeletal factors, the test can highlight a unilateral vestibular deficit, as the patient is more likely to rotate in the direction of the loss. However, whilst the test can be helpful in guiding the clinician, there is a large inter- and intrasubject variability and therefore the results must be interpreted in conjunction with all other information available.

Gait

This is a 5 m walk at normal speed first with eyes open and then with eyes closed. The examiner walks alongside the patient for safety reasons and looks out for deviation towards the side of the lesion. As with Unterberger's test, the sensitivity and specificity are low and therefore results should not be interpreted in isolation. Observe for the shuffling gait of Parkinson's disease, the broad-based or ataxic gait of central balance disorders, the erratic gait of non-organic imbalance, a slapping gait from foot drop or joint position sensory deficits (listen as well as look at the patient walking down the corridor) or the rigid gait of spasticity. Orthopaedic abnormalities should also be observed.

Tandem gait

Here the patient is asked to walk heel-to-toes in a straight line for five steps. With the eyes open this primarily tests cerebellar function as the visual inputs compensate for chronic vestibular and proprioceptive deficits. However, with eyes closed, the test assesses vestibular integrity assuming that the visual and proprioceptive inputs are intact. It is also a very non-specific test.

OTONEUROLOGICAL EXAMINATION

CLINICAL ASSESSMENTS OF EYE MOVEMENTS

The examiner should first ascertain visual acuity of both eyes. Next, cover tests should be used to determine strabismus and any latent nystagmus that may be present. The full range of gaze should be examined in both horizontal and vertical planes to 30° from the midline and conjugate eye movements ensured. Be careful not to deviate the eyes beyond the sclera as physiological nystagmus may result, and this is not pathological.

OCULAR CONTROL SYSTEMS

With the head fixed, ocular stability is maintained by sophisticated visual control systems, which include the saccadic, smooth pursuit and optokinetic system.[2] Whilst these can be assessed clinically, they are more accurately measured in the laboratory using either electronystagmography or videonystagmography.

VESTIBULAR OCULAR REFLEX AND NYSTAGMUS

During head movements a dynamic system is needed to maintain gaze. This is known as the vestibular-ocular reflex (VOR), and it converts rotational and translational movements sensed by the vestibular system into compensatory extra-ocular muscle adjustments via neural circuitry, thereby allowing the retinal image slip to be minimized. (Turn your head side-to-side whilst fixing on this page: your vision is being stabilized by your VOR.) When the amplitude of the eye movement is large, a fast eye movement in the opposite direction interrupts the slow vestibular-induced motion. The resulting eye movement is known as *vestibular nystagmus* and can be induced by rotatory chair and caloric testing. For clinical reasons the direction of the nystagmus is defined by the fast phase.

HALMAGYI HEAD THRUST

This is a test for semicircular canal paresis in which the patient is asked to fixate at a distant visual target whilst the examiner makes a small-angle, high-velocity head thrust in the plane of the canals being tested (it is best to quickly rotate the head back towards the neutral midline position).[3] Whilst these are usually the lateral canals, the manoeuvre can be conducted in the right-anterior and left-posterior canals (RALP) or the left-anterior and right-posterior (LARP) geometries also. In the presence of unilateral weakness, movements towards the lesion result in the generation of a catch-up saccade, as the vestibular system is unable to provide the corrective VOR gain. In bilateral weakness these catch-up saccades are seen on both left and right head thrusts. Quite a big deficit is needed for a positive test, and this will be seen on caloric testing.

HEAD SHAKE NYSTAGMUS

Whilst wearing Frenzel's glasses or infrared camera-based goggles, the patient is asked to pitch her head down by 30°, close her eyes and oscillate the head 20 times. Upon cessation of the head shake, the examiner observes for nystagmus. If present, this indicates vestibular imbalance. This sign may persist indefinitely after the onset of a peripheral or central vestibular deficit.

NYSTAGMUS

Spontaneous nystagmus and Alexander's law

Selective lesions in the peripheral and central vestibular pathways result in spontaneous nystagmus due to the unopposed neural activity in the intact pathway, for example the nystagmus observed immediately following vestibular neuronitis. The nystagmus is graded using Alexander's law, which states that in patients with spontaneous nystagmus due to an acute vestibular asymmetry, the slow phase velocity, or drift, of nystagmus is lower when the subject looks toward the side of the slow component of nystagmus compared with the fast phase direction.[4] Therefore, if the nystagmus is only present when the eyes are deviated in the direction of the fast phase, it is first-degree; if the nystagmus is also present in primary gaze, it is second-degree; and if it also present with the eyes deviated in the direction of the slow phase, it is known as third-degree. Furthermore, the nystagmus should become more pronounced with the removal of optical fixation (as with Frenzel's glasses).

Positional nystagmus and benign paroxysmal positional vertigo

Benign paroxysmal positional vertigo (BPPV) is a common vestibular disorder characterized by brief episodes of vertigo, which occur when the head is moved into certain positions.[5] The pathological basis of BPPV is believed to be calcium-carbonate debris that migrates from the otolith organs, where it is ordinarily present, to the semicircular canals, where it disrupts their function. There are two subtypes of BPPV, canalithiasis and cupulolithiasis, which can affect any of the three canals. In canalithiasis the debris is thought to be free-floating in the canal, and therefore there is a delay in onset between the head position being adopted and the vertigo being provoked. Furthermore, as the debris resettles, the symptoms abate. In contrast, cupulolithiasis results from the debris adhering to the cupula, thereby producing an inappropriate deflection. The result is usually sustained vertigo whilst in the provoking position, which begins immediately without delay.

A number of different manoeuvres can be used to test for BPPV depending upon the canal that is affected. The Dix–Hallpike test is used to diagnose posterior canal BPPV, which is the most common manifestation. The patient's head is turned 45° horizontally whilst he is in a sitting position. The patient then quickly lies down with the head hanging over the edge of the bed by approximately 30°. This brings the posterior canal of the downside ear into the vertical plane, allowing gravity to act fully. The patient is required to keep his eyes open throughout this procedure, and the examiner checks for nystagmus. The most commonly observed eye movement is an upbeating torsional geotropic nystagmus, which results from excitation of the posterior semicircular canal (PSC). It is to be noted that the anterior canal of the downside ear is also in a more dependent position and therefore can be triggered. In this case a down beating torsional nystagmus is observed. It is important to wait at least 30 seconds before sitting the patient up as the onset of nystagmus can be delayed in canalithiasis. The differentiation between canalithiasis and cupulolithiasis is based on the latency and duration as discussed previously. Once the patient is ready, the test is then repeated on the other side.

In lateral canal BPPV, severe horizontal nystagmus is induced on turning the head 90° to left or right with the patient lying flat. The worst most symptomatic side is best considered the affected ear. This is most commonly seen as a result of an Epley manoeuvre to treat posterior canal BPPV.

VESTIBULAR FUNCTION TESTS

Laboratory testing is an important part of the diagnostic process as it can confirm clinical suspicions as well as provide quantitative evaluation of peripheral vestibular function and the vestibular-ocular reflex. The increased sensitivity afforded by the technology can also help in cases where eye movements may be too subtle to observe in the clinical setting. However, each test asks a specific question. Simply requesting 'balance tests' is unlikely to be helpful.

ELECTRONYSTAGMOGRAPHY AND VIDEONYSTAGMOGRAPHY

Most vestibular test batteries begin by assessing the integrity of the three main ocular tracking mechanisms, which are the saccadic, smooth pursuit and the optokinetic systems. To record eye movements, many laboratories utilize videonystagmography (VNG), which is a system whereby the patient wears goggles with an inbuilt infrared camera (so that it can operate in the dark) that can track eye movements (Figure 41.1). Alternatively, electronystagmography (ENG) can still be used if VNG is not available or appropriate. ENG relies on the corneal-retinal potential (CRP) changing during eye movements. The CRP can be detected by placing recording electrodes near the eye.

Saccades

Saccades are fast eye movements (300°/s to 600°/s), which rapidly change gaze direction. It is the saccadic system that is responsible for the fast phase of vestibular nystagmus. These are tested by asking the patient to look at sets of fixation points (usually positioned straight ahead and at 30° to the left and right). Two aspects of saccades are assessed, the accuracy and the velocity. If inaccurate, the saccade can either overshoot (hypermetric) or undershoot (hypometric). These can occur with cerebellar, brain stem and other central nervous system disorders. The velocity of the saccade, if slow, can indicate neuro-degenerative disease but can also be due to internuclear opthalmoplegia (the affected eye shows impairment of adduction; when bilateral, this is typical of multiple sclerosis) as well as rarer pathologies that affect the neuromuscular junction (myasthenia gravis), and nerve conduction (such as Miller Fisher syndrome).

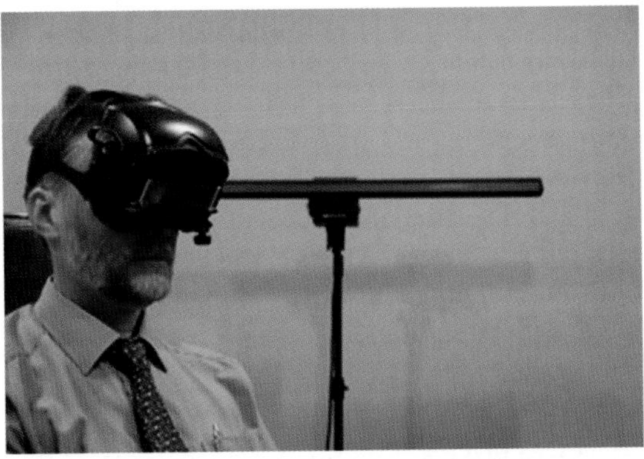

Figure 41.1 Videonystagmography (VNG). The goggles allow assessment of eye movement with vision (visor up), and with vision denied (using infrared cameras and the visor down).

Smooth pursuit

Smooth pursuit is a slow tracking movement that maintains images of small moving targets on the fovea. During the test the patient is asked to keep the head still and to use the eyes to track a target that is made to move smoothly on a screen in front. The corresponding eye movements should be smooth and not interrupted by saccades. Additionally, the gain can be calculated as the ratio between the eye and target velocities. Unilateral vestibular lesions do not impair smooth pursuit. In contrast, central lesions can cause impairment in smooth tracking in a specific direction, and degenerative changes can cause bilateral dysfunction. The most common causes are age related, and this is often seen on testing eye movement in the clinic.

Optokinetic nystagmus

Optokinetic nystagmus (OKN) is nystagmus that occurs in response to a rotation movement, which can be created by either projecting a series of moving stripes in front of a patient or using a striped curtain that is rotated around them. The patient is asked to look straight ahead, and a slow movement should result, interrupted by corrective saccades. The stripes are rotated in both directions and the results analyzed for gain and symmetry. Although acute peripheral vestibular disease may result in asymmetric OKN, abnormalities usually indicate cerebellar or other central disorders.

Caloric testing

The bithermal caloric test is a diagnostic method by which the left and right lateral semicircular canals can be stimulated independently.[6] The patient is positioned on a couch with the head at 30° to the horizontal, bringing the lateral canals into the vertical plane of gravity. A thermal stimulus is then introduced via warm and cool water or air. This temperature gradient is thought to induce convection currents in the endolymph, resulting in deflection of the cupula. Given that only one ear is irrigated at a time, an asymmetry in neural firing between the left and right sides is created, and as a result nystagmus is generated. This is then recorded using either VNG or ENG and a canal paresis (CP) and directional preponderance (DP) calculated using the following equations.

The canal paresis indicates reduction in function of one side compared to the other, whilst directional preponderance indicates the propensity of the eyes to deviate in one direction over another and indicates asymmetric neural activity in the vestibular system as a whole. Directional preponderance, however, is relatively nonspecific and does not specify the side or location of a vestibular lesion, and can occasionally be abnormal in a normal subject. For both measures it is important to generate a range of clinical normative values specific to the equipment being used.

The caloric test can result in vertigo and nausea, and as a result is not always well tolerated by patients. However, it is inexpensive and provides objective clinical information.

Rotatory chair testing

During the test the patient is seated in a chair without optical fixation (Figure 41.2). The chair can rotate in either direction, stimulating both lateral semicircular canals, and the resulting nystagmus recorded using either ENG or VNG. There are two main modalities in which the test is usually conducted. The first is a sinusoidal stimulation whereby the patient is oscillated about his or her vertical axis. The slow phase of the right- and left-beating nystagmus, which is subsequently generated, is then compared for asymmetry. Alternatively, the impulsive rotation can be used whereby the patient is rapidly moved from being stationary to a velocity of 60°/s in less than a second. Initially, nystagmus beating in the direction of rotation is created and then subsides as the chair continues to rotate at a constant velocity (the semicircular canals are only sensitive to acceleration). The chair is then brought to an abrupt stop and the nystagmus is once again measured. The whole process is repeated in the opposite direction, and all the nystagmus generated is analyzed to once again calculate a directional preponderance.

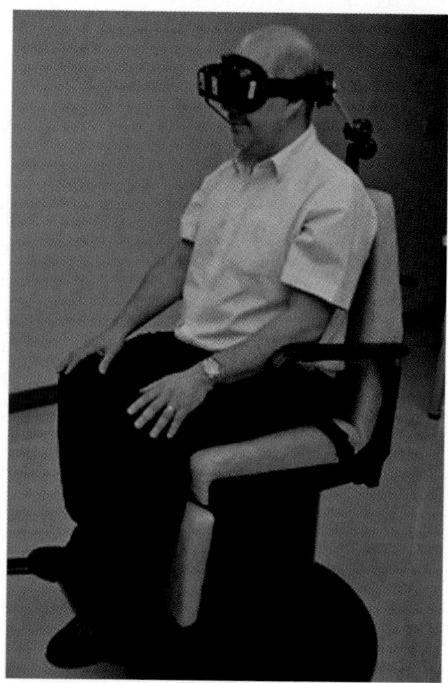

Figure 41.2 Rotating chair in conjunction with wireless VNG.

These tests are usually available only in specialist balance centres and provide a less provocative alternative to the caloric test. Hence they can be more acceptable and are tolerated well by children. They are also superior to the caloric test in cases of bilateral vestibular hypofunction. However, the localizing value of the tests is somewhat limited as both horizontal canals are stimulated simultaneously and the equipment is expensive to procure.

VESTIBULAR EVOKED MYOGENIC POTENTIALS

The vestibular evoked myogenic potential (VEMP) is a myogenic response that is generated by the otolith organs as a reaction to a number of stimuli, including air- and bone-conducted sound.[7] When recorded from the tonically contracted ipsilateral sternocleidomastoid (SCM) muscle, they are known as the cervical VEMP or cVEMP, and when the recording electrodes are placed over the contralateral inferior oblique muscle, they are referred to as the ocular VEMP or oVEMP. Both the cVEMP and oVEMP are becoming increasingly prevalent in test laboratories as they can be recorded using standard evoked potential equipment in a short time.[8] Furthermore, patients tolerate them well, which allows serial measurements to be made more easily. The cVEMP is generated by the saccule and travels via the inferior vestibular nerve. The response magnitude is measured as the difference between the p13 and n23 features. There is a large inter-subject variation of the absolute magnitudes; therefore, side-to-side differences are more useful. The origin of the oVEMP remains controversial but is most likely the utricle, and the signal travels via the superior division of the vestibular nerve. The n10 feature is used to measure the response amplitude and, as with the cVEMP, side-to-side differences are more clinically useful than the absolute magnitudes. An alternative to using the response amplitude is to determine the threshold of response onset. This is more time-consuming but can be very useful in pathologies such as superior canal dehiscence in which both cVEMP and oVEMP thresholds are significantly reduced compared to the normal population.

SUBJECTIVE VISUAL VERTICAL TEST

The subjective visual vertical (SVV) test assesses utricular function, superior vestibular nerve integrity and central connections. It is a subjective test whereby the patient orientates a projected line to his or her perceived vertical whilst in a darkened room. Usually 10 trials are completed and the mean calculated. A tilt of more than 2° is considered to be abnormal; however, the effect resolves with time as compensation occurs.

QUANTIFIED DYNAMIC VISUAL ACUITY

Quantified dynamic visual acuity (DVA) is a way of assessing the functional capability of patients with vestibular deficits.[9] During the test the patient is asked to identify a character on a screen whilst he is oscillating his head. A rate sensor on the head ensures that the character only appears if the head is moved within a set limit. This allows both the patient and the clinician to ascertain the upper limit of head movements beyond which the VOR becomes inadequate and retinal slip becomes problematic. The tool is an excellent way of monitoring progress during vestibular rehabilitation, which aims to improve VOR gain across the frequency range following a vestibular insult.

COMPUTERIZED DYNAMIC POSTUROGRAPHY

Dynamic posturography (Figure 41.3) allows postural sway to be quantified in a number of conditions where visual and somatosensory cues are either absent or altered in some way. The test is sensitive to a number of neurological disorders and is not specific for vestibular deficits, although patients with uncompensated vestibular deficits or bilateral hypofunction have difficulty maintaining

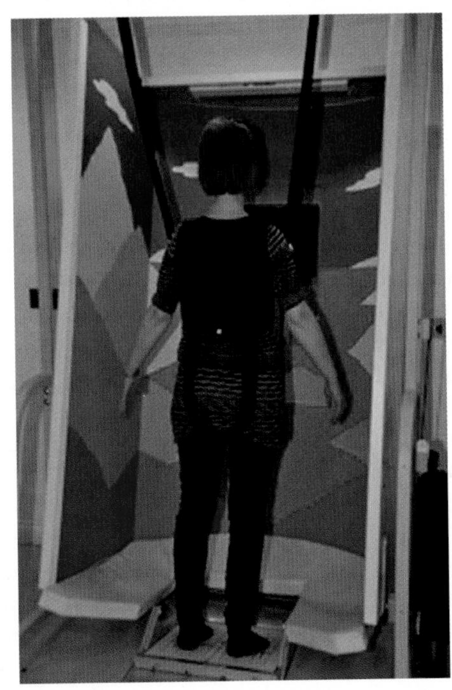

Figure 41.3 Computerized dynamic posturography.

their balance when visual and somatosensory cues are altered. The tool is very useful in establishing treatment and monitoring progress during rehabilitation. It has the added advantage that the patients can observe their own progress, which can be beneficial. It is able to characterize 'visual preference', effectively the situation where the visual system assists the injured vestibular apparatus, and so allows targeted vestibular physiotherapy. Other tests within the protocols may suggest the presence of peripheral neuropathies or musculoskeletal disorders.

ELECTROCOCHLEOGRAPHY

Electrocochleography (ECochG) measures the auditory evoked response (AER) from the cochlea and provides a direct assessment of inner ear function.[10] The AER is electrical activity generated by the auditory system in response to an acoustic stimulus such as a click or a tone burst. The ECochG provides a method of recording this electrical activity from the cochlea and VIIIth cranial nerve by placing an electrode either extratympanically (ET) in the outer ear canal so that it is close to the tympanic membrane or transtympanically (TT) and rested on the cochlear promontory. Although the TT methodology provides a better signal quality, it is more invasive compared to the ET approach and therefore is not as well tolerated by patients. The ECochG is a short latency response and is generated within a few milliseconds of the acoustic stimulus. It comprises three components: the cochlear microphonic (CM), the summating potential (SP) and the compound action potential (AP). The CM reflects the displacement of the basilar membrane and hair cells in response to the acoustic stimulus. The SP is a current response from the inner hair cells, whilst the AP is representative of usually more distal auditory fibres and is usually larger than the SP. ECochG results are normally reported as an SP/AP ratio. Whilst there are a number of specialist uses of the ECochG to monitor auditory function, it is most commonly requested for the assessment of Ménière's disease. Whilst the exact mechanism remains elusive, it is thought that the increased pressure of endolymphatic hydrops impacts the biomechanics of the basilar membrane and hair cell structures, resulting in changes in the ECochG waveform. An SP/AP ratio in excess of 0.5 is usually considered to be abnormal, with the sensitivity to Ménière's disease being reported as 60–70 per cent. To generate an ECochG there must be hearing present, and from a practical perspective, the response is difficult to elicit beyond a sensorineural hearing loss of 40 dBHL. Furthermore, the ECochG can be technically challenging and vulnerable to operator bias. However, when conducted by an experienced clinician, it can be a useful adjunct to the vestibular test battery.

SUMMARY

Clinic balance testing can incorporate many clinical skills. Whilst the history and clinical examination will provide a diagnosis in the majority of patients, increasingly sophisticated investigations are allowing a greater understanding of each part of the vestibular apparatus and its central connections, allowing for yet more accurate diagnosis and better targeted treatments.

KEY LEARNING POINTS

- The history, as always, is the key to successful assessment.
- Clinical examination should include multiple organs and systems, such as the vestibule and neurological and cardiovascular systems.
- Each laboratory test described answers a specific question; simply asking for 'balance tests' is unlikely to be helpful.
- New tests are described that assess the utricle and saccule.

REFERENCES

1. Tullio P. *Das Ohr und die Entstehung der Sprache und Schrift*. Berlin: Urban & Schwarzenberg, 1929.

2. Leigh RJ, Zee DS. *The Neurology of Eye Movements*. 4th ed. Oxford: Oxford University Press, 2006.
3. Halmagyi GM, Curthoys IS. A clinical sign of canal paresis. *Archives of Neurology*. 1988; 45: 737–39.
4. Alexander G. *Die Ohrenkrankheiten im Kindesalter*. In: *Handbuch der Kinderheilkunde*. Ed. Schlossmann A. Leipzig: Verlag von F.C.W. Vogel, 1912: 84–96.
5. Herdman SJ, ed. *Vestibular Rehabilitation*. 3rd ed. Philadelphia: F.A. Davis Co., 2007.
6. Fitzgerald G, Hallpike CS. Studies in human vestibular function: 1. Observations on the directional preponderance of caloric nystagmus resulting from cerebral lesions. *Brain*. 1942; 65: 115–37.
7. Colebatch JG, Halmagyi GM, Skuse NF. Myogenic potentials generated by a click-evoked vestibulocollic reflex. *Journal of Neurology, Neurosurgery, and Psychiatry*. 1994; 57: 190–97.
8. Sandhu JS1, Low R, Rea PA, Saunders NC. Altered frequency dynamics of cervical and ocular vestibular evoked myogenic potentials in patients with Ménière's disease. *Otology and Neurotology*. 2012 Apr; 33(3): 444–49.
9. Herdman SJ, et al. Computerized dynamic visual acuity test in the assessment of vestibular deficits. *American Journal of Otology*. 1998; 19: 790–96.
10. Gibson WP. The use of electrocochleography in the diagnosis of Meniere's disease. *Acta Otolaryngologica*. Suppl. 1991; 485: 46–52.

42

Diseases of the external ear

PATRICK M SPIELMANN AND S MUSHEER HUSSAIN

EMBRYOLOGY

The external auditory canal (EAC) is derived from the dorsal aspect of the first branchial cleft. In the ninth gestational week, the ectodermal meatal plate descends towards the tympanic cavity and forms a plug. Around the 21st week, the EAC starts to form by canalization of this ectodermal plug, a process that completes by the 28th week. The most medial aspect of the ectodermal plug persists as the lateral epithelial layer of the tympanic membrane (TM). The neonatal EAC is short and straight with an almost horizontal TM. The inferior tympanic ring is not complete, but with progressive ossification of the EAC floor during childhood, the longer adult EAC – with a near vertical tympanic membrane – becomes evident from the age of 9 years.

ANATOMY

The inner two-thirds of the EAC is formed by the tympanic bone inferiorly, the squamous temporal bone anterosuperiorly and the mastoid bone posteriorly; the outer third of the EAC is cartilaginous. The EAC is lined by keratinizing stratified squamous epithelium. The skin over the medial bony canal is thin, closely adherent to the underlying periosteum and has few subcutaneous structures. The skin over the lateral aspect is thicker with a subcutaneous layer, hair follicles, sebaceous glands and wax-secreting ceruminous glands. The bony EAC narrows at the isthmus, approximately 5 mm lateral to the TM, where the anterior wall bulges into the canal by varying degrees. Medial to this is a recess, with an acute angle between the canal wall and TM.

PHYSIOLOGY

EAR WAX (CERUMEN)

Cerumen consists of desquamated keratin mixed with lipid and peptide secretions from sebaceous and ceruminous glands, respectively. Lysosomes, immunoglobulins and hyaluronic acid are also present. It has a protective role in the EAC, forming a barrier over the skin and creating a mildly acidic environment (pH5.0–7.0). Its role in protecting against infection is unclear. Cerumen may become impacted if the migratory function of the EAC is impaired or if pushed medial in the EAC with cotton buds. The management of cerumen with otic drops is the subject of a Cochrane review: no active agent was superior to others. Ear syringing is commonly performed in primary care, with occasional complications such as otitis externa, tympanic membrane perforation or damage to the EAC. Secondary care management includes microscopic or endoscopic removal. The use of ear candles, though popular, is to be discouraged as there are reports of injury and no evidence of benefit.

SOUND CONDUCTION

The EAC is involved in sound localization and conduction to the TM. Inter-aural differences provide the most information for sound localization, but even in monaural hearing the sound pressure levels (SPLs) in the EAC at various frequencies differ in both vertical and horizontal planes. The pinna and concha concentrate the sound pressure at the external auditory meatus. The EAC acts as a chamber with a resonant frequency of 3 kHz. At this frequency approximately 10–12 dB are added to the SPL at the TM compared with the external ear.

PATHOLOGY

Conditions of the EAC can be classified according to the underlying abnormality. The important congenital anomaly to consider is atresia, and acquired pathologies are: bony, epithelial, infective or neoplastic. Otitis externa is covered in Chapter 53 and will not be addressed here.

AURAL ATRESIA

History and examination

Congenital aural atresia (CAA) has an incidence of between 0.8 and 1.6/10 000 live births. The appearance is usually sporadic, but there are associations with Treacher Collins and Goldenhar syndromes. Several grading systems have been proposed, but the most validated and comprehensive was described by Jahrsdoefer in 1992. This considers eight components of a temporal bone computed tomography (CT) scan and the appearance of the pinna. The higher the score (out of 10), the better the candidacy for atresiaplasty.

Investigations

Careful clinical examination to look for associated anomalies is mandatory. Audiometric assessment should identify whether the cochlear and eighth nerve are functional. Imaging is important to assess the middle and inner ears if surgical intervention is planned.

Management

This encompasses functional (hearing) rehabilitation and cosmesis. Hearing rehabilitation can be achieved with a bone-conduction hearing aid (such as BAHA or one of several available implantable devices); while patients report benefit, objective audiometric measures fail to show much improvement in unilateral cases. In bilateral cases audiometric rehabilitation is a greater priority and may initially be achieved by a bone conduction device applied via a headband. Implantable hearing devices such as the MeD EL vibrant soundbridge or Bonebridge provide hearing restoration and are licensed in Europe for use in children.

Atresiaplasty can be successful in reducing conductive hearing loss to 25 dB or less in well-selected cases. Cosmetic correction can be achieved with a prosthesis or a variety of surgical techniques, including complete auricular reconstruction using carved costal cartilage. This specialized process is delayed until the patient is at least 8 years of age to allow for sufficient chest wall growth.

BONY LESIONS

History and examination

Two bony lesions predominate: exostoses and osteoma. The differential diagnosis is usually achieved clinically: Exostoses are typically multiple and bilateral. They may be asymptomatic but if large and/or multiple, may occlude the EAC, resulting in otitis externa and conductive hearing loss. There is typically a history of repeated cold water exposure. The underlying pathology is a periostitis following exposure, leading to new bone formation. Osteomas are benign tumours of the bony EAC, which are typically unilateral and solitary; they arise from the tympano-squamous or tympano-mastoid suture lines. They are slow-growing, frequently asymptomatic and may be an incidental finding but, as exostoses, may cause obstructive symptoms and conductive hearing loss. Typical examples are shown in Figures 42.1 and 42.2.

Investigations

High-resolution CT scanning may be helpful in defining the extent of both pathologies, particularly when the EAC appears obstructed. The relationships with the tympanic membrane, facial nerve and temporomandibular joint (TMJ) are important to consider when planning surgery.

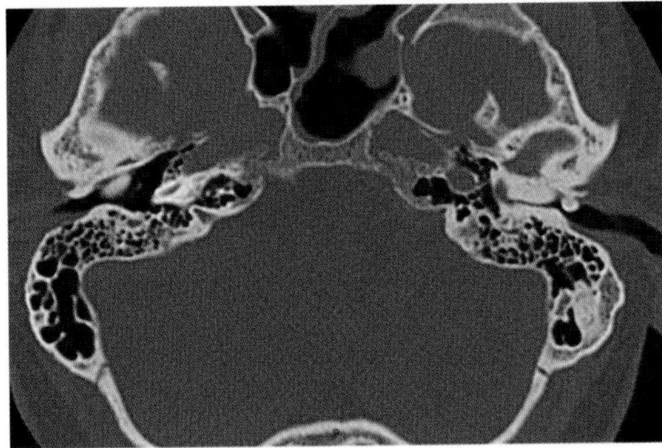

Figure 42.1 Axial CT of ear canal exostoses.

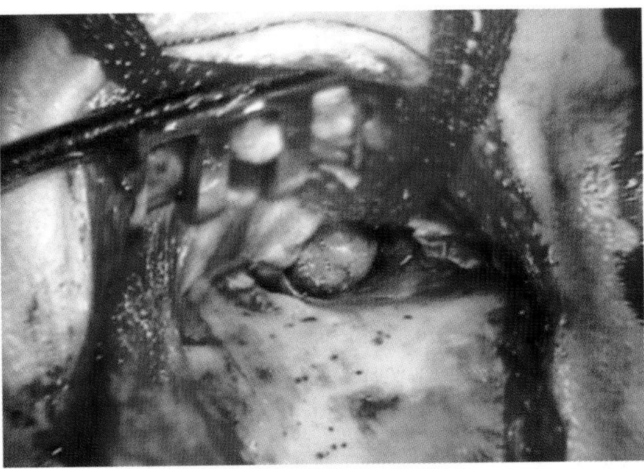

Figure 42.2 Intraoperative photograph of large ear canal osteoma.

Management

Active treatment is not necessary if lesions are asymptomatic or discovered incidentally. Conservative treatment involves regular aural toilet to prevent complications and advice to treat intercurrent otitis externa; earplugs could be recommended for continued cold-water exposure in patients with exostoses. Surgery for obstructive canal exostoses can be challenging: there may be very little space between the bony swellings, the overlying skin is thin, access can be poor, and the tympanic membrane, facial nerve and TMJ are all at risk during bone removal. The postauricular approach is favoured to remove exostoses, this provides optimum visualization – especially of the anterior exostosis – and access for drilling. The skin is elevated from lateral to medial and the anterior exostosis removed first. The bony canal wall is followed and the new bone removed, egg-shelling and collapsing the exostosis to preserve canal skin. Care must be taken to identify the TMJ, tympanic membrane and annulus. With the improved access, the skin over the remaining exostoses can be elevated and the bone removed in a similar fashion, preserving a thin layer of skin to be replaced and line the new canal. If this canal skin is lost, healing will be by secondary intention and prolonged. Osteomas may be removed by a transcanal or endaural approach since osteomas typically arise from a narrow pedicle. This pedicle can be fractured and drilled flush to the bony canal without having to elevate much skin. Exostoses may recur with continued cold-water exposure, but osteomas should not.

EPITHELIAL ABNORMALITIES

History and examination

EAC cholesteatoma (EACC) is characterized by bony erosion and invasion of squamous epithelium with localized periosteitis and bone sequestration. EACC is rare; the incidence has been calculated as 60 times less than that of middle ear cholesteatoma. The lesion is typically in the floor of the EAC, and the differential diagnosis includes skull base osteomyelitis (SBO) and squamous cell carcinoma. Keratosis obturans (KO) is characterized by a plug of organized keratin, which causes expansion of the bony EAC with obstruction of the lumen and subsequent symptoms.

Piepergedes et al. first differentiated between these two entities in 1980. They postulated that EACC was caused by periosteitis of the bony canal as opposed to an abnormality of epithelial migration, which was considered to cause KO, although the aetiology of this is not yet known.

The discriminating clinical features are shown in Table 42.1.

Investigations

The diagnosis is typically made based on clinical findings, but high-resolution CT can demonstrate middle ear and mastoid bone involvement of EACC. A typical example is shown in Figure 42.3.

Table 42.1 Comparing external auditory canal cholesteatoma (EACC) and keratosis obturans (KO)

Feature	EACC	KO
Bilateral?	No	Typically
Pain?	Dull ache and chronic	Acute and severe
Hearing?	Normal	Conductive loss
Discharge?	Common	Rare
Ear canal skin	Intact	Ulcerated with underlying osteonecrosis
Underlying pathology?	Localized periosteitis	Epithelial migration disorder

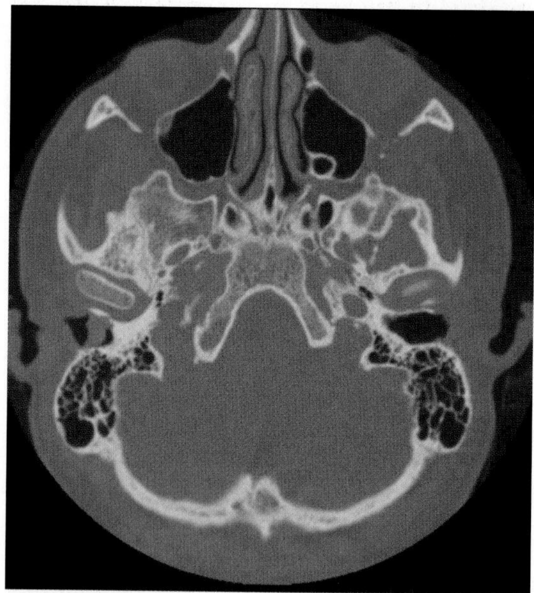

Figure 42.3 Axial CT of left ear canal cholesteatoma involving temporomandibular joint.

Management

KO can be managed effectively by removal of the keratin plug from the EAC, possibly under general anaesthesia. This procedure must be repeated at regular intervals, as the epithelial migratory defect is often chronic. The management of EACC must be tailored to the patient and the extent of disease. Local curettage with application of topical antimicrobials may be suitable for limited disease, but formal small-cavity, canal-wall-down mastoid surgery will be required for more extensive disease.

INFECTIVE LESIONS

History and examination

Skull base osteomyelitis (SBO) typically presents in an immune-compromised host with severe otalgia and unilateral otorrhea. There may be invasion of local structures and necrosis of skin, cartilage and bone. Cranial nerve palsies may ensue with involvement of the petrous apex, typically the facial nerve but the trigeminal, abducens and lower cranial nerves may also be affected. *Pseudomonas aeruginosa* is by far the most common pathogenic micro-organism, although other pathogens have been identified.

Chronic inflammation may cause progressive soft tissue stenosis of the EAC and result in a false fundus. This may cause a conductive hearing loss, but the chronic otorrhea may cease.

Investigations

Cross-sectional imaging of the skull base is helpful in achieving diagnosis and monitoring progress in SBO. High-resolution CT can demonstrate bone erosion, although magnetic resonance imaging (MRI) is more sensitive to detect skull base inflammation and cranial nerve involvement. No changes are specific for SBO, so radionucleotide investigations may be helpful: Technetium 99m bone scintigraphy is sensitive in detecting bony involvement and is therefore used for diagnostic purposes. Gallium 67 scintigraphy is used to monitor the response to treatment. Biopsy of any granulations or sequestrum is mandatory to exclude a (true) malignancy.

A CT scan can be helpful to exclude middle-ear pathology in a patient with an obstructed tympanic membrane; a typical false fundus is shown in Figure 42.4.

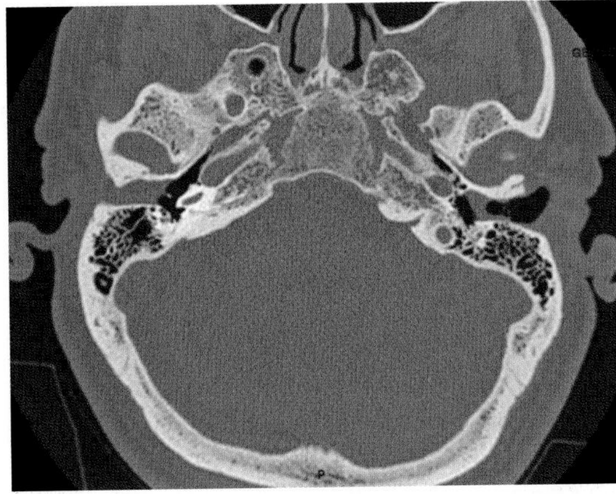

Figure 42.4 Axial CT of bilateral ear canal false fundus.

Management

Fluoroquinolones (particularly ciprofloxacin) are the treatment of choice, with a high cure rate when used for prolonged periods. Antimicrobial resistance to ciprofloxacin is emerging and must be suspected in patients with deteriorating clinical features (such as new cranial nerve palsies) or rising inflammatory markers. Hyperbaric oxygen has been used with some benefit as an adjuvant to antimicrobials, but a Cochrane review found no randomized controlled trials to support this treatment.

AURAL POLYPS

History and examination

EAC polyps typically arise from the middle ear and indicate underlying inflammatory disease: cholesteatoma is reported in up to 60 per cent of children with aural polyps. They may arise secondary to chronic inflammation such as with a foreign body (retained ventilation tube, for instance). The important distinction between granulation tissue is that a polyp has an epithelial lining. The differential diagnosis of polyps includes neoplastic and granulomatous conditions such as tuberculosis, syphilis, xanthomatosis and eosinophilic granuloma.

Investigations

CT scanning may be helpful if polyps remain refractory to medical treatment or if cholesteatoma is suspected.

Management

Conservative treatment with cautery and topical antimicrobials will often cause the polyp to regress. A thorough examination of the ear and polypectomy should be performed if the polyp persists, if necessary under anaesthesia. Polyps must not be removed blindly as they may be adherent to the stapes superstructure or facial nerve.

NEOPLASTIC LESIONS

History and examination

Primary tumours arising in the EAC are rare, and no cell type is predominant. Tumours may arise from any structure of the EAC or extend from the parotid gland anteriorly; metastases are even rarer. Common cutaneous malignancies, basal cell carcinoma (BCC) and squamous cell carcinoma (SCC), can be particularly aggressive in nature as they are not UV-light dependent. These often require more extensive surgery to achieve adequate margins, typically a sleeve excision of the canal possibly including the tympanic membrane. Glandular components of the EAC can give rise to benign and malignant tumours, including pleomorphic adenomas, adenoid cystic carcinomas and ceruminous adeno-(carcino)mas.

Investigations

High-resolution CT scanning can demonstrate tumour size, bone destruction and lymphadenopathy.

Management

In general, all lesions should be removed for histology: A small endaural incision provides adequate access for most small tumours, is quick and carries minimal morbidity. It can be difficult to achieve adequate excision margins given the close relationship with the bony canal. Benign tumours should be treated by wide local excision, while malignant tumours should receive subsequent radiotherapy, although this carries the risk of osteo-radionecrosis of the temporal bone.

Squamous carcinoma involving the temporal bone is rare and likely to recur if inadequately treated. As with all malignant disease, management should be discussed within a multidisciplinary team and, given the rarity, referral to a specialist unit should be considered. A lateral temporal bone resection is required for T1 and T2 tumours, with post-operative radiotherapy for large-volume T2 tumours. For T3 and T4 tumours, subtotal petrosectomy, parotidectomy and post-operative radiotherapy are advised. Survival rates are not improved by more extensive, debilitating surgery for this aggressive disease. Surgical resection with radiotherapy can also be useful in palliation.

KEY LEARNING POINTS

- The bony external auditory canal is incomplete inferiorly at birth.
- Congenital aural atresia affects approximately 1:10 000 births with varying degrees of severity.
- Auditory rehabilitation in ear canal atresia may be achieved by canalplasty or bone-conduction hearing devices.
- Ear canal exostoses are typically multiple and bilateral, while osteomas are typically solitary and unilateral.
- Otitis externa with cranial nerve palsy in an immunocompromised host should prompt investigation for skull base osteomyelitis.
- Resistance to fluoroquinolones in skull base osteomyelitis is increasing.

FURTHER READING

Babiatzki A, Sade J. Malignant external otitis. *Journal of Laryngology and Otology.* 1987; 101: 205–10.

Bibas AG, Ward V, Gleeson MJ. Squamous cell carcinoma of the temporal bone. *Journal of Laryngology and Otology.* 2008; 122: 1156–61.

Chaplin J, Stewart IA. The prevalence of exostoses in the external auditory meatus of surfers. *Clinical Otolaryngology.* 1998; 23: 326–30.

Dubach P, Mantokoudis G, Caversaccio M. Ear canal cholesteatoma: Meta-analysis of clinical characteristics with update on classification, staging and treatment. *Current Opinion in Otolaryngology and Head and Neck Surgery.* 2010; 18: 369–76.

Michaels L. *Ear and Temporal Bone*. In: *Pathology of the Head and Neck*. Eds. Cardesa A, Slootwig PJ. Berlin: Springer, 2006: 234–60.

Middlebrooks JC, Makous JC, Green DM. Directional sensitivity of sound-pressure levels in the human ear canal. *Journal of the Acoustical Society of America*. 1989; 86: 89–108.

Moffat DA, Wagstaff SA, Hardy DG. The outcome of surgery and post-operative radiotherapy for squamous carcinoma of the temporal bone. *Laryngoscope*. 2005; 115: 341–7.

Persaud RAP, Hajioff D, Thevasagayam MS, Wareing MJ, Wright A. Keratosis obturans and external ear canal cholesteatoma: How and why we should distinguish between these conditions. *Clinical Otolaryngology*. 2004; 29: 577–81.

Phillips JS, Jones SEM. Hyperbaric oxygen as an adjuvant treatment for malignant otitis externa. *Cochrane Database of Systematic Reviews*. 2005; 2.

Piepergerdes MC, Kramer BM, Behnke EE. Keratosis obturans and external auditory canal cholesteatoma. *Laryngoscope*. 1980; 90: 38–91.

Tay HL, Hussain SSM. The management of aural polyps. *Journal of Laryngology and Otology*. 1997; 111: 212–14.

Umeda Y, Nakajima M, Yoshiola H. Surfer's ear in Japan. *Laryngoscope*. 1989; 99: 639–41.

43

Acute otitis media

AANAND ACHARYA AND ANDREW REID

ANATOMY OF THE MIDDLE EAR CLEFT

The middle ear cleft encompasses the tympanic cavity, the eustachian tube anteriorly and the mastoid air cell system posteriorly.

TYMPANIC CAVITY

The tympanic cavity is an air-filled space within the temporal bone, which is divided into three compartments:

- Epitympanum (upper compartment, commonly referred to as the 'attic') lies above the level of the malleolar folds.
- Hypotympanum (lower compartment) lies below the inferior tympanic sulcus.
- Mesotympanum (middle compartment) lies in between these.

Its contents include the ossicles (malleus, incus, stapes), the tendons of the tensor tympani and stapedius muscles, the chorda tympani nerve and the tympanic plexus.

The lateral wall of the tympanic cavity is constituted by the bony lateral wall of the epitympanum superiorly, the tympanic membrane centrally and the bony lateral wall of the hypotympanum inferiorly. The thin, inferior border of the bony lateral wall of the epitympanum is also referred to as the outer attic wall or 'scutum': Erosion of the scutum, as identified on high-resolution computed tomography (CT) in the coronal plane, is pathognomonic of cholesteatoma.

The medial wall of the tympanic cavity comprises the osseous labyrinth. The promontory, which is the bony covering of the basal turn of the cochlea, occupies much of this. Posterosuperior to this is the oval window, which is occupied by the stapes footplate. Posteroinferiorly is located the round window. The horizontal segment of the bony facial nerve canal

(Fallopian canal) runs superior to the promontory and oval window, from the first genu anteriorly to the second genu posteriorly. The processus cochleariformis – through which the tensor tympanic runs to insert into the handle of the malleus – is a landmark for the horizontal segment of the facial nerve. At the second genu the horizontal facial canal turns 90° inferiorly to become the vertical segment, running posterior to the oval window down to the stylomastoid foramen. The pyramid – through which the tendon of the stapedius muscle passes to insert into the head of the stapes – is a landmark for the vertical segment of the facial nerve. Lateral to the vertical facial canal is a groove called the facial recess, and medial to the vertical facial canal is the sinus tympani. Posterior and superior to the second genu of the facial nerve is the bony prominence of the lateral semicircular canal.

The roof of the tympanic cavity is the tegmen tympani: a thin plate of bone separating the middle ear cleft from the middle fossa of the cranium. It is continuous posteriorly with the tegmen mastoideum, which separates the middle cranial fossa from the mastoid air cell system. The petrosquamous suture line runs through the roof of the tympanic cavity. This suture only closes in adulthood, thereby providing a route for infection to access the extradural space in children. Veins draining the tympanic cavity into the superior petrosal sinus also run through this suture line and can provide a further pathway of access for infection.

The bony floor of the tympanic cavity separates the hypotympanum from the dome of the jugular bulb, whose height is variable. This bony floor can be dehiscent, thereby rendering the jugular bulb at risk of trauma from instrumentation in this area.

The anterior wall of the tympanic cavity is a narrow convergence of the medial and lateral walls. Inferiorly is found the bony covering of the carotid artery as it enters the skull base. Above this are located the orifice to the eustachian tube and the bony canal of the tensor tympani tendon. The upper aspect of the anterior wall is made up of the anterior epitympanic space, anterior to the head of the malleus.

The posterior wall of the tympanic cavity is the aditus ad antrum – a large, irregular opening from the epitympanum anteriorly into the mastoid antrum posteriorly. Inferior to the aditus lies the fossa incudis – a shallow depression that houses the short process of the incus. The medial wall of the mastoid antrum is related to the posterior semicircular canal. The mastoid antrum communicates posteriorly with the mastoid air cell system whose roof is the tegmen mastoideum and medial wall is the bony plate separating the posterior cranial fossa and (more posteriorly) the sigmoid sinus from the mastoid air cell system. The posterior belly of the digastric muscle inserts into the base of the mastoid bone: The digastric ridge inside the mastoid bone corresponds to the insertion of this muscle and is a useful marker for the facial nerve. The outer wall of the mastoid air cell system is easily palpable behind the pinna, just below the skin. MacEwen's triangle is a direct lateral relation to the mastoid antrum.

NERVE SUPPLY

The tympanic plexus, comprising the tympanic branch of the glossopharyngeal nerve (Jacobson's nerve) and caroticotympanic nerves arising from the sympathetic plexus surrounding the internal carotid artery, provide branches to the mucous membrane lining the middle ear cleft.

BLOOD SUPPLY

Branches from both the internal and external carotid artery supply the walls and contents of the middle ear cleft with extensive variability and overlap.

MUCOSA

The tympanic cavity mucosa is mucus-secreting respiratory-type mucosa that bears cilia. It lines the bony walls and drapes over the ossicles, their supporting ligaments and the tendons of the two middle ear muscles. These mucosal folds can obstruct the ventilation pathways between the various compartments of the middle ear cleft. More posteriorly in the mastoid air cell system the mucosa is a flattened, non-ciliated epithelium without goblet cells or mucus glands.

Mucus produced by the mucosal lining of the middle ear cleft is directed by the cilia towards the tympanic orifice of the eustachian tube.

THE EUSTACHIAN TUBE

The eustachian tube connects the middle ear cleft to the nasopharynx. Its lateral third is bony, with the medial two-thirds being cartilaginous. Immature in children, it achieves adult length (36 mm) and angulation (45°) by about 7 years of age. The mucosal lining of the eustachian tube is similar to that of the middle ear: ciliated respiratory type epithelium with goblet cells and mucus-secreting glands. The tympanic orifice of the eustachian tube forms a part of the anterior wall of the tympanic cavity: At this point the carotid canal lies immediately medial and can impinge on the bony eustachian tube. The nasopharyngeal orifice of the eustachian tube is surrounded superiorly and posteriorly by the torus tubarius (eustachian tube cushion). Immediately posterior to this is the pharyngeal recess (fossa of Rosenmuller). Lymphoid tissue (adenoidal tissue) is present in this vicinity, particularly in children, and inflammation of this may impact on the patency of the nasopharyngeal orifice of the eustachian tube. The levator palati, tensor palati and salpingopharyngeus muscles are attached to the cartilaginous portion of the eustachian tube. Their action during swallowing and yawning contribute to eustachian tube function.

EMBRYOLOGY OF THE MIDDLE EAR CLEFT

The eustachian tube, middle ear and mastoid antrum are derived from the first and second branchial arches. The eustachian tube lumen and middle ear spaces are formed by 8 months' gestation, with the epitympanum and mastoid antrum developed by birth. Development of the mastoid air cell system occurs after birth and is 90 per cent complete by 6 years of age.

The malleus and incus are derived from Meckel's cartilage (first branchial arch), while the stapes superstructure is derived from Reichert's cartilage (second branchial arch). The stapes footplate embryologically is a part of the developing labyrinth. This achieves its full adult size by about 25 weeks' gestation and in the latter part of development becomes ossified. The stapes footplate eventually attaches to the stapes superstructure.

The pretrematic nerve of the first arch is the chorda tympani, and the facial nerve is the post-trematic nerve of the second branchial arch: This accounts for the close proximity of these nerves to the ossicles of the first (malleus, incus) and second (stapes) branchial arches, respectively.

The ectoderm of the first pharyngeal groove, the underlying endoderm of the primitive middle ear and intervening mesenchyme form the layers of the future tympanic membrane. The endodermal sac, which is the precursor of the middle ear, expands to drape over the ossicles and labyrinth. This eventually becomes the mucosa, which is draped over the walls, ossicles, tendons and ligaments to produce a series of mucosal folds and spaces.

RISK FACTORS FOR ACUTE OTITIS MEDIA

There is increasing evidence that genetic factors play a role in the risk of an individual patient developing acute otitis media (AOM). Racial differences, in particular in relation to the shape, size and patency of the eustachian tube, have been demonstrated with increased prevalence amongst American Indians, Eskimos and Australian Aboriginals. The influence of genetics on the immune mechanism also accounts for these variations, particularly immune deficiencies associated with low IgG2 subclasses. Atopy and maternal blood group A have also been associated with an increased risk of developing AOM.

Environmental factors are important as it may be possible to influence these and thus reduce a patient's risk of developing AOM. Low socio-economic status, particularly poor housing and overcrowding, is associated with an increased incidence of AOM. Day-care attendance, use of a pacifier and passive smoke exposure are all associated with an increased risk of AOM. Breastfeeding for 3 months confers protection against AOM.

Specific syndromes, particularly those associated with craniofacial anomalies or skull base abnormalities, are known to predispose to chronic otitis media, but whether this increases the risk of AOM is less clear. Patients with Down's syndrome and Turner syndrome suffer more frequent episodes of AOM.

EPIDEMIOLOGY AND PATHOLOGY

AOM describes a viral or bacterial infection of the middle ear and mastoid air cell system that results in mucosal inflammation, is associated with a middle ear effusion and results in a variable collection of symptoms and signs. It is one of the most common illnesses in childhood, with a peak incidence in the second 6 months of life.

Cases can be divided into four subgroups:

1. Sporadic – infrequent isolated events commonly associated with upper respiratory tract infection
2. Resistant – persistence of middle ear infection beyond a short course (3–5 days) of antibiotic treatment
3. Persistent – persistence or recurrence of symptoms or signs of AOM within 6 days of completing a course of antibiotics
4. Recurrent - three or more episodes in 6 months, or four to six episodes in 12 months

Recurrent AOM has been reported in 5 per cent of children under 2 years of age, with 25 per cent of children who have their first episode of AOM before 9 months of age going on to develop recurrent AOM.

The majority of episodes of AOM may be associated with viral infection. The typical respiratory tract viruses that are most commonly associated with AOM include respiratory syncytial virus (RSV), influenza A virus, parainfluenza viruses, adenoviruses and rhinovirus. Commonly identified bacterial pathogens include *Haemophilus influenzae, Streptococcus species, Moraxella catarrhalis* and *Staphylococcus aureus.*

The route of access of pathogens to the middle ear cleft is variable. Direct access may be acquired from the nasopharynx via the eustachian tube, although deposition in the middle ear cleft from the bloodstream may also be implicated. A third route of access is from the external auditory canal via a perforation or ventilation tube; this is most commonly associated with water exposure. Viral infection adversely affects eustachian tube function through the release of inflammatory mediators, a reduction in the number of ciliated epithelial cells and an increase in mucus production. This contributes to the development of a negative middle ear pressure and consequently AOM. Viral infection also adversely affects host immunity, increasing susceptibility to bacterial infection. Consequently, a viral upper respiratory tract infection may lead to a bacterial AOM. Bacterial adherence to nasopharyngeal epithelium may be increased by certain viruses – this may contribute to the development of biofilms, which predispose to resistant, persistent and recurrent AOM.

HISTORY AND EXAMINATION

Patients typically present with localizing ear symptoms including otalgia, hearing loss and possible otorrhoea. These may follow a preceding upper respiratory tract infection. They may also have symptoms suggestive of a more generalized systemic illness such as fever or irritability, and in children the presence of poor feeding, vomiting, ear pulling and clumsiness. Diagnosis on the basis of history alone is difficult because the condition occurs most commonly in children who may not be able to give an appropriate history, some children may have no ear symptoms and a large proportion may remain apyrexial throughout the episode.

Otoscopy can be particularly difficult in children. However, if a view of the tympanic membrane is achieved, it typically appears injected and bulging, indicating inflammation and fluid in the middle ear, which is under pressure. Mucopus in the middle ear gives the tympanic membrane a yellowish appearance. There may be evidence of mucopus in the middle ear if the tympanic membrane has spontaneously perforated, or if a ventilation tube is *in situ*.

Acute otitis media can be associated with intracranial, intratemporal and extratemporal complications. The incidence of such complications in adults in developed countries is estimated to be up to 2 per 100 000 cases per year.

The most common complication in children, occurring in up to 10 per cent of cases, is tympanic membrane perforation. This is commonly associated with a reduction in the degree of otalgia. The majority of these heal spontaneously within 3 months, although a proportion of patients develop chronic perforations, which may predispose to recurrent AOM, particularly in association with water exposure.

The most common complication in adults is acute mastoiditis (83 per cent). While it is a relatively common complication in adults, the incidence of AOM in adults is significantly lower than that in children, and acute mastoiditis is consequently predominantly a disease of childhood. There are four defined classes of mastoiditis:

1. Mucosal inflammation of the mastoid cavity that is visualized radiologically but not associated with the other signs that are typically associated with mastoiditis; this is not strictly a complication of AOM.
2. Acute mastoiditis with periostitis: Infection spreads through the cortex of the mastoid bone by emissary veins to involve the periosteum. The result is a full postauricular crease, anterior deflection of the pinna and erythema, tenderness (typically over MacEwen's triangle, palpated through the conchal bowl) and mild swelling of the postauricular region.
3. Acute mastoid osteitis: This is associated with breakdown of mastoid air cells and bone, and a subperiosteal abscess may result. Development of a zygomatic (Luc's) or cervical abscess (Bezold's or Citelli's) may also occur.
4. Subacute ('masked') mastoiditis: This may occur in incompletely treated AOM after 10–14 days. Otalgia and systemic signs such as fever may persist, but there is an absence of the postauricular signs that are typically associated with mastoiditis. While seemingly benign, this stage must be considered and excluded as it too can progress to serious complications.

About a third of adult cases of AOM are complicated by facial palsy, which should recover completely. It is much less common in childhood. Meningitis is relatively uncommon in adults and is more common in children.

Other complications include:

- Intracranial
  - Cerebritis
  - Extradural, subdural or intracranial abscess
  - Sigmoid sinus thrombosis
  - Otitic hydrocephalus
  - Intracranial complications (up to 17 per cent of cases)
- Intratemporal
  - Labyrinthitis – due to round window permeability to bacterial toxins, resulting in imbalance and sensorineural hearing loss
- Gradenigos syndrome – VI nerve palsy, severe pain in the distribution of the trigeminal nerve, middle ear discharge/otorrhoea

INVESTIGATIONS

Tympanometry can be used to confirm the presence of fluid in the middle ear, but is not usually available for the assessment of patients presenting acutely.

If acquirable a pus sample is useful for microbiological culture, particularly in cases resistant to first-line therapy or in cases where complications of AOM have occurred. Unfortunately, culture often fails to demonstrate specific bacterial growth, suggesting that in many cases middle ear inflammation persists beyond eradication of the primary organism. Nasopharyngeal swabbing for bacterial culture has a weak correlation with middle ear pathogens and is not recommended clinically.

In severe or complicated cases, blood tests including full blood count, inflammatory markers (such as CRP) and blood cultures are indicated.

Where complications of acute otitis media are suspected to have occurred, a high-resolution CT scan of the temporal bones (and neck, if required) with contrast is indicated as it may demonstrate osteitis, abscess formation and intracranial complications. The timing of this investigation is guided by the clinical status of the patient. Imaging is also indicated when mastoidectomy is to be performed and in patients who fail to improve on antibiotic therapy.

ACUTE MANAGEMENT OF ACUTE OTITIS MEDIA

The natural history of AOM is of spontaneous resolution – otalgia settles in the majority of patients within 24 hours. The question of whether treatment is required and who requires it is debated. There is no evidence to support the efficacy of antibiotics within the first 24–48 hours, although if symptoms persist beyond this time, then their use may be indicated. Nor is there any evidence that use of antibiotics reduces the progression of disease, rate of relapse of symptoms or incidence of complications.

Choice of antibiotic is governed by local microbiological protocol. A broad-spectrum antibiotic that covers the commonly encountered pathogens (e.g. amoxicillin or a macrolide such as clarithromycin) would be appropriate as a first-line choice. Antibiotic resistance is increasing, however, necessitating the increased use of higher treatment doses or the use of antimicrobials capable of eradicating beta-lactamase–producing bacteria.

Oral antibiotics successfully treat acute otitis media equally in the presence of a tympanic membrane perforation or a ventilation tube. The potential ototoxicity of aminoglycoside antibiotic drops is well recognized. Guidelines suggest that in the presence of otorrhoea, a maximum 2-week course of these drops is safe.

The use of analgesia for symptomatic control and as an antipyretic where required is advisable. There is no evidence to support the use of oral and/or intranasal antihistamines or decongestants in the management of AOM, although they may provide some relief for nasal symptoms where AOM occurs in association with an upper respiratory tract infection.

While performing a myringotomy as well as using antibiotics confers no benefit over the use of antibiotics alone, drainage of middle ear fluid (either with or without grommet insertion) is effective at reducing otalgia and can provide a sample of pus for microbiological culture in cases where this is particularly necessary and where spontaneous perforation of the tympanic membrane has not occurred. It is also indicated in high-risk patients (e.g. immunocompromised), in those who have failed to respond to conventional treatment and in patients who are seriously unwell.

The presence of complications is also an indication for surgical drainage. Management of the complications of AOM may necessitate the involvement of other specialties (e.g. neurosurgery for intracranial complications, physicians/paediatricians for meningitis). Class 2 acute mastoiditis is successfully treated in 75 per cent of cases by myringotomy (with or without grommet insertion), culture of middle ear fluid and high-dose intravenous antibiotics. Failure to improve or progression to class 3 necessitates drainage of the abscess and, ideally, cortical mastoidectomy. This can be challenging for the less-experienced surgeon as granulations make identification of landmarks difficult and the facial nerve is relatively superficial in the young child.

Where spontaneous rupture of the tympanic membrane has occurred, patients should be encouraged to keep their ears dry. The majority of such perforations will heal spontaneously within 3 months; appropriate follow-up by the general practitioner is advisable to ascertain whether closure has occurred.

LONGER-TERM MANAGEMENT OF RECURRENT ACUTE OTITIS MEDIA

Attention to risk factors for AOM is important as many of these may be modifiable. Avoidance of exposure to other children, being sat semi-upright when bottle-feeding, restricting the use of pacifiers after infancy and avoiding passive smoke inhalation are all important considerations. Increased maternal vitamin C intake and avoidance of alcohol in the third trimester is advisable, as both are weakly associated with AOM.

In patients presenting with recurrent AOM, iron deficiency anaemia and white blood cell disorders should be excluded. Immunoglobulin assay may be indicated, particularly if the patient regularly suffers other infections (e.g. urinary tract infection, lower respiratory tract infection). Typically, this includes IgG, IgG subclasses and IgM levels. Specific response to immunization (e.g. anti-haemophilus antibodies and anti-pneumococcus antibodies) can be assessed; inadequate levels of antibody should prompt consideration for repeat immunization. Similarly, immunization against Influenza A virus and pneumococcus have both been demonstrated to reduce AOM.

Where recurrent infection of ventilation tubes is associated with nasal and pulmonary symptoms, the presence of a primary ciliary dyskinesia should be considered and ruled out.

The role of prophylactic strategies is debated. A medium-term (3-month) trial of low-dose antibiotics is accepted by many as a means of attempting to alleviate recurrent AOM. Alternatively, 6 months of treatment during the winter months may be implemented. Amoxicillin or a macrolide antibiotic (e.g. clarithromycin) given as a once-daily dose may be effective at reducing the frequency and severity of the episodes, and the resultant improvement of the state of the middle ear mucosa may reduce the incidence of middle ear effusion and AOM in any individual child. If AOM develops during this course, then normal treatment should be initiated, with resumption of the low-dose course thereafter. Patients (or parents) should diarize symptoms so that any response is clearly demonstrable.

Alternative management includes the insertion of ventilation tubes. This is particularly indicated in children suffering with recurrent AOM who have persistent middle ear effusions. By providing a drainage pathway, the tubes prevent the build-up of pressure associated with AOM behind an intact tympanic membrane and thus prevent the extreme otalgia that can be associated with the condition. The compromise is that the patient will develop otorrhoea each time he or she develops AOM. On occasion the ventilation tube itself may become infected and act as a source of infection, necessitating its removal.

There is little evidence to support the efficacy of adenotonsillectomy in reducing AOM, although it may be considered in children who have failed medical therapy and continue to have recurrent AOM following the insertion of ventilation tubes.

KEY LEARNING POINTS

- Immune deficiency associated with low IgG2 subclasses, atopy and maternal blood group A have been associated with increased risk of acute otitis media.
- Environmental factors such as poor housing, attendance at day care, use of pacifier and passive smoking are associated with AOM in children.
- The most common complication of AOM in adults is acute mastoiditis; however, because AOM is much more common in children, acute mastoiditis is seen more commonly in children than in adults.

SUGGESTED READINGS

Leskinen K, Jero J. Acute complications of otitis media in adults. *Clinical Otolaryngology.* 2005; 30: 511–16.

Proctor B. The development of the middle ear spaces and their surgical significance. *Journal of Otolaryngology.* 1964; 78: 631–49.

44

Chronic otitis media

JOSEPH G TONER

Chronic otitis media can be defined as chronic inflammation of the middle ear cleft including mucosa, tympanic membrane and ossicles. It can be subdivided into non-suppurative and suppurative (Table 44.1). Chronic non-suppurative otitis media is better known as otitis media with effusion (OME) and commonly referred to as glue ear. Chronic suppurative otitis media (CSOM) has attracted a variety of subclassifications, which has caused confusion with similar terminology not always referring to the same clinical entity. The terms *tubo-tympanic* and *attico-antral* were intended to differentiate between 'safe' (central perforation) and 'unsafe' (marginal perforation) disease, respectively. The former was associated with or without persistent or intermittent discharge, and the latter associated with squamous epithelium ingrowth, i.e. cholesteatoma. While these terms were generally helpful to define the clinical picture in the majority of cases, they are not universally accurate and have fallen into disrepute. A more helpful classification of CSOM would be as follows: non-cholesteatoma ears (with the presence of either a perforation or a retraction pocket) or cholesteatoma cases with ingrowth of keratin-producing epithelium whether this is via an attic perforation or in a pars tensa perforation or retraction.

OTITIS MEDIA WITH EFFUSION

The definition of persistent (or chronic) non-suppurative chronic otitis media, or OME, is a persistent middle ear fluid and generally accepted to be persistent after an arbitrarily defined time period of 3 months (Table 44.2). There are various synonyms for OME, such as *sero-mucinous otitis media* and *chronic secretory otitis media*, although it is commonly referred to as glue ear. The peak incidence is between 2 and 5 years of age with up to 80 per cent of children having had at least one episode by the age of 10. Risk factors include attendance at day-care facilities, parental smoking and a tendency to frequent upper respiratory tract infections; syndromic risk factors include cleft palate and trisomy 21.

Table 44.1 Chronic otitis media (COM) classification

Non-suppurative (COM)
- Otitis media with effusion
Suppurative (CSOM)
Non-cholesteatoma
Tympanic membrane perforation
Retraction pockets
Tymopanosclerosis
Cholesteatoma
Attic (pars flaccid) / Middle ear
Iatrogenic

Table 44.2 Otitis media with effusion (OME)

- Common paediatric condition peak incidence age 2–5 years
- Symptoms of hearing loss/speech delay
- Management initially watchful waiting >3 months
- Medical treatments (e.g. antibiotics, steroids, otovents) of no proven value
- Surgical treatment with ventilator insertion provides definite benefits. Adenoidectomy enhances and extends benefits

PATHOGENESIS

This can be divided into conditions that cause increased mucus production or decreased clearance of normal mucus production. Infections are associated with increased mucus production, and bacterial infections can damage the cilial transport mechanism and therefore reduce clearance. The role of infective biofilms is increasingly recognized, challenging much previous research that indicated that the effusions were sterile. However, despite being strongly implicated, the exact mechanism has yet to be fully established.

Eustachian tube dysfunction may be due to an individual's specific anatomic configuration or obstructive as a result of adenoid enlargement.

SYMPTOMS

While OME can occur in adults, it is mostly encountered in the paediatric population. The most frequent presenting symptoms relate to hearing loss and/or the associated impact on speech development; this may manifest as poor attention or behavioural issues. However, the condition may be silent and therefore detected only at routine hearing screening. There may be associated otalgia if there is a supervening infection, and the presence of fluid in the ear can cause discomfort that is particularly noticeable at night when the child is lying flat.

DIAGNOSIS

The presence of middle ear fluid can be assessed on otoscopy; the tympanic membrane may be retracted and have undergone a colour change, though this is variable. Otoscopy with a magnifying otoscope is very helpful, and findings of a dull tympanic membrane or a yellow/orange discolouration are typical. Also, at times there may be fluid level evident in the middle ear (Figure 44.1). The diagnosis is confirmed on tympanometry with a Type B (a flat tracing indicating significantly reduced compliance and middle ear fluid) or C_2 tympanogram (a significant negative pressure peak) indicating reduced middle ear pressure. In the age group where pure tone audiometry is possible, a conductive hearing loss of 15 to 40 dB may

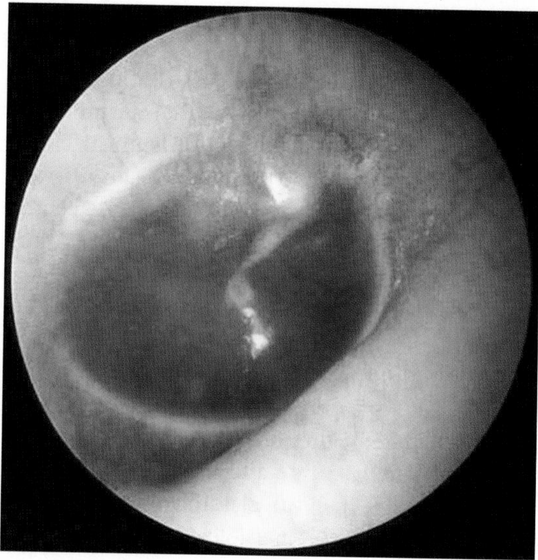

Figure 44.1 Typical appearance of glue ear.

be present; age-appropriate free field audiometry may be performed in children for whom routine audiometry is not developmentally appropriate. This will usually confirm a mild to moderate hearing loss. If a moderate to severe hearing loss is detected, then the possibility of a sensorineural loss with a superimposed conductive loss should be considered.

MANAGEMENT

In most patients with OME the effusion will resolve spontaneously, and this is most likely within the first three months. Therefore, the first line of management is a period of observation or 'watchful waiting'. There is no evidence that the various medical treatments that have been proposed enhance the natural resolution. Specifically, no benefit has been demonstrated for antibiotics, decongestants, and steroids alone or in combination; nor has the use of auto-inflation techniques been shown to confer any long-term benefit. In unilateral cases, with the context of less marked hearing symptoms afforded by the normal contralateral ear, a much longer period of observation may be appropriate. However, if the OME is persistent for longer than 3 months, then surgical management may be justified and involves myringotomy, suction clearance and insertion of a ventilating tube. There are various configurations of ventilating tube, and they can be classified as short, medium or long stay (T-tubes). Initial management is usually with either a short or medium stay tube, depending on surgical preference. T-tube use is confined to cases where repeated short or medium stay tubes fail to produce sustained resolution. Adjuvant adenoidectomy may be performed with ventilator insertion, and the Medical Research Council (MRC) Trial of Alternative Regimens in Glue Ear Treatment (TARGET) trial has confirmed that this confers benefit both in terms of prolongation of the hearing benefit of ventilator insertion and also reduction in the reinsertion rate. This must be weighed against the (admittedly low) complication rate associated with adenoidectomy. Adenoidectomy in these circumstances has a larger effect if the patient has a history of frequent upper respiratory tract infections.

CHRONIC SUPPURATIVE OTITIS MEDIA (CSOM)

CSOM NON-CHOLESTEATOMATOUS

The main subtypes of CSOM without cholesteatoma are tympanic membrane perforation and pars tensa retraction. Various time-related definitions have been applied to CSOM; however, generally a perforation present for more than 3 months is deemed chronic. This type of CSOM can be further classified into active or inactive based on the incidence of otorrhoea. The inactive group includes a persistent dry perforation (failure to heal after otitis media), and retraction pockets. Active CSOM (non-cholesteatomatous) is associated with intermittent or constant otorrhoea.

CSOM is more common in populations with poor socio-economic conditions and limited primary healthcare access. The principal symptom of inactive CSOM is hearing loss. Depending on the size and site of the perforation, the associated conductive hearing loss can vary between a minimal loss and 60 dB. The hearing loss is also influenced by the state of the ossicular chain. If the acute infective episode has caused erosion of the long process of incus, then there may be a significant conductive loss in the presence of a dry perforation. It is also possible that the tympanic membrane is retracted in addition to the presence of perforation, and this may be associated with additional conductive loss. Active CSOM presents with otorrhoea, either intermittent or constant (Figure 44.2). Common bacterial organisms are *Staphylococcus aureus* or *Pseudomonas aeruginosa*. Pain is not a significant feature of CSOM, as the discharge can drain freely from the middle ear cleft. Vertigo and tinnitus are also uncommon symptoms.

Diagnosis is confirmed on otoscopy with microscopy and suction clearance if required. Investigation includes audiometry, and the degree of conductive loss is influenced, as in the inactive category, by the size and position of the perforation and the status of the ossicular chain.

The value of imaging is debated. Plain x-ray will only indicate the degree of pneumatization and is now rarely performed. High-resolution computed comography (CT) scan provides anatomic detail

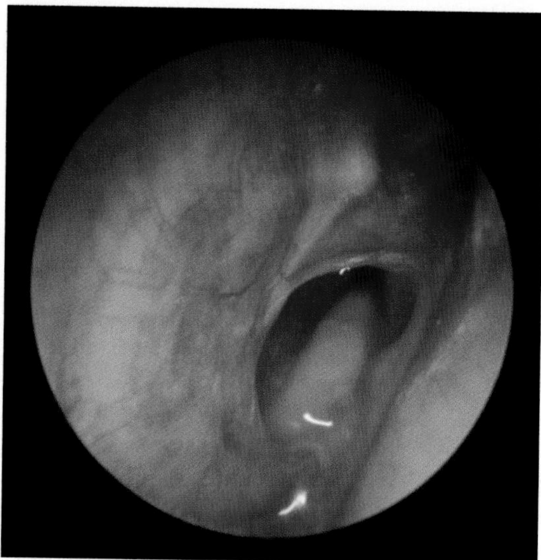

Figure 44.2 Typical appearance of active CSOM.

including the status of the mastoid air cell system and may provide information on the state of the ossicular chain, though this can often be clinically deduced from the audiogram. Imaging of the mastoid air cell system may be helpful in deciding whether or not surgical management should include mastoidectomy.

Differential diagnosis

The main differential is chronic suppurative otitis media with cholesteatoma. The presence of a relatively scanty discharge and unpleasant odour indicates chronic osteitis often associated with a pseudomonas infection and is characteristic of cholesteatoma. Other uncommon causes of chronic middle ear discharge include granulomatosis with polyangiitis (Wegener's granulomatosis), tuberculosis or malignancy, though these are rare.

Management

This initially involves conservative treatment with aural microsuction, topical antibiotics and steroids and advice to the patient to avoid external contamination of the ear when showering or bathing. Most otolaryngologists prescribe aminoglycoside antibiotics. While the potential for ototoxicity exists in clinical practice, this is regarded as an extremely rare occurrence and the therapeutic benefits of antibiotics such as gentamicin outweigh the potential risks. Surgical treatment can be considered for both restoration of hearing and provision of a carefree ear, i.e. the ability to swim, bathe without protecting the ear and improved hearing. Operative interventions are tympanoplasty with or without cortical mastoidectomy. Tympanoplasty is performed using grafts including temporalis fascia, perichondrium, or a cartilage/perichondrial composite graft. The role of cortical mastoidectomy is somewhat controversial. Definitive benefit has not been established; however, it can be considered if the otorrhoea is persistent and cannot ever be resolved despite maximal medical therapy and avoidance of external contamination. The purpose of the mastoidectomy is to clear mucosal disease from the mastoid air cell system and ensure adequate ventilation of the middle ear mastoid.

Retraction pockets

The retraction of the pars tensa is related to chronic negative pressure in the middle ear cleft and thus to eustachian tube dysfunction. There is loss of the middle fibrous layer of the tympanic membrane, and it moves medially, initially impinging on the long process of the incus and subsequently if the retraction progresses onto the promontory. While retraction pockets can be associated with hearing loss, early in the process the hearing may be relatively normal. Despite the otoscopy findings, even if the long process of incus is eroded, thus forming a natural myringostapedopexy (Figure 44.3), the hearing may still be in the 30 dB range. The grading system for retraction of the pars tensa proposed by Sade remains the mainstay of clinical assessment (Table 44.3) and ranges from slight retraction to adhesive otitis media. Treatment (or not) for retraction pockets is much debated as many are entirely stable and virtually asymptomatic; they may be an incidental finding on otoscopy performed during a consultation for an unrelated symptom. However, some undoubtedly progress to an eventual middle ear cholesteatoma (Figure 44.4). Therefore, the dilemma is in identifying those who will progress. This can be achieved only after a period of clinical observation. Serial audiometry and monitoring

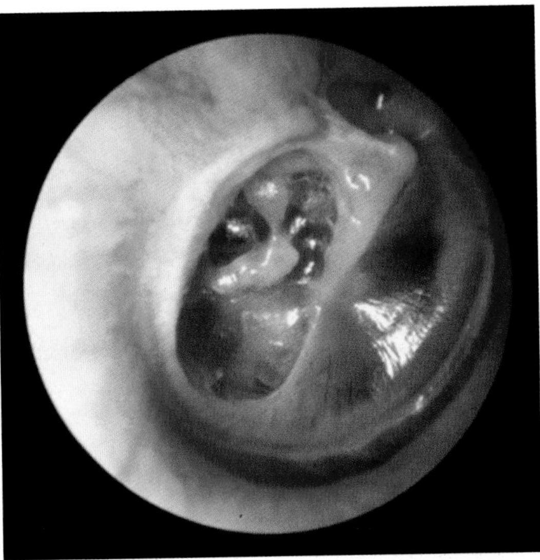

Figure 44.3 Early grade II retraction.

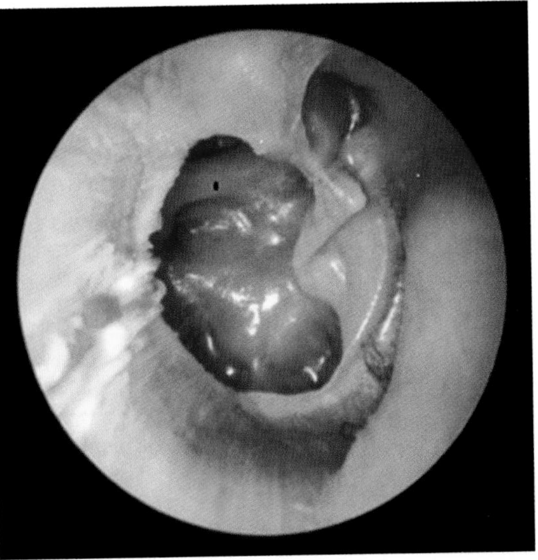

Figure 44.4 Severe grade IV retraction evidence of cholesteatoma development.

of the staging grade system and photo-documentation are valuable objective tools to augment the somewhat subjective the assessment of grade.

The spectrum of management options range from observation to reinforcement cartilage tympanoplasty. Intermediate procedures include placement of a ventilating tube, excision of the affected segment, excision and repair with fascia or perichondrium. A role for cortical mastoidectomy aimed at improving middle ear ventilation has also been proposed.

Two additional conditions associated with CSOM – cholesterol granuloma and tympanosclerosis – merit a brief discussion.

Cholesterol granulomas are cystic swellings formed with a multi-nucleated giant cell reaction to red blood cells' breakdown products, haemosiderin and cholesterol crystals. These typically affect young to middle-aged patients, often with a history of chronic otitis media. Any aerated portion of the temporal bone may develop a cholesterol granuloma; the mastoid air cells are the most common location and are the most common cystic lesion of the petrous apex.

Table 44.3 Sade classification of tympanic membrane retraction

Grade I – Mild retraction of ear drum
Grade II – Retraction touching the incus or stapes
Grade III – Tympanic membrane retraction reaching the promontory
Grade IV – Tympanic membrane adherent to the promontory

The pathogenesis is unclear but related to bleeding with the sequestrated blood undergoing degeneration and a chronic inflammatory response. On CT there is a well-defined lesion with thinned overlying bone. The appearance varies with location and in the petrous apex is more likely to be associated with bony erosion. On MR T1 there is a high signal due to the cholesterol component and a low signal rim due to haemosiderin. On T2 there is a high central signal and a peripheral low signal. If symptomatic, surgical excision is necessary and should include the cyst wall. The surgical approach depends on the location and the degree of hearing loss.

Tympanosclerosis is a very common, usually incidental, finding on otoscopy appearing as a white diffuse or thick plaque, often crescent-shaped, in the fibrous layer of the tympanic membrane. It is thought to be a complication of otitis media, where there is hyalin degeneration followed by calcification within the tympanic membrane. In most patients, the plaques are clinically insignificant with little or no hearing impairment.

It is thought to arise from recurrent bouts of otitis media or trauma and is more common in ears in which ventilator tubes have been inserted. Ossicular fixation can occur, most often affecting the heads of the malleus and incus.

Frequently, no treatment is required. In cases associated with perforation, removal may significantly enlarge the size of the perforation, thus affecting the closure rate. Ossicular tympanosclerosis can be removed, though it often recurs.

CSOM CHOLESTEATOMA

This can be classified as congenital or primary and acquired.

Congenital cholesteatoma is discussed for completeness. It is thought to be developmental in origin and a result of metaplasia or trapping of squamous epithelium in the middle ear cleft.

Acquired cholesteatoma pathogenesis is uncertain. It commonly occurs in the attic/pars flaccida (Figure 44.5), thus the previously used term *attico-antral* disease. However, it can also develop in central or marginal pars tensa perforations or in retraction pockets. There is an association with retraction of the pars tensa due to a combination of chronic inflammation and poor eustachian tube function. In adults there is an association with poor pneumatization (sclerosis of the mastoid). A retraction pocket forms and migration of the squamous epithelium layer is compromised, which leads to accumulation of a squamous epithelium in the pocket. Once this accumulation occurs, there is development of inflammation at the apex of the retraction pocket, which causes biochemical changes with osteolysis and erosion of the bony attic wall. Deepening of the retraction pocket with a further increase in squamous epithelium accumulation and the process of the incus then becomes self perpetuating, and the progressive enlargement results in bone erosion postero-superiorly, eroding the outer attic wall. Often the ossicular chain is compromised with the long process of the incus most frequently affected. Intermittent infections occur from pseudomonas, streptococcus, or *Staphylococcus aureus*. Iatrogenic cholesteatomas can occur after ventilator insertion or a tympanoplasty and also occur as a result of impaction from blast injury or other trauma.

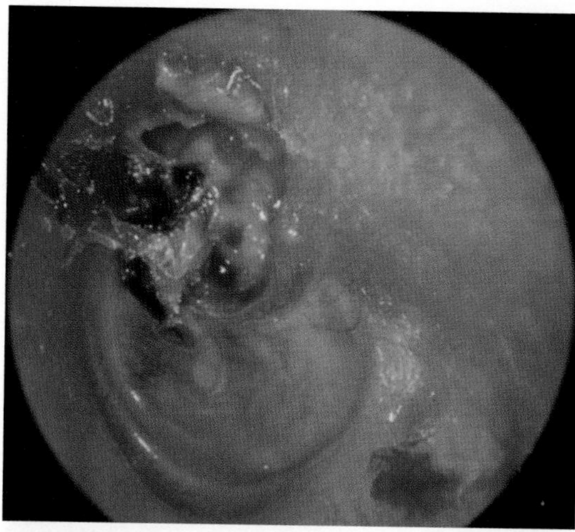

Figure 44.5 Attic cholesteatoma.

Symptoms

Symptoms include hearing loss and intermittent otorrhoea. The otorrhoea can be relatively scanty but associated with a strong odour that is unpleasant and embarrassing for the patient and is associated with pseudomonas infection. Vertigo and tinnitus can occur but are not common. Facial nerve palsy is rare but can occur in advanced disease, where there is also a higher risk of both vertigo and sensorineural loss.

Diagnosis is by otoscopy aided by microsuction. Squamous epithelium in the attic perforation is noted. Sometimes there is a crust in the attic, squamous epithelium medially or a polyp at the entrance to the back of the retraction pocket. In congenital cases there will be a white mass behind the intact tympanic membrane.

Investigation

Investigation includes a full audiometric evaluation to assess cochlear function and presence and degree of any conductive loss. The extent of conductive loss may predict the status of the ossicular chain, though the cholesteatoma sac may disguise the extent of the conductive loss by providing apparent continuity of an already deficient ossicular chain.

Imaging can be performed with magnetic resonance imaging (MRI) or CT scan. High-resolution

CT with multi-planar reconstruction enables excellent review of the bony anatomy, and while not diagnostic for the presence of cholesteatoma, it will provide some information on the likely extent of the disease and the degree of pneumatization. The cholesteatoma cannot be unequivocally distinguished from mucosal disease on CT images. It will also inform on the integrity of the labyrinth; in particular, it will demonstrate if the lateral semicircular canal has a fistula (the most common bony labyrinthine defect encountered). Diffusion weighted (DW) non-contrast MRI can be helpful. Especially for patients with previous surgery for cholesteatoma, an MRI should be performed since recurrence or residual tumour can be detected with great accuracy. Some authors suggest it can reduce the need for 'second look' surgery.

Standard T2 weighted images in the coronal and axial plane are compared with DW images, and on the latter the cholesteatoma is noted as a hyperintense area.

Management

Initial assessment will have involved otomicroscopy and suction clearance. This can be employed as a conservative management strategy with decompression of the cholesteatoma sac, by way of regular aural microsuction and treatment as required with topical antibiotic and steroid drops to resolve any infection. Aminoglycoside antibiotics, such as gentamicin, and steroid drops are often prescribed. In an elderly patient unfit for surgery, it may sometimes be appropriate to control the disease with regular aural toilet, but in most cases surgical treatment will be indicated (Table 44.4).

Table 44.4 Surgical options for CSOM cholesteatoma

Combined approach tympanoplasty (CAT)
Preserves normal ear canal anatomy, staging required, optimum technique for children
Modified radical mastoidectomy
Single-stage procedure, associated with increased post-operative care, variable cavity size
Atticoantrostomy
Single-stage procedure, cavity size dependent on disease extent, less cavity care required

Surgical treatment

The aims of surgery are to provide a safe, dry ear and maximize the residual hearing. The overlapping terminology for the range of surgical interventions is somewhat confusing. The following classification is relatively straightforward and easily understood. The surgical approach can either preserve the posterior canal wall, i.e. canal wall up (CWU) mastoidectomy (also referred to as intact canal wall tympanoplasty [ICWT]) or involve the drilling away of the canal wall, thus creating a single cavity connecting the ear canal and the mastoid air cell system, a canal wall down (CWD) mastoidectomy. These are also sometimes referred to as 'closed' and 'open' techniques, respectively. Perhaps confusingly, the CWU/ICWT surgical technique is most frequently called a combined approach tympanoplasty (CAT); the surgery involves disease removal both via a per-meatal approach to the middle ear and via an extended cortical mastoidectomy in which the surgeon also opens into the facial recess (posterior tympanotomy) between the facial nerve and the bony annulus. The CWU and CWD procedures involve creating some form of cavity and thus in effect exteriorize the disease. A cortical mastoidectomy is performed and then the posterior canal wall is removed. If (as is usual) a tympanic membrane repair is performed, the procedure is termed a *modified radical mastoidectomy* (MRM). If no reconstruction is performed, it is termed a *radical mastoidectomy*. Removal of the canal wall provides direct visualization of the facial recess and enhanced access to the other key areas of the sinus tympani and stapes, which are often poorly accessed with the CAT procedure.

The surgical steps in the canal wall procedure, following inspection of the ear, are as follows. A tympanomeatal flap is raised to access the middle ear and a postaural incision made to exposure the mastoid. A cortical mastoidectomy is performed and extended into the epitympanum, exposing the head of the malleus. A posterior tympanotomy provides surgical access to the stapes, pyramid region and facial recess. The disease is removed; a laser may be helpful in removing cholesteatoma from the stapes super-structure without excessive mobilization. If the incus is eroded, this may be removed and repositioned on malleus or drum to stapes assembly; alternatively, a prosthetic device can be used for ossicular reconstruction. The head of the malleus and body of the incus may need to be removed to allow access for disease removal. A higher rate of residual and recurrent cholesteatoma in CWU procedures provides the need for a staged or second procedure, usually at an interval of 4–6 months This increased need for a second (or subsequent) procedure is one of the major drawbacks of this technique. Attempts have been made to perform the second procedure endoscopically, but this may not be ideal if there is residual disease that requires removal. As mentioned earlier, DW MRI is not yet sufficiently reliable to replace second-look procedures.

The steps for a CWD (open cavity) procedure are as follows. Inspection and cleaning of ear canal, elevation of the tympanomeatal flap, post aural incision and cortical mastoidectomy are performed. Removal of the posterior canal wall proceeds, and then following disease removal, the cavity is contoured to minimize a facial ridge, and grafting of the tympanic membrane completes a modified radical mastoidectomy. Obliteration in these cases is optional and has been proposed with a variety of materials, including muscle flaps, bone pate, cartilage and biocompatible materials such as hydroxyapatite. If obliteration is required, the author's preference is for a combination of cartilage and bone pate.

There is an additional approach that provides the access of the CWD techniques yet minimizes the disadvantages of both CWU and CWD. This approach, originally described by Tumarkin, is termed an *atticotomy* or *atticoantrostomy* (AA) and at the prompting of Smyth (an original proponent of the CAT) has been revisited in the last couple of decades and become the default procedure in many centres. Its main advantage is that while providing the disease control of conventional CWD surgery, it tends to produce a 'small cavity'. The fact that AA results in a cavity indicates it is best to consider this operation as a variation of the CWD technique (rather than a separate entity) where the bone removal proceeds from anterior to posterior, i.e. following the disease (Figures 44.6a and 44.6b). The advantages are that with small cholesteatoma, it can result in a small, often almost normal, ear canal volume (one of the benefits of the CAT), yet the exposure is unrestricted because the removal of the outer attic wall enables direct visualization to the key areas. Drilling is kept to a minimum without the need to drill away an uninvolved often sclerotic mastoid bone. In cases of a larger cholesteatoma, the bone removal is still less than with a traditional CWD technique, and a combination of temporalis facia and perichondrial/cartilage grafts can be used to contour the cavity and can be augmented by obliteration with bone pate and or muscle flaps if required.

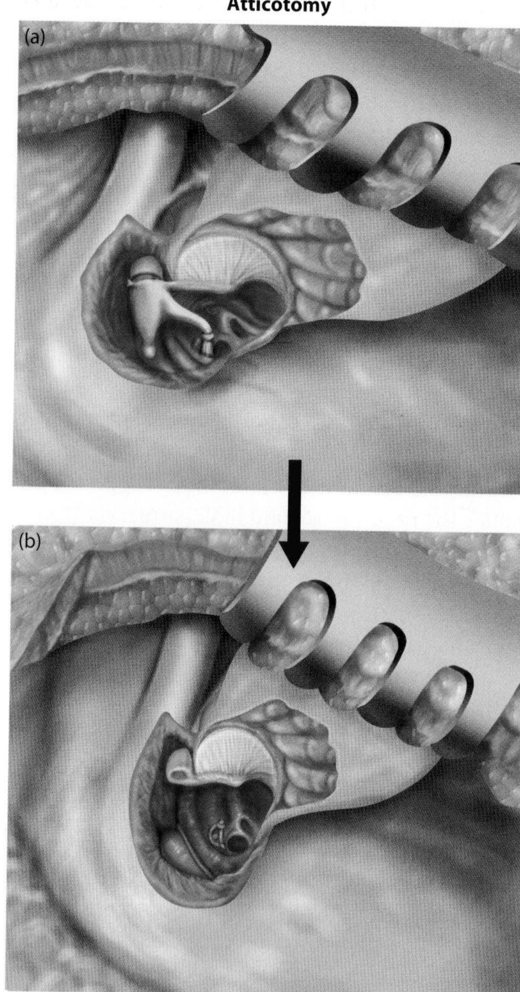

Figure 44.6 **(a)** Early stages of atticotomy – attic and intact chain exposed. **(b)** Atticotomy proceeds into antrum; incus has been removed.

The optimal technique has been much debated and is influenced by surgical experience and the clinical circumstances. For children, CWU (or CAT) would be preferred by most surgeons since the mastoid in paediatric cases tends to be pneumatized, making the end point of a small cavity more difficult. Therefore, as mastoid cavity care in children is more problematic, most surgeons accept the higher rates of recurrent and residual disease and do a staged procedure where the child will be left with a normal ear canal and acceptable hearing. Early studies with CAT suggested that better hearing outcomes were achievable. However, long-term results indicate this advantage (over other techniques) is not maintained.

In adults, the operative choice is more varied and again depends most on surgical experience and training. Some surgeons still advocate a CWU approach, others a more traditional modified radical mastoidectomy. However, increasingly the atticoantrostomy technique, which significantly reduces the post-operative morbidity associated with cavity problems, is favoured.

KEY LEARNING POINTS

- Pain is not a feature of chronic otitis media.
- Non-cholesteatomatous CSOM may be active or inactive. Retraction pockets should be observed with serial photographic documentation, staging and hearing assessment.
- Cholesteatoma needs to be treated with respect.
- Cholesterol granulomas are cystic swellings formed by multinuclear giant cell reaction to red blood cell products, haemosiderin and cholesterol crystals.
- MRI diffusion-weight imaging is useful for diagnosis of recurrent cholesteatomas.

FURTHER READING

Morris P. Chronic suppurative otitis media. *BMJ Clinical Evidence.* 2012; Aug 6: pii: 0507. http://clinicalevidence.bmj.com/x/pdf/clinical-evidence/en-gb/systematic-review/0507.pdf.

MRC Multi-Centre Otitis Media Study Group. Surgery for persistent otitis media with effusion: Generalizability of results from the UK trial (TARGET). Trial of Alternative Regimens in Glue Ear Treatment. *Clinical Otolaryngology.* 2001; 26: 417–24.

Tos M. Sequelae of secretory otitis media and the relationship to chronic suppurative otitis media. *Annals of Otololgy, Rhinology and Laryngology.* 1990; 99:18–19.

Verhoeff M, van der Veen EL, Rovers MM, Sanders EA, Schilder AG. Chronic suppurative otitis media: A review. *International Journal of Pediatric Otorhinolaryngology.* 2006 Jan; 70(1): 1–12. Epub 2005 Sep 27.

World Health Organization. Chronic suppurative otitis media. Burden of illness and management options. 2004. Available from: http://www.who.int/entity/pbd/deafness/activities/hearing_care/otitis_media.pdf.

45

Complications of otitis media

DUNCAN BOWYER

Complications of otitis media occur when infection and/or inflammation spread outside of the confines of the middle ear cleft or involve intratemporal structures such as the labyrinth or facial nerve. They are typically subclassified as either extracranial or intracranial (Table 45.1). Both acute otitis media (AOM) and chronic otitis media (COM) may lead to complications; in the pre-antibiotic era approximately half of cases were associated with AOM; today in the developed world the majority arise on a background of COM.

EPIDEMIOLOGY

Complications may occur in all age groups, but large series of cases have shown clustering between the ages of 5 and 20 years. An analysis of 268 patients presenting with otitis media complications from a rural region of South Africa[1] found 55 per cent of cases were in this demographic age group, with a further 16 per cent in children younger than 5 years. Similar findings have also been described in reports from Turkey[2] and Thailand.[3] In each, the male to female ratio was approximately 2:1. There is an increased risk in those exposed to poverty or with limited access to health care and, as a consequence, large case series often originate from the developing world. Although anticipated, there has not been a spike in case numbers in regions of the world most affected by the human immunodeficiency virus (HIV) pandemic or in other immunocompromised groups.

PATHOPHYSIOLOGY

Spread of infection with otitis media may occur by three mechanisms: bony erosion, thrombophlebitis or direct spread (Figure 45.1). Bony erosion results from an osteitic process that is poorly understood and often develops under an area of granulation that forms as part of the host inflammatory response. The intracranial venous system communicates widely with the extracranial

Table 45.1 Complications of otitis media

Extracranial	Intracranial
Acute mastoiditis	Meningitis
Subperiosteal abscess	Brain abscess
Facial nerve paralysis	Subdural empyema/ extradural abscess
Suppurative labyrinthitis	Sigmoid sinus thrombosis
Acute petrositis	Otitic hydrocephalus

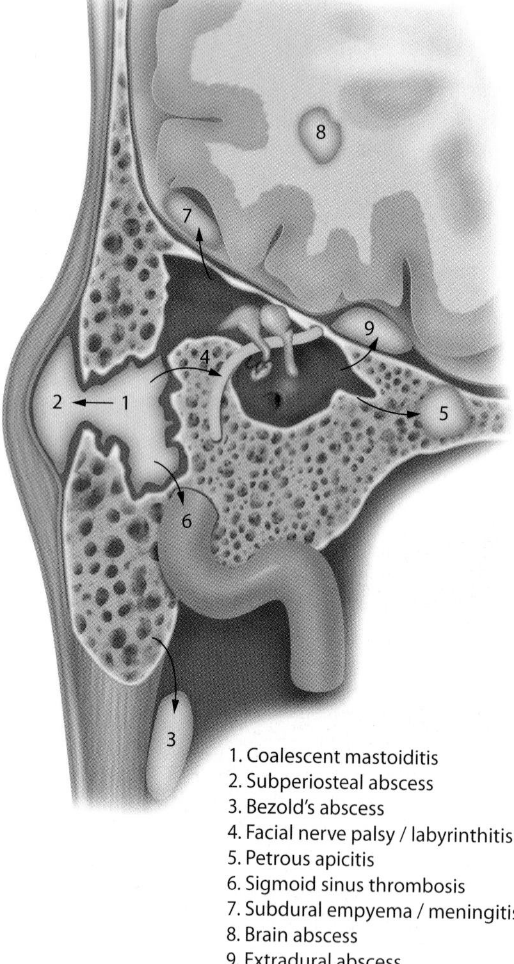

Figure 45.1 Complications of otitis media.

vasculature via the mastoid emissary veins that drain to the sigmoid sinus. Thrombophlebitis of these vessels within the temporal bone is a source of spread of infection both intracranially and extratemporally. Direct spread of infection occurs through preformed pathways, such as those resulting from previous tympanomastoid surgery and temporal bone fractures, or via anatomical points of weakness (such as the oval and round windows, a dehiscent facial canal or jugular bulb, and developmental abnormalities of the labyrinth).

The risk of developing complications from otitis media varies with the underlying ear disease. In a series of 87 patients presenting with otogenic intracranial pathology,[3] AOM was the underlying aetiology in only 5. Of the 82 patients with COM, 80 per cent had squamous epithelial disease (cholesteatoma) and 20 per cent mucosal disease. Singh and Maharaj[1] found extracranial and intracranial complications from both cholesteatomatous (53 per cent) and non-cholesteatomatous (47 per cent) ears. Intracranial complications were more common with squamous epithelial disease than with mucosal disease (59 per cent versus 41 per cent), whereas the reverse was found with extracranial complications (41 per cent versus 59 per cent).

EXTRACRANIAL COMPLICATIONS

ACUTE MASTOIDITIS/ SUBPERIOSTEAL ABSCESS

Acute mastoiditis is an acute inflammatory condition affecting the mastoid air cell system. It is closely related to AOM and represents the most common extracranial complication of otitis media. In Singh and Maharaj's series,[1] 65 of 87 patients (75 per cent) presenting with extracranial complications had acute mastoiditis. The condition is more common in males, probably reflecting the increased incidence of AOM in young boys, and has a peak incidence of 1–3 years of age.

The frequency of acute mastoiditis sharply declined following the widespread introduction of antibiotic use for AOM in the late 1940s; it now has an estimated incidence of 0.04–0.07 per cent of AOM cases.[4] This has inevitably led to a reduction in the experience of managing this life-threatening condition, and the need for prompt treatment must be emphasized to minimize the risk of the disease rapidly progressing in a previously well child.

A number of reports have suggested that the incidence of acute mastoiditis has started to rise in the past 10–15 years as clinical guidelines have restricted the routine use of antibiotics in the management of childhood upper respiratory infections (including AOM). To date, the evidence of this perceived increase in cases is conflicting,[5–8] and indeed if there are more complications, it is not known whether this is due to changing prescribing practices or variations in microbial virulence and antibiotic resistance.

In view of the close association of acute mastoiditis with AOM, the causative organisms are broadly similar. In a multicentre retrospective review of 223 cases of acute mastoiditis, Luntz et al.[9] obtained positive cultures in 92 patients. Of these, *Streptococcus pneumoniae* (15), *Streptococcus pyogenes* (14), *Staphylococcus aureus* (13), *Pseudomonas aeruginosa* (8) and a mixed flora (10) were most commonly isolated. *Haemophilus influenzae* and *Moraxella catarrhalis* were infrequently identified in this and other series,[10–12] despite their high detection rates in AOM aspirates. It has been suggested that this is due to their low affinity for bone penetration.[13]

The anatomical continuity between the middle ear and mastoid air cell system results in an episode of AOM routinely leading to mucosal inflammatory changes within the mastoid. Mastoid opacification is therefore commonly found if a patient with AOM undergoes imaging of the temporal bone. This may be incorrectly reported as mastoiditis. In a severe infection that is resistant to any early antimicrobial therapy, mucosal oedema may be sufficient to block the aditus ad antrum, trapping purulent secretions within the mastoid. Untreated, this may lead to increasing pressure and acute mastoiditis. Early clinical features consist of otalgia, postauricular pain and pyrexia with otoscopic evidence of AOM. As the condition progresses the bony trabeculae of the mastoid are destroyed by a demineralizing osteitis, creating a coalescent mastoiditis. Spread of the infection to the overlying periosteum either directly or by retrograde thrombophlebitis of the emissary veins results in the classical findings of postauricular cellulitis. Loss of the postauricular sulcus is observed, and the pinna may be displaced anteroinferiorly.

The use of plain film radiology in the investigation of acute mastoiditis has been superseded by computed tomography (CT). This imaging modality is able to demonstrate demineralization or destruction of mastoid bony septa (Figure 45.2), and the presence of a subperiosteal abscess or intracranial spread of infection.

In early, non-coalescent, mastoiditis, a conservative management approach is adopted, with the use

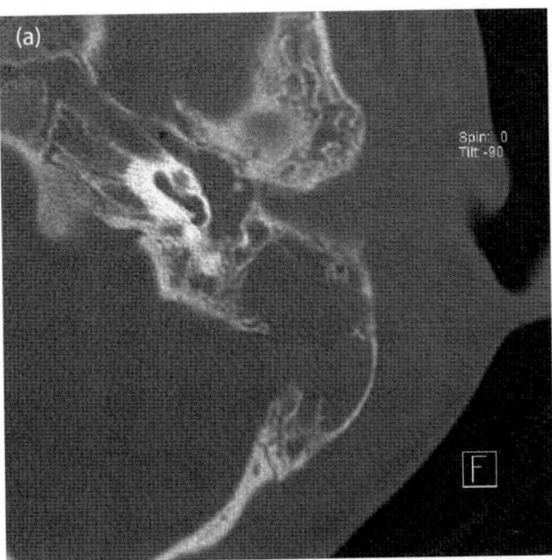

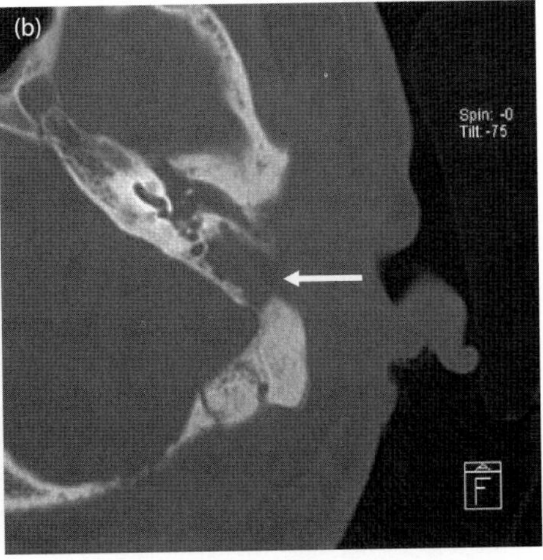

Figure 45.2 Axial CT of the temporal bone demonstrating **(a)** coalescent mastoiditis with erosion of the sigmoid sinus plate and **(b)** cortical erosion (arrow) with subperiosteal abscess formation.

of culture-directed intravenous antimicrobials, usually in conjunction with myringotomy and ventilation tube insertion. Depending on the state of the eardrum, the average duration of intravenous antimicrobial therapy is 7–10 days. Using this approach, 75–85 per cent of cases avoid cortical mastoidectomy, which remains the definitive treatment.[11,14,15]

Further clinical progression varies according to the direction of spread (Table 45.2). Lateral extension of infection results in the formation of a subperiosteal abscess. This is identified by a postauricular fluctuant swelling in a patient with acute mastoiditis (Figure 45.3) and should be managed by urgent cortical mastoidectomy, wide myringotomy and intravenous antibiotics. A Bezold's abscess occurs when there is erosion of the mastoid tip medial to the insertion of the sternocleidomastoid muscle. Purulent material extends through the digastric groove into the deep neck spaces, including the parapharyngeal space. Presentation is of a fluctuant neck mass in conjunction with mastoid tenderness; this requires surgical drainage of the neck abscess combined with a cortical mastoidectomy.

Progression of acute mastoiditis anteriorly through the zygomatic air cell tract can rarely lead to a breach in the bony cortex beneath the temporalis muscle. The resulting zygomatic abscess presents with cellulitis of the preauricular tissues. Drainage is performed through a postauricular incision with careful exenteration of the zygomatic air cells as part of a cortical mastoidectomy.

Table 45.2 Frequency of complications following acute mastoiditis

	Benito and Gorricho[5] (n = 215)	Linder et al.[10] (n = 50)	Goldstein et al.[14] (n = 72)
Subperiosteal abscess	15 (7%)	33 (66%)	10 (14%)
Bezold's abscess	0	5 (10%)	0
Zygomatic abscess	0	3 (6%)	0
Facial paralysis	1 (0.5%)	2 (4%)	3 (4%)
Labyrinthitis	0	0	0
Acute petrositis	1 (0.5%)	2 (4%)	0
Meningitis	3 (1.4%)	1 (2%)	—
Intracranial abscess	3 (1.4%)	0	—
Sinus thrombosis	2 (1%)	5 (10%)	—

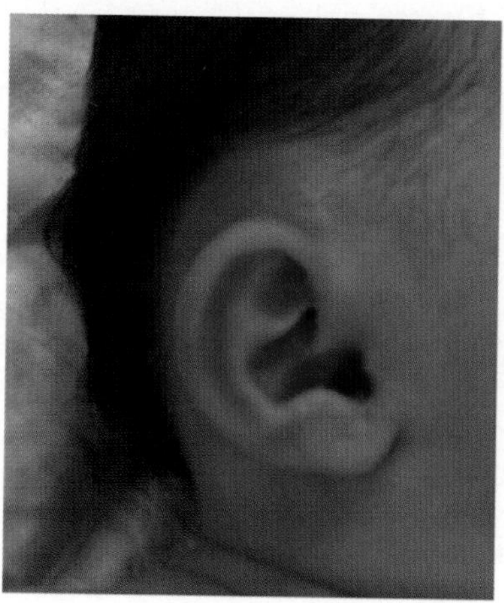
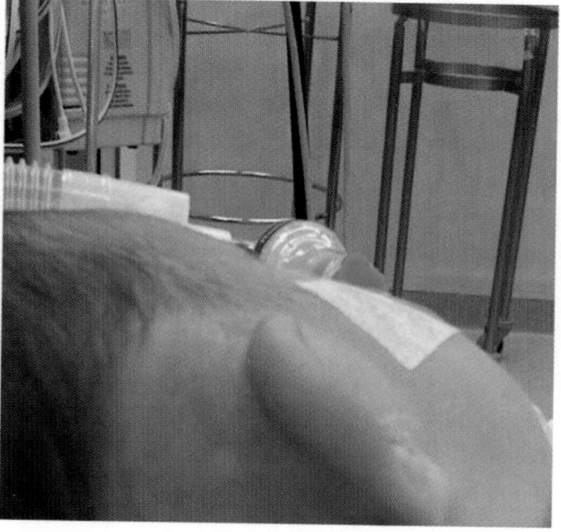

Figure 45.3 Acute mastoiditis with subperiosteal abscess. Courtesy of Dr Michel Neeff.

Anterior progression of infection within the middle ear cavity may also lead to involvement of the fallopian canal, either through bony erosion or direct spread through areas of congenital dehiscence, resulting in facial paralysis. Erosion of the bony labyrinth is also possible, presenting as acute vertigo and/or sensorineural hearing loss, although the density of the bony otic capsule offers protection to acute infection, making this complication uncommon. If the petrous apex is pneumatized, the abscess may also spread medially to form an acute petrositis.

Intracranial spread of infection in acute mastoiditis continues to be reported despite widespread use of broad-spectrum antibiotics, and the resulting rapid clinical deterioration is potentially fatal (Table 45.2). Involvement of the cerebrospinal fluid (CSF) space results in meningitis, whereas direct spread or thrombophlebitis leads to an intracranial abscess or venous sinus thrombosis.

FACIAL NERVE PARALYSIS

Facial paralysis is a rare complication of otitis media and accounts for 6–8 per cent of lower motor neuron facial palsies.[16] If presenting in the setting of AOM, this is thought to be associated with a congenital dehiscence of the fallopian canal. These are present in up to 55 per cent of temporal bones, most commonly in the tympanic segment adjacent to the oval window.[17] Bacterial toxins in an acute middle ear infection result in inflammation and oedema of the exposed nerve. In a series of 22 children with facial palsy after AOM, the presenting facial weakness was incomplete in 77 per cent and occurred on average 6 days after the onset of ear symptoms.[14] Management involves admission for intravenous antibiotics and myringotomy, with or without ventilation tube insertion. This conservative approach leads to the complete recovery of nerve function in the overwhelming majority of children, taking an average of 133 days in the above series. Children with a total palsy at presentation have a poorer prognosis, and some advocate mastoidectomy without nerve decompression in such cases if an initial conservative management fails to lead to recovery of function.

The majority of cases of facial paralysis with COM relate to squamous epithelial disease eroding the fallopian canal, with local osteitis and infection leading to neural oedema and secondary ischaemic neuropraxia.[18] Whilst the paralysis typically evolves gradually, it may also present acutely. Treatment consists of prompt mastoidectomy, cautious removal of cholesteatoma and granulations from the nerve sheath and decompression of the nerve until the proximal and distal segments appear healthy. Prognosis of the facial paralysis in this setting is poorer than when associated with AOM.

LABYRINTHITIS

Developing in the setting of either AOM or COM, labyrinthitis may be classified into serous and suppurative types.[19] Serous labyrinthitis occurs with the penetration of bacterial exotoxins into the perilymph compartment of the inner ear, leading to a partial loss of inner ear function. Suppurative labyrinthitis is a potentially life-threatening condition in which there is direct bacterial invasion and, because of the continuity of the perilymph space with the subarachnoid space through the patent cochlear aqueduct, a risk of developing meningitis. Irreversible profound hearing and vestibular loss is inevitable. The two forms may be clinically indistinguishable in the acute setting, with the diagnosis made only by the response to treatment and audiological improvement.

Bacterial invasion of the labyrinth may occur through three potential routes: (1) dehiscence of the oval or round window, (2) labyrinthine fistula, typically of the lateral semicircular canal, and (3) during meningitis through an abnormality in the fundus of the internal auditory canal or patent cochlear aqueduct.

Patients with labyrinthitis present with sudden profound hearing loss, tinnitus and severe vertigo. Initial vestibular irritation causes spontaneous nystagmus towards the affected side. As the neuroepithelium becomes irreversibly damaged by the bacterial toxins, the nystagmus shifts to the opposite ear. The initial severe vertigo lasts for 8–12 hours and gradually improves over several weeks with central compensation.

Initial management of labyrinthitis is medical and aimed at avoiding the development of meningitis. Patients are admitted for intravenous antibiotics, vestibular sedatives and possibly corticosteroids. Once the general condition has improved, definitive tympanomastoid surgery is performed to remove the source of infection.[20,21]

ACUTE PETROSITIS

Petrositis is a rare consequence of AOM in which inflammation and suppuration extend into a pneumatized petrous apex. The normally marrow-filled cells of the petrous apex prevent the spread of infection, but approximately 30 per cent of apices are pneumatized and offer no such barrier. The classic clinical syndrome associated with acute petrositis, described by Gradenigo in 1904,[22] is a triad of otorrhoea, retro-orbital pain and diplopia. Retro-orbital pain is caused by irritation of the Gasserian ganglion (trigeminal nerve) within Meckel's cave on the anterior surface of the petrous apex. Inflammation of the abducens nerve as it passes through Dorello's canal (a fold in the petroclinoid ligament) can lead to diplopia secondary to lateral rectus muscle palsy. Only a minority of patients present with the full symptom triad; in Goldstein's series of paediatric complications of otitis media,[14] all four patients diagnosed with acute petrositis had otalgia and diplopia, three reported retro-orbital pain, but none had otorrhoea.

The diagnosis of acute petrositis is confirmed by temporal bone CT, demonstrating air cell opacification and, frequently, bony destruction. Magnetic resonance imaging (MRI) is complementary, differentiating marrow from mucus, pus or CSF, and excluding associated intracranial pathology.

Traditional management consists of intravenous antibiotics and surgical drainage of the apical air cells in conjunction with mastoidectomy. The route of surgical access depends on the location of infection, and complete drainage is often not possible, necessitating prolonged post-operative antimicrobial therapy. Recent reports suggest that less aggressive surgery (mastoidectomy without drainage of apical cells) with antibiotics is also effective.[14,23]

INTRACRANIAL COMPLICATIONS

The mortality of intracranial complications of otitis media in the pre-antibiotic era was approximately 80 per cent. The introduction of broad-spectrum antimicrobial agents has significantly reduced their incidence, but they remain a devastating progression of ear disease, with recent published mortality rates of 8–26 per cent (Table 45.3). Patients often present with multiple intracranial complications (12 per cent in Singh & Maharaj's series[1]); mortality is closely related to the consciousness level on presentation rather than the type of underlying ear disease.

MENINGITIS

Otogenic meningitis is the most common intracranial complication of otitis media[2,3] and often coexists with other complications, both intracranial and extracranial. Bacterial spread from the middle ear cleft to the pia-arachnoid layer leads

Table 45.3 Mortality from intracranial complications secondary to otitis media

	Singh and Maharaj[1] (deaths/cases)	Osma et al.[2] (deaths/cases)	Kangsanarak et al.[3] (deaths/cases)
Meningitis	1/22 (5%)	12/41 (29%)	4/43 (9%)
Brain abscess	12/93 (13%)	2/10 (20%)	9/29 (31%)
Subdural/epidural abscess	2/36 (6%)	0/14	3/35 (9%)
Cerebritis/encephalitis	—	1/1 (100%)	0/16
Sinus thrombosis	0/36	0/1	4/16 (25%)
Otitic hydrocephalus	—	—	0/7
Total	15/181 (8%)	15/57 (26%)	20/123 (16%)

Sum of patient numbers exceeds totals as some patients had more than one complication.

to a rapid inflammatory response along the entire cerebrospinal axis. The otogenic origin is often missed, and a high index of suspicion is required in children with headache, fever and a history of otorrhoea or otalgia. Correspondingly, any patient with unexplained meningitis should be assessed for signs of occult otitis media.

The early stages of the illness present as a severe generalized headache and fever, progressing to neck stiffness, photophobia, vomiting and irritability. In young infants nuchal rigidity may be absent, replaced by bulging of the cranial fontanelles. Further decline of the clinical condition results in lethargy, seizures and coma.

Initial patient management involves stabilization and rehydration. CT imaging of the head and temporal bones allows exclusion of coexisting intracranial pathology and obstruction of CSF drainage, which precludes lumbar puncture. MRI is increasingly replacing CT as a diagnostic test because of its high sensitivity in detecting subtle intracranial findings and meningeal enhancement, which is diagnostic for the condition (Figure 45.4). Lumbar puncture is performed to allow CSF sampling for microbiological analysis. Meningitis is suspected if the CSF is cloudy, if there are elevated white blood cells or protein content, or reduced glucose. CSF should be sent for urgent Gram stain and culture.

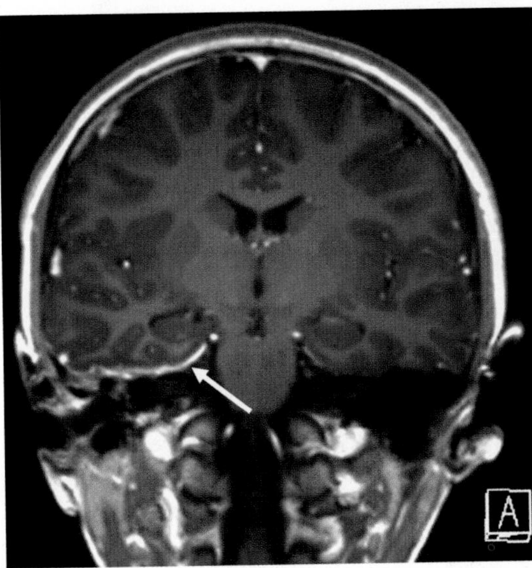

Figure 45.4 Coronal gadolinium enhanced T1-weighted MRI of a 3-year-old child with otogenic meningitis, demonstrating dural enhancement (arrow).

Broad-spectrum antibiotics are commenced promptly and modified as bacterial sensitivities are available. A recent Cochrane review[24] has recommended that corticosteroids be given before or with the first antibiotic dose and continued for 4 days. The authors report a significant reduction in hearing loss and neurological sequelae with steroid use, as well as a trend towards lower mortality. Surgical management of the underlying ear disease is performed once the patient has been stabilized. This may involve myringotomy and ventilation tube insertion (AOM), cortical mastoidectomy (mastoiditis) or tympanomastoidectomy (cholesteatoma).

BRAIN ABSCESS

In a series of 122 consecutive patients diagnosed with brain abscesses,[25] otitis media was the third most common underlying aetiology. Mortality rates from this complication have reduced substantially in the post-antibiotic era, with a current mortality of 13–31 per cent.[1–3] Otogenic brain abscesses are slightly more common in the temporal lobe than in the cerebellum (Figures 45.5 and 45.6), almost always occur on the same side as the otitis and result from squamous epithelial disease more often than AOM.

Brain abscess tends to present insidiously over several weeks that is classically divided into three distinct stages. In the initial inoculation phase there is localized encephalitis and oedema that results in an acute illness lasting several days. This is typically mild and often attributed to a viral infection. The following quiescent phase may last several weeks, during which the inflammatory response attempts to contain and encapsulate the infective focus. Symptoms during this process may be very subtle or absent. Late abscess maturation is associated with necrosis, liquefaction and expansion/rupture. This may be associated with a mass effect that results in focal neurological symptoms related to its anatomical site and more generalized symptoms of headache, vomiting, lethargy and fever.

Initial management of an otogenic brain abscess involves stabilization and broad-spectrum antibiotics. Positive cultures usually reveal polymicrobial

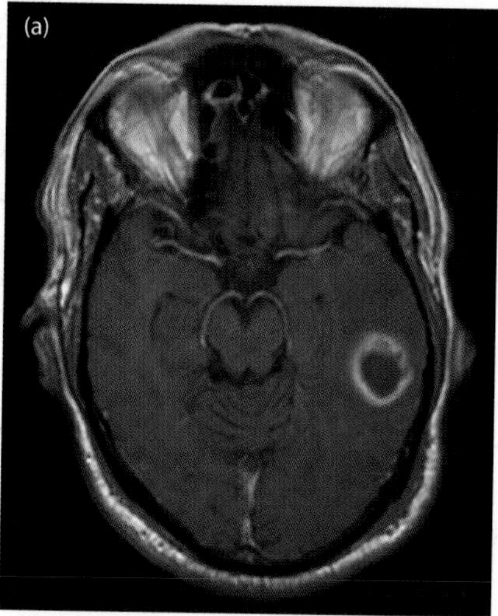

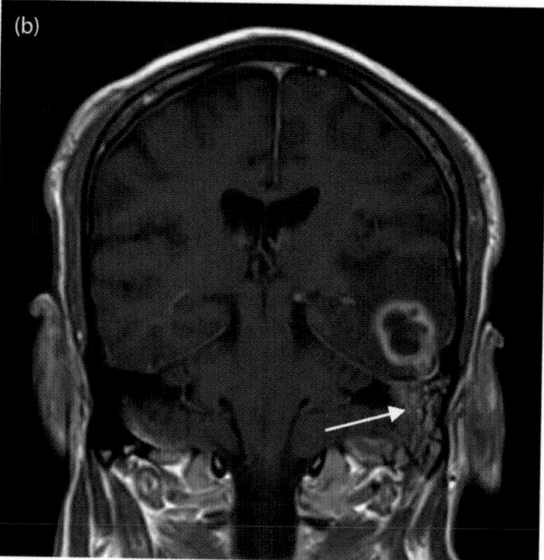

Figure 45.5 Axial **(a)** and coronal **(b)** contrast-enhanced T1 MRI demonstrating an otogenic temporal lobe abscess. Note fluid-containing mastoid air cells (arrow).

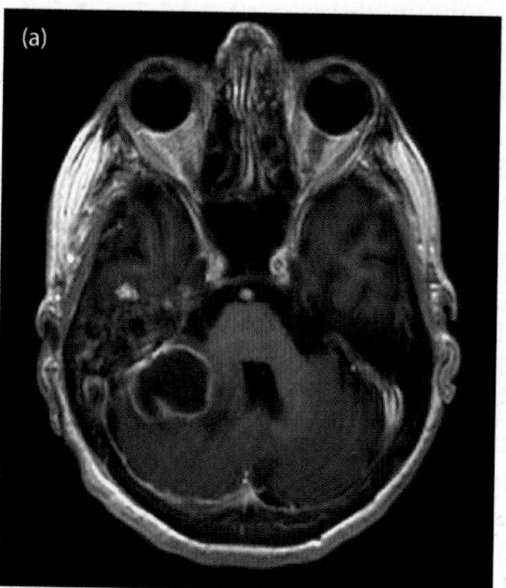

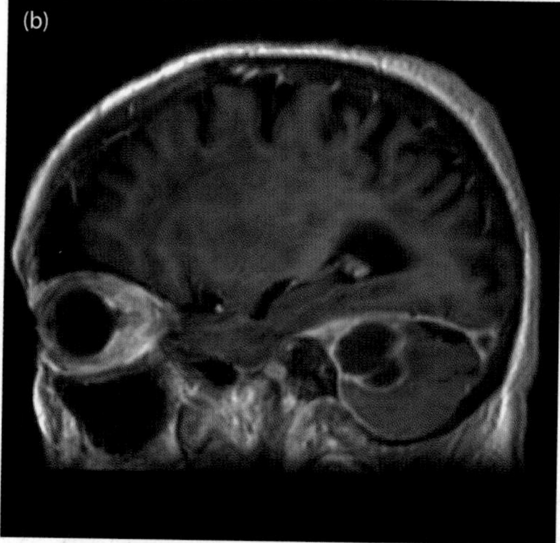

Figure 45.6 Axial **(a)** and sagittal **(b)** contrast-enhanced T1 MRI demonstrating a subdural abscess within the posterior fossa with coexisting sigmoid sinus thrombosis.

infection including anaerobes. Neurosurgical drainage of the abscess is combined with surgical management of the middle ear and mastoid disease if the patient is sufficiently stable.

SUBDURAL EMPYEMA

A subdural empyema is a collection of pus that develops in the preformed space between the dura and pia-arachnoid layers. It is a rare complication of otitis media. Infection may spread readily once it enters the subdural layer, limited only by anatomical barriers such as the tentorium cerebelli, falx cerebri or foramen magnum. The expanding mass presents as a rapidly deteriorating clinical picture, commencing with severe headache, fever, vomiting and malaise, progressing to falling consciousness level and focal neurological signs. Confirmation of the diagnosis is made with CT or MRI, and lumbar puncture is contraindicated owing to the risk of brain herniation. Emergency neurosurgical drainage is performed and culture-directed intravenous antibiotics given. Management of the underlying ear disease is addressed only once the patient has been stabilized.

EXTRADURAL ABSCESS

Extradural (epidural) collections occur when infection spreads directly through defects in the middle or posterior fossa bony plates. Granulation tissue and bony erosion lead to a localized abscess forming between the dura and surrounding temporal bone. These collections are usually asymptomatic and are often discovered coincidently on imaging or during mastoid surgery. Epidural abscesses frequently coexist with other intracranial complications, particularly sigmoid sinus thrombophlebitis. Surgical management involves the removal of granulation tissue and drainage of pus through a mastoidectomy with post-operative intravenous antibiotics.

SIGMOID SINUS THROMBOSIS

Thrombosis of the sigmoid (lateral) sinus occurs either with direct spread of infection or from retrograde thrombophlebitis of the veins that drain the middle ear cleft. Initial intimal inflammation of the vessel wall leads to mural thrombus formation. As this becomes infected, the resulting attraction of fibrin, blood cells and platelets causes enlargement of the thrombus and eventually venous occlusion. The thrombus may then propagate into the internal jugular vein (IJV) or, retrograde, towards the cavernous sinus. Dislodgement of clot at the leading edge of the thrombus produces septic emboli, characterized by spiking fever and metastatic abscess formation.

The classical clinical description of sigmoid sinus thrombosis is a 'picket-fence' spiking temperature coinciding with septic embolization. Widespread use of antibiotics often masks this feature and pyrexia is no longer a reliable sign.[26] Patients often complain of otalgia and neck pain. Propagation of the clot into the IJV may be palpated as a cord-like structure in the neck. The presence of severe headache, vomiting or depressed conscious level should alert the clinician to the possibility of additional intracranial pathology, particularly otic hydrocephalus, cerebral oedema or cavernous sinus thrombosis. MRI with magnetic resonance venography (MRV) has high sensitivity in detecting sigmoid sinus thrombosis and may delineate the extent of the clot and any associated intracranial complications (Figure 45.7).

Sigmoid sinus thrombosis is managed with intravenous antibiotics and surgical debridement, although the extent of surgery remains controversial. A cortical mastoidectomy is performed to remove infected tissue, particularly granulations

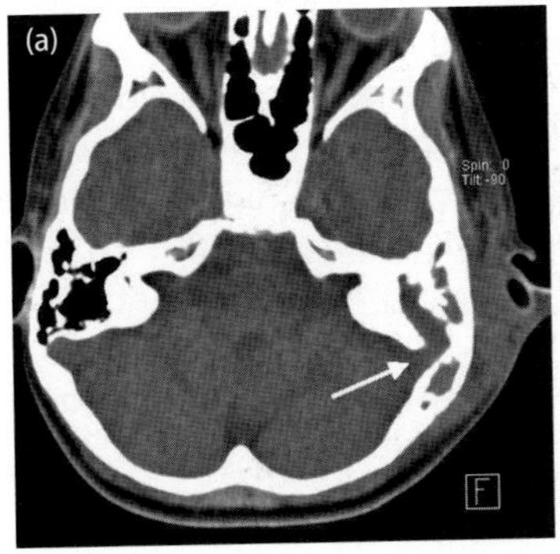

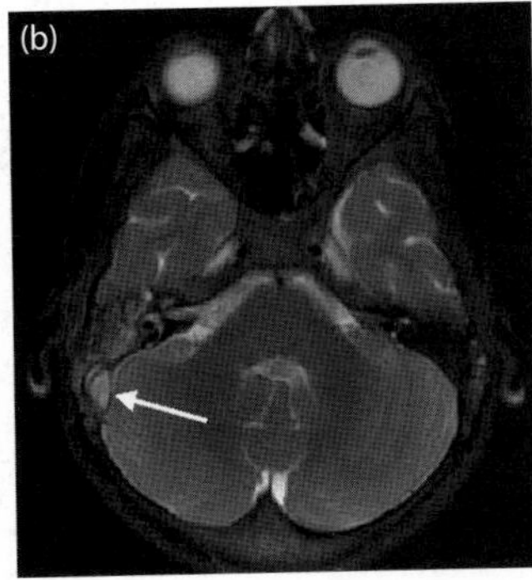

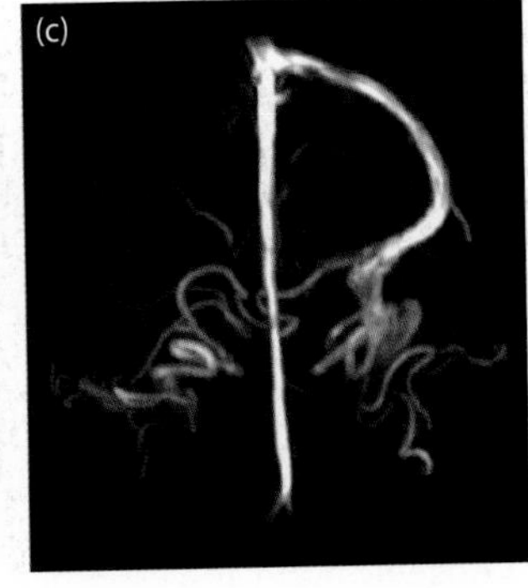

Figure 45.7 **(a)** Axial CT demonstrating a breach in the sigmoid sinus plate and probable sinus thrombosis (arrow). Thrombosis was confirmed intraoperatively. **(b)** Axial T2 MRI provides superior diagnostic imaging in suspected sigmoid sinus thrombosis. **(c)** Magnetic resonance venography (MRV) identifies absent venous flow in the right sigmoid and transverse sinuses due to thrombosis.

overlying the sinus. Routine opening of the sinus and removal of the infected clot has been advocated by some, although others aspirate from the vein and only open the sinus if frank pus is evacuated. A review of otogenic sigmoid sinus thrombosis has suggested that complications of embolization and sepsis are lower in this cohort than in non-otogenic thrombosis and that anticoagulation is only used in selected cases.[27]

OTITIC HYDROCEPHALUS

Otitic hydrocephalus is a very rare complication of otitis media and has a poorly understood aetiology. The condition is often associated with sigmoid sinus thrombosis, and it has been postulated that this is a key factor in the development of raised intracranial pressure, possibly by preventing CSF reabsorption into the cranial venous sinuses. Patients complain of a diffuse headache in the early stages, progressing to lethargy, blurred vision (from retinal vein occlusion) and diplopia (abducens palsy). MRI scanning demonstrates normal ventricular volume, but a raised intracranial pressure is discovered on lumbar puncture. Management is high-dose intravenous corticosteroids, diuretics and hyperosmolar agents such as mannitol. Surgical correction of the underlying ear disease is performed only once the patient has become neurologically stable.

KEY LEARNING POINTS

- Complications of otitis media occur when infection/inflammation spreads outside of the middle ear cleft.
- Complications are most common in children.
- Acute mastoiditis is the most common extracranial complication.
- Intracranial complications often co-exist and continue to carry a significant mortality rate.
- Otogenic brain abscesses may present insidiously, and detection requires a high index of suspicion.

REFERENCES

1. Singh B, Maharaj TJ. Radical mastoidectomy: Its place in otitic intracranial complications. *Journal of Laryngology and Otology.* 1993; 107: 1113–18.
2. Osma U, Cureoglu S, Hosoglu S. The complications of chronic otitis media: Report of 93 cases. *Journal of Laryngology and Otology.* 2000; 114: 97–100.
3. Kangsanarak J, Navacharoen N, Fooanant S, Ruckphaopunt K. Intracranial complications of suppurative otitis media: 13 years' experience. *American Journal of Otology.* 1995; 16: 104–9.
4. Ghaffar FA, Wordemann M, McCracken GH. Acute mastoiditis in children: A seventeen-year experience in Dallas, Texas. *Pediatric Infectious Disease Journal.* 2001; 20: 376–80.
5. Benito MB, Gorricho BP. Acute mastoiditis: Increase in the incidence and complications. *International Journal of Pediatric Otorhinolaryngology.* 2007; 71: 1007–11.
6. Sharland M, Kendall D, Yeates A, et al. Antibiotic prescribing in general practice and hospital admissions for peritonsillar abscess, mastoiditis and rheumatic fever in children: Time trend analysis. *BMJ.* 2005; 331: 328–29.
7. Van Zuijlen DA, Schilder AG, Van Ballen FAM, Hoes AW. National differences in incidence of acute mastoiditis: Relationship to prescribing patterns of antibiotics for acute otitis media? *Pediatric Infectious Disease Journal.* 2001; 20: 140–44.
8. Kvaerner KJ, Bentdal Y, Karevold G. Acute mastoiditis in Norway: No evidence for an increase. *International Journal of Pediatric Otorhinolaryngology.* 2007; 71: 1579–83.
9. Luntz M, Brodsky A, Nusem S, et al. Acute mastoiditis – The antibiotics era: A multicenter study. *International Journal of Pediatric Otorhinolaryngology.* 2001; 57: 1–9.
10. Linder TE, Briner HR, Bischoff T. Prevention of acute mastoiditis: Fact or fiction? *International Journal of Pediatric Otorhinolaryngology.* 2000; 56: 129–34.

11. Vera-Cruz P, Farinha RR, Calado V. Acute mastoiditis in children – Our experience. *International Journal of Otorhinolaryngology*. 1999; 50: 113–17.
12. Hoppe JE, Köster S, Bootz F, Niethammer D. Acute mastoiditis – Relevant once again. *Infection*. 1994; 22: 178–82.
13. Ginsburg CM, Rudoy R, Nelson JD. Acute mastoiditis in infants and children. *Clinical Pediatrics*. 1980; 19: 549–53.
14. Goldstein NA, Casselbrant ML, Bluestone CD, Kurs-Lasky M. Intratemporal complications of acute otitis media in infants and children. *Otolaryngology – Head and Neck Surgery*. 1998; 119: 444–54.
15. Tarantino V, D'Agostino R, Taborelli A, et al. Acute mastoiditis: A 10-year retrospective study. *International Journal of Pediatric Otorhinolaryngology*. 2002; 66: 143–48.
16. Fisch U. Current surgical treatment of intratemporal facial palsy. *Clinical Plastic Surgery*. 1979; 6: 377–88.
17. Baxter A. Dehiscence of the fallopian canal. An anatomical study. *Journal of Laryngology and Otology*. 1971; 85: 587.
18. Antoli-Candela F Jr, Stewart TJ. The pathophysiology of otologic facial paralysis. *Otolaryngology Clinics of North America*. 1974; 7: 309–30.
19. Schuknecht HF. *Infections*. In: *Pathology of the Ear*. Philadelphia: Lea and Febiger, 1993: 211–16.
20. Sanna M, Zini C, Gamoletti R, et al. Closed versus open technique in the management of labyrinthine fistulae. *American Journal of Otology*. 1988; 9: 470–75.
21. Manolidis S. Complications associated with labyrinthine fistula in surgery for chronic otitis media. *Otolaryngology – Head and Neck Surgery*. 2000; 123: 733–37.
22. Gradenigo G. Ueber circumscripte leptomeningitis mit spinalen symptomen. *Arch Ohrenheilk*. 1904; 51: 60–62.
23. Tutuncuoglu S, Uran N, Kavas I, Ozgur T. Gradenigo syndrome: A case report. *Pediatric Radiology*. 1993; 23: 556.
24. Van de Beek D, de Gans J, McIntyre P, Prasad K. Corticosteroids for acute bacterial meningitis. *Cochrane Database of Systematic Reviews*. 2010; Issue 9. doi: 10.1002/14651858.CD004405.pub3.
25. Yen PT, Chan ST, Huang TS. Brain abscess: With special reference to otolaryngolgic sources of infection. *Otolaryngology – Head and Neck Surgery*. 1995; 113: 15–22.
26. Manolidis S, Kutz JW Jr. Diagnosis and management of lateral sinus thrombosis. *Otology and Neurotology*. 2005; 26: 1045–51.
27. Bradley DT, Hashisaki GT, Mason JC. Otogenic sigmoid sinus thrombosis: What is the role of anticoagulation? *Laryngoscope*. 2002; 112: 1726–29.

46

Otosclerosis

DAVID E C BARING AND IAIN R C SWAN

DEFINITION

Otosclerosis is a disease affecting the otic capsule, resulting in foci of increased bone turnover. Disorganized bone remodelling causes a predominately conductive hearing loss by reducing movement of the stapes footplate in the oval window. It can also have a direct effect on the cochlea, resulting in a sensorineural hearing loss.

EPIDEMIOLOGY

Clinical otosclerosis is most commonly found in the Caucasian population, and is decreasingly common through the Asian, Native American and black populations. The UK National Study of Hearing conducted by the Medical Research Council in the 1980s showed a population prevalence of 2.1 per cent. Male-to-female ratios were not statistically different in those with an air–bone gap (ABG) <30 dB, but females were three times more likely to have otosclerosis where ABG >30 dB. Hence the female population seems to be more prone to more severe disease and tends to present as better potential surgical candidates. The rates of histological otosclerosis, where foci of otosclerotic disease are identified in cadaveric studies are nearly equivalent (7:6 female to male). Histological otosclerosis is identified in 8.3–11 per cent of the Caucasian population on unselected cadaveric studies.

PATHOLOGY

The otic capsule and ossicles undergo endochondrial ossification, and this process is complete by the end of the first year of life. Thereafter, there is minimal remodelling of this bone with few osteoclasts and osteoblasts present. Otosclerosis occurs with excessive remodelling in otosclerotic foci exclusively confined to the temporal bone, predominately related to the otic capsule and ossicles.

In otosclerosis two phases are described. In the active phase, well-vascularized bone undergoes excessive remodelling with increased osteoclast and osteoblast activity, vascular proliferation and a stroma of fibroblasts and histiocytes, giving a spongy appearance (hence the continental name of *otospongiosis* for this disease). The inactive phase is characterized by dense hypercellular mineralized sclerotic bone. The remodelled bone extends outwith the confines of the margins of the normal endochondrial bone into the middle ear and perilymphatic process, leading to alteration of normal function.

Light microscopy reveals the most common area for these foci is the fissula ante fenestrum in the otic capsule, just anterior to the oval window. Histological examination shows involvement of the anterior oval window in 80–96 per cent of cases, posterior oval window 11–28 per cent and the round window 30–36 per cent. This has the effect of fixing the stapes in the oval window, resulting in the conductive deficit that progresses as the degree of fixation advances.

Other areas of the otic capsule can be affected, resulting in the concept of histological otosclerosis with otosclerotic foci without clinical effects. This is more common than clinically apparent otosclerosis as described above. Where foci abut the cochlea, a sensorineural hearing loss is observed; this tends to be as a mixed loss but can occur as an isolated sensorineural loss, or 'cochlear otosclerosis'. This is reported to be due to two mechanisms: involvement of the endosteal portion of the cochlea and hyalinization of the spiral ligament adjacent to a focus.

AETIOLOGY

No discrete aetiology has been identified for this disease, and it is likely that it is multifactorial with genetic, autoimmune/inflammatory, hormonal and infective factors all proposed as involved in the development and progression of otosclerosis.

GENETIC FACTORS

Otosclerosis was recognized to have an autosomal dominant inheritance with a penetrance of 40 per cent and 50 per cent of cases being sporadic. To date, family linkage studies have identified eight genes internationally.

INFECTIVE FACTORS

Measles virus has been suggested as a factor in the development of otosclerosis. It has been noted that the incidence of otosclerosis is decreasing in the German population vaccinated against measles. Measles IgG has been identified in perilymph samples in otosclerotic patients. In addition viral matrix protein and nucleoprotein have been identified in otosclerotic foci samples. Measles viral RNA has also been found in the stapes footplate.

AUTOIMMUNE/INFLAMMATORY FACTORS

Immunohistochemistry has been used to investigate autoimmunity and inflammation in otosclerotic foci. Autoantibodies to collagen subtypes present in the otic capsule have been identified. Similar autoimmune reactions induced in rats cause lytic bone lesions of the otic capsule that resemble otosclerosis. Osteoprotegerin (OPG) deficient mice have been shown to have otosclerotic-like bone remodelling.

HORMONAL FACTORS

The sex hormones have been implicated in the pathophysiology of otosclerosis due to the relatively increased severity of disease seen in females. Oestrogen has an effect on the RANK (receptor activator of nuclear factor kappa-β) system by decreasing the response of osteoclasts to RANK-ligand complex and inducing apoptosis. In addition prolactin, itself increased by oestrogen and progesterone, decreases effects of OPG, resulting in increased osteolysis and affecting calcium metabolism, resulting in decreased bone mineral density. These effects may explain why pregnancy has been reported to induce or aggravate otosclerosis, and in rarer cases established otosclerosis has deteriorated with the combined oral contraceptive. However, the effects do not seem to be universal, and in the otosclerotic population as a whole, there is no hearing difference between females with and without children. In addition, the hormone levels in modern oral contraceptives are tiny in comparison to the hormone levels in maternal blood during pregnancy. Although concerns have been raised about the use of hormone replacement therapy (HRT) in otosclerotic patients, there is no evidence to support this.

Many areas affect this disease process. As understanding improves, potential avenues for disease-modifying treatment may become clear.

CLINICAL FEATURES

The following features need to be examined in the patient's history:

HEARING LOSS

- Side: 70 per cent of cases are bilateral, although initially there may only be a unilateral problem.
- Onset: Otosclerosis most commonly presents in the third decade. If congenital, other causes need to be considered (e.g. congenital stapes ankylosis). Ask the patient if there has been any significant head trauma related to onset (suggesting ossicular dislocation rather than otosclerosis).
- Tinnitus: This will be present in 75 per cent of cases and is increasingly common in those with a sensorineural hearing loss.
- Vertigo: This is rarely troublesome and is not a major feature. However, if patients describe vertigo in response to loud noises and to Valsalva's manoeuvre, consider 'third window lesions', e.g. superior semicircular canal dehiscence.
- Family history: Up to two-thirds of patients have a positive family history.
- Previous ear surgery: If the patient has had previous successful stapes surgery on the other side, it makes the diagnosis clearer and suggests a good surgical prognosis.
- Occupational history: This will have ramifications if surgery is undertaken owing to the potential for vertigo. A conservative approach may be more appropriate for those who work at a height or scuba dive.

EXAMINATION

OTOSCOPY

This is essential to exclude external ear or middle ear pathology causing hearing loss. Classically the tympanic membrane should be intact with no signs of middle ear disease (e.g. retraction or effusion). Mobility of the tympanic membrane can be assessed with a pneumatic otoscope or via a Valsalva/Toynbee manoeuvre. Tympanosclerosis, if extensive, may suggest an alternative cause for conductive hearing loss. Schwartz sign (a flamingo pink blush) is supposed to represent increased vascularity over the promontory due to active otosclerosis.

FISTULA TEST

Although the sensitivity of the fistula test is low, it should be performed where there is a history of vertigo as a positive test suggests some pathology other than otosclerosis.

TUNING FORK TESTS

Both Weber and Rinne tests are described in the assessment of otosclerosis. However, modern pure tone audiometry is significantly more sensitive. The Weber and Rinne tests may have a role in those cases where pure tone audiometry and clinical assessment do not match.

INVESTIGATION

AUDIOMETRY

Pure tone audiometry

Clinical otosclerosis initially starts with a low-frequency conductive hearing loss. As the disease progresses and the footplate is increasingly fixed, a flat maximal conductive hearing loss is seen (Figure 46.1). Bone conduction is artificially reduced by 5–15 dB, the Carhart effect, maximal at 2 kHz, which is near the resonant frequency of the ossicular chain. This occurs because in bone conduction audiometry, some of the vibration is transferred to the ossicular chain and to the external ear canal and reaches the inner ear by the air conduction route. In an abnormal middle ear, this energy will be lost. Successful surgery can, therefore, improve bone conduction thresholds by restoring this transfer.

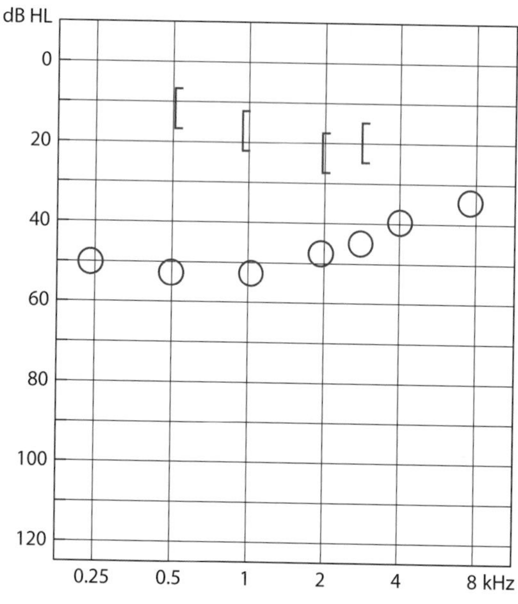

Figure 46.1 Typical pure tone audiogram in otosclerosis.

Speech audiometry

Speech audiometry is not routinely used in UK practice. However, with appropriate aiding, scores should be high.

Stapedial reflex

Stapedial reflex again is less frequently used but may be useful in indicating when alternative diagnoses should be sought. The stapedial reflex can be absent in the presence of 5 dB of conductive hearing loss, and at a 15 dB conductive hearing loss is absent in 50 per cent of cases; where it is present, the possibility of conditions such as superior semicircular canal dehiscence remains.

Tympanometry

In classic otosclerosis, tympanic membrane mobility should be normal, though compliance is rarely high. However, where the suspicion of other middle ear disease exists, a tympanogram can be of assistance.

IMAGING

High-resolution scanning provides good sensitivity (84–95.1 per cent) and specificity (99.5 per cent) in a cohort of 200 clinical otosclerosis patients who went on for surgery (examination under anaesthetic being the gold standard investigation). It is worth noting that in the 5 per cent of cases that were negative on computed tomography (CT) scanning, there was a significant increase in footplate incidents (e.g. floating footplate, fractured stapes, and so forth). It is worth bearing in mind that CT scanning is more helpful in active disease, with hypodense lesions visible on scans, rather than inactive sclerotic disease, which is less apparent around the dense otic capsule (Figure 46.2).

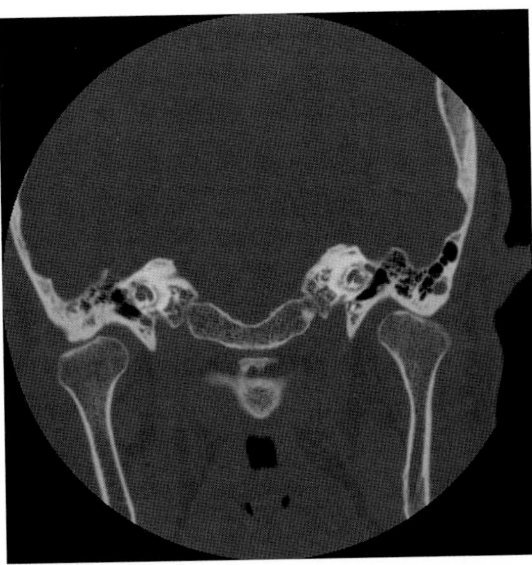

Figure 46.2 CT in otosclerosis.

DIFFERENTIAL DIAGNOSIS (AND KEY FEATURES/ INVESTIGATIONS)

- Superior semicircular canal dehiscence (SSCD): Relative conductive gain, autophonia, conductive hyperacusis, Tullio's phenomenon
- Tympanosclerosis: Previous history of middle ear disease, pale plaques on tympanic membrane
- Ossicular dislocation: History of trauma, excessive compliance on tympanometry, CT findings
- Congenital footplate/ossicular fixation: Non-progressive history from birth, CT findings
- Paget's disease: Producing a mixed hearing loss, later presentation, CT findings
- Osteogenesis imperfecta: Brittle bones, blue sclera, unusual to be undiagnosed at presentation of conductive hearing loss secondary to footplate fixation due to micro-fractures
- Congenital cholesteatoma: Features of chronic otitis media or 'pearl' seen through tympanic membrane, CT findings or diffusion weighted magnetic resonance imaging (MRI) scanning

TREATMENT

The treatment of otosclerosis is based on the patient's symptoms and wishes. For the hearing deficit there are three main options – observation, aiding and surgery – and these will be discussed below. Medical interventions have also been proposed and utilized predominately against the remodelling process seen in otosclerotic foci. These should be considered separately from the treatment of the hearing disability.

OBSERVATION

This is most appropriate in unilateral or early bilateral disease, where the patient has a minimal functional hearing disability that can be successfully managed with hearing tactics. Two approaches can be adopted: either serial audiometric follow-up or the patient representing when he or she feels there has been a deterioration requiring additional input.

AIDING

This should be tried in all patients with a hearing disability with an appropriate aiding appliance. The options are for unilateral or bilateral aiding depending on disability. It is recommended that a hearing aid trial is undertaken prior to surgical intervention. Where hearing aids are not tolerated or accepted, be it for comfort, utility or, more commonly, cosmesis, surgical intervention can be considered.

SURGERY

Stapes surgery

Surgery for otosclerosis has developed over the last two centuries. Initial attempts to improve hearing involved mobilizing the fixed stapes. The results were mixed, with early recurrence in those that were successful and a significant risk of profound hearing loss. The next evolution was to provide an alternative window that could conduct sound waves into the inner ear via a fenestration procedure to the lateral semicircular canal. This produced hearing improvement in 50 per cent of patients. Stapes surgery proper emerged in the 1950s with Rosen initially mobilizing the stapes and then Shea developed the stapedectomy procedure with initial removal of the whole stapes footplate. This technique progressed to partial removal of the footplate. Recently, stapedotomy has become the more common type of surgery where a small fenestra is created in the footplate. Over the last 50 years, stapes surgery has been refined; however, there are some areas of difference between surgeons.

SUITABILITY

The ideal case is a fit adult with bilateral ABG of >20 dB who has tried hearing aids but would prefer to have a surgical intervention (having discussed the risks and potential benefits) and has no relative contraindication to surgery for social/occupational reasons (flying, diving and working at height).

Unilateral or second-side surgery can be performed, but the risks remain the same as first-side surgery, while the benefits are reduced owing to the relatively lower hearing disability in unilateral hearing loss and the need to achieve similar air conduction thresholds (i.e. within 10 dB) to the good ear for the patient to perceive significant benefit.

Those cases with severe or profound mixed hearing loss may find surgery beneficial by elevating their air conduction thresholds to a range that is more amenable to hearing aid use.

Prospective audit of surgical outcomes is mandatory in stapes surgery. It is desirable that a surgeon performing stapes surgery maintains regular practice. The aim is to achieve closure of the air–bone gap to within 10 dB in 90 per cent of cases and a have a dead ear rate of <1 per cent.

The procedure can be divided into three distinct phases:

1. **Confirmation of diagnosis (tympanotomy).** Access is achieved by an endaural or permeatal incision. A tympanomeatal flap is elevated with the annulus freed from 8 o'clock (4 o'clock in the left ear) to 12 o'clock. The corda tympani is identified and preserved. Bone is curetted from the ear canal to expose the pyramid and stapedius tendon to ensure adequate exposure. The ossicular chain is inspected and the stapes palpated, looking for footplate fixation to confirm the diagnosis. Other conditions (e.g. malleus fixation) need to be excluded. There should be no technical contraindications (relative or otherwise) to proceeding with stapes surgery (e.g. prolapsed facial nerve, persistent stapedial artery, round window obliteration).
2. **Dealing with the stapes fixation.** A prosthesis is selected to be 0.25 mm longer than the distance from the underside of the incus to the footplate. The incudo-stapedial joint is mobilized. The stapedius tendon is divided. The posterior crus is divided, with a laser if used, and the anterior crus is weakened until the superstructure is removed. A hole (stapedotomy) is made in the footplate with a laser, a microdrill or cold steel.
3. **Prosthesis insertion**. The premeasured prosthesis is then placed round the long process of the incus and into the hole created with soft tissue to obliterate potential leaks of perilymph. It is then secured by crimping around the long process. The soft tissue used can be in the form of a vein graft (especially in large window procedures) or fibrous tissue. The position is then confirmed and the ossicular chain palpated to ensure continuity. The tympanomeatal flap is replaced and the ear canal dressed.

VARIATIONS

Anaesthetic

General anaesthetic is the norm in current UK practice, permitting good hypotensive anaesthesia to optimize operative field and a stationary patient.

Local anaesthetic is more common in Europe and North America. It avoids the deleterious effects of general anaesthetic and allows the patient to report symptoms perioperatively (i.e. vertigo or hearing improvement). This patient feedback can be useful in revision surgery where vertigo will give some warning of potential problems.

Incision

Permeatal incision is more cosmetic but allows no access to fibrous tissue for placing around the piston. Endaural incision gives better access plus allows harvesting of fibrous tissue. Stapedotomy and prosthesis can be placed prior to removal of the superstructure. This is more stable with less risk of footplate issues but depends on the width of the oval window.

Dissection tools

Lasers are expensive but are very easy to use and minimize trauma to the inner ear. Microdrills are less expensive and do not require special theatre precautions.

Size of stapedotomy

The aim is to achieve a small enough hole in which a prosthesis can securely sit without being caught on the lateral margins of the hole. The smallest prosthesis is 0.4 mm in diameter and normally 0.2 mm is added to ensure mobility.

Prosthesis material

There are a multitude of prostheses and materials available, and it is beyond the remit of this chapter to discuss their relative merits except to say it is more likely that the surgeon, his or her experience and skill will have a greater effect on the hearing outcome than which appropriately sized and placed prosthesis is used.

Stapedotomy plug

Vein graft is the traditional material and is robust and malleable. However, when placed over the stapedotomy, it obscures it, which can make prosthesis insertion more troublesome. Fibrous tissue is readily available, and small particles can be placed around the prosthesis base and the stapedotomy once satisfactory placement is achieved.

POST-OPERATIVE CARE

The patient should be cautiously mobilized in the post-operative period. The patient can be discharged once ambulant and established on oral intake. If day surgery is to be undertaken, the patient should have rapid access to the ear, nose and throat (ENT) unit in the event he or she experiences problems overnight and should stay locally. Stitches and dressings should be removed 5–7 days postoperation. Audiometry should be performed 4–6 weeks after the operation once the ear has fully healed. The ear should be kept dry until this point.

COMPLICATIONS

Immediate

- Tympanic membrane perforation: Should this occur, it should be repaired at the time with an underlay graft and the stapes surgery should continue as planned.
- Corda tympani division: It is desirable for the corda to be preserved. Patients may complain of an alteration of sense of taste or a metallic taste following surgery even when the corda is preserved. These symptoms tend to settle over a few months irrespective of the nerve's integrity.
- Facial nerve injury: Ten per cent of facial nerves are reported to be dehiscent and at greater risk during surgery. This is particularly true in revision surgery where adhesions can complicate safe dissection. However, this should not preclude surgery unless nerve prolapse grossly obscures the oval window. The risks to the nerve should be much less than 1 per cent during the operation.
- Bleeding: Vascular anomalies can confound attempts at surgery with persistent stapedial arteries or dehiscent internal carotid arteries. Caution should be taken with larger stapedial vessels that can have a segmental supply to the facial nerve or brain stem.
- Gusher: A perilymphatic gusher occurs where there is a dilated cochlear or vestibular aqueduct or an internal auditory canal defect. On opening the footplate, perilymph gushes out, filling the middle and external ear. This is treated at surgery by elevating the head of the operating table and placing a tissue graft anchored by a prosthesis +/- a lumbar drain. The incidence of hearing loss is high.

Early

- Profound hearing loss: The dead ear rate in larger series should be low with <1 per cent in uncomplicated primary cases. This rate rises to more than 4 per cent in revision cases.
- Vertigo: Mild transient unsteadiness is common post-operatively. Profound prostrating

vertigo suggests there has been trauma to the inner ear structures, and it should be treated symptomatically with vestibular sedatives. The hearing should be assessed. Mild vertigo can occur in the first week post-operatively with an associated sensorineural hearing loss. It tends to resolve and is ascribed to a labyrinthitis as a response to surgery.
- Tinnitus: Many patients with otosclerosis will have tinnitus preoperatively. Five per cent are reported to have deterioration in their tinnitus postoperation, with 34 per cent reporting an improvement in their tinnitus levels.
- Facial nerve palsy: Delayed palsy is reported associated with higher energy laser dissection. This is thought to be due to thermal injury. Recovery is to be expected but may take months.
- Reparative granuloma: This complication is due to granulations forming around the oval window and prosthesis. These granulations can extend into the vestibule. It occurs more commonly with gelfoam or fat (as opposed to fascia, vein or perichondrium). The main symptom is of hearing loss and can also include vertigo (30 per cent), pain and tinnitus. It presents 2–6 weeks post-operatively. Treatment is controversial, ranging from surgical exploration with removal of inflamed tissue +/- prosthesis to more conservative steroids and antibiotics, reserving surgery for those who fail to settle.

Late

- Perilymph fistula: The initial stapes surgery intentionally creates a fistula, which should rapidly heal in the post-operative period. A secondary fistula can develop months or years later, presenting with fluctuating hearing loss, vertigo, tinnitus and aural fullness. A fistula test is positive in two-thirds of cases. Definitive treatment is exploration and soft tissue obliteration.
- Hyperacusis: This presents as discomfort with loud noises and is reported in 40 per cent of post-operative patients. It is thought to be related to the loss of the stapedius reflex due to division of the stapedius tendon. Attempts at reconstruction, although strongly advocated by some, have not proven to be beneficial.
- Prosthesis failure: This results in a conductive hearing loss that can occur at any stage post-operatively. It most commonly occurs as a result of the prosthesis falling out of the oval window or necrosis of the long process of incus resulting in loss of continuity of the ossicular conduction path.
- Sensorineural hearing loss: Cochlear otosclerotic pathology may coexist in these patients, and the bone conduction thresholds may deteriorate more than the 1 dB every 2 years normally seen in the ageing non-otosclerotic population.

OTHER TREATMENTS

Bone-anchored hearing aids

Bone-anchored hearing aids (BAHA) are ideally placed to address the hearing deficit from otosclerosis and are viewed as a viable alternative. The major advantage is there is no risk of a dead ear from the implantation surgery. In cases of an only hearing ear with otosclerosis, this may be an attractive option.

Cochlear implantation

There are unfortunate patients who have profound hearing loss due to otosclerotic disease. Cochlear implantation remains a viable option providing the cochlea has not been obliterated.

Medical

The two medical agents used most commonly are fluoride and bisphonphonates. At present, medical therapy for otosclerosis is not proven and more research is needed to establish if effective modulation of the disease process can be achieved. It is worth noting that only a minority of UK stapes surgeons will attempt medical intervention.

Fluoride therapy is suggested to work by a variety of mechanisms. It is reported to modify enzymatic action causing inflammation in the perilymph of otosclerotic patients, reduce the intensity of the active phase of otosclerosis, and inhibit diastrophic dysplasia sulphate transporter that is involved in the sulphation of bone matrix glycosaminoglycans (raised levels correlate with increased sensorineural hearing loss in otosclerosis). Epidemiological studies of otosclerosis comparing areas with high-fluoride and low-fluoride drinking water have shown conflicting results with regards to hearing and disease activity between the two groups. Clinical studies, as yet, have not shown fluoride therapy to be conclusively beneficial in the long term.

Bisphosphonates (etidronate, risedronate, alendronic acid) are alalogues of pyrophosphates and reduce bone turnover, and are thought to act on the osteolytic foci in otosclerosis. It has been suggested their use can have an adjuvant effect to the use of sodium fluoride. Side effects relate to demineralization of bone and gastro-intestinal disturbance, renal failure and hypocalcaemia.

FUTURE DEVELOPMENTS

Implantable hearing aids have been used to amplify sound at the round window in those who have failed conventional stapes surgery. The floating mass transducer of the Soundbridge has been placed in the round window niche with good effect. This may hold future promise for those with more complex disease.

KEY LEARNING POINTS

- Otosclerosis is the likely diagnosis in progressive conductive hearing loss with a normal tympanic membrane.
- It can be managed by provision of a hearing aid or by surgery.

SUGGESTED READINGS

Chole RA. Pathophysiology of otosclerosis. *Otology and Neurotology*. 2001; 22: 249–57.

Ealy M. Genetics of otosclerosis. *Hearing Research*. 2009; 266: 70–74.

Layleyre S. Reliability of high resolution CT scan in the diagnosis of otosclerosis. *Otology and Neurotology*. 2009; 30: 1152–59.

Lippy W. Pearls on otosclerosis. *Ear, Nose and Throat Journal*. 2008; 326–28.

Schuknecht H. Histologic variants in otosclerosis. *Laryngoscope*. 1985; 95(11): 1307–17.

Uppal S. Otosclerosis 2: The medical management of otosclerosis. *International Journal of Clinical Practice*. 2010; 64(2): 256–65.

47

Sensorineural hearing loss

DAVID K SELVADURAI

SENSORINEURAL HEARING LOSS

Previously termed *nerve deafness*, sensorineural hearing loss (SNHL) is due to impairments in the function of the cochlea or auditory nerve. The majority of cases are due to acquired causes, but congenital cases have many implications for childhood development and merit detailed discussion. Sensorineural hearing loss may coexist with conductive loss, as mixed hearing loss.

The degree of loss can be classified in various ways (Table 47.1) and may range from mild to profound.

CLINICAL FEATURES

Clinical presentations of SNHL depend on the age of the patient, the degree of hearing loss and whether it is bilateral. The hearing needs of the patient determine the nature of the presenting complaints. In childhood delayed acquisition of speech and language, inattentive behaviour and the need to listen to sound sources at a raised volume predominate.

In adults the demands of speech perception in working and business life often determine the nature of the symptoms. SNHL creates specific difficulties in speech perception that merit mention.

1. Recruitment: The ability to hear low-volume sounds in detail is largely conferred by the amplification function of the outer hair cell (OHC) system of the cochlea. As sound intensity increases, this function becomes less important. In most cases of SNHL, outer hair

Table 47.1 Scale of hearing loss

Threshold (dBHL)	Degree of impairment
<20	Normal hearing
21–40	Mild hearing loss
41–70	Moderate hearing loss
71–95	Severe hearing loss
>95	Profound hearing loss

cell function is reduced, leading to a lack of sensitivity at low volumes. However, higher volumes are perceived as normal, and so volume perception becomes non-linear, with quiet sounds barely audible and loud sounds seemingly very loud. This phenomenon is termed *recruitment.*

2. Loss of frequency resolution: In addition to amplification, the OHC system allows fine frequency selectivity in the cochlea, with each frequency stimulating a different region of the basilar membrane in a tonotopic way. If this ability is lost, then adjacent frequencies in the basilar membrane become overlapping in their responses. When this occurs and the degree of outer hair cell loss is different in adjacent areas (e.g. in a sloping or 'cookie bite' audiogram), then the more-sensitive frequencies will mask the adjacent less-sensitive areas. In noise-induced hearing loss (NIHL) this occurs around the 4 kHz area and increases difficulties in speech perception.

Unilateral losses are often asymptomatic in early childhood. However, binaural hearing is important for hearing performance in noise, with multiple sound (or speech) sources and for sound localization. Patients with unilateral losses notice difficulties in noisy environments, including the classroom, and aiding may be appropriate. The problems are more pronounced in sudden unilateral losses where other coping strategies have not developed.

AUDIOMETRIC TYPES

The pattern of SNHL may be pan frequency (flat) with equal loss at all tested frequencies, downward sloping (high-frequency losses predominate), upward sloping (low-frequency losses predominate) or *U*-shaped ('cookie bite'). This last form is seen in NIHL and some congenital losses (Figures 47.1 to 47.3).

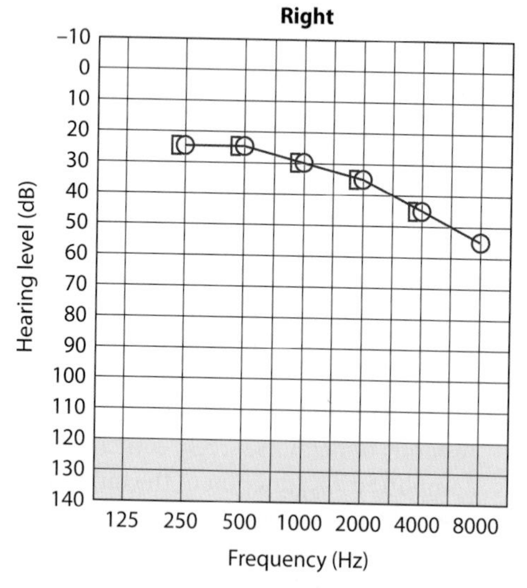

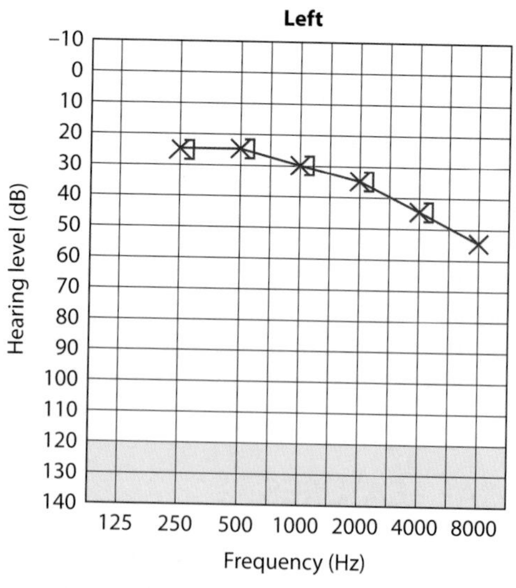

Figure 47.1 Audiogram of high-frequency loss typical of presbycusis.

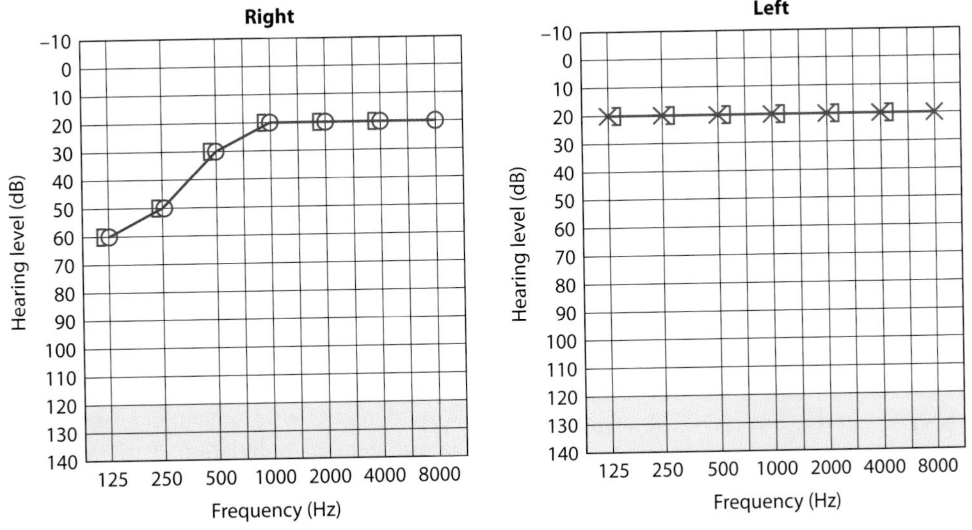

Figure 47.2 Audiogram of right-sided Ménière's disease.

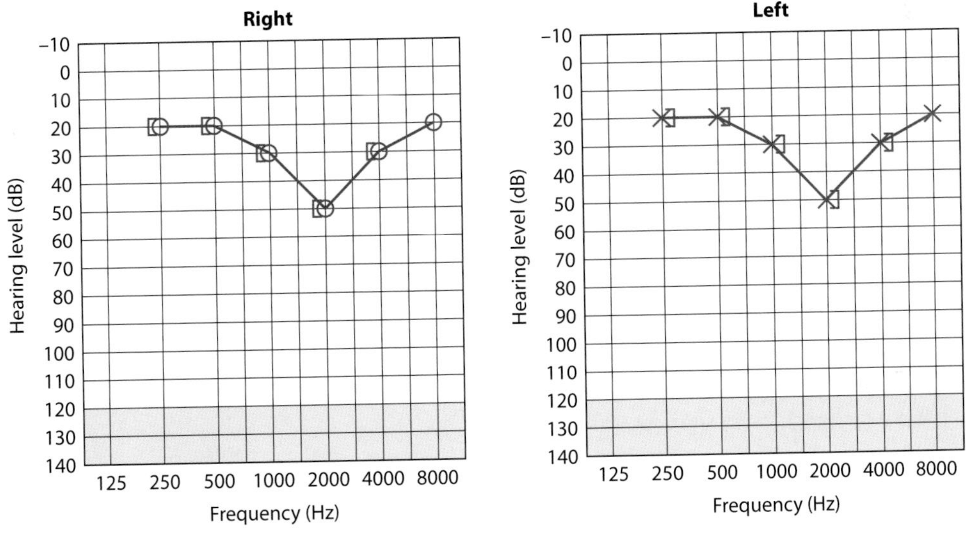

Figure 47.3 Audiogram of U-shaped loss seen in some congenital causes.

CONGENITAL, HEREDITARY AND ACQUIRED DEAFNESS

Congenital hearing loss is present at birth. Many cases are due to genetically inherited causes and are therefore also hereditary, but other causes exist. Some acquired cases are also due to inherited genetic defects which present later in life or predispose to hearing loss in the presence of other factors. Even 'normal' age-related hearing loss, or presbyacusis, has a genetically determined component.

CONGENITAL SENSORINEURAL HEARING LOSS

About 1.1 per 1000 children born in the UK have a bilateral hearing loss greater than 40 dB. Fifty per cent of these are in the severe to profound range. It should be remembered that this number will be higher in populations in less-developed countries and those communities where inherited diseases are more common.

Genetic hearing loss

Genetically determined loss accounts for approximately 60 per cent of all permanent childhood hearing impairment (PCHI). Approximately a third of cases are part of a clinical syndrome, and most are non-syndromic. More than 400 syndromic causes are now known, but only a few are common. Genetically determined loss may be inherited in an autosomal recessive (AR), dominant (AD) or sex (X-linked) pattern. Approximately 70 per cent of cases are AR, 25 per cent AD and 5 per cent X-linked.

Autosomal recessive syndromic

USHER'S SYNDROME

This syndrome leads to both hearing impairment and visual loss. Three types are recognized, and all are associated with the development of retinitis pigmentosa. The hearing loss is most pronounced in type 1, where it can be profound. Vestibular function is absent in this sub-type. A number of genetic abnormalities have now been described for this condition.

PENDRED'S SYNDROME AND LARGE VESTIBULAR AQUEDUCT SYNDROME

There is a close association between this form of inherited deafness associated with thyroid abnormalities and large vestibular aqueduct syndrome (LVAS). Thyroid function testing is often normal, but a goitre may develop during childhood. Hearing loss is variable at birth but is usually progressive. Minor head injuries are associated with sudden worsening of SNHL and vestibular symptoms in LVAS, which may temporarily respond to steroid treatment. Ultimately, many cases progress to bilateral profound loss. Both conditions appear linked to defects on chromosome 7, explaining their common coexistence.

JERVELL AND LANGE-NEILSEN SYNDROME

This rare condition displays SNHL that can be profound and electrocardiogram (ECG) abnormalities. The most common abnormalities include QT prolongation and T-wave inversion. Screening for this condition using ECG is required in all PCHIs, as these individuals may develop dangerous arrhythmias under anaesthesia.

Autosomal dominant syndromic

Waardenburg syndrome affects about 1 in 40 000 of the general population. Patients have various phenotypic characteristics, including white forelock, heterochromis iridis, dystopia canthorum and bushy eyebrows that meet in the midline. Expression is highly variable.

Branchio-oto-renal syndrome has a similar prevalence to Waardenburg syndrome. As a defect of the first and second branchial arches, a variety of physical abnormalities are seen, including cochlear dysplasia, pre-auricular pits, sinuses and branchial fistulae. The renal dysplasias seen include polycystic kidneys, abnormal calyces and aplasia.

The phenotypic features of Stickler syndrome also appear highly variable. About 40 per cent of such patients show SNHL, but there is also cleft palate, abnormal growth, vertebral abnormalities and ocular abnormalities. Mitral valve prolapse is frequently seen. When present, the hearing loss is high-frequency and progressive.

X-linked syndromic

Alport's syndrome shows glomerulonephritis with variable SNHL in about 50 per cent. Norrie's syndrome consists of optic atrophy and SNHL (progressive).

Chromosomal disorders

SNHL is also seen in some chromosomal disorders including trisomy 21 (Down's syndrome), trisomy 18 (Edwards' syndrome), trisomy 13 (Patau syndrome) and Turner's syndrome (XO).

Non-syndromic hearing loss

Approximately 70 per cent of inherited hearing loss is non-syndromic. The nomenclature of these conditions is most easily considered in relation to their genetic inheritance pattern. Thus the genetic loci involved are termed DFN (deafness), and subdivided into DFNA (AD), DFNB (AR) and DFNX.

The disorder DFNB1, which leads to a defective protein connexin 26 through mutation in the GJB2 gene and defective protein connexin 30 through defect in GJB2, is the most common, accounting for about 50 per cent of AR non-syndromic cases. *It is worth noting that the GJB 2 mutation is carried by approximately 1 in 33 of the general population.*

DFNA defects usually cause post-lingual deafness and can also affect connexin 26 and other similar proteins.

DFNX is much less common and is associated with moderate to profound loss that can be progressive. It may also present post-lingually.

Mitochondrial mutations can also be associated with SNHL, which can be syndromic or non-syndromic and of various severities. It is worth noting that mitochondrial mutation A1555G predisposes an individual to extreme aminoglycoside susceptibility.

ACQUIRED SNHL

Acquired SNHL in childhood

Events during pregnancy and the early neonatal period can lead to pre-lingual acquired SNHL of various severities. The causes to be considered are as follows.

FETAL INFECTION

Rubella

In utero, infection leads to the development of congenital rubella syndrome. The degree of disability reflects the gestational stage at the time of infection, with early infections leading to multi-system disease. Eye disease, SNHL and cardiac defects are most commonly seen, with up to 60 per cent showing SNHL. This is usually severe/profound and may be progressive.

Cytomegalovirus

Maternal cytomegalovirus (CMV) infection is often associated with very mild symptoms, but the fetus can suffer multisystem disease including SNHL, which again can be progressive and severe. There is current interest in early neonatal anti-viral treatment to reduce disability.

Toxoplasmosis

Infection with the protozoal parasite *Toxoplasma gondii* is important in developing countries. In Brazil, incidence has been estimated at 1 case per 1000 births with up to 40 per cent having SNHL. Early treatment may significantly reduce the disability and prevent the hearing loss.

Other neonatal factors may cause the development of SNHL. Jaundice, low birthweight, mechanical ventilation, hypoxia and neonatal sepsis have all been linked to SNHL. Prematurity is linked to all of the above and is associated with a heightened risk of SNHL. Most newborn screening programmes therefore target extra surveillance on neonatal unit patients.

CHILDHOOD INFECTION

Meningitis

These infections remain the most common cause of acquired childhood deafness despite extensive vaccination programmes. Bacterial infections with *Streptococcus pneumonia*, *Haemophilus influenza* and *Neisseria meningitidis* can cause profound SNHL. Inflammation within the cochlea can lead to cochlear duct obliteration and even ossification within a few weeks of illness. This can make cochlear implantation difficult, and early implantation is often advised.

Measles can be associated with SNHL. The hearing loss is often bilateral and of varying severity. Some cases of SNHL have been reported after live vaccination. There is also work suggesting that some cases of otosclerosis are linked to the measles virus present in the otic capsule around the footplate of the stapes. Mumps is a similar virus, rarely causing a unilateral hearing loss.

Bacterial otitis media is dealt with in the adult infection section.

ADULT SENSORINEURAL HEARING LOSS

Hearing loss is considered the most common disability affecting the adult population. Approximately 7.5 per cent of the population between 60 and 70 years of age have a hearing loss of more than 45 dBHL. We have discussed many of the congenital genetic causes, but it is worth mentioning those genetic causations that typically present after the early infant, pre-lingual period or display a progressive pattern.

The great majority of the non-syndromic cases are due to an AD pattern of inheritance. They fall into various DFNA types (e.g. DFNA 1–5, 6, 8, 9). It is usually progressive from the first decade of life and is low frequency in distribution. Other DFNA types display different ages of onset, progression and audiometric characteristics.

The syndromic cases are generally diagnosed in childhood but display progression. Progression has been defined as >15 dB change in the pure tone audiometry (PTA) average over a 10-year period.

ACQUIRED SNHL

The majority of cases of SNHL are acquired through disease and ageing in adulthood. In many cases multiple risk factors interact to cause the hearing loss. The most common cause is presbyacusis.

Presbyacusis

Sensorineural hearing loss associated with the ageing process is termed *presbyacusis*, or age-related hearing loss. Typically, it manifests a bilateral, symmetrical high-frequency loss. It is more common in men at all ages, and its progression accelerates with increasing age. Subclassification into sensory, neural, strial and mechanical types was suggested by Schuknecht but has not gained acceptance.

It is difficult to separate the effects of other ototraumas, especially environmental noise, from the genesis of presbyacusis, although by definition they should be excluded.

As the population ages, the importance of this subgroup will rise.

SUDDEN SENSORINEURAL HEARING LOSS

Sudden sensorinerual hearing loss (SSNHL) syndrome is defined as a loss of 30 dBHL in three contiguous frequencies over a 72-hour period. It most often affects a single ear but is bilateral in about 1 per cent of cases. It is an uncommon condition with an incidence of about 1 in 5000.

Audiology on presentation will demonstrate the level of loss, which may be moderate to profound and display flat, downsloping or even low-frequency characteristics.

In more than 90 per cent of cases no cause is found, and it is postulated that the condition is due to a microvascular deficiency in the cochlear circulation. Nonetheless, examination and investigation are mandatory to exclude treatable causes.

Examination must exclude concomitant middle ear infection or disease, and elicit neurological signs if present. It is important to establish if vertigo and accompanying nystagmus is present.

Investigations include magnetic resonance imaging (MRI) scanning to exclude a cerebropontine angle lesion. Blood tests for autoimmune disease, inflammatory markers and syphilis are required.

Approximately half of patients will improve spontaneously over 10–14 days. Early treatment using high-dose steroids, either orally or transtympanically, may further improve prognosis, but the evidence for this is limited. Indicators of a poor prognosis include delay in diagnosis and treatment beyond 72 hours of onset, more severe losses, vertigo and high-frequency hearing loss (downward sloping).

A variety of viral infections have been associated with the development of sudden hearing loss. There is evidence to support that the following are linked with SSNHL: mumps, CMV, herpes zoster, measles, rubella and Lassa fever.

Despite these links, a systematic review has not demonstrated benefit from concurrent use of antiviral medication, and there also is no clear evidence to support the use of hyperbaric oxygen, dextran infusions or betahistine.

MÉNIÈRE'S SYNDROME, DISEASE AND ENDOLYMPHATIC HYDROPS

The characteristics of these conditions are detailed in Chapter 49, but they are important causes of acquired hearing loss. As previously described, these conditions lead to episodes with vertigo, tinnitus and hearing loss. The hearing loss is characteristically low-frequency SNHL in the early stages of the disease, and initially recovers to a normal level after the attacks. As the condition progresses, the hearing loss becomes increasingly permanent, with partial recovery and ultimately no recovery. Over time the low-frequency loss spreads to include mid- and high-frequency areas. Patients often describe qualitative changes in their hearing prior to attacks, and in later stages loudness recruitment is seen.

Treatment of the hearing loss itself is with hearing aids, some of which are user-tuneable to allow changes in amplification for hearing fluctuation. In a small number of cases the hearing loss may reach profound levels and render the patient a candidate for cochlear implantation.

AUTOIMMUNE INNER EAR DISEASE

Autoimmune inner ear disease (AIED) is a rare condition accounting for at most 1 per cent of acquired hearing loss. It is characterized by fluctuating, bilateral, progressive hearing loss over weeks to months. The time course of the progression is too rapid for presbyacusis, and too indolent for SSNHL. Currently, there are no truly diagnostic tests, and the previously used 68kDa Otoblot test has fallen out of favour owing to low specificity and sensitivity, and doubt over its target antigen. Currently, tests for other auto-antibodies (positive in 30 per cent of cases), a typical clinical course and response to steroids are used to support the diagnosis. The absence of clear diagnostic tests and a specific aetiological auto-antibody are, however, problematic, and this diagnosis is still controversial.

TUMOURS PRESENTING AS SNHL

The most common tumour presenting with hearing loss is the vestibular schwannoma (often erroneously termed an *acoustic neuroma*). This tumour arises from the Schwann cells that cover the superior and inferior vestibular nerves. This benign tumour usually grows initially within the internal acoustic meatus and exerts pressure on the vestibular and auditory nerves, leading to hearing loss and balance disturbance. The growth may extend (or start) in the cerebello-pontine angle and hence exert pressure effects on the brain stem and eventually cause a rise in intracranial pressure. Untreated, this space-occupying tumour can grow to sufficient size to cause death.

Except in neurofibromatomosis type 2 (NF2) the lesion is unilateral, and so the hearing loss is asymmetric, often high frequency. Speech discrimination testing is useful and may be unexpectedly poor. Investigation of asymmetric SNHL is mandatory, and the investigation of choice is the gadolinium-enhanced MRI scan. Treatment is covered elsewhere.

TOXICITY-INDUCED SNHL

A variety of drugs have the potential to be toxic to the auditory and vestibular systems. These are termed *ototoxic* and may display cochleotoxic, vestibulotoxic or mixed effects. Individual patients will display particular susceptibilities.

The most important drug groups are:

- Aminoglycoside antibiotics
- Cytotoxic chemotherapy
- Quinine, salicylates and nonsteroidal anti-inflammatory drugs (NSAIDs)
- Loop diuretics

Physiological factors that may increase the risks of ototoxcity include concomitant renal or liver dysfunction, dehydration and genetic predisposition. The clinical scenario will also exert an effect through dose, duration and concurrent ototrauma, including other drugs, noise, hypoxia and cochlear hypoperfusion.

Aminoglycoside antibiotics

These include gentamicin, neomycin, streptomycin, kanamicin and amikacin. All interfere with mitochondrial energy production. Mitochondrial DNA mutations are associated with increased susceptibility to ototoxicity.

It is problematic that topical ear drops often contain aminoglycosides, which in theory may cause otoxicity. This is not a concern if the tympanic membrane is intact but represents a potential risk if there is a perforation. Non-ototoxic alternatives are available and are gaining popularity in this situation.

Cytotoxic chemotherapy

Cisplatin is commonly used in a variety of chemotherapeutic regimens. It can induce a high-frequency SNHL that is permanent and dose dependent. A variety of studies have looked at otoprotection against this effect, but this has not reached general clinical practice yet.

Quinine, salicylates and NSAIDs

All these drugs are capable of causing a reversible SNHL. The mechanism is dose dependent and probably relates to alterations in outer hair cell function. Tinnitus is often seen in association with the hearing loss.

Loop diuretics

The agents furosemide and bumetanide are used extensively in the treatment of cardiac failure and hypertension. They can induce a reversible SNHL but may also act synergistically with concomitant aminoglycoside therapy to cause a permanent SNHL.

NOISE-INDUCED HEARING LOSS

Noise-induced hearing loss (NIHL) has characteristically been due to exposure to either industrial noise or military noise. Increasingly, recreational noise exposure may reach sufficient levels to induce NIHL as well. Tinnitus commonly accompanies NIHL.

The principal site of noise damage in the cochlea is the outer hair cell. These structures are directly damaged by very high sound levels but also suffer metabolic damage leading to cell death by extended exposure to less-elevated sound levels. In addition, there is damage at both the auditory neurone and inner hair cell level.

NIHL usually causes a symmetrical bilateral SNHL affecting the high frequencies but centred on a notch at around 4 kHz. Asymmetric loss can be seen in asymmetric exposure, such as with rifle shooting.

There is a considerable variation in an individual's susceptibility to noise exposure, but industrial noise levels are regulated to ensure safety at work. European guidance in 1989 stipulated that employers take precautionary measures when sound levels exceed 80 dB(A). Below this level, NIHL risk is very small, above 85 dB(A) it may affect susceptible individuals and regular exposure above 90 dB(A) is very likely to cause NIHL.

Establishing the diagnosis is largely through history and audiometry, but for medico-legal reasons strict protocols have been developed. A full review is available from Coles et al., 2000. These guidelines must also be interpreted in light of other confounding causes of hearing loss, especially presbyacusis.

INFECTIOUS CAUSES OF SNHL

We have already mentioned the role of prenatal and perinatal infections in generating childhood hearing loss, but other specific examples exist.

Hearing loss is seen occasionally after acute otitis media. In this scenario it may follow the spread of toxin into the cochlea from the infected middle ear. This is termed a *serous labyrinthitis* and can be of varying severity, often accompanied by some balance disturbance.

More serious is direct bacterial invasion of the labyrinth. This suppurative labyrinthitis is also seen in association with cholesteatoma if a labyrinthine fistula is present, and can lead to devastating hearing loss and balance disturbance.

Viral infection leading to balance disorder (viral labyrinthitis) is well recognized, and sometimes hearing loss is seen after such episodes. More specific examples include:

1. Patients with Ramsay Hunt syndrome, which is caused by the herpes zoster virus (hence also called herpes zoster oticus), present with lower motor neurone type facial weakness, associated with marked otalgia. This is the same virus that causes chickenpox, and careful examination often demonstrates the presence of virally induced vesicles in the pinna, ear canal, tympanic membrane or even intraorally. Many patients also demonstrate a SNHL, tinnitus and balance disturbance. Early urgent treatment with antivirals and steroids is essential to reduce long-term disability from the facial weakness, and post-herpetic neuralgia.
2. Hearing loss, tinnitus and vertigo are all common findings in human immunodeficiency (HIV) infected adults. HIV infection predisposes individuals to many viral and bacterial infections that may affect the audiovestibular system. In addition, the effect of the often ototoxic medication used to treat these infections must be considered.
3. Syphilitic otitis media is caused by *Treponema pallidum*. It is now a rare condition, which initially causes a suppurative middle ear infection, but can lead to SNHL. Late onset deafness is seen in some congenitally infected individuals.

DISORDERS OF BONE

A variety of disease processes affecting the temporal bone can lead to SNHL. Otosclerosis (see Chapter 46) may affect sensorineural levels in approximately 15 per cent of cases. In these individuals the hearing loss may even progress to profound levels, resulting in consideration of cochlear implantation. The bone dysplasias may also cause SNHL, predominantly by compression of the auditory nerve in the temporal bone.

TRAUMA

Fractures of the temporal bone that traverse the cochlea or internal auditory meatus can lead to sudden SNHL, which may be complete or partial. Both longitudinal and transverse fractures are seen, but profound loss is more often associated with transverse fractures.

KEY LEARNING POINTS

- Sensorineural hearing loss is a common disability of varying severity affecting all age groups.
- Prelingual speech and language acquisition are compromised, potentially severely.
- There are genetic and acquired causes, and both types can present in childhood or later life.
- All forms of inheritance are seen, and many new genetic defects are being discovered.
- SNHL may be seen in a variety of syndromic conditions.
- Some causes are preventable, while others require treatment with hearing aids.
- When severe enough, cochlear implantation may be appropriate.

FURTHER READING

Coles RR, et al. Guidelines on the diagnosis of noise-induced hearing loss for medicolegal purposes. *Clinical Otolaryngology and Allied Sciences*. 2000; 25(4): 264–73.

Bovo R, et al. The diagnosis of autoimmune inner ear disease: Evidence and critical pitfalls. *European Archives of Otorhinolaryngology*. 2009; 266(1): 37–40.

Graham JM, Baguley D. *Ballantyne's Deafness*. Chichester: Wiley-Blackwell, 2009.

Gray RF, Hawthorne M. *A Synopsis of Otolaryngology*. Oxford: Butterworth-Heinemann, 1992.

Luxon LM, et al. *Textbook of Audiological Medicine: Clinical Aspects of Hearing and Balance*. London: Martin Dunitz, 2003.

Marlow ES, et al. Sensorineural hearing loss and prematurity. *Archives of Disease in Childhood, Fetal and Neonatal Edition*. 2000; 82(2): F141–144.

Stew, BT, et al. Sudden sensorineural hearing loss. *British Journal of Hospital Medicine (London)*. 2012; 73(2): 86–89.

Smith RJH, et al. *Nonsyndromic Hearing Loss and Deafness, DFNA3*. In: *GeneReviews*. Eds. Pagon RA, Bird TD, Dolan CR, Stephens K, Adam MP. Seattle, WA: University of Washington, 1993.

48

Tinnitus

JULIAN A GASKIN, OWEN JUDD AND HENRY PAU

INTRODUCTION

The word *tinnitus* originates from the Latin *tinnire*, which means 'ring, jingle or clink'. Tinnitus can be categorized into subjective or objective. Subjective tinnitus can be described as a perception of sound in the absence of an external stimulus. Objective tinnitus (accounting for only 1 per cent of tinnitus presentations[1]) is a perception of sound caused by an internal stimulus, such as vascular abnormalities, especially if the tinnitus is described as pulsatile. Tinnitus affects around 15 per cent of the population,[2] but this percentage appears to be on the increase, with some reports nearer to 20 per cent. Theories for this include the increased use of headphones, particularly from a younger age, and an increased awareness about tinnitus and higher health expectations.[3]

PATHOPHYSIOLOGY

The pathophysiology of subjective tinnitus is unknown. However, there have been several theories, which include abnormalities with the subcortical auditory pathways, cochlear dysfunction and a genetic predisposition. Also, crossover with the auditory and other higher centre pathways has been postulated, involving pain, emotion and vision. The neurophysiological model described by Jastreboff[4] suggested a processing disorder in the auditory system was the likely cause of tinnitus. This occurs before the signal is perceived centrally. Persistence then ensues as a result of autonomic or emotional stimulation.

AETIOLOGY

There are several causes for tinnitus, which can be categorized initially into subjective and objective, and then subcategorized. The history and examination should be targeted towards eliciting any of the following aetiologies.

OBJECTIVE

- Vascular
  - Hypertension
  - Atherosclerosis
  - Arterial stenosis
  - Arteriovenous malformation (AVM)
  - High jugular bulb
  - Glomus tumours
  - Persistent stapedial artery
  - Benign intracranial hypertension
- Neuromuscular
  - Palatal myoclonus
  - Tensor tympani myoclonus
  - Stapedial myoclonus
- Other
  - Patulous eustachian tube
- Audible spontaneous otoacoustic emissions

SUBJECTIVE

- Otological
  - Hearing loss
  - Noise exposure
  - Barotraumas
  - Ménière's disease
  - Cerebellopontine angle (CPA) lesions (i.e. vestibular schwannoma, meningioma)
- Medication
  - Aminoglycosides
  - Nonsteroidal anti-inflammatory drugs (NSAIDs)
  - Cisplatin
  - Thiazide diuretics
  - Salicylates
  - Antihypertensives
- Psychological
  - Stress
  - Heightened emotion
  - Anxiety
  - Depression
- Neurological
  - Head injuries
  - Meningitis
  - Multiple sclerosis
  - Cerebellar pathology
- Metabolic
  - Diabetes mellitus
  - Hyper- and hypothyroidism
  - Hyperlipidemia
- Vitamin deficiency (A, B, zinc)

ASSESSMENT OF THE PATIENT

As tinnitus can often be variable in its presentation, a careful focused history is essential. This will allow differentiation between objective and subjective tinnitus, and direct further examination or investigation modalities.

FOCUSED HISTORY

The history from the patient is the most important first step in the management. After the patient clearly describes tinnitus as defined above, it is important to ask the patient to describe the sound if possible. Most patients can, and those with subjective tinnitus can usually be categorized as describing ringing, white noise, rushing, machinery or a pure tone. In objective tinnitus a pulsatile noise may be suggestive of an aberrant blood vessel or paraganglioma (i.e. glomus tympanicum or glomus jugulare), whereas a fluttering or thumping noise may be related to stapedial, tensor tympani or palatal myoclonus. Bilateral tinnitus is much more common and also more reassuring to the clinician than unilateral tinnitus, which may represent a vestibular schwannoma or other cerebellopontine angle lesion. It is important to ascertain whether the tinnitus is constant or intermittent. If intermittent, the duration and frequency of episodes should be identified along with any aggravating or relieving factors, helping to determine a potential cause. Tinnitus tends to be more intrusive in quiet environments and therefore worse at night, but this is not always the case for everyone.

The patient's occupation is important, especially if it relies on the patient using headsets or speaking in public. If this is the case, the patient may be unable to perform effectively at work, potentially creating further anxiety. A stressful job or period in someone's life where there is heightened emotion may also result in worsening tinnitus. Any vertiginous symptoms should be excluded. If present, further questioning should look into potential diagnoses of a vestibular schwannoma or Ménière's disease.

FURTHER HISTORY

The past medical history needs to include questioning on co-morbidities such as diabetes, meningitis or previous middle ear disease or surgery. Within the drug history, particular attention should be drawn to any known ototoxic medications or treatments received currently or in the past. These must include the use of NSAIDs, aminoglycosides, or chemotherapeutic agents (such as cisplatin). It can often be elicited that the onset of tinnitus can be linked with commencing certain medication. A family history of early hearing loss is important. Activities that could result in hearing loss, for example scuba diving and exposure to loud noise, should be included for a comprehensive history. Finally, it is vitally important to gauge the impact of the tinnitus on the patient's life. Any suicidal thoughts, albeit in rare circumstances, must prompt an urgent psychiatric opinion.

EXAMINATION

A full neuro-otological examination is required. This should involve inspection of the ears, particularly looking for any scars to suggest trauma or surgery. Any congenital abnormalities such as fistulae or skin tags could represent branchial arch abnormalities and may require further investigation. Otoscopy needs to assess again for any evidence of fistulae in the external auditory canal or otitis externa. The tympanic membrane should be assessed for perforation, myringosclerosis, middle ear effusion, vascular lesion or cholesteatoma. A free field hearing test and Rinne's and Weber's tuning fork tests will assess for hearing loss. A full cranial nerve examination completes the neuro-otological examination. In cases of pulsatile tinnitus, auscultation of the neck, temporal and mastoid regions is required to listen for bruits, which may indicate a vascular lesion.

INVESTIGATIONS

A pure tone audiogram (PTA) will confirm the presence and type of any hearing loss. Serum testing will be able to investigate for conditions of anaemia, diabetes, hyperthyroidism, hypothyroidism and hyperlipidaemia. Syphilis serology should be included as this is a rare cause of tinnitus. It has been reported that up to 10 per cent of patients with a vestibular schwannoma have unilateral tinnitus. A magnetic resonance imaging (MRI) scan of the internal auditory meati would be required to exclude this. In cases of pulsatile tinnitus, radiological imaging must be performed to exclude a vascular abnormality within the head and neck. This is most commonly done with MRI and magnetic resonance angiography (MRA). Raised serum and urine catecholamine levels are indicative of paragangliomas. For rhythmic, fluttering or thumping tinnitus, tympanometry and stapedial reflexes may be helpful to diagnose tensor tympani or stapedial myoclonus. This is done by using a tympanogram run over 30 seconds, at a single frequency, looking for rhythmic changes in impedance. Tinnitus matching, although not strictly an investigation for tinnitus, can be performed at the same time as the PTA. This may determine the intensity and frequency of the tinnitus and allow future planning of sound therapy in the form of masking.

MANAGEMENT

OBJECTIVE TINNITUS

In objective tinnitus the management revolves around the treatment of the underlying cause.

The patient's blood pressure should be screened, and if it is found to be elevated on three separate occasions, antihypertensive medication should be commenced in accordance with local health guidelines. This would improve tinnitus caused directly by hypertension but may also reduce the tinnitus from atherosclerosis, an arteriovenous malformation (AVM), a high jugular bulb, a glomus tumour or a persistent stapedial artery. If the tinnitus remains unchanged despite the controlled hypertension, these other vascular causes will need to be addressed. This may require vascular surgical input to treat artherosclerosis. Intracranial vascular pathology would need neurosurgical input or a neurological interventional radiologist to consider embolization. Glomus tumours and persistent stapedial arteries may require surgery. Benign intracranial hypertension often requires involvement from the neurosciences team.

Persistent tinnitus related to tensor tympani or stapedial myoclonus, refractory to conservative measures (such as avoidance of loud sounds), rarely requires surgical intervention. This would be in the form of sectioning of the affected tendon via a tympanotomy. Palatal myoclonus causing tinnitus may respond to simple relaxation techniques or muscle relaxant medication. A patulous or widely open eustachian tube has been described as a cause for tinnitus with associated autophony. At present there is no consensus on treatment for this.

SUBJECTIVE TINNITUS

Current management strategies of subjective tinnitus include psychological therapies, the use of hearing aids or masking devices and, less commonly, pharmaceutical treatments. Management should ideally be guided via a multidisciplinary setting, including otolaryngologists, audiovestibular physicians, audiologists, hearing therapists and psychologists. Patient support groups are often invaluable to many tinnitus sufferers.

Devices

When tinnitus is associated with a hearing loss, and conditions such as CPA lesions have been excluded, aiding the hearing is a commonly accepted treatment. This allows not only improvement of overall communication as a result of amplified hearing thresholds, but studies have shown relief of tinnitus in around 80 per cent of patients.[5] Traditionally, tinnitus masking devices have been thought to be useful because patients reported their tinnitus usually was less intrusive around noise. White noise generators were therefore used, sometimes in conjunction with hearing aids. However, a systematic review from 2009 concluded there was insufficient evidence to prove the effectiveness of tinnitus masking devices.[6] More accessible ways to mask tinnitus, often found within the home, include the use of a radio, television or fan to generate noise. In many cases this is the easiest and most successful way to distract the patients' focus from their tinnitus.

Psychological therapies

Within the remit of psychological therapies, tinnitus retraining therapy (TRT) is the most commonly used. This relies upon habituation to the tinnitus and involves a combination of counselling to reassure the patient as to the benign nature of the tinnitus with the use of a white noise generator. This was shown to be more effective than tinnitus masking alone.[7] In cases of severe intrusive tinnitus causing significant psychological distress, cognitive behaviour therapy (CBT) has been used. CBT addresses and aims to change distorted or negative beliefs surrounding tinnitus and has been shown to be effective.[8] Hypnosis or hypnotherapy has been used as an adjunctive treatment for tinnitus, and whilst not treating the tinnitus directly, it is thought that inducing a relaxed state of mind allows the tinnitus to become more manageable. There is insufficient evidence in the current literature to support the use of alternative therapies previously tried. These include the use of Ginkgo biloba, acupuncture and homeopathy, amongst others.

Surgical treatments

As the most common cause for subjective tinnitus is hearing loss, surgical treatment of certain forms of hearing loss have been shown to improve the tinnitus. In otospongiosis or otosclerosis there is a conductive or mixed hearing loss which is often associated with concurrent tinnitus in up to 80 per cent of patients.[9] Surgery for this condition involves a stapedotomy procedure by forming a fenestration in the stapes footplate. This has been shown to improve or in some cases abolish tinnitus in up to 90 per cent of patients.[10] This has often been related to an improvement in the post-operative hearing thresholds. However, improvements in tinnitus have also occurred after surgery for otosclerosis without improved hearing, and the exact mechanism for this is as yet unclear.[11]

Middle ear implants to improve conductive hearing loss are increasing in popularity. These newer techniques may have a positive influence on tinnitus. Cochlear implants are used in patients with profound sensorineural hearing loss, but those same patients with associated tinnitus have had improvement in their tinnitus symptoms. However, there are cases where cochlear implantation has been used as the treatment for patients with intractable tinnitus as their primary symptom, and it has been shown to be beneficial in 95 per cent of cases in a small study.[12] Microvascular decompression is a common treatment for trigeminal neuralgia caused by a vascular loop compressing the fifth cranial nerve. The technique has been used in patients with tinnitus found to have a vascular loop compressing the eighth cranial nerve. However, controversy surrounds this intervention as vascular loops have been incidental findings in asymptomatic patients.

Pharmaceutical therapies

When discussing pharmaceutical therapies, it is important to begin by highlighting the point that no medicines are currently approved specifically for the treatment of tinnitus. Although many studies have been undertaken to assess a wide range of pharmaceutical agents, numbers often remain small and it is difficult to determine a significant effect on the improvement or cure of tinnitus with these agents. The fact that so many therapies have been assessed bears testament that no one treatment has been found to be of significant benefit. Particular groups studied include glutamate receptor antagonists, gamma-amino butyric acid (GABA) receptor agonists and local anaesthetic agents.

GLUTAMATE RECEPTOR ANTAGONISTS

Glutamate is one of the most prevalent excitatory neurotransmitters, and over-expression of glutamate can lead to excess synaptic activity. This can result in the destruction of the glutamate receptors N-methyl-D-aspartate (NMDA) and has been thought to be a contributing factor to reduced hearing and tinnitus. For this reason, NMDA receptor antagonists, such as acamprosate and neramexane, have been trialled. One study of acamprosate in 2007 found a significant difference in the improvement of tinnitus over the control group,[13] but these results have never been replicated. A randomized double-blind control trial using neramexane was studied in 2011 and not found to have a significant difference in improving tinnitus.[14]

GABA RECEPTOR AGONISTS

GABA is one of the main inhibitory neurotransmitters in the central nervous system. It has been postulated that a reduction in GABA in the auditory system secondary to acoustic trauma may result in an increase in tinnitus.[15] Benzodiazepines, as GABA agonists, have been used and shown to be effective in up to 77 per cent of cases;[16] however, it would appear difficult to separate out its effects as an anxiolytic, and side effects, potential dependence and subsequent withdrawal effects must not be forgotten with this form of medication.

LOCAL ANAESTHETIC AGENTS

There have been several studies looking at the effects of local anaesthetic agents, which have shown variable results. A double-blinded randomized control trial using intravenous lidocaine revealed 40 per cent of subjects reported a decrease in their tinnitus, with 30 per cent reporting an increase after its administration.[17] However, the risk of cardiac complications with intravenous local anaesthetics must not be forgotten.

Other areas of pharmaceutical interest in the alleviation of tinnitus symptoms continue to be studied and include the use of tricyclic antidepressants, antiepileptics and lipoflavinoids.

EMERGING RESEARCH

Because of the relative lack of knowledge as to the exact cause of subjective tinnitus, coupled with the inability to find a consistent treatment, research into tinnitus remains active and varied. Areas of interest in the recent literature include the use of positron emission tomography (PET) to help identify a cause. This has suggested abnormalities in the auditory and also emotional processing regions of the brain. Further areas of research examine crossover of the auditory system with the somatosensory, limbic, motor and visual systems.

KEY DEFINITIONS

cognitive behavioural therapy (CBT) addresses and aims to change distorted or negative beliefs surrounding tinnitus

objective tinnitus a perception of sound caused by an internal stimulus

tinnitus originates from the Latin *tinnire*, which means 'ring, jingle or clink'; can be categorized into subjective or objective

tinnitus matching determines the intensity and frequency of the tinnitus and allows future planning of sound therapy in the form of masking

tinnitus retraining therapy (TRT) habituation to the tinnitus involving a combination of counselling with the use of a white noise generator

subjective tinnitus a perception of sound in the absence of an external stimulus

KEY LEARNING POINTS

- Tinnitus can be categorized into subjective or objective.
- A neuro-otological examination is required for all cases of tinnitus.
- Unilateral tinnitus has been shown to be the only presenting symptom of a vestibular schwannoma, and MRI imaging may wish to be considered.
- It is important to address the psychological impact the tinnitus may be having on the patient.
- The mainstay of management in subjective tinnitus remains sound therapy (such as aiding any underlying hearing loss) and psychological therapy (such as TRT or CBT).

REFERENCES

1. Folmer RL, Hal Martin W, Shi Y. Tinnitus: Questions to reveal the cause, answers to provide relief. *Journal of Family Practice.* 2004; 53(7): 532–40.
2. Coles RR. Epidemiology of tinnitus: (1) Prevalence and (2) Demographic and clinical features. *Journal of Laryngology and Otology Supplement.* 1984; (9): 7–15, 195–202.
3. Nondahl DM, Cruickshanks KJ, Huang GH, Klein BE, Klein R, Tweed TS, Zhan W. Generational differences in the reporting of tinnitus. *Ear and Hearing.* 2012; 33(5): 640–44.
4. Jastreboff PJ, Hazell JWP. A neurophysiological approach to tinnitus: Clinical implications. *British Journal of Audiology.* 1993; 27(1): 7–17.
5. Kochkin S, Tyler R. Tinnitus treatment and the effectiveness of hearing aids: Hearing care professional perceptions. *Hearing Review.* 2008; 15(13): 14–18.
6. Savage J, Cook S, Waddell A. *Tinnitus.* In: *BMJ Clinical Evidence.* London: BMJ Publishing Group, 2009.
7. Henry J, Schechter M, Zaugg T, Griest S, Jastreboff P, Vernon J, Kaelin C, Meikle M, Lyons K, Stewart B. Clinical trial to compare tinnitus masking and tinnitus retraining therapy. *Acta Otolaryngologica Suppl.* 2006; (566): 64–69.
8. Andersson G, Stromgren T, Strom L, Lyttkens L. Randomised controlled trial of Internet-based cognitive behavioural therapy for distress associated with tinnitus. *Psychosomatic Medicine.* 2002; 64(5): 810–16.

9. Cawthorne T. Otosclerosis. *Journal of Laryngology and Otology.* 1955; 69(7): 437–56.
10. Oliveira CA. How does stapes surgery influence severe disabling tinnitus in otosclerosis patients? *Advances in Otorhinolaryngology.* 2007; 65: 343–47.
11. Szymański M, Golabek W, Mills R. Effect of stapedectomy on subjective tinnitus. *Journal of Laryngology and Otology.* 2003; 117(4): 261–4.
12. Van de Heyning P, Vermeire K, Dieb IM, Nopp P, Anderson I, DeRidder D. Incapacitating unilateral tinnitus in single-sided deafness treated by cochlear implantation. *Annals of Otology, Rhinology and Laryngology.* 2008; 117(9): 645–52.
13. Azevedo AA, Figueiredo RR. Treatment of tinnitus with acamprosate: Double-blind study. *Brazilian Journal of Otorhinolaryngology.* 2005; 71(5): 618–23.
14. Suckfüll M, Althaus M, Ellers-Lenz B, Gebauer A, Görtelmeyer R, Jastreboff PJ, Moebius HJ, Rosenberg T, Russ H, Wirth Y, Krueger H. A randomized, double-blind, placebo-controlled clinical trial to evaluate the efficacy and safety of neramexane in patients with moderate to severe subjective tinnitus. *BMC Ear Nose and Throat Disorders.* 2011; 11: 1.
15. Dong S, Mulders WH, Rodgers J Woo S, Robertson D. Acoustic trauma evokes hyperactivity and changes in gene expression in guinea-pig auditory brainstem. *European Journal of Neuroscience.* 2010; 31(9): 1616–28.
16. Johnson RM, Brummett R, Schleuning A. Use of alprazolam for relief of tinnitus. A double-blind study. *Archives of Otolaryngology – Head and Neck Surgery.* 1993; 119(8): 842–45.
17. Duckert LG, Rees TS. Treatment of tinnitus using intravenous lidocaine: A double-blind randomized trial. *Otolaryngology – Head and Neck Surgery.* 1983; 91(5): 550–55.

FURTHER READING

Ceranic B, Luxon LM. *Tinnitus and Other Dysacuses* (Chapter 238f). In: *Scott-Brown's Otorhinolaryngology, Head and Neck Surgery.* 7th ed., Volume 3. Ed. Browning GG. London: Hodder Arnold, 2008: 3594–3628.

Pasha R. *Otolaryngology Head and Neck Surgery – Clinical Reference Guide.* 3rd ed. San Diego: Plural Publishing, 2011.

Roland NJ, McRae RDR, McCombe AW. *Key Topics in Otolaryngology.* 2nd ed. London: Taylor & Francis, 2005.

Warner G, Burgess A, Patel S, Martinez-Devesa P, Corbridge R. *Oxford Specialist Handbook in Surgery – Otolaryngology and Head and Neck Surgery.* Oxford: Oxford University Press, 2009.

49

Disorders of balance

RAHUL KANEGAONKAR

INTRODUCTION

Dizziness and vertigo are common symptoms. Epidemiological studies have shown that vertigo and balance disorders affect 30 per cent of the general population before the age of 65 years, rising to 60 per cent at 85 years.[1] Annually, five out of every thousand patients present to their general practitioner complaining of symptoms classified as vertigo, with another 10 per thousand with symptoms of dizziness or giddiness. In the elderly a balance disorder may result in a fall, a leading cause of death in this age group.

Irrespective of age, a separate but relevant issue is that of the adverse psychological impact of those with a balance disorder.[2] Two-thirds of patients develop psychiatric disturbances, including depression and anxiety. These clearly limit social and occupational activities and may lead to chronic invalidism, which in turn may lead to a worsening of the vertiginous symptoms experienced.

THE BALANCE SYSTEM: AN OVERVIEW

Normal balance function relies on sensory information from the visual, peripheral vestibular and somatosensory systems, as well as hearing. This sensory information is integrated, modulated and 'interpreted' within the central nervous system to enable gaze stabilization and postural control and provide information regarding self- and environmental movement (Figure 49.1). 'Interpretation' requires comparing relayed sensory information with preformed templates within the central nervous system. Absence of a suitable template, or a mismatch between the two, results in symptoms of dizziness, vertigo or unsteadiness.

The relative importance of the sensory information used is likely to vary depending on one's environment. Over-reliance on one particular sensory input may result in disequilibrium and dizziness even in normal subjects (e.g. vision in subjects with motion sickness).

In general, a unilateral static deficit affecting one sensory input may through central compensation result in little or no functional deficit, but abnormalities in more than one sensory input or concomitant central pathology may lead to profound and debilitating vertigo and dizziness. Hence, the assessment of the vertiginous patient requires a thorough general clinical assessment supplemented with audiovestibular tests and radiological imaging. As symptoms are often due to peripheral vestibular pathology, particular

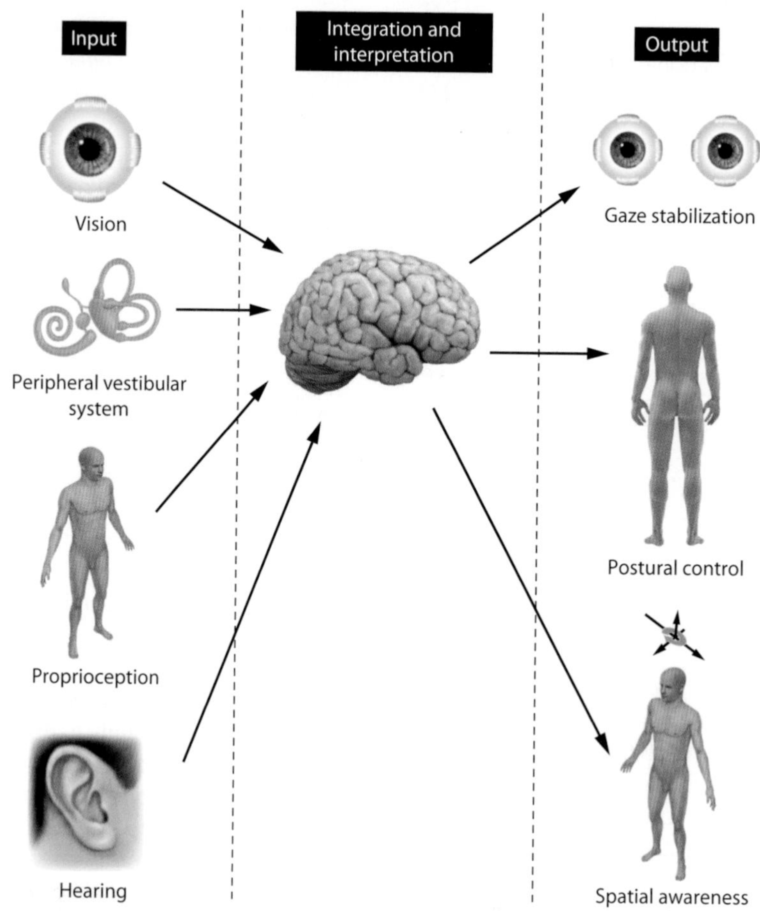

Figure 49.1 Overview of the balance system illustrating the pathway of input from the visual, balance and auditory senses, which are processed to maintain postural control and vision and spatial awareness.

emphasis should be placed on the assessment of this sensory pathway.

PERIPHERAL VESTIBULAR SYSTEM

The peripheral vestibular system consists of five confluent chambers. The maculae of the utricle and saccule are responsible for detecting linear acceleration and static head tilt (horizontal and vertical, respectively), and the lateral semicircular canals for angular head acceleration (Figures 49.2 to 49.4).

The neuroepithelium of the maculae of the utricle and saccule consist of elaborately arranged hair cells that project into a fibro-calcareous plate, the otoconial membrane. As this membrane is denser than the surrounding endolymph, head movement results in hair cell deflection and depolarization.

The neuroepithelium of the semicircular canals is limited to a crest within the dilated segment, the ampulla. Hair cells project into a gelatinous mass, the cupula, which is deflected as a result of head rotation. This results in an increased firing rate in one semicircular canal and a reduced firing rate of the same semicircular canal on the contralateral side. This allows gaze stabilization on head

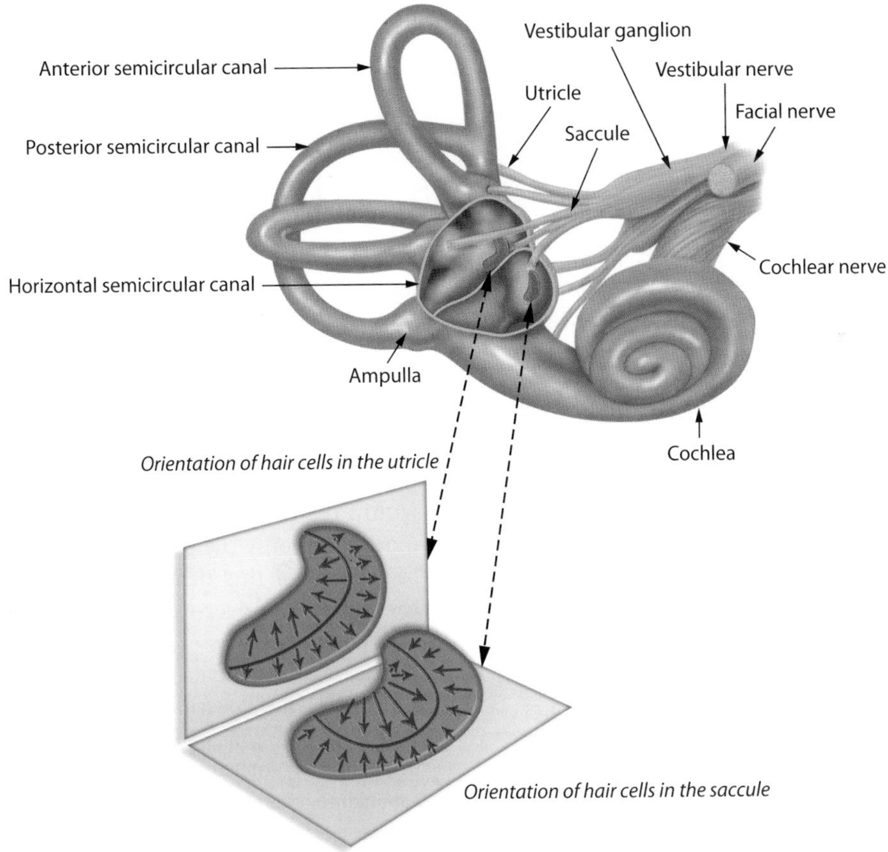

Figure 49.2 The membranous labyrinth. The maculae of the saccule and utricle are orientated at 90° to each other to detect vertical and horizontal movement. Hair cells are arranged around a curvilinear depression of the otoconial membrane, the striola. Arrows indicate the direction of maximal stimulation for both neuroepithelial regions.

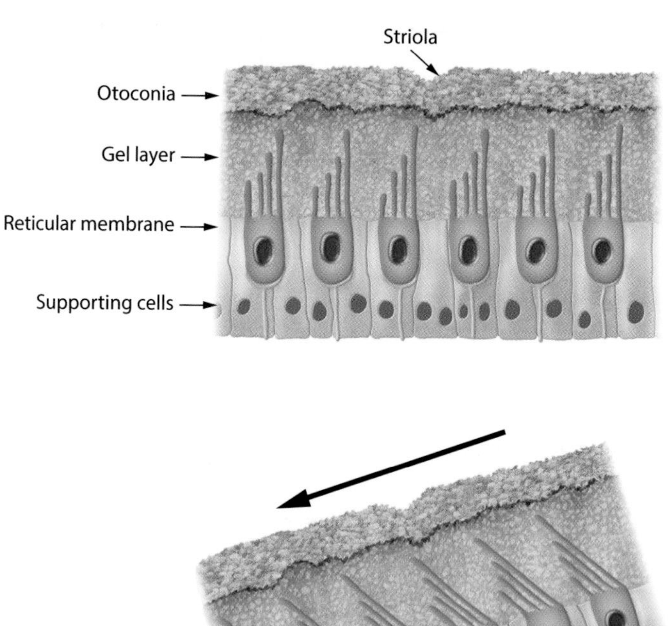

Figure 49.3 The otoconial membrane. Static head position and movement result in a relative movement of the comparatively denser otoconial membrane (2.7 c.f. endolymph). Deflection of the stereocilia results in depolarization of the hair cells.

rotation and is the basis of the vestibulo-ocular reflex illustrated in Figure 49.4.

BENIGN PAROXYSMAL POSITIONAL VERTIGO

HISTORY AND CLINICAL EXAMINATION

Benign paroxysmal positional vertigo (BPPV) is characterized by brief intense bouts of rotatory vertigo associated with nausea and vomiting. With a lifetime prevalence of 2.4 per cent, this is the most common cause of vertigo.[3] The posterior canal is involved in the majority of cases (85–95 per cent) with the lateral canal affected in 5–15 per cent. The superior canal is rarely involved.

Otoconial debris from the degenerating uricular macula is thought to be responsible. When prone, these calcium carbonate crystals settle within the most dependent part of the inner ear, most commonly the posterior semicircular canal. Movement of this debris results in deflection of the cupula with over-excitation of the semicircular canal hair cells.

Classically, patients wake and on rolling out of bed experience severe rotatory vertigo. Although this lasts seconds, patients are left with marked unsteadiness for several hours thereafter. There is associated nausea and vomiting, but no hearing loss nor tinnitus. Some may also experience diarrhoea. For most, this is an extremely frightening experience with many patients fearing they are suffering a 'stroke'. A tumbling or rolling vertigo may also be experienced when looking down or up suddenly ('top shelf syndrome'). As a result

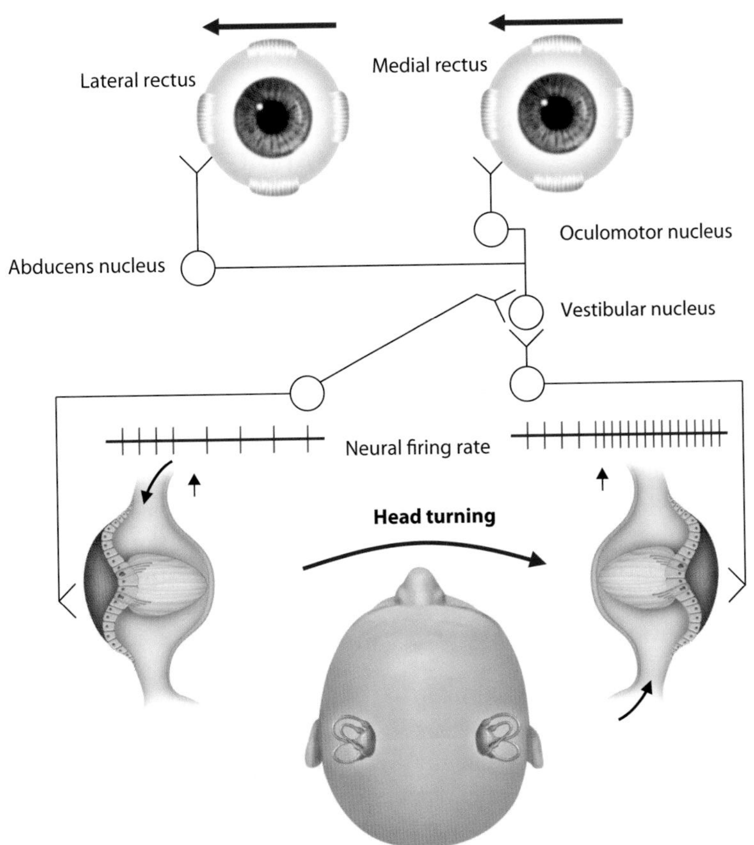

Figure 49.4 The vestibulo-ocular reflex. As a result of head rotation, endolymph flow within the semicircular canals causes movement of the cupulae within the ampullae of the lateral semicircular canals and relative shearing of the underlying stereocilia. Neural impulses increase on the right and decrease on the left. Neural connections to the third and sixth cranial nuclei result in contraction of the left lateral rectus and right medial rectus stabilizing gaze (↑ = start of head rotation).

patients are cautious when moving, in particular when rising or rolling over in bed when waking.

A Dix–Hallpike manoeuvre is used to confirm a diagnosis, with posterior canal BPPV resulting in a short latency followed by geotropic torsional nystagmus that completely settles. Lateral canal BPPV produces a rapid, intense high-frequency nystagmus that abates completely. Persistent, vertical, or direction-changing nystagmus is, however, in keeping with central pathology, and these patients require urgent magnetic resonance imaging (MRI).

INVESTIGATIONS

A thorough neuro-otological examination is required to exclude concomitant pathology. A pure tone audiogram should be performed, but no additional investigations are required.

MANAGEMENT

Treatment involves moving the otoconial debris into the utricle where it is believed to be reabsorbed. Manoeuvres to address posterior canal BPPV include the Epley, Semont and Brandt-Daroff exercises. Each has its merits, with the Semont and Brandt-Daroff particle positioning manoeuvres performed by patients at home. The Epley manoeuvre is immediately curative in more than 85 per cent of patients, but recurrence is common within the first year. A barbeque roll may be used to treat lateral canal BPPV.

Rarely, surgical intervention may be required in those with recurrent or unresponsive particle repositioning manoeuvres. Procedures used include posterior canal plugging, gentamicin ablation and surgical labyrinthectomy.

ACUTE PERIPHERAL VESTIBULAR LOSS

HISTORY AND CLINICAL EXAMINATION

There are various terms used to describe acute peripheral vestibular loss (APVL). These include *vestibular neuritis*, *vestibular neuronitis* and *labyrinthitis*. Although these terms are used interchangeably, the term *labyrinthitis* should be reserved for cases where there is simultaneous vestibular and sensorineural hearing loss.

An abrupt peripheral vestibular loss results in profound continuous and severe rotatory vertigo. Nausea and vomiting are common, and frequently patients are bed bound for several days after the initial insult. Any movement will result in worsening of symptoms.

Signs include horizontal ocular nystagmus with the slow component towards the affected ear and skew deviation of the eye towards the affected ear in the initial phase.

The cause of APVL remains obscure, although both viral and vascular causes have been suggested.[4] The superior vestibular nerve pathway is generally affected with relative sparing of the inferior vestibular nerve pathway.

A full neuro-otological examination is required to exclude central pathology and ear microscopy to exclude chronic suppurative middle ear disease. Nystagmus is present in the initial phase and patients are markedly unsteady. Central compensation allows patients to gradually mobilize. Unterberger testing may demonstrate rotation towards the affected side, and a head thrust test may show catch-up saccades.

INVESTIGATIONS

Full audiovestibular testing is required. An isolated vestibular loss will result in a caloric confirmed unilateral canal paresis, whilst true labyrinthitis results in a concomitant sensorineural hearing loss.

MANAGEMENT

The initial vestibular loss is managed with prochlorperazine, but the use of this peripheral vestibular sedative should be limited to 7 days. Prolonged use hinders central compensatory pathways and slows rehabilitation.

Whilst some patients recover fully without intervention, many continue to complain of disequilibrium on rapid head movement. Some develop imbalance when presented with visually rich patterns or crowds owing to an over-dependence on visual information (*visual vertigo*).

Mainstay treatment is customized vestibular rehabilitation that has replaced the generic exercises previously recommended (e.g. Cawthorne-Cooksey exercises). This physiotherapy-led intervention involves encouraging patients to undertake increasingly more difficult exercises to promote central compensation, often in a group setting. Visual vertigo may be treated by simultaneously presenting subjects with a visually rich environment (e.g. projected moving dots on a screen). Any associated psychological complications should also be addressed.

VESTIBULAR MIGRAINE

HISTORY AND CLINICAL EXAMINATION

Vestibular, or vertiginous migraine, accounts for approximately one-third of patients presenting to a tertiary referral balance service. Although the aetiology of this condition remains obscure, symptoms are likely to be due either to a rapid change in blood flow within certain territories of the brain or to a spreading wave of hyper-excitability.

Patients classically present in their late 30s and 40s. Women generally describe an initial 2- to 3-day spell of vertigo and marked disequilibrium that then settles completely. Subsequent spells are less intrusive, lasting 1 to 2 days. There is no associated hearing loss, nor tinnitus, but patients often describe photophobia and phonophobia. Most will rest in a dark, quiet room. In women, spells occur just prior to their periods.

In men symptoms are insidious, and most patients complain of a pervasive sense of disequilibrium. There is often a family or personal history of migraine.

Clinical examination is entirely unremarkable.

INVESTIGATIONS

Vestibular migraine is a diagnosis of exclusion, and full audiovestibular testing and MRI of the brain are required to exclude any central pathology.

MANAGEMENT

Initial treatment requires removal of classic dietary migraine triggers such as chocolate, cheese, caffeine, red wine, bananas, citrus fruits and processed meats. Should symptoms persist, serotonin 5HT agonists (triptans) may be used for acute spells and beta blockers, sodium valproate, topiramate and tricyclic antidepressants such as amitryptiline and pizotifen as prophylactic medication. Those who fail to settle may benefit from a neurology referral.

MÉNIÈRE'S DISEASE

HISTORY AND CLINICAL EXAMINATION

Ménière's disease is a relatively uncommon cause of vertigo, with an estimated incidence of 5 per 100000 per year. Patients experience spontaneous, unpredictable bouts of severe rotatory vertigo. Episodes are often preceded by aural fullness in the affected ear and associated with hearing loss and roaring tinnitus.

Although the exact aetiology is uncertain, postmortem studies have demonstrated expansion of the scala media compartment of the inner ear. Symptoms are thought to arise owing to either rupture of Reissner's membrane and toxic overstimulation of the neuroepithelial elements of the inner ear, or an abnormality in endolymph drainage, with longitudinal drainage of endolymph to the endolymphatic sac hindered. Once a critical level is reached, endolymph drains into the utricle, stretching the cristae of the semicircular canals and resulting in profound vertigo.

INVESTIGATIONS

Serial pure tone audiograms demonstrating a fluctuating sensorineural hearing loss (initially in the low frequencies) in the affected ear is characteristic of this condition. Caloric testing will reveal a peripheral vestibular deficit as the disease process progresses. Electrocochleography may demonstrate an increase in the ratio between the amplitudes of the summating and action potentials.

An MRI of the internal auditory meatii is required to exclude central pathology (e.g. a vestibular schwannoma).

MANAGEMENT

Management is influenced by the level of hearing and vestibular function in the affected and non-symptomatic ear. Destructive treatments should be undertaken with caution as Ménière's disease may affect both inner ears in approximately 50 per cent of patients.

Medical

Medical treatment in the form of lifestyle changes (e.g. adopting a low-salt diet; avoiding alcohol, caffeine and stress) and medication is effective in controlling vertigo in approximately 85 per cent of patients.

Medication includes betahistine, which has no proven benefit but is thought to prevent symptoms by vasodilatation in the inner ear. The drug is harmless. Thiazide diuretics, thought to reduce the volume of the endolymph compartment, and antiemetic agents such as prochlorperazine are prescribed for acute spells.

Surgery

If first-line treatments fail to control the attacks, surgery may be appropriate. If functional hearing exists in the affected ear, grommet insertion in isolation or combined with the Meniett device may be appropriate. The evidence base is poor for both these procedures. The device has been approved by the National Institute for Health and Care Excellence (NICE) for monitored usage.

Endolymphatic sac decompression has been used in the management of Ménière's disease for many years. This is achieved via a cortical mastoidectomy, exposure of the posterior fossa dura and incision of the sac and/or insertion of a silastic tube. This has been a controversial procedure but has proponents, and indeed patients, who find it helpful.

Ablative treatments should be reserved for those cases failing to respond to conservative surgical measures. Gentamicin ablation has been popularized recently and involves injecting gentamicin into the middle ear until symptoms resolve. Usually, one injection is sufficient; a small percentage may require two, and rarely three injections are needed. If used judiciously, hearing is preserved, though a small risk of hearing loss is well recognized. The use of steroid injection into the middle ear has been gaining momentum, but there is a paucity of evidence for this. Surgical labyrinthectomy (removal of all vestibular neuro-epithelium) or vestibular nerve section is reserved for those with intractable vertigo.

Customized vestibular physiotherapy

The vestibular hypofunction associated with Ménière's disease results in episodic dysequilibrium. Periods of decompensation may be misinterpreted as further attacks and should be distinguished by taking a careful history. Hence, vestibular rehabilitation is also of benefit.

SUPERIOR SEMICIRCULAR CANAL DEHISCENCE

HISTORY AND CLINICAL EXAMINATION

Superior semicircular canal dehiscence syndrome was first described by Llyod Minor and colleagues in 1998.[5] It is a rare condition characterized by bony dehiscence of the superior semicircular canal. As a result, this third window allows pressure transmission into the inner ear from the middle cranial fossa, resulting in dizziness, and an apparent conductive hearing loss because sound pressure energy is diverted through a path of lesser resistance.

Sound-induced vertigo (Tullio's phenomenon) is a common complaint due to stapes footplate movement following activation of the stapes reflex. This results in a pressure wave through the inner ear. Momentary vertigo may also be triggered by pressure changes (e.g. when straining). Patients often describe autophony (e.g. joint and eye movement, pulsatile tinnitus) and oscillopsia.

Microscopy is unremarkable, whilst pneumatic otoscopy or tragal pressure may elicit nystagmus (Hennebert's sign). Tuning fork testing may suggest a conductive hearing loss in the affected ear.

INVESTIGATIONS

A pure tone audiogram typically suggests an apparent conductive hearing loss. Stapedial reflex testing, although normal, may elicit an episode of disequilibrium.

A significant amplitude asymmetry on vestibular-evoked myogenic potential testing may also be suggestive of a superior semicircular canal dehiscence.

A high-resolution computed tomography (CT) scan of the temporal bones is the radiological imaging of choice, although a dehiscence may be apparent on T2-weighted fast spin echo MRI imaging of the inner ear structures.

MANAGEMENT

Most patients can be managed through education and avoidance of triggers. The minority suffer significant symptoms and benefit from surgical intervention. A middle fossa approach and resurfacing with fascia, bone or cartilage may be undertaken, although a transmastoid approach with blue lining of the anterior and posterior limbs of the superior semicircular canal and subsequent plugging is preferred by some surgeons.[6] Irrespective of the approach used, vestibular physiotherapy is indicated post-operatively owing to the inevitable imbalance experienced.

VESTIBULAR SCHWANNOMA

HISTORY AND CLINICAL EXAMINATION

Vestibular schwannomas are benign tumours. With an estimated incidence of 1 in 100 000, they are a rare cause of vertigo and dizziness. More than 90 per cent are unilateral and sporadic, most commonly arising from the superior vestibular nerve. Bilateral schwannomas are associated with neurofibromatosis type 2 (NF2), owing to an autosomal dominant mutation of the NF2 tumour suppressor gene.

The most common presentation is that of a hearing loss that may be associated with a general sense of imbalance. Rotation towards the affected ear may be apparent on Unterberger testing.

INVESTIGATIONS

An asymmetric sensorineural hearing loss on pure tone audiometry should raise the suspicion of an underlying vestibular schwannoma. Prior to MRI, auditory brain stem reflexes were used as an aid in making a diagnosis (an increased wave V latency suggestive of a cerebellopontine lesion), but imaging has superseded this audiological investigation.

MANAGEMENT

The majority of patients are often initially managed conservatively, with serial imaging to assess the rate of growth of the tumour. Surgical intervention or stereotactic radiotherapy is reserved for tumours that continue to enlarge. Vestibular rehabilitation exercises are of benefit in those with static lesions or in the post-operative period following surgical excision.

PERILYMPH FISTULA

HISTORY AND CLINICAL EXAMINATION

Perilymph fistulae are rare. They represent an abnormal communication between the perilymph of the inner ear and spaces surrounding the otic capsule. Frequently misdiagnosed, acquired fistulae most commonly arise as a result of barotrauma, penetrating or blunt head trauma, or rapid changes in intracranial pressure. An iatrogenic fistula may occur following ear surgery for chronic ear disease or stapedectomy. Presentation is variable, with most patients describing fluctuating audiovestibular symptoms, including vertigo. Nystagmus may be evident on pneumatic otoscopy in 25 per cent of patients.

INVESTIGATIONS

A pure tone audiogram is mandatory and may demonstrate a fluctuating sensorineural hearing loss. Imaging is of limited value, although a pneumolabyrinth may be seen.

MANAGEMENT

In the acute setting, conservative measures such as bed rest and head elevation are appropriate. Surgical exploration or injection of either autologous blood or fibrin glue into the middle ear is reserved for those with persistent symptoms.[7,8]

KEY LEARNING POINTS

- Vertigo and dizziness are common symptoms.
- Assessment of the dizzy patient requires a thorough neuro-otological assessment supported by specialist vestibular investigations.
- In those with an acute peripheral vestibular loss, the use of proclorperazine should be limited to 1 week.

- Customized vestibular physiotherapy is of benefit in many patients with vestibular asymmetry.

REFERENCES

1. Shepard NT, Telian SA. *Balance Disorder Patient*. In: *Basic Anatomy and Physiology Review*. San Diego: Singular Publishing Group, Inc., 1996: 1–16.
2. McKenna L, Hallam RS, Hinchcliffe R. 1991. The prevalence of psychological disturbance in neuro-otology outpatients. *Clinical Otolaryngology*. 1991; 16, 452–56.
3. Fife TD. *Benign paroxysmal positional vertigo*. In: *Seminars in Neurology*. 2009; 29(5): 500–8.
4. De Ciccio M, Fattori B, Carpi A, Casani A, Ghilardi P, Sagripanti A. Vestibular disorders in primary thrombocytosis. *Journal of Otolaryngology*. 1999; 28(6): 318–24.
5. Minor LB, Solomon D, Zinreich JS, et al. Sound- and/or pressure-induced vertigo due to bone dehiscence of the superior semicircular canal. *Archives of Otolaryngology – Head and Neck Surgery*. 1998; 124: 249–58.
6. Agrawal SK, Parnes LS. Transmastoid superior semicircular canal occlusion. *Otology and Neurotology*. 2008; 29(3): 363–67.
7. Shinohara T, Gyo K, Murakami S, Yanagihara N. Blood patch therapy of the perilymphatic fistulas – An experimental study. *Nihon Jibiinkoka Gakkai kaiho*. 1996; 99: 1104–9.
8. Garg R, Djalilian HR. Intratympanic injection of autologous blood for traumatic perilymphatic fistulas. *Otolaryngology – Head and Neck Surgery*. 2009; 141: 294–95.

FURTHER READING

Kanegaonkar R, Tysome J (eds.). *Vertigo and Dizziness: An Introduction and Practical Guide*. Boca Raton, FL: CRC Press, 2013.

50

Cerebellopontine angle tumours

CHRISTOPHER J SKILBECK AND SHAKEEL R SAEED

INTRODUCTION

Tumours of the cerebellopontine angle (CPA) account for approximately 10 per cent of all intracranial tumours. Of these, the majority (80 per cent) are vestibular schwannomas. The remainder comprise tumours originating from the structures within the CPA, embryological remnants, lesions extending from the brain and skull base, and metastatic deposits.

ANATOMY

The cerebellopontine angle is defined as a space within the posterior fossa of the cranial cavity, immediately medial to the petrous temporal bone (Figure 50.1). It serves as a potential space, usually only containing cerebrospinal fluid (CSF), cranial nerves, blood vessels and their associated arachnoid layer. Medial to this space lies the brain stem, posteriorly and laterally the cerebellum, and

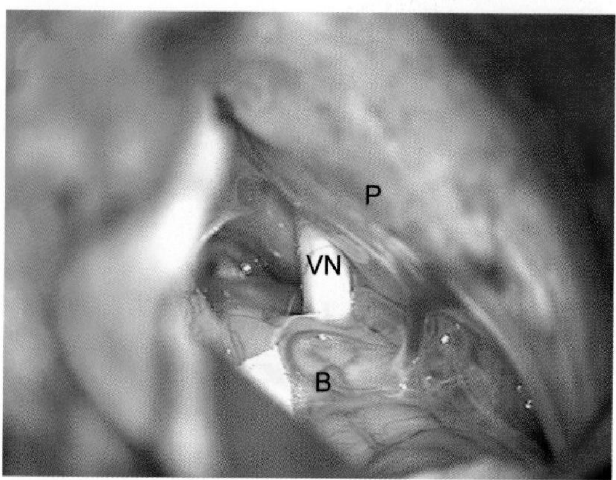

Figure 50.1 View of the right cerebellopontine angle viewed through a retrosigmoid approach for a vestibular neurectomy. The superior and inferior vestibular nerves (VN) are shown entering the porus acousticus. The brain stem (B) and posterior petrous ridge (P) are labelled.

anteriorly the petrous apex. The tentorium cerebelli forms the roof. Cranial nerves originating from the pons, the ponto-medullary junction and medulla traverse the CPA. The trigeminal (V) runs anterosuperiorly whilst the lower cranial nerves, glossopharyngeal (IX), vagus (X) and accessory (XI), are located postero-inferiorly. The facial (VII) and vestibulocochlear (VIII) nerves lie together in the centre of the CPA entering the temporal bone via the internal auditory canal (IAC) at the porus acousticus. The major vascular supply of the CPA is derived from the antero-inferior cerebellar artery (AICA), which is a branch of the basilar artery. The labyrinthine artery (a branch of the AICA) is an end artery, and therefore occlusion of this vessel is likely to result in audiovestibular dysfunction, with sensorineural hearing loss, tinnitus, vertigo with nausea and vomiting.

SYMPTOMS OF CEREBELLOPONTINE ANGLE TUMOURS

Patients with cerebellopontine angle tumours may present with minor and irritating symptoms when the tumour is small with slow progression as the tumour grows. Even moderately large tumours may only give rise to unilateral tinnitus. This is due to the space available to accommodate the growing tumour. However, once the tumour begins to significantly indent the brain stem and cerebellum, the constellation of symptoms it may produce increases. The so-called CPA syndrome comprises tinnitus, sensorineural hearing loss, facial sensory loss and lower motor neurone facial weakness, ataxia, speech and swallowing problems and, finally, symptoms and signs of raised intracranial pressure leading to death if untreated.

IMAGING THE CEREBELLOPONTINE ANGLE

Both computed tomography (CT) and magnetic resonance imaging (MRI) are of value when investigating the skull base patient. Although lesions of the CPA are diagnosed by their MRI characteristics, CT scans are contributory, particularly when considering surgery (Table 50.1).

Table 50.1 Imaging characteristics of CPA lesions

Lesion	T1 appearance	T2 appearance	Defining features
Vestibular schwannoma	Low	Low	Enhances
Meningioma	Intermediate	Intermediate	Durally based with 'tail'
Epidermoid cyst	Low	High	Diffusion-weighted MRI helpful
Cholesterol granuloma	High	High	
Paraganglioma	Intermediate	Intermediate	'Salt and pepper', avid enhancement
Lipoma	High	Low	No enhancement
Arachnoid cyst	Low	High	Isointense to CSF

VESTIBULAR SCHWANNOMAS

These tumours are commonly termed *acoustic neuromas*, an inappropriate term as they are schwannomas originating from the sheath of one of the two vestibular nerves rather than the neuronal tissue itself. They are benign and usually slow-growing, although the growth rate is unpredictable and can occur at any time. Vestibular schwannomas (VS) arise in the medial internal auditory canal where their growth is restricted by the bony limits of the canal. They develop at the site of the transition zone from central to peripheral myelin. As progressive growth ensues, the tumour enlarges medially along the canal, eventually reaching the opening into the CPA – the porus acousticus. Once growing in the CPA, the tumour can enlarge freely without restriction. At this point the facial nerve is stretched over the anterosuperior surface of the tumour and is often thinned. Further growth results in the tumour touching the brain stem, which begins to be displaced by the mass (Figure 50.2). As the brain stem is compressed, the fourth ventricle can become obstructed and hydrocephalus develops.

The incidence of VS is quoted as 2 in 100 000 per year, apparently increasing. However, it is clear that many tumours went undiagnosed before widespread access to high-resolution MRI. In this same period the average size of tumours at the time of diagnosis has been reducing.

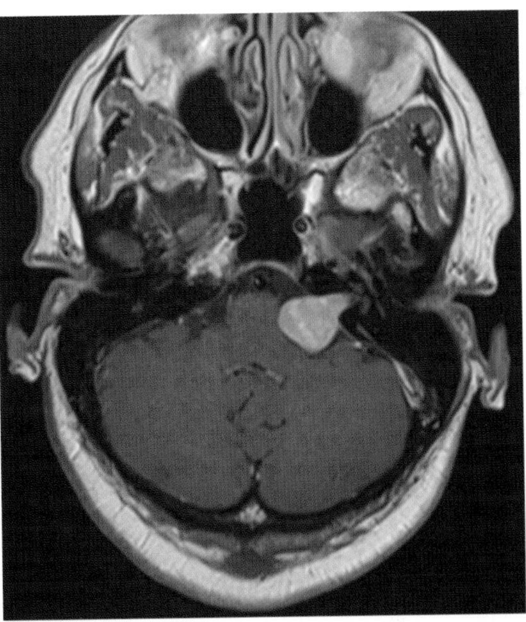

Figure 50.2 Contrast enhanced axial T1-weighted MRI scan of a left vestibular schwannoma. There is evidence of widening of the porus and compression of the brain stem.

PATHOPHYSIOLOGY AND NEUROFIBROMATOSIS TYPE 2

The majority of vestibular schwannomas arise *de novo* from a mutation in the merlin gene on chromosome 22q. The same genetic defect occurs in families with neurofibromatosis type 2 (NF2), which is inherited in an autosomal dominant fashion. In the sporadic form the schwannoma typically develops in middle age, whereas in NF2 the patient will invariably present with his or her first tumour by the age of 20. Although the genetic defect is now known, the diagnostic criteria for diagnosis of NF2 should be fulfilled. Defining features are bilateral VS, unilateral VS with a positive family history, unilateral VS and two other tumours (e.g. meningioma, glioma, neurofibroma, schwannoma). Tumours commonly affect the spine; these are often asymptomatic and should be treated only when and if they become symptomatic.

SIZE AND GROWTH

Approximately 60 per cent of vestibular schwannomas do not grow from the time of diagnosis. Of those that do grow, the rate of growth is slow and has been shown to be at approximately 2 mm per year. When measuring the size of a VS, it is conventional to disregard the intracanalicular portion of the tumour to give consistent and reproducible data collection. The maximal intracranial tumour diameter is measured in the axial plane (Table 50.2).

PRESENTING SYMPTOMS

The most common symptoms at presentation include unilateral or asymmetric hearing loss and

Table 50.2 Classification of tumour size by maximal intracranial tumour diameter

	Size in mm
Small	1–10
Medium	11–20
Moderate	21–30
Large	31–40
Giant	>40

tinnitus. The majority of patients will also have experienced vertigo, though this is usually not persistent. Owing to the slow progression of the tumours, there is likely central compensation, meaning that the patient will often not appreciate his or her deterioration in balance. The hearing loss is likely to affect the high frequencies, and on speech audiometry the patient demonstrates the 'rollover' phenomenon. Approximately 5 per cent of patients will have a sudden deterioration in their hearing.

Later symptoms include those due to facial and trigeminal nerve compression. The corneal reflex may be diminished before the patient notices any sensory loss. Facial weakness is relatively rare, although we know that up to 90 per cent of facial neurones can be non-functioning owing to compression, whilst the facial function is clinically normal.

INVESTIGATION

Historically, a multitude of audiological tests and imaging with ventriculography (insertion of air into the subdural space) were required to characterize CPA tumours. Thankfully, for the patients, unilateral audiovestibular symptoms and asymmetry on pure-tone audiometry should alert the physician to order a high-resolution MRI of the internal auditory meati. The initial sequence should include a heavily T2-weighted scan. In addition, pre- and post-gadolinium enhanced T1 sequences should help differentiate between other causes of CPA symptoms.

MANAGEMENT

The management of vestibular schwannomas relies on working within a multidisciplinary team (MDT). The core team comprises doctors from radiology; ear, nose and throat (ENT); oncology and neurosurgery as well as clinical nurse specialists. In addition, contributions from allied specialists, including those from audiology and physiotherapy, is important in making decisions regarding which of the three management options is most appropriate for the patient.

Conservative

The majority of small to moderate tumours can be managed conservatively with no risk of significant harm to the patient. Conservative management entails regular imaging with gadolinium-enhanced MRI of the internal auditory meati and cerebellopontine angle. It also relies upon willingness of the patient to subscribe to this course of treatment. A clear explanation of the condition, the natural history including likely changes over time, and how to contact the team is vital. Unless the tumour is large at the time of diagnosis, it is commonplace to organize the first interval scan at 6 months. On review, if the tumour is unchanged in size, it would be appropriate to continue this conservative approach with annual scanning and clinical review of symptoms. Local policy dictates the frequency of subsequent scans. The authors recommend annual scans for 5 years, followed by scans every 2 years until 10 years from diagnosis. At this point the patient is advised to have a scan every 5 years.

Surgery

The goal of surgery is total tumour removal whilst minimizing the neurological impact to the patient. To maintain normal or near-normal function, a compromise position may be adopted such that a small tumour remnant is left behind (near-total excision). In a few cases the surgical team feels that the risk to neurological function is threatened, whilst a more substantial proportion of the tumour remains (sub-total excision). The structures at risk are the same as those that give rise to the symptoms of the tumour, namely the facial and cochlear nerves (the vestibular nerves are removed with the tumour), the trigeminal and lower cranial nerves, the cerebellum and the vessels in the CPA.

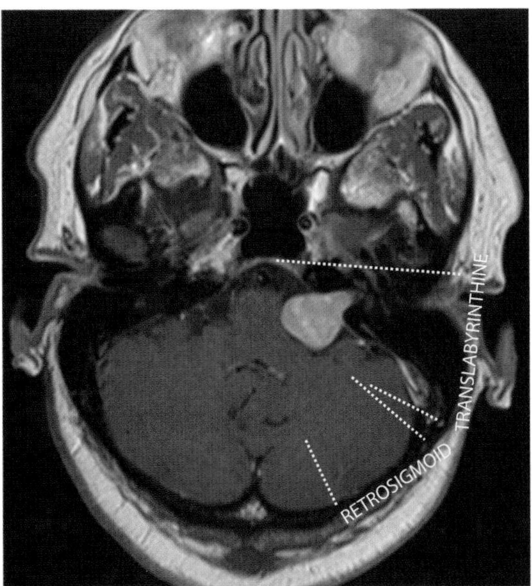

Figure 50.3 The translabyrinthine and retrosigmoid approaches to the cerebellopontine angle.

The surgery is performed under general anaesthesia with expert anaesthetists in a neurosurgical centre with specialist high-dependency and intensive care unit (ICU) provision. The surgical team comprises both ENT and neurosurgeons. Three surgical approaches to the CPA are described; the translabyrinthine, retrosigmoid and middle fossa. In practice in the United Kingdom, the middle fossa approach is very seldom used in vestibular schwannoma surgery. There are advantages to both of the commonly used approaches, and surgical teams should be acquainted with both (Figure 50.3).

The retrosigmoid approach offers the possibility of hearing preservation whereby the cochlear nerve is identified and left *in situ* at the time of tumour dissection. The main disadvantages of this approach are of cerebellar retraction, poor access to the fundus (lateral-most end) of the internal auditory canal and the increased incidence of chronic post-craniectomy headache. There is no limit in the size of tumour this approach can be utilized for.

The main advantage of the translabyrinthine approach is the excellent view that is afforded of the fundus, allowing early identification and subsequent preservation of the nerves within the IAC. Again, any size of tumour can be removed through this approach, although no cerebellar retraction is required. The incidence of cerebrospinal fluid (CSF) fistula is reported to be higher in the translabyrinthine approach, though this is not the experience of the authors. A consequence of the removal of the vestibular apparatus is not only the loss of the ipsilateral peripheral (usually already failing) balance function, but also the loss of any residual hearing.

During the surgery, electromyography of the orbicularis oris and orbicularis oculi is performed to confirm the location and function of the facial nerve and to aid in decision making with regard to the amount of tumour remnant left *in situ*. It is also possible to monitor other cranial nerves to provide guidance regarding the preservation of hearing, and speech and swallowing function.

Radiotherapy

Unlike surgery, the goal of treating the patient with radiotherapy is not to ablate the tumour but to arrest its growth. It therefore follows that it is seldom considered appropriate to offer radiotherapy as an intervention unless demonstrable growth has occurred following a period of observation.

A discussion of radiobiology is beyond the remit of this chapter, but it should be appreciated that the effect of radiotherapy on pathological tissue differs from that on the nearby normal tissue. Given that vestibular schwannomas are slow-growing benign tumours, their cellular response to irradiation is not vastly different to the surrounding local tissues. In addition, because the structures closely related to the tumour are functionally so important, a method of delivering the radiation that is extremely precise with a steep 'shoulder' or 'fall-off' away from the tumour is vital.

Unlike conventional radiotherapy techniques that deliver the dose through up to three overlapping fields, or even intensity-modulated radiotherapy (IMRT) that uses up to seven fields, the most common method of radiotherapy delivery in the treatment of vestibular schwannoma is using stereotactic radiotherapy. This is also known as gamma knife stereotactic radiosurgery. The term *surgery* is used simply because the treatment is a 'one-off' not because an operation is involved, although a titanium frame is fixed to the patient's head to allow a precise reference point. Approximately 200 individual sources of photons (usually Cobalt-60) are arranged with a common focus point. By varying which sources are active in relation to the position of the patient, a very precise target can be treated. Complex planning software is required to match the MRI scan data to the treatment plan and subsequently deliver the single-shot treatment.

The benefits of stereotactic radiotherapy over surgery are that the treatment is administered without general anaesthesia, with a brief stay in hospital (less than 24 hours) and a much shorter recovery time. Other advantages include the possibility of preserving any residual hearing, which though theoretically possible using middle fossa and retrosigmoid approaches is practically seldom achieved at the same peroperative level. The risk profile is less than that of surgery, with the likelihood of adverse events including facial nerve palsy, dizziness, stroke and death being significantly lower. The disadvantages of stereotactic gamma knife radiosurgery in the treatment of vestibular schwannoma include the inability to treat lesions greater than 30 mm in maximal diameter, because of the likelihood of tumour swelling in the post-treatment period and the theoretical risk of inducing malignant change in the irradiated field.

Long-term data regarding the efficacy and risks of gamma knife radiotherapy are available and suggest tumour control rates of approximately 95 per cent with adverse events occurring in less than 5 per cent. Post-treatment imaging is usually performed.

MENINGIOMAS

Meningiomas are the second most common type of tumour in the CPA after vestibular schwannoma. They account for approximately 10 per cent of all CPA lesions. They are twice as common in women than in men. Compared to vestibular schwannomas, meningiomas are less likely to cause symptoms in general and, in particular, the audiovestibular symptom constellation is less prevalent.

PATHOPHYSIOLOGY

Meningiomas arise from the dura, specifically from cells at the tip of the arachnoid villi (also known as arachnoid granulations), where they project into the dural venous sinuses and around the skull base neurovascular foramina. The multitude of foramina and intracranial vasculature in the CPA explains the propensity of meningiomas to arise in this area. Other intracranial sites in addition to spinal deposits are well described. CPA meningiomas may be located on the dural folds around the trigeminal nerve – Meckel's cave, around the internal acoustic meatus (IAM), in continuity with the lower cranial nerves at the jugular foramen or along the vessels and venous sinuses.

Compared to vestibular schwannomas, meningiomas are generally firmer in texture and more vascular. They tend to invade the neighbouring bone with increased vascular supply. Immunohistopathology has demonstrated hormone receptors within meningiomas, particularly for the female sex hormones. This explains the preponderance in women as well as the well-known rapid growth that may be witnessed in pregnancy and with certain contraceptive medication.

As described earlier, meningiomas are associated with NF2, and a diagnosis should be considered in a young patient or those presenting with multiple tumours.

INVESTIGATIONS

MRI scanning again provides the best method of differentiating meningiomas from other lesions (Figure 50.4). Classically, meningiomas are broad-based and show a thin enhancing strip of dura – the dural tail – emanating from the edge of the bulk of the tumour. There is often calcification within the tumour, shown as low signal on T1- and T2-weighted scans. This is more evident on CT scanning.

MANAGEMENT

Meningiomas, like vestibular schwannomas, can be managed with a conservative approach and the patient subjected to regular interval scanning and treated if symptoms dictate. The growth of these tumours is generally slow, but some are exquisitely

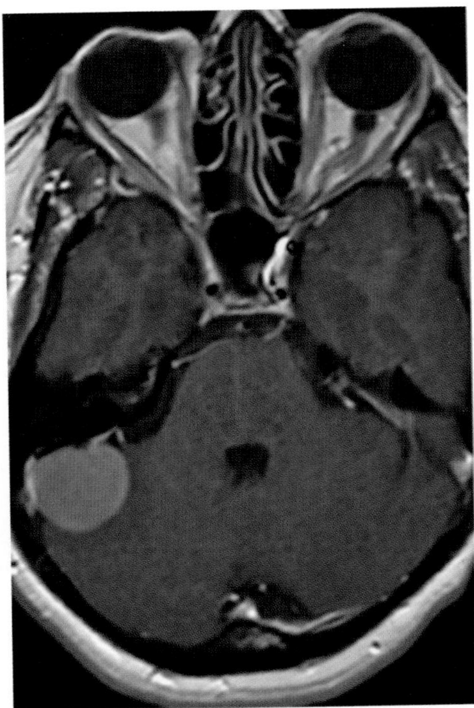

Figure 50.4 An axial gadolinium-enhanced T1-weighted MRI of right petrous ridge meningioma.

sensitive to hormonal stimulation and can grow rapidly, occasionally making for a difficult discussion regarding termination with a pregnant woman and her family.

Surgical resection via the approach with least morbidity and with preservation of cranial nerves is considered the aim if an intervention is required. Surgery is best performed on smaller tumours, meaning less extensive dural and skull base resection, and therefore it can be argued that earlier intervention is in the patient's best interest.

Radiotherapy, either through gamma knife stereotactic radiosurgery or with traditional external beam administration, has a role in the management of meningiomas. Like in vestibular schwannomas, the morbidity tends to be less significant compared to surgery, although meningiomas seem to be less effectively treated this way. One of the issues is that the tumours are often considered too large for radiotherapy at the time of presentation. Radiotherapy therefore offers a good option when used as an adjunctive treatment, following sub-total resection.

EPIDERMOIDS/CHOLESTEATOMA

Epidermoids are congenital lesions that arise from the inclusion of ectodermal tissue during embryonal development. A sac of keratin that is produced by the squamous epithelium surrounding it grows gradually along a low-resistance path, becoming adherent to the dura, cranial nerves and vessels. The lesion is otherwise identical to cholesteatoma formed secondarily in the middle ear. It appears as a pearly white, irregularly shaped soft mass.

Patients with epidermoids are likely to present with a relatively long and slowly evolving history. Facial and trigeminal nerve involvement is more common than in VS with audiovestibular symptoms less likely.

The imaging characteristics show the tumour to appear similar to the CSF within the CPA (Figure 50.5). The lesion appears as high-signal intensity on T2-weighted sequences, low on T1 and does not enhance with gadolinium.

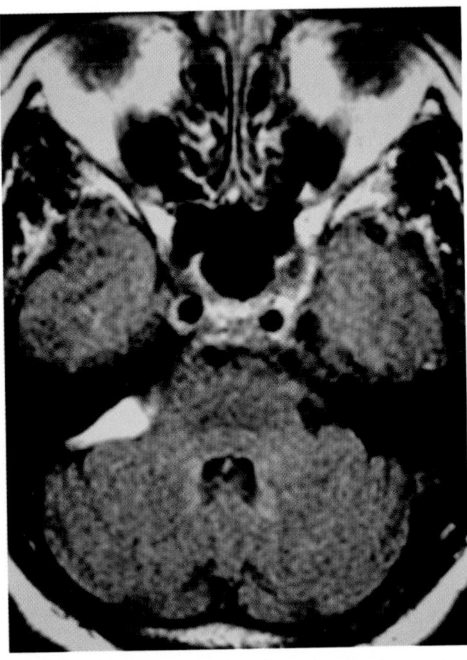

Figure 50.5 An axial FLAIR (fluid attenuated inversion recovery) sequence MRI of a right cerebellopontine epidermoid cyst.

Careful surgery is the treatment of choice, accepting that total removal is near-impossible without risking permanent cranial nerve deficits. In view of the extremely slow growth of these lesions, leaving residual tumour that may require revision surgery long into the future is an acceptable stance to take.

NON-VESTIBULAR SCHWANNOMAS

Schwannomas can occur on any nerve with schwann cells present on the surface. These cells produce myelin, which acts as an insulator, increasing conduction velocity along the axon. They are present on all the cranial nerves apart from the olfactory (I) and optic (II), whose myelin is produced by another glial, or supporting cell, the oligodendrocyte. Therefore, schwannomas can occur on any of the remaining 10 pairs of cranial nerves. In the CPA, nerves V to XI can develop schwannomas, the most common being vestibular (see earlier discussion).

FACIAL SCHWANNOMAS

Although facial schwannomas are likely to present with similar characteristics to the closely anatomically related vestibular schwannoma, they are more likely to be associated with facial nerve symptoms. The symptom may not be facial weakness but twitching and spasm. Facial schwannomas most commonly arise at the geniculate ganglion and slowly enlarge the fallopian canal, moving laterally as well as medially into the CPA (Figure 50.6). Because of this, CT scanning is useful in addition to the more commonly utilized MRI. Thus, the middle ear extent can be ascertained giving some guidance in preoperative planning. Unless CPA symptoms dominate, the decision on timing of surgery is controversial. Over time the facial function will deteriorate. Of course, tumour (and nerve) resection will render the patient paralyzed on the affected side. Waiting for this to occur naturally is tempting; however, the motor end plates and muscles require neural stimulation to remain viable. Surgical resection would normally be combined with some attempt at facial reanimation, either primary repair or cable grafting. Therefore, a compromise between dwindling facial function and potential success of the reanimation is usually sought. In addition, the level of conductive hearing loss often plays a part in the decision making. The authors' approach to the patient with a facial schwannoma is to offer surgery if either the tumour is of a size that gives rise to concern about the patient's neurological well-being or if, with non-threatening tumours, the facial function has deteriorated to grade 3 or worse on the House–Brackmann scale. This is because a cable-grafted facial nerve should allow facial function to recover to grade 3.

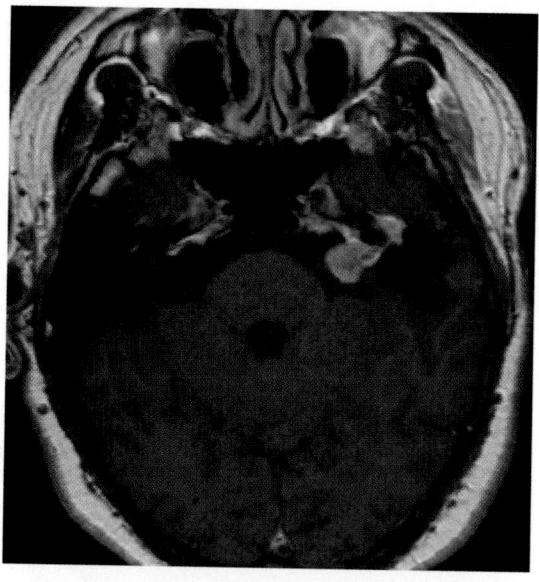

Figure 50.6 An axial gadolinium-enhanced T1-weighted MRI of a left facial nerve schwannoma extending into the CPA.

TRIGEMINAL SCHWANNOMAS

Trigeminal schwannomas arise at the Gasserian ganglion in Meckel's cave, and because of this location can involve both the middle and posterior cranial fossa (Figure 50.7). Patients present with unilateral facial hypaesthesia, neuralgia and later

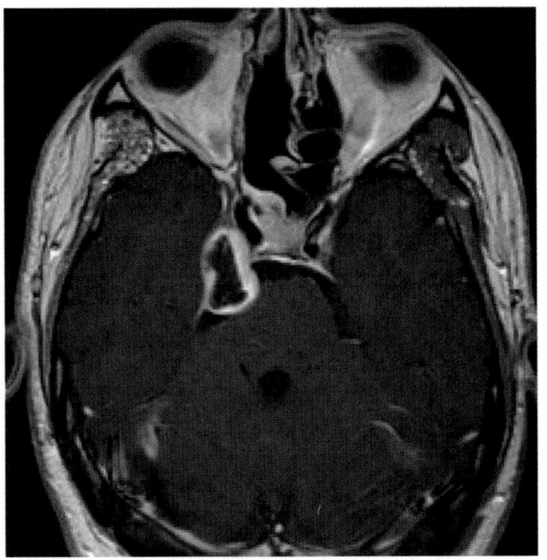

Figure 50.7 An axial gadolinium-enhanced T1-weighted MRI of a right cystic trigeminal schwannoma.

weakness in the muscles of mastication. If necessary, surgery may require a combined middle fossa and CPA approach.

LOWER CRANIAL NERVE SCHWANNOMAS

Schwannomas of the glossopharyngeal (IX), vagus (X) and accessory (XI) nerves are rare and arise at the jugular foramen, from where they may expand into the CPA or inferiorly into the parapharyngeal space. Patients present with the associated cranial neuropathy. Management depends upon the extent of the tumour and the deficit, particularly in speech and swallowing function. Surgery, including rehabilitation, is sometimes required.

CHOLESTEROL GRANULOMAS

Cholesterol granulomas arise at the apex of the petrous bone. In approximately one-third of people, the petrous apex is pneumatized. Inflammation in

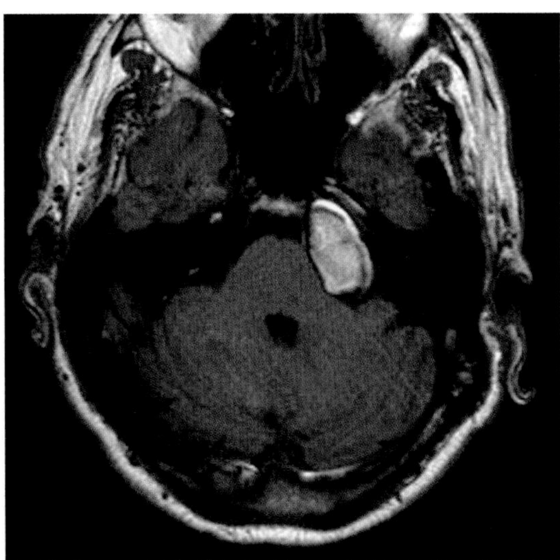

Figure 50.8 An axial T1-weighted MRI of a left cerebellopontine angle cholesterol granuloma.

these air cells can lead to deposition of cholesterol and a chronic inflammatory reaction. The patient may present with CPA symptoms but classically presents earlier with abducens (VI) nerve palsy. The MRI appearance of cholesterol granulomas is pathognomic. On both T1- and T2-weighted sequences the lesion appears hyperintense (Figure 50.8). The aim of treatment is decompression of the cyst, which may be achieved through a transmastoid or endoscopic endonasal approach. Because of the incomplete nature of the surgery, symptoms usually recur, requiring revision surgery. This is often performed more than a decade later; during that period the patient has enjoyed no or minimal neurological sequaelae.

PARAGANGLIOMAS

These neuroendocrine tumours arise from the neural crest cells and may be found throughout the body located near the autonomic nerves. They are most common in the abdomen and are rarest in the head and neck. However, they are most symptomatic in this location. Jugular paragangliomas, or *glomus jugulare*, arise at the jugular bulb and expand from here with increasing symptoms. They are vascular tumours and classically present with pulsatile tinnitus and hearing loss. Cranial neuropathies occur later. The tumour may expand into the CPA. Because of their vascular nature, they enhance avidly on both CT and MRI. The classical 'salt-and-pepper' appearance seen on MRI relates to the varying flow of blood within the tumour. Complete surgical removal is curative, although conservative management, maintaining neurological function, is considered. Radiotherapy is proving to be useful for these tumours too.

LIPOMAS

Lipomas are extremely rare and are usually identified incidentally. They are very rarely symptomatic. MRI scanning shows a hyperintense lesion on T1-weighted sequencing that does not become any brighter with the addition of contrast (Figure 50.9). Once they are identified, the authors do not recommend further investigation and the patient should be reassured.

ARACHNOID CYSTS

Arachnoid cysts account for approximately 1 per cent of all intracranial lesions and are again often asymptomatic, although they can cause CPA symptoms. Their MRI characteristics are in direct contrast to those of lipomas, being hypointense on

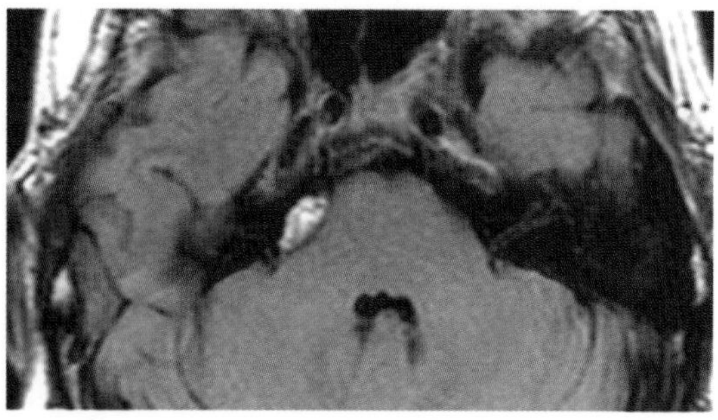

Figure 50.9 An axial T1-weighted MRI of a right cerebellopontine lipoma.

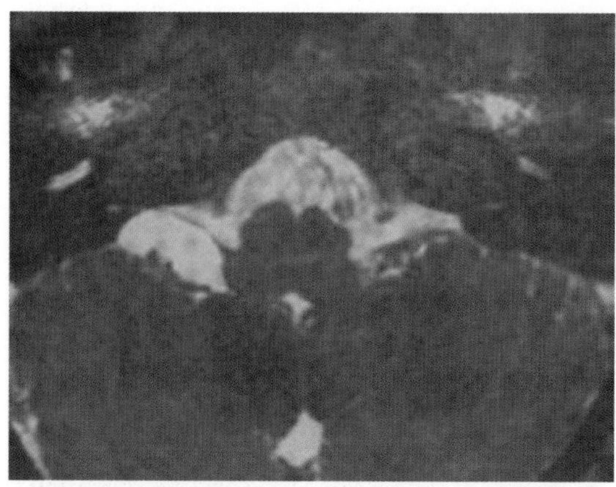

Figure 50.10 An axial T2-weighted MRI scan of a right cerebellopontine arachnoid cyst.

T1 and hyperintense on T2-weighted sequences (Figure 50.10). There is no enhancement. Should treatment be deemed necessary, it is usually acceptable to decompress the cyst, opening it into the surrounding CSF space rather than removing it in total.

CHORDOMAS

These aggressive tumours, which arise from notochord remnant, are found most commonly at the clivus. They can expand to involve the CPA. Treatment is by surgical resection and usually requires post-operative radiotherapy, ideally in the form of a proton beam.

CHONDROSCARCOMAS

Chondrosarcomas also arise at the clivus, although more laterally than chordomas. They usually behave in a more benign fashion than chordomas (Figure 50.11).

METASTASES

Metastasis to the CPA from lung, breast, prostate and skin malignancy is likely to occur only with

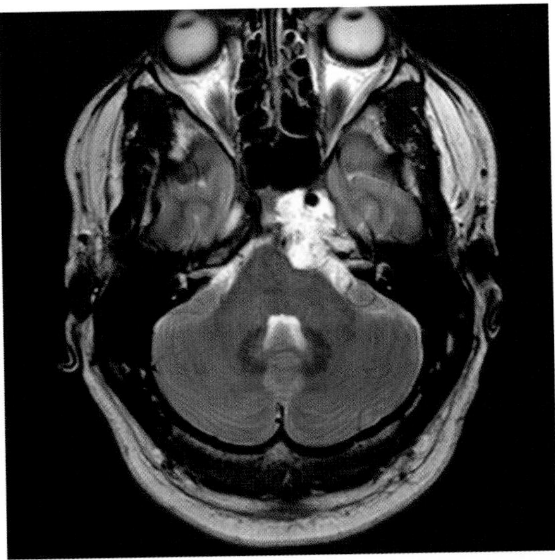

Figure 50.11 An axial T2-weighted MRI of a left clival chondrosarcoma extending to the cerebellopontine angle.

relatively widespread disease, although the lesion may be responsible for some of the patient's symptoms. In this circumstance there are likely to be several skull base and intra-axial metastases as well. Treatment is guided by the oncological team looking after the patient's primary disease and should be palliative and symptomatically focused.

ACKNOWLEDGEMENTS

The authors would like to thank Dr S. E. J. Connor, consultant neuroradiologist, Guy's & St Thomas' and King's College Hospitals, London, for his invaluable help and guidance with the imaging for this chapter.

KEY LEARNING POINTS

- CPA tumours account for 10% of intracranial tumours.
- Vestibular schwannomas account for the majority (80%) of CPA tumours.
- Diagnosis is made on MRI characteristics.
- Conservative management with serial imaging is often appropriate.
- Surgery and radiotherapy both have roles when treatment is necessary.

FURTHER READING

Cushing H. *Tumours of the Nervus Acousticus and the Syndrome of the Cerebellopontine Angle* (reprinted 1963). New York: Hafner Publishing Company, 1917.

Evans DG, Baser ME, O'Reilly B, Rowe J, Gleeson M, Saeed S, King A, Huson SM, Kerr R, Thomas N, Irving R, MacFarlane R, Ferner R, McLeod R, Moffat D, Ramsden R. Management of the patient and family with neurofibromatosis 2: A consensus conference statement. *British Journal of Neurosurgery*. 2005 Feb; 19(1): 5–12.

Gleeson M. *Skull Base (Part 20)*. In: *Scott-Brown's Otolaryngology, Head and Neck Surgery*. Eds. Gleeson M, Browning GG, Burton MJ, Clarke R, Hibbert J, Jones, NS, Lund VJ, Luxon LM, Watkinson JC. Boca Raton: CRC Press, 2008.

House WF. Transtemporal bone microsurgical removal of acoustic neuromas. Report of cases. *Archives of Otolaryngology*. 1964; 80: 617–67.

Lalwani AK. Meningiomas, epidermoids, and other nonacoustic tumors of the cerebellopontine angle. *Otolaryngology Clinics of North America*. 1992 Jun; 25(3): 707–28.

Rowe J, Radatz M, Walton L, Hampshire A, Seaman S, Kemeny A. Gamma knife stereotactic radiosurgery for unilateral acoustic neuromas. *Journal of Neurology, Neurosurgery and Psychiatry*. 2003 November; 74(11): 1536–42.

Stangerup SE, Tos M, Thomsen J, Caye-Thomasen P. True incidence of vestibular schwannoma? *Neurosurgery*. 2010 Nov; 67(5): 1335–40.

51

Otological trauma

NASHREEN BANON OOZEER AND JOHN CROWTHER

INTRODUCTION

The external, middle and inner ear structures are liable to be affected by trauma in isolation or in combination, depending on the type and severity of the injury. The most common cause is a blunt head injury as a result of road traffic accidents (RTAs) and falls, usually in association with temporal bone fracture and often combined with other injuries. Penetrating injuries of the temporal bone are less common. Damage to the tympanic membrane and middle ear can also be caused by objects inserted through the ear canal, a blow to the pinna or blast injuries. Iatrogenic injury is usually the result of inadvertent surgical trauma to the labyrinth or facial nerve. Other mechanisms of injury to the ear include barotrauma and noise.

TRAUMA TO THE PINNA

PINNA LACERATION

History and examination

Trauma with a sharp object, e.g. a knife, results in a laceration of the skin and/or cartilage of the pinna. Trauma with a blunt object or a bite (animal or human) tends to produce an irregular laceration. There can be loss of tissue or a degloving injury. If the cartilage of the pinna is exposed, there is a risk of necrosis due to loss of blood supply. There is also a risk of infection, pinna cellulitis or perichondritis with resultant deformity ('cauliflower ear').

Investigations

A microbiology swab is advised in the presence of suppuration or contamination.

Management

The wound should be washed thoroughly and any necrotic tissue debrided. It may be necessary to trim exposed cartilage or use a local skin flap to provide soft tissue cover. A tetanus booster is recommended in those whose vaccination schedule is unknown or immunoglobulin in the vaccine naive. In the presence of a human bite, Hepatitis B accelerated or hyperaccelerated vaccination is generally provided.[1] Broad-spectrum antibiotics are prescribed in the context of delayed presentation and/or bites.

PINNA HAEMATOMA

History and examination

A subperichondrial or pinna haematoma is a collection of blood between the auricular perichondrium and cartilage normally occurring as a result of a shearing action on the pinna, tearing the perichondrial capillaries. This type of blunt injury can occur with contact sports or assaults. Cartilage does not have an innate blood supply and relies on the blood vessels in the overlying perichondrium for oxygen and nutrients. Deprived of the latter, the cartilage will necrose, resulting in a deformed ear. Untreated, there is the risk of abscess formation and subsequent necrosis of cartilage.

Investigations

No investigation is required.

Management

Drainage of the haematoma either by aspiration or by incision, usually under local anaesthetic, forms the mainstay of treatment. Compression to prevent recurrence can be provided by a head bandage for 48 hours, sutures or a hearing aid mould (in the case of a conchal bowl haematoma). Broad-spectrum antibiotics are prescribed if there is delayed presentation and high risk of infection.

TRAUMA VIA THE EXTERNAL AUDITORY MEATUS

Trauma via the external auditory meatus (EAM) can produce injury to the external auditory canal (EAC), a tympanic membrane (TM) perforation or damage to the ossicles depending on the extent of the injury.

EXTERNAL AUDITORY CANAL INJURY

History and examination

The EAC skin can be traumatized by insertion of an object into the ear canal. There is usually some bleeding from the canal and associated otalgia, and the injured area can become infected. Other causes of direct trauma to the EAC include a chemical burn from a hearing aid battery.

Investigations

No routine investigation is indicated, but a microbiology swab may be helpful if there are signs of infection.

Management

Any foreign object should be removed. Hearing aid batteries should be removed with some urgency as these will cause progressive damage. The EAC should be kept dry until the skin has healed. Aural toilet and topical antibiotic/steroid drops are recommended in the presence of infection (refer to Chapter 53).

MIDDLE EAR INJURY: TYMPANIC MEMBRANE PERFORATION

History and examination

A defect in the TM (Figure 51.1) can be produced by direct trauma from a foreign body inserted into the EAC or indirectly from a relative change in pressure between the external and middle ear, e.g. from a slap to the ear or a blast injury (refer to the section on barotrauma later in this chapter). Patients are likely to complain of otalgia, hearing loss (characteristically conductive), and may have blood-stained otorrhoea.

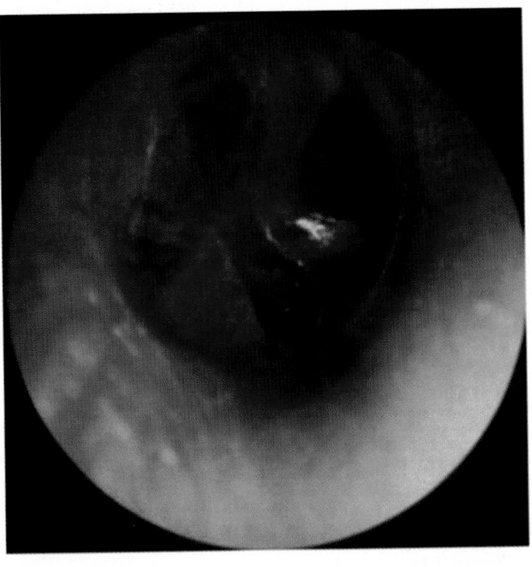

Figure 51.1 Right tympanic membrane showing an irregular inferior tympanic membrane perforation secondary to a slap to the ear. Courtesy of Professor Brian O'Reilly.

Investigations

Pure tone audiometry (PTA) is obtained to document the degree of hearing loss. An air–bone gap of more than 30 dB should raise the suspicion of ossicular damage.

Management

In the majority of cases, a traumatic perforation will heal spontaneously within 10 weeks of the injury,[2] thus conservative management is advocated. Patients should be advised to keep the affected ear dry. If the TM perforation shows no sign of healing after 3 to 6 months, surgical repair should be considered. Persistent conductive hearing loss (CHL) after the TM has healed is suggestive of ossicular damage (refer to the section on ossicular chain injury later in this chapter).

TEMPORAL BONE TRAUMA WITH FRACTURE

HISTORY AND EXAMINATION

Falls, assaults and RTAs may cause a temporal bone fracture. An inner ear–penetrating injury can also occur secondary to a sharp object, e.g. a patient assaulted with an axe, a knife or a gunshot wound to the temporal bone. The force of trauma will determine the magnitude of temporal bone injury and the severity of intracranial injury. Often only a limited or no history is available. Temporal bone fractures may be obvious in the presence of a step deformity or penetrating wound to the lateral skull but should be suspected in the presence of Battle's sign (Figure 51.2a), blood in the EAC, haemotympanum (Figure 51.2b), TM perforation, cerebrospinal fluid (CSF) otorrhoea and a lower motor neuron facial nerve palsy.

INVESTIGATIONS

A computed tomography (CT) scan of the brain with high-resolution CT scan of the temporal bone is obtained (Figure 51.3). Traditionally,

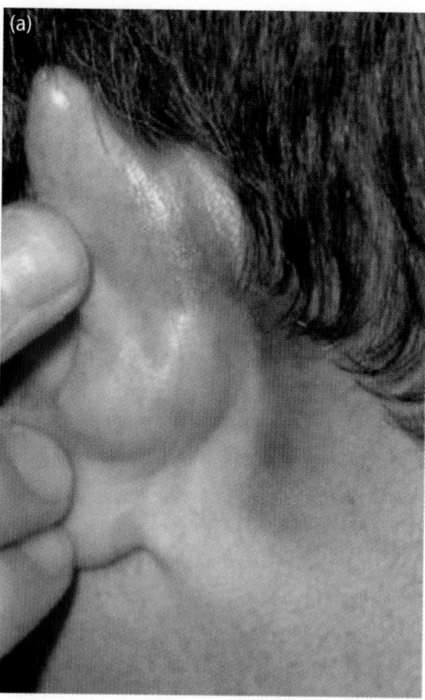

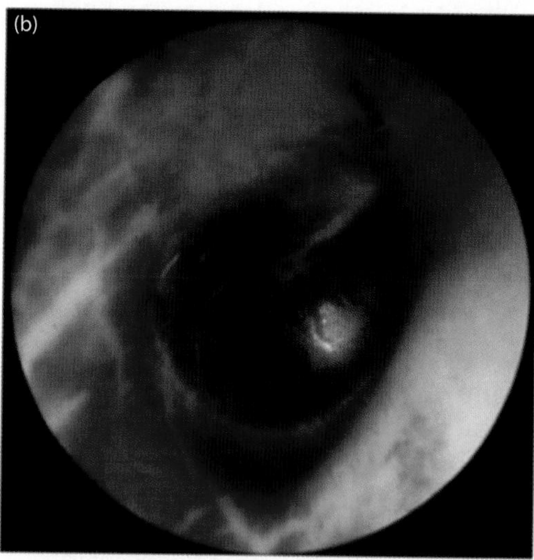

Figure 51.2 **(a)** Left post-auricular bruising, also known as Battle's sign; **(b)** right haemotympanum and evidence of dried blood in the external auditory canal. Courtesy of Professor Brian O'Reilly.

fractures are classified as longitudinal or transverse, but most tend to be mixed. Eighty per cent are predominantly longitudinal fractures where the fracture line runs along the longitudinal axis of the petrous temporal bone, from the lateral skull along the EAC roof towards the petrous apex. The mechanism of injury tends to be a blow to the squamous part of the temporal bone. Less commonly, the fracture line is transverse to the longitudinal axis and may run through the otic capsule. These are usually secondary to a blow to the frontal or occipital bone. In addition, PTA and tympanometry are obtained to assess hearing when the patient has recovered enough to cooperate with these tests.

MANAGEMENT

Treatment is directed by the patient's symptoms and clinical signs. Concomitant intracranial and cervical spine injury takes precedence over the temporal bone injury, and the patient should be initially managed according to advanced trauma life support (ATLS) protocols. A multidisciplinary approach is often required, which may involve a neurotologist, intensivist and neurosurgeon.

EXTERNAL AUDITORY CANAL INJURY

A laceration can occur if the temporal bone fracture extends into the EAC and a step deformity of the bony canal may be visible on otoscopy. This is managed conservatively, but blood clots and debris may need to be removed from the EAC to visualize the TM.

MIDDLE EAR INJURY

Haemotympanum

Any fracture involving the middle ear will cause bleeding and, in the presence of an intact TM, a haemotympanum. This will produce a temporary CHL. Conservative management is advocated as blood will be absorbed within 2 to 3 weeks.

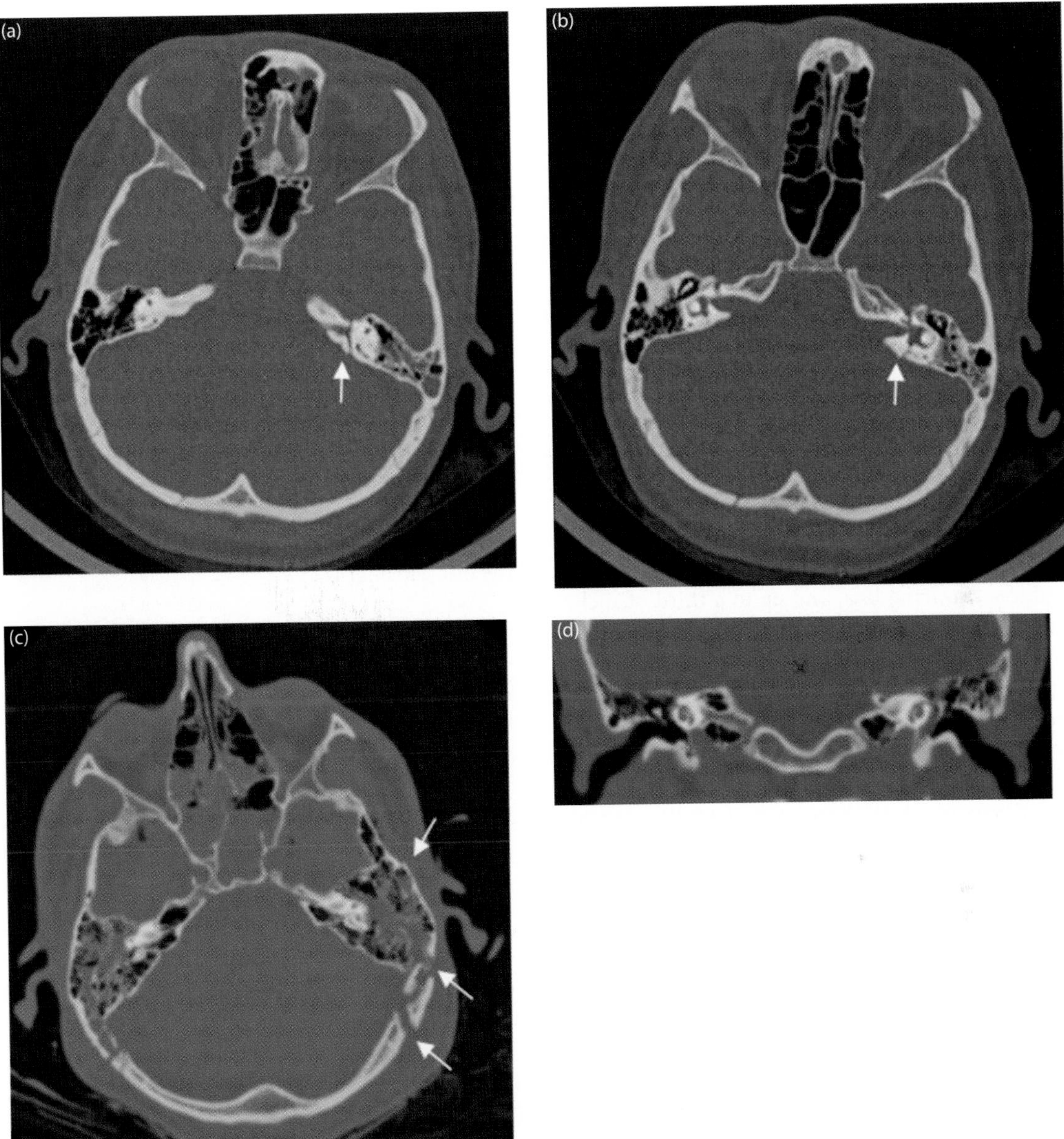

Figure 51.3 **(a)** Axial CT scan of left temporal bone, arrow showing transverse fracture through the otic capsule at superior semicircular canal level; **(b)** at lateral semicircular canal level; **(c)** comminuted fracture of left temporal bone in a pedestrian road traffic accident (arrows showing multiple fracture lines); **(d)** coronal CT scan, 1 year post-injury, showing the presence of cerebrospinal fluid in left middle ear.

TM perforation

A fracture through the tympanic ring will produce a TM perforation and can disrupt the ossicular chain. TM perforations will cause a CHL. They are initially managed conservatively as the majority will heal spontaneously, but consider surgical repair if the perforation persists 3 to 6 months after the injury.

Ossicular chain injury

Dislocation of the incus (62 per cent) is most common (Figure 51.4a), with fracture of the stapes, long process of incus, handle of malleus and ossicular fixation secondary to scar tissue in the attic constituting the majority of the remaining cases of ossicular injury found at tympanotomy.

Around 22 per cent of temporal bone trauma produces a hearing loss, and up to a third of such cases are conductive in nature.[3] A haemotympanum may be seen at the initial stage of injury. A persistent CHL, approximately 6 weeks to 3 months after the injury when the haemotympanum has resorbed and the TM healed, is highly suspicious of ossicular chain injury. PTA will confirm a CHL with a maximum air–bone gap of 60 dB, with a Type A_d tympanogram in ossicular discontinuity (Figure 51.4b) and a Type A_s in ossicular fixation. Modern fine-cut CT scans of the temporal bone should be able to identify the type of ossicular damage, which can be confirmed at exploratory tympanotomy. Ossicular reconstruction can be carried out using a prosthesis or preferably the patient's own ossicles. Ossiculoplasty results tend to be better than those achieved in patients with chronic otitis media in view of the normal eustachian tube (ET) function, provided no ET injury has been caused by the fracture. The literature shows a 54–78 per cent closure of the air–bone gap to less than 10 dB in head injury patients.[4–5]

INNER EAR INJURY

Damage to the inner ear is more severe with transverse fractures as they are more likely to involve the otic capsule.

Sensorineural hearing loss

Sensorineural hearing loss (SNHL) occurs as a result of trauma to the inner ear. Pure tone audiometry is performed when possible. Elevated thresholds in the high frequencies (≥ 4 KHz) in patients with temporal bone fractures are seen[6] with an estimated 17 per cent of patients losing

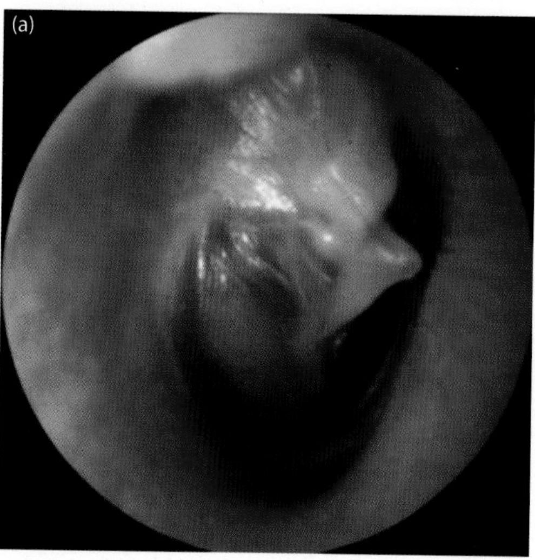

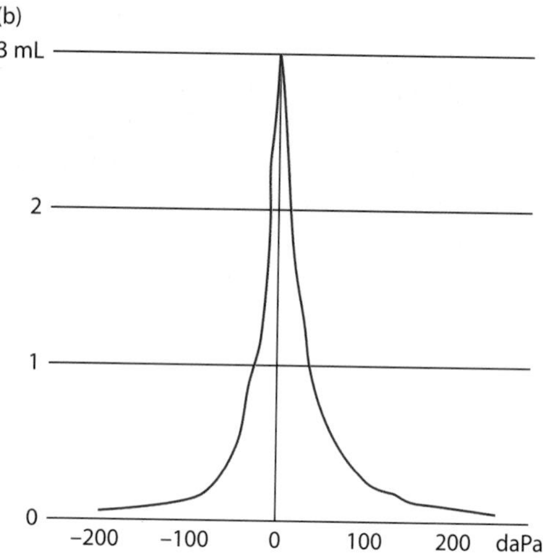

Figure 51.4 **(a)** Right tympanic membrane showing dislocation of the malleus head; **(b)** right ear, Type A_d tympanogram. **(a)** Courtesy of Professor Brian O'Reilly.

all ipsilateral hearing.[7] Post-traumatic SNHL may be unilateral or bilateral and is not reversible. Management with hearing aids is instituted as appropriate.

Vestibular disturbance

Balance disturbance following a temporal bone injury is common and may be secondary to diffuse brain injury or damage to the peripheral vestibular apparatus. Vestibular testing is usually performed in the presence of a persistent sensation of imbalance and vertigo. Caloric testing will confirm ipsilateral vestibular hypofunction. A magnetic resonance imaging (MRI) scan is helpful to exclude any coexisting retrocochlear lesion in those with intractable symptoms. In addition, a perilymph leak can occur following a head injury (or barotrauma) and tends to be at the oval window (60 per cent), round window (20 per cent), both windows (20 per cent) and bilaterally (20 per cent). Patients may complain of unexplained fluctuating or progressive SNHL with or without vertigo or tinnitus.[8] Vestibular sedatives initially help control symptoms but should be discontinued as early as possible and replaced by vestibular rehabilitation to aid central compensation.

CEREBROSPINAL FLUID OTORRHOEA

A persistent watery discharge from the ear following a temporal bone fracture is highly suspicious of CSF otorrhoea. This occurs in up to a third of patients in some series.[9] In the presence of an intact TM, diagnosis may be delayed with patients presenting with presumed otitis media with effusion (OME), or with CSF rhinorrheoa due to CSF flowing from the middle ear, via the ET into the nasal cavity. Previously asymptomatic patients may rarely present with episodes of meningitis weeks to months after the original injury. A persistent clear fluid from the ear is sent for β_2-transferrin level to confirm the presence of CSF. Up to 60 per cent of patients will have a CHL of >20 dB within 3 days of the injury, which drops to 17 per cent at 6 weeks.[7] Use of prophylactic antibiotics in the presence of CSF otorrhoea or rhinorrheoa is not favoured, with the literature showing similar incidence of meningitis (2 per cent) with or without prophylactic antibiotics.[10] In the authors' practice, antibiotics are only given in the presence of concurrent local infection. We also advocate a single dose of pneumococcal polysaccharide vaccine, which protects against 23 different strains of pneumococcus, to reduce the risk of meningitis.[11] The vast majority of CSF otorrhoea cases will stop spontaneously usually within 5 days of the injury. Persistent ones will require further investigation with a skull base CT and/or MRI to determine the site of dural defect. Surgical repair of persistent leaks can be performed via a transmastoid or craniotomy approach. Dural defects are repaired with fascia, and larger associated bony defects in the tegmen may require autologous tragal cartilage or cranial bone to support soft tissue repair. Fibrin glue is a useful adjunct, and a temporary lumbar drain to reduce CSF pressure can be beneficial.

FACIAL NERVE INJURY

Seven per cent of temporal bone fracture cases are associated with an injury to the intratemporal portion of the facial nerve. The two most important prognostic indicators of cranial nerve (CN) VII recovery following a temporal bone fracture were found to be the time of onset (immediate or delayed) and the severity of the palsy (complete/total or incomplete/partial).[12] The dilemma arises in those who have been unconscious or intubated for days following a head injury. The facial nerve function of the conscious patient is assessed and documented with the commonly used House–Brackmann grading system. Routine eye care as for all patients with facial paralysis should be commenced early. Electroneuronography (ENoG) may identify those patients with more severe nerve trauma with poorer prognosis, i.e. those who may benefit from surgical exploration. In departments without access to ENoG, a decision to explore should be based on whether the CN VII palsy is complete and immediate together with radiological findings. The site of nerve trauma, hence the area to be explored, will be guided by radiological appearances. Transmastoid exploration will access the horizontal and vertical portions of CN VII. The supra-labyrinthine nerve will require middle fossa approach if hearing is still present and translabyrinthine approach in the presence of total hearing loss. Bony spicules should be removed from the nerve and, if intact, the nerve sheath should be incised proximally and distally. If the nerve has been transected, the proximal and distal ends usually retract away from each other and cannot be anastomosed without tension. Cable grafting using the greater auricular nerve is ideal as it can be harvested by limited anterior extension of the post-aural incision. A vein sleeve should be placed around the anastomosis. Nerve exploration does carry a risk of iatrogenic palsy and ideally should be carried out by an experienced otologist. There is only limited evidence of the benefit of surgical exploration of CN VII partly because the overall recovery rate is generally good. Brodie et al. showed complete or almost complete recovery of the partial and delayed traumatic CN VII palsy group to a HB 1-2 function spontaneously, whilst only 60 per cent of the immediate palsy group recovered facial function.[11] A management algorithm is proposed in Figure 51.5.

MAJOR HAEMORRHAGE

Bleeding from the EAC is a common feature due to skin lacerations or can arise from the middle ear via a TM perforation. Major haemorrhage is rare but can be secondary to injury to the jugular bulb or carotid artery. The patient should be resuscitated according to the ATLS protocol first and, once stabilized, angiography is indicated to identify the source with interventional radiology to control haemorrhage.

TEMPORAL BONE TRAUMA WITHOUT FRACTURE

INNER EAR INJURY: LABYRINTHINE CONCUSSION/POST-TRAUMATIC VERTIGO

History and examination

Trauma can produce temporary or permanent damage to the delicate neural tissue of the vestibular and auditory apparatus. Even with permanent damage to the peripheral vestibular system, balance tends to improve as a result of central compensation. Benign paroxysmal positional vertigo (BPPV) is the cause of approximately two-thirds of post-traumatic vertigo, occurring secondary to displaced otolithic particles in the posterior semicircular canal. A Dix–Hallpike test helps confirm the diagnosis of BPPV.[13,14] There may be bilateral signs. Damage to the cochlea leads to SNHL.

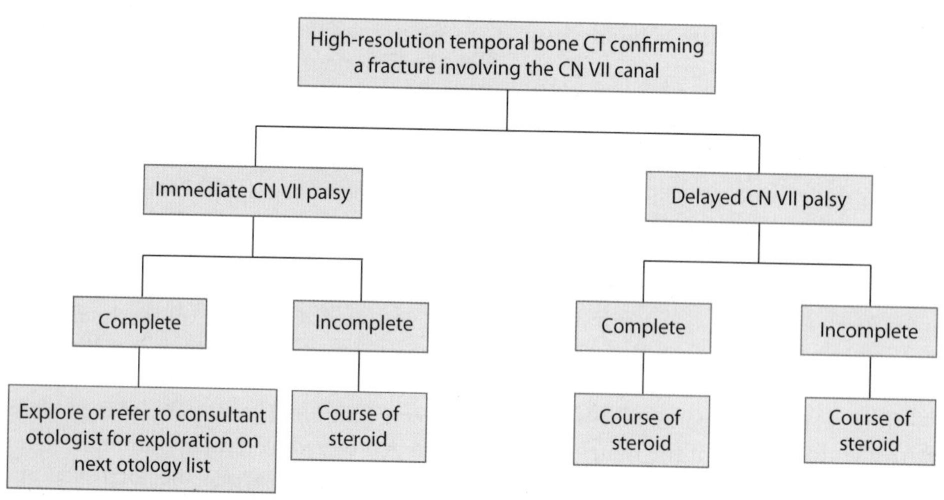

Figure 51.5 Algorithm for the management of post-traumatic facial nerve palsy.

Investigations

Audiometry will assess hearing loss, and caloric test may reveal vestibular hypofunction.

Management

A particle repositioning manoeuvre should be attempted in post-traumatic BPPV, and all persistent cases of post-traumatic vertigo should be referred for vestibular rehabilitation to aid central compensation.

IATROGENIC/SURGICAL TRAUMA

HISTORY AND EXAMINATION

Inadvertent damage to the middle and inner ear structures may occur during otologic and neuro-otologic surgery. Displacement or fracture of the stapes footplate from excessive manipulation of the ossicles, or transmission of energy from the surgical drill via the ossicular chain to the inner ear may result in SNHL. Removal of cholesteatoma from the lateral semicircular canal in the presence of a fistula may cause SNHL and vertigo as a result of vestibular damage. The facial nerve may be traumatized during otologic and neuro-otologic surgery.

INVESTIGATIONS

Intraoperative facial nerve monitoring may reduce the risk of iatrogenic CN VII injury.

MANAGEMENT

Sensorineural deafness is permanent, but balance disturbance should gradually improve with central compensation, aided by vestibular rehabilitation. Iatrogenic CN VII injury seems to be reducing in frequency, possibly as a result of the use of preoperative cross-sectional imaging showing the relationship of disease with respect to CN VII in addition to intraoperative nerve monitoring. Unless the operating surgeon is certain that the nerve is definitely intact, CN VII should be explored within 24–48 hours of immediate, complete post-operative palsy. Oral steroids for a week may be beneficial.

BAROTRAUMA

HISTORY AND EXAMINATION

Barotrauma is produced by mechanical forces arising from pressure changes. Middle ear barotrauma is more common than external ear or inner ear barotrauma. Boyle's law states that the pressure of a confined ideal gas is inversely proportional to its volume at a constant temperature ($V = k/P$, where V stands for volume, P for pressure and k is a constant). Examples of large changes in pressure include the rapid increase in external ambient pressure (EAC and nasopharyngeal pressure) with respect to the middle ear during descent of an airplane, from scuba diving or a blast injury. Barotrauma can cause TM retraction or, in more severe cases, an accumulation of fluid within the middle ear (OME) with or without haemorrhage. A middle ear pressure of –30 mm Hg for 15 minutes starts producing a middle ear transudate. Patients initially complain of the sensation of blocked ear, with otalgia developing as the plane descends and compression occurs. The risk of otitic barotrauma is maximal during the first 10 metres of diving and the first 1000 metres of altitude. Middle ear barotrauma can result in a perforated TM (500 mm Hg pressure) with an associated CHL. The patient often experiences severe otalgia. Perilymph fistula can occasionally be caused by barotrauma and will lead to SNHL and balance disturbance. The fistula test may be positive in such cases. Decompression sickness occurs when a reduction in ambient pressure (as occurs when ascending from depth) causes the formation and release of bubbles of inert gases within the tissues of the body. This mainly affects divers who have been breathing gas at a higher pressure. Bubbles of gas can occur anywhere in the body, but when these occur in the inner ear, the resulting damage causes hearing loss, tinnitus and balance disturbance.

INVESTIGATIONS

PTA confirms a CHL, and tympanogram will show a negative middle ear pressure (Type B or C, Figure 51.6) or a high middle ear volume in the presence of a TM perforation. SNHL may be present as a result of perilymph fistula or decompression sickness.

MANAGEMENT

Prevention by oral or topical nasal decongestants or chewing gum prior to air travel, during the flight and prior to descent is aimed at improving ET function. Evidence in the literature favours the use of oral decongestants, e.g. 120 mg of oral pseudoephedrine, prior to flying.[15] When diving, pressure in the ears must be regularly equalized prior to further descent. In patients with known ET malfunction, grommet insertion will prevent the pressure gradient across the TM that may occur during air travel. Decompression sickness can be prevented by divers limiting their ascent to a rate of 10 metres per minute. When decompression sickness occurs, the initial treatment should be 100 per cent oxygen until hyperbaric

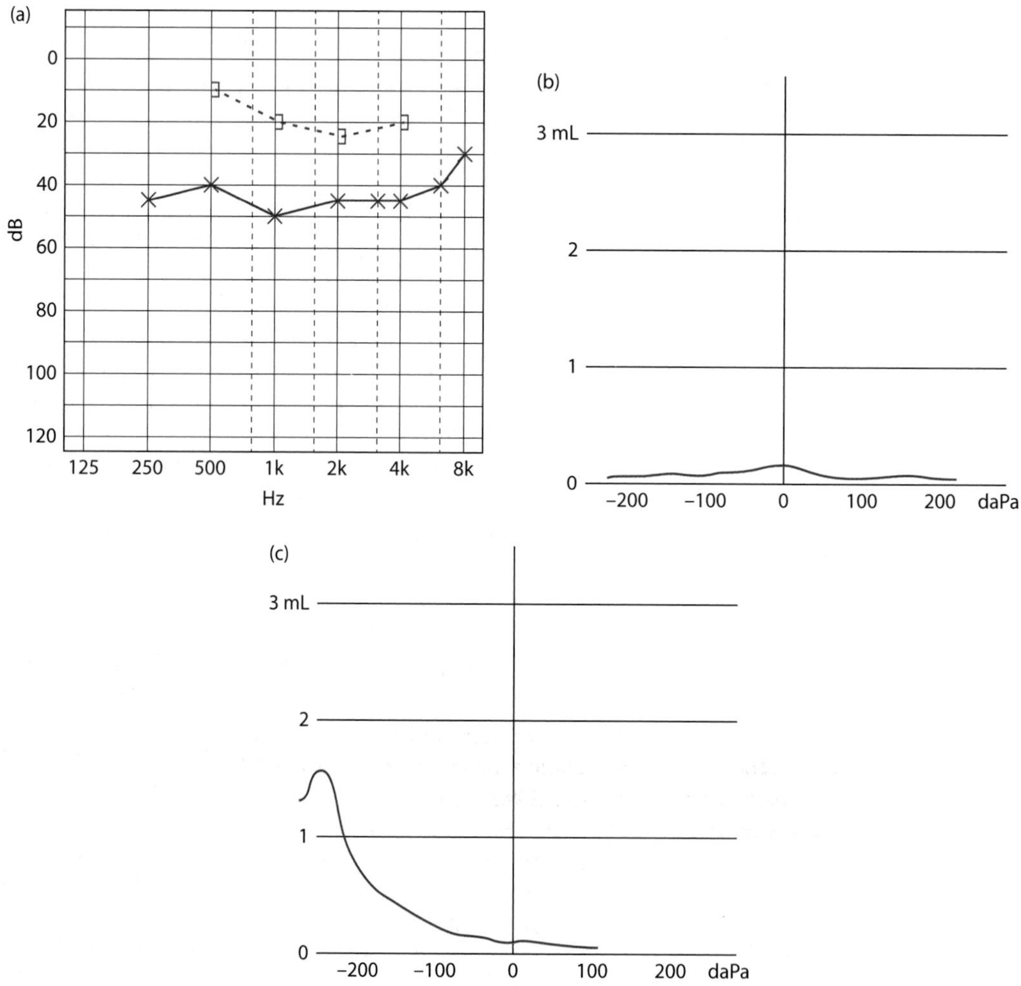

Figure 51.6 **(a)** Left CHL; **(b)** type B; and **(c)** type C tympanogram.

oxygen therapy can be provided in a high-pressure chamber.

ACOUSTIC TRAUMA

HISTORY AND EXAMINATION

Acoustic trauma is also known as noise-induced hearing loss. Tinnitus is often a prominent symptom. A temporary threshold shift occurs initially after exposure to loud sounds (>85 dB), which tends to recover after the stimulus has been taken away. A permanent threshold shift can occur if there is constant or repeated exposure to loud sounds, e.g. working in a noisy factory or being near gunfire or loud music. Individuals vary in their susceptibility to noise. Hearing loss results from damage to the outer hair cells of the organ of Corti. Inner hair cells seem to be more resistant to acoustic trauma. Above a certain noise level, there may be permanent damage to the outer hair cells, inner hair cells, Reissner's membrane and spiral ganglion cells producing a SNHL. There is reduced speech discrimination, especially in background noise. Extremely loud sounds >180 dB can produce an acute acoustic trauma.

INVESTIGATIONS

The external auditory canal resonates at a frequency of 3 KHz. There is maximal damage to the outer hair cells at the basal turn of the cochlea, where the high tones are tonotropically represented, producing a 3–6 KHz dip on the audiogram (Figure 51.7).

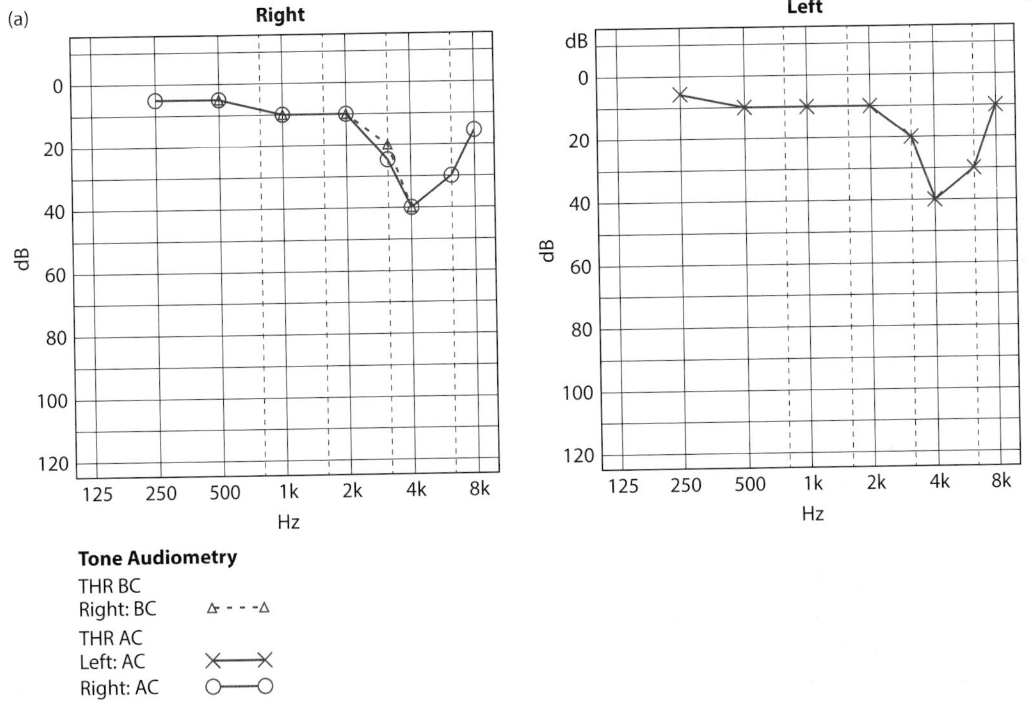

Figure 51.7 **(a)** Symmetrical moderate sensorineural hearing loss (SNHL) in the 4 KHz section following noise exposure; **(b)** worsening SNHL from increased loud noise exposure; **(c)** symmetrical high-tone SNHL in a right-handed soldier shooting a rifle from the right shoulder. *(Continued)*

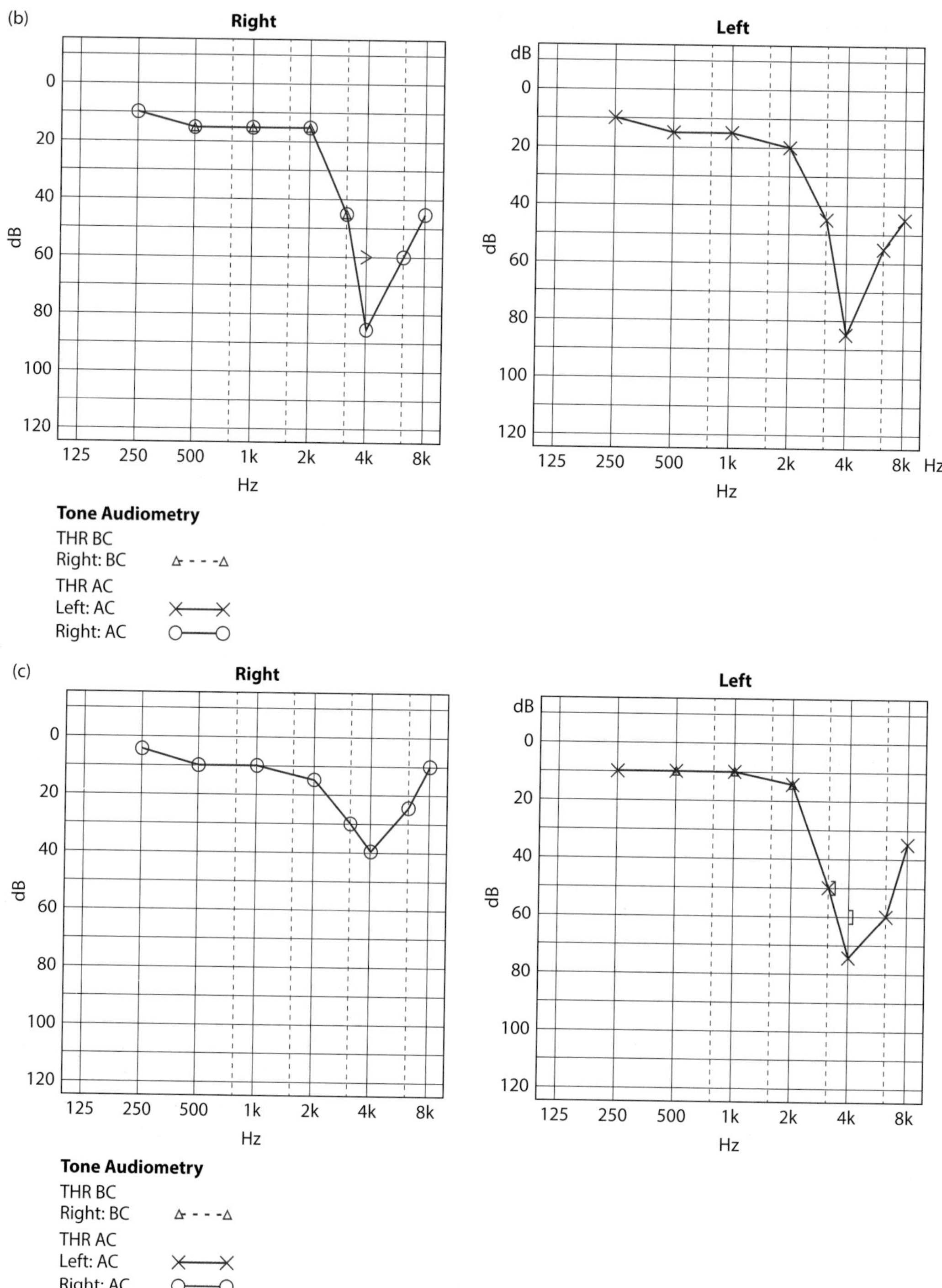

Figure 51.7 (Continued) **(a)** Symmetrical moderate sensorineural hearing loss (SNHL) in the 4 KHz section following noise exposure; **(b)** worsening SNHL from increased loud noise exposure; **(c)** asymmetrical high-tone SNHL in a right-handed soldier shooting a rifle from the right shoulder.

MANAGEMENT

A temporary threshold shift will be reversed with no further loud sound exposure. A permanent threshold shift results in an irreversible SNHL. Acoustic trauma can be prevented by use of well-designed ear defenders. Ear protection in the form of ear plugs or earmuffs are a legal requirement in industries with high background noise levels. Industries should also ensure employees are exposed to a maximum daily noise level of 85 dB(A) for less than 8 hours. In those with permanent but serviceable SNHL, hearing aid provision should be available.

KEY LEARNING POINTS

- The external, middle and inner ear structures are liable to be affected by trauma in isolation or in combination, depending on the type and severity of the injury.
- Mechanisms of injury can be broadly divided into blunt or penetrating direct trauma and indirect blast injury, barotrauma or acoustic trauma.
- The majority of tympanic membrane perforations will heal spontaneously within 3 months of the injury.
- A persistent conductive hearing loss with a healed tympanic membrane is suspicious of ossicular chain fracture/discontinuity or fixation.
- Major head and neck trauma should be managed and stabilized according to the ATLS protocol prior to management of temporal bone injury.
- The majority of CSF otorrhoea will heal spontaneously within a week of the injury and do not require any prophylactic antibiotics.
- The two most important prognostic factors in traumatic facial nerve recovery are the delay in onset and the severity of the palsy.
- Balance tends to improve secondary to central compensation despite permanent damage to the peripheral vestibular system.
- Sounds above 180 dB can produce an acute acoustic trauma with an irreversible SNHL.

REFERENCES

1. Health Protection Agency North West 2010. Guidance for the management of human bite injuries. Available from: www.hpa.org.uk.
2. Tos M. Course of and sequelae to 248 petrosalfractures. *Acta Otolaryngologica.* 1971; 85: 1147–59.
3. Podoshin L, Fradis M. Hearing loss after head injury. *Archives of Otolaryngology.* 1975; 101: 15–18.
4. Hough JVD. Restoration of hearing loss after head trauma. *Annals of Otology, Rhinology and Laryngology.* 1969; 78: 210–25.
5. Mills RP, Starritt N. Management of dislocation of the incus by physiological repositioning. *Journal of Laryngology and Otology.* 2002; 116: 589–92.
6. Browning GG, Swan IRCS, Gatehouse S. Hearing loss in minor head injury. *Archives of Otolaryngology.* 1982; 108: 474–77.
7. Nosan DK, Benecke JE, Murr AH. Current perspective on temporal bone trauma. *Otolaryngology – Head and Neck Surgery.* 1997; 117: 67–71.
8. Glasscock ME 3rd, Hart MJ, Rosdeutscher JD, Bhansali SA. Traumatic perilymphatic fistula: How long can symptoms persist? A follow-up report. *American Journal of Otology.* 1992; 13: 333–38.
9. McGuirt WF Jr., Stool SE. Temporal bone fractures in children: A review with emphasis on long-term sequelae. *Clinical Pediatrics.*1992; 31:12–18.
10. Rathmore MH. Do prophylactic antibiotics prevent meningitis after basilar skull fracture? *Pediatric Infectious Disease Journal.* 1991; 10: 87–88.
11. Department of Health. Immunisation against infectious diseases. Chapter 25:

Pneumococcal. August 2006. Available from: http://www.dh.gov.uk/prod_consum_dh/groups/dh_digitalassets/@dh/@en/documents/digitalasset/dh_4137924.pdf.
12. Brodie HA, Thompson TC. Management of complications from 820 temporal bone fractures. *American Journal of Otology*. 1997; 18: 188–97.
13. Davies RA, Luxon LM. Dizziness following head injury: A neuro-otological study. *Journal of Neurology*. 1995; 242: 222–30.
14. Katsarkas A. Benign paroxysmal positional vertigo (BPPV): Idiopathic versus post-traumatic. *Acta Otolaryngologica*. 1999; 119: 745–49.
15. Jones JS, Sheffield W, White LJ, Bloom MA. A double-blind comparison between oral pseudoephedrine and topical oxymetazoline in the prevention of barotrauma during air travel. *American Journal of Emergency Medicine*. 1998; 16: 262–64.

FURTHER READING

Bove A. *Bove and Davis' Diving Medicine*. 3rd ed. Toronto: WB Saunders Company, 1997.
DeHart RL, Davis JR. *Fundamentals of Aerospace Medicine*. 3rd ed. Baltimore, MD: Lippincott Williams & Wilkins, 2002.

52

The facial nerve

SOMIAH SIDDIQ AND RICHARD IRVING

The facial nerve is the most common cranial nerve to be involved in functional deficit. Its long and complex course, commencing intra-cranially and then located in a non-expandable bony canal, the parotid gland and superficial tissues, may account for its vulnerability to involvement by trauma, inflammation or neoplasia. The nerve contains motor, sensory and parasympathetic fibres; however, it is the motor component that predominates and produces the greatest morbidity associated with conditions affecting the nerve.

EMBRYOLOGY

The facial nerve develops during the time closely adjacent derivatives of the first arch give rise to the external and middle ear components, hence anomalies of the facial nerve should be anticipated where malformations of the external or middle ear are present.[1]

The facial nerve is derived from the second branchial arch. Development of the facial nerve begins at 3 weeks of gestation, becoming fully developed approximately 4 years following birth. At 3 weeks the facioacoustic primordium appears, and by the fourth week of gestation the facial nerve splits into the caudal and rostral trunks.

During weeks five and six, the geniculate ganglion is identifiable. There is complete separation of the facial and acoustic nerves, and the nervus intermedius develops. The distal branches of the facial nerve are a loose network at this stage. During week seven, the nervus intermedius enters the brain stem between the eighth and motor root of the facial nerve. At this stage the parotid bud gives rise to the parotid gland, and the development of multiple facial muscles begins. The fallopian canal develops around week eight.

By 16 weeks, all definitive communications of the facial nerve are complete with ossification of the sulcus into the fallopian canal. At birth, the facial nerve approximates to that found in adults, except that it exits through the more superficially located stylomastoid foramen with ongoing development of the mastoid tip following birth.

ANATOMY

The facial nerve is a mixed nerve comprising upper and lower motor neurons with the lower having intracranial, intratemporal and extracranial segments (Figure 52.1).

Corticobulbar fibres from the precentral gyrus project to the internal capsule, then to the lower brain stem, synapsing in the pontine facial nerve nucleus. The corticobulbar fibres cross to the contralateral side with bilateral contribution to the upper part of the facial nerve nucleus. This bilateral cortical representation results in forehead sparing in upper motor neuron lesions involving the motor cortex or internal capsule, resulting in weakness of the contralateral lower facial muscles. In contrast, lower motor neuron lesions will result in ipsilateral paralysis of the both upper and lower face.

From the pontine facial motor nucleus, the facial nerve loops around the abducent nerve nucleus before exiting the ventral surface of the pons antero-inferior to the vestibulooccular nerve and nervus intermedius. It then crosses the cerebellopontine angle to enter the fallopian canal via the internal auditory meatus.

The course of the nerve through the temporal bone measures approximately 3 cm and can be divided into the labyrinthine, tympanic and mastoid segments.

The labyrinthine segment courses anterolaterally from the internal auditory meatus to the geniculate ganglion. This segment of the nerve lies immediately posterior and superior to the cochlea

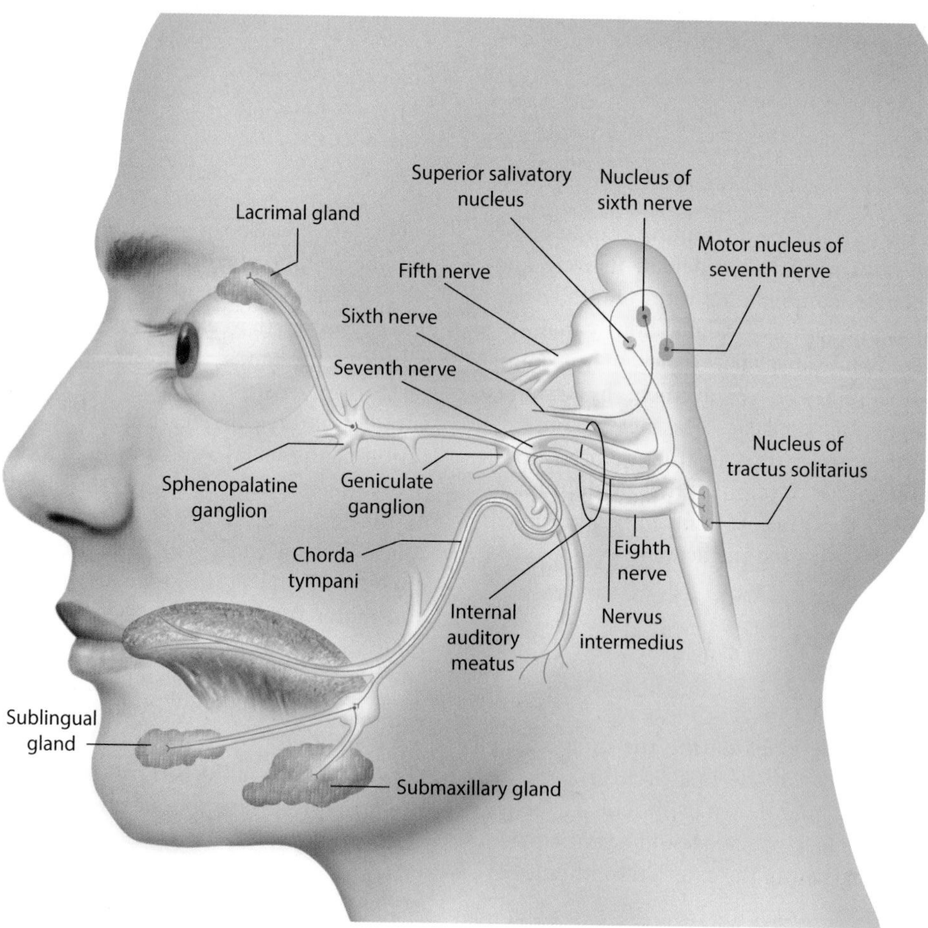

Figure 52.1 Facial nerve anatomy.

and posterolateral to the ampulla of the horizontal and superior semicircular canals. This is the narrowest segment of the facial nerve canal and therefore is susceptible to compression secondary to inflammation and to vascular insults, as it lacks epineurium and anastomosing arterial cascades.

The first genu marks the location of the geniculate ganglion, which contains the cell bodies of the somatic sensory component of the nerve. The nerve at this point gives a branch, the greater superficial petrosal nerve (GSPN). The GSPN contains parasympathetic fibres from the nervus intermedius. They then join the deep pterosal, synapse in the pterygopalntine ganglion and innervate the lacrimal gland and mucus glands of the nasal and oral cavities.

The tympanic or horizontal segment passes from the geniculate ganglion to the second genu. The nerve here lies medial to the cochleariform process and tensor tympani against the medial wall of the tympanic cavity, above the oval window and stapes, and below the lateral semicircular canal. Of note, the fallopian canal may be dehiscent in up to 50 per cent of cases, especially if congenital ear malformations coexist. The distal portion of the facial nerve then exits the middle ear between the posterior wall of the external auditory canal and lateral semicircular canal, marking the second genu just distal to the pyramidal eminence.

The mastoid or vertical segment runs from the second genu to the stylomastoid foramen.

The nerve continues vertically down where it lies in front of and lateral to the ampulla of the posterior semicircular canal and medial to the tympanic annulus within the mastoid. The mastoid segment of the nerve gives rise to three branches, the nerve to the stapedius muscle, chorda tympani nerve and the sensory auricular branch. The chorda tympani runs through the middle ear between the incus and handle of malleus and exits through the canal of Huguier to join the lingual nerve. It carries parasympathetic fibres to the sublingual and submandibular glands and the anterior two-thirds of the tongue.

Important surgical landmarks for identifying the intratemporal facial nerve include the cochleariform process, lateral semicircular canal, fossa incudis and digastric ridge.

The facial nerve exits the stylomastoid foramen, passing inferiorly and laterally around the styloid process, and enters the parotid gland. Within the gland the nerve divides into two major divisions, the temporalofacial and cervicofacial branches, going on to form five major branches: temporal, zygomatic, buccal, marginal mandibular and cervical. Variation may exist where the nerve may divide prior to exiting the stylomastoid foramen with further variation in the peripheral branches.

Surgical landmarks to identify the extracranial facial nerve include the tympanomastoid suture line (6–8 mm lateral to the stylomastoid foramen) and the tragal pointer (approximately 1 cm inferior and medial to the tragal pointer). The posterior belly of the digastric muscle is arguably the most useful, with the nerve lying immediately above this where the muscle joins the mastoid and at the same depth.

PHYSIOLOGY

Each facial nerve has approximately 10 000 fibres of which two-thirds are motor and the remaining one-third sensory.

The use of topodiagnostic tests to assess function of a branch of the facial nerve to determine the site of the lesion is of historical significance only. Routinely, taste, salivary flow, Schirmer and stapedial reflex tests are not done, as they have no prognostic value and provide limited clinical correlation.

Electrophysiology tests evaluate the degree of facial nerve dysfunction and potential recovery and can guide ongoing management, in particular timing of surgical decompression and facial reanimation procedures. Currently, the two most common objective tests used are electroneuronography (ENoG) and electromyography (EMG).

ENoG relies on a functional contralateral nerve and is mainly of value in acute onset complete facial nerve paralysis. The amplitude of nerve conduction velocity stimulated at the stylomastoid foramen and detected with a surface electrode at the nasolabial fold, correlates with a poor prognosis if greater than 95 per cent reduction in amplitude occurs on the affected side within 3 to 21 days. It takes up to 3 days for Wallerian degeneration to occur, and after 3 weeks, owing to concurrent degeneration and regeneration, ENoG is of less value.

EMG studies are useful in delayed paralysis and cases of bilateral facial nerve palsy and are used in conjunction with ENoG. EMG measures voluntary motor unit potentials (the patient is asked to make forceful contractions) using needle electrodes placed in the orbicularis oris and orbicularis oculi muscles. Fibrillation potentials suggest Wallerian degeneration and arise 2 to 3 weeks following injury, whilst polyphasic potentials indicate early signs of reinnervation, which can precede clinical signs of recovery by 3 months. Electrical silence is a poor prognostic indicator and argues against attempts at facial reanimation designed to use the native facial musculature.

Both Seddon and Sunderland classifications of nerve injury (Table 52.1) are commonly used and aid a fuller appreciation of electrophysiological studies.

Several facial grading systems attempt to objectively quantify facial function. Facial grading scales are used in measuring recovery, potential deterioration and comparison of facial nerve outcomes across therapeutic modalities. The House–Brackmann (HB) score (Table 52.2), first described in 1985, is widely used clinically to measure the degree of facial motor weakness. It consists of six grades from normal (HB I) to total paralysis (HB VI).

Table 52.1 Nerve injury classification

Pathology	Sunderland	Seddon	Prognosis
Conduction block No anatomical disruption	First degree	Neurapraxia	Reversible with full recovery
Division of axon	Second degree	Axonotmesis	Reasonable recovery
Division of axon and endoneurium	Third degree	Axonotmesis/ Neurotmesis	Incomplete recovery
Complete transection of nerve but epineurium intact	Fourth degree	Neurotmesis	Poor recovery
Complete transection of nerve	Fifth degree	Neurotmesis	No recovery

Table 52.2 House–Brackmann grading

Grade	Gross	Resting tone	Forehead	Eye closure	Mouth
I		Normal function			
II	Slight weakness Very slight synkinesis	Normal	Moderate to good function	Complete closure with minimal effort	Slight asymmetry
III	Obvious weakness Noticeable but not severe synkinesis, contracture, and/or hemi-facial spasm	Normal	Slight to moderate function	Complete closure with full effort	Slight weakness with maximum effort
IV	Disfiguring	Normal	None	Incomplete closure	Asymmetric with maximum effort
V	Barely perceptible motion	Asymmetric	None	Incomplete closure	Slight movement
VI		Total paralysis			

PATHOLOGY

Facial nerve paralysis can result from numerous causes, some of which are listed in Table 52.3, the most common being idiopathic or Bell's palsy, trauma, infection and neoplasia. Cases of bilateral facial palsy should alert the clinician to underlying systemic or neurological pathology, such as syphilis, Lyme disease or Guillain–Barré syndrome.

BELL'S PALSY

Named after Sir Charles Bell, who first described the syndrome, Bell's palsy is an idiopathic peripheral nerve lesion with some evidence to support a viral aetiology. Annual incidence is 20 to 30 cases per 100 000 people per year,[2] with an equal sex incidence and a peak incidence of 40 years, although it can occur in all age groups. Patients who have had an episode of Bell's palsy have an 8 per cent risk of recurrence. Although Bell's palsy is the most common cause of unilateral facial paralysis, accounting for 60–70 per cent of all cases,[3] it is a diagnosis of exclusion. The majority of patients will show partial recovery within 3 weeks of onset, and all patients get some recovery. Poor prognostic factors include complete facial palsy at onset, age over 60 years, severe pain, no recovery by 3 weeks, and associated conditions, e.g. hypertension and diabetes.

Table 52.3 Differential diagnoses of facial nerve palsy

Idiopathic	Bell's palsy
Infection	Otitis media Cholesteatoma Skull base osteomyelitis Lyme disease Syphilis Varicella zoster HIV
Trauma	Temporal bone fracture Gunshot/penetrating injuries Traumatic delivery Iatrogenic
Tumour	Schwannoma Meningioma Haemangioma Parotid malignancy
Neurological	Lacunar/brain stem infarct Guillain–Barré syndrome
Congenital	Mobius syndrome CHARGE syndrome
Other	Sarcoidosis

Bell's palsy normally presents with sudden onset of unilateral lower motor nerve facial palsy over a course of 24–48 hours. It is frequently preceded by periauricular paresthesia or otalgia. A viral prodome may exist and dysgeusia, hyeracusis and facial numbness may be present. The tearing mechanism is affected, but paradoxically the patient may complain of excess tears owing to loss of lower lid control. Examination includes assessment of facial nerve function, remaining cranial nerves, otoscopy and palpation of the parotid. Specifically, the degree of eye closure and presence of Bell's phenomenon should be determined, to quantify corneal risk.

A baseline pure tone audiogram should be obtained, especially if the patient complains of hearing loss, as this is not typical in Bell's palsy.

Ocular care takes precedence, in cases where there is incomplete eye closure, to prevent sight-threatening complications. Regular topical lubricants throughout the day with thicker viscosity lubricant at night should be prescribed with taping of eye shut at night. Referral to ophthalmology should be considered in complete facial palsy.

Controversy still exists in relation to corticosteroids and antivirals versus corticosteroid alone. The use of antivirals is still of questionable value;[3,4] however, the use of corticosteroids has a good evidence base, especially if taken within the first 24 hours. A typical treatment for an adult would be prednisolone 1 mg/kg[3] with maximum of 60 mg a day for 7 days if no medical contraindications exist. Follow-up should be arranged in 3 weeks following onset to document recovery. In cases where progressive loss occurs over weeks; recovery is not seen within 3 weeks; or the patient has twitching, other cranial nerve deficits or recurrence, then imaging should be arranged. In such cases it is essential to rule out a tumour, and enhanced magnetic resonance imaging (MRI) combined with computed tomography (CT) of the course of the facial nerve is the best technique.

The role of surgical decompression in the management remains controversial, largely owing to the lack of randomized trials comparing surgery with medical therapy. However, surgical decompression may have a role in recurrent facial palsy either secondary to Bell's palsy or associated with Melkersson–Rosenthal syndrome.[5]

INFECTION

Bacterial causes for facial nerve paralysis include acute or chronic otitis media and skull base osteomyelitis. Facial paralysis secondary to acute otitis media is rare and tends to be more common in young children. Middle ear cholesteatoma is associated with facial paralysis in less than 1 per cent of cases; however, when the disease is in the petrous apex, this increases to close to 50 per cent. Most cases of facial paralysis secondary to acute otitis media resolve with conservative management in the form of systemic antibiotics. Surgical options of myringotomy with or without ventilation tube may be indicated when spontaneous perforation of the tympanic membrane is not present. A mastoidectomy may be indicated for suppurative complications, lack of clinical improvement or worsening of the facial palsy. Rarely, surgical decompression of the facial nerve is necessary.

The converse generally is true for chronic otitis media or cholesteatoma or the delayed onset of facial paralysis, as this is probably secondary to erosion of the facial nerve canal and early surgical intervention is warranted in the form of a mastoidectomy. Recovery can occur even if treatment is delayed for several months in facial paralysis secondary to cholesteatoma.[6]

Lyme disease and Ramsay Hunt syndrome are uncommon infections causing facial palsy.

Lyme disease is a multisystemic illness caused by the spirocheate *Borrelia burgdorferi*. The disease is transmitted by tick bites and can give rise to both unilateral and bilateral facial nerve paralysis. Erythema migrans is evident in the early stages of the disease with associated joint pain, fever and later symptoms of fatigue and neck stiffness. Enquire regarding the patient's recent travel or certain outdoor activities such as hiking or camping. The diagnosis is confirmed by serology, and first-line treatment in adults of early Lyme disease without neurological or cardiac involvement is doxycycline (100 mg twice daily) or amoxicillin (500 mg three times daily) for 2 to 3 weeks.[7]

Ramsay Hunt syndrome is caused by the varicella-zoster virus and is characterized by vesicles in the external ear, soft palate or tongue. It may be misdiagnosed as Bell's palsy as the classic vesicles may not appear or may be delayed. Varicella-zoster virus polymerase chain reaction (PCR) may help to distinguish between Ramsay Hunt syndrome and Bell's palsy patients. If the diagnosis is suspected, prompt treatment with steroids and antivirals is recommended. However, despite treatment the prognosis is poor with fewer than half of patients achieving complete recovery of facial function.[2]

TRAUMA

Both blunt and penetrating mechanisms of injury may result in facial nerve paralysis. Causes of injury include motor vehicle accidents, assault, stab and gunshot injuries and iatrogenic injury.

Temporal bone fractures account for 18–22 per cent of skull fractures in patients treated for head trauma.[8] Common sequelae of temporal bone fractures include facial nerve injury, damage to the cochleovestibular apparatus with associated sensorineural hearing loss, conductive loss, balance disturbance, tinnitus, vertigo and cerebrospinal fluid (CSF) leak.

Traditional classification systems of longitudinal, transverse and mixed temporal bone fractures are still used but poorly correlate to clinical complications. More recently, petrous or otic capsule sparing versus non-petrous or otic capsule violating classifications have been suggested to provide improved clinical correlation, aiding early recognition of potential complications and guiding management.

Facial nerve injury is more common in transverse compared to longitudinal temporal bone fractures and less common in children.

Gunshot-related temporal bone injury results in extensive injury to adjacent structures, with a much higher incidence of facial nerve paralysis compared to closed head injury.[9] As a result, gunshot injuries are more likely to require surgical exploration than blunt temporal bone fractures.

In middle ear surgery, iatrogenic injury of the tympanic segment of the facial nerve is the most common site of injury, owing to the prevalence of facial canal dehiscense or exposure secondary to cholesteatoma. The nerve can also be damaged in the cerebellopontine angle during acoustic neuroma surgery or when operating on the parotid gland.

Owing to the nature of force required, the majority of patients with temporal bone fractures will have multiple injuries, including possible intracranial and cervical spine injury. Therefore, initial assessment follows advanced trauma life support (ATLS) protocols with multidisciplinary involvement. Once stabilized, a complete neuro-otological examination of the patient is required, including otoscopy for haemotympanum/perforated eardrum, evidence of postauricular ecchymosis (Battle's sign), CSF leak from the ear or nose and, in the conscious patient, assessment of facial nerve function, nystagmus and hearing loss (bedside tuning fork tests and formal audiometric testing at the earliest opportunity).

In the critically ill patient, rapid imaging with high-resolution CT is essential to evaluate the temporal bone but also the intracranial contents and potential cervical spine injury.

Delayed onset or incomplete paresis almost always recovers, the majority within the first 3 months. Treatment involves high-dose corticosteroids and eye care. The decision to explore a facial nerve following trauma is complex. Factors favouring exploration and indicating a severe injury to the nerve are a penetrating injury, immediate onset of paralysis, CT evidence of nerve canal disruption or bony spicule, loss of inner ear function, persistent CSF leak and 90 per cent or greater degeneration on ENoG. Iatrogenic injury should be repaired at the time of surgery if noticed or re-explored within days and the nerve repaired.

Patients with persistent facial paralysis are observed for at least a year before considering reanimation and reinnervation techniques, to allow for natural recovery.

TUMOURS

Tumours account for an estimated 5 per cent of patients with facial nerve paralysis. Schwannomas form the majority of intrinsic facial nerve tumours and can occur anywhere along the course of the facial nerve. Haemangiomas are extremely rare benign vascular tumours and tend to arise around the geniculate ganglion and internal auditory canal, reflective of the rich blood supply at these sites.

Malignant involvement includes direct perineural spread via the facial nerve into the temporal bone by parotid mucoepidermoid and adenoid cystic carcinoma and squamous cell carcinoma.

Facial nerve tumours manifest with facial weakness, hearing loss, tinnitus, imbalance, vertigo or pain. Symptoms are dependent upon the site of tumour along the course of the facial nerve. Eliciting a history of slowly progressive facial nerve paresis over a number of weeks, absence of recovery after 6 months, presence of facial spasms or twitching and ipsilateral recurrence are suggestive of a tumour. Hearing loss may be sensorineural with associated tinnitus or vertigo with tumours in the labyrinthine segment, or conductive with tumours in the horizontal segment. Examination should include assessment of facial nerve function, otoscopy, and palpation of parotid and neck.

The diagnosis of facial nerve tumours is often missed or delayed owing to the small size of these tumours and difficulties of achieving a diagnosis on standard imaging.[10] Thin-sectioned contrast-enhanced MRI in combination with high-resolution CT of the temporal bone is advised. The facial nerve course must be imaged from the brain stem to the terminal branches.

Benign intrinsic tumours with good facial motor function should be observed and managed conservatively. Facial nerve schwannomas tend to reach a relatively large size by the time they become symptomatic. However, facial nerve haemangiomas may cause severe neural deficit while they are still relatively small and hence early resection offers the best chance of good facial nerve recovery.[11] Care must be taken to avoid biopsy of a middle ear mass noted on exploratory tympanotomy for conductive hearing loss, as this may represent a facial nerve schwannoma (Figure 52.2).

Tumour location, size and level of residual hearing will dictate the surgical approach. A middle fossa approach may be considered in small tumours at the geniculate ganglion in patients with good hearing, translabyrinthine in larger tumours

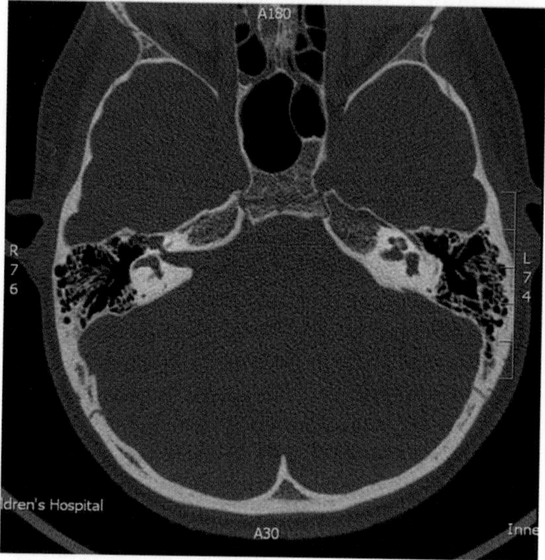

Figure 52.2 Schwannoma of the geniculate ganglion on the right.

or in poor hearing and transmastoid for involvement of the horizontal or vertical facial nerve.

FACIAL REANIMATION

Facial nerve paralysis is a devastating event even in its partial form, resulting in both a very evident deformity as well as functional problems of eyelid closure, oral continence and speech. Any patient with a persisting weakness should be offered treatment aimed at improving cosmesis and restoring function. This may include facial therapy, Botox or surgical reanimation techniques.[12]

The main factor in deciding the surgical approach to facial nerve reconstruction is the status of the facial musculature. Successful muscle unit survival is unlikely beyond 18–24 months after nerve injury. Techniques utilizing the native musculature typically give better results, so early referral for reanimation is critical.

FACIAL MUSCULATURE VIABLE

Primary neurorrhaphy with accurate end-to-end facial nerve repair is recommended in facial nerve transection following oncologic resection, temporal bone fracture and iatrogenic injury. Where the nerve defect cannot be overcome by rerouting, interposition nerve grafts can be used. The most common graft sources are the greater auricular and the sural nerves.

Where the proximal nerve stump is not available, nerve transfer using an end-to-side hypoglossal-facial nerve anastomosis (XII–VII) or end-to-end facial masseteric anastomosis remains the most popular technique. Cross-facial nerve grafts are an alternative and can enable more symmetrical movement. This involves anastomosing redundant facial branches on the normal side to branches on the paralyzed side with use of an interposition nerve graft.

FACIAL MUSCULATURE NON-VIABLE

In late presentation where the onset of the facial palsy is more than 24 months old, as well as in congenital cases, muscle units are either non-viable or non-existent, and facial reanimation is achieved with muscle transposition or free muscle importation. Both of these techniques are mainly used for the animation of the lower third of the face.

Muscle transposition involves the usage of regional muscles such as the temporalis or masseter. Free muscle transfer provides soft tissue coverage of a defect and involuntary, mimetic facial movements. The preferred muscles are the gracilis, latissimus dorsi and pectoralis minor, and the microneurovascular muscle transfer is a two-stage procedure.

STATIC PROCEDURES

Static techniques do not achieve spontaneous dynamic movement but try to achieve static or resting symmetry, with the correction of abnormal postures, eye protection and oral continence. They can be used either as single procedures or in conjunction with the more complex nerve and muscle techniques described above.

Gold and platinum weights to the upper lid can be used in lagophthalmos and medial and lateral canthoplasty to correct lower lid ectropion.

Static slings in the form of facia lata, plantaris tendon or alloplastic material such as Gore-Tex or

Alloderm can be used to suspend the nasolabial fold or the perioral muscles and can achieve good resting symmetry. Facelift and brow lift procedures and Botox injections into the non-paralyzed side to reduce asymmetry have a place in selective cases.

KEY LEARNING POINTS

- The facial nerve is the most common cranial nerve to be affected by disease.
- Imaging is critical to diagnosis and exclusion of alternative pathology.
- Bell's palsy always recovers to some extent.
- Early referral for reanimation is critical to outcome.

REFERENCES

1. Sataloff RT, Selber JC. Phylogeny and embryology of the facial nerve and related structures. Part II: Embryology. *Ear Nose and Throat Journal*. 2003; 82(10): 764–6, 769–72, 774 passim.
2. Holland NJ, Weiner GM. Clinical review. Recent developments in Bell's palsy. *BMJ*. 2004; 329: 553–7.
3. Gilden DH. Clinical practice. Bell's palsy. *New England Journal of Medicine*. 2004; 351(13): 1323–31.
4. Sullivan FM, Swan IR, Donnan PT et al. Early treatment with prednisolone or acyclovir in Bell's palsy. *New England Journal of Medicine*. 2007; 357(16): 1598–607.
5. Doshi J, Irving R. Recurrent facial nerve palsy: The role of surgery. *Journal of Laryngology and Otology*. 2010; 124(10): 1202–4.
6. Siddiq MA, Hanu-Cenat LM, Irving RM. Facial palsy secondary to cholesteatoma: Analysis of outcome following surgery. *Journal of Laryngology and Otology*. 2007; 121(2): 114–17.
7. The epidemiology, prevention, investigation and treatment of Lyme borreliosis in United Kingdom patients: A position statement by the British Infection Association. *Journal of Infection*. 2011; 62(5): 329–38.
8. Johnson F, Semaan MT, Megerian CA. Temporal bone fracture: Evaluation and management in the modern era. *Otolaryngology Clinics of North America*. 2008; 41: 597–618.
9. Moore PL, Selby G, Irving RM. Gunshot injuries to the temporal bone. *Journal of Laryngology and Otology*. 2003; 117(1): 71–74.
10. Alaani A, Hogg R, Saravanappa N, Irving RM. An analysis of the diagnostic delay in unilateral facial palsy. *Journal of Laryngology and Otology*. 2005; 119(3): 184–88.
11. Salib RJ, Tziambazis E, McDermott AL, Chavda SV, Irving RM. The crucial role of imaging in detection of facial nerve haemangiomas. *Journal of Laryngology and Otology*. 2001; 115(6): 510–13.
12. Ramakrishnan Y, Alam S, Kotecha A, Gillett D, D'Souza A. Reanimation following facial palsy: Present and future directions. *Journal of Laryngology and Otology*. 2010; 124: 1146–52.

53

Otitis externa

SIMON A MCKEAN AND S MUSHEER HUSSAIN

INTRODUCTION

Otitis externa can be acute or chronic, diffuse or localized; and can be caused by infection, allergy, irritation or inflammation. It includes all inflammatory conditions of the auricle, external ear canal and outer surface of the tympanic membrane. It is a common problem, and although only 3 per cent of cases are referred from general practice to secondary care, it still constitutes one in six new patient referrals and 30 per cent of people seen in an ear, nose and throat (ENT) emergency clinic. There are very few good quality trials of treatment for acute otitis externa. A Cochrane review published in 2010[1] found 19 randomized controlled trials, only three of which were good quality.

CLINICAL FEATURES

HISTORY

Acute diffuse otitis externa affects up to 10 per cent of the population at some time in their lives. It generally develops within 48 hours and can last up to 3 weeks. The common symptoms are itching or pain (which can be severe) with variable discharge and a feeling of blockage, with a conductive hearing loss noted due to occlusion of the external canal. Any chemical or physical irritation (including syringing and cotton bud abuse) can predispose to infection. Any cause of immunosuppression, including diabetes, can be a predisposing factor for otitis externa. Swimming[2] may underlie otitis externa, or 'swimmers' ear'. Any history of skin complaints should be noted. Contact dermatitis, eczema and psoriasis can affect the skin of the external canal. If there is any bony tenderness over the mastoid, or the pinna is protruding, consider mastoiditis as a differential diagnosis.

EXAMINATION

Look for any surrounding cellulitis and/or lymphadenitis. It may be important to demarcate the edge of the cellulitis to monitor treatment. With regards to the external canal, look for tenderness, erythema, oedema or narrowing. Obstruction of the ear canal may necessitate aural toilette, wick placement or even the use of systemic antimicrobial agents. Stenosis of the canal causes considerable difficulties. Examine to ensure there is not currently anything in the ear canal. Cotton buds, hearing aids, middle ear ventilation tubes, excess ear wax and foreign bodies can traumatize the external canal skin, increasing susceptibility to infection. Look for discharge and note any smell, colour, blood staining, keratin or mucoid element. A green, offensive-smelling discharge may indicate infection with *Pseudomonas aeruginosa.* Fungal hyphae may sometimes be identified. The presence of a mucoid discharge suggests an open middle ear. The tympanic membrane must be fully examined before discharge from clinic, although this may not be possible on the first visit. Look for the presence of grommet, T tube or a tympanic membrane perforation and active middle ear. These may change the management, because of either the primary cause of the problem or its subsequent treatment (i.e. the use of potentially ototoxic medications). Cranial nerves (VII–XII) should be tested since a palsy, although rare, may indicate deep extension of infection, such as malignant otitis externa.

DIFFERENTIAL DIAGNOSES

Other causes of otalgia, otorrhoea and inflammation of the external ear canal should be excluded. It is worth remembering that otalgia is commonly a referred pain from the teeth, tonsils, temporomandibular joint, larynx, neck or even sphenoid sinus. Cranial nerves V, IX and X transmit sensation from the middle and external ear.

Chronic otitis externa causes a continued sensation of itch with mild discomfort. It may be caused by repeated trauma, repeated exposure to infection (i.e. from an open middle ear), inadequate aural toilette, allergy, irritation or otomycosis. On examination the external canal skin is often dry and flaky, with a lack of cerumen. Cerumen itself has some antimicrobial effect on *Staphylococcus aureus*, *Pseudomonas aeruginosa* and *Candida albicans.*[3] It is worth educating many patients about this. The canal itself may become stenosed, aggravating the condition. Chronic otitis externa may be very difficult to treat.

Otomycosis is most commonly caused by *Aspergillus* or *Candida* species. There are anecdotal reports of fungal infection after repeated topical antimicrobial treatments. At least 10 per cent of otitis externa is caused by fungal infection. It is best treated by repeated careful microsuction and topical antifungals for no less than 2 weeks.

Abscesses can develop (furunculosis) in the lateral third of the canal. This leads to severe pain, and the abscesses may rupture or need to be incised and drained to give relief. They are usually caused by *Staphylococcus aureus.*

Herpes zoster oticus consists of severe neuralgic otalgia with cutaneous vesicles and an acute peripheral facial palsy. The vesicles are found on the meatal and pre-auricular skin, along the canal itself and sometimes on the soft palate.

Myringitis means inflammation of the tympanic membrane. Primary myringitis can be due to trauma, infection or sudden pressure changes. Bullous myringitis, due to infection, is seen as bubbles filled with blood on the surface of the tympanic membrane that can burst; however, the tympanic membrane itself is not perforated. Secondary myringitis occurs as a result of adjacent inflammation of the middle ear or the external canal. Granular myringitis is sometimes seen after there has been loss of the epidermal layer of the tympanic membrane.

Malignant (necrotizing) otitis externa is a rare but dangerous extension of infection into the mastoid and temporal bones. It is more common in immunocompromised patients, such as the elderly diabetic, and is often caused by Gram negative bacilli such as *Pseudomonas aeruginosa.* The patients often have severe deep otalgia and may develop cranial nerve palsies. Malignant otitis externa is diagnosed by high-definition computed tomography (CT) or magnetic resonance imaging (MRI) scans of the temporal bones. Isotope bone scans may also be useful. Treatment is with long courses of appropriate antibiotics, which may need to be given intravenously. Unfortunately, resistance of *Pseudomonas aeruginosa* to ciprofloxacin is now being reported, and this will have a significant impact on the management of these patients. These patients also need nutrition, blood sugar control (if diabetic) and analgesia.

Benign necrotizing otitis externa is also rare and is characterized by itching and pain with a variable discharge. Examination reveals focal bone exposure in the canal with minimal surrounding inflammation. It is not associated with any co-morbidities.

Perichondritis in the younger population is often due to piercing of the pinna cartilage and can lead to widespread cellulitis. The combination of the crush injury to the cartilage and *Pseudomonas aeruginosa* is likely to be the cause. Relapsing perichondritis is the severe, episodic and progressive inflammation of the cartilage of the ear, nose and tracheobronchial tree, and has an autoimmune pathogenesis.

Keratosis obturans, which is of unknown aetiology, is characterized by a large amount of cerumen and keratin filling a ballooned external ear canal, which produces otalgia, otorrhoea and conductive hearing loss. It is usually bilateral and leads to erosion of the external canal.

Neoplasms of the external canal skin are rare, but any non-healing ulcer should be biopsied.

INVESTIGATIONS

Ear swabs are not routinely taken at a first appointment, but for treatment failures or chronic cases[4] they might be helpful. The most commonly identified pathogens in a UK series were *Pseudomonas aeruginosa* (45.1 per cent), followed by *Staphylococcus aureus* (9 per cent), anaerobes (6.3 per cent), *Streptococcus* species (4.9 per cent), *Candida* species (9.7 per cent) and *Aspergillus* species (4.2 per cent).

Blood glucose testing may reveal previously undiagnosed diabetes mellitus.

Potential allergens and irritants include neomycin, benzalkonium chloride, propylene glycol and hearing aid mould materials. Up to one-third of patients may develop[5] sensitivity to either the carriers (i.e. propylene glycol) or the antibiotics themselves (i.e. neomycin). Nickel can cause sensitivity reactions. Also, household chemicals such as hairsprays or perfumes can be very irritant. In chronic or recurrent disease, involvement of dermatologists may be very beneficial, with regards to allergy testing and further treatment.

TREATMENT

Aural toilette (especially anterior recess)[6] may be treatment enough and is necessary for diagnosis and visualization of the tympanic membrane to exclude perforation.

Instillation of 3 per cent hydrogen peroxide (H_2O_2) can be useful to help clear the external canal, but is recommended only if the tympanic membrane is intact. Previously, it was commonly used in the cleaning of open wounds. It helps with both the mechanical, physical clearance of debris and also has oxidizing, antimicrobial effects. Although it is not ototoxic if used for brief periods in the middle ear, it does form a significant volume of gas. This could cause problems in the confines of the middle ear.

Analgesia is important. Pain symptoms are often overlooked but must be addressed and managed by appropriate analgesia, which may necessitate admission to hospital.

Patients are often advised to keep the ear dry. Cotton wool with petroleum jelly may be effective in keeping the ear dry while showering.

Patients should be advised not to scratch the ear or use cotton buds.[7] Any trauma to the skin can reduce its protective ability, therefore allowing initiation or extension of infection.

Patients should be shown how to effectively insert ear drops. If possible, an assistant should administer the drops while the patient is lying on his or her side. The patient should remain in this position for 5 minutes. The anti-tragus can be gently massaged to encourage drops deeper into the canal.

Topical acetic acid 2 per cent spray can be bought without prescription and has both antifungal and antibacterial action, but it can have high rates of adverse effects. The external canal is less acidic whilst it is inflamed owing to otitis externa. A good-quality randomized controlled trial found acetic acid alone to be less beneficial than antibiotic-steroid combination drops. It is, however, still recommended for mild acute diffuse disease and may be particularly useful in granular myringitis.

Topical antibacterial medications should be used for the initial treatment of diffuse, uncomplicated acute otitis externa. A systematic review concluded that topical antimicrobial therapy is highly effective for acute otitis externa, with clinical cure rates of 65–80 per cent within 10 days. In randomized controlled trials, a significant number of patients preferred the use of a neomycin-dexamethasone-acetic acid spray (Otomize) compared to drops and rated their outcome as 'good' compared to those treated with framycetin-dexamethasone-gramicidin (Sofradex) or neomycin-hydrocortisone-polymyxin B sulphate (Otosporin). However, neomycin does not cover *Pseudomonas aeruginosa*, which is a common pathogen in otitis externa. It is also clear that aminoglycosides have measurable vestibulotoxic and ototoxic effects. Fluroquinolones do not pose these threats and will treat both *Pseudomonas aeruginosa* and *Staphylococcus aureus*. Combination drops of 0.3 per cent ciprofloxacin and 0.1 per cent dexamethasone (Ciprodex) are available in some countries. However, in the United Kingdom, only 0.3 per cent ciprofloxacin eye drops are currently available. Other quinolone eye drops are also available (e.g. 0.3 per cent ofloxacin).

Metronidazole gel can be useful if there is an otitis externa where anaerobes have been cultured.

In difficult cases a broad therapeutic approach may need to be taken. Tri-Adcortyl ointment (a substitute is now made by Mandeville Medicines in the United Kingdom) contains steroid, neomycin and gramicidin and also an antifungal medication. After thorough microsuction, this ointment can be instilled into the ear canal and left until the next appointment. There has been one reported case of ototoxicity in use with a perforated tympanic membrane.

There is no clear therapeutic 'best option' for topical antibiotics in otitis externa, but choices can be made with regards to potential for ototoxicity, microbial resistance or sensitivity, cost, availability and dosing schedule.

Topical steroid drops alone may be useful for patients that have inflammation secondary solely to allergy or sensitization rather than infection. They are not as effective as antibiotic-steroid combination therapy.

An external ear canal wick, such as the Pope otowick (Xomed), expands into the canal, improving delivery of topical medicines.

Glycerine and ichthammol impregnated ribbon gauze has a hygroscopic effect to reduce canal oedema and good antibacterial effect against *Staphylococcus aureus* and *Streptococcus pyogenes*, but not *Pseudomonas aeruginosa*. 'Glyc and Ic' ribbon is a cheap option that may be useful for those with allergies to pharmaceutical carriers in drops or those who cannot manage to use drops effectively.

Topical aluminium acetate drops are as effective as antibiotic drops but are expensive, difficult to obtain and need to be freshly prepared. They can be useful in diffuse, chronic disease.

Systemic antibiotics are unnecessary unless there is extension outside the ear canal, immunosuppression, or local factors that hinder the delivery of topical preparations.

Topical antifungal drops such as clotrimazole solution should be combined with regular aural toilette.

Early reassessment is important, and may be essential for further microsuction.

THE FUTURE?

Chronic otitis externa can be frustrating for both the patient and the doctor treating it. Chemical ear peeling has been suggested for these cases. This consists of a polyvinylic acid film formed by a combination of a specific antibiotic and steroid drop along with acetic acid. The film is then removed under the microscope after 2 weeks. The benefit may be due to the removal of the bacterial biofilm, giving longer-term results.

An alternative strategy in antibiotic-resistant chronic otitis externa may be a single dose of therapeutic bacteriophage preparations. These are viruses that can break down the biofilm to specifically destroy bacteria and then self-replicate until that bacteria is no longer present.

KEY LEARNING POINTS

- Preventative measures should include avoiding both mechanical trauma and water ingress.

- Aural toilette is a cornerstone of treatment.
- Topical antibiotics are of benefit.
- Choice of topical antibiotic drop shows little difference in resolution of symptoms, except in the case of microbial resistance, and with the increased recognition of *Pseudomonas aeruginosa*, infection the topical use of quinolones is likely to be important.
- Remember potential allergens and the possibility of fungal infection in those ears that have already had prolonged treatment.
- Patients may have significant pain that needs to be managed.
- Effective delivery of medication is important; therefore, microsuction and the use of an ear wick can be beneficial.
- Intravenous antibiotics may be necessary.

KEY DEFINITIONS

furuncle a 'boil'; a deep infection of the hair follicle in the lateral ear canal
malignant otitis externa extension of external ear infection causing temporal bone or skull base osteomyelitis
myringitis inflammation of the tympanic membrane
otomycosis a fungal infection of the external ear

REFERENCES

1. Kaushik V, Malik T, Saeed SR. Interventions for acute otitis externa. *Cochrane Database of Systematic Reviews*. 2010; 20(1): CD004740.
2. Springer GL, Shapiro ED. Fresh water swimming as a risk factor for otitis externa: A case control study *Archives of Environmental Health*. 1985; 40(4): 202–6.
3. Lum CL, Jeyanthi S, Prepageran N, et al. Antibacterial and antifungal properties of human cerumen. *Journal of Laryngology and Otology*. 2009; 123(4): 375–8.
4. Bluestone C, Casselbrandt M, Dohar J. *Targeted Therapies in Otitis Media and Otitis Externa*. Ontario: BC Decker, 2003.
5. Rasmussen PA. Otitis externa and allergic contact dermatitis. *Acta Otolaryngologica*. 1974; 77(5): 344–7.
6. Sander R. Otitis externa: A practical guide to treatment and prevention. *American Family Physician*. 2001; 63(5): 927–36.
7. Yelland M. Otitis externa in general practice. *Medical Journal of Australia*. 1992; 156(5): 325–26.

FURTHER READING

McKean SA, Hussain, SSM. 12-minute consultation for otitis externa, evidence based guideline article. *Clinical Otolaryngology*. 2007; 32: 457–59.

54

Tumours of the middle ear

ANIL R BANERJEE

Tumour (derived from the Latin *tumere*, 'to swell') is defined as an abnormal swelling or a mass of tissue formed by a new growth of cells, independent of the surrounding structures.[1] Tumours of the middle ear therefore take various forms, both benign and malignant.

Cholesteatoma is the most common tumour found in the middle ear but will not be discussed further given the detailed description given elsewhere in this textbook.

BENIGN MIDDLE EAR TUMOURS

For the inexperienced ear, nose and throat (ENT) surgeon, diagnosing any form of middle ear disease can be challenging and particularly so in the case of a tumour. Myringosclerosis of the tympanic membrane can make visualization of a lesion difficult, and imaging is often vital to ensure a correct diagnosis and treatment plan is made. Hearing loss, tinnitus and balance disorders are common symptoms, but one must remember that benign lesions can also produce cranial nerve palsies.

GLOMUS TUMOURS

Glomus tumours are paragangliomas. (The term *glomus* is a misnomer and refers to the originally held belief that their origin was vascular.) After cholesteatomas, these are the most common form of middle ear tumour and are classified as one of two forms depending upon their location:

1. *Glomus tympanicum* arises from the area of Jacobsen's nerve typically on the promontory.
2. *Glomous jugulare* arises from the jugular bulb and tends to be larger, involving the jugular foramen and adjacent structures.

Glomus tumours are more common in females and tend to present in adults over the age of 40. There are classification systems based upon their location and size, the most widely used being that of Fisch and Oldring.[2]

The Fisch classification is used to categorize the tumour spread, which in turn influences the surgical approach necessary.

- A – Tumour limited to the middle-ear cleft (glomus tympanicum)
- B – Tumour limited to the tympanomastoid area with no infra-labyrinthine compartment involvement
- C – Tumour involving the infra-labyrinthine compartment of the temporal bone and extending into the petrous apex
  - C1 – Tumour with limited involvement of the vertical portion of the carotid canal
  - C2 – Tumour invading the vertical portion of the carotid canal
  - C3 – Tumour invasion of the horizontal portion of the carotid canal
- D – Tumour with intracranial extension
  - D1 – Tumour with an intracranial extension less than 2 cm in diameter
  - D2 – Tumour with an intracranial extension greater than 2 cm in diameter

Glomus tympanicum

SYMPTOMS

The most common symptom – described in more than half of all patients presenting with this condition – is pulsatile tinnitus. Between one-third and one-half of patients also complain of hearing loss.

In a patient presenting with a history of these symptoms otoscopy is essential.

DIAGNOSIS

In addition to the characteristic symptom history, otoscopy may reveal a pulsing red mass in the middle ear sometimes described as a 'setting sun' or 'rising sun' in that it often appears to arise from the floor of the hypotympanum. In other cases, however, the lesion may arise from the promontory, in which case a rounded red lesion is seen. In more advanced cases the lesion may have extruded into the ear canal, producing a friable polyp prone to bleeding.

INVESTIGATIONS

Before any intervention is considered, a pure tone audiogram is mandatory to appraise any conductive hearing loss on the affected side and also to ensure that normal or better hearing exists in the other ear.

A computed tomography (CT) or magnetic resonance imaging (MRI) scan of the middle ear will show the extent of the soft tissue lesion and also the extent to which it has interfered with the ossicles. It is important to obtain imaging of the lesion to differentiate a glomus tumour from

1. a high jugular bulb, visible arising through a dehiscent bony floor to the middle ear, or
2. an abnormally placed internal carotid artery.

The radiologist reporting on the CT scan should be asked to comment on the bony floor of the middle ear to ensure it is intact before diagnosing a glomus tympanicum. An MRI scan can be useful in assessing the relationship of the tumour to surrounding structures if the lesion is thought to have produced bony erosion.

MR angiography can be used in larger lesions to identify feeding vessels. If required, feeding vessels may be embolized radiologically shortly before any planned surgery.

Although rare, some glomus tumours in the middle ear will secrete catecholamines. This must be evaluated preoperatively to avoid catastrophic hypertensive changes that can ensue when removing the tumour.

TREATMENT

In many patients, watchful waiting is sufficient as smaller tumours may not grow and reassurance once a diagnosis has been established is sometimes enough. If this route is followed it is important to properly stage the tumour and monitor progress indefinitely.

Excision of a glomus tympanicum can be a bloody affair unless preoperative planning is adequate.

Resection of a glomus tympanicum can usually be performed by an endaural route, sometimes with only a permeatal incision. A KTP laser is often very useful for shrinking the tumour and reducing blood loss. It may be necessary to stage the tumour resection in some cases if excessive bleeding occurs as visualization of the fallopian canal is important to avoid laser damage to the facial nerve. Recurrence can occur from remnants left *in situ*.

Glomus jugulare

Although these tumours are derived from the same tissue as tympanicum tumours – neural crest cells – they are more difficult to treat owing to their association with the jugular bulb. They are rarely familial. Larger tumours may present with cranial nerve involvement, with facial nerve and vagus nerve palsies being the most common associated neuropathies.

The highly invasive nature of these tumours, together with their insidious and slow growth along paths of least resistance, means that resection tends to occur late and can be associated with significant morbidity.

NEURALLY ASSOCIATED TUMOURS

Middle ear schwannomas are the most common form of neurally associated middle ear tumours. Although more common in the internal acoustic meatus and cerebellopontine angle, they can occasionally be found along the horizontal course of the facial nerve. Rarely, they will be found on Jacobsen's nerve. They tend to be extremely slow-growing and may be chanced upon when operating for other pathology such as cholesteatoma. A conductive loss mimicking otosclerosis is sometimes seen, and the temptation to biopsy a middle ear lesion found to be interfering with the ossicular chain during stapedectomy should be resisted until imaging or better exposure can rule out a facial nerve lesion.

Otic capsule bone may be eroded, but despite facial nerve compression, the majority of patients do not have facial palsy. Nevertheless, the most common presenting symptom is facial nerve dysfunction.

Diagnosis

Patients with an initial diagnosis of Bell's palsy who fail to show signs of improvement or who suffer slowly worsening facial nerve function should be investigated with MRI scanning with contrast. The reporting radiologist should be asked to comment on the whole of the facial nerve. Although the facial nerve is extremely resistant to slowly increasing pressure, some patients may present with intermittent or worsening facial twitch. Intermittent facial paralysis is also seen. Later manifestations include pain, sensorineural hearing loss and vertigo.

Treatment

Treatment is likely to produce significant morbidity and despite interposition grafts following resection, a House–Brackmann Grade III–IV facial nerve function is the most that can be achieved. Most facial nerve schwannomas are therefore monitored rather than removed. Surgery becomes an option when the facial nerve function has fallen below what could be expected post-operatively following resection, or if growth of the tumour medially is putting the patient at risk.

MIDDLE EAR MENINGIOMA

This is most commonly seen in women over the age of 40. It is a benign tumour arising from the arachnoid cells. A middle ear meningioma can be an extension from a middle cranial fossa lesion or a primary middle ear tumour. It is more common in neurofibromatosis and may mimic otitis media with effusion. Survival following surgical excision is the usual outcome.

ADENOMAS

Middle ear adenomas include a diverse range of tumours. They encompass a variety of lesions with a mixture of epithelial and neuroendocrine components.

Diagnosis

Diagnosis is not usually made on symptoms as these tend to be non-specific, including hearing loss (conductive), aural fullness, tinnitus and vertigo. The group includes the carcinoid neuro-endocrine tumours, but despite their ability to produce catecholamines, it is extremely rare for them to act in a similar fashion to gastro-intestinal carcinoids with flushing and palpitations. CT imaging is non-specific for a middle ear soft tissue mass. Diagnosis is usually made on exploratory tympanotomy with confirmation following biopsy and histological analysis. Full tumour excision often requires removal of ossicles to prevent remnants being missed.

GIANT CELL TUMOURS

Although usually associated with long bones, rare case reports of giant cell tumours of the middle ear exist.[3]

MIDDLE EAR CHORISTOMAS

These are masses of histologically normal tissue occurring in an abnormal location. Salivary gland choristomas are most common, but even these are extremely rare. Conductive hearing loss may be described, but most are discovered by chance during exploratory surgery. Association with the facial nerve has been described in a significant number of cases, and therefore resection can lead to partial facial palsy. Diagnosis and monitoring is usually sufficient in these slow-growing lesions.

HAEMANGIOMAS

These tumours vary widely in both size and associated morbidity. They tend to present in children, and some may completely involute so that no intervention is required. Although extremely rare, each needs to be managed depending upon the symptoms produced and likelihood of further growth.

EOSINOPHILIC GRANULOMA OF THE MIDDLE EAR

These granulomas are rare and form part of the group known as granulomatous diseases. They represent nodular inflammatory reactions to an irritant – usually an infecting organism. They tend to present with otorrhoea as the primary symptom.

EXTREME RARITIES

Melanoma and endolymphatic sac tumours are rare types of benign tumours found in the middle ear.

MALIGNANT TUMOURS OF THE MIDDLE EAR

In addition to hearing loss, tinnitus and balance disturbance, patients may describe symptoms of pain and bleeding, both of which should alert the attending doctor to the possibility of a malignant lesion. Facial paralysis is sometimes a presenting feature, in which case examination may reveal other associated cranial nerve palsies. Imaging is mandatory.

PRIMARY MALIGNANT NEOPLASMS OF THE MIDDLE EAR

Squamous cell carcinoma

This is the most common primary malignant lesion of the middle ear. Like most malignant lesions in this area, it is often confused with chronic suppurative otitis media and may therefore be quite advanced before treatment is instituted.

DIAGNOSIS

Lack of response to conservative treatment with increasing associated morbidity should be enough to prompt urgent imaging with both high-resolution CT and MRI scanning being employed. Many cases are treated conservatively for years before an ENT opinion and imaging is sought.

TREATMENT

The disease tends to spread locally, invading the eustachian tube and mastoid initially.

Treatment is primarily surgery with adjunctive radiotherapy, but in those who are medically unfit, radiotherapy is used as a single modality. Mortality is high, with the majority of patients succumbing to their disease within 5 years of diagnosis. In one series of 13 patients, only two survived irrespective of treatment.[4]

Adenocarcinoma

These extremely rare tumours arise from the middle ear mucosal cells. Although they do not appear to metastasize, they tend to slowly extend intracranially. It is important to exclude a primary disease site elsewhere in the body before diagnosing a primary lesion in the middle ear. Treatment of middle ear adenocarcinoma is with wide surgical resection.

Aggressive papillary tumour is a variant that has an association with von Hippel-Lindau syndrome.

Langerhans cell histiocytosis

These rare lesions are most commonly found in the temporal bone. Treatment options include surgical curettage, low-dose radiotherapy and – in systemic cases – chemotherapy.

Rhabdomyosarcoma

This tends to be a disease of children. The lesion is usually noted in the outpatient clinic to be a unilateral, friable painless aural polyp that fails to respond to the usual conservative measures. Lack of treatment response should lead to suspicion and subsequent CT imaging, but many patients are simply listed for an aural polypectomy. At surgery the disease is found to be far more extensive than previously thought. Even at this point it may be diagnosed as middle ear granular disease, so it is important that a biopsy is taken once the facial nerve has been identified.

At the point of presentation to an ENT specialist, the lesion has usually started to invade surrounding structures.

Prognosis is linked to tissue type.

- I – Superior prognosis (botyroid and spindle cell types)
- II – Intermediate prognosis (embryonal type)
- III – Poor prognosis (alveolar and undifferentiated types)
- IV – Unknown prognosis (rhabdoid features)

METASTATIC MIDDLE EAR NEOPLASMS

Sarcomas of various types, including haemangiosarcoma and rhabdomyosarcoma, have been rarely described in the middle ear. The most common sites of primary lesions are breast, lung and kidney; and also prostate and skin, respectively.

Local head and neck cancers can also metastasize to the middle ear. Descriptions of secondary deposits as well as direct tumour spread have been described from the pharynx, salivary glands and central nervous system.

The tumour type together with the extent of the disease lead to a customized treatment regimen comprising components of surgery, radiotherapy and chemotherapy as required.

KEY LEARNING POINTS

- Cholesteatoma is the most common middle ear tumour.
- Benign middle ear tumours can cause cranial nerve palsies.
- Pulsatile tinnitus should alert the examiner to the possibility of a glomus tumour.
- Rhabdomyosarcomas often present as painless polyps in children.

REFERENCES

1. Tumour. In: *Collins English Dictionary*. Available from: http://www.collinsdictionary.com/dictionary/english/tumour?showCookiePolicy=true.
2. Oldring D, Fisch U. Glomus tumors of the temporal region: Surgical therapy. *American Journal of Otology*. July 1979; 1(1): 7–18.
3. Rosenwasser H. Giant cell tumor involving the middle ear. *Archives of Otolaryngology – Head and Neck Surgery*. 1969; 90(6): 726–31.
4. Savić DL, Djerić DR. Malignant tumours of the middle ear. *Clinical Otolaryngology and Allied Sciences*. 1991; 16: 87–89.

FURTHER READING

Jackson CG, Glasscock ME 3rd, Harris PF. Glomus tumors. Diagnosis, classification, and management of large lesions. *Archives Otolaryngology*. July 1982; 108(7): 401–10.

55

Implants in otology

E MARY SHANKS AND PETER WARDROP

COCHLEAR IMPLANTS

INTRODUCTION

The ability to restore hearing function for the profoundly deaf by direct electrical stimulation of the auditory nerve is one of the most important advances in medical science to date.

It is made possible using an implanted intracochlear electrode array. In profoundly deafened human adults, unlike other species, the auditory nerve survives and remains viable for many years. In congenitally deaf infants, cochlear implantation is also very successful, but only if implantation occurs before the age of 4. After this, if the cortical language centres receive no stimulation, they lose the ability to organize and function. The currently agreed optimal age of implantation in the United Kingdom is around 1 year, though in other countries, such as Canada, implantation is routine in children as young as 6 months. Below this age there are still doubts about accurate diagnosis of profound deafness and the safety of surgery, though this may change as technology improves.

HISTORY

In 1800, Alessandro Volta placed electric rods in his ears as an experiment and reported a bubbling sound. In 1957, Djourno and Eyries in Paris reported the first therapeutic hearing implant. A patient deafened by bilateral cholesteatomas had a wire inserted into one of the auditory nerve stumps and reported hearing the sound of chirping crickets. Later the patient identified basic words such as *allo* and *papa*. In the 1960s, William House in Los Angeles pioneered a single-channel device that stimulated the cochlea externally to produce a tone that fluctuated with speakers' voices, which could be used as an aid to lip-reading. In the 1970s, Clarke in Melbourne produced the first intracochlear multichannel implant, and truly open set speech discrimination (understanding speech regardless of context and without lip-reading) became possible. Since then there have been many ingenious innovations and improvements with better performance, battery life, miniaturization, reliability and even waterproofing of processors. Electrodes have become less traumatic and better designed for the cochlea. Appreciation of music and better performance in noisy conditions (important for school, work and social life) are current areas of intense research.

ASSESSMENT AND SELECTION

Current UK adult and child selection criteria are shown in Table 55.1. Patients must be judged better off with implantation than with optimal hearing aiding. It must be established that there is insufficient functional aidable hearing. There are four main criteria: linguistic, audiometric, functional and medical. Adults must have intelligible speech. They must be profoundly deaf (i.e. thresholds of 90 dB or worse) at 2 and 4 kHz. They must also score 50 per cent or less on Bamford-Kowal-Bench (BKB) sentence scores without lip-reading, in optimally aided conditions, i.e. in quiet and with the best available hearing aiding.

Children must have had at least 3 months' hearing aid trial and shown not to make significant progress in spoken language or preverbal sounds. They should also be shown to be profoundly deaf by objective measurement, such as auditory brain stem responses (ABR). If they are more than 4 years old, they must have acquired functional spoken language through previously aidable hearing. All adults currently have a computed tomography (CT) scan to exclude middle ear disease, cochlear ossification or dysplasia. Children usually have magnetic resonance imaging (MRI) as well as CT, as MRI is more sensitive for cochlear occlusion and confirms the presence of auditory nerves (which are occasionally absent – a contraindication to cochlear implantation).

Universal neonatal hearing screening (UNHS) is now standard in many Western countries, allowing identification of profoundly deaf babies within a few weeks of birth. In the United Kingdom, binaural hearing aiding is usually commenced at 3 months of age with cochlear implant assessment completed at 10–12 months and implantation surgery at 10–18 months. It can be difficult to decide whether a child has severe (but serviceable) or profound hearing loss. If there is any doubt, the child should be referred to the cochlear implant centre so the opportunity is not missed, as if the child passes 4 years of age without functional spoken language, the chance of implantation is lost forever and the child must be educated and live in a sign language environment.

Currently, children are usually implanted bilaterally, owing to improved localization of sound and better performance in noise. Adults are usually implanted unilaterally in the better ear or occasionally in the poorer ear if a contralateral hearing aid may add to the result. Adults with coexistent blindness or who have been deafened by meningitis are implanted bilaterally. Profound deafness from meningitis, particularly pneumococcal meningitis, is an emergency, requiring implantation as

Table 55.1 Current UK selection criteria

	Adults	Children <4 years	Children >4 years
Audiometric	Worse than 90 dB at 2 and 4 kHz	No response to 90 dB Clicks on ABR	No response to 90 dB Clicks on ABR
Functional	<50 per cent keywords in BKB sentences	No progress with >3 months hearing aids	Limited speech perception on age appropriate speech tests
Linguistic	Functional spoken language	Emerging communication skills	Functional spoken language
Medical	Fit for surgery No infection in ear No cochlear occlusion	Fit for surgery No infection in ear No cochlear occlusion Auditory nerves present	Fit for surgery No infection in ear No cochlear occlusion

soon as the patient has sufficiently recovered, as the cochlea can become occluded and ossified in as little as a few weeks.

TECHNOLOGY

The basic structure of a cochlear implant is shown in Figure 55.1. The external part of the device resembles a hearing aid but instead contains a battery pack, microphone and a processor that selects and codes useful elements of speech and sound. The information and power are conveyed through intact scalp skin by a transmitter coil to a similar receiver coil in the internal part of the device. The transmission is via a radio inductive link much like a mobile phone signal. The information is then carried in the lead through to the intracochlear array where auditory nerve fibres are stimulated, and this is perceived as sound by the auditory cortex. After activation ('switch-on'), patients require regular tuning of the device(s) for life. This is carried out by clinical scientists and involves adjustment of current levels across the intracochlear electrode array to maximize comfort and clarity of perception. Reliable patient feedback is required to achieve this. Appointments are frequent in the first year and eventually become annual as the patient's settings (known as the programming 'map') stabilize.

SURGERY

In 95 per cent of cases the gross anatomy is normal, so the procedure is very standardized. The procedure takes 1 to 2 hours per side and uses a transmastoid approach via the facial recess, with the electrode array inserted into the scala tympani through the round window, or near it. Direct round window insertion is least traumatic and is becoming increasingly popular and practical with more flexible electrode arrays. The surgical route is shown superimposed on the axial CT image in Figure 55.2.

A postauricular incision is performed and the pinna dissected forward up to the margin of the bony ear canal. A cortical mastoidectomy is used to identify the incus short process. The triangular space between the descending facial nerve and corda tympani (facial recess) is dissected open to allow a view of the stapes and the round window (Figure 55.3). Depending on the make of electrode, the array is inserted through the round window itself after exposing it by drilling away the bony overhang (niche), or the round window is enlarged

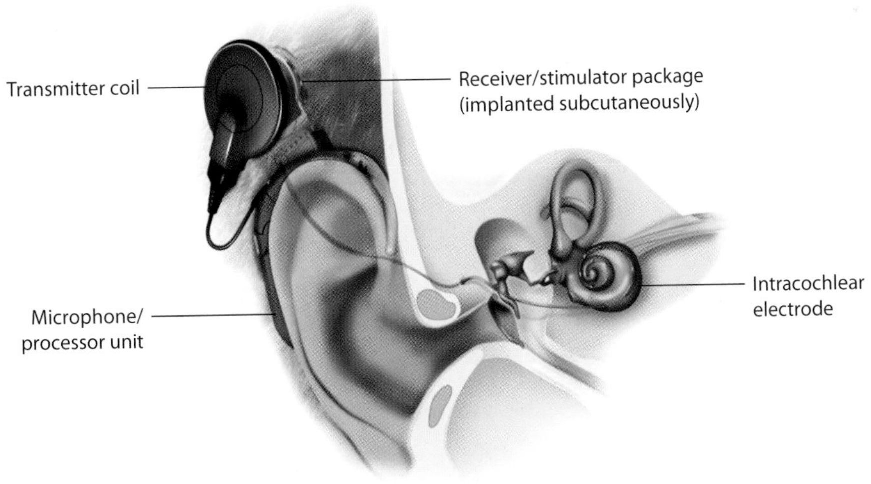

Figure 55.1 Basic structure of device. The microphone/processor/battery pack and transmitter coil are worn externally while the receiver/stimulator package and intracochlear and electrode lead are surgically implanted. (Courtesy of MED-EL.)

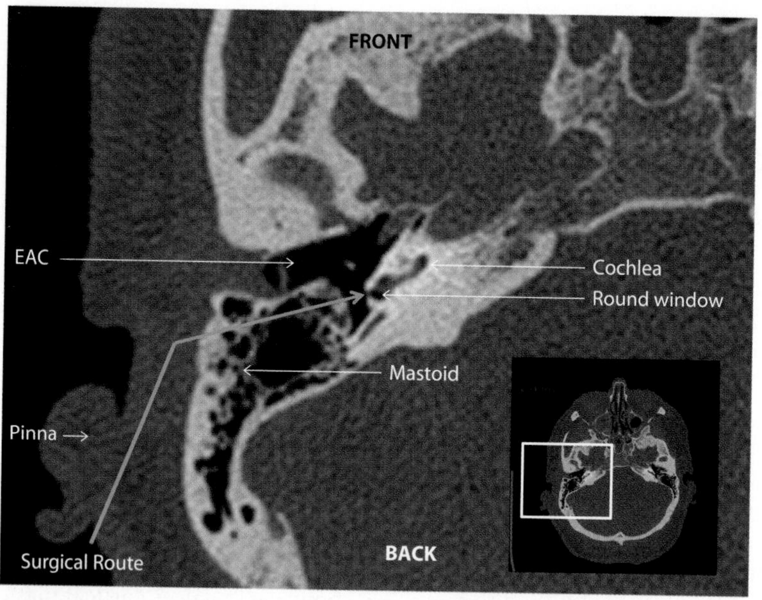

Figure 55.2 Axial CT right temporal bone with surgical route to round window of cochlea (green arrow).

antero-inferiorly or a separate cochleostomy is drilled anterior to the round window. Efforts should be made to avoid sucking intracochlear fluids directly or allowing bone dust or blood into the cochlea, as these actions can injure surviving auditory neurons or increase intracochlear scarring. Figure 55.4 is a schematic of the electrode *in situ* in the right cochlea, as viewed from below.

The package is inserted postero-superiorly under the scalp. Traditionally, it was fixed to bone

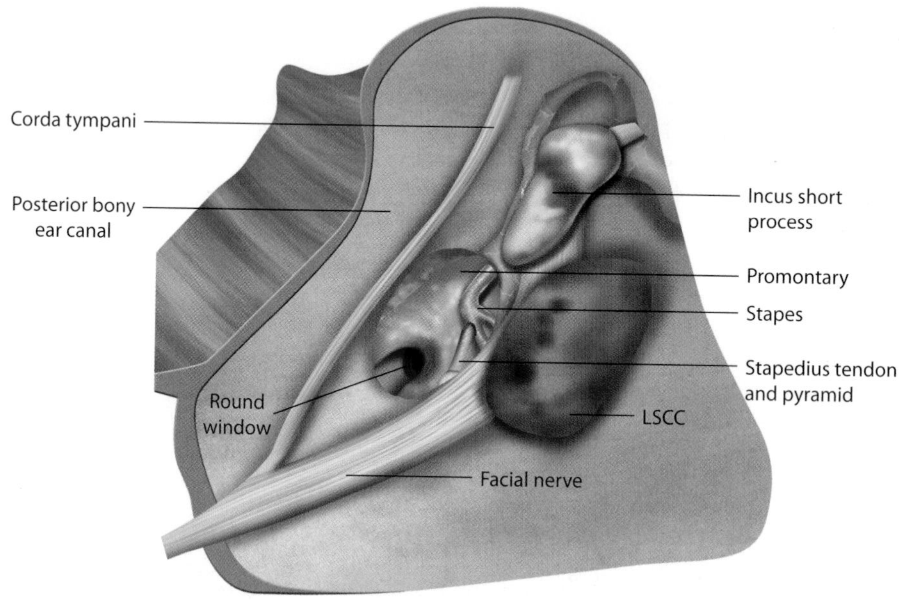

Figure 55.3 View through left facial recess to show round window and niche. LSCC = lateral semicircular canal.

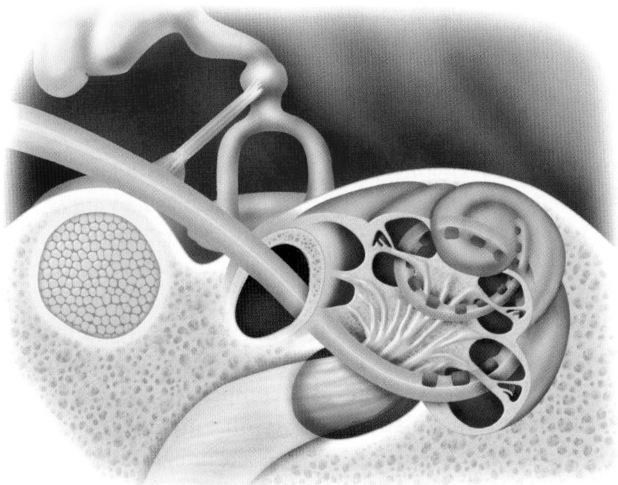

Figure 55.4 Schematic showing electrode array *in situ* in the right cochlea, seen from below (courtesy of Advanced Bionics). The round window is enlarged antero-inferiorly to allow insertion of the array into the scala tympani. The auditory nerve cell bodies are seen within the modiolus. The descending facial nerve is seen in cross section on the extreme left of the picture.

to prevent movement and subsequent wire fatigue, but increasingly surgeons are simply placing the package in a tight periosteal pocket on the bone and relying on scarring to fix the package. This reduces operating time by about half an hour.

OUTCOMES

Most adults require 6 to 9 months to become fully accustomed to their implant.

Fifty to 60 per cent of adult implant recipients regain the ability to use the telephone, which is important for social life and especially for employment. Most are able, with practice, to converse effortlessly in a quiet environment, and with moderate effort in competing noise.

Almost all regain sufficient speech recognition to lip-read more effectively.

Outcomes are measured either by speech perception tests, e.g. BKB sentence scores (percentage of keywords identified in standard sentences), or by what level of communication they achieve (e.g. categories of auditory performance, or CAP, Table 55.2). There are more challenging tests, including recognition of speech in various levels of competing noise.

Table 55.2 Categories of auditory performance (CAP)

1. Can detect environmental sounds
2. Can understand common phrases when lip-reading
3. Can understand conversation when lip-reading
4. Can identify at least five environmental sounds
5. Can understand common phrases without lip-reading
6. Can understand conversation without lip-reading
7. Can use the telephone with a familiar caller
8. Can use the telephone with an unfamiliar caller

Children require 1 to 4 years to make up for the prior auditory deprivation, with more time being required the older they are at implantation. This 'catch-up' time is roughly equal to their age at implantation. For best results, they must be 'immersed' in spoken language (i.e. encouraged to speak, and exposed to as much spoken language as possible). Sign language should not be used as a substitute. They should also wear the device(s) all of their waking hours. Children then have onward learning in speech and language as for normal-hearing children. All receive speech therapy and teacher of the deaf (TOD) support. Roughly 80 per cent go on to attend mainstream schools, with TOD support. This figure drops to 20 per cent for those children implanted at or near the age of 4.

FUTURE DEVELOPMENTS

In the United Kingdom, bilateral cochlear implantation is routine for children and some adults and may become routine for all adults in future. Battery life, currently 2 to 3 days, is increasing and may one day be superseded by solar- or even motion-powered processors; however, these technologies do not currently provide enough power. The radio inductive link between internal and external parts of the device consumes 90 per cent of the power of the battery and may be improved, allowing these innovations to become reality. Routine programming, once the patient's tuning 'map' is stable, may become possible remotely using the Internet.

Patients with residual hearing, especially in lower frequencies (below 1 kHz), can benefit from a hybrid device that utilizes this hearing (amplified if necessary) while electrically stimulating neurons serving the lost high-frequency hearing. As the technology advances, patients who have aidable hearing losses may perform better instead with cochlear implantation. As mentioned, music appreciation and performance in competing noise are significant challenges but will undoubtedly improve further. Currently, processors sample the overall sound wave form (the 'envelope'). However, with improvements that allow processors to interpret the minute oscillations (fine structure) of the sound wave, these difficulties may be overcome.

The totally implantable cochlear implant (TICI) has been used in a small number of patients but has problems with microphone placement and power supply. Simplification of cochlear implant surgery has reduced operating time from 4–5 hours to around 1.5 hours, and day case surgery is a possibility. Surgery under local anaesthetic is surprisingly well tolerated and makes the procedure possible for frailer and older patients.

ACOUSTIC HEARING IMPLANTS

BONE-ANCHORED HEARING AIDS

A bone-anchored hearing aid transmits sound to the inner ear by means of a skin-penetrating titanium fixture inserted into the skull. Bone conduction stimulates the cochlea in three ways: vibrating bone radiating into the external ear and through the middle ear, the inertial response of the middle ear ossicles and the inner ear fluids, and direct compression of the inner ear fluids that deflects the basilar membrane. Once the fixture is implanted, osseo-integration takes place between the titanium surface and surrounding osteocytes, creating a stable fixation to bone. This direct transmission of sound avoids the disadvantages of conventional transcutaneous bone-conduction hearing aids, which are less efficient and give inconsistent sound quality. They can also cause patients discomfort or skin problems owing to continuous pressure on the temporal bone.

Indications

1. *Sensorineural hearing loss.* Patients who are unable to wear conventional air-conduction hearing aids owing to recurrent otitis externa or skin reactions associated with hearing aid moulds. Pure tone average bone-conduction thresholds should be no worse than 60 dBHL.
2. *Congenital atresia and acquired stenosis of the external auditory meatus.* Malformations of the external canal may be combined with middle ear malformations but inner ear function is often normal.
3. *Chronic otitis media with persistent otorrhoea or large mastoid cavities that are unsuitable for conventional hearing aids.*
4. *Conductive hearing loss.* Bone-anchored hearing aids may be considered in patients with otosclerosis and other causes of conductive hearing loss as an alternative to surgery, particularly if they have unilateral hearing. Bone-conduction aids tend to give better quality sound than air-conduction aids when inner ear function is normal and there is a large conductive loss.

5. *Unilateral sensorineural hearing loss.* In patients with unilateral hearing loss due to congenital or acquired causes, for example following acoustic neuroma surgery, binaural hearing can be restored by fitting a bone-anchored hearing aid behind the deafened ear. Sound is transmitted transcranially and perceived by the healthy contralateral cochlea.

Surgery

Insertion of the bone-anchored hearing aid fixture with an abutment for attaching the hearing aid can be performed as a one-stage procedure under local anaesthesia in most adults. The position behind the ear is planned using a template to ensure the hearing aid is not touching spectacles or the pinna. It is important when drilling to keep the bone as cool as possible to encourage osseo-integration. The hearing aid is fitted 2 to 3 months after surgery.

In children, surgery is carried out under general anaesthesia, usually between the ages of 3 and 6 years old, once the skull thickness is sufficient. Surgery may be performed in two stages with insertion of one and often a second back-up fixture. Three months later, once osseo-integration has occurred, the abutment is attached under general anaesthesia. Very young children can wear a bone-anchored hearing aid attached to a softband, which can be fitted when they are only a few months old.

Bilateral bone-anchored hearing aids can be fitted in suitable patients with a symmetrical hearing loss to restore binaural hearing (Figure 55.5).

Complications

1. Failure of osseo-integration resulting in the loss of the fixtures
2. Skin reactions and thickening around the abutment, which may require revision of the skin flap

Patients and parents need to be aware that the skin flap surrounding the implant requires regular cleaning to reduce the risk of infection and other skin problems.

BONEBRIDGE HEARING IMPLANT

This is a semi-implantable bone-conduction hearing aid system consisting of an external audio processor that magnetically attaches to an implant inserted under intact skin (Figure 55.6). The vibrating bone conductor is embedded in the temporal bone and attached by two screws. The audio processor consists of a battery, microphone and digital signal processor. Once sound has been processed it is transmitted to the implant, causing mechanical vibrations that are then transmitted to the inner ear.

The Bonebridge avoids the skin problems associated with transcutaneous bone-anchored hearing aids and enables earlier fitting of the audio processor as osseo-integration is not required. However, it requires a more complex surgical procedure and a mastoid cavity with no active infection that is of sufficient depth to embed the implant.

ACTIVE MIDDLE EAR IMPLANTS

Active middle ear implants are designed to mechanically stimulate the vibratory structures of the middle ear. Most types of middle ear implant do not occlude the external auditory canal. Implants can be partially or totally implantable and are powered by either piezoelectric or electromagnetic devices. Ideally, the implant should

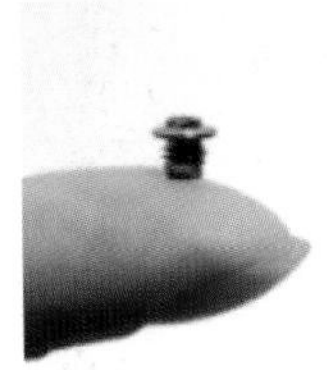
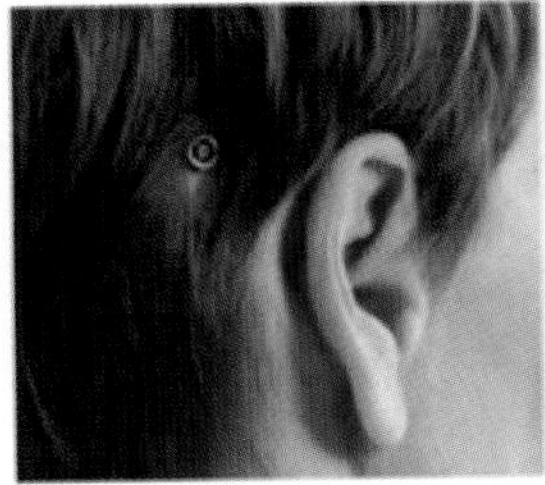
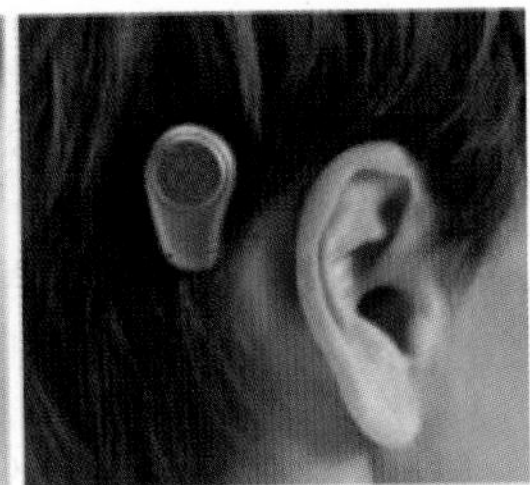

Figure 55.5 Bone-anchored hearing aid. Courtesy of Oticon Ponto.

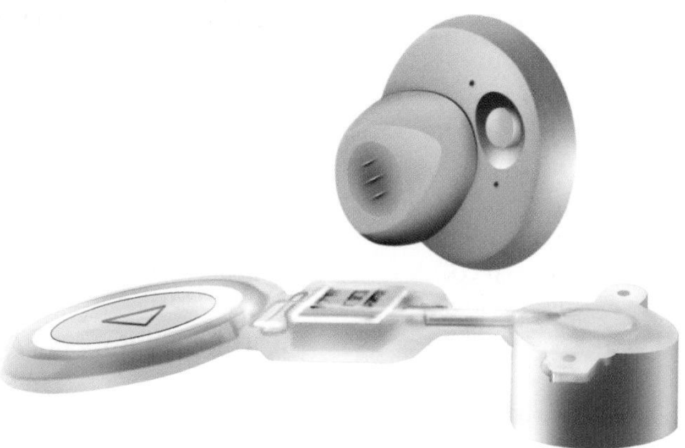

Figure 55.6 Bonebridge. Courtesy of MED-EL.

be fixed securely to one of the middle ear structures without disruption of the ossicular chain or impairment of existing middle ear function.

Indications

1. *Patients with mild to severe sensorineural hearing loss.* Indications have recently been extended to include conductive hearing loss owing to the development of round window implantation.
2. *Recurrent otitis externa and other skin conditions that prevent the use of conventional air-conduction hearing aid moulds.* Some patients without skin problems find the occlusive effect of hearing aid moulds very unpleasant.
3. *Meatal atresia and acquired stenosis of the external auditory canal.*
4. *Improvement of sound quality, especially at high frequencies, and reduction of feedback.*
5. *Cosmesis.* The audio processor is small and easily concealed. For swimmers and athletes, a totally implantable device is both practical and cosmetic.

Surgery

Three devices are currently available, all requiring surgery, which usually includes cortical mastoidectomy and may also require posterior tympanotomy to access the middle ear.

1. The Vibrant Soundbridge (MED-EL) is a semi-implantable electromagnetic device that consists of an implanted receiver that is surgically inserted under the skin behind the mastoid, similar to a cochlear implant (Figure 55.7). A lead from the receiver is attached to a transducer, which consists of a coil wrapped round a magnet called a floating mass transducer (FMT)

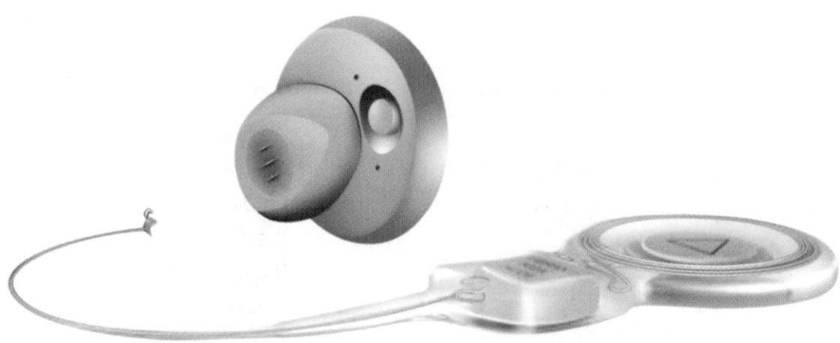

Figure 55.7 Vibrant Soundbridge. Courtesy of MED-EL.

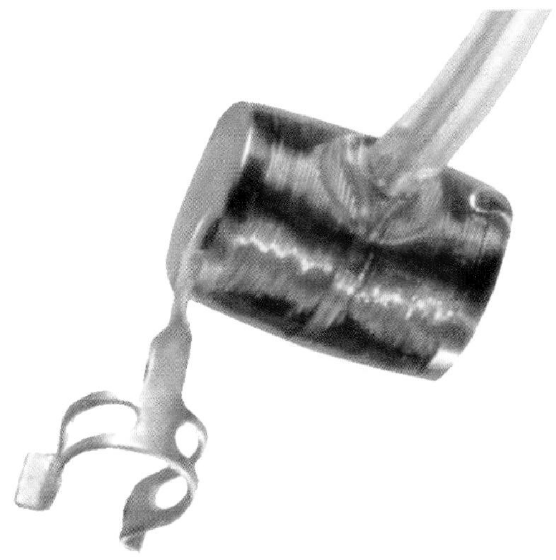

Figure 55.8 Close-up of floating mass transducer (FMT).

(Figure 55.8) The FMT is attached to the long process of the incus by a clip. The FMT can also be attached to the stapes footplate by using specially designed couplers or placed adjacent to the round window. The external auditory processor is attached to the receiver magnetically and transmits processed sound to the internal receiver. The receiver then transmits an electrical signal to the FMT, which mechanically vibrates the ossicular chain or round window.

2. The Esteem (Envoy) is a totally implantable piezoelectric device placed under the skin behind the ear. It uses the tympanic membrane as a microphone and picks up sound signals via a sensor attached to the body of incus. The sound is processed and transmitted to a piezoceramic crystal within the transducer that is attached to the head of stapes. When stimulated by an electrical current, the piezoceramic crystal vibrates the head of stapes. The lenticular process of the incus has to be removed to prevent feedback. The Esteem is programmed and can be controlled by the patient using a remote control device. The implanted battery has a life of 5 to 7 years. Replacement batteries can be inserted under local anaesthesia.
3. The Carina (Otologics) is a totally implantable electromagnetic device with a microphone situated under the skin. The transducer is inserted into a laser-drilled hole in the body of the incus. The battery is recharged by placing an external coil attached to a charger over the implanted device.

Surgical complications are uncommon, but revision surgery to re-position devices is occasionally required.

Middle ear implants are an option for a small number of patients who do not benefit from conventional air-conduction aids and are unsuitable for bone-anchored hearing aids because their bone-conduction hearing levels are too poor. Middle ear implants are also an attractive option for patients who do not wish to be seen wearing conventional hearing aids because they are totally implanted or because the sound processor can be worn discreetly, hidden by the patients' hair.

TRANSCUTANEOUS BONE-ANCHORED HEARING AID

This is a magnetic bone conduction implant system that avoids the skin complications associated with a percutaneous abutment (Figure 55.9). A preoperative trial of a sound processor on a Softband is essential to give patients a realistic experience of hearing benefit for both percutaneous and transcutaneous bone-anchored hearing aid candidates. A further Softband trial is also recommended if patients are transitioning from a percutaneous to a transcutaneous system.

Surgery

Surgery is usually carried out under general anaesthesia. A C-shaped incision is made in the skin at least 15 mm anterior to the anterior edge of the magnet. The titanium fixture is inserted into the skull bone and a circular magnetic plate attached. The plate should not be in contact with bone, and the periosteum should remain intact. The skin above the magnet should be 3–6 mm thick. If less than 3 mm thick, then the magnet may cause discomfort and skin problems. If more than 6 mm thick, then the sound processor magnet may fall off.

The sound processor can be fitted 4 weeks after surgery. The magnet must be temporarily

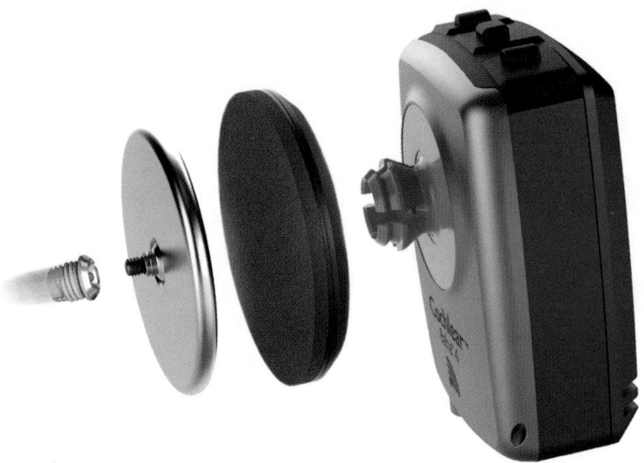

Figure 55.9 Cochlear Attract System. (Courtesy of Cochlear Limited.)

removed if the patient requires MRI scanning. The magnet can be replaced with a percutaneous abutment attached to the same titanium fixture if hearing deteriorates and additional amplification is required.

ACKNOWLEDGEMENT

Peter Wardrop would like to thank Miss Agnes Allan, scientific head of service of the Scottish Cochlear Implant Programme, for her many helpful suggestions on his manuscript.

KEY LEARNING POINTS

Introduction:

- Cochlear implantation involves electrical stimulation of the auditory nerve in profoundly deafened adults, which restores the ability to recognize speech and environmental sounds.
- In young children, cochlear implantation allows the *de novo* development of speech and recognition of environmental sounds.

History:

- Cochlear implantation has been routine since the 1980s and has revolutionized the treatment of profound deafness.
- Cochlear implants significantly improve quality of life together with education and employment prospects.
- Open set speech understanding is the ability to interpret speech without lipreading and regardless of context.

Selection:

- Patients must be shown to have no serviceable hearing.
- Adults and children over the age of 4 must have intelligible speech indicating functional auditory cortex and speech centres.
- Children must be implanted before the age of 4 unless they have functional spoken language.
- Congenitally deaf children implanted younger do better.
- The optimal age of implantation for profoundly deaf infants is currently 10–18 months.
- Universal neonatal hearing screening (UNHS) has improved the chances of early implantation.
- Profound deafness after meningitis requires emergency cochlear implant assessment and surgery.

Technology:

- There are internal and external parts of the device, which communicate by radio frequency link through intact skin.
- Cochlear implants require lifelong maintenance and tuning by clinical scientists.
- For patients, regular device programming requires a substantial lifetime commitment in terms of hospital visits and travelling time.
- Bone-anchored hearing aids are an effective alternative for children and adults unable to wear conventional hearing aids because of chronic middle or external ear infections and for patients with meatal atresia or stenosis.
- Bone conduction thresholds should be better than 60 dB for bone-conduction hearing aids to be effective.
- Bone-anchored hearing aids can also be used in the management of single-sided deafness.
- Active middle ear implants are an option for patients with sensorineural or mixed hearing losses who do not benefit from conventional air-conduction aids and are unsuitable for bone-anchored hearing aids.

Surgery:

- Surgery is standardized, is well tolerated and has an excellent safety record.

Outcomes:

- With careful selection almost all patients benefit from implantation.
- Most patients regain open set speech and about half regain telephone use.
- The main purpose of implantation in children is that they can communicate in spoken language.
- Most children implanted before the age of 2 go on to attend mainstream school.

Future:

- Cochlear implantation technology and surgery are advancing rapidly in all aspects, and results may approach or even surpass normal hearing function during the twenty-first century.

FURTHER READING

Arunachalam PS, Kilby D, Meikle D, Davison T, Johnson IJ. Bone-anchored hearing aid quality of life assessed by Glasgow Benefit Inventory. *Laryngoscope*. 2001 July; 111(7): 1260–3.

Dumon T, Gratacap B, Firmin F, Vincent R, Pialoux R, Casse B, Firmin B. Vibrant Soundbridge middle ear implant in mixed hearing loss, indications, techniques, results. *Revue de Laryngologie Otologie, Rhinologie*. (Bord). 2009; 130(2): 75–81.

Green K. The role of active middle ear implants in the rehabilitation of hearing loss. *Expert Review of Medical Devices*. 2011 July; 8(4): 441–7.

Luxon L (ed.). *Textbook of Audiological Medicine*. London: Martin Dunitz, 2003.

Macnamara M, Phillips D, Proops DW. The bone anchored hearing aid (BAHA) in chronic suppurative otitis media (CSOM). *Journal of Laryngology and Otology Suppl*. 1996; 21: 38–40.

National Institute for Health and Care Excellence (NICE). www.nice.org.uk.

National Institute for Health and Care Excellence (NICE). Cochlear implants for children and adults with severe to profound deafness. Available from: http://publications.nice.org.uk/cochlear-implants-for-children-and-adults-with-severe-to-profound-deafness-ta166

The Ear Foundation. www.earfoundation.org.uk.

Wilson BS, Dorman MF. Cochlear implants: A remarkable past and a brilliant future. *Hearing Research*. 2008; 242: 3–21.

SECTION IV

Paediatrics

56

Tonsils and adenoids

PETER J ROBB

INTRODUCTION

The 'tonsils' are correctly termed the palatine tonsils, forming paired structures developing from the second pharyngeal pouch. The covering stratified squamous epithelium typically dips into the tonsillar surface forming tonsillar crypts. The adenoid is the nasopharyngeal tonsil, and both form part of Waldeyer's ring of lymphoid tissue in the upper respiratory tract, the first point of immunological contact for inhaled and ingested antigens.

The tonsils and adenoid can be identified during the third month of gestation. From the adenoid, lymph drains to the retropharyngeal lymph nodes and upper deep cervical nodes, particularly the posterior triangle of the neck. The tonsils drain predominantly to the jugulodigastric and upper deep nodes in the mid-cervical region.

The adenoid starts to involute in later childhood and by early adulthood, the adenoid has largely disappeared. In the absence of recurrent infections, the tonsils become smaller and less prominent.

The tonsils and adenoid produce B-cells, which give rise to production of immunoglobulins, predominantly IgA. Exposure to antigens through the mouth and nose contributes to part of natural acquired immunity in early childhood. Evidence supports the view that adenoidectomy should be avoided in young children. This produces a small but detectable negative effect on the development of serum IgG antibodies, resulting in impaired immunity to pneumococcus.

The adenoid may become infected in upper respiratory tract infections leading to acute or chronic adenoiditis. This may lead to rhinitis, rhinosinusitis, otitis media and otitis media with effusion. Recurrent rhinosinusitis will generally resolve after adenoidectomy without the need for endoscopic sinus surgery.

The tonsils are subject to recurrent bacterial infections, typically streptococcal, but may also become acutely inflamed and enlarged during infection with viral mononucleosis (glandular fever). In chronically inflamed tonsils, actinomyces is frequently identified in the tonsil when submitted for histological examination.

OTITIS MEDIA

Adenoidectomy (but not tonsillectomy) is effective (together with insertion of ventilation tubes) in the management of both otitis media with effusion (OME) and recurrent acute otitis media. While traditionally the size of the adenoid causing eustachian tube obstruction was believed to be important, it is probable that the chronic infective biofilm in the adenoid leads to a cascade of inflammatory mediators causing upregulation of the mucin genes in the middle ear mucosa. Subsequent changes in the mucosa, including reduced mucociliary clearance, contribute to the development of the biofilm infection, resulting in middle ear effusion. Adenoidectomy with ventilation tube insertion in children over the age of 3 is helpful in managing OME. Where low-dose prophylactic antibiotic treatment has failed for recurrent acute otitis media, adenoidectomy may be helpful at the time of grommet insertion.

RECURRENT ACUTE TONSILLITIS

Recurrent bacterial tonsillitis, occurring frequently over a prolonged period, with interference with normal functioning (e.g. school attendance) is a common indication for tonsillectomy. It is important to explain to parents or patients that tonsillectomy is ineffective in managing recurrent viral sore throats, coughs and colds or ear infections. In older children and young adults without a history of frequent tonsillitis, glandular fever sometimes leads to frequent and recurrent infections in association with symptoms of post-viral fatigue. While tonsillectomy will not directly address the fatigue symptoms, it will abolish the debilitating attacks of recurrent tonsillitis. Current guidance is to recommend tonsillectomy following seven episodes in a 12-month period, five or more episodes each year in the preceding 2 years or three or more episodes in the preceding 3 years. With stricter criteria for surgery, the rate of tonsillectomy in the United Kingdom has fallen by more than 35 to 44 per cent in the past 15 years. However, admissions to hospital for tonsil-related illnesses (e.g. quinsy) have increased by up to 310 per cent since 1991, perhaps indicating that the pendulum has swung too far and that we are now removing too few tonsils.

SLEEP-DISORDERED BREATHING

The term *sleep-disordered breathing* (SDB) covers all degrees of upper airway obstruction during sleep, up to and including obstructive sleep apnoea syndrome (OSAS). Despite the widespread acceptance of the benefits of adenotonsillar surgery in these children, a Cochrane review of adenotonsillectomy for obstructive sleep apnoea found no randomized trials addressing the efficacy of surgery in managing OSAS in children. Despite this lack of evidence, in the United Kingdom, approximately 25 per cent of tonsil and adenoid operations are now for symptoms of SDB. There is uncertainty at what level of SDB intervention is effective and when benefits outweigh potential hazards of surgery and anaesthesia. Snoring and disturbed sleep may not reach the level of obstructive sleep apnoea, but an increasing body of evidence supports daytime neurocognitive disadvantage from poor-quality sleep in childhood.

Consider adenotonsillectomy for children with SDB with clinical evidence of upper airway obstruction. Children with significant sleep apnoea will develop poor growth with failure to gain weight. This is partly due to difficulty eating a normal diet owing to the obstruction caused by the tonsils and adenoid during swallowing; gagging and choking is a common feature. These children also breathe against an obstruction all night and are effectively exercising to breathe, burning many calories. The disruption to cyclical (REM/non-REM) sleep interferes with the normal release of endocrine growth factors.

TUMOURS

Tumours of the tonsils and adenoid in childhood are rare. Where unusual adenoidal enlargement with no infection is present, or where there is smooth asymmetrical enlargement of one tonsil, consider lymphoma. Following imaging, send biopsy material as a fresh specimen to allow full immunohistochemistry.

OTHER INDICATIONS FOR ADENOIDECTOMY AND/OR TONSILLECTOMY

Adenoidectomy is sometimes indicated alone for nasal obstruction with hyponasal speech and mouth breathing with subsequent poor dental hygiene and disordered development of the palate and mid-face.

Tonsillectomy is helpful in the management of recurrent guttate psoriasis. In the United Kingdom, post-streptoccal nephritis is uncommon, but occasionally children are referred by renal physicians for tonsillectomy for this condition.

In the United Kingdom, consideration of tonsillectomy would follow two or more admissions to hospital with severe tonsillitis and/or peritonsillar abscess (quinsy).

Deep crypts on the surface of the tonsils can lead to trapping of fetid mucosal debris with severe and unpleasant halitosis. The debris can sometimes organize into small tonsil stones (tonsilloliths). Other than gargling to clear the crypts of debris, the only effective remedy is tonsillectomy.

HISTORY AND EXAMINATION

Include a full ear, nose and throat (ENT), developmental paediatric and family history. Specific attention to nasal obstruction, possible atopy and rhinitis, sleep disturbance and eating are important. A family history of atopy may be relevant. Difficulties with speech, articulation and eating may be due to a large adenoid and large, obstructing tonsils. Enquire about specific sleep disturbance, arousals and daytime naps. Parents will sometimes bring a video clip of their child sleeping, and this is very helpful supporting information. Some children with SDB develop secondary enuresis, having previously been dry at night.

Enquire about infective episodes of tonsillitis, including the frequency, severity, time off school or nursery and need for medication, both analgesics and antibiotics.

A full history of medication, prescribed, over the counter and alternative or complementary is important. Family history, perinatal history, development and growth should be documented. Where adenoidectomy and/or tonsillectomy is being considered, it is essential to *positively exclude* a history or family tendency of unusual bleeding or bruising, as a routine clotting screen may not confirm mild von Willebrand's disease. If this is suspected, refer to a haematologist for full coagulation and clotting assessment.

Examine the ears and neck, looking particularly for clinical evidence of OME and for glands or masses in the neck.

Examine the external nose, looking for a skin crease in the supra-tip region that may indicate frequent nose rubbing due to irritation secondary to rhinitis, causing nasal obstruction.

In children, anterior rhinoscopy is easier using a halogen light auriscope with a large ear speculum. Children tolerate this better than examination with a Thudicum's speculum. Use a cold Lack's tongue depressor or large laryngeal mirror to assess the nasal airway. Older children may tolerate nasendoscopy with topical intranasal local anaesthetic spray, such as co-phenylcaine, to assess adenoidal size. (Topical cocaine *must not* be used in children.)

When examining the mouth and pharynx, some children will not tolerate a tongue depressor. It is, however, generally possible to assess the form and size of the tonsils with a bright light and no depressor. Confirm or exclude tongue tie and assess the palate and uvula looking for a high-arched palate and bifid uvula (Figure 56.1).

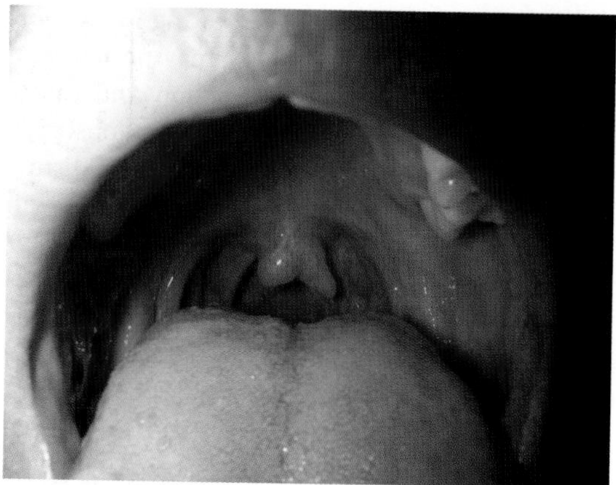

Figure 56.1 Bifid uvula – possible underlying submucous cleft.

INVESTIGATIONS

The child should be weighed in the clinic. Children with severe SDB, with significant co-morbidity and under 15 kg weight and/or 2 years of age are more safely managed in a regional centre with on-site access to a paediatric intensive care unit (PICU) and ventilation, should this be required post-operatively. Approximately 1–2 per cent of small children with severe SDB will develop post-operative pulmonary oedema following the sudden reversal of the positive end expiratory pressure (PEEP) that the airway obstruction has produced. Some children with SDB may be ventilating with a CO_2 respiratory drive. Both these groups may require temporary post-operative ventilation. While preoperative polysomnography is the gold standard for assessing children with SDB, this is rarely available outside specialist centres. Evidence from the history, examination and domicillary, overnight pulse oximetry are helpful in triangulating the evidence to confirm both the diagnosis and severity of the SDB. For very small (<15 kg) children with severe SDB, intracapsular Coblation tonsillectomy (tonsillotomy) is the surgical option least associated with pain and post-operative haemorrhage.

In fit and well ASA (American Society of Anesthesiologists) 1 or 2 children having tonsillectomy, adenoidectomy or adenotonsillectomy, no routine preoperative investigations are indicated.

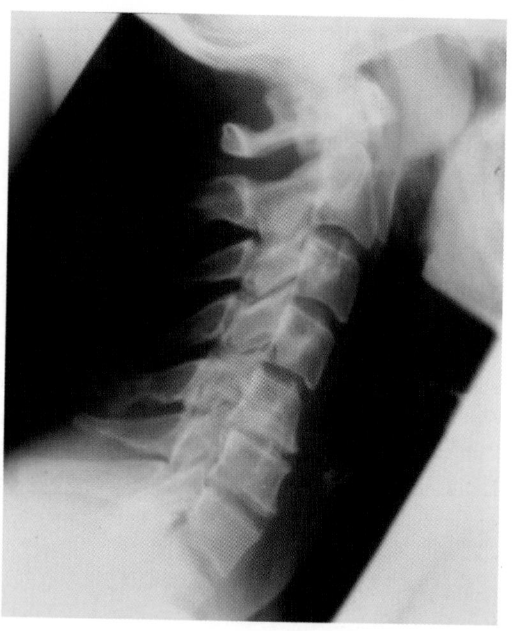

Figure 56.2 Lateral soft tissue radiograph of the nasopharynx. Adenoidal hypertrophy with loss of postnasal airway.

Specific investigations for sickle-cell disease, thalassaemia, Down's syndrome and congenital heart disease are indicated as appropriate. Management of type 2 diabetes mellitus should follow local paediatric guidelines for diabetic children undergoing elective surgery. When von Willebrand's disease is suspected, a routine clotting screen *will not* confirm or exclude the diagnosis, and referral for full investigation of clotting and coagulation should be made.

If a child requires only adenoidectomy and endoscopic examination in clinic has not been possible, a plain lateral soft tissue radiograph of the nasopharynx is helpful (Figure 56.2). While the image gives only a two-dimensional view of the nasopharynx, reduction of the postnasal airway in the context of the history supports the diagnosis of adenoidal hyperplasia.

MANAGEMENT

Where social and geographical factors allow, the majority of children may be safely discharged home within 3 hours of adenoidectomy and 6 hours after tonsillectomy. Safe day case surgery for this group relies on appropriate surgical and anaesthetic skills and techniques, pre-emptive fluid replacement, anti-emetics and analgesia, avoiding narcotic analgesia and emetic anaesthetic.

ADENOIDECTOMY

Adenoidectomy has traditionally been performed under general anaesthesia with the child in the tonsillectomy position using the blind technique of curettage. Assessment of the adenoid is made digitally prior to curetting the adenoid from the nasopharynx, and haemostasis achieved with gauze swab tamponade. Techniques employing direct vision have the advantage of reduced blood loss (<4 mL vs. >50 mL) and the ability to remove adenoid tissue from the choanae, avoiding trauma to the eustachian cushions (Figure 56.3). The largest clinical experience is with the suction coagulator and microdebrider (Figure 56.4). While the microdebrider is faster than curettage, the suction coagulator is significantly cheaper. The Coblator is also suitable for adenoidectomy, but the cost of the device precludes its use unless tonsillectomy is carried out at the same time. The KTP laser is associated with a high incidence of post-operative nasopharyngeal stenosis and should not be used for adenoidectomy. Where a bifid uvula is noted or a submucous cleft identified, a partial adenoidectomy, sparing the tissue at the lower part of the nasopharynx, reduces the risk of velopharyngeal insufficiency.

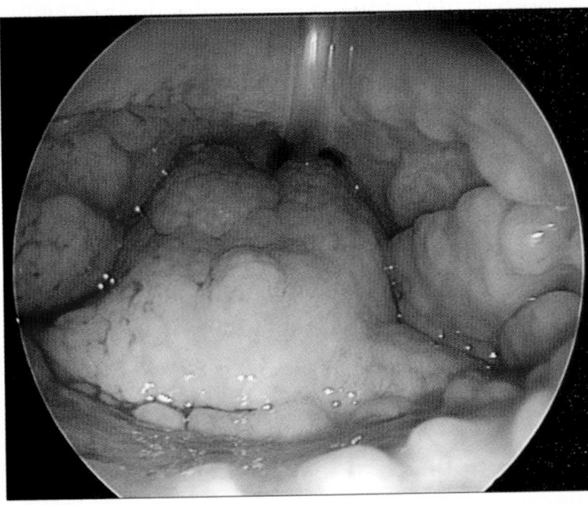

Figure 56.3 Operative view of adenoid with catheter visible in choana retracting palate. Courtesy of P. Valentine.

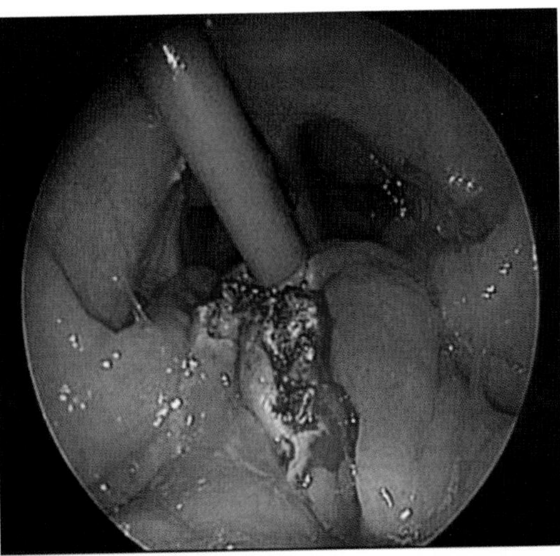

Figure 56.4 Operative view of suction diathermy adenoidectomy. Courtesy of P. Valentine.

TONSILLECTOMY

In the tonsillectomy position, and usually following adenoidectomy, if this is being performed, the tonsils can be removed using various techniques. Where the tonsils are enormous, it can be helpful to remove these prior to adenoidectomy. Special care is needed to avoid damage to the teeth and lips. If using diathermy or Coblation, care must be taken to avoid burns around the mouth and face. Paraffin or petroleum jelly should never be used as a lubricant for the lips prior to surgery. Both are inflammable, and are a hazard when using diathermy; using these to lubricate the lips may also cause slippage of the mouth gag and risk damage to the teeth.

Tonsillectomy may be carried out using cold steel dissection, hot bipolar diathermy, a combination of these or radiofrequency Coblation dissection. Diathermy should *never* be combined with Coblation because of the higher risk of severe secondary haemorrhage. Overall, cold steel dissection is less painful, but the blood loss is generally

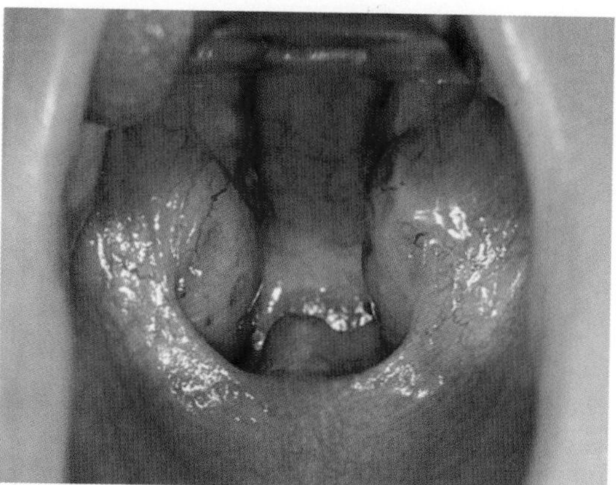

Figure 56.5 Hypertrophied tonsils – operative view with gag extended and flexible laryngeal airway in place.

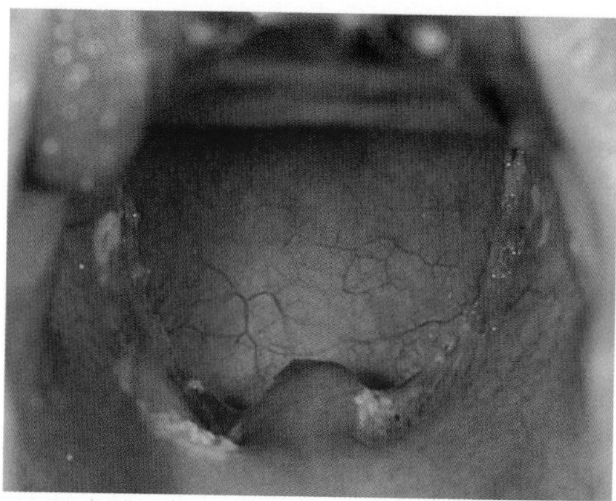

Figure 56.6 Same operative view at the conclusion of Coblation tonsillectomy.

higher during the operation. The secondary haemorrhage rate is statistically lower. Diathermy dissection causes less blood loss but is more painful with a slightly higher secondary haemorrhage rate. Coblation tonsillectomy in children is generally a near bloodless procedure, with less post-operative pain, but with the reputation for a higher secondary haemorrhage rate. The data from the UK National Prospective Tonsillectomy Audit were collected at the time Coblation was being introduced into the United Kingdom, and there were many new, inexperienced users. Some combined Coblation and diathermy in the same patient, resulting in a very high secondary haemorrhage rate. Data published by experienced users since then confirms the safety and efficacy of Coblation with less intraoperative blood loss and lower post-operative pain than other techniques (Figures 56.5 and 56.6).

COMPLICATIONS

HAEMORRHAGE

The reactionary haemorrhage rate, that is bleeding following adenoidectomy within 6–12 hours of operation, is less than 0.7 per cent, and for tonsillectomy reported between 1 per cent and 2 per cent. If severe enough to require a return to theatre, diathermy or postnasal packing to the adenoid bed may be required. Ties, diathermy or Coblation may be used to control a reactionary tonsil bleed.

Secondary haemorrhage after adenoidectomy is rare. It may be due to bleeding from an aberrant ascending pharyngeal artery. Secondary haemorrhage should raise the possibility of a clotting or coagulation defect. Following tonsillectomy, the secondary bleed rate is typically between 1 per cent and 4 per cent. The peak time of haemorrhage is during the second week following surgery. While the bleeding may stop spontaneously, return to theatres to arrest the haemorrhage should not be delayed, particularly in a child, where the blood volume (approximately 80 mL/kg body weight) and reserve are correspondingly smaller. Where ties, diathermy or Coblation do not achieve haemostasis, oversewing the faucal pillars may be necessary. Systemic antifibrinolytic treatment (e.g. tranexamic acid) is helpful. Transfusion is uncommonly required, but always establish intravenous access, administer fluids (avoiding dextrose-saline) and send blood for a full blood count and cross-match at the time of presentation.

DENTAL TRAUMA

Damage to the teeth may be accidental owing to slippage of the gag or supports. In older children, particular care is needed, particularly if the secondary incisors have erupted. These incisors are large but the mandible immature, and it is safer to use an adult gag, which will rest lateral to the incisors. When taking consent for surgery, it is mandatory to include a warning about possible damage to teeth. However, damage to the teeth will usually be considered negligent. Where there are loose deciduous teeth, take consent preoperatively to remove these under anaesthetic, avoiding the possibility of inhalation during the operation or during recovery from anaesthesia.

RETAINED SWAB

It is *mandatory* to confirm that if swabs are opened or used, the count is correct at the end of the operation before the gag is removed and anaesthesia reversed. A swab hidden from view may be retained in the nasopharynx, tonsillar fossa or laryngo-pharynx.

NASOPHARYNGEAL BLOOD CLOT

Blood may pool and clot in the nasopharynx during the procedure. The nasopharynx should be gently suctioned to clear any clot before removing the gag. Using a nasal suction catheter can cause bleeding from the adenoid bed. It is better to use an angled rose-tipped sucker in the mouth and through the nostrils to clear the nasopharynx. Failure to do so may lead to the clot falling onto the larynx during recovery and causing potentially fatal acute airway obstruction.

INFECTION

Infection in the nasopharynx following adenoidectomy is clinically uncommon, although many parents report fetor from the child in the week following surgery. This is more common following suction diathermy adenoidectomy, and many surgeons prescribe a short course of antibiotics, which abolishes this fetor. Rarely, retropharyngeal and mediastinal abscesses may occur as a result of trauma and secondary infection of the adenoid bed.

Following tonsillectomy, slough forms on the tonsil bed as it heals by secondary intention. While this is superficially infected, there is no compelling evidence that prophylactic antibiotics reduce infection and the risk of secondary haemorrhage. Chest infection is now much less common with contemporary anaesthetic techniques, when aspiration of blood and debris is unlikely.

CERVICAL SPINE

Non-traumatic atlanto-axial subluxation (Grisel syndrome) is rare but associated with overuse of diathermy either for removal of the adenoid or following curettage when used for haemostasis. Minimum, effective power settings for diathermy should always be used. Children with Down's syndrome may have atlanto-axial instability. Routine plain imaging of the cervical spine prior to surgery is not considered necessary in uncomplicated cases. Care and attention to the child's neck position during intubation and surgery is essential.

VELOPHARYNGEAL INCOMPETENCE

Following adenoidectomy, severe velopharyngeal incompetence is rare, estimated to occur in between 1:1500 and 1:10 000 procedures. It may lead to significant problems with hypernasal speech and swallowing, severe enough to cause nasal regurgitation of fluids. It is mandatory to assess the palate and uvula for submucous cleft of the palate prior to surgery, as surgery often unmasks pre-existing palatal dysfunction in a child with a bifid uvula with or without a submucous cleft about to undergo adenoidectomy. Using a direct-vision technique, it is possible to perform a partial adenoidectomy, clearing the choanal airway but leaving the adenoid intact at the velopharyngeal junction. In children with SDB and very large tonsils and adenoid, temporary, mild velopharyngeal insufficiency is not uncommon for some weeks after surgery as the palate movement and function return to normal. This should be discussed and explained to parents preoperatively. Long-term velopharyngeal insufficiency is rare.

ADVERSE DRUG EFFECTS

While nonsteroidal anti-inflammatory drugs pose a theoretical risk of increased post-operative haemorrhage, evidence supports the safe use of these during the post-operative period with no increased risk of bleeding.

At the time of writing, the US Food and Drug Administration (FDA) issued a Drug Safety Communication about the use of codeine in children as an analgesic following tonsillectomy and/or adenotonsillectomy for obstructive sleep apnoea syndrome. In some groups, particularly those of African origin, nearly 30 per cent are ultra-rapid metabolizers of codeine, producing a higher than therapeutic range and the effects of morphine toxicity. Three fatalities were reported. Codeine should NOT be used in children under the age of 18 years following tonsillectomy. If a 'rescue' analgesic is required, a small supply of soluble morphine (e.g. 3 days) at 1 mg/kg qds prn is a safe option. Soluble morphine is not a controlled drug at the standard concentration. Preparations combined with other drugs (e.g. paracetamol) should not be used. Narcotic anaesthesia should be avoided.

KEY LEARNING POINTS

- Tonsillectomy remains effective surgical intervention for recurrent tonsillitis and SDB.
- Adenoidectomy is effective as adjunct treatment when ventilation tubes are indicated for OME in children older than 3 years.
- The decreasing use of tonsillectomy has produced a very large increase in admission rate to the hospital for complications of tonsillitis.
- In very young children with SDB requiring surgery, Coblation tonsillotomy and suction diathermy adenoidectomy are associated with the lowest risk of postoperative bleeding.
- Codeine should never be used as analgesia for children undergoing tonsillectomy because of their unpredictable metabolism of morphine with potential toxicity.

KEY REFERENCES

Brockmann PE, Bertrand P, Pardo T, Cerda J, Reyes B, Holmgren NL. Prevalence of habitual snoring and associated neurocognitive consequences among Chilean school aged children. *International Journal of Pediatric Otorhinolaryngology*. 2012; 76(9): 1327–31.

MRC Multi-centre Otitis Media Study Group 2012. Adjuvant adenoidectomy in persistent bilateral otitis media with effusion: Hearing and revision surgery outcomes through 2 years in the TARGET randomised trial. *Clinical Otolaryngology*. 37: 107–16.

Mattila PS, Hammarén-Malmi S, Saxen H, Kaijalainen T, Käyhty H, Tarkkanen J. Adenoidectomy in young children and serum IgG antibodies to pneumococcal surface protein A and choline binding protein A. *International Journal of Pediatric Otorhinolaryngology*. 2012; 76: 1569–74.

Robb PJ, Ewah BN. Post-operative nausea and vomiting following paediatric day-case tonsillectomy: Audit of the Epsom protocol. *Journal of Laryngology and Otology*. 2011; 125: 1049–52.

Lock C, Wilson J, Steen N, Eccles M, Mason H, Carrie S, Clarke R, Kubba H, Raine C, Zarod A, Brittain K, Vanoli A, Bond J. North of England and Scotland Study of Tonsillectomy and Adeno-tonsillectomy in Children (NESSTAC): A pragmatic randomised controlled trial with a parallel non-randomised preference study. *Health Technology Assessment*. 2010 Mar; 14(13): 1–164, iii–iv. doi: 10.3310/hta14130.

Robb PJ. Childhood tonsillitis and tonsillectomy. *Otolaryngologica*. 2009; 59: 229–239.

Hesham A. Bipolar diathermy versus cold dissection in paediatric tonsillectomy. *International Journal of Pediatric Otorhinolaryngology*. 2009; 73(6): 793–95.

Robb PJ, Bew S, Kubba H, Murphy N, Primhak R, Rollin A-M, Tremlett, M. Tonsillectomy and adenoidectomy in children with sleep related breathing disorders: Consensus statement of a UK multidisciplinary working party. *Clinical Otolaryngology*. 2009; 34: 61–63.

Robb PJ. Adenoidectomy: Does it work? *Journal of Laryngology and Otology*. 2007; 121: 209–14.

Belloso A, Chidambaram CS, Morar P, Timms MS. Coblation tonsillectomy versus dissection tonsillectomy: Postoperative hemorrhage. *Laryngoscope*. 2003; 113(11): 2010–13.

FURTHER READING

Burton MJ, Glasziou PP. 2009. Tonsillectomy or adeno-tonsillectomy versus non-surgical treatment for chronic/recurrent acute tonsillitis. Cochrane Ear, Nose and Throat Disorders Group. Available from: http://onlinelibrary.wiley.com/doi/10.1002/14651858.CD001802.pub2/abstract.

FDA Drug Safety Communication. 2012. Codeine use in certain children after tonsillectomy and/or adenoidectomy may lead to rare, but life-threatening adverse events or death. Available from http://www.fda.gov/Drugs/DrugSafety/ucm313631.htm.

Lim J, McKean MC. 2009. Adenotonsillectomy for obstructive sleep apnoea in children. Cochrane Airways Group. Available from: http://onlinelibrary.wiley.com/doi/10.1002/14651858.CD003136.pub2/abstract.

National Institute for Health and Clinical Excellence. *Suction Diathermy Adenoidectomy (IPG 328)*. 2009. Available from: http://publications.nice.org.uk/suction-diathermy-adenoidectomy-ipg328.

National Institute for Health and Clinical Excellence. *Systematic review of the safety and efficacy of electrosurgery for tonsillectomy (IP 324)*. 2005. Available from: http://www.nice.org.uk/ip_324review.

Scottish Intercollegiate Guidelines Network, Royal College of Physicians. *Management of sore throat and indications for tonsillectomy.* National Clinical Guideline No 117. 2010. Available from http://www.sign.ac.uk/guidelines/fulltext/117/index.html.

The Royal College of Surgeons of England. National Prospective Tonsillectomy Audit. May 2005. Available from: http://www.rcseng.ac.uk/publications.

van den Aardweg MTA, Boonacker CWB, Rovers MM, Hoes AW, Schilder AGM. Effectiveness of adenoidectomy in children with recurrent upper respiratory tract infections: Open randomised controlled trial. *BMJ*. 2011; 343:d5154.

57

Acute rhinosinusitis and complications

MARY-LOUISE MONTAGUE

Acute rhinosinusitis (ARS) in adults is covered in Chapter 4, but in children it is anatomically, immunologically and clinically different, hence the need for a separate chapter. Its diagnosis and treatment in the paediatric population has undergone dramatic changes in the last few decades.

DEFINITION

ARS in children is defined as sudden onset of two or more symptoms of nasal blockage/congestion, nasal discharge and cough at daytime and night-time for less than 12 weeks with complete resolution of symptoms.[1] The term *rhinosinusitis* is used in preference to *sinusitis* to reflect that the inflammatory response involves the nasal mucosa and mucosa of at least one adjacent sinus cavity simultaneously.

CLASSIFICATION

ARS is classified as viral, post-viral or bacterial.

VIRAL ARS

ARS is most often viral in aetiology. As in adults, viral ARS or the 'common cold' is defined as symptoms of rhinosinusitis for less than 10 days. Children can have six to 10 common colds each year compared to two or three per year in adults. The usual causative viral agents are:

- Rhinovirus (>50 per cent)
- Coronavirus (15–20 per cent)
- Adenovirus
- Respiratory syncytial virus (RSV)
- Influenza virus

POST-VIRAL ARS

This is defined as an increase in symptoms after 5 days or persistent symptoms after 10 days.

ACUTE BACTERIAL RHINOSINUSITIS

In acute bacterial rhinosinusitis (ABRS), there are at least three symptoms/signs of discoloured discharge (with unilateral predominance) and purulent secretions in the nasal cavity, severe local pain (with unilateral predominance), fever (>38°C), elevated erythrocyte sedimentation rate/C-reactive protein, and a clinical picture of deterioration after an initial milder illness.[1] Recurrent ABRS involves discrete episodes of bacterial infection of the paranasal sinuses separated by asymptomatic intervals of at least 10 days. The most common pathogens causing ABRS in children are:

- *Streptococcus pneumoniae*
- *Haemophilus influenzae*
- *Moraxella catarrhalis*
- *Staphylococcus aureus*
- *Streptococcus pyogenes*
- Anaerobic bacteria

ANATOMY

The paediatric skull differs from the adult skull in a number of ways. The paranasal sinuses in children are significantly smaller in size compared to those in an adult. In toddlers the maxillary sinus floor lies at a higher level than in an adult and never extends lower than the floor of the nose. The

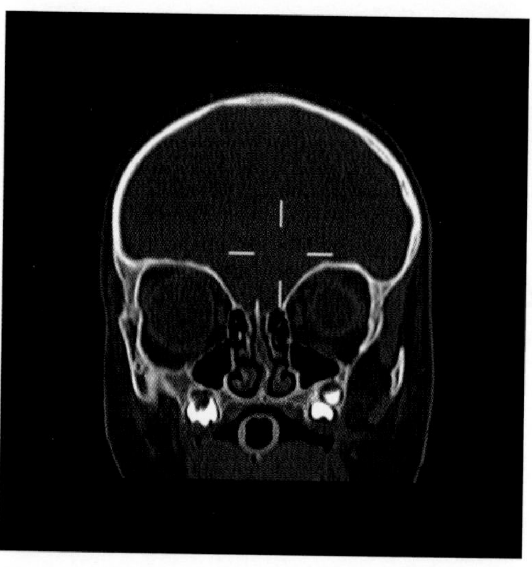

Figure 57.1 Coronal CT in a young child demonstrating level of the floor of the maxillary sinuses, absent alveolar recesses and narrow ethmoid infundibula.

ethmoid bone is longer than the maxillary sinus as the alveolar process has not yet developed. The infundibulum is relatively short and narrow. There are only a few millimetres between the medial wall of the infundibulum and the lamina papyracea. The lamina papyracea is particularly thin in children, facilitating the spread of infection to the orbit. In addition, the ophthalmic venous system is valveless and communicates with the ethmoid veins, providing a path for infection to enter the orbit. Whilst ethmoid and maxillary sinusitis may occur at any age, frontal sinusitis is rarely seen before the age of 6 years as pneumatization of the frontal sinus does not commence until the age of 4 years (Figure 57.1).

EMBRYOLOGY OF THE PARANASAL SINUSES

The paranasal sinuses develop as outpouchings of the nasal cavity pre-natally. Their overall growth is slow in the first 6 years of life. Their development is summarized in Table 57.1.[2]

Table 57.1 Embryological development of the paranasal sinuses

Sinus group	Neonatal period	Age visible on plain x-rays	Growth in childhood	Age permanent size attained	Average final volume
Maxillary	Present 7 mm deep 3 mm wide 7 mm high	4–5 months	Usually very small until age 7	15–18 years	5 mL
Ethmoid	2 or 3 ethmoid cells present bilaterally	1 year	3–4 cells to 10–15 cells per side by age 12 years	15–16 years	14–15 mL
Sphenoid	Present 4 mm high 2 mm wide	>3 years	Usually pneumatized by age 5	15 years	0.5–3 mL
Frontal	Absent	>6 years	Gradual development from the anterior ethmoid cells into the cranium commences at age 4 years Usually pneumatized by age 7–8 years	Second decade of life	4–7 mL

PATHOGENESIS

The primary sinus abnormality for initiation of rhinosinusitis is osteomeatal complex obstruction by mucosal oedema or mechanical obstruction. Various local, regional or systemic factors can cause obstruction of the osteomeatal complex. Local and regional factors include a deviated nasal septum, nasal polyps, concha bullosa, choanal atresia, nasal foreign bodies and oedema due to viral infections, allergic and non-allergic rhinitis. Systemic factors include ciliary dyskinesia syndromes, cystic fibrosis, and immunological deficiencies. Air pollution, gastro-oesophageal reflux, use of day nursery care and adenoid hypertrophy have also been implicated in paediatric rhinosinusitis. Viral upper respiratory tract infections (URTIs) and allergy are by far the most frequent causes in children. Ostial obstruction results in sinus hypoxia, which leads to ciliary dysfunction and abnormal clearance of mucus from the sinus. Stasis of secretions allows bacteria in the upper respiratory tract to multiply with subsequent invasion of the mucosa of the obstructed sinus.

DIAGNOSIS

Diagnosis of ARS in children is based on the history, examination and nasal endoscopy. Allergy testing, microbiology studies and assessment of immune status may also be useful investigations.

HISTORY

In children, ARS most often presents as a severe URTI with fever >39°C, as purulent rhinorrhoea and facial pain or, more commonly, as a prolonged URTI with chronic cough and nasal discharge. The symptoms in infants and toddlers are often nonspecific and generalized with fever and lymphadenitis predominating.

A diagnosis of ABRS can be made after a viral URTI when children have persistent symptoms for more than 10 days without improvement (nasal discharge, daytime cough worsening at night) or an abrupt increase in severity of symptoms after initial improvement of symptoms, or an URTI that seems more severe than usual (high fever, copious purulent nasal discharge, periorbital oedema and pain).

For completeness, enquire about allergic symptoms of sneezing, watery rhinorrhoea, nasal itching and itchy, watery eyes.

EXAMINATION

Nasal examination in children should begin with anterior rhinoscopy examining the middle meatus, inferior turbinates, nasal mucosa and presence of purulent discharge. This is usually achieved using a well-illuminated otoscope with a large speculum. An alternative is to use a head light and nasal speculum. Topical decongestion can be used to improve visualization. Usually there is erythema of the nasal mucosa and purulent rhinorrhoea. Nasal endoscopy affords superior visualization of the middle meatus, adenoids, and nasopharynx and can usually be successfully performed in children using a 2.7 mm rigid nasendoscope or fine fibreoptic endoscope. This allows exclusion of other pathology including nasal polyps, foreign bodies, a deviated nasal septum and tumours. In very young children nasal endoscopy may require recourse to general anaesthesia. Examination of the oropharynx and oral cavity may reveal purulent postnasal discharge, erythema and cobblestoning of the posterior pharyngeal wall, tonsillar hypertrophy or dental caries. Cervical lymph nodes may be enlarged and tender.

INVESTIGATIONS

MICROBIOLOGICAL CULTURE

This is not usually necessary in children with uncomplicated ARS. It might be useful in the following situations:

- Failed response to medical treatment within 48–72 hours
- Immunocompromised children
- Presence of suppurative complications (intraorbital or intracranial)
- Children with severe illness who appear toxic

As antral puncture requires general anaesthesia in children, middle meatal cultures are generally accepted as a reasonable surrogate as they correlate well with antral cultures.[3]

ALLERGY TESTING

Skin-prick allergy tests or specific IgE measurement should be performed if there is any doubt about a possible allergic cause.

IMAGING

ARS in children is generally a clinical diagnosis. Plain radiographs are not sufficiently sensitive to justify the radiation exposure in children. Computed tomography (CT) scanning is the imaging of choice, but it should be reserved for children with symptoms persisting after 10 days of medical therapy, children with suspected intraorbital or intracranial complications, or if surgery is planned after failed medical therapy.

ASSESSMENT OF IMMUNE FUNCTION

Young children have a physiological immune deficiency. This usually resolves by the age of 10 years. Common variable immune deficiencies may present with recurrent ABRS. Preliminary investigation of this group of children should include full blood count (FBC), differential white cell count, immunoglobulin levels including IgG subclasses, and vaccine responses to pneumococcus, *Haemophilus influenzae* type B and tetanus toxoid.

DIFFERENTIAL DIAGNOSIS

When a child presents with symptoms of ARS, the differential diagnosis must include intranasal foreign body and unilateral choanal stenosis. In these entities, the symptoms are usually unilateral and can be relatively easily differentiated clinically from ARS by history and physical examination, including nasal endoscopy. ARS will usually not manifest with purulent discharge as part of the clinical presentation. Adenoiditis can have a very similar clinical presentation, including anterior and posterior purulent discharge and cough, and is very relevant in the differential diagnosis in the paediatric age group.

MANAGEMENT

MEDICAL TREATMENT

Uncomplicated viral rhinosinusitis usually resolves without treatment in 7 to 10 days. ABRS may also resolve without treatment, though antibiotic therapy hastens recovery. Treatment is therefore symptomatic in most cases, with isotonic saline nose drops, humidification of warm air, simple analgesia and antipyretics.

The indications for antibiotic therapy and the antibiotics of choice are outlined in Table 57.2. The recommended duration of treatment is 10–14 days in children.[4] Children allergic to penicillin should receive a suitable alternative antibiotic such as clarithromycin or azithromycin. Clindamycin is useful if anaerobic organisms are suspected but provides no coverage against Gram-negative organisms.

Table 57.2 Indications for antibiotic therapy in ARS in children and appropriate agent.

Indication	Appropriate antibiotic
Severe ARS	Oral amoxicillin-potassium clavulanate or second-generation cephalosporin, e.g. cefuroxime
Children with concomitant disease that may be exacerbated by ARS, e.g. asthma, chronic bronchitis	Oral amoxicillin (45 mg/kg/day, doubled if <2 years or risk factors for resistance)
Children with a suspected or proven suppurative complication	Intravenous amoxicillin-potassium clavulanate or ceftriaxone + flucloxacillin

Topical nasal steroids might have a beneficial ancillary role in the treatment of ARS when allergy is involved. Antihistamines are helpful in reducing coexisting allergic symptoms of watery rhinorrhoea, itch and sneezing. Mucolytic agents, e.g. acetyl-cysteine, have not been proven to be helpful.

Topical decongestants (xylo- and oxymetazoline) can give rapid relief of nasal blockage and can be considered for up to 5 days (to avoid potential rebound) in children aged 6–12 years. They should not be used in children under 6 years because of their toxic side effects. There is little evidence to support the use of systemic decongestants in children.

PREVENTION

High-risk groups of children need pre-seasonal flu vaccination according to national guidelines.

COMPLICATIONS OF ARS

Complications of ARS are typically classified as orbital (60–75 per cent), intracranial (15–20 per cent) and osseous (5–10 per cent).[5] Orbital complications are more common in children than in adults, because of the thinness of the lamina papyracea. Intracranial complications are less common in children but can occur at any age, with a predilection for the second and third decades of life. Boys are more frequently affected than girls. ARS is the main precipitating factor in children, while chronic rhinosinusitis (CRS) with or without nasal polyps is more important in adults. There is a clear seasonal pattern of complications, mirroring the higher incidence of URTIs during the winter months.

Prompt recognition and management of complications is vital to avoid long-term sequelae. All of the potential orbital, intracranial and osseous complications of ARS are listed in Table 57.3.

ORBITAL COMPLICATIONS

These are the most common complications and occur much more frequently in children than in

Table 57.3 Complications of ARS

Periorbital complications	Preseptal cellulitis Orbital cellulitis Subperiosteal abscess Intraorbital abscess
Intracranial complications	Epidural abscess Subdural abscess Brain abscess Meningitis Encephalitis Superior sagittal sinus thrombosis Cavernous sinus thrombosis
Osseous complications	Pott's Puffy tumour Frontocutaneous fistula

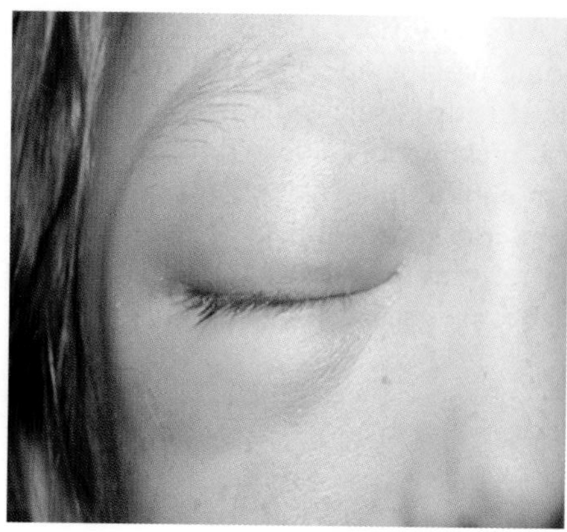

Figure 57.2 Right preseptal cellulitis with eyelid oedema and erythema.

adults. They are associated in order of decreasing frequency with the ethmoid, maxillary, frontal and rarely the sphenoid sinus. Microbiology specimens usually grow *Haemophilus influenzae, Streptococcus pneumoniae* or *Staphylococcus.* It is important to note that orbital complications in children may occur without pain.

Orbital complications have been classified by Chandler in a stepwise sequence as follows[6]:

- Stage I: Preseptal cellulitis
- Stage II: Orbital cellulitis
- Stage III: Subperiosteal abscess
- Stage IV: Orbital abscess
- Stage V: Cavernous sinus thrombosis

Preseptal cellulitis

This refers to inflammation of the eyelid and conjunctiva (i.e. tissues anterior to the orbital septum). It presents with non-tender eyelid oedema and erythema but no associated proptosis and no limitation of eye movement. This can be difficult to assess, especially in small children. It is usually a clinical diagnosis and does not require a CT scan (Figure 57.2).

Orbital cellulitis

As the inflammation progresses to involve the orbit, conjunctival oedema (chemosis), proptosis, ocular pain and tenderness and restricted painful eye movement (ophthalmoplegia) develop.

Subperiosteal abscess

Abscess forms between the periorbita and the sinuses and is located out with the ocular muscles (extraconal). The clinical features are oedema, erythema, chemosis, proptosis, ophthalmoplegia and diminished visual acuity. High fever and raised white cell count are strongly associated with subperiosteal and orbital abscess formation.

Orbital abscess

Abscess forms within the space defined by the ocular muscles (intraconal). It is characterized by severe globe displacement, ophthalmoplegia and progressive visual loss due to optic neuropathy. Pupil reactions may be abnormal and a relative afferent pupillary defect (RAPD) may be present.

Cavernous sinus thrombosis

Spread of infection to the veins around the sinuses can lead to cavernous sinus thrombosis. Although strictly an intracranial complication, it is described here alongside the other stages in Chandler's classification of orbital complications. It is characterized by sudden onset of bilateral lid drop, exophthalmos, ophthalmic nerve neuralgia, retro-ocular headache with deep pain behind the orbit, complete ophthalmoplegia, papilloedema and signs of meningeal irritation, multiple cranial nerve involvement and sepsis associated with swinging pyrexia. A 30 per cent mortality rate and 60 per cent morbidity rate remain in the adult population. No data are available for children in whom the mortality rate for intracranial complications is 10–20 per cent.

Management

In most paediatric centres management is multidisciplinary with the paediatrician, ophthalmologist, otolaryngologist, radiologist and microbiologist all having a role to play. Ophthalmology assessment should be sought early.

Preseptal cellulitis usually responds to oral antibiotic therapy. Any child who cannot be assessed clinically and those with proptosis, reduced or painful eye movement, or diminished visual acuity (initially manifesting itself with colour vision impairment) or a relative afferent pupillary defect should have a contrast-enhanced CT scan with orbital detail to distinguish between orbital cellulitis and subperiosteal or orbital abscess (Figure 57.3). If an intracranial complication is suspected, magnetic resonance imaging (MRI) adds valuable information.

Orbital cellulitis requires aggressive treatment with intravenous antibiotics. The antibiotics should cover aerobic and anaerobic bacteria. Ophthalmology assessments of visual acuity should take place at regular intervals. Intravenous antibiotic therapy may be converted to oral antibiotics when the child has remained afebrile for 48 hours and the eye symptoms and signs are resolving.

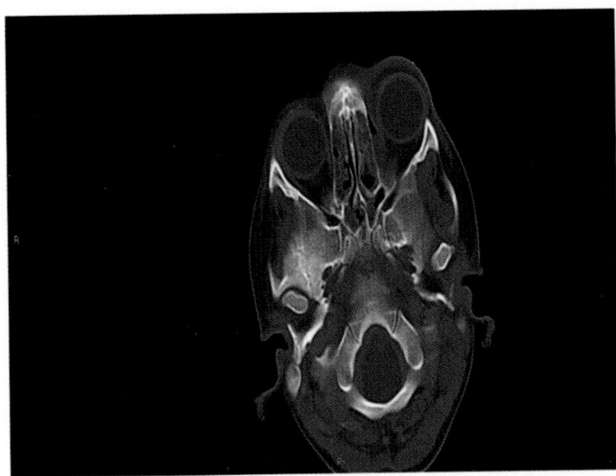

Figure 57.3 Axial CT of orbits showing left postseptal orbital cellulitis with a focal collection abutting the medial wall of the left orbit and displacing the left medial rectus muscle laterally.

CT evidence of abscess, progressive orbital signs or impaired visual acuity (especially colour vision) after initial (24–48 hours) intravenous antibiotic therapy are indications for surgical exploration and drainage of the orbit and offending sinus. Endoscopic drainage of the abscess by opening the lamina papyracea and endoscopic ethmoidectomy are favoured nowadays. External approaches to medial, superior and superolateral orbital abscesses can also be used if the operative field and childhood anatomy are such that an endoscopic approach is not feasible.

Some recent studies have shown good outcomes with intravenous antibiotics in small children with subperiosteal abscesses. Children were carefully selected, this approach being confined to those under 5 years old with small-volume (<0.5–1.0 mL), medially located subperiosteal abscesses with normal visual acuity and no systemic involvement.

Cavernous sinus thrombosis is fortunately rare. The use of anticoagulants in these children is controversial but is probably indicated provided imaging shows no evidence of any intracerebral haemorrhagic changes. Steroids may help to reduce inflammation and are likely to be helpful, administered with concomitant antibiotics. Drainage of the offending sinus (almost always the sphenoid) is indicated.

INTRACRANIAL COMPLICATIONS

Infection can spread intracranially from the sinuses via the diploic veins, by eroding the bone of the sinus or by haematogenous spread. Intracranial complications are most often associated with frontoethmoid or sphenoid rhinosinusitis. They may present with non-specific symptoms and signs (fever and headache), or even be silent. As such, their diagnosis requires a high index of suspicion. The majority of patients present with more specific symptoms and signs (nausea and vomiting, neck stiffness and altered conscious level). Organisms most commonly involved in the pathogenesis of intracranial complications are *Streptococcus*, *Staphylococcus* species and anaerobes.

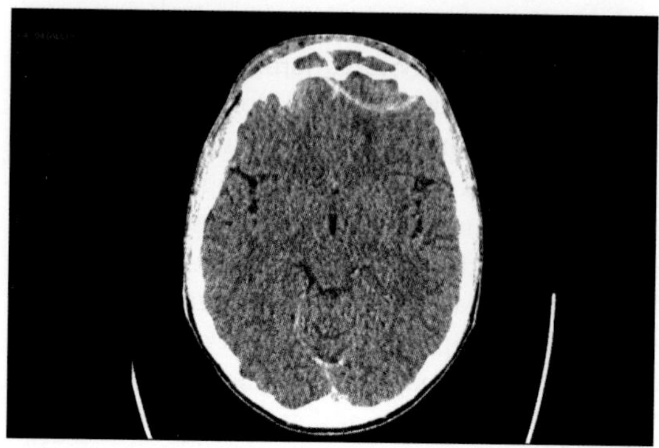

Figure 57.4 Contrast CT demonstrating frontal subdural abscess secondary to frontal sinusitis.

Intracranial abscesses may be multiple and are most often frontal. They are often heralded by signs of raised intracranial pressure, meningeal irritation and focal neurologic deficits, including third, sixth or seventh cranial nerve palsies. An axial CT with contrast is essential for diagnosis (Figure 57.4). This is combined with MRI venography to exclude associated venous sinus thrombosis.[7]

High-dose, long-term intravenous antibiotic therapy followed by burr hole drainage, craniotomy or image-guided aspiration as needed are usually required for successful treatment. Drainage of the paranasal sinuses (often the frontal sinus) may also be required. The mortality associated with intracranial abscess remains high (20 per cent).

As for orbital complications of ARS, the management of intracranial complications should also be multidisciplinary, with input from a paediatric neurologist and neurosurgeon being essential.

OSSEOUS COMPLICATIONS

Osteomyelitis of the anterior table of the frontal sinus presents with 'doughy' oedema of the skin over the frontal bone producing a subperiosteal abscess referred to as Pott's puffy tumour (Figure 57.5). Contrast-enhanced CT scan confirms the diagnosis. The infection can proceed anteriorly by breaching the skin, resulting in a frontocutaneous fistula. Treatment includes broad-spectrum antibiotics combined with adequate drainage of the involved sinus, debridement of sequestered bone and drainage of the abscess.

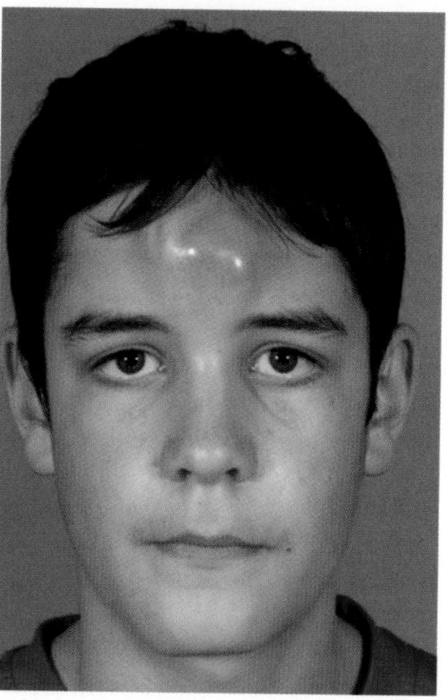

Figure 57.5 Pott's puffy tumour complicating acute left frontal sinusitis in a 13-year-old boy.

Osteomyelitis of the posterior table of the frontal sinus may spread directly or via the diploic veins to cause intracranial complications.

KEY LEARNING POINTS

- Rhinosinusitis is common in children and is different from adult rhinosinusitis.
- In most instances, acute bacterial rhinosinusitis in children follows a viral upper respiratory infection.
- The pattern of sinus involvement is determined by the child's age: Younger children will present with ethmoid and maxillary disease, whilst older children will also have frontal disease.
- Many children do not require treatment, and very few need surgery.
- Complications of ARS are typically classified as orbital (60–75 per cent), intracranial (15–20 per cent) and osseous (5–10 per cent). Although rare, these must be considered in any child with severe or protracted symptoms.

KEY DEFINITIONS

acute bacterial rhinosinusitis at least three symptoms/signs of purulent discharge (with unilateral predominance), severe local pain (with unilateral predominance), fever (>38°C), elevated ESR/CRP and a clinical picture of deterioration after an initial milder illness

acute rhinosinusitis sudden onset of two or more symptoms of nasal blockage/congestion, nasal discharge, and cough at daytime and night-time for less than 12 weeks with complete resolution of symptoms

Pott's puffy tumour osteomyelitis of the anterior table of the frontal sinus presenting with oedema of the skin over the frontal bone and producing a subperiosteal abscess

relative afferent pupillary defect a medical sign observed during the swinging-flashlight test where the patient's pupils constrict less (therefore appearing to dilate) when a bright light is swung from the unaffected eye to the affected eye. The affected eye still senses the light and produces pupillary sphincter constriction to some degree, albeit reduced.

REFERENCES

1. Fokkens WJ, Lund VJ, Mullol J, Bachert C, et al. European position paper on rhinosinusitis and nasal polyps 2012. *Rhinology.* 2012; Supplement 23: 1–298.
2. Wolf G, Anderhuber W, Kuhn F. Development of the paranasal sinuses in children: Implications for paranasal sinus surgery. *Annals of Otology, Rhinology and Laryngology.* 1993; 102: 705.
3. DeMuri GP, Wald ER. Acute bacterial sinusitis in children. *New England Journal of Medicine.* 2012; 367: 1128–34.
4. American Academy of Pediatrics, Subcommittee on Management of Sinusitis and Committee on Quality Improvement. Clinical practice guideline: Management of sinusitis. *Pediatrics.* 2001; 108: 798–808.
5. DeMuri GP, Wald ER. Complications of acute bacterial sinusitis in children. *Pediatric Infectious Disease Journal.* 2011; 30: 701–2.
6. Chandler JR, Langenbrunner DJ, Stevens ER. The pathogenesis of orbital complications in acute sinusitis. *Laryngoscope.* 1970; 80: 1414–28.
7. Reid JR. Complications of pediatric paranasal sinusitis. *Pediatric Radiology.* 2004; 34: 933–42.

FURTHER READING

Wald ER. *Rhinitis and Acute and Chronic Sinusitis.* In: *Paediatric Otolaryngology.* 2nd ed. Eds. Bluestone CD, Stool SE, Sheetz MD. Philadelphia: Saunders, 1990.

58

Stridor and airway endoscopy

DAVID ALBERT AND YOGESH BAJAJ

INTRODUCTION

The safe management of the stridulous child is one of the core skills for all ear, nose and throat (ENT) surgeons. It is assessed at the exit examination and will be reassessed at revalidation. ENT surgeons must have an understanding of the common causes of acute and chronic stridor and be able to practise safe initial management. Most acutely stridulous children are initially managed by paediatricians and emergency physicians. By the time an ENT surgeon becomes involved in the acute situation, the stridor may be well established. Usually, medical treatment alone will suffice, but occasionally a child will need to be taken to the operating theatre for controlled intubation. In many institutions an ENT surgeon is in attendance in case an emergency tracheostomy is needed, but in reality this is rarely required.

Another situation that an ENT surgeon may be called to respond to is a child with an inhaled foreign body. All ENT surgeons should be able to assess the child to see if he or she is stable or struggling. Most of these children are actually relatively stable and should be transferred to a specialist centre. There is considerable debate about how to manage the rare case where the child with a foreign body is struggling. Airway endoscopy in a compromised child with a foreign body is extremely challenging, and a careful assessment must be made about the relative risks of endoscopy versus transfer. All units need to discuss in advance how to deal with these rare emergencies and have an agreed protocol. At present it seems as though all ENT surgeons may need to be aware of how to use paediatric endoscopy equipment as part of revalidation in the United Kingdom and as an extreme emergency measure. Routine paediatric endoscopy would not be a requirement and indeed would be unsafe due to the small caseload.

In chronic stridor the history and examination, whilst suggestive, are rarely sufficient for a firm diagnosis. Deciding which patients require further investigation may be difficult. Even after appropriate noninvasive investigations, such as imaging, there may still be a number of possible diagnoses. Flexible endoscopy in the office is useful but gives limited information beyond the glottis. The definitive diagnostic tool of laryngo-tracheobronchoscopy requires highly specialized equipment and an experienced surgical, anaesthetic and nursing team.

This chapter describes a current and safe approach to assessing and treating the airway of the stridulous child and how to perform endoscopy if required. The diagnostic workup is examined in detail.

DEFINITION AND PHYSICAL PRINCIPLES

Stridor is an audible respiratory noise derived from turbulent airflow due to narrowing or obstruction of the upper airway. Stridor may be inspiratory, biphasic or expiratory in nature. It is classically a harsh sound, which can vary in quality from a squeak to a whistling noise. *Stertor* describes the snoring-like noise, which typically originates from nasopharyngeal or oropharyngeal obstruction. Clinically, however, the supraglottic larynx can occasionally produce this quality of noise. Obstruction from all levels of the airway should thus be considered when approaching the differential diagnoses of airway obstruction (Table 58.1).

It is helpful to review the physical principles of tubular flow according to Poiseuille's law, which states that $Q = [\pi r^4(P_1 - P_2)]/8\eta L$, where Q is flow, r is radius, P is pressure, η is viscosity and L is length of tube. From this law, resistance is inversely proportional to the radius to the fourth power. From a practical viewpoint, this explains why a minor narrowing of the airway in a child is of much greater consequence than in an adult. For example, 1 mm of edema in a 4 mm diameter paediatric airway will reduce the cross-sectional area by 75 per cent (16-fold increase in resistance), whilst in a 12 mm adult airway, the same 1 mm of edema will reduce the airway area by just 30 per cent (twofold increase in resistance), as demonstrated in Figure 58.1.

Even so a child can cope with quite a severe narrowing if the airflow is laminar (determined by the Reynolds number Re). It may only take a small amount of additional narrowing to dramatically increase the resistance as the flow becomes turbulent. In a compliant structure such as a child's larynx, collapse on inspiration is the third factor that can create a sudden and catastrophic increase in airway resistance. This is the Bernoulli effect (Figures 58.2 and 58.3).

ASSESSMENT

It is important to perform a rapid initial evaluation of the stridulous child to assess his or her degree of respiratory distress and thus the urgency with which the child's clinical presentation must be dealt with. If the patient has acute airway obstruction with significant respiratory distress, then the history, examination and initial resuscitation take place simultaneously. If the child is stable, then a thorough assessment can be conducted.

Stridor may be *characteristic* of a particular pathology but is never *diagnostic*. The diagnosis can be confirmed with certainty only after endoscopy. However, the combination of a thorough history, examination and investigation can in some conditions (e.g. mild laryngo-malacia) provide sufficient diagnostic probability to avoid initial rigid endoscopy. It is important to note that infants with laryngo-malacia on flexible endoscopy may have a synchronous lesion.

HISTORY

Features of the stridor, including the timing of onset, progression, variability and presence of exacerbating or relieving factors, should be carefully established. Stridor present from birth suggests an underlying anatomical cause. This generally denotes a fixed congenital narrowing such as a laryngeal web, subglottic stenosis or tracheal narrowing. The important exception is congenital vocal cord palsy, which is typically evident with the first breath. Dynamic conditions such as laryngo-malacia typically become evident in the first few weeks of life. A gradual increase in severity of stridor or airway

Table 58.1 Differential diagnosis of airway obstruction

	Supra-laryngeal	Laryngeal	Tracheobronchial
Congenital	Choanal atresia Choanal/midnasal/piriform aperture stenosis Benign tumour Nasal glioma Encephalocoele Meningocoele Nasopharyngeal mass (e.g. hairy polyp, teratoma) Structural Midface hypoplasia (e.g. Apert's, Crouzon's, Down syndrome) Micrognathia (e.g. Pierre Robin, Treacher-Collins) Macroglossia (e.g. Down syndrome, cystic hygroma, lingual thyroid) Cysts Dermoid Thyroglossal duct cyst Neurological dysfunction	Laryngo-malacia Vocal cord palsy Laryngeal atresia Laryngo-tracheal stenosis Laryngeal web Posterior laryngeal cleft Cysts Vallecular cyst Laryngeal cyst	Tracheomalacia/bronchomalacia Tracheal stenosis Extrinsic compression Vascular compression (e.g. aberrant brachiocephalic, double aortic arch, vascular ring, pulmonary artery sling) Mediastinal tumour Tracheal atresia Complete tracheal rings Tracheal cysts
Acquired	Adenotonsillar hypertrophy Infection Tonsillitis Adenoiditis Infectious mononucleosis Retropharyngeal abscess Ludwig's angina Rhinitis Foreign body	Trauma Intubation trauma (e.g. subglottic stenosis) Cricoarytenoid joint fixation Surgical trauma (e.g. laser) Thermal and caustic burns Infection Croup Epiglottitis Reflux laryngitis	Post-intubation/instrumentation Tracheal stenosis Foreign body Reflux Infection Croup Bacterial tracheitis Post-surgical malacia (e.g. tracheostomy, post-TEF repair)

(Continued)

Table 58.1 (Continued) Differential diagnosis of airway obstruction

Supra-laryngeal	Laryngeal	Tracheobronchial
Thermal and caustic burns	Benign tumour Papillomatosis Hemangioma Cystic hygroma Malignant tumour (e.g. rhabdomyosarcoma) Foreign body	Extrinsic compression Mediastinal tumour (e.g. hemangioma, cystic hygroma, lymphadenopathy, thyroid mass)

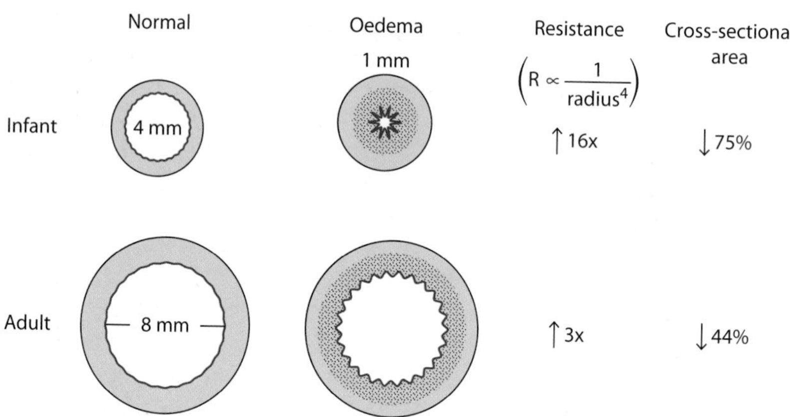

Figure 58.1 Effect of airway narrowing upon airway cross-section and resistance in the paediatric and adult airway.[2]

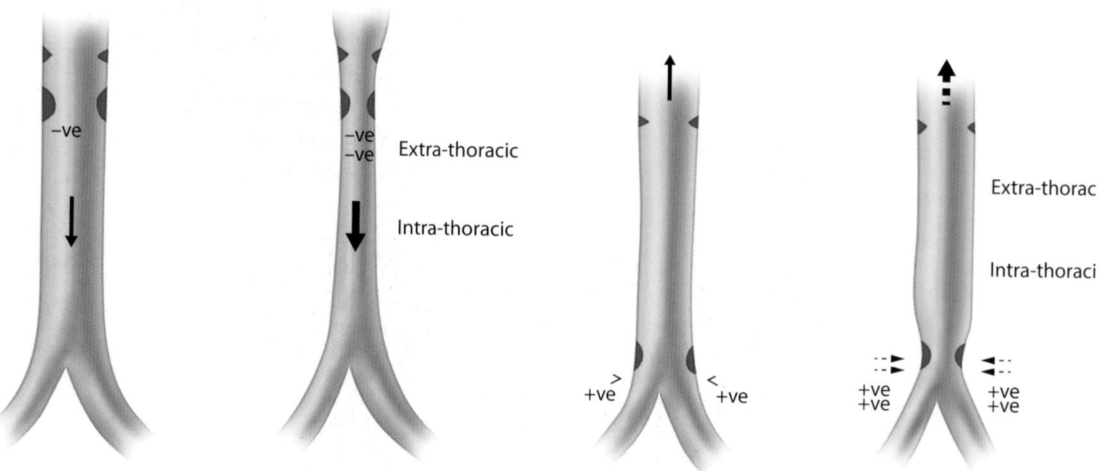

Figure 58.2 Intrathoracic obstruction.

Figure 58.3 Extrathoracic obstruction.

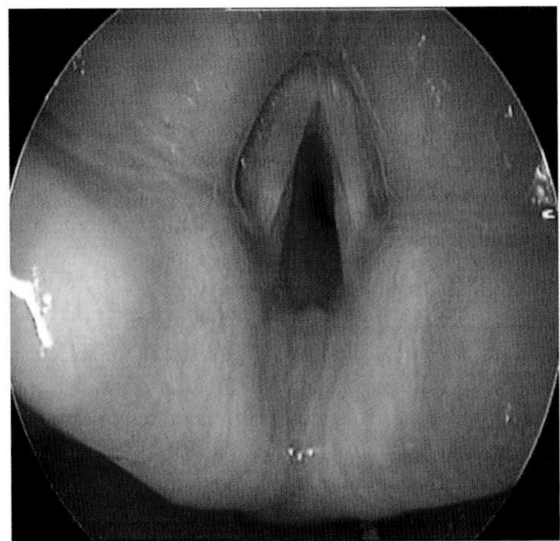

Figure 58.4 Endoscopic view of subglottic haemangioma presenting with increasing stridor.

compromise implies progressive obstruction. The obstruction may be luminal (as in a subglottic hemangioma, Figure 58.4) or extrinsic (as with a mediastinal mass or vascular anomaly, Figure 58.5). Alternatively, over a longer period of time, increasing stridor may coincide with increased respiratory demands of the child as he or she becomes more active. Typically, laryngo-malacia improves during rest or sleep but is worsened by crying, feeding or physical activity. Airway obstruction associated with supine positioning may occur with supra-laryngeal obstruction, such as micrognathia where there is associated airway obstruction by the tongue

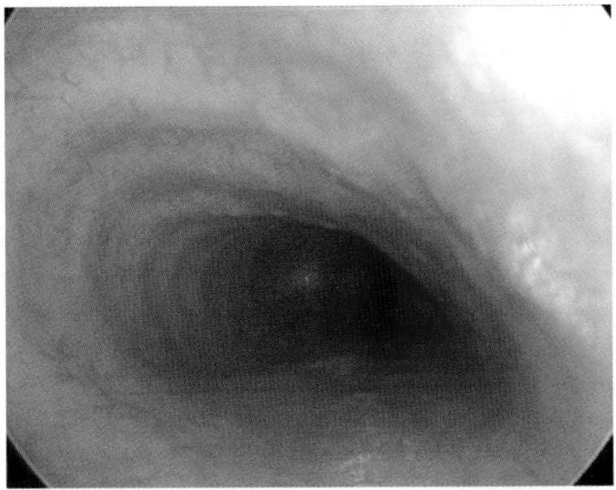

Figure 58.5 Extrinsic vascular compression of trachea.

base. More rarely, a pedunculated laryngeal mass, for example a vallecular cyst, can give positional variation in the stridor as it is displaced in and out of the airway. Improved airway obstruction with crying may occur in gross nasal obstruction such as bilateral choanal atresia.

Airway obstruction produces a number of associated symptoms (Table 58.2), which may be useful in formulating a differential diagnosis. Parents have often observed signs of increased respiratory work, including tracheal tug, subcostal recession, suprasternal or sternal indrawing. Apneas with cyanosis may occur, and parents will often attempt resuscitation if these are severe. These episodes are typical of severe tracheobronchomalacia and are sometimes termed *dying spells*. The differential diagnosis includes underlying congenital cardiac disease; hence these episodes should be investigated further. Cough is typical of tracheoesophageal fistula and tracheomalacia (Figure 58.6), and raises the possibility of aspiration. Hoarseness suggests laryngeal pathology such as laryngeal papillomatosis (Figure 58.7), whilst supra-laryngeal pathology may give a muffled voice. Voice change may also occur in vocal cord palsy, although these children can also present with airway compromise and a normal voice. Tachypnea and dyspnea are not limited to upper airway obstruction, but a clear description of exertional dyspnea in an older child may provide a useful functional assessment of severity.

The baby may feed slowly due to airway obstruction and 'run out of breath' or 'come up for air' during feeds. Bottle-fed babies may require thickened feeds or a 'slow teat' (i.e. one with small holes). Uncomplicated slow feeding, whilst often a source of significant maternal anxiety, is not necessarily of concern in isolation. However, if there is failure to thrive and documented poor weight gain on the centile growth chart, further investigation and possible intervention should be considered. Laryngo-malacia commonly gives rise to feeding difficulties, but it is important to consider other causes. Choking episodes, documented aspiration or recurrent chest infections may occur with vocal cord palsy, tracheoesophageal fistula (Figure 58.6) or, rarely, a laryngeal cleft (Figure 58.8). Gastro-esophageal reflux is also common in infants with stridor and may exacerbate airway obstruction via oedema.

Table 58.2 Features of history and examination in the stridulous child

Symptoms	Signs

Stridor
  Timing of onset
  Progression
  Variability
  Exacerbating/relieving factors
Features of systemic infection
Apnoeas/cyanosis (dying spells)
Parental observation of recession
Shortness of breath, respiratory rate
Cough
Feeding difficulties
Aspiration/reflux
Cry/hoarseness
Specific questioning re: foreign body aspiration
Past history:
  Perinatal
  Intubation history
  Recurrent/persisting croup or bronchiolitis
  Co-morbidities, e.g. neurological – Arnold Chiari, vascular malformation, cardiac disease/surgery, "birth marks"
	Characteristics of stridor
	  Quality, duration, timing
	General appearance/syndromic features
	Work of respiration:
	  Respiratory rate, distress, fatigue, accessory muscle use, recession, nasal flaring, tracheal tug
	Positioning for optimal airway
	Drooling
	Quality of cry
	Observation chart: temperature, pulse rate
	Nasal patency
	Oropharynx – mandible, tongue, tonsils
	Neck – fullness/masses, torticollis
	Auscultation of upper airway and chest
	Remainder of ENT assessment (ears etc.)

The possibility of foreign body aspiration (Figure 58.9) should always be raised with the parents, although it is an unusual cause of isolated stridor. The clinician must, however, maintain a high index of suspicion to avoid missing this diagnosis, particularly if there is a history of a choking episode.

Caustic ingestion or thermal injury to the hypopharynx or supraglottis sustained by the infant drinking from microwave-heated bottles are other potential sources of upper airway obstruction.

The clinician should determine whether the child has been systemically unwell, possibly

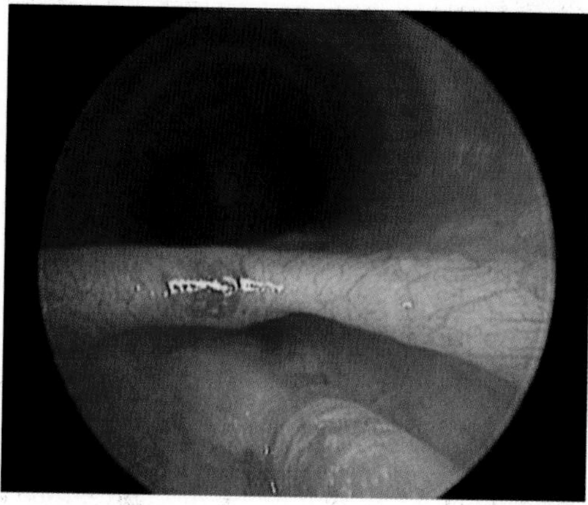

Figure 58.6 Tracheo-oesophageal fistula.

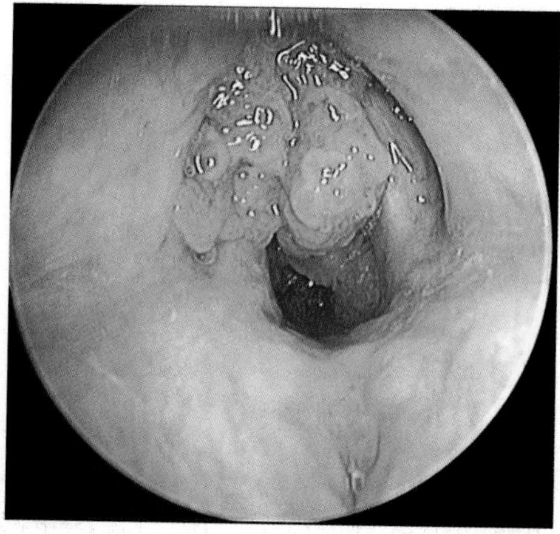

Figure 58.7 Laryngeal papillomatosis.

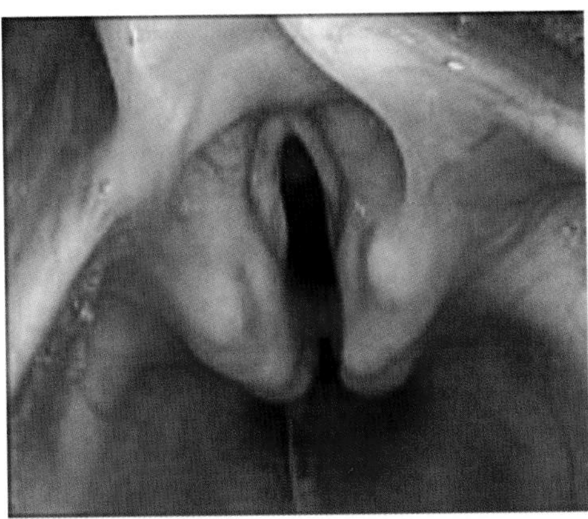

Figure 58.8 Endoscopic view of type 3 laryngeal cleft.

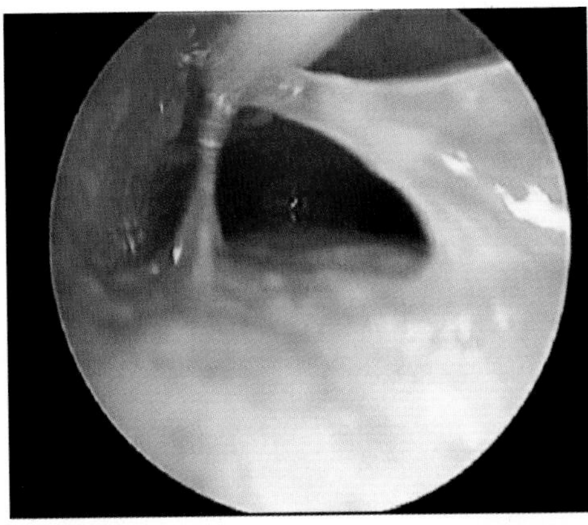

Figure 58.10 Bacterial tracheitis.

with high temperatures. Acute episodes of airway infection will cause acute inflammation and obstruction. Viral laryngo-tracheitis (croup) classically has a barking cough with low-grade fever and a preceding prodromal upper respiratory tract infection. Epiglottitis typically produces rapidly progressive upper airway obstruction in association with drooling, marked odynophagia and a 'muffled' voice. It is now very rare due to a dramatic reduction in incidence with *Haemophilus influenzae* type b (Hib) immunization. Bacterial tracheitis (Figure 58.10) has a variable onset with a toxic appearance, high fevers, cough and stridor.

Parents should be specifically asked about neonatal intubation, which has an increased risk of acquired subglottic stenosis (Figure 58.11). This history must be taken carefully, as the passage of nasogastric tubes for feeding or nasal/oral mucous suctioning may be mistaken for intubation.

Other co-morbidities may predispose to airway obstruction, for example vocal cord palsy in Arnold–Chiari malformation or birth injury, neurological disease giving hypotonia, or iatrogenic injury following cardiac surgery. A previously diagnosed syndrome may alert the clinician to potential pathology that is recognized as a component of the syndrome, for example laryngeal webs in velo-cardio-facial syndrome. Vascular malformations, congenital cardiac disease or vascular

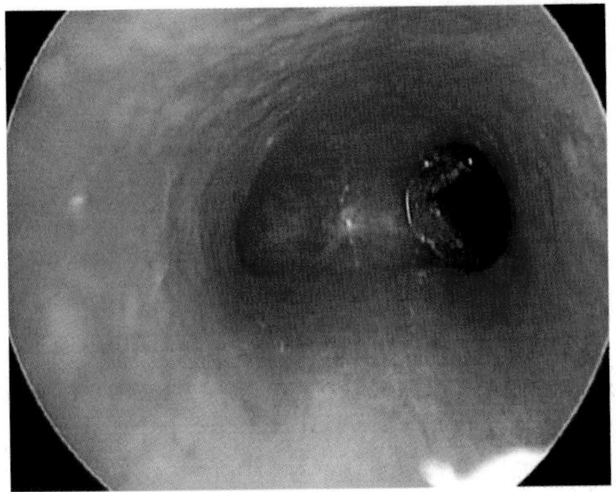

Figure 58.9 Foreign body right main bronchus.

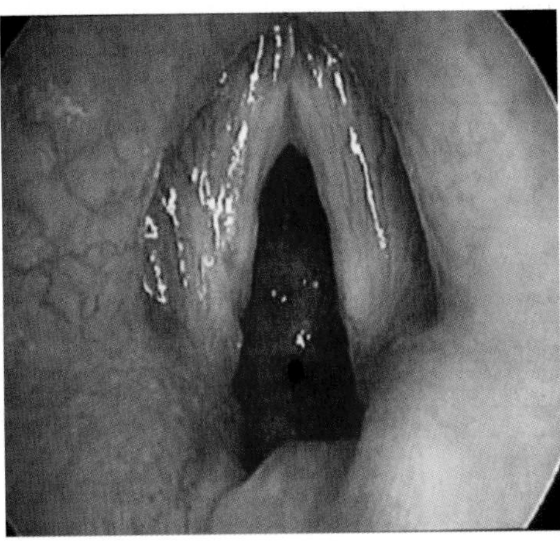

Figure 58.11 Acquired subglottic stenosis.

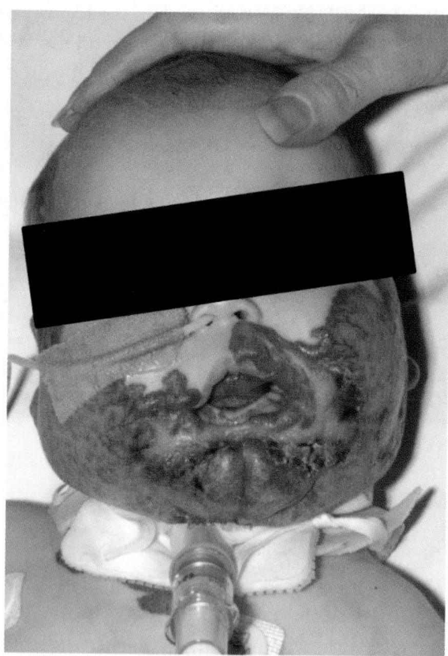

Figure 58.12 Extensive cutaneous cervicofacial haemangioma in a 'beard' distribution in an infant with transglottic, tracheal and mediastinal haemangioma.

anomalies may give extrinsic compression of the airway and subsequent tracheomalacia. Parents should be asked about the presence of any 'birthmarks' as 50 per cent of children with a subglottic haemangioma (see Figure 58.4) have a cutaneous lesion at the time of diagnosis (Figure 58.12). There is a markedly increased risk for children with cutaneous hemangiomas in a 'beard' distribution (Figure 58.12). Some of these children present with a history of recurrent episodes of laryngo-tracheitis or bronchiolitis that has been slow to settle.

EXAMINATION

An overall assessment of the degree of respiratory distress and airway compromise should be expedited in the acute situation and a full examination completed if the child is stable (Table 58.2). Observation of the child at rest in the parent's arms provides an initial assessment of the degree of respiratory distress, the characteristics of any stridor and whether the child appears systemically unwell. It also allows time to gain the child's confidence before any further examination. A careful general examination is necessary to avoid missing subtle features of related syndromes or of other general paediatric disease. Syndromic features, if present, may suggest likely sources of airway obstruction associated with the particular syndrome, for example micrognathia in Pierre Robin sequence, macroglossia in Beckwith–Weidemann syndrome or anterior glottic webs in velo-cardio-facial syndrome (see Figure 58.15).

Simple inspection of the child will reveal valuable information regarding the work of breathing and degree of obstruction. Potential findings of increased respiratory work include suprasternal or sternal recession, subcostal indrawing, 'see-saw' or paradoxical abdominal movement during respiration, nasal flaring, tracheal tug, anxiety, irritability or evidence of fatigue. The amount of recession is a better indicator of the severity of airway compromise than the degree of stridor. Stridor can paradoxically become quieter and less apparent as the obstruction worsens due to the diminishing airflow, and may be a sign of impending respiratory arrest. Pallor and subsequent cyanosis are late events in paediatric patients, and no comfort should be taken from the fact that a child still appears pink. The child may position himself to optimize his own airway as is classically described in epiglottitis where the child prefers to sit upright with his head in a 'sniffing' position. Pectus excavatum may be seen in children with chronic airway obstruction due to negative intrathoracic pressure in their highly compliant rib cage.

The observation chart should be checked for elevated temperatures, tachycardia or tachypnea. Drooling may occur in epiglottitis, severe oropharyngeal inflammation or deep neck space infection. Any cough or change in voice or cry should be noted. The clinician should listen carefully to the audible respiratory noise to differentiate between inspiratory stridor, biphasic stridor, expiratory stridor or wheeze and stertor. This can be useful in determining the likely anatomical site of the pathology, although this is not absolute and is only useful as a guide.

Inspiratory stridor typically occurs due to obstruction at the level of the supraglottis or glottis. Obstruction arising in the bronchi or lower trachea classically produces an expiratory stridor or prolongation of the expiratory phase. Biphasic stridor can occur with obstruction anywhere in the laryngo-tracheobronchial tree but is classically associated with either upper tracheal or subglottic pathology where it is attributed to the fixed luminal diameter of the cricoid. The characteristic sound of stridor, even in a common condition such as laryngo-malacia, is so variable as to be of little diagnostic use in isolation. Laryngo-malacia has been traditionally described as having stridor that is of a musical quality, whilst stridor in vocal cord palsy has a breathy quality, viral laryngo-tracheitis has a barking cough and tracheomalacia has a brassy cough. It is important to recognize that these descriptions are highly subjective and their assessment is not reliably reproducible.

Nasal patency is assessed via fogging of a mirror or metal tongue depressor. Nasal airflow may also be detected via a wisp of cotton wool, or using the bell end of a stethoscope. This is particularly relevant if supra-laryngeal obstruction is suspected. The clinician should also make a conscious assessment of jaw and tongue size. Stridor and recession will vary as the child rests, cries and sleeps. It can be useful to observe the child whilst he or she is feeding, particularly if poor feeding or aspiration has been reported. Auscultation may be used to aid in localizing the site of maximal obstruction, but the transmission of sound through the thorax is variable, often making this technique difficult. Auscultation is useful to detect heart murmurs and wheeze.

The nose, throat, neck and ears should also be examined (Figure 58.13). The oropharynx is examined to assess the size and appearance of tonsils and palate and to check for oropharyngeal swelling or fullness. The neck is also inspected and palpated to identify swelling or masses. The usual caution should be used in examining a child with possible epiglottitis where sudden airway obstruction may be precipitated. In this situation, equipment for immediate intubation must be present if examination is to be attempted. It is also acceptable to make a provisional diagnosis of epiglottitis on the basis of the history and appearance of the child, with formal examination performed in the safety of the operating theatre under endoscopic control.

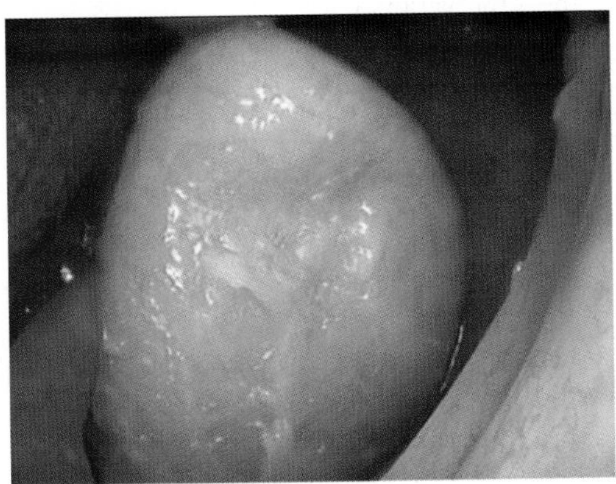

Figure 58.13 Hairy polyp presenting in postnasal space.

NON-ENDOSCOPIC INVESTIGATIONS

Investigations should not be routinely conducted, but judicious use may be helpful. Selection of investigations should be tailored to the clinical presentation on the basis of the history and examination findings and are not necessary in every patient.

O_2 SATURATION MONITORING

O_2 saturation monitoring is noninvasive and readily accessible, although considerable airway obstruction may occur without desaturation, providing the child is not tiring and continues to have the energy to overcome the obstruction. Care should be taken in administering supplemental oxygen as this can maintain O_2 saturations whilst masking raised levels of CO_2. Arterial blood gases are useful in this situation. From a clinical viewpoint, cyanosis occurs very late in paediatric respiratory distress.

RADIOLOGY

Soft tissue lateral neck x-rays demonstrate the airway outline from the nasopharynx to the subglottis. Posterioanterior (PA) chest x-ray shows the lungs' fields and mediastinum. Persistent air trapping may be demonstrated on the side of a bronchial foreign body in inspiratory/expiratory views. A decubitus view may be useful in young children, where normally the dependent lung deflates. A Cincinnati (high-kilovoltage filter) view enhances the tracheal air column whilst de-emphasizing the bony cervical spine to demonstrate the major airways. These x-ray techniques may be useful as screening investigations. Careful consideration of the stability of the child's airway is mandatory, and radiology should not be undertaken if there is any potential for acute airway deterioration. Policy for suspected epiglottitis differs between centres; however, the result of the x-ray may not influence management and may be associated with significant risk to the child. Further imaging should be performed according to the endoscopy findings.

Videofluoroscopy is an excellent way of demonstrating tracheomalacia and can be combined with a contrast swallow to exclude vascular compression, tracheoesophageal fistula or aspiration. It may demonstrate diaphragmatic immobility on the side of a foreign body airway obstruction.

Bronchograms using safe nonionic contrast media are useful for outlining the luminal surface of the lower airway, demonstrating tracheobronchial stenosis and malacia. Opening pressures of the collapsed bronchi and lower trachea can also be measured, to determine the level of airway support needed.

Computed tomography (CT) and magnetic resonance imaging (MRI) continue to lack sensitivity in assessing airway stenoses and cannot replace endoscopic assessment. They are useful in demonstrating vascular anomalies and extrinsic compression of the airway. Virtual endoscopy uses radiological data to create computer simulations that may be viewed as one would conventional endoscopy. Helical CT with multiplanar reconstruction provides 3D images, which are utilized in real time to simulate endoscopy views. It is noninvasive and allows retrograde luminal airway views. Although it demonstrates some fixed airway stenoses, it is not helpful in detecting obstruction during dynamic movement as occurs in tracheomalacia or vocal cord palsy. There is also a lack of detail, with airway pathology such as glottic webs being poorly demonstrated.

OTHER INVESTIGATIONS

Vocal cord ultrasound and laryngeal electromyography (EMG) sometimes have a place in the management of vocal cord immobility.

Airway obstruction that worsens during sleep is usually a feature of pharyngeal obstruction, such as adenotonsillar obstruction or craniofacial anomaly. Laryngo-tracheal pathology at any level, including laryngo-malacia, may, however, occasionally worsen during sleep, thus requiring sleep study investigation.

Paediatric lung function tests are not usually useful in the evaluation of stridor. Stridor is often associated with reflux, and tests for reflux such as double-probe pH studies, contrast studies, milk scan or oesophagoscopy should be considered.

Echocardiography detects congenital heart disease but does not demonstrate all abnormal vasculature. Thus it cannot be used to exclude vascular anomalies.

ENDOSCOPY

Paediatric airway endoscopy requires a full range of specialized paediatric endoscopy equipment and an experienced team. An inadequate evaluation will need to be repeated and referral to an experienced centre should be made as required, to ensure a single comprehensive and definitive evaluation. A systematic approach will provide a diagnosis in most cases.

FLEXIBLE ENDOSCOPY IN THE OFFICE OR WARD

The introduction of ultra-thin endoscopes in a range of diameters and with good optics has allowed even neonates to be endoscoped without the need for a general anaesthetic. This is usually considered a screening procedure, as the view of the larynx may be suboptimal. Rigid endoscopy of the airway is superior in examining the airway for structural abnormalities. Flexible endoscopy is very useful in assessing the dynamic airway for vocal cord movement or features of laryngomalacia. A systematic approach must be adopted, observing first the nasal cavity followed by the postnasal space, oropharynx, supraglottis and glottis during dynamic respiration and phonation. It is difficult to reliably obtain good views of the subglottis. This is purely a diagnostic procedure, with no opportunity for therapeutic procedures, in contrast to a rigid laryngo-tracheobronchoscopy. Flexible endoscopy under sedation in an endoscopy suite is widely practised by paediatricians and pulmonologists and is also used by otolaryngologists as an adjunct to rigid endoscopy. Rigid endoscopy is helpful if the diagnosis remains unclear despite flexible endoscopy, if there is clinical suspicion of a second airway lesion or subglottic/tracheal or bronchial pathology is suspected.

LARYNGO-TRACHEOBRONCHOSCOPY

Laryngo-tracheobronchoscopy is the gold standard in the evaluation of the stridulous child. It enables a thorough assessment to be performed whilst the airway is maintained and allows findings to be visually recorded for future reference. The airway may be formally sized to grade any narrowing that is present. It also may incorporate therapeutic procedures, including foreign body removal or the endoscopic management of airway pathology. It requires an experienced team skilled in airway assessment, including the surgeon, anaesthetist and nursing assistant, who work closely to ensure an optimal and safe examination. The use of a video is essential to facilitate training and allows the anaesthetist and nurse to follow the procedure and status of the airway on the monitor.

It is vital that accurate records are kept in a standardized form within a department. Digital prints provide a valid record of static conditions, whilst video clips record dynamic findings. Digital images and video recordings should be saved and archived. This provides an invaluable source of information for sequential clinical comparisons, teaching and medicolegal purposes.

Anaesthetic considerations

This procedure requires a cooperative approach to airway management, with both the anaesthetic team and surgeon sharing the control of the airway. The use of atropine premedication provides a dry surgical field and improves the efficacy of topical anaesthesia. It is most effective via intramuscular injection. Anaesthesia is often induced using inhalational anaesthesia with sevofluorane or intravenous agents (total intravenous anaesthesia). Topical lignocaine is applied to the airway to minimize airway stimulation during the procedure and help avoid laryngospasm. The lignocaine dose needs to be carefully measured to avoid overdosage and the risk of fits.

Spontaneous respiration allows assessment of dynamic conditions. Ideally, the endoscopist has a view of the airway before intubation. A transnasal endotracheal tube may be positioned with the tip in the hypopharynx to optimize delivery of anaesthetic gases and oxygen without obstructing the view of the airway. Airway control can be regained at any stage via intubation or through the use of a bronchoscope.

ENDOSCOPY TECHNIQUE

The most controlled examination is with the larynx in suspension, but as this tends to splint the larynx, many paediatric endoscopists use the anaesthetic laryngoscope instead. This has the disadvantage of not leaving two hands free for any manipulation.

Preparation and positioning

It is essential to anticipate equipment requirements so all equipment can be checked and prepared prior to commencement. A range of Hopkins rod telescopes should be available that includes all lengths and diameters that may be required, so the endoscopist is fully prepared for all eventualities. Charts that predict age-appropriate sizes of bronchoscopes should be consulted and be readily available in the operating theatre. The appropriate bronchoscope (Figure 58.14) needs to be checked and assembled, and at least one size smaller must be on hand. A 30° telescope may be utilized to enable assessment of the supraglottis without splinting. It may also assist assessment of an anteriorly placed larynx. A small sandbag is placed under the child's shoulders, with supporting lateral sandbags in children with long, thin heads, as is typically seen in ex-premature neonates.

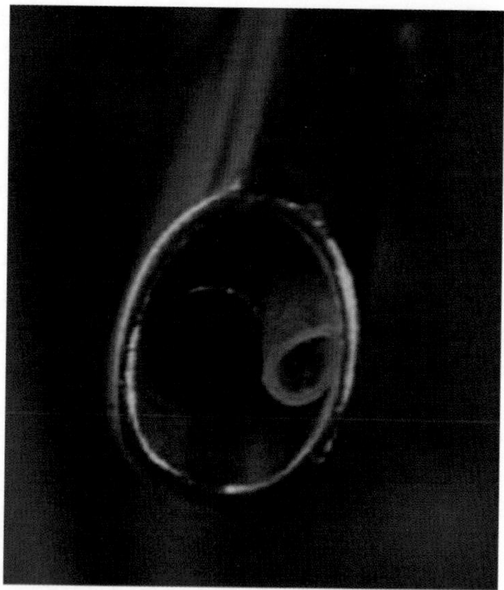

Figure 58.14 Ventilating bronchoscope, telescope and sucker.

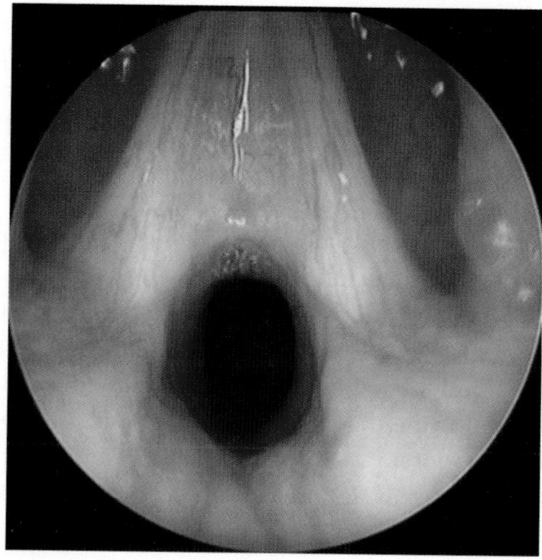

Figure 58.15 Laryngeal web.

Telescope-only technique

A suspension straight-blade laryngoscope is gently inserted whilst assessing the overall appearance of the laryngopharynx, taking care to protect the teeth, lips and oral mucosa whilst keeping the tongue midline to provide a well-centred view. The laryngoscope is placed in the vallecula and the epiglottis is carefully lifted forward. The larynx should be examined ideally without intubation but with an endotracheal (ET) tube in the nasopharynx and the child breathing spontaneously. A probe may be used to independently palpate the arytenoids to assess the mobility of the cricoarytenoid joints and any limitation in joint movement. An absence of independent arytenoid movement on palpation is indicative of interarytenoid scarring. A posterior laryngeal cleft should be excluded by passing the probe between the arytenoids to allow comparison of the inferior limit of the interarytenoid groove with the posterior commissure. The subglottis should also be inspected from above (Figure 58.15). Topical decongestion and vasoconstriction of the airway may be helpful, particularly in the presence of low-grade inflammation or oedema (Figure 58.16). Any airway narrowing should be formally sized. The largest ET that permits a leak at less than 30 cm H_2O pressure provides a measure of the airway diameter. Subglottic stenosis may then be graded using the Cotton-Myer grading system, thus allowing reproducible assessment of the stenosis and aiding in treatment selection.

Bronchoscopy technique

Traditionally, a ventilating bronchoscope has been used to assess the distal airway, which provides a means of actively ventilating the patient during the procedure, if required. A smaller diameter rigid Hopkins rod telescope can be used as an alternative to examine the airway in a spontaneously breathing child, particularly if there is significant

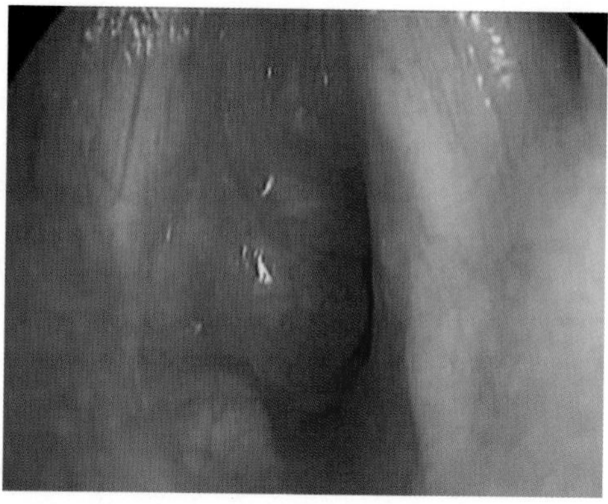

Figure 58.16 Subglottic cyst.

subglottic stenosis. The rigid telescope may reduce local airway trauma and lessen airway splinting, whilst allowing the distal airway to be visualized. An age-appropriate sized bronchoscope is used unless stenosis is suspected.

Evidence of tracheomalacia should be sought in the absence of positive airway pressure to avoid splinting of the airway and using a small bronchoscope withdrawn from the area being assessed. The ratio of cartilage to trachealis is significant in recording the type of malacia. The presence of complete tracheal rings is of importance when considering slide tracheoplasty for the treatment of long segment tracheal stenosis. Extrinsic compression and prominent transmitted pulsation may be evident where there is an underlying vascular anomaly, which can be confirmed with imaging.

DYNAMIC AIRWAY ASSESSMENT

A dynamic assessment of the larynx may be performed as the child lightens and is observed whilst recovering from the anaesthesia. Dynamic views can be achieved by placing a 0° or 30° telescope so it is positioned just posterior to the tip of the epiglottis. This allows a good view of the vocal cords to exclude vocal cord immobility. It is useful if the anaesthetist calls the phase of respiration, thus allowing the endoscopist to check for paradoxical cord movement. The arytenoids and adjacent mucosa can also be visualized to check for evidence of laryngo-malacia. Anterior collapse of the epiglottis may, however, be masked.

An excellent technique for dynamic assessment of vocal cord movement utilizes a laryngeal mask with a fibre-optic bronchoscope passed through to visualize the airway. The flexible endoscope is positioned just proximal to the laryngeal inlet to observe airway dynamics.

COMPLICATIONS

Possible complications include oral injury, subglottic injury, pneumothorax, cardiac complications, loss of control of the airway and bleeding.

POST-OPERATIVE CARE AND PLANNING

Airway obstruction may increase following the procedure due to underlying pathology, oedema, blood, secretions or postintubation croup. Oedema is usually maximal within 4 hours and settles by 24 hours. Humidified oxygen by mask is initially trialed. Nebulized epinephrine (1:1000) may be trialled, but the child must be kept under observation and reviewed within an hour for recurrence due to its limited duration of action. The patient may be given intraoperative dexamethasone if there is a potential for oedema from instrumentation of the airway. Steroids may be continued in the post-operative period depending on the endoscopy findings and underlying airway pathology. The patient must be recovered by nursing staff experienced in the care of paediatric airways and remain as an inpatient for close observation until the airway is adequately stable for discharge.

The operative record should clearly record the endoscopy findings, ideally with a photographic record of the findings. Using the endoscopic assessment, a plan of management can then be decided upon and discussed with the parents on the post-operative ward round.

KEY LEARNING POINTS

- The quality of stridor may be characteristic of a particular pathology but is never diagnostic; the diagnosis can only be confirmed with certainty after endoscopy.
- Improvement in stridor can paradoxically be due to worsening airway obstruction and reduced airflow.
- Laryngo-tracheobronchoscopy is the gold standard in the assessment of the stridulous child. It is now a highly technical procedure and the whole team (surgeon, anaesthetist and nursing assistant) needs to work closely together to perform the examination safely and to optimize the assessment.

- Children with croup who demonstrate increased work of breathing in the clinic or emergency department should be treated with glucocorticoids.
- The risk with low tracheobronchial obstruction is that neither intubation nor tracheostomy will relieve the obstruction, though positive pressure will tend to improve malacia and, to a lesser extent, stenosis.
- A difficult and potentially dangerous situation occurs if a tracheotomy is attempted for tapering long segment tracheal stenosis. Not only is it not possible to insert a normal neonatal size tracheotomy tube, but the tracheotomy itself severely limits the therapeutic options for surgical reconstruction of the stenosis.
- Medical therapy with steroids, anti-reflux treatment, nebulized adrenaline (epinephrine), heliox and antibiotics (in some cases) may avert the need for more invasive measures such as tracheotomy.
- Therapeutic surgical options to manage the stridulous child include tracheotomy, endoscopic and open laryngeal surgery. Treatment is individualized depending on the underlying pathology, associated co-morbidity and social circumstances.

FURTHER READING

Benjamin B. Prolonged intubation injuries of the larynx: Endoscopic diagnosis, classification, and treatment. *Annals of Otology, Rhinolology and Laryngology Suppl.* 1993; 160: 1–15.

Bent J. Pediatric laryngotracheal obstruction: Current perspectives on stridor. *Laryngoscope.* 2006; 116-7: 1059–70.

Gonzalez C, Reilly JS, Bluestone CD. Synchronous airway lesions in infancy. *Annals of Otology, Rhinolology and Laryngology.* 1987; 96-1 Pt 1: 77–80.

Hartnick CJ, Cotton, RT. *Stridor and Airway Obstruction.* In: *Pediatric Otolaryngology.* Vol. 2, 4th ed. Ed. Bluestone CD. Philadelphia: Saunders, 2003.

Rahbar R, Nicollas R, Roger G, Triglia JM, Garabedian EN, McGill TJ, Healy GB. The biology and management of subglottic hemangioma: Past, present, future. *Laryngoscope.* 2004; 114-11: 1880–91.

59

Tracheostomy

ANN-LOUISE MCDERMOTT AND JOE GRAINGER

DEFINITION

Trachesotomy is defined as 'the creation of an opening into the trachea through the neck'.

BACKGROUND

Tracheostomy is not a new procedure. Egyptian tablets dating back to 3600 BC depicting tracheostomy have been discovered,[1] and Asclepiades was recorded as performing a tracheostomy in 100 BC. There are many references of tracheostomy being performed for children with diphtheria in the nineteenth century, and, by 1887, approximately 20,000 tracheostomies had been reported in Western Europe and the United States.[2] The indications for tracheostomy expanded in the early 1950s. Tracheostomy was then advocated for patients with poliomyelitis who required long-term ventilation respiratory care.[3]

INDICATIONS AND CONTRAINDICATIONS

The indications for paediatric tracheostomy are summarized in Table 59.1. In recent years long-term ventilation and congenital abnormalities of the airway have become more prevalent, and infective/inflammatory indications for tracheostomy have decreased partly as a result of better vaccination programmes. Tertiary paediatric centre reviews have demonstrated tracheostomy for prolonged ventilatory support to be the most common indication.[4,5,6] With the advent of improved endoscopic airway procedures and improved anaesthetic skills, upper airway obstruction is less likely to require tracheostomy. However, this depends on the experience of and facilities available to the surgeon,[2–6] as demonstrated by results from different centres.[4,7,8] Conditions for which tracheostomy is now used less frequently include subglottic haemangiomas and laryngeal clefts.[9] Relative contraindications to tracheostomy include

Table 59.1 Indications for paediatric tracheostomy

1. Airway obstruction
   - Congenital anomalies
   - Failed extubation with severe subglottic oedema and mucosal damage
   - External trauma
   - Acute infection
   - Tumours
   - Functional obstruction, e.g. bilateral vocal cord palsy
   - Tracheomalacia or extrinsic compression of the trachea
2. Prolonged respiratory support
3. Airway protection for surgical procedures
4. Clearance of secretions

severe bleeding diatheses and congenital tracheal stenosis.

ANATOMICAL CONSIDERATIONS

The surgeon should be mindful that the neck of a child differs from that of an adult in the following ways:

- The neck is short with limited space between the thyroid cartilage and the sternal notch.
- The domes of the pleura are very easily pulled into the neck with minimal neck extension.
- The trachea is very soft and pliable and can be easily displaced laterally with retraction.
- The cricoid is very soft and may be difficult to distinguish.

CHOICE OF TRACHEOSTOMY TUBE

The correct choice of tracheostomy tube is extremely important.[10] Ideally, the tracheostomy tube should be small enough to allow voice but large enough for adequate ventilation. Use of a tube with too large a diameter will cause damage to the tracheal mucosa with granulations and bleeding. The use of a low-pressure cuffed tracheostomy tube should be avoided if possible but may be required with mechanical ventilation. A cuffed tube may cause mucosal injury and later long-term tracheal stenosis if overinflated for prolonged periods of time. Most paediatric tracheostomy tubes are cuffless.

Tracheostomy tube size can be determined by various methods:
Calculation based on patient age:[11]

- Inner diameter (mm) = (age in years/3) + 3.5
- Outer diameter (mm) = (age in years/3) + 5.5

Calculation based on patient age and weight:[12]

- Premature neonates who weigh less than 1000 g: 2.5 mm
- Premature neonates who weigh 1000–2500 g: 3.0 mm
- Neonates or infants aged 1–6 months: 3.0–3.5 mm
- Infants aged 6 months to 1 year: 3.5–4.0 mm
- Child aged 1–2 years: 4.5–5.0 mm
- Children older than 2 years: (age in yrs + 16)/4

As the child grows, the tracheostomy tube needs to be adjusted accordingly.

SURGICAL PROCEDURE

The majority of paediatric tracheostomies are performed under general anaesthesia as an elective or semi-elective procedure. Ideally, the child will have an endotracheal tube or a ventilating bronchoscope in place during the procedure, which will provide ventilation during surgery.

The recommended surgical steps for a paediatric tracheostomy are:

- Head extension facilitated by a chin strap and a small shoulder roll/suction head ring (Figure 59.1).
- Vertical incision at midpoint between thyroid cartilage and sternal notch.

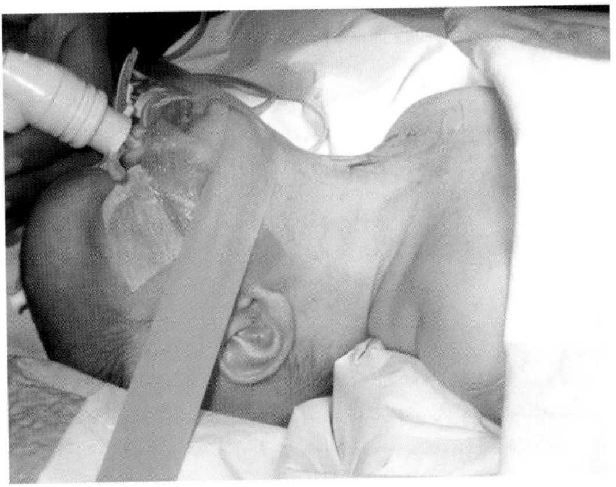

Figure 59.1 Use of a chin strap to provide good neck exposure.

- Removal of subcutaneous fat from midline of the neck to improve visibility and facilitate healing of the stoma.
- Division and retraction of strap muscles in the midline.
- Division of thyroid isthmus using bipolar diathermy.
- Lateral 'stay sutures' using non-resorbable sutures, typically polypropylene. These 'stay sutures' can be used to apply traction and expose the trachea during the surgery and they can also be lifesaving should accidental decannulation occur before the tracheostomy stoma is fully established.
- Vertical tracheal incision in midline through tracheal rings 2–4.
- Stomal maturation sutures: tracheal edge to skin edges, typically using resorbable sutures.
- Tracheostomy tube secured with twill ties. Velcro straps are not used until the stoma is mature and fully established.
- The 'stay sutures' are labeled 'left' and 'right' and should be taped on the corresponding side of the chest. These should not be removed until the stoma is established.
- A post-operative chest radiograph to evaluate the position of the tube and ensure there is no pneumothorax.
- Post-operative management in a location able to provide adequate post-operative care.

Percutaneous tracheostomy is not regularly performed in children, but no increase in morbidity has been reported from those centres that do perform this technique.[13,14]

POST-OPERATIVE TRACHEOSTOMY CARE

Many centres provide the initial post-operative care of children with a tracheostomy tube in the intensive care unit. A spare tracheostomy tube the same size and one smaller should be available by the patient's bedside. Regular suction should be performed in the first 24 hours and thereafter, as required, and humidification should be maintained. Tapes should be changed daily, and the tracheostomy tube should be changed one week following the surgery. At this time, the stoma should be fully established.

COMPLICATIONS

EARLY

1. **Pneumomediastinum and pneumothorax** are potential risks as the domes of the pleura can easily extend into the neck, especially with an over-extended position. Pneumothorax has been reported following high-pressure ventilation in neonates.[15,16] A post-operative chest radiograph can be used to exclude these complications; however, there is some debate as to whether this should be performed routinely.[16]
2. **Haemorrhage.** Typically, this arises from inadequate division and cautery to the thyroid isthmus. Skin edges may also cause troublesome bleeding.
3. **Surgical emphysema.**
4. **Accidental decannulation.** This is a life-threatening complication. Tracheostomy tapes must be securely fastened. Stay suture placement and stomal maturation sutures facilitate replacement of the tracheostomy tube. Creation of a false passage is more likely if a tracheostomy tube has to be replaced in an emergency situation.

INTERMEDIATE

Infection at the tracheostome can cause difficulty with tube changing. Granulation tissue and fibrosis may develop.[17]

LATE

1. **Stomal scarring and granulations.** The granulations may occur within the trachea and are commonly seen at the position of the distal end of the tracheostomy tube.[18]
2. **Inability to decannulate.** Formal laryngotracheobronchoscopy is recommended prior to any attempt to decannulate to ensure there are no adverse anatomical factors[18] (Table 59.2).
3. **Tracheocutaneous fistula** occurs in 19–42 per cent of children.[19]
4. **Delayed speech and language skills.** The age at which the child has the tracheostomy and the duration of tracheostomy are influencing factors.[20]
5. **Death.** There remains a mortality rate of 1–2 per cent in children with a tracheostomy.[21–24]

DISCHARGE PLANNING

The child's family and any other carers must undergo a structured training programme in both the management of the tracheostomy as well as basic life support. Suction equipment and a supply of tracheostomy tubes should be provided for use at home.

Table 59.2 Causative factors for failure of decannulation

1. Tracheal granulations
2. Suprastomal collapse
3. Subglottic stenosis secondary to a high placement of tracheostomy tube through the cricoid ring
4. Tracheal stenosis
5. Psychological dependence on the tracheostomy tube
6. Tracheomalacia

DECANNULATION

Successful decannulation following tracheostomy depends first on resolution of the primary disorder and the absence of any secondary complications of the tracheostomy[18] (Table 59.2).

KEY LEARNING POINTS

- The most common indication is prolonged ventilatory support.
- Remember the anatomical differences in the paediatric neck.
- The correct size tracheostomy tube must be carefully selected.
- The key differences in children are use of a vertical tracheal incision and stomal maturation sutures.
- Paediatric tracheostomy is associated with a mortality rate of 1 to 2 per cent.

REFERENCES

1. Pahor AL. Ear, nose and throat in Ancient Egypt. *Journal of Laryngology and Otology.* 1992; 106: 773–79.
2. Rogers JH. *Tracheostomy and Decannulation.* In: *Scott-Brown's Otolaryngology.* Eds. Adams DA, Cinnamond MJ. Oxford: Butterworth-Heinemann, 1997: 6/26/1–6/26/16.
3. Graamans K, Pirsig W, Biefel K. The shift in the indications for the tracheotomy between 1940 and 1955: An historical review. *Journal of Laryngology and Otology.* 1999; 113: 624–27.
4. Hadfield PJ, Lloyd-Faulconbridge RV, Almeyda J, Albert DM, Bailey CM. The changing indications for paediatric tracheostomy. *International Journal of Pediatric Otorhinolaryngology.* Jan 2003; 67(1): 7–10.
5. Primuharsa Putra SH, Wong CY, Hazim MY, Megat Shiraz MA, Goh BS. Paediatric tracheostomy in Hospital University

Kebangsaan Malaysia – A changing trend. *Medical Journal of Malaysia*. Jun 2006; 61(2): 209–13.

6. Pérez-Ruiz E, Caro P, Pérez-Frías J, Cols M, Barrio I, Torrent A, et al. Paediatric patients with a tracheostomy: A multicentre epidemiological study. *European Respiratory Journal*. 2012; 40(6): 1502–07.
7. Midwinter KI, Carrie S, Bull PD. Paediatric tracheostomy: Sheffield Experience 1979–1999. *Journal of Laryngology and Otology*. 2002; 116; 7: 532–35.
8. Trachsel D, Hammer J. Indications for tracheostomy in children. *Paediatric Respiratory Review*. Sep 2006; 7(3): 162–8.
9. Perez-Ruiz E, Caro P, Perez-Frias J, Cois M, Torrent A, et al. Paediatric patients with a tracheostomy: A multicentre epidemiological study. *European Respiratory Journal*. 2012; 40: 1502–07.
10. Tweedie DJ, Skilbeck CJ, Cochrane LA, Cooke J, Wyatt ME. Choosing a paediatric tracheostomy tube: An update on current practice. *Journal of Laryngology and Otology*. 2008; 122: 161–69.
11. Behl S, Watt JW. Prediction of tracheostomy tube size for paediatric long-term ventilation: An audit of children with spinal cord injury. *British Journal of Anaesthesia*. Jan 2005; 94(1): 88–91.
12. Wetmore RF. *Tracheotomy*. In: *Pediatric Otolaryngology*. Eds. Bluestone CD, Stool SE, Alper CM, Arjmand EM, Casselbrant ML, Dohar JE, Yellow RF. Philadelphia: Saunders, 2003: 1583–98.
13. Rao BK, Pande R, Sharma SC, Ray S, Lakshmi B, Singh VK, et al. Percutaneous tracheostomy. *Annals of Cardiac Anaesthesia*. Jan 2003; 6(1): 19–26.
14. Toursarkissian B, Fowler CL, Zweng TN, Kearney PA. Percutaneous dilational tracheostomy in children and teenagers. *Journal of Pediatric Surgery*. Nov 1994; 29(11): 1421–24.
15. Albert D, Leighton S. *Managing the Stridulous Child*. In: *Cummings Otolaryngology Head and Neck Surgery*. Ed. Richardson MA. Philadelphia: Elsevier Mosby, 2005: 4241–65.
16. Genther DJ, Thorne MC. Utility of routine postoperative chest radiography in pediatric tracheostomy. *International Journal Pediatric Otorhinolaryngology*. Dec 2010; 74(12): 1397–400.
17. Prescott CA. Peristomal complications of paediatric tracheostomy. *International Journal of Pediatric Otorhinolaryngology*. Mar 1992; 23(2): 141–49.
18. Leung R, Berkowitz RG. Decannulation and outcome following pediatric tracheostomy. *Annals of Otology, Rhinology and Laryngology*. Oct 2005; 114(10): 743–48.
19. Tasca RA, Clarke RW. Tracheocutaneous fistula following paediatric tracheostomy. A 14-year experience at Alder Hey Children's Hospital. *International Journal of Pediatric Otorhinolaryngology*. 2010; 74: 711–12.
20. Jiang D, Morrison GA. The influence of long-term tracheostomy on speech and language development in children. *International Journal of Pediatric Otorhinolaryngology*. Dec 2003; 67 Suppl 1: S217–20.
21. Messineo A, Giusti F, Narne S, Mognato G, Antoniello L, Guglielmi M. The safety of home tracheostomy care for children. *Journal of Pediatric Surgery*. Aug 1995; 30(8): 1246–48.
22. Caussade S, Paz F, Ramírez M, Navarro H, Bertrand P, Zúñiga S, et al. Clinical experience in home care of children with tracheostomy. *Revista Médica de Chile*. Nov 2000; 128(11): 1221–26.
23. Reiter K, Pernath N, Pagel P, Hiedi S, Hoffmann F, Schoen C, et al. Risk factors for morbidity and mortality in pediatric home mechanical ventilation. *Clinical Pediatrics* (Phila). Mar 2011; 50(3): 237–43.
24. Oberwaldner B, Eber E. Tracheostomy care in the home. *Paediatric Respiratory Review*. Sep 2006; 7(3): 185–90.

60

Subglottic stenosis

PETER BULL AND NEIL BATEMAN

INTRODUCTION

Subglottic stenosis (SGS), whether congenital or acquired, presents a significant challenge to the paediatric otolaryngologist. Despite efforts on the part of neonatologists to reduce the incidence of acquired paediatric SGS in the preterm neonatal population, this condition continues to affect a small but significant proportion of babies intubated at birth.

SGS is strictly defined as stenosis within the laryngeal subglottis, that is, below the vocal folds and above the trachea. This narrow definition overlooks the fact that most cases of SGS will also involve a degree of narrowing at the glottic and tracheal level, and might more accurately be termed *laryngo-tracheal stensosis*. All aspects must be recognized and corrected to achieve a satisfactory outcome for the patient.

While in previous years the main challenges have been to reconstruct the airway and allow decannulation of the tracheostomy, more recently interest has focused on the avoidance of tracheostomy where possible and the adoption of endoscopic procedures as an alternative to open surgery. Paediatric otolaryngologists are also focusing on laryngeal function (airway and voice) following interventions, rather than exclusively regarding decannulation as the only objective measure of success when examining treatment outcomes for these children.

APPLIED ANATOMY

The lamina and arch of the cricoid cartilage form the subglottis, the narrowest portion of the paediatric airway and the only complete ring of cartilage within the airway. When a neonate undergoes endotracheal intubation, the tube selected should be of a size that fits the subglottis with a small air leak. As the subglottic airway is the narrowest part of the larynx and trachea, no cuff is required. This is in contrast to adults and older children, where the narrowest part of the airway is the glottis and a cuff is required to provide an airtight seal below this.

When a child is intubated for any length of time, or with an inappropriately sized tube, with excessive tube movement or in the presence of acute airway inflammation, there is a potential for damage to the subglottis.

BASIC PHYSICAL PRINCIPLES OF AIRFLOW

Airflow through the larynx and trachea is governed by certain fundamental laws of physics. Poiseuille's law states that flow through a tube is proportional to the fourth power of the radius of the tube (as well as to the length of the tube, the pressure difference across the length, and the viscosity of the fluid or gas). Relatively small changes in the diameter of the airway result in correspondingly large changes in airflow. If the normal neonatal subglottic diameter is 4 mm, 1 mm of oedema in this area causes a reduction in airflow by a factor of 16.

Resistance to airflow is greater for turbulent than for laminar airflow. Whether airflow is laminar or turbulent is dependent on the physical dimensions of the airway and the gas flowing through it. As the airway becomes narrower, the switch from laminar to turbulent flow may cause a significant worsening in clinical airway obstruction. This switch can occur relatively suddenly and account for rapid clinical deterioration. The point at which the switch from laminar to turbulent flow occurs is determined by the Reynolds number, a ratio of inertial forces to viscous forces. Turbulent flow is dominated by inertial forces that slow the flow against the vessel wall.

Bernoulli's principle states that when a fluid, such as air, flows through a tube, such as the larynx or trachea, then as flow increases so the pressure within the lumen decreases. This has an implication in the relatively soft paediatric airway, in that it may cause some part to collapse if there is malacia of the structure of the airway or an increase in the work of breathing.

The use of heliox (79 per cent helium, 21 per cent oxygen) replaces nitrogen with helium, changes the flow properties of the gas within the airway and correspondingly reduces the work of breathing. The density of helium is less than that of nitrogen. The reduction in the viscosity and resistance to flow makes laminar flow more likely when compared to breathing air, with a corresponding reduction in resistance. Heliox has been used for many years for relief of respiratory distress and is an important tool for the paediatric airway surgeon in the acute situation.

CAUSATION OF SUBGLOTTIC STENOSIS

CONGENITAL

A small number of instances of SGS are congenital. The cricoid ring is often elliptical in such cases and narrowed side to side. Congenital SGS is not usually as severe as the acquired form, though severe degrees of atresia may occur. The diagnostic difficulty comes once a baby has been intubated. It then becomes all but impossible to know whether the stenosis was congenital or has been caused by the intubation. Only if diagnostic laryngoscopy was performed prior to intubation can a confident diagnosis of congenital SGS be made.

Some conditions have a known association with congenital stenosis, such as Down's syndrome. Other conditions, such as laryngo-malacia, are often associated with minor degrees of congenital SGS. Congenital stenosis usually occurs sporadically, but there are reports of siblings with congenital stenosis.

ACQUIRED

The majority of cases of SGS encountered in clinical practice are acquired as the result of endotracheal intubation, usually for the purpose of positive pressure ventilation. In the late 1970s and early 1980s, prior to the clinical introduction of surfactant, small birthweight babies could need prolonged ventilation because of lung immaturity and a lack of naturally occurring surfactant. The introduction of surfactant treatment made ventilation much easier because of reduced alveolar surface tension, and the need for prolonged ventilation was lessened. SGS is not, however, restricted to premature babies and can be a complication of prolonged intubation in older children, usually for ventilation purposes following trauma or surgery.

Acquired stenosis is rare and has become less common in the last 20 years.[1] It is interesting to note that while many neonates are intubated for relatively long periods of time, the development of stenosis is now rare among this group of patients. Incidences of less than 2 per cent of SGS requiring intervention have been reported in children following intubation for more than 48 hours.[2]

It is important to recognize that the pathological processes leading to SGS may also affect the glottis and cause glottic webs and crico-arytenoid joint fixation, as well as other pathologies in this area. For this reason the term *laryngo-tracheal stenosis* is probably more appropriate for this condition.

CLINICAL PRESENTATION

There are several well-recognized clinical scenarios by which SGS may present.

FAILURE TO TOLERATE EXTUBATION IN THE INTUBATED INFANT

Failure to tolerate extubation may indicate an acquired or 'acquired-on-congenital' SGS. It is important to elicit a clear history of airway obstruction and, as far as possible, to eliminate other pathologies, such as pulmonary disease, that can cause failure to tolerate extubation. Often in this situation the inflammatory process in the larynx is evolving, and an established scar has not been produced. This gives the opportunity for attempts to modify this process and prevent progression to an established, fibrotic stenosis.

CHILD WITH AN EXISTING TRACHEOSTOMY

A child may present to the paediatric otolaryngologist with a tracheostomy already performed, often undertaken as a result of a failure to tolerate extubation. Commonly, under these circumstances the stenosis is firm and established.

STRIDULOUS CHILD

Older children with previously undiagnosed SGS may present with stridor. This may occur following previous intubation or in those with congenital stenosis. There may be severe stridor with respiratory distress and failure to thrive or stridor only on exertion. The stridor may be episodic and related to periods of respiratory tract infection; mild SGS is one of the causes of recurrent croup.

The possibility of SGS should be considered in any child presenting with progressive stridor, even without a history of intubation, since congenital SGS may not be immediately evident at birth.

ASSESSMENT AND STAGING

Where there is a clinical suspicion of SGS, the definitive investigation is endoscopy of the complete airway – laryngoscopy, tracheoscopy and bronchoscopy – performed under general anaesthesia. The subglottis can be visualized, probed, measured and photographed.

The limitations of awake flexible fibre-optic laryngoscopy (often referred to erroneously as nasendoscopy) are the relatively poor image from fibre bundles and the difficulty of seeing past the vocal cords with any element of a leisurely and detailed view. The image quality is now much improved with the introduction of distal chip endoscopes, but the drawback of not seeing past the cords persists.

Flexible fibre-optic laryngoscopy is a highly useful tool in the assessment of the paediatric airway, can be carried out in an outpatient setting and gives good views of the supraglottis and vocal cords (allowing vocal cord movements to be assessed, for instance). Its use in assessing SGS is limited.

Imaging, in the form of plain x-rays, computed tomography (CT) or magnetic resonance imaging (MRI) scanning, may be useful in assessing lower respiratory disease but has little role to play in the assessment of upper tracheal and laryngeal stenosis and is not in general use.

TECHNIQUE OF AIRWAY ENDOSCOPY

Safe and controlled airway endoscopy requires close cooperation between an appropriately trained and experienced paediatric otolaryngologist and anaesthetist. Ideally, the child should be breathing spontaneously to allow a dynamic visualization of the upper airway. Achieving this state of anaesthesia is greatly facilitated by the use of topical local anaesthetic spray on the larynx and vocal cords. Anaesthesia may be maintained either by the use of volatile agents or by total intravenous anaesthesia delivered by an infusion pump. Oxygenation may be accomplished by the use of a nasopharyngeal airway or through the laryngoscope. Meanwhile the larynx, trachea and main bronchi may be examined by the use of a telescope. This approach also allows endoscopic procedures to be performed on the larynx and trachea.

It is usual to start with detailed examination of the larynx using a Storz telescope. This can be of a relatively large size, say 4 mm, even in a small baby. It can be introduced either directly or using an anaesthetic-type laryngoscope, or can be used after the introduction of a rigid Benjamin-Lindholm laryngoscope held in suspension. In setting up the suspension, it is important not to splint the larynx and thereby impede the movement of the cords. With the suspension maintained, a telescope of a suitable size is passed through the cords to examine the subglottis, trachea and main bronchi. Even if the initial examination confirms the presence of SGS, the examination is not complete until the rest of the airway has been assessed.

The recording of both still and video images is now easy with the introduction of digital recording equipment, and a record of the findings, including hard copy images, should be made and stored.

ASSESSMENT OF THE STENOSIS

SGS may be classified on the basis of the degree of stenosis (Figures 60.1 to 60.4). It may also be described as either evolving (or soft) or established. The Myer-Cotton staging system is universally accepted (Table 60.1).

The staging can be made either by direct visualization to estimate the degree of stenosis, or by sizing the subglottis with an endotracheal tube. With this technique, the size of the largest tube that gives an air leak when a ventilation pressure of 25 cm H_2O is applied gives the dimension of the subglottis. This is the preferred method when

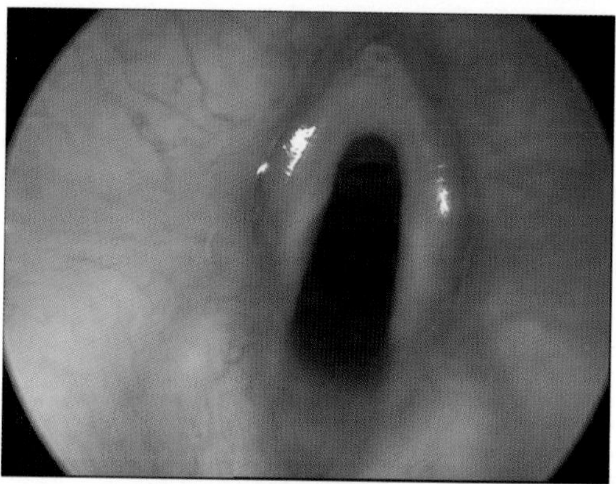

Figure 60.1 Grade 1 subglottic stenosis.

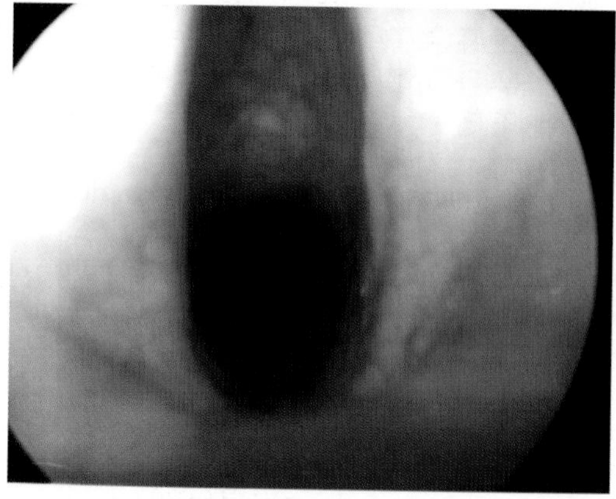

Figure 60.2 Congenital grade 2 subglottic stenosis.

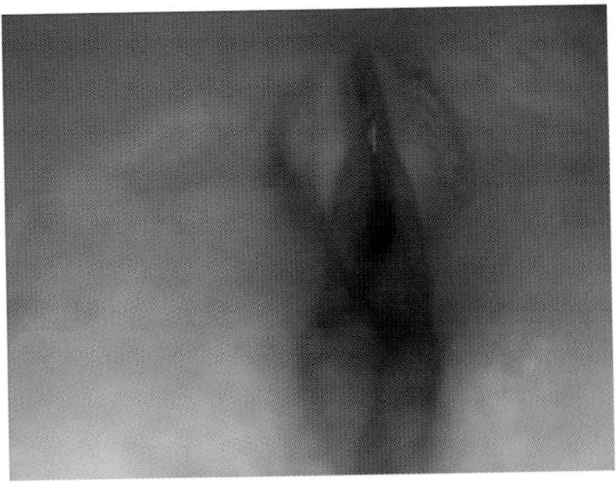

Figure 60.3 Grade 3 subglottic stenosis with active inflammation, which settled after fundoplication.

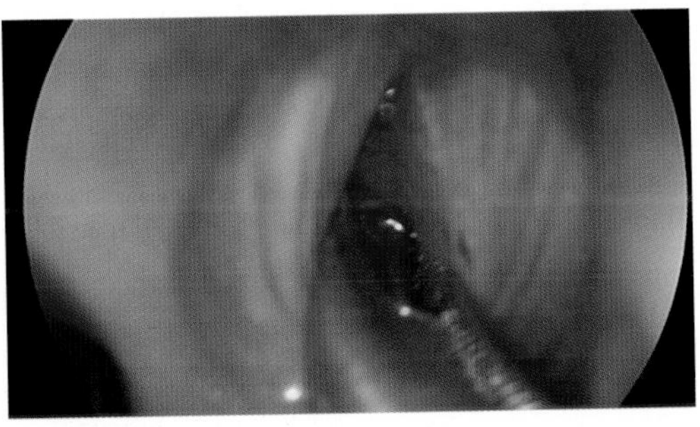

Figure 60.4 Grade 4 congenital subglottic stenosis.

assessing the degree of anything but the most severe stenoses. The Myer-Cotton system relies on the reduction in cross-sectional area. As this is a function of the square of the diameter, it is very easy to underestimate the degree of reduction in the area when simply visualizing the subglottis.

Table 60.1 The Myer-Cotton grading system for subglottic stenosis

Grade	Reduction in proportion of cross-section area of subglottis
1	0–50 per cent
2	51–70 per cent
3	71–99 per cent
4	No lumen

TREATMENT OPTIONS

In recent years there has been a move towards tracheostomy avoidance and endoscopic techniques of airway management where possible.

OBSERVATION

Mild degrees of SGS (Grade 1, sometimes Grade 2) causing little in the way of symptoms can be safely observed and may not need surgical intervention. Any deterioration will require more active intervention. Such children may be more susceptible to attacks of croup with upper respiratory infections and should have easy access to appropriate inpatient facilities.

BALLOON DILATATION

Radial dilatation of the subglottis can be achieved using a balloon. Angioplasty balloons provide a radially disposed force, which is less traumatic to the mucosa than the shearing force of a tube or bougie and is more easily controlled. In the child this can be carried out with the patient apnoeic and the airway completely occluded for 1 to 2 minutes. The use of a balloon when completely occluding the airways requires close cooperation with the anaesthetist.

Balloon dilatation can be supplemented by radial incisions in the soft tissue made with a laryngeal knife.

Even in the case of a child with a tracheostomy, similar durations of dilatation are used to avoid damaging pressure necrosis to the area.

SURGERY, ENDOSCOPIC AND OPEN

Anterior cricoid split

This is a technique to be considered in the evolving stenosis, usually where there is failure to tolerate extubation in the preterm infant. Often a period of laryngeal rest will have been undertaken prior to this, and a cricoid split is undertaken if this is unsuccessful. Cotton et al.[3] have specified criteria for patients suitable for this procedure (Table 60.2).

Table 60.2 Criteria for anterior cricoid split in a neonate

- Failure of extubation on two occasions due to subglottic pathology
- Weight greater than 1500 g
- No ventilator support for 10 days prior to procedure
- Supplementary oxygen requirement less than 30 per cent
- No congestive heart failure for 1 month prior to procedure
- No acute respiratory infection
- No antihypertensive medication for 10 days prior to procedure

Following an endoscopy to assess the stenosis, the patient is intubated and positioned as for tracheostomy. A horizontal incision is made at the level of the cricoid cartilage, and the cricoid and thyroid cartilages exposed as well us the upper tracheal rings. The cricoid is completely divided in the midline as is the first tracheal ring and the lower portion of the thyroid cartilage (although not extending beyond the anterior commissure). Many surgeons make it their practice to graft the cricoidotomy with autologous cartilage from either thyroid ala[4] or the auricle.

The patient is re-intubated with an age-appropriate tube and a trial of extubation performed after 5–10 days, during which treatment with antibiotics, anti-reflux agents and steroids can be used.[5]

Endoscopic cricoidotomy

The cricoid split may be accomplished endoscopically (Figure 60.5).[6] This is carried out using a sickle knife to divide the cricoid arch in the midline and can often be combined with a balloon dilatation of the subglottis. The patient is then intubated in a similar fashion as for the open procedure and extubation attempted after 5–10 days. It has been the authors' experience that this procedure has been successful only when the Cotton criteria for open cricoid split have been satisfied and the cricoid arch has been completely divided (i.e. when the same objectives are achieved endoscopically as through an open approach). Success rates of more

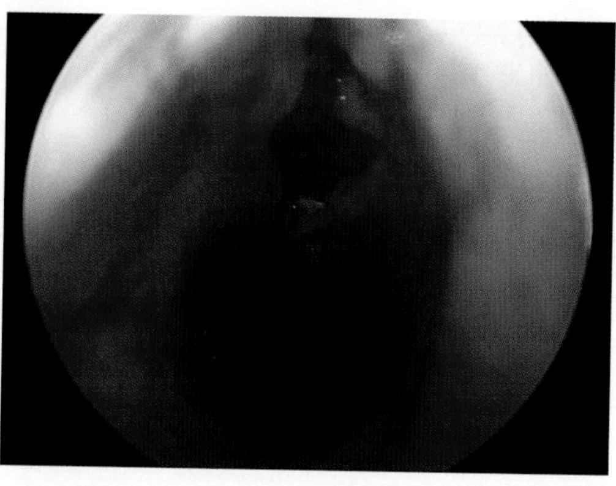

Figure 60.5 Endoscopic cricoid split.

than 80 per cent have been reported when combined with post-operative intubation and serial endoscopies with balloon dilatation.[6]

Endoscopic placement of cartilage grafts

The endoscopic placement of posterior grafts has been described[7] and is becoming more widespread. Patients with posterior glottic stenosis are particularly suited to this approach, which involves endoscopic division of the cricoid lamina (either with sharp instrumentation or with the laser) and placement of a graft harvested from the rib. The area is then stented, with a period of endotracheal intubation if necessary. This is a technique particularly suited to posterior glottic stenosis but probably has limited application for the majority of patients with SGS.

Other endoscopic treatments

In the acute stage the removal of granulations or subglottic retention cysts may be helpful. This may be accomplished by the use of microlaryngoscopy instruments.

It is acknowledged that the stenotic process involving the subglottis may extend to the glottis, and thus there is sometimes a need to deal with glottic stenosis or crico-arytenoid joint fixation in addition to the SGS. The airway surgeon must therefore be familiar with endoscopic treatments to manage these problems, including laser arytenoidectomy, cordotomy and suture lateralization.

Laryngo-tracheal reconstruction

Established SGS causing symptoms will require open corrective surgery. There are several different techniques, and the choice will be determined by the patient's clinical condition and the degree and site of the stenosis. The aim of surgery is to expand the laryngeal framework to allow decannulation of the tracheostomy.

Laryngo-tracheoplasty uses autologous cartilage grafts, usually from the rib. The larynx is opened vertically in the midline from the lower border of the thyroid cartilage to the upper trachea, and a boat-shaped graft is placed to widen the subglottis. If there is also posterior stenosis, a posterior graft will be placed first, after dividing completely the posterior cricoid lamina and distracting its edges to provide posterior enlargement. Surgical closure of the tracheostomy may be undertaken at the same time – the single-stage laryngo-tracheal reconstruction (LTR) (Figure 60.6). The frequent complication from tracheostomy of supra-stomal indentation can be corrected at the same time using cartilage graft reinforcement. Otherwise, the larynx is splinted with some form of stent, which is removed a week or 10 days later, and the tracheostomy retained until the subglottis has healed and the airway is confirmed to be adequate (two-stage LTR).

If there is no pre-existing tracheostomy, the operation can be performed as a single-stage procedure as described earlier but using a period of intubation as a stent.

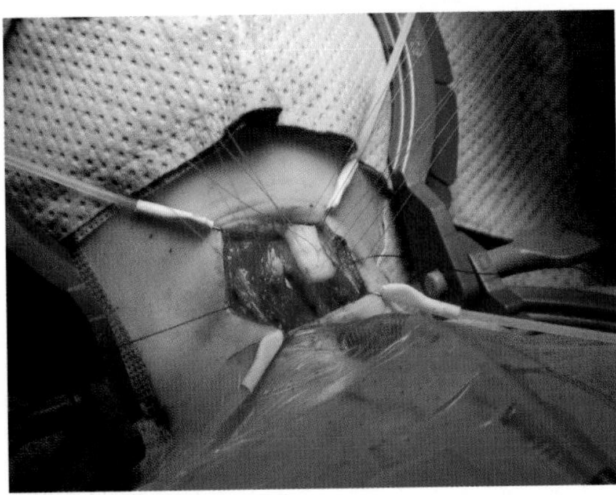

Figure 60.6 Placement of anterior graft at laryngo-tracheal reconstruction.

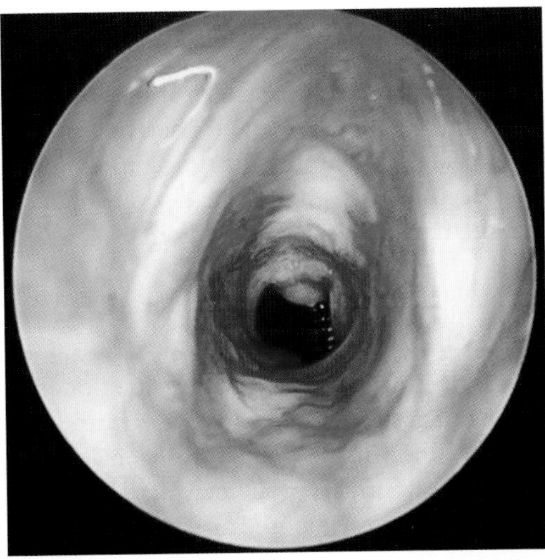

Figure 60.7 Laryngo-tracheal reconstruction – post-operative view immediately following removal of the stent.

If there is a tracheostomy, the LTR can be done as a staged procedure with a period of luminal stenting for two to three weeks (see Figure 60.4; Figure 60.7).

The operation is traditionally performed as a staged procedure with a period of stenting, but the single-stage approach has become the preferred method of treatment where possible.

Laryngo-tracheal reconstruction is suitable for surgical treatment of Grade 2–3 SGS. Most patients with Grade 2 stenosis would be suitable for a single-stage procedure, usually with an anterior graft only. Patients with Grade 3 stenosis often require anterior and posterior grafting, which may be carried out as a single-stage or staged procedure.

Most published series report overall success rates for both staged and single-stage procedures in between 83 and 96 per cent.[8,9,10]

Cricotracheal resection

Cricotracheal resection was described by Philippe Monnier.[11] The anterior arch of the cricoid is excised, leaving the posterior lamina, which is burred down. The trachea and the larynx are then joined in an end-to-end anastomosis. This is a technique best employed for Grade 3 and 4 stenoses where there is sufficient clearance below the vocal cords to allow resection. There is some evidence to suggest that it is the procedure of choice in Grade 4 stenosis, giving a higher rate of decannulation than LTR.[12]

ADJUNCTIVE TREATMENTS

Steroids may be useful in the acute situation in the evolving stenosis, especially to cover an attempt to extubate either in the premature neonate or following airway surgery. They may also have a role where there is superimposed airway inflammation in an existing stenosis.

Mitomycin C is used following surgical interventions in the airway, either open or endoscopic, to prevent re-scarring and stenosis. It is used by topical application in a dose of 400 mcg/mL. Although it is still used by paediatric airway surgeons, there is limited high-quality evidence to support its use.

There is a general acceptance of the role of reflux in SGS and its potential to complicate reconstructive surgery. There is a paucity of well-controlled studies in SGS, largely due the relative scarcity of the condition. There are reports, however, implicating reflux disease in surgical failures. In the authors' practice, all children undergoing reconstructive surgery are treated with a proton pump inhibitor and an alginate empirically. Where there is endoscopic evidence of active airway inflammation despite the use of this treatment regimen, a full diagnostic workup is undertaken after referral to a paediatric gastroenterologist.

FOLLOW-UP

Following successful treatment of SGS, with or without surgery and with or without prior tracheostomy, children should be followed carefully for some years. A number will have periodic croup associated with the effects of acute infection on a marginal airway. Others may continue to have voice and feeding problems, and some will require further laryngeal intervention because of worsening airway limitation as they grow.

FUTURE DEVELOPMENTS

While recent advances in tissue engineering have provided solutions to more extensive tracheal problems, interest in the management of laryngotracheal stenosis in the future will probably focus on the biology of scarring in these patients, to determine if this can be modified in any way. While in the past, decannulation has been seen as the primary outcome measure in these patients, paediatric otolaryngologists in the coming years are likely to focus their efforts on achieving decannulation while preserving good phonation and limited long-term airway morbidity.

KEY LEARNING POINTS

- Acquired sub-glottic stenosis usually results from endotracheal intubation.
- Congenital SGS may be associated with other congenital anomalies.
- Where there is a suspicion of SGS, endoscopic examination of the *whole* airway is required.
- Gastro-oesophageal reflux must be considered and controlled.
- Current management of upper airway obstruction is to try to avoid tracheostomy and to correct the airway narrowing.
- Some reconstructive surgery of the upper airway can now be performed endoscopically.
- Outcome measures include both airway function and voice.

REFERENCES

1. Walner DL, Loewen MS, Kimura RE. Neonatal subglottic stenosis – Incidence and trends. *Laryngoscope*. 2001; 111(1): 48–51.

2. Choi SS, Zalzal GH. Changing trends in neonatal subglottic stenosis. *Otolaryngology – Head and Neck Surgery*. 2000; 122(1): 61–63.
3. Cotton RT, Myers CM, Bratcher GO, et al. Anterior cricoid split 1977–1987: Evolution of a technique. *Archives of Otolaryngology – Head and Neck Surgery*. 1998; 114(11): 1300–02.
4. Forte V, Chang MB, Papsin BC. Thyroid ala cartilage reconstruction in neonatal subglottic stenosis as a replacement for the anterior cricoid split. *International Journal of Pediatric Otorhinolaryngology*. 2001; 59(3): 181–86.
5. Eze NN, Wyatt ME, Hartley BEJ. The role of the anterior cricoid split in facilitating extubation in infants. *International Journal of Pediatric Otorhinolaryngology*. 2005; 69(6): 843–46.
6. Mirabile L, Serio PP, Baggi RR, Couloigner VV. Endoscopic anterior cricoid split and balloon dilation in pediatric subglottic stenosis. *International Journal of Pediatric Otorhinolaryngology*. 2010; 74(12): 1409–14.
7. Inglis AF Jr., Perkins JA, Manning SC, Mouzakes J. Endoscopic posterior cricoid split and rib grafting in 10 children. *Laryngoscope*. 2003; 113(11): 2004–09.
8. Gustafson LM, Hartley BE, Liu JH, Link DT, Chadwell J, Koebbe C, Myer C M 3rd, Cotton RT. Single-stage laryngotracheal reconstruction in children: A review of 200 cases. *Otolaryngology – Head and Neck Surgery*. 2000; 123(4): 430–34.
9. Younis RT, Lazar RH, Bustillo A. Revision single-stage laryngotracheal reconstruction in children. *Annals of Otology, Rhinology and Laryngology*. 2004; 113(5): 367–72.
10. Agrawal N, Black M, Morrison G. Ten-year review of laryngotracheal reconstruction for paediatric airway stenosis. *International Journal of Pediatric Otorhinolaryngology*. 2007; 71(5): 699–703.
11. Monnier P, Savary M, Chapuis G. Partial cricoid resection with primary tracheal anastomosis for subglottic stenosis in infants and children. *Laryngoscope*. 1993; Nov:103(11 Pt 1): 1273–83. doi: 10.1288/00005537-199311000-00011.
12. Gustafson LM, Hartley BE, Cotton RT. Acquired total (grade 4) subglottic stenosis in children. *Annals of Otology, Rhinology and Laryngology*. 2001; 110(1): 16–19.

61

Tumours and cysts of the head and neck

FIONA B MACGREGOR

Neck lumps in children are common and are mostly secondary to reactive lymphadenopathy. These swellings are usually self-limiting but may progress to abscess formation requiring aspiration or incision and drainage. Chronic infections are less common, and congenital abnormalities can present as a neck swelling at birth or frequently later in childhood following an acute infective episode. Head and neck malignancies in children are rare. Many present with an asymptomatic swelling in the head and neck region. Survival rates have improved significantly over the last 20 years. It is particularly important to detect these malignancies at an early stage when prognosis will be more favourable.

HEAD AND NECK ANATOMY

In the neck, the sternomastoid muscle in each side divides the neck into the anterior and posterior triangles. The submandibular triangle lies superior to the digastric muscle and below the mandible. Lymph nodes are distributed throughout the neck, but the main deep cervical chain runs down, almost parallel to and deep to the sternomastoid muscle. The site of any swelling can indicate the likely underlying diagnosis.

CERVICAL LYMPHADENOPATHY

Children are predisposed to frequent upper respiratory tract infection, and subsequent enlargement of lymph nodes is very common. Serious pathology is rare. Features that are associated with a higher risk of serious pathology include lymph nodes that measure more than 3 cm, enlarged lymph nodes in the supraclavicular area, and children with a history of malignancy and who have other findings, such as hepatosplenomegaly, generalized lymphadenopathy, weight loss or night sweats. In these cases, urgent excisional biopsy is recommended.

When the diagnosis is less clear, a number of investigations may be useful. These include a chest x-ray and bloods: full blood count, infectious mononucleosis, bartonella (cat scratch), toxoplasmosis and cytomegalovirus. A human immunodeficiency virus (HIV) test should also be considered, and a Mantoux test may be indicated. An ultrasound scan can be useful in determining whether the lymph node has maintained a normal internal architecture suggesting a reactive process. Fine-needle aspirate cytology is generally avoided in the paediatric setting; when there is reasonable concern, excision biopsy is recommended.

Acute infective lymphadenopathy is usually self-limiting and settles with antibiotic therapy, but abscess formation may occur, requiring aspiration or incision and drainage.

Atypical mycobacterial infection resulting in chronic cervical lymphadenopathy is not uncommon in children. Initially, children present with painless enlarging neck nodes (lymphoma may be suspected), but with time the overlying skin becomes red and indurated, and subsequent abscess formation and a persistent discharging sinus may develop. Diagnosis is often made clinically, but a fine-needle aspirate or excision biopsy may be required where there is doubt. A chest x-ray and Mantoux test should be performed.

Ideally, complete surgical excision is performed to eradicate the disease. When access is limited or surgery is contraindicated because of significant risk of damage to surrounding structures (e.g. the facial nerve), then the use of antituberculous therapy can be considered.

CONGENITAL CYSTS AND OTHER DEVELOPMENTAL ANOMALIES

Developmental anatomy of the head and neck region is complex. Failure of this process to proceed normally predisposes children to cysts, sinuses and fistula formation in the neck.

THYROGLOSSAL DUCT CYST

At approximately 7 weeks *in utero* the thyroid gland descends from the foramen caecum at the base of the tongue to sit anterior to the primitive foregut. The duct that descends behind this should involute with time, but when this does not occur, then a cyst may develop anywhere along this pathway. Consequently, children or young adults present with a midline smooth, fluctuant swelling in the neck usually closely associated with the hyoid bone. This can become infected and present with abscess or fistula formation. Typically, the cyst will move on swallowing and protrusion of the tongue.

Any infection should be treated, and an ultrasound scan should be performed to confirm that there is a normal thyroid gland separate to the cyst (to avoid the possibility of excision of the only functioning thyroid tissue of the neck). Histological sections have confirmed that the duct or tract may be very closely associated with the hyoid bone, and therefore excision should include the cyst plus the middle portion of the hyoid bone and a wedge of muscle extending up to the foramen caecum. This is called a Sistrunk's procedure, after the surgeon who initially described it.

DERMOID CYSTS

Dermoid cysts in the neck are often mistaken for thyroglossal duct cysts. They are formed by fusion of midline epithelial elements *in utero*. They are smooth, discrete, mobile cysts filled with sebaceous material and often found superficially in the midline of the anterior neck. Simple excision is the treatment of choice.

BRANCHIAL APPARATUS ANOMALIES

In early embryological development, a series of arches with external clefts and internal pouches become apparent, and failure of these to develop normally can result in a cyst, fistula or sinus occurring in the head and neck region. Often these do not become apparent until infection occurs. Because these lesions are rare, there can be a delay in diagnosis and some children have undergone multiple surgical interventions before the underlying problem is recognized.

First branchial arch anomalies

These often present with a cyst, mass or sinus in the periauricular area or upper neck just anterior to sternomastoid. A tract leading the external auditory canal may be present, and a child can present with a discharging sinus in the external auditory canal. Diagnosis is often delayed. Investigations can include a computed tomography (CT) or magnetic resonance imaging (MRI) scan, and treatment is excision after infection has settled. These lesions can be closely associated with the facial nerve; therefore, surgery should be carried out by an experienced surgeon. The use of a facial nerve monitor is recommended.

Third and fourth branchial pouch anomalies

These are rare and are often diagnosed late. More commonly, older children present with an anterior neck abscess or recurrent thyroiditis. There is an internal sinus extending down from the pyriform fossa towards the upper pole of the thyroid gland. Management includes treatment of infection and a barium swallow to confirm the presence of the sinus. The treatment of choice is direct cautery to the sinus opening or, in recurrent cases, excision of the tract.

Second branchial arch anomalies

Second branchial cleft sinuses extend from an external skin opening in the mid- or lower neck along the anterior border of sternomastoid and run superiorly along the carotid sheath, passing over the hypoglossal nerve and beneath the belly of the digastric muscle between the external and carotid artery. A cyst can recur anywhere along its length. The sinus will usually end in a blind sac along this course, while a true fistula will continue upwards and open into the tonsil fossa.

These commonly present in early childhood and may be asymptomatic. However, patients may experience recurrent pain and discharge. The diagnosis is usually clinical, but a sinogram provides a good demonstration of the course of any tract.

In symptomatic cases, sinuses are excised. An elliptical skin incision should be made around the external opening and the tract followed up to the tonsil fossa if necessary. In young children one horizontal skin incision is usually adequate, but in older children or adults a stepladder incision may be required.

PAROTID SWELLINGS

The majority of these are infective, with mumps being the most common. Serology will confirm the diagnosis. Bacterial infection also occurs. The most common are staphylococcal and streptococcal infection, and antibiotic may be required. On occasion incision and drainage of an abscess may be necessary. Recurrent parotitis can occur in childhood but nearly always resolves by puberty. Atypical mycobacterial infection may also affect the parotid gland. Benign tumours, such as pleomorphic adenomas, are rare but are managed in a similar way to adults.

LYMPHATIC MALFORMATIONS

Lymphatic malformations or cystic hygromas can occur at birth or develop during childhood. The swelling consists of dilated channels and associated epithelial-lined cysts. The cyst may be large (macrocystic) or small (microcystic), or a combination of the two. They are commonly associated with venous malformations. These can occur in the neck, floor of mouth, tongue, parotid region, cheek or lip (and can extend through several regions). An upper respiratory tract infection or trauma can result in a sudden increase in size, and upper airway obstruction may occur, necessitating tracheostomy. Involvement of the tongue may result in macroglossia, and there is often significant cosmetic and functional disability. The diagnosis is usually clinical but may be assisted with imaging techniques such as MRI or CT. Sclerotherapy under ultrasound control can be effective in macrocystic lesions, but surgical intervention may be more appropriate. This can be challenging and is often subtotal in practice as these lesions often can be closely associated with vital structures, i.e. nerves and vessels. Children with lymphatic malformations often have facial disfigurements; therefore, psychological support in addition to input from speech and language therapists and dieticians is required.

HEAD AND NECK MALIGNANCIES

Fortunately, these are rare. They often present as an asymptomatic swelling in the neck. Sinister symptoms include pain, dysphagia, haemoptysis, diplopia and proptosis. The incidence of head and neck malignancies in children appears to be increasing, but this may be in part due to better data collection. In parallel, children are now surviving these tumours in much greater numbers. Malignant tumours are managed in centralized paediatric cancer units by specialized multidisciplinary teams. A number of treatment protocols have been developed and implemented. The type of tumour varies with age and sex. For example, neuroblastomas are most common in infants, and thyroid carcinoma is usually seen in adolescent females.

HODGKIN'S LYMPHOMA

Hodgkin's lymphoma (HL) is distinguished morphologically by the presence of Reed–Sternberg cells. Nodular sclerosing is the most common type in children and young adults. There is an association with previous Epstein–Barr virus infection. HL most commonly presents with lymphadenopathy in the neck. Systemic upset – fever, night sweats and weight loss – is present in approximately 30 per cent of patients and associated with a poorer prognosis. Diagnosis is usually made by excision of a lymph node. Multimodality treatment is common in children, and the survival rate is more than 90 per cent in many series.

NON-HODGKIN'S LYMPHOMA

Approximately 60 per cent of paediatric lymphomas are non-Hodgkin's lymphoma (NHL), and these tend to be more aggressive than in adults. Classification is complex, but there are three main types: lymphoblastic lymphoma (predominantly T cell origin), small non-cleaved cell lymphoma (Burkitt's and non-Burkitt's subtype of B cell origin) and large cell of T or B origin.

The frequency, subtype and incidence of NHL varies considerably from country to country. In some parts of the world, such as Africa, many of these tumours are positive for Epstein–Barr virus. Forty-five per cent of children will have cervical lymphadenopathy at the time of presentation, and Waldeyer's ring including the tonsils and adenoids is a common site of extra-nodal spread. Children with endemic Burkett's often present with involvement of the jaw. Staging investigations include relevant blood tests, bone marrow biopsy and cerebrospinal fluid examination. CT and MRI are also used in staging. The treatment of choice is multiagent chemotherapy, while radiotherapy plays a limited role. Survival depends on histological subtype and extent of disease, but the outlook for most children is good.

RHABDOMYOSARCOMA

Forty per cent of rhabdomyosarcomas occur in the head and neck region, and nearly half of these tumours present before the age of 5 years. In the head and neck region, these tumours are most frequently found in the orbit, paranasal sinuses, nose, nasopharynx and middle ear. Consequently, a child may present with a proptosis or a mass within the nose or ear, which may be associated with pain and bloody discharge. Lymph node involvement is reported to be between 3 and 30 per cent.

A thorough examination of the head and neck region must be performed, including the cranial nerves. An MRI scan should be performed to assess the primary lesion and to detect metastases. A CT scan is a useful complementary tool.

Treatment protocols employ multiagent chemotherapy and radiotherapy. Surgery is usually performed for diagnostic purposes only.

Before 1960 only 10 per cent of children with rhabdomyosarcoma survived 5 years. Now the 5-year survival rate is more than 80 per cent in early disease but still relatively poor in advanced disease.

THYROID CANCER

Thyroid carcinoma is rare in children. It is most common in adolescent females. In the paediatric population the majority are differentiated tumours (papillary and follicular). Children usually present with an asymptomatic solitary mass in the anterior lateral neck (cervical metastases) or with a thyroid nodule. At presentation there is often lymph node involvement (74 per cent) or distant metastases (25 per cent). Medullary carcinoma is rare and must be suspected in children with multiple endocrine neoplasia (MEN).

Investigations should include an ultrasound, usually in conjunction with a fine-needle aspirate biopsy, as these are older children who will often tolerate such an investigation. Plasma calcitonin levels should be measured where medullary carcinoma is suspected. Treatment remains controversial and similar to that in adults, and usually includes total thyroidectomy and radiodine ablation therapy. Children with a family history of multiple endocrine neoplasia should have their plasma calcitonin levels checked and should be genetically screened for the RET proto-oncogene on chromosome 10. If positive, prophylactic total thyroidectomy is recommended.

NASOPHARYNGEAL CARCINOMA

Nasopharyngeal carcinoma is uncommon in children in Europe and the United States but common in other locations such as parts of Africa. This is associated with the Epstein–Barr virus. Children tend to have more advanced local and regional disease and distant metastases. Children can present with asymptomatic cervical lymphadenopathy. Others complain of nasal blockage, epistaxis, otitis media with effusion, headache or cranial nerve palsy. Up to 60 per cent may have lymph node involvement at presentation. Treatment is similar to that for adults.

NEUROBLASTOMA

Neuroblastoma is the most common malignancy in those under the age of 1 year. It arises from undifferentiated sympathetic nervous system precursor cells of neurocrest origin. The adrenal gland is the most common site, but tumours can arise in the sympathetic chain, posterior mediastinum and cervical region. Lymph nodes are involved at presentation in up to 35 per cent of patients. The symptoms and signs reflect the primary site and location of the metastases. Children with neuroblastoma in the head and neck region can present with a firm mass in the lateral neck, occasionally associated with Horner's syndrome. Ophthalmological manifestations include proptosis and periorbital ecchymosis, and bilateral periorbital haematomas are a classical sign ('racoon eyes'). An appropriate tissue biopsy is usually obtained for diagnosis, and MRI and CT imaging are usually performed for staging. A metaiodobenzylguanidine (MIBG) scan is a useful method of assessing the metastases.

Treatment is tailored for the individual at the sites involved within the neck. Surgical resection may be possible and can be combined with multiagent chemotherapy. Survival rates greater than 90 per cent can be achieved in early disease. Primary neuroblastoma in the head and neck region carries a better prognosis than neuroblastoma in other sites.

KEY LEARNING POINTS

- Swellings in the head and neck region are common in children.
- The majority are due to benign reactive lymphadenopathy.
- Excision biopsy of a lymph node is the investigation of choice when malignancy is suspected.
- Survival rates are improving, and patients with malignancy should be managed in specialized paediatric centres.
- Consider the diagnosis of an underlying congenital cyst, sinus or fistula in recurrent infection or abscess formation in the head and neck region in children.

62

The deaf child

S J PROWSE AND C H RAINE

INTRODUCTION

To be blind is to be isolated from the world; to be deaf is to be isolated from other people. Hearing impairment can have an immense impact on psychosocial well-being whatever an individual's age, but the implications for deaf children are particularly profound.

A child's first experience of the world is the perception of environmental noise whilst still a fetus. By 20 weeks' gestation the human ear is sufficiently developed to support hearing, and it perceives environmental sounds by 27 weeks.[1] Once born, children are continually exposed to sound and, more importantly, speech, which immediately begins to shape the development of the hearing centres within the brain stem and auditory cortex. By their first birthday, children with normal hearing are already accomplished linguists able to recognize common words and discern subtle differences in voice tone. By their fourth birthday, hearing children will have developed a sophisticated vocabulary of several thousand words and be able use this to interact effectively with their peers and adults.

Without external stimulation the development of central auditory pathways and speech centres is severely curtailed, and language, social and academic milestones will fail to be met. In the United Kingdom, 2.05 out of every 1000 children have a significant hearing loss, defined as being greater than 40 dBHL in their better hearing ear.[2] In developing countries the prevalence is significantly higher owing to the lack of universal immunization programmes and poorer provisions for perinatal care. For many children around the world, a hearing impairment leads to a life of exclusion, of dependence and of wasted potential.

SCREENING FOR HEARING LOSS

The plasticity of the central auditory pathways decreases with age, and there is increasing awareness that a deaf child's potential for normal language acquisition is improved by early intervention. Of course, early intervention relies on correctly identifying children with hearing problems as soon as possible after they are born. Many countries have introduced universal hearing screening programmes for all neonates. In the United Kingdom this consists of an automated otoacoustic emissions (AOE) test soon after birth. This painless test involves exposing the child to a series of high-tone clicks. The screening equipment listens for the 'echo' generated by a healthy cochlea in response to this stimulus. The test has a sensitivity of around 80 per cent for detecting moderate to profound hearing loss. False positives can arise owing to obstruction of the ear canal or excessive ambient noise and, for this reason, children who fail are followed up with further audiometric testing. In the United Kingdom, this consists of an automated auditory brain stem response (AABR) test.

Hearing loss can be progressive or may result from insults sustained later in childhood. Therefore, it is important to remain vigilant for signs of hearing loss, even in children who have passed early screening tests. In the United Kingdom, the majority of children undergo a health-check prior to school entry at age four. This includes a screening pure tone audiogram. Other children come to the attention of health services because of parental or school concerns regarding poor hearing or speech.

Degrees of hearing loss are defined as:

- 25–39 dBHL, mild
- 40–69 dBHL, moderate
- 70–89 dBHL, severe
- 90 > dBHL, profound

CAUSES OF CHILDHOOD DEAFNESS

As with adult hearing loss, deafness in children can be due to either a sensorineural or a conductive loss (or a mixture of both). It is useful to divide aetiologies into three categories – prenatal, perinatal and postnatal – based on the timing of the insult that resulted in hearing damage. The common aetiological factors are summarized in Table 62.1.

GENETICS AND CHILDHOOD DEAFNESS

Hearing loss is termed *syndromic* when it is associated with other anomalies. Several hundred syndromes are associated with hearing loss, and some of the most important are listed in Table 62.2. Although it is important to be aware of these syndromic associations, in the majority of children

Table 62.1 Causes of childhood deafness

Cause	Conductive loss	Sensorineural loss
Prenatal (congenital)	Atresia of external ear canal Ossicular anomalies Congenital cholesteatoma	Genetic – Syndromic and non-syndromic. Inherited and sporadic Infection – Rubella, cytomegalovirus (CMV), herpes simplex, syphilis
Perinatal		Prematurity Hypoxia Jaundice (Kernicterus)
Postnatal	Infection – Sequela of otitis media and otitis media with effusion (OME)	Infection – Measles, meningitis, mumps, CMV Ototoxicity – Aminoglycosides, cytotoxics

Table 62.2 Important genetic syndromes associated with childhood deafness

Syndrome	Inheritance	Important manifestations
Pendred syndrome	AR	Sensorineural loss and thyroid goitre +/- enlarged vestibular aqueduct
Usher syndrome	AR	Sensorineural loss and retinitis pigmentosa
Jervell Lange-Nielson syndrome	AR	Sensorineural loss and prolonged Q-T interval on electrocardiogram
Waardenburg syndrome	AD	Sensorineural loss, heterochromia iridis, white forelock
Crouzon syndrome	AD	Conductive loss and external ear anomalies. Craniosynostosis and exopthalmos
Apert syndrome	AD (majority sporadic)	Conductive loss due to fixation of stapes. Craniosynostosis and syndactyly
Alport syndrome	X-linked or AR	Glomerulonephritis and sensorineural loss
Down syndrome	Sporadic	Increased risk of senorineural loss and glue ear. Increased risk of middle ear anomalies
CHARGE syndrome	Sporadic	Coloboma, heart defects, atresia of choana, retardation of growth, genital anomalies, ear anomalies – abnormal pinna, ossicular anomalies, malformed cochlea (Mondini dysplasia)
Cleft palate	Variable	Almost universal glue ear due to poor eustachian tube function

born with hearing loss, the condition is due to a non-syndromic genetic anomaly. Non-syndromic hereditary hearing loss is usually autosomal recessive in nature, accounting for four-fifths of all cases. The implication is that a significant number of children will be born to normally hearing parents with a 25 per cent chance that subsequent siblings could have a similar hearing impairment. Autosomal dominant inheritance accounts for most of the rest, although both X-linked and mitochondrial transmission have also been implicated in rare cases.

Connexin 26 is a transmembrane protein responsible for the transport of potassium ions between the hair cells of the inner ear. The protein is coded for by the GJB2 gene, located on chromosome 13. Mutations in both copies of this gene result in varying degrees of deafness and are the most common cause of non-syndromic hereditary hearing loss.[3] Around 1:51 Caucasian Europeans are believed to be carriers.[4] It is possible to analyze the GJB2 gene for the presence of mutations and determine if this is the cause of deafness. This allows for the genetic counselling of affected families.

CLINICAL EVALUATION OF A CHILD WITH SUSPECTED DEAFNESS

Many children come to the attention of clinicians because of parental concerns regarding poor hearing or speech development or because of a failed hearing test. It is important to appreciate the anxiety that a potential diagnosis of deafness can cause within families. Parents are likely to have many questions and concerns, and it is important that these are addressed.

The assessment begins with a comprehensive medical history. Details should be sought regarding pregnancy, birth, the perinatal period and infancy with reference to common aetiological factors (see Table 62.1). Children who have received care on an intensive care unit are particularly at risk of hearing loss, and many centres recommend more detailed hearing assessments in these children as a matter of routine. Although most cases of congenital hearing loss are sporadic, a genetic pedigree should be drawn up to evaluate any potential inheritable component. If this is likely, then the opinion of a medical geneticist should be sought.

INVESTIGATIONS

These are performed with three primary aims: to investigate the cause of hearing loss, to assess for associated morbidity (e.g. syndromic associations) and to assess the child's suitability for hearing rehabilitation, including cochlear implantation if appropriate.

AUDIOLOGY

If screening tests or history suggest the possibility of a hearing impairment, this should be confirmed with formal audiology. The method employed will depend on the age and ability of the child.

RADIOLOGY

A magnetic resonance imaging (MRI) scan of the inner ear and internal acoustic meati is the first-line radiological investigation in children with profound congenital hearing loss. It provides high-resolution images of the inner ear and VIIIth cranial nerve and does not expose the child to radiation. However, assessment of any abnormality of the ossicles is more difficult. The scan takes 30 minutes, which makes it more suitable for neonates who can be scanned whilst they sleep.

High-resolution computed tomography (CT) scan of the temporal bones is superior when assessing the bony structures of the outer, middle and inner ear and is quicker to perform than an MRI scan. However, CT provides less information about the nerves and involves a significant radiation exposure for young children. Its primary role is when contemplating cochlear implantation in a child who may also have anomalies of the inner ear (e.g. Mondini dysplasia).

GENETIC TESTING

The decision to proceed to genetic testing will depend on the presentation of the child. If a syndromic cause is suspected, then this will guide investigations. In the case of non-syndromic hereditary hearing loss, it is common practice to assess for the presence of mutations coding for the Connexin proteins. It is essential that any genetic testing be preceded by a consultation with a clinical geneticist who can provide families with information regarding the likelihood of further siblings being affected.

SPECIAL TESTS

- **Electrocardiogram (ECG):** A 12-lead ECG can be performed to exclude conduction anomalies. These manifest as a prolonged Q-T interval in children with Jervell Lange-Nielsen syndrome and can cause syncopal attacks or sudden fatal arrhythmias.
- **Renal ultrasound scan:** This is indicated if syndromes such as branchio-oto-renal or Alport's are suspected or if there are multi-system anomalies.
- **Ophthalmology:** Ophthalmic conditions coexist in 40 per cent of children with congenital hearing loss, and all should be reviewed by a paediatric ophthalmologist. Problems include squint and refractive errors as well as syndromic associations such as seen in Usher's, Waardenburg and CHARGE syndromes, congenital rubella and cytomegalovirus (CMV).

MAXIMIZING THE POTENTIAL OF THE DEAF CHILD

Once a child is identified as having a hearing impairment, a number of interventions can be employed to either maximize residual hearing or provide alternative means for communication. The specific methods chosen will depend on the severity of the hearing loss and the presence of any additional issues. It is important that measures are instigated as soon as possible after a hearing impairment is confirmed; this is particularly important in children with a bilateral profound hearing loss. However, even children with a relatively mild unilateral hearing loss can have problems with sound localization or when listening in noisy situations and will derive great benefit once appropriate support is provided.

EDUCATIONAL SUPPORT

The most important aspect of managing any child with a hearing impairment is creating an environment in which the child's ability to hear can be maximized. This will require close coordination between family, medical, audiological and educational services. Communication will be easier if background noise can be minimized and people made aware that the child's hearing is poor. Nonverbal cues take on added importance, and it is therefore essential that the child can clearly see the speaker. With adequate support many deaf children can be educated with their hearing peers, but extra provision is often required.

CONVENTIONAL AIR-CONDUCTION HEARING AIDS

A hearing aid acts to amplify sound so that the sound level presented to the eardrum is greater. In its most basic form it consists of a microphone, an amplifier, a power source and a speaker. Modern hearing aids also contain sophisticated microprocessors that allow for tailored amplification of selected frequencies and prevent over-amplification of loud sounds and excessive feedback. The supply and fitting of hearing aids in young children is demanding and requires skilled audiologists and perseverance from parents to achieve appropriate use. Evidence exists that hearing aids should be provided prior to 6 months of age to maximize language acquisition. With bilateral hearing impairment, bilateral aids should be fitted unless there are contraindications. Binaural hearing has numerous benefits, some of which include better sound localization, improved speech recognition in quiet and noise and general ease of listening.

BONE-CONDUCTING HEARING DEVICES AND ACTIVE MIDDLE EAR IMPLANTS

Bone-conducting hearing implants (BCHDs) work on the same principle as the more familiar acoustic aids, but the amplified signal is transmitted to the cochlea by vibration through the temporal bone. This can be achieved by initial wearing of the auditory processor held in place over the mastoid with either a tight-fitting headband or a softband. When the child is old enough, a permanent percutaneous osseointegrated abutment can be inserted surgically into the bone.

BCHDs are useful in children who cannot wear a conventional hearing aid. This could be due to atresia of the ear canals, microtia or recurrent ear infections that would interfere with an air conduction aid.

Transcutaneous BCHDs and active middle ear implants (AMEIs) offer similar benefits and avoid cutaneous issues that can be associated with percutaneous devices.

COCHLEAR IMPLANTS

These are sophisticated transducers; they convert sound energy to electric impulses, which directly stimulate the auditory nerve via an electrode array inserted into the cochlea. The criteria for cochlear implantation are children with severe to profound hearing loss who have derived little or no benefit from conventional hearing aids. Originally, only a single ear was implanted, but it is now accepted that bilateral simultaneous implantation has many benefits, including improved speech recognition in noisy environments and better sound localization.[5] Since the first children were implanted with cochlear implants in the late 1980s, technology has advanced significantly. Originally envisioned as a means to allow recognition of environmental sound and as an aid to lip-reading, today cochlear implants allow users to understand speech and music without needing visual clues. Early implantation is to be encouraged with children with congenital hearing loss.

KEY LEARNING POINTS

- Early detection of hearing loss is important.
- Permanent childhood hearing losses require comprehensive assessment.
- Early amplification and stimulation are important.
- Maintain vigilance for progressive hearing losses.

- Early cochlear implantation should be considered for children with severe to profound hearing loss.

REFERENCES

1. Hall JW. Development of the ear and hearing. *Journal of Perinatology.* 2000 Dec; 20(8): 12–20.
2. Fortnum HM, Summerfield AQ, Marshall DH, Davis AC, Bamford JM. Prevalence of permanent childhood hearing impairment in the United Kingdom and implications for universal neonatal hearing screening: Questionnaire based ascertainment study. *BMJ.* 2001 Sep; 323: 536–40.
3. Lefebvre PP, Van De Water TR. Connexins, hearing and deafness: Clinical aspects of mutations in the connexin 26 gene. *Brain Research.* 2000 Apr; 32(1): 159–62.
4. Gasparini P, Rabionet R, Barbujani G, Melçhionda S, Petersen M, Brøndum-Nielsen K, et al. High carrier frequency of the 35delG deafness mutation in European populations. Genetic Analysis Consortium of GJB2 35delG. *European Journal of Human Genetics.* 2000 Jan; 8(1): 19–23.
5. Steffens T, Lesinski-Schiedat A, Strutz J, Aschendorff A, Klenzner T, Rühl S, et al. The benefits of sequential bilateral cochlear implantation for hearing-impaired children. *Acta Oto-laryngologica.* 2008 Feb; 128(2): 164–76.

FURTHER READING

United Kingdom Newborn Hearing Screening Programme, www.hearing.screening.nhs.uk.

63

Acute otitis media and mastoiditis

GAVIN MORRISON

ACUTE OTITIS MEDIA

CLASSIFICATION, DEFINITION AND PATHOLOGY

Acute otitis media (AOM) is an inflammation of recent onset, of part or all of the mucoperiosteal lining of the middle ear cleft. This can include the eustachian tube, tympanic cavity and mastoid antrum and air cells. If the infection spreads beyond the soft tissue lining as an osteitis of the mastoid, then mastoiditis is diagnosed. Uncomplicated AOM is diagnosed when the eardrum remains intact and there is no spread of infection. Complicated AOM includes cases with eardrum perforation or further spread of infection. Severe AOM is often a term used when the pyrexia is 39°C or over.

AOM is very common in infants and young children, most commonly from the age of 3 months to 3 years. The greatest incidence is in the second 6 months of life. By the age of 6 to 7, attacks have usually stopped. It is the most common reason for prescribing antibiotics to children in the United States.

Boys are slightly more likely to get AOM. Climate, socio-economic status and racial background are also probably predisposing factors. Children with a cleft palate, Down syndrome or craniofacial anomalies or immune deficiencies are also more prone to AOM. Siblings of those with recurrent AOM are more likely to be affected, with genetic as well as environmental factors being responsible. Attending day care at an early age, passive smoking and use of dummies (pacifiers) are also associated with a greater risk of AOM.

Table 63.1 Viruses causing AOM

Respiratory syncytial virus (RSV)
Human rhinovirus (HRV)
Human coronavirus (HCV)
Influenza (IV) type A
Adenovirus

Table 63.2 Bacteria in AOM (descending order of frequency)

Streptococcus pneumoniae
Non-typeable *Haemophilus influenzae*
Moraxella catarrhalis
Streptococcus pyogenes
Staphylococcus aureus

Exclusive breastfeeding appears to be protective for attacks of AOM.

Viral AOM can occur with the common cold viruses, adenoviruses or influenza viruses, but respiratory syncytial virus (RSV) is the most common viral isolate from the middle ear in viral AOM (Table 63.1). The inflammatory reaction will produce erythema engorgement and sometimes exudation. Bacterial AOM, usually from pyogenic bacteria, can result in suppuration in the middle ear. About 30 per cent of AOM is viral alone, but co-infection with bacteria is much more common. The pathogenesis of AOM involves an interplay between viruses, bacteria and the host's inflammatory response. The origin of the infective organisms is usually via the eustachian tube from the nasopharynx. Tubal infection leads to inflammatory swelling and occlusion of the eustachian tube. Mucociliary drainage from the eustachian tube will be arrested and oxygen within the middle ear cleft will be absorbed or metabolized. The inflammatory reaction leads to a fluid effusion behind the eardrum, which can initially be retracted and then bulge from the exudate and suppuration. The resultant bulging eardrum may burst with the bloodstained muco-purulent discharge draining from the ear canal.

Allergic AOM can occur and is more likely to result in a clear or pale mucus effusion behind the eardrum.

Otitis media can be classified as (1) acute suppurative otitis media (ASOM); (2) acute non-suppurative otitis media (otitis media with effusion or OME); (3) specific otitis media, such as tuberculous otitis media and (4) adhesive otitis media.

ASOM OR BACTERIAL AOM

ASOM is an acute infection of the mucoperiosteal lining of the middle ear cleft by pyogenic organisms. It is very common, and by the age of 3 years, 50–85 per cent of children have had AOM. It will typically cause measurable hearing loss of up to 30 dB.

Bacterial organisms most commonly responsible for acute otitis media are shown in Table 63.2. However, it remains very difficult clinically to distinguish between viral AOM and bacterial AOM in the early phase of infection.

Tuberculous OM can start with AOM but runs a chronic course, and classically is said to be associated with multiple drum perforations. Adhesive OM represents an end stage of recurrent OM where there has been protracted eustachian tube dysfunction, a collapsed eardrum and subsequent healing with adhesive scar tissue obliterating the middle ear space.

AOM HISTORY AND EXAMINATION

The infant or child presenting with early AOM will initially touch the ears or complain of earache, and may be irritable. Examination at this early stage of tubal occlusion will show a retracted eardrum, which is pink, and there may be evidence of a middle ear effusion with fluid behind the eardrum. In the stage of pre-suppurative OM, the blood vessels on the eardrum will be more prominent, radiating from the circumference inwards and from the handle of the malleus, and the drum will be bulging (Figure 63.1). The child may develop a fever, and pain will be much more apparent. If the disease progresses to a stage of true suppuration with pus formation, there is a greater potential for spontaneous perforation of the tympanic membrane or other complications. The patient may experience throbbing pain or pulsatile tinnitus.

As soon as the drum perorates, the mucopus and a little blood will often be seen coming from the ear canal, and the pain instantly subsides.

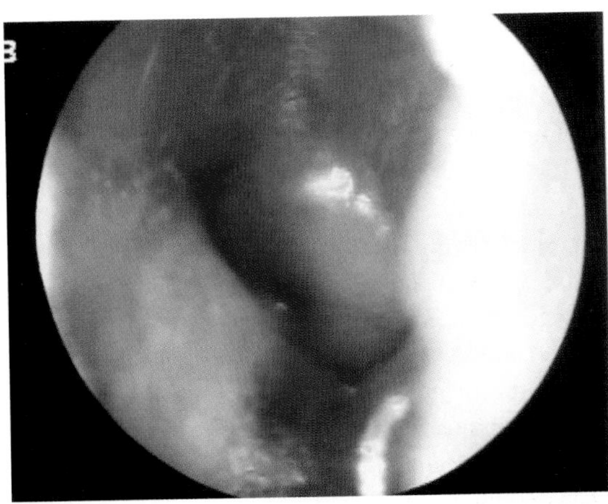

Figure 63.1 Acute otitis media.

Differential diagnoses of the child presenting with an acutely painful ear are: mastoiditis, acute haemorrhagic viral bullous myringitis, a furuncle in the ear canal, acute bacterial otitis externa (often *Pseudomonas* infection), acute fungal otitis externa or, rarely, herpes zoster oticus.

The history of pain subsiding when the discharge develops is most suggestive of AOM, whilst an increasing blockage, discomfort or pain, itching, and a moist scanty discharge with swelling seen in the ear canal strongly suggests an otitis externa.

For viral AOM and many bacterial AOM infections, the process will be self-limiting with or without perforation. Through the immune response, natural resolution and reversal of the inflammatory phases occurs, with drainage of the middle ear fluid and re-aeration of the middle ear cleft. The natural history of AOM is for resolution within 4 to 7 days in the majority of cases. About 1 per 1000 cases treated without antibiotics, however, is estimated to develop mastoiditis.

INFANTILE AOM

Infants have a relatively short, wide and straight eustachian tube. Aetiological factors that predispose to infant middle ear infections are therefore bottle-feeding with regurgitation, vomiting and teething. The infant presents in some discomfort with distress crying or rolling the head from side to side, sleeping badly and perhaps vomiting. Examination of the infant's tympanic membrane can be difficult. The drum tends to be thicker so bulging is not always apparent, but there will be a dull and reddened appearance.

Investigations

Tympanograms, if attempted, will show a flat type B trace. Audiometry, if undertaken, will confirm a conductive hearing impairment. Pneumatic otoscopy will show an immobile eardrum. However, for an acute infection the diagnosis is largely a clinical one and treatment is started without any specific investigations. Purulent discharge can be swabbed for microbiology culture and sensitivity.

Treatment of AOM

As a first-line treatment, simple analgesics, paracetamol and/or ibuprofen can be prescribed for non-severe uncomplicated AOM. When the triad of earache, fever over 39°C and an inflamed bulging tympanic membrane is apparent, then suppurative otitis media (bacterial) is likely and broad-spectrum antibiotic therapy is advisable for 1 week to 10 days. AOM in children under 2 years old tends to be more severe and is more likely to become complicated, so antibiotic treatment is probably more important in these young children. For children under 6 months of age, all AOM cases should be treated with antibiotics. Otherwise, if the AOM is not clearly improving after 48–72 hours, antibiotics also indicated. The first choice of antibiotic in primary care is usually amoxicillin (80–90 mg/kg/d). For penicillin-allergic patients, erythromycin or azithromycin is prescribed. If the child has had amoxicillin recently or has AOM with conjunctivitis, then beta-lactamase–producing organisms are more likely and co-amoxiclav (amoxicillin/clavulanate) is advised. Sometimes the infection is with a resistant *Haemophilus influenzae* or penicillin-resistant *Streptococcus*, and in secondary care co-amoxiclav is usually prescribed. It will usually lead to resolution of almost all AOM infections except those caused by *Pseudomonas*. A 10-day course of antibiotics by mouth is advised for children 5 years old or younger. Older children may be given 7 days of treatment. Details of the current clinical practice guidelines from the American Academy of Pediatrics can be accessed via the Internet.[1]

If AOM with perforation does not resolve quickly on the chosen broad-spectrum antibiotic and the ear continues to discharge mucopus, then an ear swab should be taken for microbiology, culture and sensitivity.

There remains a debate in primary care about when to prescribe antibiotics for AOM.[2] Viral AOM does not require antibiotic therapy. The desire to avoid over-prescription of antimicrobials, and thereby keep antibiotic-resistant organisms to a minimum in the community, has led to a tendency by doctors to prescribe simple analgesics only. However, there is some evidence to suggest that the incidence of acute bacterial mastoiditis has increased in the last two decades. It is possible, but not proven, that these events are causally related.

Acute suppurative otitis media usually resolves within a few days on antibiotics. The bulging eardrum is likely to reduce, but if it has perforated already, complete healing is highly likely. The drum will remain pink and become retracted, and the middle ear effusion will probably take some time (typically 2–6 weeks) to completely resolve. If the middle ear effusion does not resolve and OME continues after 3 months of active surveillance, and there is a significant hearing loss or disability, then grommet insertion is indicated.

Rarely, with modern antimicrobials, a middle ear empyema with a bulging drum that becomes thickened and chronically reddened persists after two or even three courses of antibiotics. A short general anaesthetic for myringotomy, aspiration of the mucopus and insertion of ventilation tube (grommet) is then indicated at this earlier stage.

RECURRENT OTITIS MEDIA, GROMMETS AND ADENOIDS

Ten to 20 per cent of infants and children with AOM develop repeated attacks. In the very young, and when AOM coincides with teething, then treatment of each episode should be on its merits. Recurrent otitis media with perforation and discharge, however, can risk tympanosclerosis or a chronic eardrum perforation as well as some permanent hearing impairment. Middle ear biofilms are implicated in the causation. Low-dose, once-daily prophylactic antibiotic treatment for a 2- to 3-month period can be prescribed. Amoxicillin, erythromycin, trimethoprim or a second-generation cephalosporin could be selected.

If such treatment is ineffective, then insertion of ventilation tubes (grommets) has been shown to be very successful. This applies even to the child who has a well-ventilated middle ear without OME in between attacks.

The child with recurrent acute otitis media who is 2 years of age or over might well have enlarged adenoid tissue, which is a focus for infection from a chronic *Haemophilus influenzae* or other bacterial colonization. If the adenoids are enlarged, especially when there are concomitant symptoms of nasal obstruction and rhinorrhoea, an adenoidectomy can be undertaken. In this case the use of diathermy techniques by 'sterilizing' the residual adenoid bed might have added benefit.

Recurrent AOM in the presence of ventilation tubes is associated with swimming and upper respiratory tract infections (URTIs) and presents with discomfort, blockage and copious ear discharge. The spectrum of organisms differs from the child without a ventilation tube and is principally *Streptococcus pneumoniae, Pseudomonas sp., Haemophilus influenzae* and *Moxarella sp.* Treatment is with oral antibiotics or, for a light discharge, with antibiotic ear drops with or without steroids. Quinolone ear drops are safe, but the potentially ototoxic aminoglycoside ear drops should be given for no more than 2 weeks, ideally for 1 week.

VACCINATION

In the United Kingdom, the standard vaccination regimen uses the 7-valent Prevnar vaccine, (pneumococcal conjugate vaccine (PCV)) given at 2, 4 and 12 months of age. The 23-valent Pneumovax II, a polysaccharide vaccine against pneumococcus (*Strep. pneumonia*), covers 90 per cent of all known infections and does reduce pneumococcal otitis media. However, it is not recommended for use in patients under 2 years old. The overall incidence of AOM in Pneumovax-vaccinated children can be reduced, but the effect is not very marked as other pathogens show an increased frequency of infections.

OTHER VARIANTS OF AOM

Acute necrotic otitis media

In more debilitated children, a profuse and foul-smelling odour ear can develop in association with measles, scarlet fever or influenza, for example. Examination reveals a large tympanic membrane defect, and the rapid necrosis of the membrane is usually the result of an aggressive beta-haemolytic *Streptococcus*. Healing can be with fibrosis, and chronic suppurative ear disease may result.

Haemorrhagic otitis media

This is a primary otitis media, also seen with influenza, that may be associated with bullous eruption of the tympanic membrane but is principally established by the presence of a bloodstained middle ear effusion. Haemolytic *Streptococcus* is generally the causative organism. This condition differs from a bullous myringitis in which there can be a haemorrhagic bullous otitis externa. The bloodstained blisters are confined to the drum and meatus, and a viral aetiology is responsible.

Barotraumatic otitis media

Acute barotrauma from rapid air pressure changes (when the eustachian tube cannot open to equalize) can result in a haemotympanum or bloodstained middle ear effusion. It is usually managed expectantly and will clear, but grommet insertion can be undertaken for failed 'watchful waiting'.

COMPLICATIONS OF AOM

Apart from tympanic membrane perforation, complications are usually caused by the spread of infection to adjacent areas, and are listed in Table 63.3.

Bacterial infection can spread directly to the regions in continuity with the middle ear, by retrograde venous spread, or by distant blood borne spread. Thus intracranial abscesses may be in the cerebellum from incontinuity spread or supratentorially in the hemisphere by distal embolic spread. These complications are discussed further under the mastoiditis section of this chapter.

Table 63.3 Complications of ASOM

Facial palsy
Sensorineural (cochlear) hearing loss
Acute mastoiditis
Thombosis of the lateral or sigmoid venous sinus
Petrositis (petrous apex infection)
Gradenigo's syndrome
Zygomatic process abscess
Medial soft tissue mastoid tip abscess (Bezold's abscess)
Labyrinthitis
Meningitis
Intracranial abscess
Ossicular erosion (of long process of incus)
Non-healing perforation (CSOM)
Atelectasis of the TM
Retraction pocket
Scarring/retraction leading to cholesteatoma

Labyrinthitis can be a non-suppurative one caused by toxic effects via the round window membrane and will cause vertigo and nystagmus. A degree of permanent high-frequency sensorineural hearing loss can also result. Much more rarely, a severe infective labyrinthitis or cochlear infection will result in moderate to profound permanent deafness.

Facial palsy in AOM

Facial palsy is usually the result of pressure from pus on the VII nerve in its horizontal tympanic segment, where there is a natural bony dehiscence in up to 10 per cent of ears. It is treated with antibiotics, but in addition a short course of systemic steroids can be considered. Wide myringotomy (often with insertion of a ventilation tube) to drain the middle ear pus is also recommended.

ACUTE MASTOIDITIS

DEFINITION AND PATHOLOGY

Acute mastoiditis occurs when an otitis media infection spreads directly to involve the bone

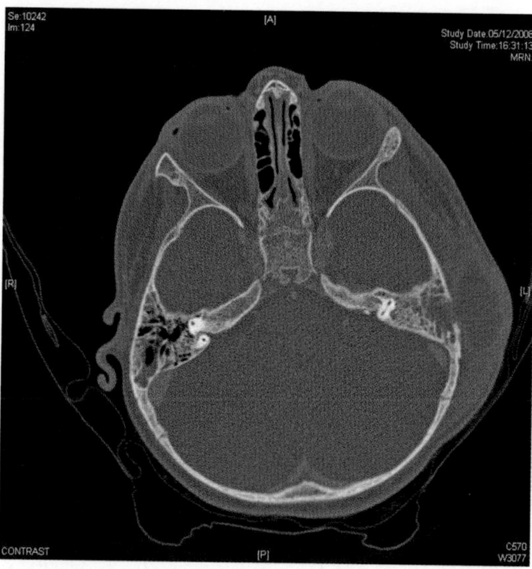

Figure 63.2 Axial CT showing coalescent mastoiditis and subperiosteal abscess.

of the mastoid air cell system as an osteitis. This typically leads to breakdown of some of the fine bony trabeculae of the mastoid cells, producing a coalescent mastoiditis (often seen on a computed tomography, or CT scan) with an empyaema in the mastoid antrum (Figure 63.2). In other areas, such as the mastoid tip, cells will remain intact but infected. As the pus is under pressure, the infection causes localized bone necrosis and resorption and can spread to form a sub-periosteal abscess. This is found either directly behind the upper part of the pinna (over MacEwen's triangle and the underlying mastoid antrum) or higher, superior to the pinna towards the zygomatic process, or over the squamous temporal bone without obvious direct continuity with the mastoiditis itself.

The infecting organism is usually a *Streptococcus pneumoniae* (up to 60 per cent) but can be *Streptococcus pyogenes* (Group A *Streptococci*), *Haemophilus influenzae, Staphylococcus aureus, Klebsiella pneumonia, Pseudomonas* or other organisms. Microaerophilic organisms such as *Streptococcus milleri* and other anaerobes are less common but can occur, and will require metronidazole in addition. *Fusobacterium necrophorum* causes a mastoiditis associated with a high likelihood of venous thrombosis (Table 63.4).

Table 63.4 Organisms causing acute mastoiditis

Streptococcus pneumoniae (60 per cent)
Streptococcus pyogenes
Haemophilus influenzae
Staphylococcus aureus
Klebsiella pneumonia
Pseudomonas aeruginosa
Escherichia coli
Streptococcus milleri
Fusobacterium necrophorum

INCIDENCE, HISTORY AND EXAMINATION

Three-quarters of cases of acute mastoiditis occur in children under two years of age, and in this age group the likelihood of complications of mastoiditis is greatest. The estimated incidence in the Western world is varied but may be three to four per 100 000 per year. Some, but not all, reports suggest an increase in the incidence over the past two decades.[3,4] Nevertheless, if antibiotics are given for an AOM, the chance of the child developing mastoiditis is reduced by 50 per cent. It is argued that more than 4000 cases of AOM need to be treated with antibiotics to prevent one case of acute mastoiditis.

The patient will have otalgia, a blocked or deaf ear and usually a pyrexia. The fever can be swinging (picket fence pyrexia). Examination can show a red bulging eardrum, some oedema of the posterior and superior part of the deep ear canal and tenderness behind the pinna, especially over MacEwen's triangle. Not infrequently, however, especially if the child has been commenced on antibiotics, the eardrum itself may not be bulging or perforated. However, it is never normal. The infection and empyaema can be sealed off in the mastoid antrum and air cells, sparing the middle ear somewhat. If the overlying post-aural skin is thickened and erythematous in addition, the diagnosis is certain (Figure 63.3). The pinna can be pushed forwards by the swelling and appear more prominent.

COMPLICATED MASTOIDITIS

About 50 per cent of children presenting with mastoiditis will have been given prior antibiotics for

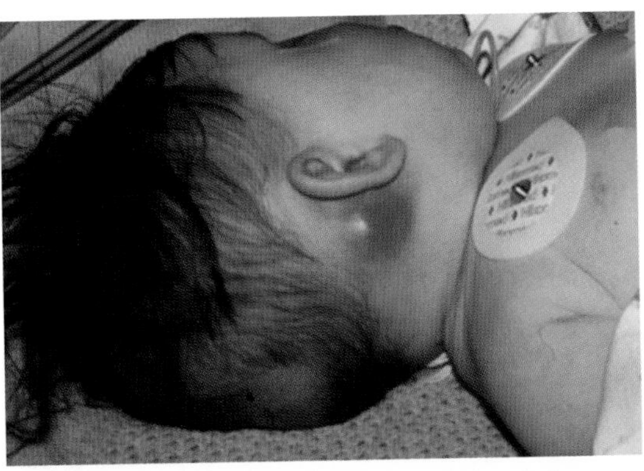

Figure 63.3 Acute mastoiditis with post-aural swelling and erythema.

AOM. If subperiosteal abscess is included as a complication, then about 60 per cent of cases become complicated; if it is not, then about 20 per cent do so. Thirty per cent of paediatric patients presenting with mastoiditis have a sub-periosteal abscess. Twelve per cent have lateral sinus thrombosis. The incidence of *intracranial* complications is reported between 4 and 18 per cent of children admitted with mastoiditis. Figure 63.4 summarizes spread of infection causing the various complications.

Masked mastoiditis occurs when antibiotics have been given but have not controlled the mastoid infection fully. The acute symptoms are largely masked, so there may be malaise but little pain, no fever and no bulging red eardrum on examination. The illness is more insidious, and it usually presents with one of the complications of mastoiditis.

INVESTIGATIONS

Ear swab

If the ear is discharging or a post-aural subperiosteal abscess is oozing, then a swab must be sent for microbiology, culture and sensitivity. Blood tests may show a leucocytosis and will show raised inflammatory markers (C-reactive protein and/or erythrocyte sedimentation rate). Tympanometry is seldom required. Audiometry, if practical to undertake, will typically show a conductive hearing loss.

CT scan and MRI scan

A CT scan with contrast of the brain and mastoid system is required in all but the most straightforward cases of simple, uncomplicated mastoiditis. The CT scan will help to confirm the diagnosis with a high level of confidence, showing osteitis, the possible appearance of a coalescence of the

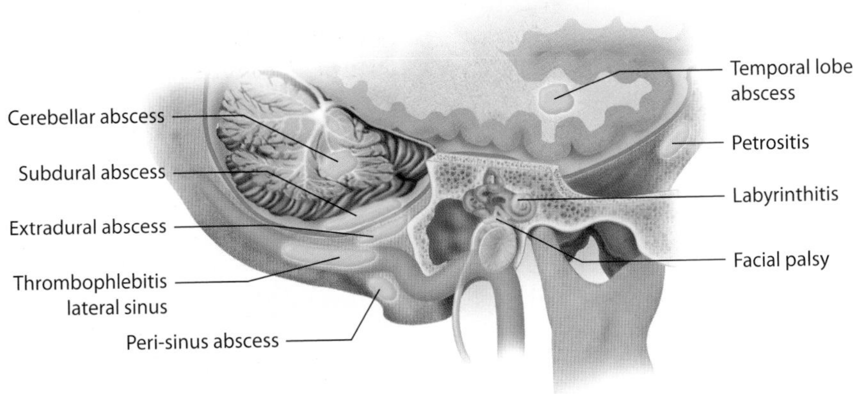

Figure 63.4 Schematic drawing of spread of infection causing complications of mastoiditis.

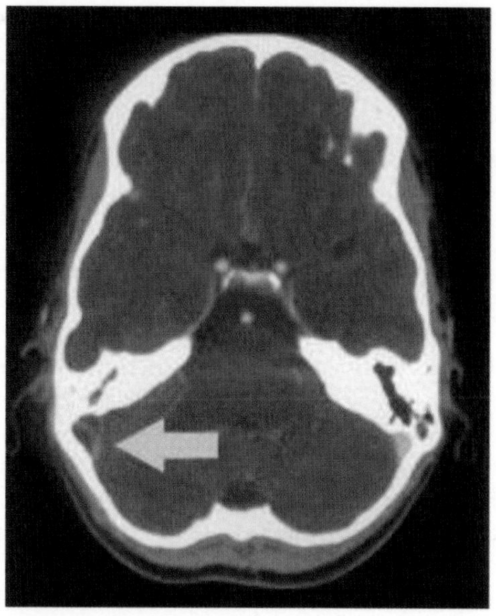

Figure 63.5 Axial CT with contrast; lateral sinus thrombosis marked by arrow.

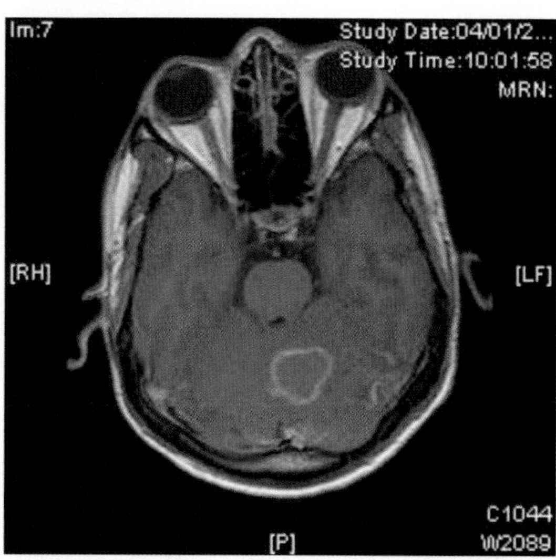

Figure 63.6 Axial CT with contrast showing brain abscess.

mastoid air cells, and an opaque mastoid and middle ear. It may also show overlying soft tissue thickening or a sub-periosteal abscess (see Figure 63.2). It can also show or exclude intracranial complications of extradural or subdural pus, venous thrombosis (Figure 63.5) or brain abscess (Figure 63.6). The so-called delta sign on CT or magnetic resonance imaging (MRI) with enhancement is the empty triangle of the thrombosed sigmoid/lateral venous sinus and its surrounding enhancement.

The advantage of CT over MRI scanning is that the images can be acquired very quickly, so scanning after a feed or under sedation is often possible and avoids the need for a general anaesthetic.

However, MRI scanning under general anaesthesia in younger children is helpful in cases of complicated mastoiditis because of its higher sensitivity for detection of extra-axial fluid collections and associated vascular problems. It can demonstrate intracranial abscess formation, extradural and subdural collections, adjacent cerebellar oedema (Figure 63.7) and propagation of venous thrombosis (Figure 63.8), better that CT alone. Magnetic resonance venography (MRV) imaging will best identify thromboses.

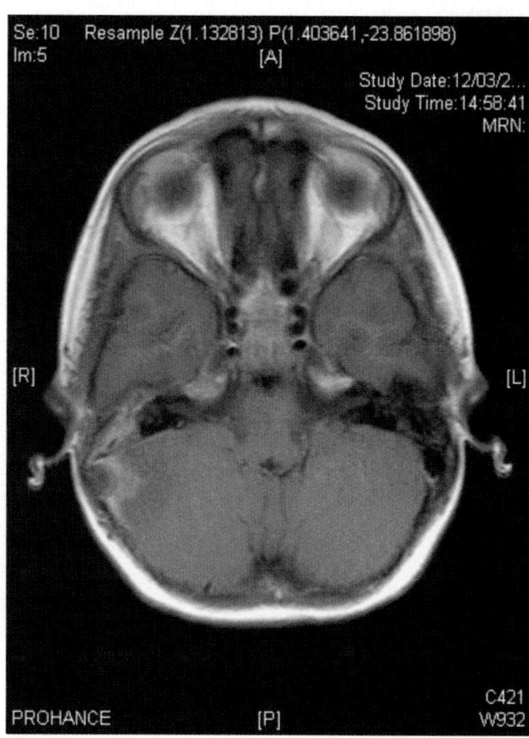

Figure 63.7 Axial MRI showing right lateral sinus thrombosis, subdural pus and adjacent cerebellar oedema with mastoiditis.

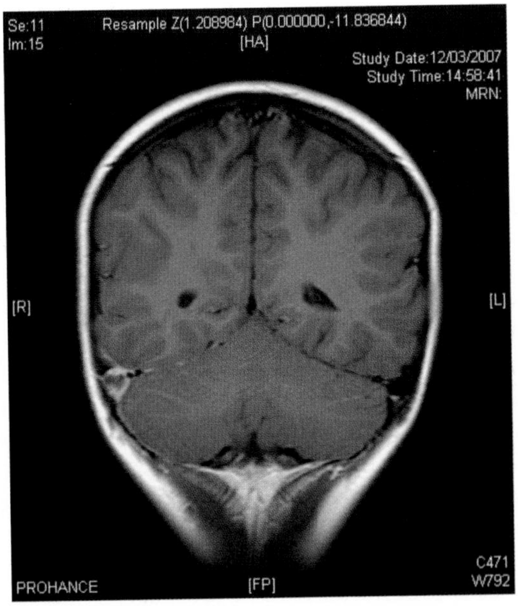

Figure 63.8 Coronal MRI with gadolinium contrast showing right lateral sinus thrombosis.

Audiometry

Clinical tests for hearing should be recorded. The child is often too young and too ill to allow behavioural audiometry for thresholds.

Lumbar puncture

If meningitis is suspected, the CT scan may be helpful, but a lumbar puncture (LP) to analyze the cerebrospinal fluid (CSF) and obtain microbiology gives the definitive diagnosis. This should be discussed with paediatricians (see discussion later in this chapter).

DIFFERENTIAL DIAGNOSES

These are the same as the differential diagnoses given earlier for AOM, but if there is post-aural or mastoid swelling, then differential diagnoses include an infected pre-auricular sinus, or infected or inflamed post-aural lymph node. Very rarely, conditions such as Langerhans cell histiocytosis or rhabdomyosarcoma of the ear have to be considered as causes of malaise with mastoid swelling and radiological opacity.

TREATMENT OF ACUTE MASTOIDITIS

The initial treatment of acute mastoiditis is with intravenous antibiotics as an inpatient. If the infection appears uncomplicated, without marked malaise and no subperiosteal abscess, then this conservative treatment is often sufficient and surgery is not required.

The first choice of intravenous antibiotics should be agreed locally but must cover the likely causative organisms, including *Streptococci* and *Staphylococcus aureus*. Either high-dose co-amoxiclav or a third-generation cephalosporin, such as ceftriaxone, is usually chosen. Because of resistant organisms, a third-generation cephalosporin alone might be insufficient and newer antibiotics may be required. For IgE-mediated penicillin-allergic patients (who may not be given cephalosporins), advice from the microbiologists is required, but clindamycin can be considered instead. If a *Pseudomonas* species is suspected, an antipseudomonal penicillin should be used.

If the child is recovering and the pyrexia has settled, then switching to oral antibiotics for a further 14 days is usually sufficient.

SURGERY FOR ACUTE MASTOIDITIS

Depending on the published series, between 10 and 60 per cent of admitted patients with acute mastoiditis require surgery. There is still some controversy about both the place for surgery in acute mastoiditis and extent or nature of surgery required. In general, if apparently simple, uncomplicated mastoiditis is slow to improve clinically after 48 hours on intravenous antibiotics, then surgical drainage is indicated. A continuing pyrexia, malaise and persistent post-aural erythema and soft tissue swelling are all signs that surgical drainage will be beneficial.

If there is a soft, boggy post-aural swelling from a subperiosteal abscess, drainage under general anaesthesia should be undertaken. Some would consider needle aspiration of the pus, and some a simple incision and drainage in the post-aural soft tissue, but the author prefers to recommend a formal cortical mastoidectomy to fully open the mastoid antrum and drain the infection. When this is undertaken, there is usually no need to insert a post-operative drain (which might lead to a discharging sinus).

Under the anaesthetic, myringotomy and drainage of the middle ear pus is worthwhile. Insertion of a ventilation tube can be undertaken, but it frequently blocks with dry blood or discharge and is not essential.

If the mastoiditis is considered complicated (i.e. to have spread further), then formal post-aural cortical mastoidectomy is required with extension of the surgery to adjacent areas as required to achieve complete open drainage of the infection. Where there is pus extradurally or around the sigmoid sinus, this should be exposed. If the venous sinus is involved, it may be thrombosed. Needling it and aspirating on a syringe may confirm this. If blood is drawn out, nothing more is done; if the sinus seems thrombosed without aspirate, it should not be opened. If pus is aspirated from within the sinus, it should be opened and drained out. In this latter case, however, there is very little likelihood of effective re-canalization for the sinus. If it is a dominant sinus, otitic hydrocephalus/benign intracranial hypertension can ensue. Preoperative scanning is therefore invaluable in these situations.

Technique for mastoidectomy

A post-aural skin incision is made and then the periosteum, if intact, is incised as an anterior based *U*-shaped flap to allow wide exposure of the surface of the mastoid bone. Drilling is commenced to open air cells over the area of any discharging pus, which can be followed towards the antrum. A wider exposure, making crescentic drilling, parallel to the posterior canal wall, rather than a 'pothole', is recommended. The mastoid antrum is sited over the MacEwen's triangle and is said to lie at a depth of 1 mm medial to the cortical bone for each year of life. It is frequently found higher (superior) than one would imagine. To avoid damage to the usually low-lying middle fossa dura, it is safer to expose and open it working upwards from mastoid air cells at a lower level – that is, from the level of the midpoint of the external canal. The extent of the surgery depends on whether there is peri-sinus or extradural pus or probable lateral venous sinus thrombosis. After full drainage of the pus, closure is undertaken without leaving a drain *in situ*.

Acute mastoiditis in the presence of cholesteatoma

Sometimes the child presenting with acute mastoiditis is noted to have an underlying congenital or acquired cholesteatoma. In this case the acute infection should be managed as described above and surgery initially limited to achieving drainage of pus from the mastoid system from a post-aural approach. This might include removal of a volume of cholesteatoma matrix from the mastoid antrum but not definitive surgery of the cholesteatoma. That is better achieved as a secondary tympano-mastoid exploration a few weeks later when the acute infection has been treated.

COMPLICATIONS OF ACUTE MASTOIDITIS

Table 63.5 lists many of the common complications of acute mastoiditis.

Table 63.5 Complications of acute mastoiditis

Facial palsy
Sensorineural (cochlear) hearing loss
Labyrinthitis
Petrositis (petrous apex infection) Gradenigo's syndrome
Zygomatic process abscess
Citelli's abscess
Medial soft tissue mastoid tip abscess (Bezold's abscess)
Thrombosis of the lateral or sigmoid venous sinus
Otitic hydrocephalus/*pseudotumour cerebri*
Lemierre syndrome
Peri-sinus abscess
Extradural abscess
Subdural abscess
Meningitis
Intracranial (cerebellar or cerebral) abscesses

Facial palsy

This was discussed earlier as a complication of AOM. The most likely cause is from middle ear infection in the presence of a dehiscent facial nerve in its horizontal tympanic segment. Insertion of a ventilation tube and simple cortical mastoidectomy is probably indicated in most cases, but facial nerve decompression in its entire course is not indicated. However, if there is a large erosive cholesteatoma as well, then the second genu or descending portion of the nerve may be damaged. In that case, mastoid surgery to explore or decompress the facial nerve is essential to optimize nerve recovery.

Labyrinthitis

This was discussed earlier as a complication of AOM. However, if there is a fistula to the inner ear from a coexisting cholesteatoma, surgery is essential.

Bezold's abscess

As listed in Table 63.2, this is an abscess in the soft tissue medially and below the mastoid tip, extending into the neck. It involves the sternocleidomastoid fascial sheath.

Citelli's abscess

This is also a spread of abscess infection into deep neck soft tissues, but via the posterior belly of the digastric muscle into the posterior triangle of the neck (high-level V region).

Zygomatic abscess

This is an abscess in the soft tissue at the root of the zygomatic process of the mastoid bone and can involve the upper part of the superficial parotid gland. If infection tracks more inferomedially to the sub-temporal region, it is a Luc's abscess.

Gradenigo's syndrome

This syndrome comprises a discharging ear, a VI cranial nerve (abducens) palsy and facial or retro-orbital pain. It results from spread of infection to the petrous apex and adjacent dura. It seems to occur in children 6 to 7 years old and requires imaging. Surgical drainage without loss of hearing is sometimes possible through a well-pneumatized bone, but usually the mainstay of treatment is prolonged intravenous antibiotics and more superficial conservative surgery.

Lateral sinus thrombosis/ thrombophlebitis

This is estimated to occur in 12 per cent of cases of complicated acute mastoiditis. The presentation is with headache, spiking fever, vomiting, possible torticollis, papilloedema or seizures. It needs to be diagnosed with imaging, a CT with contrast, or an MRI/MRV. A less invasive study is to undertake a high neck Doppler ultrasound to identify if there is good flow in the internal jugular vein at the skull base. If the dominant sinus is on the side of the infection and thomboses, then otitic hydrocephalus (pseudotumour cerebri)/benign intracranial hypertension (BIH) can ensue with headaches and risk of visual loss. Paediatric neurology and haematology opinions should be sought. Sometimes steroids and acetazolamide are required to lower the CSF pressure.[5] Anticoagulation therapy has been a topic of debate, but certainly in cases of retrograde propagation of the thrombus back along the lateral sinus or even to the straight sinus or cavernous sinus, and where there is raised CSF pressure, it is strongly indicated. Blood clot within the vein without pus should not be opened or evacuated surgically as the venous wall is friable, easily damaged and later re-canalization is far less likely.

Initially a low molecular weight heparin followed by warfarin for 6 months is one regimen; alternatively, a prolonged course of low molecular weight heparin injections is sometimes chosen.

Lemierre's syndrome

This represents the occurrence of liberated infected clots spreading as a distal thrombo-embolism,[6] typically to the lungs but possibly a more distant metastasis. The causative organism is usually *Fusobacterium necrophorum,* as it induces haemagglutinin-mediated platelet aggregation. The organism can be identified by anaerobic culture or 16s rDNA PCR sequencing.

Anticoagulation is probably indicated, although some consider the theoretical risk that this might increase the likelihood of clots breaking away and embolizing distally.

Extradural and peri-sinus abscess formation

This is suspected in the child who continues to spike a fever and remains unwell. There may be vomiting. The diagnosis is made at surgery, on CT scan with contrast or from MR scanning. Surgical drainage is undertaken by exposing the abscess as part of the mastoidectomy.

Meninigitis

Meningitis as an isolated complication of mastoiditis, as distinct from brain abscess is not especially common. Diagnosis can be difficult. The features are headache, vomiting, fever, irritability or lethargy, sensitivity to light and sometimes seizures and a rash. The signs in the infant are not as clear as in older children – neck stiffness and a positive Kernig sign might not be apparent. Definitive diagnosis is ideally on lumbar puncture, but if there is lateral sinus thrombosis and raised CSF pressure, this may be dangerous. CT and MRI scanning can assist, showing mild ventriculomegaly, sulcal effacement on CT and leptomeningeal enhancement on contrast MRI scanning. Management should involve the paediatric intensive care unit or paediatricians, and intravenous antibiotics are given.

Subdural empyaema

The ill, febrile vomiting child with mastoiditis requires imaging. Posterior fossa subdural pus with adjacent cerebellar oedema can be seen on MRI and less easily on CT scanning with contrast (Figure 63.7). The mastoid should be widely explored, including the infected dura, and neurosurgeons should be consulted.

Cerebellar and temporal lobe brain abscesses

The presentation is the same as that for the other complications of mastoiditis already described. The diagnosis needs to be confirmed with CT or MRI scanning. The latter is more sensitive. Posterior fossa cerebellar abscesses can be the result of direct spread from the dura and are then in continuity with extradural pus. Discussion with neurosurgery is helpful, but the experienced neurotologist or skull base surgeon can sometimes needle and drain the abscess directly, intraoperatively from the opened mastoid.

The abscess can also occur more distally from blood-borne spread and be located in the temporal lobe or hemispheres. In this case, neurosurgeons must be involved and drainage is via a separate burr hole.

Longer-term aftercare of complicated mastoiditis

All the complications of infection beyond the mastoid and intracranially that have been described will require a prolonged course of oral antibiotics after the child has recovered and is fit to discharge. A 6-week treatment on the appropriate antimicrobial in full treatment dosage is usually sufficient. Where anticoagulation is undertaken, a 6-month course is suggested, and even if there is no re-canalization of the lateral venous sinus after this time, it can be stopped.

The ear and mastoid will require outpatient review to assess for a dry ear with an intact eardrum, to exclude a missed cholesteatoma and to assess and mange any resultant hearing loss.

KEY DEFINITIONS

AOM the rapid onset of signs and symptoms of inflammation in the middle ear

ASOM acute suppurative otitis media

MacEwen's triangle also suprameatal triangle, a bony landmark and surface marking for the mastoid antrum, between the posterior wall of the external acoustic meatus and the posterior root of the zygomatic process

non-severe AOM AOM with the presence of mild otalgia and a temperature below 39°C

OME (otitis media with effusion) inflammation of the middle ear with liquid collected in the middle ear; the signs and symptoms of acute infection are absent

otitis externa an infection of the external auditory canal

otorrhea discharge from the ear

recurrent AOM three or more well-documented and separate AOM episodes in the preceding six months *or* four or more episodes in the preceding 12 months with at least one episode in the past six months

severe AOM AOM with the presence of moderate to severe otalgia *or* fever equal to or higher than 39°C

tympanogram measure of acoustic immittance (transfer of acoustic energy) of the ear as a function of ear canal air pressure

uncomplicated AOM AOM without otorrhea

KEY LEARNING POINTS

Acute otitis media:

- AOM is most common in the first year of life.
- It is infrequent in children older than 6 years of age.
- Only 30 per cent of AOM cases are viral.
- Antibiotics are given if:
  - under 6 months old.
  - 39°C, earache and red or bulging tympanic membrane.
  - uncomplicated but symptoms persist after 48–72 hours.
- 10 days of antibiotics are given if child is 5 years old or under.
- Amoxicillin/co-amoxiclav/clarithromycin can also be used.

Acute mastoiditis:

- Admit to hospital.
- Take ear swab, WCC and CRP.
- Commence intravenous antibiotics.
- Low threshold for CT scan with contrast of brain and mastoid.
- MRI scan head if suspect complicated mastoiditis.
- Surgery – cortical mastoidectomy if:
  - subperiosteal abscess.
  - failure to improve after 48 hours.
  - any complication of mastoiditis.

REFERENCES

1. Lieberthal AS, Carroll AE, Chonmaitree T, Ganiats TG, Hoberman A, Jackson MA, Joffe MD, Miller DT, Rosenfeld RM, Sevilla XD, Schwartz RH, Thomas PA, Tunkel DE. The diagnosis and management of acute otitis media. Clinical Practice Guideline, American Academy of Pediatrics. *Pediatrics*. 2013; 131(3): e964–e999 (doi: 10.1542/peds.2012-3488). Available from: http://pediatrics.aappublications.org/content/131/3/e964.long.
2. Hoberman A, Paradise JL, Rockette HE, Shaikh N, Wald ER, Kearney DH, Colborn DK, Kurs-Lasky M, Bhatnagar S, Haralam MA, Zoffel LM, Jenkins C, Pope MA, Balentine TL, Barbadora KA. Treatment of acute otitis media in children under 2 years of age. *New England Journal of Medicine*. 2011; 364: 105–15. doi: 10.1056/NEJMoa0912254.
3. Anthonsen K, Høstmark K, Hansen S, Andreasen K, Juhlin J, Homøe P, Caye-Thomasen P. Acute mastoiditis in children. A 10-year retrospective and validated multicenter study. *Pediatric Infectious Disease Journal*. 2013; 32(5): 436–40. Epub http://www.ncbi.nlm.nih.gov/pubmed/23380667, PMID:23380667.
4. Niv A, Nash M, Slovik Y, Fliss DM, Kaplan D, Leibovitz E, Katz A, Dagan R, Leiberman A. Acute mastoiditis in infancy: The "soroka" experience: 1990–2000. *International Journal of Pediatric Otorhinolaryngology*. 2004; 68(11): 1435–39. Accession Number 2004442097.
5. Sébire G, Tabarki B, Saunders DE, Leroy I, Liesner R, Saint-Marti C, Husson B, Williams AN, Wade A, Kirkham FJ. Cerebral venous sinus thrombosis in children: Risk factors, presentation, diagnosis and outcome. *Brain*. 2005; 128(3): 477–89.
6. Le Monnier AP, Jamet A, Carbonnelle E, Barthod G, Moumile K, Lesage F, Zahar R, Mannach Y, Berche P, Couloigner V. Fusobacterium necrophorum middle ear infections in children and related complications: Report of 25 cases and literature review. *Pediatric Infectious Disease Journal*. 2008; 27(7): 613–17.

64

Otitis media with effusion

MATT ROLLIN AND ANTONY A NARULA

Otitis media with effusion (OME) is chronic inflammation of the middle ear mucosa, and accumulation of mucus in the middle ear space, with no signs of infection. Both mucosal inflammatory change and mucus accumulation can potentially extend to involve the mastoid cells. The typical presentation is with hearing loss, possibly following an upper respiratory illness, with or without otalgia. The usual definition of 'chronic' in this context is 12 weeks.

The common term is *glue ear*, and several medical terms have now passed out of use, including *secretory otitis media*, *serous otitis media* and *chronic nonpurulent otitis media*, all of which were considered to lack sufficient precision.

The effusion that accumulates in this condition is similarly ambiguous: Surgically recovered middle ear fluid shows a full spectrum of viscosity, from serous to mucoid, dependent on its mucin content.

AETIOLOGY

The respiratory-type ciliated mucus-producing epithelium that lines the nasal cavity extends up the eustachian tube to the level of the anterior middle ear cavity, at which point it gives way to the flat, dry cuboidal mucosa, which lines the remainder of the middle ear and mastoid cavities. OME is characterized by chronic inflammation of both types of epithelium, and eventually by disorganized replacement of normal middle ear mucosa with thickened, pseudostratified de-ciliated epithelium, which is inefficient at moving secretions. This inefficiency, combined with inflammation of the submucosa, eventually results in retention of secretions within the middle ear space.

The current generally accepted theory of pathogenesis considers that the initial mucosal damage comes from a viral upper respiratory infection. If bacteria then secondarily infect stagnant secretions, acute suppurative otitis media is the result. Hypoxia is increasingly being seen as a necessary concomitant.

The incidence of pathogens isolated from middle ear fluid is greater in younger children, and in those suffering from frequent infections. *Streptococcus pneumoniae* and *Moraxella catarrhalis* (*Branhamella catarrhalis*) are the two most commonly isolated organisms, but a negative culture is much more common than either of these, and no study has ever reported isolating pathogens from an effusion present for 6 months or more.

There have been several other proposed theories of pathogenesis, including a role for allergy and irritation from cigarette smoke, but none of these has convincingly been shown to be important. The reported incidence of allergy in patients with OME varies between centres worldwide, but it has been independently shown not to be a risk factor for development of OME in children of any age.

Pharyngeal acid reflux has been widely demonstrated radiographically in children, and pepsin has been discovered in up to 80 per cent of middle ear effusions, but causation is not clear and this area remains under investigation.

EPIDEMIOLOGY

Combining prevalence data from several European studies gives a bimodal age-distribution, with peak prevalence of approximately 20 per cent at 2 years of age and a secondary peak (approximately 16 per cent) at around 5 years of age. It is worth noting that the first is approximately the age when most European children first attend nursery, and the second approximates to the age when most start school.

The association of these peaks of prevalence with bursts of new social interaction lends support to the theory that infection is an important factor causing initial damage to the upper respiratory mucosa. Furthermore, in temperate regions of the world, where upper respiratory illnesses are very much more common in cold, damp winter months, there is a strong association between prevalence of childhood OME and season, with approximately twice as many diagnoses in the winter as compared to the summer.

RISK FACTORS

The fact that there is no standard, universally applicable diagnostic test for OME has complicated the identification of standard risk factors by making several large studies incompatible. However, Table 64.1 shows risk factors for development of OME in children under 3 years of age from published multivariate analyses.

Other multivariate analyses have suggested that there is a doubling of risk from attendance at nursery or day care with four or more other children under 3.5 years of age. The possibility of a genetic component has been raised by a twin study, in which monozygotic twins showed significantly greater concordance in episodes of OME during the first 2 years of life than dizygotic twins.

Race and sex have not clearly been shown to be significant risk factors. There is currently no consensus in the literature on whether or not irritation from cigarette smoke is a significant risk factor for development of OME, but maternal smoking has been shown to be a risk factor for persistence of existing childhood effusions.

In one study of 2253 children, 91 per cent had suffered an episode of OME by the age of 2 years. A 2003 Cochrane review that posed the question of whether universal screening of young children for OME would be efficacious identified three suitable studies for inclusion, and concluded that it would not.

Table 64.1 Risk factors for development of OME in children under 3 years of age

Factor	Odds ratio
History of acute otitis media	1.7
Age	1.0 per month
Number of older siblings	1.6 per sibling
Family history of OME	1.4

DURATION AND RESOLUTION OF OME

In young children, the median duration of an episode of OME is approximately 3 months, but the distribution is highly skewed, with the 95th centile at 12 months. Prospective studies of large cohorts have shown that although half of affected ears resolve after 3 months, half of those will suffer a further episode of OME. Other work suggests that severely affected children tend to suffer in the form of multiple short episodes, rather than fewer, longer ones.

Episodes of OME in older children follow a similar pattern, with the majority resolving and a small but significant percentage of episodes proving persistent. One study of children between 5 and 8 years of age reported a resolution rate of 91 per cent at 1 year follow-up, and another study of 7-year-old children reported that only 12 per cent of episodes lasted longer than 6 months. Episodes of OME diagnosed in colder and wetter seasons tend to last longer than those diagnosed in warmer or drier seasons. Apart from this seasonal effect, risk factors for persistence of OME episodes are presence of upper respiratory illness, significant hearing loss and maternal smoking.

DIAGNOSIS

There is no formal and universally accepted diagnostic test. Diagnosis in secondary care will typically involve a combination of otoscopy, pneumatic otoscopy, tympanometry and pure-tone audiometry. A careful history of hearing loss and language development should be taken, eliciting other related symptoms such as snoring, blocked nose, respiratory illnesses, mouth-breathing and so on.

In primary care, diagnostic options are more limited, and more emphasis is placed on history and otoscopy. Parental report of a child's hearing ability has been shown – somewhat surprisingly – to be a poor discriminator. However, parental report of hearing loss in association with frequent upper respiratory illnesses, snoring and mouth breathing does make a diagnosis of OME more likely. Common sense would suggest that a schoolteacher, who has the ability to compare many children of a similar age, would be a more effective judge of an individual child's hearing ability; however, this has not been subjected to formal examination.

It must be stressed that all children in whom there is a suspicion of hearing loss must undergo formal hearing evaluation to exclude sensorineural hearing loss, which may require a hearing aid.

NATURAL OUTCOMES OF OME IN CHILDHOOD

Studies across many years and many different countries have shown that the great majority of middle ear effusions will resolve given enough time. The key question is therefore not whether this will happen, but rather what harm may be caused by the child's hearing loss in the meantime.

HEARING LOSS

Levels of hearing loss in bilateral OME vary between effusions and between children. In studies of children aged 2 to 11 years, mean pure-tone thresholds were 21 dBHL in the better-hearing ear, and 31 dBHL in the poorer-hearing ear (standard deviations 10 and 13, respectively). It has also been shown that viscosity of recovered middle ear fluid does not correlate with severity of hearing loss.

However, measurement of dBHL hearing thresholds using pure-tone audiometry is by definition performed under ideal conditions. These methods provide very accurate measurements of the thresholds of hearing but are only useful as far as they can predict 'real-world' hearing disability.

Such disability is better analyzed by questionnaires such as the Reported Hearing Disability (RHD) questionnaire. It contains nine questions answerable by adults in close contact with a child, four of which have been shown to predict hearing disability (Table 64.2).

Table 64.2 Questions to predict hearing disability

Question	Responses
How would you describe your child's hearing?	normal, slightly below normal, poor, very poor, not sure
Has he/she misheard words when not looking at you?	no, rarely, often, always, not sure
Has he/she had difficulty hearing when with a group of people?	no, rarely, often, always, not sure
Has he/she asked for things to be repeated?	no, rarely, often, always, not sure

A theoretical ideal measure would be able to make an objective direct assessment of hearing disability. 'Speech-in-noise' audiometry is a variant of speech audiometry occasionally used in adult practice, and it tests ability to recognize words in the presence of background noise. It provides a good objective measurement of 'real-world' hearing ability but is more difficult to administer in a child.

Evidence exists that there are long-term sequelae from effusions – or possibly from the infections and inflammatory response that precipitate them. In one cohort followed up until the age of 18, those suffering recurrent otitis media (without any differentiation between acute otitis media and OME) had a mean air-conduction hearing deficit of 4 dB, and a mean bone-conduction deficit of 2 dB, compared to unaffected individuals.

LANGUAGE AND INTELLECTUAL DEVELOPMENT

Language development in children is complex and incompletely understood, and therefore standard assessments use comparison against standardized milestones within acceptable time frames. Using these measures, prospective studies and meta-analyses have suggested that OME does have a deleterious impact on language development. There is a correlation between the number of days in early childhood spent with bilateral effusions and an adverse impact on speech production and language development. However these children have largely caught up with their unaffected peer group in terms of spoken language by the age of 8 years. It has not been determined how much this 'catch-up' effect relies on extra effort from parents and input from specialist therapeutic services, or whether it is a spontaneous phenomenon.

The effect of OME on cognition and intellectual development is harder to determine and quantify, and most investigations have studied early childhood development. Cohort studies have suggested that the effects of OME are concentrated during a child's early intellectual development – typically 3 to 4 years of age – and that mitigation of the delay occurs by the age of 8. None of the studies persisted beyond that age.

In contrast to this, however, the subtler effects of a mild delay in development appear to be much more persistent.

Evidence from a long-term birth-cohort study suggests that the OME-related deficit in IQ testing scores remains significant as far as 13 years of age, and that the OME-related deficit in reading ability remains significant as far as 18 years, with the worst cases of persistent bilateral OME in childhood showing a long-term 2-year delay in mean reading scores, compared to unaffected peers.

Furthermore, evidence from this cohort suggests that diagnosis and treatment at 5 years of age comes too late to prevent such effects on language development and reading ability.

Two questionnaires are commonly used to quantify a child's behaviour: the MRC Behaviour Questionnaire and the Rutter score. Studies have shown that significantly higher proportions of young children with bilateral persistent OME and mild hearing loss have abnormal behaviour scores, compared to their unaffected peer group.

Children with OME suffer significantly more clumsiness and balance problems than the general child population, both on parental report and after formalized assessment. It is possible that this phenomenon represents an effect of inflammation surrounding middle ear structures, but no formal investigation has been made.

MANAGEMENT OF OME

If the problem is not too severe, counselling and hearing tactics can be very helpful. Hearing tactics include the following:

- Get the child's attention before starting to talk.
- Reduce background noise as much as possible.
- Face the child directly, so that the child can see you speaking.
- Speak in a normal voice, as close to the child as possible.
- Avoid unusual volume, speed or emphasis.

If a child has only a mild hearing loss, these tactics may be all that are required to mitigate the disability while waiting to see if the effusion resolves. However, it is not clear how successful these tactics are when the affected child is the youngest of three – or indeed, the youngest in a class of 30.

No medical therapy has been adequately shown to be beneficial, including local steroids, systemic steroids, mucolytics, antibiotics and decongestants. Most investigations into the efficacy of these therapies have been weakened by poor methodology, and so meta-analyses have not so far been possible. Autoinflation of the middle ear can be helpful, but the procedure is not simple to perform, relies heavily on compliance and is not practical in young children.

Surgical treatment without ventilation tubes (i.e. myringotomy and aspiration of effusion only) is not effective. Ventilation tubes (VTs) designed for long-term placement are associated with higher complication rates; therefore, short-term designs are recommended for use in children.

The natural history of VTs has been investigated in many published studies from all regions of the world. Typical findings are that at 6-month follow-up, 55 per cent of short-term VTs are functioning, and anywhere from 30–55 per cent have extruded from the tympanic membrane.

Following published outcome analyses of surgical technique, it is generally recommended that ventilation tubes are placed in the antero-inferior tympanic membrane, via a radial or circumferential incision.

OUTCOMES OF INTERVENTIONS FOR OME

Children undergoing VT placement (without adenoidectomy) spend on average 32 per cent less time with effusions in the year following the procedure. VTs have been shown to improve hearing thresholds by approximately 10 dB at 6-month follow-up, after which the benefit over untreated children diminishes, possibly as the effusions in untreated children resolve and VTs begin to extrude.

A recent large multi-centre study, the Trial of Alternative Regimens in Glue Ear Treatment (TARGET), examined a cohort of 3831 children aged between 3 and 7 years with proven OME and 20 dB hearing loss bilaterally. Ventilation tubes conferred an improvement in hearing thresholds over non-surgical cases of 12 dB on average, for the first year after treatment. After this time, the differences between the two groups were negligible.

Although this benefit (as measured by pure tones) may seem modest, the effects are certainly measurable. Other studies have found that children with untreated 'mild' OME-related hearing loss were on average 3.2 months behind their surgically treated peers in their objective speech and language development at 9-month follow-up.

TARGET also compared VTs against VTs plus adjuvant adenoidectomy. This further procedure conferred no additional benefit after 3 or 6 months of follow-up; however, after both 12 and 24 months of follow-up, when the benefit of VTs alone had diminished, adenoidectomy provided an additional 4.2 dB of hearing benefit, and significantly reduced the requirement for revision surgery.

The Reported Hearing Disability questionnaire was also included in the study, and there was a large difference on this measure between VTs and non-surgical management, even when the results were statistically adjusted to take account of the 'expectation effect' that parents experience with surgery. As might be expected, the additional benefit of surgery on hearing disability was more modest when measured over the 2 years following surgery; however, parental report of children's hearing ability showed continued benefit of VTs well into the second year of observation, even when there was ostensibly no further benefit as measured by pure-tone thresholds.

It seems that although the absolute improvement in pure-tone thresholds conferred by ventilation tubes is modest by the standards of adult audiology, it is sufficient to produce a major improvement in hearing disability scores. Possibly this may represent the difference between 'real-world' and idealized measures of a child's hearing ability and language development. Or possibly a 10–12 dB hearing improvement has a more significant impact at this young age than a similar improvement would have at 18 years of age, when patterns of language reception and production are firmly established.

It is an accepted principle that children with early language delay are at risk for later low intelligence scores, poor reading attainment and behavioural difficulties. Children suffering with OME in early childhood are disadvantaged in their language development and schooling, and at risk of falling behind. The disadvantages arising from under-treated OME linger well into the teens, secondary education and the threshold of working life.

SUMMARY

- Otitis media with effusion (OME) is chronic inflammation of the middle ear mucosa, and accumulation of mucus in the middle ear space, with no signs of infection.
- The great majority of episodes will resolve spontaneously, given time. The key challenge is to identify and intervene on those which do not.
- Both hearing deficit and improvement with treatment may be mild as measured with pure-tone audiometry, yet have a dramatic impact on a child's development.
- Both untreated effusions and surgery can have long-term consequences on hearing ability and educational attainment.
- Mild cases can be successfully managed with hearing tactics and extra effort; surgery is an effective treatment for selected cases.

KEY DEFINITIONS

AET artificial eustachian tube, an alternative term for ventilation tube

glue ear otitis media with effusion

grommet alternative term for ventilation tube

OME otitis media with effusion

TARGET Trial of Alternative Regimens in Glue Ear Treatment, a recent multi-centre trial

ventilation tube a cannulated plastic tube, placed into the tympanic membrane to allow equalization of pressure in the middle ear cleft

KEY LEARNING POINTS

- Aetiology is thought to be an initial infective insult causing disorganized epithelial metaplasia.
- Risk factors include history of middle ear infection, family history, number of siblings and attendance at day-care nursery. Maternal smoking is a risk factor for persistence of OME.
- All children with a suspicion of hearing loss *must* have a formal evaluation of hearing to diagnose the small number with a sensorineural loss who require a hearing aid.
- Level of hearing deficit on pure-tone audiometry does not necessarily predict real-world hearing ability. In this context audiometry alone is a poor surrogate for disability.
- Adjuvant adenoidectomy with VT placement may confer additional benefit in children older than 3.5 years.

FURTHER READING

Bennett KE, Haggard MP, Silva PA, Stewart IA. Behaviour and developmental effects of otitis media with effusion into the teens. *Archives of Disease in Childhood*. 2001; 85: 91–95.

Maw R, Wilks J, Harvey I, Peters TJ, Golding J. Early surgery compared with watchful waiting for glue ear and effect on language development in preschool children: A randomized trial. *Lancet*. 1999 Mar 20; 353(9157): 960–63.

McGee R, Prior M, Willams S, Smart D, Sanson AJ. The long-term significance of teacher-rated hyperactivity and reading ability in childhood: Findings from two longitudinal studies. *Child Psychology and Psychiatry*. 2002 Nov; 43(8): 1004–17.

MRC Multicentre Otitis Media Study Group. Adjuvant adenoidectomy in persistent bilateral otitis media with effusion: Hearing and revision surgery outcomes through 2 years in the TARGET randomized trial. *Clinical Otolaryngology*. 2012 Apr; 37(2): 107–16.

MRC Multicentre Otitis Media Study Group. Surgery for persistent otitis media with effusion: Generalizability of results from the UK trial (TARGET). Trial of Alternative Regimens in Glue Ear Treatment. *Clinical Otolaryngology and Allied Sciences*. 2001 Oct; 26(5): 417–24.

Roberts JE, Rosenfeld RM, Zeisel SA. Otitis media and speech and language: A meta-analysis of prospective studies. *Pediatrics*. 2004 Mar; 113(3 Pt 1): e238–48.

Rovers MM, Black N, Browning GG, Maw R, Zielhuis GA, Haggard MP. Grommets in otitis media with effusion: An individual patient data meta-analysis. *Archives of Disease in Childhood*. 2005 May; 90(5):480–85.

Tos M. Pathogenesis and pathology of chronic secretory otitis media. *Annals of Otology, Rhinology and Laryngology Suppl*. 1980 May–Jun; 89(3 Pt 2): 91–97.

65

Chronic otitis media

C MARTIN BAILEY

INTRODUCTION

Chronic otitis media is a chronic inflammation of the mucosa and submucosa of the middle ear cleft, which may cause damage to the tympanic membrane and ossicles. Chapter 44 covers this condition as it relates to adult practice; the purpose of this chapter is to highlight specific issues relevant to children.

CHRONIC SUPPURATIVE OTITIS MEDIA: PERSISTENT TYMPANIC MEMBRANE PERFORATION

In chronic suppurative otitis media (CSOM) there is by definition a perforation of the tympanic membrane, which has been prevented from healing by chronic inflammation and has persisted for more than 3 months, with a history of discharge for at least 6 weeks. In children this most commonly follows an episode of acute otitis media (AOM) with discharge.

HISTORY AND EXAMINATION

The cardinal symptoms of CSOM are otorrhoea (which may be intermittent or continuous) and hearing loss (which is usually mild unless there is associated ossicular erosion). These symptoms are shared with cholesteatoma, so the most important aspect of examination is to visualize the tympanic membrane.

The tympanic membrane may be obscured by discharge, and to obtain a clear view this must be cleared by mopping and a course of antibiotic ear drops. If this fails to afford a good view, then the ear should be examined under anaesthesia, as outpatient microsuction is not well tolerated by young children, and the opportunity should be taken to thoroughly irrigate the ear with saline and then quinolone antibiotic drops.

INVESTIGATIONS

A swab of the discharge should be sent for microbiology to guide topical antibiotic therapy, especially if the otorrhoea proves refractory to treatment. Age-appropriate audiometry should be undertaken when the ear is dry, ideally a pure-tone audiogram with masked bone conduction. This gives a measure of hearing disability, indicates the possibility of associated ossicular discontinuity if the air–bone gap is large, and provides a baseline prior to any surgical intervention.

TREATMENT

The initial goal is to render the ear dry, which may well result in almost complete loss of symptoms and enable tympanic membrane repair to be deferred (especially if the child is very young). Careful precautions should be taken to prevent ingress of water during hair-washing and swimming by use of silicone putty ear plugs (combined with a neoprene headband for swimming). In some children recurrent discharge can only be prevented by avoiding swimming altogether, but this does present a safety hazard if the child is consequently unable to learn to swim.

Nevertheless, young children are prone to recurrent discharge through a perforated tympanic membrane, especially in association with colds, and occasional courses of medical treatment will be required. Topical antibiotic therapy is more successful than systemic antibiotic treatment, and quinolone ear drops are preferable to aminoglycoside drops because they are more effective and carry no risk of ototoxicity.[1,2]

Frequent otorrhoea can remain a problem in some children, especially at a young age, and other measures may need to be considered. Immune function tests are seldom helpful (unless there is other evidence to suggest an immunodeficiency). Adenoidectomy may be beneficial in some children by improving eustachian tube function and removing a focus of recurrent infection with colds.

Tympanic membrane repair (myringoplasty)

Spontaneous healing of chronic tympanic membrane perforations in children is uncommon, especially if present for more than 2 years. Myringoplasty using a temporalis fascia graft may be undertaken with a high closure rate in adults, but the failure rate is greater in children. Furthermore, children are more liable than adults to develop otitis media with effusion (OME) postoperatively, and to suffer from AOM with the risk of re-perforation. Meta-analysis of published outcomes has shown that success increases with age from 6 to 13 years,[3] although subsequent papers have claimed that cartilage reinforcement of the temporalis fascia graft can prevent this higher rate of graft failure in younger children.

There is thus a compromise to be struck between the morbidity incurred by leaving the perforation open, and the increased rate of success as the child grows older. In unilateral perforations the other ear can provide some guidance, and myringoplasty should not generally be attempted unless the contralateral ear is healthy and well-ventilated.

Occasionally, despite all efforts an ear will continue to discharge. In this situation it may be necessary to undertake a myringoplasty with cortical mastoidectomy under antibiotic cover, preceded by an intensive period of medical treatment in an effort to render the ear dry at the time of surgery.

TYMPANIC MEMBRANE ATROPHY AND RETRACTION POCKETS

Loss of the middle fibrous layer of the tympanic membrane results in a flimsy, atrophic 'dimeric membrane' that is liable to retraction if there is a negative middle ear pressure.

Children are particularly prone to generalized tympanic membrane atrophy and retraction (sometimes termed *atelectasis*) as a sequel to long-standing otitis media with effusion, and to localized atrophy and retraction at the site of grommet insertion for OME. Of particular concern is that there is a definite relationship with subsequent development of cholesteatoma, especially where the atrophy and retraction involves the posterosuperior quadrant of the tympanic membrane. In some cases retraction onto the ossicular chain can result in erosion, initially of the lenticular process of the incus, but sometimes progressing to erosion of the incus long process and the stapes superstructure. Some retraction pockets progress while some remain stable, and only an extended period of active monitoring will distinguish between them. Various classifications have been devised to aid surveillance of retraction pockets, of which the most well-known and widely used is that of Sadé.[4] Children's eustachian tube function can be expected to improve with increasing age, but while this may stabilize retraction, it cannot reverse atrophic change or ossicular damage.

HISTORY, EXAMINATION AND INVESTIGATIONS

Pars tensa atrophy and retraction may cause minimal symptoms, unless there is underlying OME or associated infection. Hearing loss is slight unless there is significant ossicular erosion. Pneumatic otoscopy will permit assessment of the tympanic membrane and categorization according to Sadé's classification, and serial audiometry is an important part of follow-up.

TREATMENT

Because some retraction pockets stabilize, and either do not progress or revert to normal, surgical treatment may not be required. However, it is impossible to reliably predict which pockets will progress and which will not. There is therefore controversy as to whether it is better to operate early to prevent disease developing, or to watch and wait until it is clear that disease is progressing, by which time the surgery will be more difficult.

Grommet insertion will temporarily re-ventilate the middle ear, but may not influence progression of tympanic membrane retraction in the long term. Furthermore, a grommet may induce further atrophic change, the tube may not be retained by the flimsy tympanic membrane for very long and there is an increased risk of residual perforation following grommet extrusion.

Simple permeatal excision of a retraction pocket can result in spontaneous healing of the tympanic membrane with resolution of the pathology, and is an attractively minor procedure.

Alternatively, the pocket may be excised and the tympanic membrane repaired by grafting, often using cartilage reinforcement in an effort to prevent further retraction, but this is a more major undertaking and a second-look procedure will be required if there is suspicion that any squamous epithelium may have been left behind in the middle ear.

Unfortunately, evidence is lacking as to which of these procedures ultimately offers the best results. However, whatever management approach is taken, there is no doubt that long-term follow-up is required.

ATTIC RETRACTION POCKETS

Attic retraction pockets, which arise in the pars flaccida of the tympanic membrane and may be very small, are liable to develop into cholesteatoma and so should be regarded with the greatest suspicion. An attic crust or polyp often obscures an underlying attic cholesteatoma, and in children an examination under anaesthesia is usually necessary to establish the diagnosis.

CHOLESTEATOMA

Cholesteatoma is the accumulation of keratin in the middle ear cleft following ingress of keratinizing squamous epithelium. It may be congenital or acquired.

CONGENITAL CHOLESTEATOMA

Congenital cholesteatoma develops as an epidermal cyst behind an intact tympanic membrane from an epithelial cell rest in the middle ear (the so-called epidermoid formation). It accounts for 4–24 per cent of cholesteatomas in children: most (77 per cent) arise on the promontory anterosuperiorly, but some (22 per cent) are located posterosuperiorly, and they take the form of keratin 'pearls' with an intact surrounding matrix.[5] To be classified as a congenital cholesteatoma, there must be a white mass medial to a normal, intact tympanic membrane, with no previous history of ear discharge, perforation or otological surgery.[6]

Congenital cholesteatoma presents most frequently at around the age of 5 years. Most small congenital cholesteatomas are incidental findings at otoscopy, or are found at grommet insertion for OME. However, a large congenital cholesteatoma may present with hearing loss, and if the matrix ruptures into the middle ear or through the tympanic membrane, then it will behave in the same way as an acquired cholesteatoma.

ACQUIRED CHOLESTEATOMA

The aetiology of acquired cholesteatoma is discussed in Chapter 44. Presentation is typically later than for congenital cholesteatoma, often at around the age of 10 years. There are important differences between cholesteatoma in children and in adults: In children the incidence is higher, there is a greater rate of pars tensa cholesteatoma, it behaves more aggressively in the child's more pneumatized mastoid and spreads more readily to the extremes of the middle ear cleft, there is a higher rate of recurrence after treatment and there is a higher risk of complications.

HISTORY, EXAMINATION AND INVESTIGATIONS

Congenital cholesteatoma may be an incidental finding at otoscopy or may present with hearing loss. Acquired cholesteatoma may likewise present with hearing loss, but more typically in children there is secondary infection with persistent or recurrent offensive discharge that obscures the otoscopic view of both the tympanic membrane and the underlying disease. Young children do not tolerate outpatient microsuction well, finding the sensation and the noise alarming, and it is best to proceed directly to an examination under anaesthesia: a microbiology swab can be taken for culture and sensitivity, careful microsuction allows a thorough assessment of the disease and topical antibiotic therapy with drops may then render the ear dry prior to definitive surgery (which is appreciated by the patient, but also makes the surgery easier and improves surgical outcomes).

Age-appropriate audiometry must be undertaken to show the baseline hearing preoperatively; ideally a pure-tone audiogram with air conduction and masked bone conduction. A large air–bone gap may indicate ossicular discontinuity, but sometimes cholesteatoma can bridge the gap between the eroded ossicles and maintain surprisingly good sound transmission (which is then worse postoperatively, after the disease has been removed).

A computed tomography (CT) scan is mandatory to show the anatomy and degree of pneumatization (which may influence the surgical approach), and to assess bone erosion, which will give an indication of the extent of disease (which may occasionally reach as far as the petrous apex), as well as the degree of damage to middle ear structures (ossicles, horizontal semi-circular canal, tegmen and facial nerve canal). The scan may require a general anaesthetic in young children.

TREATMENT

Treatment consists of surgical removal of the cholesteatoma, to achieve a 'safe' ear free from risk of complications, to prevent further cholesteatoma from developing, to give the patient a dry and trouble-free ear and if possible to improve the hearing.

The range of surgical techniques for removal of cholesteatoma is more fully discussed in Chapter 44. Small, intact congenital cholesteatomas may be removed by tympanotomy, for which an endaural incision is recommended as it allows good access without a speculum, with elevation of a posterior, superior or anterior tympanomeatal flap as appropriate.

Small or localized acquired cholesteatomas may sometimes be managed by limited surgery, but this is seldom appropriate in children. Occasionally, a cholesteatoma arising from the posterosuperior pars tensa may be locally excised, with repair and reinforcement of the tympanic membrane defect. Infrequently, it may be possible to remove a small attic cholesteatoma by means of an atticotomy, with or without repair of the scutum defect.

However, for extensive cholesteatoma a mastoidectomy is required, using either an 'open' technique (a 'canal wall down' or 'modified radical' mastoidectomy), or a 'closed' technique (a 'canal wall up' or 'combined approach' tympanomastoidectomy). There are enthusiastic proponents of both techniques, the advantages and disadvantages of which have been discussed in Chapter 44, but in fact the surgeon should be able to tailor the surgery to the needs of the individual patient and use either technique as the situation demands. A post-aural transmastoid approach gives greatest flexibility, as it allows for either an open or a closed technique depending upon the operative findings. A canal wall up procedure is done where possible, if the mastoid bone is cellular and the disease is limited; but a canal wall down procedure can be done when necessary, if the mastoid bone is sclerotic (especially if there is a forward sigmoid sinus or low dura), if the disease is extensive or if there are poor prospects for follow-up.

Canal wall up technique

For this technique to be successful, it is essential to have good exposure of the disease. A widely bevelled transmastoid approach is employed, with a 'superior tympanotomy' to extend the cortical mastoidectomy anteriorly and open the attic above the intact canal wall. A generous 'posterior tympanotomy' is created to open the facial recess, following which removal of the incus and malleus head should permit meticulous removal of all cholesteatoma. The incus may be 'banked' in the mastoid for future use in an ossicular reconstruction.

A 'second-look' re-exploration should be undertaken after 9–12 months to ensure that there is no residual or recurrent cholesteatoma. This interval is intended to be long enough to allow any cholesteatoma to grow large enough to be easily found, but not so long that it becomes extensive and difficult to remove. It is a shorter interval than is typically employed in adults, because cholesteatoma re-accumulates faster in children.

New techniques include use of the KTP laser to vapourize adherent cholesteatoma, and this can result in a 10 times lower rate of residual disease.[7]

Diffusion-weighted magnetic resonance imaging (MRI) has been used to identify residual or recurrent cholesteatoma but is not yet able to reliably replace second-look surgery. An endoscopic second-look has been used successfully in adults, but is difficult in children because of the speed at which the mastoid cortex regrows.

Canal wall down technique

In this technique a similar widely bevelled transmastoid approach is used, following which the posterior canal wall is taken down, the incus and malleus head are removed and the cholesteatoma meticulously dissected out. To achieve a stable, dry and trouble-free ear, it is essential to lower the facial ridge and create a round cavity that is as small as possible, to graft the tympanic membrane remnant and line the cavity with a generous temporalis fascia graft, and to fashion a large meatoplasty that is in proportion to the size of the cavity. In children it is recommended to change the bismuth, iodoform and paraffin paste (BIPP) pack under general anaesthesia as a day case 3 weeks later, which allows an opportunity to clean the cavity and cauterize any meatal granulations with silver nitrate. The second (looser) pack can then be removed 3 weeks after that in the outpatient clinic.

Techniques to reduce cavity size include bevelling the edges to allow soft-tissue blunting, and removal of the mastoid tip to allow soft tissue to fall in. Obliteration of the cavity carries the risk of trapping and hiding residual cholesteatoma, but if the risk of residual disease is low, then obliteration can be achieved by a variety of methods such as soft-tissue flaps, bone pate or hydroxyapatite. Conchal cartilage (removed in creation of the meatoplasty) covered with a musculo-periosteal flap can work well in older children in whom the piece of cartilage is sufficiently large. Alternatively, the wall of the external auditory meatus can be reconstructed, usually using bone or cartilage, although this is a technically demanding technique.

There are several potential causes of failure to achieve a trouble-free cavity: in particular, residual cholesteatoma; a high facial ridge (resulting in a bean-shaped cavity); a perforation with consequently open middle ear and eustachian tube; an inadequate meatoplasty; a cavity that is too large (commonly because of a cellular mastoid bone); and inadequately intensive post-operative care.

Residual disease

The risk of residual cholesteatoma is increased if there is erosion of the ossicular chain, if there is cholesteatoma in the posterior mesotympanum (especially the sinus tympani and facial recess), if the middle ear mucosa is inflamed and if the operator is inexperienced. The incidence of both residual and recurrent disease is higher for canal wall up than canal wall down procedures.

Ossicular reconstruction

Cholesteatoma may cause erosion of any of the ossicles, but most commonly the long process of the incus is eroded, sometimes with loss of the stapes superstructure as well. If the stapes crura are missing, then successful hearing reconstruction is much more difficult.

In the canal wall up technique, ossicular reconstruction should be deferred until the second-look procedure. If the ear is free of cholesteatoma, then an ossiculoplasty may be performed, typically using the previously 'banked' incus or a titanium prosthesis. For canal wall down surgery, ossiculoplasty may be undertaken at the primary operation if feasible, using the incus if available or else a titanium prosthesis.

The results of ossicular reconstruction are highly dependent upon the expertise of the surgeon.

COMPLICATIONS OF CSOM

Complications of CSOM in children are uncommon, but are serious and potentially life-threatening. Youngs[8] has usefully classified them into those within the temporal bone (facial nerve palsy, suppurative labyrinthitis, labyrinthine fistula, acute mastoiditis, subperiosteal abscess, postauricular fistula, petrositis) and those within the cranial cavity (extradural abscess, subdural abscess, sigmoid sinus thrombophlebitis, meningitis, cerebral abscess, otitic hydrocephalus).

Treatment is with antibiotic therapy, mastoid surgery and neurosurgical intervention as required. The most common complication in childhood is acute mastoiditis, which often can be treated successfully with intravenous antibiotics alone, supplemented by myringotomy and grommet insertion if necessary, with cortical mastoidectomy held in reserve for those cases which fail to respond. A subperiosteal abscess may be managed in most cases by incision and drainage of the abscess under antibiotic cover together with myringotomy and grommet insertion, again holding cortical mastoidectomy in reserve.

KEY DEFINITIONS

cholesteatoma an accumulation of keratin in the middle ear cleft following ingress of keratinizing squamous epithelium

chronic otitis media chronic inflammation of the mucosa and submucosa of the middle ear cleft

chronic suppurative otitis media (CSOM) chronic otitis media that has produced a chronic tympanic membrane perforation (present for more than 3 months) with at least 6 weeks of otorrhoea

myringoplasty surgical repair of the tympanic membrane

ossiculoplasty surgical reconstruction of the ossicular chain

KEY LEARNING POINTS

- Chronic otitis media is more aggressive and unrelenting in children than in adults.
- The success rate for myringoplasty in children increases with age.
- Pars tensa atrophy is more common in children than in adults.
- Cholesteatoma in children is more aggressive than in adults, tends to spread more widely, and has a higher rate of recurrence and incidence of complications.

- Myringoplasty, ossiculoplasty and mastoid surgery for cholesteatoma are all difficult, and successful outcomes are therefore highly dependent upon the expertise of the surgeon.

REFERENCES

1. Acuin J, Smith A, Mackenzie I. 2003. Interventions for chronic suppurative otitis media (Cochrane Review). *The Cochrane Library*. CD000473.
2. Couzos S, Lea T, Mueller R, Murray R, Culbong M. Effectiveness of ototopical antibiotics for chronic otitis media in Aboriginal children: A community-based, multicentre, double-blind randomised controlled trial. *Medical Journal of Australia*. 2003; 179: 185–90.
3. Vrabec JT, Deskin RW, Grady JJ. Meta-analysis of pediatric tympanoplasty. *Archives of Otolaryngology – Head and Neck Surgery*. 1999; 125: 530–4.
4. Sadé J, Avraham S, Brown M. Atelectasis, retraction pockets and cholesteatoma. *Acta Otolaryngolica*. 1981; 92: 501–12.
5. Kazahaya K, Potsic WP. Congenital cholesteatoma. *Current Opinion in Otolaryngology and Head and Neck Surgery*. 2004; 12(5): 398–403.
6. Derlacki EL, Clemis JD. Congenital cholesteatoma of the middle ear and mastoid. *Annals of Otology, Rhinology and Laryngology*. 1965; 74: 706–27.
7. Hamilton JW. Efficacy of the KTP laser in the treatment of middle ear cholesteatoma. *Otology and Neurotology*. 2005; 26(2): 135–9.
8. Youngs R. *Complications of Suppurative Otitis Media*. In *Diseases of the Ear*. Eds. Ludman H, Wright A. London: Arnold, 1998: 398–415.

FURTHER READING

Hamilton J. *Chronic Otitis Media*. In: *Pediatric ENT*. Eds. Graham JM, Scadding GK, Bull PD. Berlin: Springer, 2007: 421–40.

Hamilton J. *Chronic Otitis Media in Childhood*. In: *Scott-Brown's Otorhinolaryngology, Head and Neck Surgery*. Eds. Gleeson M, Clarke R. London: Hodder Arnold, 2008: 928–64.

Niparko JK (ed.). *Middle Ear, Mastoid, and Temporal Bone*. In: *Cummings Otolaryngology Head & Neck Surgery*. Ed. Flint PW, et al. Vol. 2, Part 7, Section 4. Philadelphia: Mosby Elsevier, 2010: 1963–2016.

66

Balance disorders in children

KATHERINE HARROP-GRIFFITHS

Balance is a complex function comprising the awareness of orientation in space and the ability to control stance, movement and visual stability. It requires central integration of input from the vestibular system, vision and proprioception moderated by previous learnt experience with output through control of muscles (ocular and skeletal) and joints.

The ability to balance well is essential for normal child development. Not only is it a prerequisite for normal locomotor development as evidenced by a child's ability to sit, walk and run, but it is also important for normal learning, social integration and independence.

DEVELOPMENT OF BALANCE IN CHILDREN

The vestibular system is the first sensory system to develop and is fully functional by 32 weeks' gestation. However, central connections are immature at birth and require input from vision and gravity as well as experience and feedback in order to mature. Maturation of the vestibular system occurs throughout childhood and is evidenced by the locomotor milestones of childhood and increasing stability with age.

SYMPTOMS

Vertigo is usually defined as a sensation of rotation or movement. The term *dizziness* can refer to light-headedness or vertigo, and it can be difficult to distinguish between the two, particularly in children. Pathology of the vestibular system will give rise to vertigo if it is acute or changing. Where pathology is fixed and significant, it can lead to chronic imbalance.

EPIDEMIOLOGY

Vertigo in children is common. Epidemiological studies have shown that between 5.7 and 8 per cent[1,2] of children experience vertigo/dizziness, with 2–3 per cent having to stop their activity because of the severity of the episode.

Imbalance is more difficult to quantify because of the many causes. Studies of the deaf population have found that between 30 per cent and 40 per cent of the severe to profoundly deaf population have significant vestibular hypofunction or 'areflexia'.

CLINICAL APPROACH

The physiology of the vestibular system is the same in children and adults, and pathology has similarities. The main differences are in children's ability to describe their symptoms, their compliance with examination and testing, and interpretation of the test results, which themselves are affected by maturation and attention. Examination must include a full neurological examination and assessment of development, as well as a detailed examination of the ears, head and neck, and eye movements (Table 66.1). Testing is as for adults with allowance made for maturation and compliance. Normative data is not readily available.

Magnetic resonance imaging (MRI) is a valuable investigation in cases where there is hearing loss accompanying the presentation or where the child has central neurological signs or significant recent onset headache.[3] However, it is mostly unnecessary in cases of vertigo in children; a good history and thorough neurological examination are of more diagnostic worth.

Computed tomography (CT) scan is used to identify bony abnormalities and is of value in cases of trauma where fractures are likely, or when a perilymph fistula or dehiscence of the superior semicircular canal is suspected.

Table 66.1 Investigations

Audiological
Behavioural tests of hearing, e.g. VRA, PTA (routine)
Tympanometry (routine)
Stapedial reflexes – ipsi and contralateral (if indicated)
OAE with OAE suppression (if indicated)
ABR for latencies (if indicated)
Blood – rarely needed
Genetic tests (only if indicated)
FBC, TFTs (only if indicated)
Autoimmune profile (only if indicated)
Serology for CMV, *Borrelia* (only if indicated)
Other
Electrocardiography (ECG) (only if indicated)
Electroencephalography (EEG) (only if indicated)
Imaging (see text)
MRI (only if indicated)
CT scan (only if indicated)

CAUSES OF BALANCE DISORDER

There are many causes of dizziness and imbalance in children, and the following will dwell only on the more common or important of these. Division into central and peripheral is dependent on the site of pathology; migraine presents as a peripheral pattern with discrete episodes of rotatory vertigo although the pathology is central.

PERIPHERAL VESTIBULAR DISORDERS

Peripheral vestibular disorders are listed in Table 66.2.

MIDDLE EAR DISORDERS

Otitis media with effusion (OME) is commonly (about 50 per cent of cases)[4] associated with poor balance and can present with dizziness or vertigo. Increased sway is found on posturography, and grommet insertion has been found to lead to a significant improvement in sway. Imbalance or delayed motor milestones with OME is considered by some as an indication for grommet insertion.

Cholesteatoma can lead to erosion of the lateral semicircular canal in about 10 per cent of cases. The symptoms of vertigo are exacerbated by exertion because of the effect of fistula formation. Otorrhoea is common. Hearing loss is usually conductive, but with erosion a sensorineural element is superimposed and can be progressive. Treatment is surgical.

INNER EAR DISORDERS

Congenital with inner ear dysplasia

Malformation of the inner ear, especially where the vestibule or semicircular canals are affected, can be associated with vestibular hypofunction. The usual cause is genetic, although rarely acquired causes such as thalidomide and congenital rubella can lead to structural abnormalities of the labyrinth. Examples include:

- **Dysplastic semicircular canals.**
- **Absent semicircular canals.**
    - CHARGE association (Coloboma, Heart defects, choanal Atresia, growth

Table 66.2 Peripheral vestibular disorders

- Middle ear pathology
    - OME (v/d/i +HL)
    - Cholesteatoma (v, +HL)
- Inner ear pathology
    - Genetic
        - With labyrinthine dysmorphology, e.g. WVA (v/i, +HL)
        - With normal labyrinthine morphology (i, +HL)
    - Infective
        - Congenital, e.g. CMV, rubella, syphilis (v/i +HL)
        - Acquired
            - Meningitis (v/i, +HL)
            - Viral labyrinthitis (v, +HL)
            - Vestibular neuronitis (v, –HL)
            - BPPV (v, –HL)
            - Other: Lyme disease (v, +HL)
    - Traumatic
        - Direct trauma, factures, barotrauma, iatrogenic trauma (v/i, +HL)
        - Perilymph fistula (v, +HL)
            - Vascular, e.g. sickle cell disease (v, +HL)
            - Ototoxic – drugs (v/i, +HL)
            - Autoimmune, e.g. Cogan's syndrome (v/i, +HL)
            - Neoplastic, e.g. vestibular schwannoma (i, +HL)
            - Dehiscence of the superior semicircular canal (v, –HL)
            - Unknown aetiology, e.g. Ménière's disease (v, +HL)

d = dizziness, v = vertigo, i = imbalance, +/–HL = with/without hearing loss.

  Retardation, Genital abnormalities and Ear deformities). These children usually have absent semicircular canals. There is a variable macular function in these children and often a sensorineural hearing loss, which can be profound.
  - Michel deformity, complete absence of the inner ear structures, or the presence of primitive otocysts without differentiation is rare.
- **Widened or large vestibular aqueducts (WVA or LVA).** The vestibular aqueduct is normally a narrow *J*-shaped channel between the vestibule and the posterior cranial fossa that contains the endolymphatic duct and sac. When dilated it is associated with hearing loss and balance disorders. Classically, the history is of minor trauma giving rise to a fluctuation or step-wise progression in hearing loss. Coincident with trauma, vestibular function can also be compromised with the patient describing vertigo. Vestibular hypofunction is common. WVA occur commonly in Pendred syndrome when they are associated with large endolymphatic sacs. They are also seen in CHARGE association and branchio-oto-renal syndrome and can occur in non-syndromic causes of hearing loss.
- **Aplasia or hypoplasia of the CVIII.** A recognized cause of hearing loss, this defect can be associated with vestibular hypofunction. The aetiology is unknown.

Congenital with normal inner ear morphology

There are a number of genetic conditions associated with vestibular hypofunction where the labyrinth has normal morphology. Some of these are dominantly inherited, and it is not uncommon in a deaf family for affected members to display delayed motor milestones as part of the phenotype. Two recognized syndromes are important to identify early, and both present as vestibular hypofunction in severe to profoundly deaf babies:

- **Usher I syndrome.** The Usher syndromes are caused by recessively inherited genetic mutations giving rise to deafness and retinitis pigmentosa (RP). Usher I gives rise to considerable morbidity in that individuals are profoundly deaf, have no vestibular function and become blind in adulthood. Early diagnosis is important to give families choice about future pregnancies and may dictate management options: early cochlear implantation, the potential need for Braille and deaf-blind sign language. Diagnosis is confirmed by early electroretinogram (ERG). Genetic testing is helpful, although there are a number of genotypes giving rise to the Usher I phenotype.
- **Jervell and Lange-Nielsen syndrome (JLN).** This recessively inherited condition is due to a defect in the potassium-conducting channels in the inner ear and in the conduction system of the heart, giving rise to a prolonged QT interval. It is usually caused by a mutation in the KCNQ1 gene on chromosome 11p15 or in the KCNE1 gene on chromosome 21q22. The child is severely to profoundly deaf and susceptible to the sudden onset of ventricular arrhythmias, leading to episodes of syncope, and is at high risk of sudden death. Early identification is important as active management with beta-blockers or defibrillators can be life saving.
- **Other.** Other conditions include Usher III, Waardenburg syndrome, Alport syndrome, Alström syndrome, mitochondrial disorders and more.[5,6,7]

INFECTION

Congenital infections

Congenital infections affecting the labyrinth can give rise to vestibular pathology, e.g. rubella, syphilis and cytomegalovirus (CMV). CMV is the most common congenital infection currently seen and gives rise to a sensorineural hearing loss that can progress throughout the first decade. Vestibular function is variably affected and can progress as the hearing drops. Treatment (ganciclovir and valganciclovir) is available if the infection is identified early and can prevent progression of the hearing loss. Inadequate information is available about the effect of treatment on vestibular function.

Acquired infections

Bacterial labyrinthitis can arise from middle ear sepsis (otogenic) as a sequel of acute otitis media, mastoiditis or cholesteatoma, or as a consequence of haematogenous spread from a distant site of infection, as well as from meningitis. The consequence of bacterial labyrinthitis is commonly deafness and vestibular loss associated with labyrinthitis ossificans. Reports suggest that between 40 and 80 per cent of children develop vestibular hypofunction following meningitis; those with profound losses are invariably affected.

Vestibular neuronitis is probably as common in children as in adults but rarely presents. The pathology is probably of a viral infection or reactivation of a latent herpes simplex virus type 1 (HSV-1) infection affecting the vestibular ganglion. The onset is sudden, often after a mild upper respiratory tract infection, and of rotatory vertigo with vomiting and instability. The illness is short in children (2–3 days), and because of their innate desire to play, they compensate quickly. Older children can present much as adults, with a more drawn-out illness and difficulty compensating from the resultant canal paresis. They may require a rehabilitative approach.

The presentation for viral labyrinthitis is as for a vestibular neuronitis, with the addition of hearing loss that is permanent. Specific causes include mumps and herpes zoster reactivation (Ramsay Hunt syndrome).

Lyme disease can lead to vertigo with a sensorineural hearing loss as a consequence of infection by the spirochete *Borrelia* carried by deer ticks. A history of travel to an endemic area with perhaps an erythematous rash at the site of a tick bite indicates the need to test for specific antibodies. Treatment with antibiotics is effective and prevents chronic neurological sequelae.

TRAUMA

Direct trauma, blows to the ear or significant acoustic trauma, such as explosion, can disrupt the tympanic membrane and displace stapes, leading to hearing loss and vertigo. Fractures of the petrous temporal bones can be associated with hearing loss and vestibular disturbance because of damage either to the labyrinth or to the CVIII nerve. The history is usually clear and fractures will be evident on CT scan. Management is expectant unless a perilymph fistula is present and symptoms of vertigo persist.

Iatrogenic trauma needs to be considered after middle ear surgery and especially after cochlear implantation when vertigo is a reasonably common sequel.

Barotrauma can give rise to balance problems. This usually occurs as the consequence of a dive without ear pressure equalization, leading to perilymph fistula, or as the result of rapid decompression, giving rise to the 'staggers' as a consequence of nitrogen gas bubbles within the brain stem or inner ear. Prevention is important, but if damage has occurred, surgery is indicated in the case of perilymph fistula and hyperbaric oxygen in the case of decompression sickness.

Perilymph fistulae can present with fluctuating vertigo and progressive hearing loss associated with straining and stooping or other actions that change pressure across the fistula. These usually occur as a consequence of trauma. Spontaneous perilymph fistulae can occur in congenitally deformed inner ears. Whether spontaneous perilymph fistulae arise in anatomically normal ears is a subject of debate, but the general consensus is that they do not. Treatment is surgical for persistent cases.

Benign paroxysmal positional vertigo (BPPV) is rare in children and only occurs as a consequence of trauma sufficient to detach the otoconia from the maculae. The pathology is considered to be caused by shifting of loose otoconia into a semicircular canal, usually the posterior, with stimulation of the cupula and resultant short-lived vertigo on postural change, particularly lying on one side. The Dix–Hallpike positioning test will provoke both symptoms and rotatory nystagmus towards the downmost ear. The nystagmus is delayed in appearance, resolves after about 40 seconds and is reversed on sitting up again. Repetition of the manoeuvre leads to a reduction in severity of both the symptoms and the nystagmus. Treatment is with particle positioning manoeuvres.

AUTOIMMUNE DISEASE

Autoimmune disease, as a cause of labyrinthine pathology, is rare in children and can be difficult to diagnose. The presentation is usually of a progressive hearing loss with vestibular disturbance. Additionally, there are usually other symptoms or signs of autoimmune disease, such as eye inflammation (e.g. Cogan's syndrome), joint pain and inflammation, or rash (e.g. systemic lupus erythematosus, Raynaud's phenomenon). MRI scan can show evidence of labyrinthine fibrosis. Blood tests for inflammatory markers and autoantibodies are helpful. Treatment is with steroids and other immunosuppressants, and management should be joint with a paediatrician.

NEOPLASTIC CAUSES

The most common neoplasm to produce both hearing loss and vertigo/imbalance is the vestibular schwannoma. Although much more common in adulthood, this tumour can present in childhood in cases of neurofibromatosis 2 (NF2), which is a dominantly inherited condition characterized by multiple schwannomas, meningiomas and other intracranial tumours. As with most dominantly inherited conditions, *de novo* mutations occur reasonably frequently (~50 per cent). Cases can present in the first decade, although this is uncommon. The clinician should always be aware of the possibility of a schwannoma, and MRI scan, as a routine for all cases of unilateral hearing loss, is important in excluding this rare condition. Vestibular function is compromised, but the onset is gradual and with unilateral tumours, symptoms of vertigo and imbalance are rare.

OTOTOXIC DRUGS

A number of drugs can affect hearing and balance. Aminoglycosides are ototoxic, and some, such as streptomycin and gentamicin, are highly vestibulotoxic. The use of aminoglycosides in sick neonates is common and the effect on the vestibular system largely unknown. Monitoring the levels of aminoglycosides during treatment and avoiding high serum levels is useful in prevention of both hearing loss and vestibular damage. Cisplatin is a chemotherapeutic agent used widely in the treatment of sarcomas, lymphomas and germ cell tumours. It is known to give rise to a dose-dependent high-frequency hearing loss, and there are variable reports of the effect of the drug on the vestibular system.

UNKNOWN AETIOLOGY

Ménière's disease is rare in children and is not a diagnosis to be made lightly. The only cases seen by the author are those with a strong family history, raising the question of a genetic mutation. Symptoms are of episodic vertigo with tinnitus and a feeling of pressure in the ear with a fluctuating low-frequency sensorineural hearing loss. Full investigation should be conducted for other causes of these symptoms, such as migrainous vertigo, WVA, automimmune disease, congenital syphilis and Lyme disease. Management is with a low-salt diet and the use of thiazide diuretics as in adults, with more radical treatments used with considerable caution.

Dehiscent superior semicircular canals are a recognized cause of Tullio phenomenon (vertigo induced by noise) in adults but are rarely seen in children.

CENTRAL VESTIBULAR DISORDERS

Central vestibular disorders are listed in Table 66.3.

Migraine and migraine equivalents

Migrainous pathology is the most common cause of episodic vertigo in children and can present at any age. Three main presentations are recognized in children, outlined as follows. Nevertheless, there are common patterns running through all. Children may progress from one condition to another.

The vertigo is episodic and usually short lived, particularly in younger children, there are no interictal phenomena of note and there is a family history in 50 per cent or more of cases. The presentation is dependent on age and headache is a rare accompaniment in the younger child, although may become more of a problem in the second decade. Investigation can reveal subtle signs of central vestibular dysfunction, but generally most measures of audiological or vestibular function are within the normal range for the age of the child. In most cases with a good clear history and normal findings on

Table 66.3 Central vestibular disorders

Migraine and migraine equivalents (v/d, +/–HL)
Benign torticollis of infancy
Benign paroxysmal vertigo of childhood
Migrainous vertigo
Epilepsy (v, –HL)
Episodic ataxia 2 – channelopathy (v/i, –HL)
Infections, e.g. meningitis, encephalitis, cerebral abscess (v/d/i, +/–HL)
Head trauma (d/i +/–HL)
Congenital abnormalities of the skull base – Chiari type 1 (v/d, –HL)
Neoplasia – posterior fossa tumours, brain stem tumours (v/d/i, –HL)
Heredodegenerative diseases, e.g. Refsum, DIDMOAD (d/i, +/–HL)
Demyelination, e.g. multiple sclerosis (v/d/i, +/–HL)
Vestibular processing disorder (i, –HL)

d = dizziness, v = vertigo, i = imbalance, +/–HL = with/without hearing loss.

neurotological examination, there is no need for detailed vestibular testing, nor for MRI.

- Benign paroxysmal torticollis of infancy is an accepted migrainous variant, and criteria are included in the International Classification of Headache Disorders (ICHD-II). Presenting in the first year of life, it includes episodes of torticollis usually accompanied by distress, pallor and instability with occasionally vomiting. The duration of an episode is from a few minutes to days. It is a self-limiting condition resolving between the ages of 3 and 5 years.
- Benign paroxysmal vertigo of childhood (BPV or BPVC) is characterized by brief episodes of vertigo of sudden onset that present within the first 3 years of life and resolve spontaneously between the ages of 5 and 7 years. The child is often frightened and will hold onto the cot sides or his mother's legs. The episode lasts a few minutes, during which the child is pale and unwell, and the cessation of the episode is sudden and complete. Older children will describe vertigo. Sometimes these episodes are predictable or occur in clusters, in which case medication can help. Antihistamines have been found to be of value.
- Migrainous vertigo, a common cause of episodic vertigo in children, accounts for a third or more cases of vertigo presenting to a balance clinic. The vertiginous episodes occur in clusters and can be predictable in their periodicity. They can last from a few minutes to several hours and are usually accompanied by other migrainous phenomena such as visual or olfactory aura, photophobia, phonophobia and prostration. These episodes are not usually accompanied by headache (acephalgic) in children, although when they are it can help with the diagnosis. Children often give a history of travel sickness. A fluctuating, mild low-frequency sensorineural hearing loss can be found in the author's experience.

Also related are abdominal migraine, which can present with abdominal pain and vomiting, and cyclical vomiting.

Treatment is as for migraine. Explanation and reassurance are powerful tools as is avoidance of precipitants. Common precipitants include caffeine, chocolate, cheese, citrus fruits and monosodium glutamate, and keeping a diary often identifies these. Simple analgesics such as ibuprofen or paracetamol are useful with the addition of an antihistamine if nausea or vomiting are significant features. Occasionally, the use of prophylactic medication such as pizotifen or propranolol can be used if episodes are frequent. Advice from, or joint working with, a paediatric neurologist is recommended.

Usually the episodes of vertigo will subside with treatment. The essence of management is ensuring that the child has strategies to call upon should the symptoms reoccur. Migraine can be a lifelong problem with periods of exacerbation often precipitated by stress, such as examinations, or hormonal changes.

EPILEPSY

There are thought to be three presentations of vertigo in the epileptic patient. The most common is when vertigo forms part of the aura preceding a grand mal seizure, and in these cases the main seizure is usually recognized.

An uncommon presentation is that of vertiginous epilepsy where the symptoms of the seizure are those of vertigo. The focus of epileptic activity is usually in the parietal or fronto-parietal region, although other areas have been implicated. These cases can present to a balance clinic because the diagnosis is usually unclear. The episodes are often accompanied by a change in level of consciousness. The vestibular function tests are usually normal, but an electroencephalogram (EEG) may identify the focus of epileptic activity. Referral to a neurologist is indicated.

The third type of epilepsy is that of vestibulogenic epilepsy, when a seizure may be precipitated by vertigo such as that induced by bithermal caloric stimulation. This is fortunately rare.

EPISODIC ATAXIA 2 (EA2)

EA2 is an uncommon cause of vertigo that usually presents in the first or second decade. It is a dominantly inherited channelopathy due to a mutation in the CACNA1A gene on chromosome 19, which encodes a calcium channel strongly expressed in the cerebellum.

The symptoms are of vertigo and of ataxia during the episode. Headache can be a symptom. The episodes last from an hour to a day or two with resolution and can be precipitated by stress or exercise. During the interictal period, signs of cerebellar dysfunction persist, in particular, downbeat nystagmus. The electronystagmogram (ENG) is central in type indicating cerebellar pathology. MRI scan is indicated, and atrophy of the vermis may be reported. Treatment with acetazolamide is effective. Most cases have good control, while resistant cases can often be managed with 4-aminopyridine.

CHIARI MALFORMATION TYPE 1

This condition is a congenital malformation in which the cerebellar tonsils prolapse (tonsillar ectopia) through the foramen magnum. It is often asymptomatic but can present with short-lived vertigo, particularly with neck extension, and with accompanying headache. Examination may identify cerebellar signs and, in particular, downbeat nystagmus, which can be more marked on performing the Dix–Hallpike test with the head back in the midline. Investigation will include an MRI scan with views of the craniocervical junction and upper cervical spine because of the chance of identifying an accompanying syringomyelia. Referral to a neurosurgeon is indicated and consideration given to decompression if symptoms are severe or deteriorating.

POSTERIOR CRANIAL FOSSA TUMOURS

Although vertigo can be a presenting symptom in intracranial tumours occurring in 7 per cent of posterior cranial fossa tumours,[8] it is far more common for children to present with imbalance and disorders of gait, which can occur in 60 per cent of those with posterior cranial fossa tumours and 78 per cent of those with brain stem tumours. The onset of unsteadiness is progressive and usually fairly rapid, with ataxia and cerebellar signs being the hallmark for medical concern. There are usually additional symptoms such as headache, lethargy and visual symptoms. Here a thorough neurological examination is of the essence, and urgent MRI scan is indicated. Delay in the identification of an intracranial tumour in a child leads to increased morbidity and a reduced chance of effective treatment.

NON-VESTIBULAR CAUSES OF DIZZINESS OR INSTABILITY

Non-vestibular causes of dizziness or instability are listed in Table 66.4.

Psychological

Dizziness or light-headedness can be caused by psychological factors and can be common in children who do not have the resources to manage stressful situations nor the ability or opportunity to express fears and worries. Hyperventilation as a consequence of anxiety is a common cause of dizziness and will exacerbate other causes of vertigo. It is always difficult to understand whether vertigo

Table 66.4 Non-vestibular causes of balance problems

Psychological – psychosomatic, hyperventilation, abuse (v/d/i, –HL)
Cardiac arrhythmias, e.g. long QT interval, bradycardias (d, –HL)
Visual disorder – vergence (d, –HL)
Vasovagal (d, –HL)
Drugs – recreational drugs, alcohol and caffeine (v/d/i, –HL)
Metabolic, e.g. hypoglycaemia (d, –HL)
Musculo-skeletal, e.g. Still's disease, muscular dystrophy (i, –HL)
Other: breath-holding attacks, night terrors (i, –HL)

d = dizziness, v = vertigo, i = imbalance, +/–HL = with/without hearing loss.

due to organic pathology has caused anxiety or whether anxiety is the root cause of dizziness.

A careful history that does not establish a pattern indicative of other causes of vertigo suggests that a psychological cause may be the precipitant. A psychological assessment has value in identifying any psychological issues. Of particular note is that abuse can present as vertigo in children, and it is imperative that the underlying factors are explored fully. Joint management with a psychologist or paediatrician is recommended.

Cardiac arrhythmias

Arrhythmias can present as dizziness or 'funny turns'. A history of syncope, drop attacks, palpitations or dyspnoea should raise awareness, and cardiovascular examination may reveal an abnormality. An electrocardiogram (ECG) may illustrate an arrhythmia or conduction defect such as a prolonged QT interval. Referral for a cardiological opinion is indicated in appropriate cases. Of particular concern is that Jervell and Lange-Nielsen syndrome can present with dizziness owing to cardiac arrhythmia; see earlier discussion.

Visual disorder

Ophthalmological abnormalities, particularly of vergence, are considered to be the cause of dizziness in about 5 per cent of cases. It is reported that ophthalmological exercises can overcome the feelings of dizziness and instability.[9,10]

Vasovagal episodes

Feeling faint or light-headed is common, particularly in teenagers. Episodes with pallor, sweatiness, loss of consciousness with an aura of lightheadedness, visual or auditory disturbance especially on standing quickly, prolonged standing in a warm environment or with stress are suggestive of vasovagal episodes. Blood pressure readings indicating a low blood pressure or a postural drop on standing can aid diagnosis. Management consists of advice to maintain hydration and to avoid other precipitants when possible. Lying or sitting with the head below the heart when dizzy can abort the episode. It is important to exclude cardiological causes of these episodes.

Drugs

Dizziness is a common side effect of prescribed medication and can occur in children as in adults. More commonly the use of recreational drugs amongst older children, particularly alcohol, glue sniffing and ecstasy, can lead to symptoms of vertigo. Caffeine in large doses, as in coffee or in soft drinks such as cola, can give rise to heightened anxiety and dizziness and can also precipitate migrainous vertigo in susceptible individuals.

VESTIBULAR PROCESSING DIFFICULTIES

Vestibular processing difficulties are recognized by occupational therapists rather than by medics.[11] The presentation may be with early onset and severe motion sickness or frequent falls with a poor saving reflex. It is likely that the child is unable to process the different sensory inputs required for balance. The child is otherwise well but may have subtle central signs such as hypotonia, poor reflexes, visual problems and other processing difficulties, such as dyslexia or dyspraxia (Table 66.5). Vestibular tests are usually within normal ranges,

Table 66.5 Pathology in children

Common causes of vertigo/dizziness in children
Migrainous vertigo and migraine equivalents
Psychogenic
Otitis media with effusion
Visual disorders
Common pathologies in adults and rare in children
Benign paroxysmal positional vertigo (BPPV)
Ménière's disease
Vestibular schwannoma

and referral to an occupational therapist for sensory integration assessment and exercises is recommended.

MANAGEMENT

In most cases an accurate diagnosis with an explanation is invaluable. Some pathologies respond well to specific treatment, such as migrainous vertigo, EA2 and BPPV as outlined earlier in this chapter. General management includes vestibular rehabilitation to promote central compensation. Children with vestibular areflexia benefit from physiotherapy to build up strength in core muscles and to develop balance function. Psychological input may be required, and a multidisciplinary team approach is recommended.

KEY LEARNING POINTS

- The diagnosis is reached by a careful history and is supported by examination.
- MRI scan is unnecessary in the majority of cases of dizziness or vertigo in children.
- Migraine is common in children but presents differently to adults. Treatment is effective.
- Psychological causes of vertigo in children are fairly common and need active management.
- Abuse – physical, emotional and sexual – can cause dizziness and vertigo in children.
- Caffeine, particularly in fizzy drinks, can give rise to vertigo.
- BPPV is rare in children. Positional vertigo is more likely to be due to an intracranial tumour or Chiari I malformation.
- Explanation and reassurance can be very effective management strategies.

REFERENCES

1. Niemensivu R. Vertigo and balance problems in children – An epidemiologic study in Finland. *International Journal of Pediatric Otorhinolaryngology*. 2006; 70(2): 259–65.
2. Humphriss RL, Hall AJ. Dizziness in 10 year old children – An epidemiological study. *International Journal of Pediatric Otorhinolaryngology* 2011; 75(3): 395–400.
3. Niemensivu R, Pyykkö I, Valanne L, Kentala E. Value of imaging studies in vertiginous children. *International Journal of Pediatric Otorhinolaryngology*. 2006; 70(9): 1639–44.
4. Jones NS, Radomskij P, Pritchard AJN, Snashall SE. Imbalance and chronic secretory otitis media in children: Effect of myringotomy and insertion of ventilation tubes on body sway. *Annals of Otology, Rhinology and Laryngology*. 1990; 99 (6 Pt 1): 477–81.
5. Pikus A. Heritable vestibular disorders. *Seminars in Hearing*. 2002; 23: 113–20.
6. Bitner-Glindzicz M. Hereditary deafness and phenotyping in humans. *British Medical Bulletin*. 2002; 63(1): 73–94.
7. Eppsteiner RW, Smith RJ. Genetic disorders of the vestibular system. *Current Opinion in Otolaryngology and Head and Neck Surgery*. 2011; 19(5): 397–402.
8. Diagnosis of Brain Tumours in Children Guidelines, RCPCH publication. Available from: http://www.rcpch.ac.uk/sites/

default/files/Diagnosis%20of%20Brain%20Tumours%20in%20Children%20Guideline%20-%20Full%20report.pdf

9. Anoh-Tanon MJ, Bremond-Gignac D, Wiener-Vacher SR. Vertigo is an underestimated symptom of ocular disorders: Dizzy children do not always need MRI. *Pediatric Neurology*. 2000 Jul; 23(1): 49–53.
10. Bucci MP, Kapoula Z, Yang Q, Wiener-Vacher S, Bremond-Gignac D. Abnormality of vergence latency in children with vertigo. *Journal of Neurology*. 2004; 251(2): 204–13.
11. Ayres AJ. Learning disabilities and the vestibular system. *Journal of Learning Disabilities*. 1978; 11(1): 18–29.

67

Choanal atresia

HAYTHAM KUBBA

EMBRYOLOGY

Choanal atresia occurs in about 1 in 7000 births, so it is not rare. It occurs when the nasobuccal membrane of Hochstetter fails to involute, leaving a plate of tissue across the back of the nose, closing it off completely and separating it from the pharynx. The nose looks normal from the outside, but it is completely blocked to airflow on one or both sides. The atretic plate is made of bone, thick at the edges but quite thin in the middle. The central part may in fact be membranous rather than bony in 70 per cent of cases, although this membranous part is often quite small. Just over half of all cases are unilateral (Figure 67.1), the rest bilateral (Figure 67.2).

Choanal atresia often presents as an airway emergency soon after birth. It is such a serious problem because newborn babies are unable to breathe through their mouths by choice; they are obligate nasal breathers. This occurs because the larynx of the neonate is positioned very high, so that it is in line with the back of the nose. The uvula and epiglottis sit on top of one another, directing the food stream around the sides of the larynx to the piriform fossae, while the air goes in the midline through the nose to the larynx.[1] This allows the infant to suckle and breathe at the same time. Subsequent descent of the larynx into its normal adult position is a uniquely human phenomenon that facilitates mouth-breathing and speech.

ASSOCIATED CONDITIONS

Around 75 per cent of children with choanal atresia have other congenital abnormalities, and in half there is a named syndrome[2] The most common of these is CHARGE (coloboma, heart defects, choanal atresia, retarded growth and development, genital hypoplasia, ear anomalies and deafness), which is present in approximately 25 per cent of children with choanal atresia.

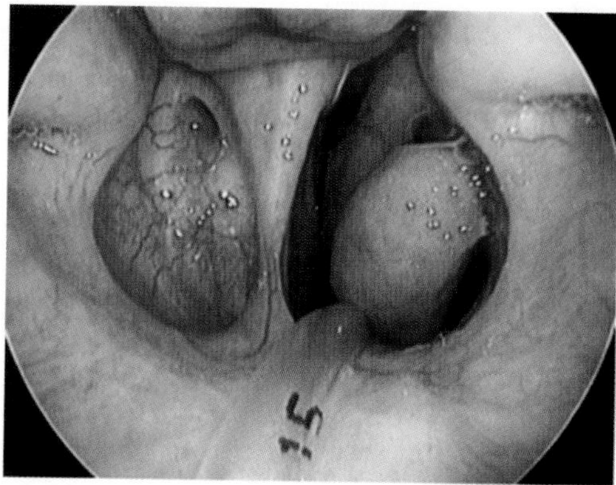

Figure 67.1 Left unilateral choanal atresia, as seen from the nasopharynx looking forward into the back of the nose using a 120° endoscope.

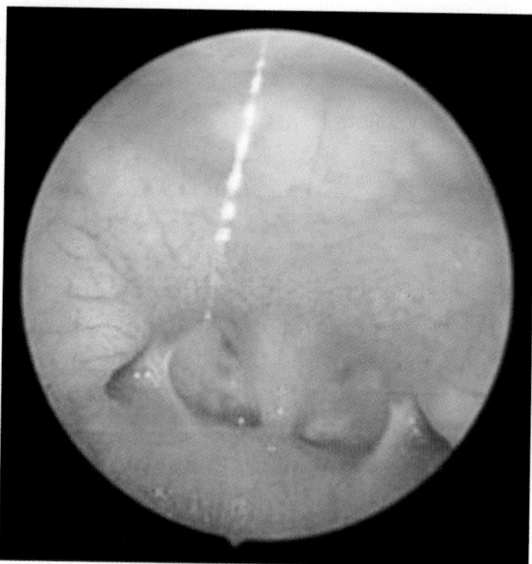

Figure 67.2 Bilateral choanal atresia, as seen from the nasopharynx looking forward into the back of the nose using a 120° endoscope.

CLINICAL PRESENTATION

Infants with nasal obstruction will be very snuffly and may have difficulties with feeding, leading to a referral to the otolaryngologist in the neonatal period. Most bilateral cases and some unilateral ones present in this way.

The classical presentation of choanal atresia is with cyclical hypoxia: The baby cries, taking in air through the mouth (which relieves the hypoxia) but then settles down, closes the mouth, struggles to breathe and becomes hypoxic again. Repeated oxygen desaturations occur with consequent growth failure and effects on brain development. In many cases, the presentation is the same as for any airway emergency with noisy breathing (stertor), respiratory distress and persistent hypoxia.

Some children with unilateral (and occasionally bilateral) atresia will make it through the neonatal period without any intervention. They present in their preschool (toddler) years with unilateral nasal discharge, or complaining of nasal obstruction in later childhood.

PHYSICAL EXAMINATION

It is important to make an assessment of the urgency of the situation based on signs of respiratory distress, including stertor, intercostal recession, sternal recession, tracheal tug, respiratory rate, peripheral perfusion, conscious level and oxygen saturation.

Clinical examination of the infant's nose is easy, and in most cases the diagnosis can be made by means of a few simple manoeuvres. First, examine the nose with an otoscope. This gives excellent illumination and magnification and will allow you to see if there is a nasal mass causing obstruction. Next, look for airflow through both nostrils by holding a cold metal spatula under the nose. Misting excludes choanal atresia affecting that nostril. Finally, attempt to pass a nasogastric tube through each nostril in turn. Failure to get past the nostril suggests piriform aperture stenosis (see discussion that follows), while a tube that passes into the nasal cavity but stops at the back of the nose suggests choanal atresia.

DIFFERENTIAL DIAGNOSIS

NASAL MASSES

These can cause nasal blockage and therefore present in the same way as choanal atresia. The most common nasal masses in infants are meningoencephalocoeles and gliomas, which develop from herniations of meninges and brain tissue through the anterior skull base down into the nose. Meningoencephalocoeles are still connected to the meninges and brain, while nasal gliomas are isolated lumps of brain tissue in the nose, cut off from the brain by the formation of the anterior skull base. They should be obvious on clinical inspection of the nose. The important point is to remember that congenital nasal masses may be connected to the brain, so they should always be scanned before any kind of surgical intervention such as a biopsy. Transnasal excision with repair of the skull base is the approach of choice.[3]

Haemangiomas (strawberry naevi) can occur in the nose and may cause nasal obstruction and poor feeding. They are obvious on nasal examination. It may be worth getting a scan to define the extent of the lesion. Without any treatment they grow, plateau and then eventually disappear, usually over 2 to 5 years, but if they are causing symptoms they may need treatment. Corticosteroids, propranolol and surgery all have a role, depending on the site and size of the lesion.

PIRIFORM APERTURE STENOSIS

This is a rare abnormality of midline structures producing narrowing at the bony entrance to the nose (Figure 67.3).[4] It is often associated with a single central mega-incisor tooth and abnormalities of the pituitary gland and brain. It presents like choanal atresia, but on examination the nostrils are narrow and slit-like, and it is difficult to pass a nasogastric tube into the front of the nose. The single central incisor tooth may be seen or palpated through the upper gum. Computed tomography (CT) scans are helpful in diagnosis. An endocrine specialist should assess pituitary function. The stenosis can be easily drilled wider through a sublabial incision, and it may be worth stenting the nose for a few weeks.

True bony stenosis of the nasal cavity is rare. Stenosis at the level of the nasopharynx occurs largely as part of a syndrome where the maxilla is hypoplastic, such as the syndromic craniosynostoses (Crouzon's, Apert's, Pfeiffer's and Saethre–Chotzen syndromes).

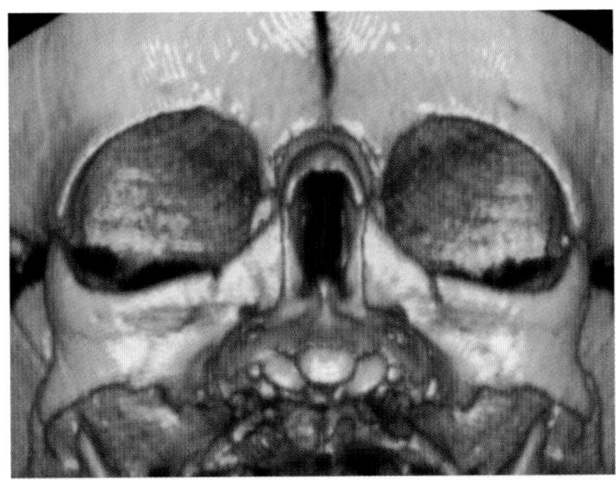

Figure 67.3 3D reconstruction from a CT of the face of an infant with congenital piriform aperture stenosis. Note the bony projections from the maxilla narrowing the nostrils and the single central incisor tooth.

NEONATAL RHINITIS

This is by far the most common cause of a snuffly nose in a baby. The diagnosis is made if there is evidence of nasal congestion with noisy breathing and feeding difficulties, but air can be seen passing through both sides of the nose (bilateral misting of a cold metal spatula, for example), or nasogastric tubes can be passed through both sides, and there is no bony narrowing of the nostrils or nasal mass on examination. The cause is usually unclear, although some cases may be caused by congenital infection with chlamydia.[5] Snuffly babies are very common, and most settle quickly with no specific treatment. Saline douches may be helpful, as may regular suction with a handheld rubber bulb syringe. Corticosteroid drops and decongestants are effective but prone to side effects. They should be used very rarely, very sparingly and for a very short time.

INVESTIGATIONS

Examination with a paediatric flexible laryngoscope can be helpful if secretions are removed with suction first. If you can pass the scope through the nose and see the larynx, there is no choanal atresia on that side.

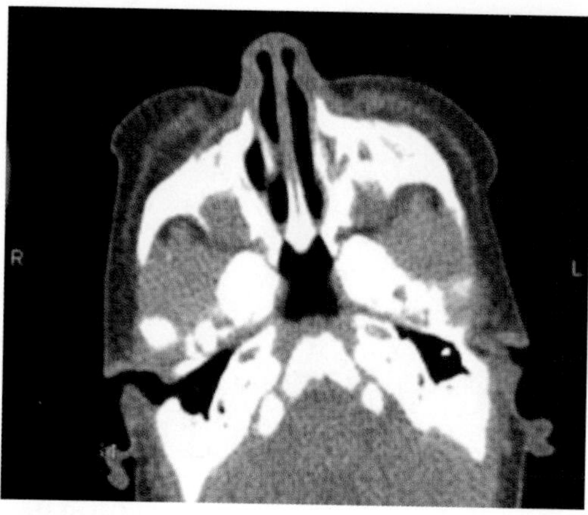

Figure 67.4 Axial CT scan of the face showing bilateral choanal atresia.

The definitive investigation for choanal atresia is an axial CT scan (Figure 67.4). This will reliably confirm or exclude the diagnosis, and it will also exclude piriform aperture stenosis. The best pictures are achieved by suctioning secretions from the nose and applying a few drops of decongestant immediately prior to the scan; otherwise, secretions pool in the nose against the atretic plate, making it difficult to make out. Good scans give the surgeon useful information about the amount of bone that needs to be removed.

It is vital to arrange a series of investigations, known as a CHARGE screen, for every child with choanal atresia. Of these, the cardiac assessment is the only one that is urgent enough to need doing before choanal atresia surgery; the rest can be done in the post-operative period.

MANAGEMENT

An infant who is struggling to breathe through the nose will need something to hold the mouth open. In many cases, an orogastric feeding tube is enough. If not, a Guedel oropharyngeal airway works very well as a short-term measure but can cause palatal ulceration if left in more than a couple of days. A McGovern nipple is a softer alternative that resembles somewhat the teat of a feeding bottle.

Remember that these children are small and vulnerable, and often also medically complex, so the role of the otolaryngologist is to work as part of a wider team including neonatologists, geneticists, cardiologists and others.

The surgery of choanal atresia involves perforating the central, thin, often membranous part of the atretic plate, then widening the hole with a drill. It is important to be able to see what you are doing so as to avoid injury to the palate or skull base. There are various ways of achieving this. Using a zero-degree Hopkins rod telescope in the nostril together with instruments, as in sinus surgery, is fine in older children, but space is very limited in neonates. A better view is obtained using a mouth gag on suspension as for tonsillectomy and a 120° telescope passed through the mouth, looking up behind the soft palate (Figure 67.5).[6] Instruments passed into the nose will appear to be coming towards you on screen. The palate should be retracted out of the way with a retraction suture at the base of the uvula.

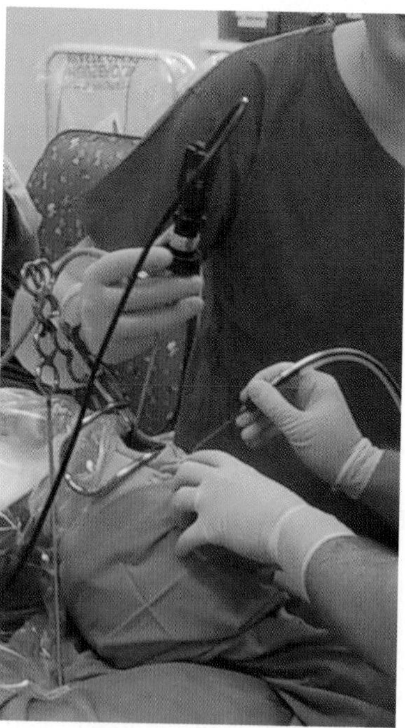

Figure 67.5 The setup for choanal atresia surgery. The 120° endoscope is held by an assistant in the mouth, directed to look up behind the soft palate into the nasopharynx. The operator passes instruments into the nose.

However the surgery is done, the choanae will restenose to some extent. It helps to make the choanae as large as possible by removing plenty of bone laterally and by removing the back of the vomer with back-biting forceps (Figure 67.6). It is also helpful to warn parents at the outset that some degree of restenosis is inevitable and to schedule at least one procedure to dilate the choanae with a balloon over the first few weeks. Regular balloon dilatation should keep the choanae from closing completely and forming a stable opening.

Nasal stents can be bought pre-formed or made from cut endotracheal tubes held in place with a polypropylene suture encircling the septum. They provide a patent nasal airway for infants during the early neonatal phase when they are obligate nasal breathers. It is important that they are sized and placed very carefully: too large and they will cause pressure necrosis of the alar cartilage, too small and they won't provide an adequate airway, too tight and they cause necrosis of the columella, too loose and they cause difficulties with suction. The stents are prone to block with dried secretions, so very frequent suction and instillation of saline drops are required. Six to eight weeks of stenting is usually enough (Figure 67.7).

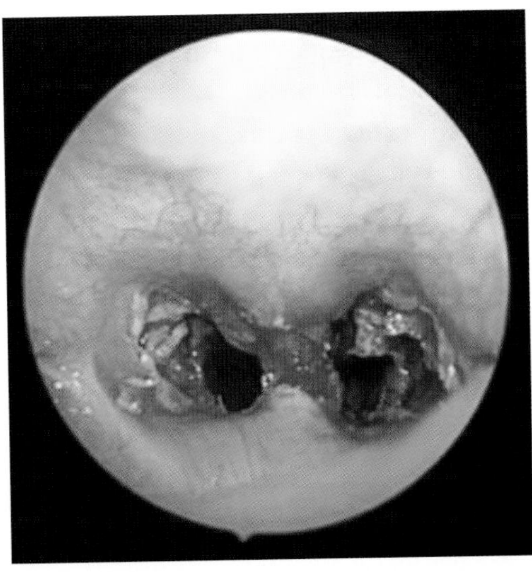

Figure 67.6 The same patient as in Figure 67.2, at the end of the procedure. The atretic plate has been drilled away on each side and the back of the septum removed with back-biting forceps.

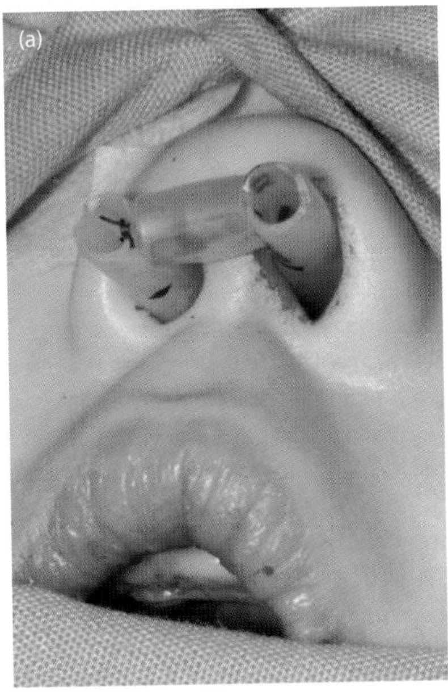

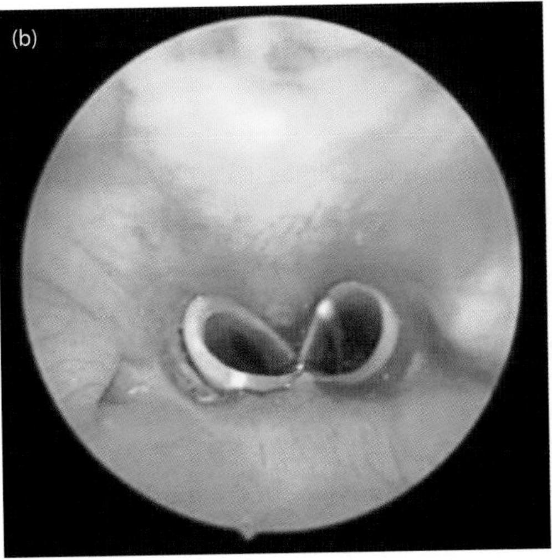

Figure 67.7 **(a)** Nasal stents in place. Note the spacer protecting the columella from pressure damage. **(b)** Nasal stents as seen from the nasopharynx. **(a)** Courtesy of Mr W Andrew Clement.

KEY LEARNING POINTS

Presentation of nasal obstruction in neonates:

- Babies cannot choose to breathe through their mouths if their noses are blocked.
- This can cause severe respiratory distress.
- If not diagnosed at birth, choanal atresia may cause symptoms in childhood such as unilateral nasal discharge and obstruction.

Physical examination:

- Look for signs of respiratory distress.
- A clinical diagnosis can be reached in most cases with nothing more than an otoscope, a cold metal spatula and a nasogastric tube.

Nasal masses:

- Never biopsy a nasal mass in a young child without first getting a scan.
- MRI scans give the best views of the anterior skull base and brain.
- Transnasal excision and skull base repair is the approach of choice.
- Detailed imaging and the advice of a neurosurgeon are essential.

CHARGE screen:

- Cardiac assessment with echocardiogram (urgent).
- Hearing test.
- Ophthalmology assessment for coloboma.
- Renal ultrasound.

Choanal atresia surgery:

- Pre-operative planning with CT scan.
- Good endoscopic visualization.
- Adequate lateral bone removal with the drill.
- Remove the vomer with back-biting forceps.
- Insert stents for 6 to 8 weeks in neonatal cases.
- Careful sizing and fixation of stents to prevent alar stenosis.
- Early, regular balloon dilatation until choanae are stable and patent.

REFERENCES

1. Kubba H, Moores T. Developmental anatomy of the airway. *Anaesthesia and Intensive Care*. 2006; 7(5): 158–60.
2. Burrow TA, Saal HM, de Alarcon A, Martin LJ, Cotton RT, Hopkin RJ. Characterization of congenital anomalies in individuals with choanal atresia. *Archives of Otolaryngology – Head & Neck Surgery*. 2009; 135(6): 543–47.
3. Kanowitz SJ, Bernstein JM. Pediatric meningoencephaloceles and nasal obstruction: a case for endoscopic repair. *International Journal of Pediatric Otorhinolaryngology*. 2006; 70(12): 2087–92.
4. Devambez M, Delattre A, Fayoux P. Congenital nasal pyriform aperture stenosis: diagnosis and management. *Cleft Palate-Craniofacial Journal*. 2009; 46(3): 262–7.
5. Iskandar NM, Naguib MB. *Chlamydia trachomatis*: an underestimated cause for rhinitis in neonates. *International Journal of Pediatric Otorhinolaryngology*. 1998; 42(3): 233–7.
6. Kubba H, Bennett A, Bailey CM. An update on choanal atresia surgery at Great Ormond Street Hospital for Children: preliminary results with mitomycin C and the KTP laser. *International Journal of Pediatric Otorhinolaryngology*. 2004; 68(7): 939–45.

68

Obstructive sleep apnoea

RAY CLARKE

It is not surprising that children suffering from adenoidal obstruction should be mentally dull and apathetic, and incapable of sustained attention even when at play. This condition is traditionally termed 'aprosexia'. Fortunately, it is susceptible of marked improvement following operation.

Wilson, 1955

INTRODUCTION

Obstructive sleep apnea (OSA) is part of a spectrum of sleep-related breathing disorders (SRBDs) characterized by episodic reductions (hypopnoeas) – or brief cessations (apnoeas) – in respiratory airflow during sleep. Simple or primary snoring (PS) is the mildest form of SRBD, with OSA as the most severe manifestation. Nocturnal apnoeas in children may be due to a variety of aetiologies, including malfunction of the respiratory centre in the brain stem and reduced respiratory drive, but the defining characteristic of obstructive sleep apnoea is that reduction of airflow occurs despite normal or even increased respiratory effort.

OSA in children is more difficult to define using precise measurements – even with good sleep studies – than its adult counterpart. Adults with repeated apnoeas and hypopnoeas insufficient to fulfill the diagnostic criteria for OSA are often described as having upper airway resistance syndrome, but this is not a useful term in children who are best considered to have primary snoring or OSA, which can vary from mild to severe.

Good quality clinical research studies in paediatric SRBDs have been hampered by uncertainties around definitions and a poor understanding of the pathophysiology of sleep in children. There is variation in normal sleep physiology in children depending on the child's age and maturation, and sleep patterns can vary from night to night. The adverse effects of disturbed sleep and the response to intervention are also very different in children. It is best to regard childhood OSA as a discrete clinical entity.

PREVALENCE AND NATURAL HISTORY

Most children will snore at some times, and otherwise healthy children may have brief periods of nocturnal apnoeas during respiratory tract infections. It is estimated that about 12 per cent of 4- to 5-year-old children in the United Kingdom have habitual snoring or PS. The incidence of obstructive sleep apnoea – despite some variation in diagnostic criteria – is estimated between .7 per cent and 1.8 per cent of the paediatric population. There are racial differences, with higher incidences in black and Hispanic children. Boys are affected more often than girls. The peak age of onset is from 2 to 5 years. OSA is uncommon in very young children and in adolescence unless there is co-morbidity – e.g. craniofacial dysmorphism – and tends to improve as pharyngeal lymphoid tissue atrophies after the age of 7 or 8 years.

AETIOLOGY AND PREDISPOSING FACTORS

The majority of children who present with obstructive sleep apnoea are otherwise healthy children with no significant co-morbidity. Any pathology that predisposes the child to airway obstruction will exacerbate a tendency to OSA. Children with allergic rhinitis, adenotonsillar enlargement (Figure 68.1), nasal polyposis, nasal septal deformity, macroglossia and micrognathia are especially susceptible. Midfacial hypoplasia such as occurs in Down syndrome and many varieties of craniofacial dysmorphism can cause severe airway compromise. Children with neuromuscular dysfunction, such as cerebral palsy and muscular dystrophy, may have marked hypotonia, particularly during sleep, and can develop severe OSA as a result. Both local factors in the airway and systemic disorders can predispose children to OSA as listed in Tables 68.1 and 68.2.

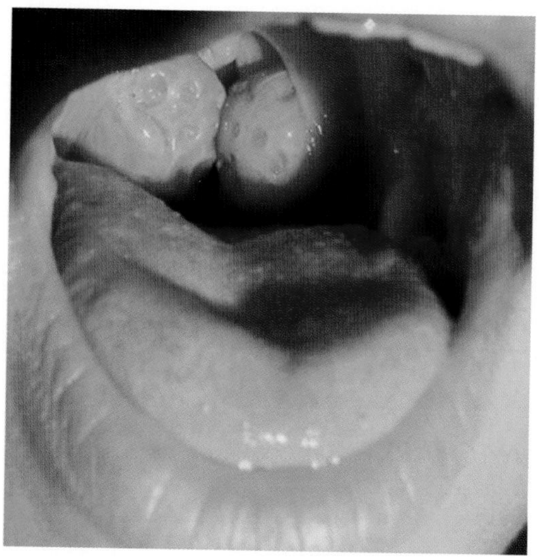

Figure 68.1 Large obstructing tonsils.

Table 68.1 Local causes of OSA in children

Oropharyngeal	Nasal/nasopharyngeal
Enlarged tonsils	Rhinitis
Retrognathia	Adenoids
Macroglossia	Septal deviation
Glossoptosis	Nasopharyngeal masses

PATHOPHYSIOLOGY

A newborn baby will typically sleep for 16–18 hours per day, falling to around 11 hours at age 5 years. Many young children will have a short 'nap' during the day. Sleep physiology is complex but

Table 68.2 Systemic causes of OSA

Diseases	Syndromes – craniofacial dysmorphism
Cerebral palsy/ muscular dystrophy	Down syndrome
Reticuloses	Prader–Willi syndrome
Sickle cell disease	Apert syndrome
Mucopolysaccharidosis	Treacher–Collins syndrome
Achondroplasia	Crouzon syndrome

a simplistic division of the types of sleep is into two main categories, quiet sleep or 'non-REM' and 'REM' (rapid eye movement) sleep. Each has a series of different functions, REM sleep being particularly important to neuronal maturation. Newborns spend some 60 per cent of their sleep time in REM sleep, with the proportion falling as the child gets older. During REM sleep there is marked inhibition of muscle tone, including the intercostal and the pharyngeal muscles – e.g. genioglossus – that maintain airway patency. Mild airway obstruction with intercostal recession and snoring due to partial obstruction of the pharyngeal airway during REM sleep is common in children especially up to the age of 3 years. This is greatly exacerbated in children with macroglossia (e.g. in Down syndrome) or micrognathia. The ventilatory response to mild hypoxia is more marked during non-REM sleep, and in a child with marked OSA repeated arousals in response to cyclical hypoxia will prevent the child passing from quiet to REM sleep. This deprivation of REM sleep is probably the basis of most of the adverse consequences of OSA.

OSA is essentially a manifestation of pharyngeal airway obstruction. Snoring and stertorous breathing is due to vibration of the pharyngeal structures, including the soft palate. The patency of the pharyngeal airway is maintained in part by muscle tone, hence the tendency for this type of obstruction to worsen during sleep as muscles relax and the pharyngeal walls become flaccid. This is exacerbated by the tongue falling back into the oropharynx, especially in the recumbent position. Continued respiratory efforts give rise to cyclical vibrations of the pharyngeal walls (snoring) interspersed with episodes of partial (hypopnoea) and complete (apnoea) closure of the pharyngeal airway. Hypoxaemia causes reflex wakening (arousal) and the cycle is repeated. Hypoxaemia triggers the respiratory centre to respond with an 'arousal'. Parents will often describe a pattern of increasingly loud snoring followed by cessation of breathing and then a rapid tachypnoeic response with vigorous respiratory effort as the child 'wakes himself up'.

EFFECTS OF OSA

The adverse effects of OSA are due to a combination of factors: hypoxaemia and hypercarbia, prolonged respiratory muscle effort and the cognitive and neuropsychological deficits brought about by poor-quality sleep. Frequent arousals result in fragmentation of the sleep. Repeated hypoxaemia leads to a rise in sympathetic output, causing peripheral vasoconstriction, with tachycardia and a rise in blood pressure. Effectively, the child has a combination of intermittent hypoxia and sleep deprivation. The cognitive and neuropsychological consequences of OSA are now well known. OSA children have demonstrable deficits in attention span and general intellectual ability when compared with age-matched controls. There is some evidence of poorer school performance in children who snore but do not have a clear-cut clinical history of sleep apnoea when compared with age-matched controls, and it is now accepted that clinical history alone underestimates the true prevalence of OSA. School performance improves following adenotonsillectomy in appropriately selected cases. Neurocognitive deficits in primary snoring are now increasingly reported, and the traditional advice that snoring in children – particularly if it is prolonged – is entirely benign may need to be revised.

The daytime somnolence so characteristic of adult OSA may manifest in children as hyperactivity, irritability, behaviour disorders and fatigue. This as well as a disturbed sleep pattern contributes to the often profound adverse effect of OSA on quality of life for both the child and family. This effect is particularly marked in the families of children with special needs where sleep patterns are often disturbed independent of airway obstruction. Adequate treatment of OSA can bring about marked improvement in quality of life.

OSA may be a factor in some children who have been considered in the past to have attention deficit hyperactivity disorder (ADHD). Untreated OSA may lead to failure to thrive and recurrent upper respiratory infections. In children with neurodevelopmental delay, the hypoxic episodes can be compounded by aspiration with repeated chest infections. Prolonged hypoxaemia and hypercarbia may give rise to pulmonary oedema, pulmonary hypertension and right-sided heart failure – cor pulmonale. There is evidence to link childhood OSA with hypertension that may persist into adult life (Marcus et al. 1998). Pectus excavatum secondary to chronic sternal recession is nowadays rarely seen. The plethoric facies of polycythaemia secondary to prolonged hypoxaemia is also rarely seen. In *The Posthumous Papers of the Pickwick Club* (1837), Charles Dickens provides a classic description of a boy with OSA: a 'fat and red-faced boy in a state of somnolency'.

Prolonged untreated OSA may contribute to hypoplasia of the mid-face. The 'adenoidal facies' characteristic of pharyngeal airway obstruction may persist into adulthood. There is some evidence to link untreated childhood OSA with snoring and SRBDs in adults.

CLINICAL PRESENTATION AND ASSESSMENT

Often the only abnormal clinical findings relate to the history. It is important to have a structured approach to history taking. Ask the parent to describe the child's sleep pattern and enquire in particular about snoring, posture, periods of 'stopping breathing', sweating and enuresis. Enquire about daytime symptoms, and in younger children ask to see the child's medical records showing a graph of the growth pattern to determine if there is any evidence of failure to thrive. In clinical practice the term OSA is used imprecisely. A typical history will include snoring, gasps, short episodes of apnoea, a poor sleep pattern with increased work of breathing and repeated arousals as the child 'wakes himself up'. Often the child will have an unusual sleeping posture and may change position frequently during the night. Early morning headaches, sweating and irritation may be related to nocturnal CO_2 retention. Very rarely, the parents may report that the child is cyanotic. Tiredness, poor school performance, irritability, listlessness and behaviour issues are common daytime problems. The child may have features of airway obstruction during the day. These include mouth breathing, adenoidal facies and sometimes nasal speech. If there is a clear-cut history, then treatment can be planned on this basis, but there is growing unease about offering surgery – with its attendant morbidity – to children with only clinical evidence of OSA. Moreover, it is now accepted that clinical history underestimates the frequency of OSA, and an increasing number of children require both screening and more definitive investigations.

Many parents will record the child's sleep on a mobile phone video sequence, or as a short audio clip. Examine these carefully as they can provide useful preliminary evidence of OSA. On clinical examination the child may be mouth breathing during the consultation. There may be features of rhinitis, retrognathia, high arched palate, mid-face hypoplasia or nasal septal deviation. Examine the oropharynx and the nasal airway carefully, observe the position of the chin and the tongue and note the architecture of the palate and the mid-face. Many ear, nose and throat (ENT) surgeons grade the tonsils according to how much of the oropharyngeal airway is occupied by tonsil tissue, with grade 1 being 25 per cent; grade 2, 26–50 per cent; grade 3, 51–75 per cent and grade 4 in excess of 75 per cent. Adenoid and tonsillar size is variable, but the relationship with OSA is uncertain and tonsil size is a poor predictor of response to surgery. The principal differential diagnoses are PS and central apnoea. PS is not associated with apnoeas and can be difficult to differentiate from OSA on clinical grounds alone. Occasional snoring in children is physiological, but there is mounting evidence that persistent snoring may be a marker for prolonged airway obstruction. In particular there may be adverse neuropsychological effects, and otolaryngologists need to be alert to the possibility of undiagnosed OSA in these children. Pulse oximetry or polysomnography (PSG) may be needed to make a definitive diagnosis.

The much less common 'central' apnoeas are caused by reduced drive in the respiratory centre rather than by airway obstruction. They may be a feature of global neuro-developmental delay. Mixed patterns occur with obstructive and central components and detailed respiratory investigations may be needed to unravel the exact pattern.

INVESTIGATIONS

Most ENT surgeons in the United Kingdom and the rest of Europe will make a diagnosis based on a clear-cut history and clinical assessment and will recommend intervention – often adenotonsillectomy – on this alone. In the United States, insurance companies will typically authorize surgery only if there is objective evidence of repeated nocturnal hypoxia on a 'sleep study' of one sort or another. With changes in hospital reimbursement patterns in the United Kingdom, an increasing number of ENT units are now being asked to provide similar objective evidence before undertaking surgery. Children with severe OSA or significant co-morbidity may require specific investigations, such as electrocardiography/echocardiography, chest imaging, haematological tests and metabolic screening, depending on the pathology. Respiratory assessment including PSG or 'sleep studies' to measure respiratory function during sleep is useful in two situations – where there is diagnostic doubt and to predict which children are at increased risk of post-operative respiratory complications and may therefore need surgery and perioperative care in a different setting. The identification and management of children with OSA has been bedeviled by diagnostic uncertainty, variation in thresholds for intervention among clinicians, and inadequate provision of diagnostic facilities even in specialist children's hospitals.

The two modalities of respiratory assessment in common use are overnight pulse oximetry (Figure 68.2) and formal PSG. Pulse oximetry involves the sequential measurement of oxygen saturation and heart rate. The family can be given portable oximetry equipment to take home. The test is non-invasive, relatively inexpensive and a useful screening tool. It has a high positive predictive value but is less good at excluding OSA in marginal cases as apnoeas are not always accompanied by desaturations. The tracings need to be interpreted by a suitably trained assessor. Desaturations are considered significant if there are more than four per hour, each exceeding 4 per cent, or there are abnormal clusters or prolonged desaturations exceeding 90 per cent. Table 68.3 summarizes the recommendations of a UK Multidisciplinary Working Party listing the categories of children who ideally should have more thorough investigations before considering surgery.

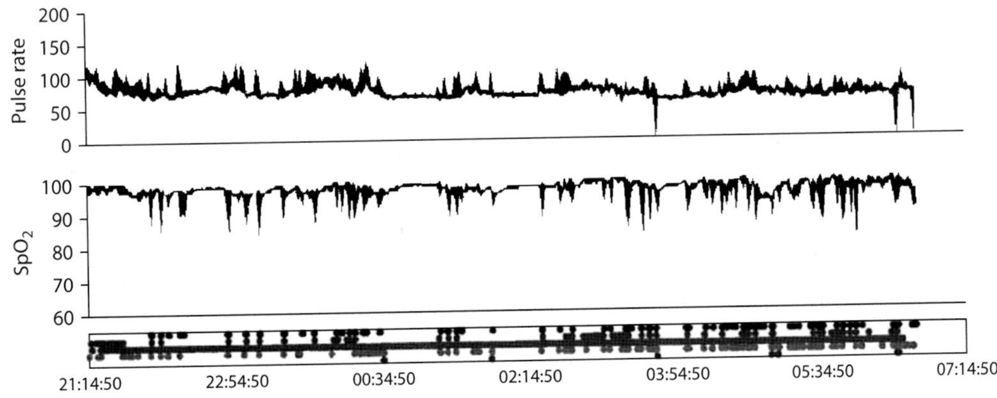

Figure 68.2 Pulse oximetry trace.

Table 68.3 Indications for paediatric respiratory investigations

- Diagnosis of OSA uncertain
- Age <2 years
- Weight <15 kg
- Down syndrome
- Cerebral palsy
- Hypotonia or neuromuscular disorders
- Craniofacial anomalies
- Mucopolysaccharidosis
- Obesity
- Significant co-morbidity
- Residual symptoms after adenotonsillectomy

Formal sleep studies such as PSG are far less widely used in children and are usually available only in specialized units. Provision in the United Kingdom is patchy, and there is a good deal of variability in what is measured. A reasonable minimum standard includes – in addition to pulse oximetry – respiratory airflow measurements, electrocardiography (ECG), thoraco-abdominal muscle movements, video and sound recording and arousal detection via, for example electroencephalography (ENG). End-tidal CO_2 to detect hypercarbia and oesophageal pH monitoring to correlate hypoxic events with gastro-oesophageal reflux are more sophisticated and less widely available measurements. PSG studies require a quiet room or cubicle rather than an open ward and need skilled interpretation by a physician with a specific interest in paediatric sleep medicine.

TREATMENT

GENERAL PRINCIPLES

Current evidence does not support the use of surgery for snoring alone (PS). Bear in mind that a clinical history alone may not be adequate to exclude OSA, and if there is doubt, overnight oximetry with PSG in selected cases may be appropriate. Children with very mild OSA – particularly if they are improving – can be managed expectantly. It is important to address causative factors such as rhinitis, which is common in children but often unrecognized and undertreated. Even if there is adenotonsillar hypertrophy, there may be coexistent rhinitis; it may be sensible to give the child a therapeutic trial of intra-nasal steroids. Both systemic steroids and prolonged antibiotic therapy have been advocated for children with tonsillar enlargement, but the safety of adenotonsillectomy and the morbidity of systemic steroids is now such that surgery will usually be preferable.

ADENOTONSILLECTOMY

Adenotonsillectomy is by far the most widely performed procedure for OSA in children. Symptomatic improvement is rapid. In judiciously chosen cases the procedure will bring about marked improvement in quality of life measures for parent and child. Childhood OSA is generally a rewarding and simple condition to treat.

PERIOPERATIVE CARE AND INVESTIGATIONS

OSA children by definition have airway obstruction. This can make for challenges in perioperative management. Otherwise healthy children rarely present endotracheal intubation difficulties, but they may be difficult to extubate, slow to recover from anaesthesia and show a marked sedating response to opioid analgesia. Severe cases may have segmental atelectasis or incipient right heart failure. They may have an impaired ventilatory response to carbon dioxide and are at increased risk of respiratory complications.

An experienced anaesthetist skilled in the management of children is an essential member of the team treating these children. Perioperative glucocorticoids may help reduce post-operative morbidity. Children with severe OSA tend to do best when they have surgery in the morning rather than later in the day.

Most children with OSA can have surgery in their local ENT unit without the need for a paediatric intensive care unit (PICU) or high-dependency unit (HDU) bed. Very young (under 2 years) patients and children with severe OSA or significant co-morbidity are best managed in a specialist centre where HDU

Table 68.4 Children at risk from respiratory complications where treatment should ideally take place in a specialist children's centre

- Age under 2 years
- Weight under 15 kg
- Failure to thrive
- Obesity
- Severe cerebral palsy
- Moderate or severe hypotonia or neuromuscular disorders
- Significant craniofacial anomalies
- Mucopolysaccharidosis
- Syndromes associated with difficult airway
- Significant co-morbidity (e.g. ASA 3 or above)
- ECG or echocardiographic abnormalities
- Severe OSA

and PICU facilities are readily available. Local protocols vary, but Table 68.4 summarizes the recommendations of the UK Multidisciplinary Working Party in regard to which OSA children need referral to a specialist unit.

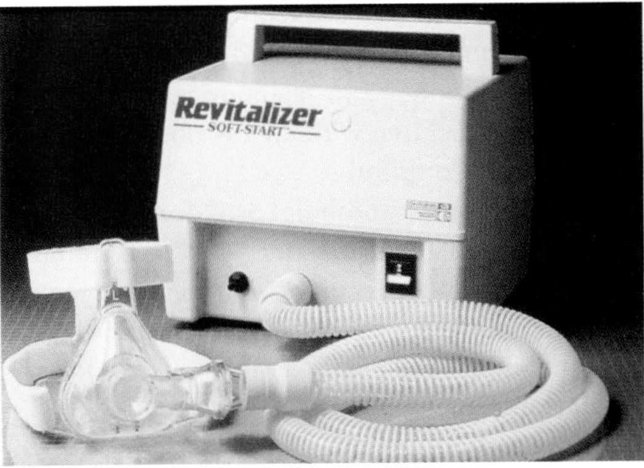

Figure 68.3 CPAP machine.

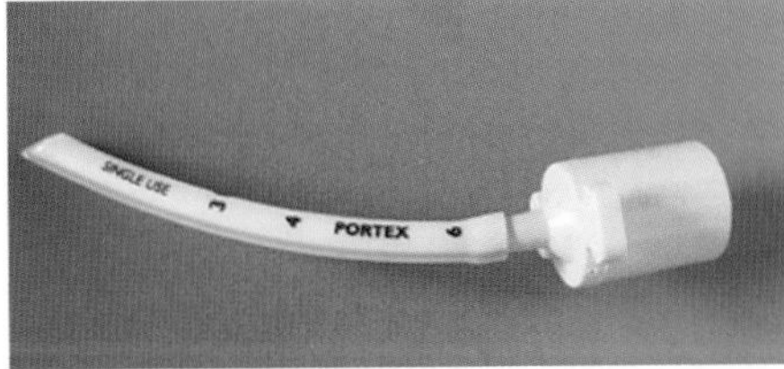

Figure 68.4 A size 3.5 (newborn) endotracheal tube makes an excellent nasopharyngeal airway for an infant, e.g. with Pierre Robin sequence. It can be cut to about 6 cm, lubricated and gently inserted into the nasal cavity so that the end projects into the nasopharynx. The nasal end can then be anchored to the skin of the cheek with adhesive strapping or secured with ribbon gauze tied at the back of the baby's head. In many cases parents learn to manage the nasopharyngeal airway so the child can go home.

CPAP

Continuous positive airway pressure (CPAP) is widely used in the management of nocturnal airway obstruction in adults. The principle relies on a continuous stream of air usually delivered through a face mask to act as a pneumatic splint and maintain patency of the otherwise flaccid pharyngeal airway (Figure 68.3). There may be compliance problems in children, but the device can be used at home and is particularly useful in children with complex medical needs or in those with severe OSA who have had a poor response to surgery. Many children's hospitals and clinics now manage home CPAP programmes. The help of a respiratory physician or anaesthetist is invaluable. CPAP is not without side effects and can cause nasal drying, vestibulitis headaches and epistaxis.

NASOPHARYNGEAL AIRWAY

A modified endotracheal tube introduced transnasally with the distal end positioned just below the free margin of the soft palate may maintain a patent nasopharyngeal airway (NPA) in children with glossoptosis. If parents are adequately trained to clean and change such an airway, the child can often be discharged home and monitored for weeks or even months until the retrognathia improves and he or she can manage without airway support (Figure 68.4).

MAXILLOMANDIBULAR SURGERY

Maxillofacial and paediatric craniofacial surgeons are getting better results with the technique of 'distraction osteogenesis'. This involves the placement of an interposed prosthesis into the growing facial skeleton, which is then sequentially expanded over a period of months. Often used for aesthetic reasons, this technique can facilitate reversal of tracheotomy in children with airway obstruction due to craniofacial syndromes.

Maxillary and mandibular osteotomies are used in the management of adult OSA, but this modality of treatment is not part of the routine management of OSA in children except on a carefully considered individual basis in a designated craniofacial surgical unit.

TRACHEOTOMY

Tracheotomy is a tried-and-trusted technique to bypass upper airway obstruction. It is very rarely considered for uncomplicated OSA, but in children with severe multisystem disease, it may be a last resort. Tracheotomy is sometimes requested in children with severe neurological dysfunction. It should be considered an extreme measure, and the implications and potential complications (see Chapter 59) need to be discussed in detail with the parents or caregivers, the child's medical attendants and – if he or she is old enough – with the child.

KEY LEARNING POINTS

- OSA in children is common but not well defined.
- The diagnosis is clinical, with confirmatory tests needed only in selected cases.
- Intervention – typically adeno-tonsillar surgery – is highly effective
- Peri-operative management of severe or difficult cases is best undertaken in centres with specialist paediatric facilities and expertise.
- Continuous positive airway pressure (CPAP) is increasingly available for home use.

FURTHER READING

Brietzke SE, Gallagher D. The effectiveness of tonsillectomy and adenoidectomy in the treatment of pediatric obstructive sleep apnea/hypopnea syndrome: A meta-analysis. *Otolaryngology – Head and Neck Surgery.* 2006; 134: 979–84.

Brouilette RT, Morielli A, Leimnais A, Waters KA, Luciano R, Ducharme FM. Nocturnal pulse oximetry as an abbreviated testing modality for pediatric obstructive sleep apnea. *Pediatrics.* 2000; 105: 405–12.

Gozal D, O'Brien LM. Snoring and obstructive sleep apnoea in children: Why should we treat? *Paediatric Respiratory Reviews.* 2004; 5 Suppl A: S371–6.

Guilleminault C, Lee JH, Chan A. Pediatric obstructive sleep apnea syndrome. *Archives of Pediatrics and Adolescent Medicine.* 2005; 159(8): 775–85.

Lim J, McKean MC. Adenotonsillectomy for obstructive sleep apnoea in children. *Cochrane Database of Systematic Reviews.* 2009; (2): CD003136.

Powell S, Kubba H, O'Brien C, Tremiett M. Paediatric obstructive sleep apnoea. *BMJ.* 2010; 340: c1918.

Robb PJ. Bew S. Kubba H. Murphy N. Primhak R. Rollin AM. Tremlett M. Tonsillectomy and adenoidectomy in children with sleep-related breathing disorders: Consensus statement of a UK multidisciplinary working party. *Annals of the Royal College of Surgeons of England.* 2009; 91(5): 371–3.

Royal College of Paediatric and Child Health Working Party on Sleep Physiology and Respiratory Control Disorders in Childhood. Standards for services for children with disorders of sleep physiology. 2009. Available from: www.rcpch.ac.uk/Research/ce/Guidelines-frontpage/Guideline-Appraisals-by-Organisation/RCPCH-Working-Party. (This is a comprehensive review of children's sleep disorders, including obstructive sleep apnoea.)

Sohn H, Rosenfeld RM. Evaluation of sleep-disordered breathing in children. *Otolaryngology – Head and Neck Surgery.* 2003; 128: 344–52.

Wilson TG. *Diseases of the Ear, Nose and Throat in Children.* London: Heinemann, 1955.

69

Drooling

S MUSHEER HUSSAIN AND MUHAMMAD SHAKEEL

Drooling can be defined as an involuntary spillage of saliva over the lower lip. It is important to clarify the definition of drooling, as *sialorrhea* is an increased salivary flow but typically with a normal volume of saliva produced and *hypersalivation* is increased saliva production.

Drooling in healthy infants and toddlers is normal and may be associated with teething. Drooling beyond 4 years of age in normal children is generally regarded as abnormal, but it is normal in children up to 6 years of age with neuromuscular disorders like cerebral palsy as neuromuscular control may take longer in these children. The prevalence of drooling can be between 37 to 58 per cent in children with cerebral palsy.[1]

Drooling can be classified as acute and chronic. Acute drooling can occur in oropharyngeal infections such as quinsy, retropharyngeal abscess or epiglottitis. Medications such as clonazepam can cause increased saliva production.

More often, the condition is chronic and is seen in children with general physical disability or oral motor control impairment. Common conditions include cerebral palsy, severe mental retardation, facial paralysis or encephalopathy.[2]

The drooling may be predominantly anterior when the saliva is lost from the front of mouth or posterior when saliva flows over the back of tongue and spills through the faucial isthmus, creating a risk of aspiration.

PATHOPHYSIOLOGY

Saliva is produced by the salivary glands, and its production is controlled by the autonomic nervous system (primarily parasympathetic). The nervous control is regulated by external somatic stimuli such as vision, smell and taste. The unconscious swallowing of saliva is a complex procedure and requires coordination of more than 25 pairs of bulbar muscles.[3] Drooling can be caused by excess production of saliva, inability to retain saliva within the mouth, or problem swallowing the saliva caused by dysphagia and odynophagia.

Chronic drooling primarily results from in-coordination of the oral phase of swallowing, allowing pooling of saliva in the anterior mouth and spillage secondary to poorly synchronized inadequate lip closure, disorganized tongue movements, impaired oral and perioral sensory function, head-down posture and reduced frequency of swallowing.

PROBLEMS CAUSED BY DROOLING

For the child, the anterior drooling can cause: perioral dermatitis, skin breakdown, malodour, recurrent infections, impaired masticatory function, interference with speech and social embarrassment and isolation. Dehydration and electrolytes disturbance can result from severe drooling. The posterior drooling can potentially cause cough, gagging, vomiting and aspiration with resultant pneumonia.

A drooling child may require frequent clothes and bib changing because of soiling. The child also may need increased educational efforts as teaching materials and communicative devices become wet.

Drooling has significant social implications for both parents and the child, with a drooling child being less likely to receive normal physical reassuring contact from parents and carers.

ASSESSMENT OF A CHILD WITH DROOLING

Assessment should ideally be carried out in a multidisciplinary team setting. Such a team should consist of a speech and language therapist, otolaryngologist, occupational therapist, paediatrician and dentist with input available from an interventional radiologist, neurologist, plastic surgeon, physiotherapist, specialist nurses and teachers.

Detailed history is taken to assess the frequency and severity of drooling. This includes consideration of the secondary effects of drooling. Every effort should be made to identify the factors that may increase the problems of drooling, such as posture; dental health; ear, nose and throat (ENT) symptoms and neurological status. It is essential to establish whether there is any evidence of chronic aspiration. This should be suspected if there is coughing and choking on saliva, especially at night. Check if the child suffers from chest infections or is on home oxygen. Ask about symptoms of gastro-oesophageal reflux. Reflux, if severe, may cause hyperstimulation of the salivary glands and thus genuine hypersalivation. Reflux is common in children with neuromuscular conditions. Ask about feeding, speech and general development. Children with oral motor dyspraxia may have speech problems and difficulty manipulating food in the mouth as well as drooling. Drooling may also be a feature of general developmental delay. Review current medication to identify anything that may have an adverse effect on saliva control. Medication with cholinergic effects, such as anticonvulsants, may cause genuine hypersalivation.

The drooling severity can be quantified to some degree by means of counting bibs or clothing changes during the day. Objective assessment of drooling can be accomplished using severity ratings such as Blasco's scale[4] and the Teachers' Drooling Score.[5]

The effects of drooling on the child and family can be assessed using the Drooling Impact Scale (DIS). Any potential benefits to the family must carefully be weighed against the risks and discomforts suffered by the child as a possible complication of interventions for drooling management.

Carry out a general assessment of the patient's physical health with a view to assess fitness for anaesthesia. Observe the child when feeding, drinking and swallowing and when performing a simple task that requires concentration, appropriate to the child's neurological status.[3]

A clinical examination is then performed, focusing on the dental health, adenotonsillar hypertrophy, nasal obstruction, postural control and the neurology of the tongue, cranial nerves, bulbar region, swallowing and the respiratory system.[3]

MANAGEMENT

A comprehensive, individualized management plan is formulated in consultation with the child and parents depending upon the aetiology. It is based on improving the child's quality of life without compromising oral health. The treatment plan follows an incremental approach (Table 69.1) and may include the following.

PHYSICAL THERAPIES TO IMPROVE POSTURE

Optimize the posture control of head, neck and trunk to prevent anterior drooling. Posture is particularly important in children who are wheelchair-dependent. The chair may need to be adapted to give the child a slightly reclined position. A small platform can be used on top of a desk to raise the working position for a child who has a particular problem when leaning forward over a computer keyboard or written homework.

CORRECTION OF REVERSIBLE CAUSES OF DROOLING

Correct the malocclusion, caries and gum disease accordingly. Prevention of excessive mouthing of fingers or objects helps reduce the stimulus of saliva production and encourages lip closure. It is best to avoid fizzy drinks and very acidic foods to minimize saliva production. Adenotonsillectomy can be considered if adenotonsillar hypertrophy is causing the child to mouth-breathe, contributing to drooling.

Table 69.1 Managing the drooling – an incremental approach

	Management option
1	Physical therapies to improve posture
2	Correction of reversible causes of drooling
3	Conservative measures to improve drooling
4	Acupuncture to improve drooling
5	Behavioural interventions to improve drooling
6	Specific oral-motor exercises to improve drooling
7	Intraoral devices to improve drooling
8	Pharmacotherapy to improve drooling
9	Botulinum toxin A to improve drooling
10	Surgical interventions to improve drooling

CONSERVATIVE MEASURES

Use sports towelling wristbands in older children who are able to wipe their mouth. 'Dabbing' rather than 'wiping' across the mouth and chin causes less local stimulation to the salivary glands. Use absorbent neckerchiefs and bandanas in children with profuse drooling to protect clothes.[3]

ACUPUNCTURE

Tongue acupuncture is an innovative technique in traditional Chinese medicine and has been used in the treatment of drooling in children with neurological impairment. It involves acupuncture performed daily to five points of the tongue for 30 sessions.[6] This could be used as an adjunctive or alternative treatment for a child with drooling problems before subjecting the patient to invasive surgical procedures on the salivary glands.

BEHAVIOURAL INTERVENTIONS

These interventions aim to enforce target behaviours such as swallowing, wiping, head control, mouth closure, nondrooling and performing self-control of drooling behaviour. They can be categorized into (1) instruction, prompting, and positive social reinforcement; (2) negative social reinforcement and declarative procedures; (3) cueing techniques; and (4) self-management. Behavioural treatment has been shown to be effective to increase swallowing and wiping and to decrease drooling.[7]

SPECIFIC ORAL-MOTOR EXERCISES

These aim to improve lip and jaw closure as well as increase tongue control, reduce tongue thrust, normalize tone, and normalize facial and oral sensation. For children who are aware enough to obey commands and cooperate with training, this is the keystone of non-surgical intervention for drooling, and should usually be trialled for at least 6 months before considering surgical intervention. Initial manoeuvres include improving the child's seating position and a programme of improving lip and jaw closure and tongue movements. In its simplest form, it consists of exercises that are presented as part of play, such as presenting different textures around the mouth (ice cubes, electric toothbrush and so forth) to stimulate sensory awareness and exercises to improve lip seal and tongue movement (blowing through a drinking straw, making lipstick kisses on paper, blowing party blowers and so forth). It is important to remember that children with severe developmental delay will not be able to comply.[2,8] Based on the results of a recent evidence-based systematic review, there is insufficient evidence to determine the effects of oral-motor exercises on children with oral sensorimotor deficits and swallowing problems.[9]

INTRAORAL DEVICES

These appliances aim to modify and improve oral motor function to prevent drooling of saliva. These devices have a potential role as an intermediate step, following failed oral motor therapy, before considering surgical intervention. These appliances vary according to shape, position within the oral cavity and the length of time that the person must wear the appliance.[1] Examples include the Exeter Lip Sensor, palatal training appliances and the Innsbruck Sensorimotor Activator and Regulator (ISMAR). The palatal training appliances encourage active lip, tongue and palatal movements, moving saliva to the back of the oral cavity for swallowing rather than passive spill from the front. The risk of aspiration or airway blockage means they are not suitable for children or young people with severely limited control of tongue movement, and epilepsy is a contraindication.[3]

PHARMACOTHERAPY

Anticholinergic medications are used with an aim to reduce the volume of saliva produced in the oral cavity and in the gastro-intestinal tract. The common agents used are atropine, benztropine, glycopyrrolate bromide, benzhexol hydrochloride (also known as trihexyphenidyl) and scopolamine. Medications can be administered orally, intravenously, topically as dermal patches, intramuscularly and via nebulization. Anticholinergic medication is by far the most common treatment used, especially by community paediatricians. Side effects do occur, but anticholinergics should still be tried, in conjunction with provision of information to the parents on potential side effects. Hyoscine patches are a reasonable first-line choice because they are convenient (change every 3 days), but skin reaction to the adhesive is common. Oral hyoscine given four times a day is also effective. Trihexyphenidyl syrup (benzhexol) is helpful for those who are gastrostomy dependent.[2]

The side effects from anticholinergic medications include: xerostomia, thick mucoid secretions, dehydration, urinary retention, urinary tract infections, constipation, facial flushing, skin rash, fever, dizziness, drowsiness, headache, dilated pupils, blurred vision and epilepsy.[1]

BOTULINUM TOXIN A

Botulinum toxin A is the most common neurotoxin used to treat drooling. The submandibular and sub-lingual salivary glands contribute most of basal salivary secretion, and therefore are targeted for botulinum therapy. Ultrasound guidance can potentially lower the side-effect profile of botulinum toxin injection by facilitating targeted injection into the salivary glands rather than accidentally into surrounding tissues. When injected directly, this potent neurotoxin is taken up into the parasympathetic end plate and irreversibly blocks release of acetylcholine (ACh), thereby reducing the amount of saliva produced by the salivary glands. The dosage varies according to the product and weight of the child, but use a lesser amount of botulinum toxin if the glands look small. Quantitative and qualitative benefit are greatest at 4 to 6 weeks post-injection. The injections can be repeated every 3 to 6 months, dependent on response. Most children require repeated injections for long-term control. Although minimally invasive, children with neurological disabilities may tolerate the procedure after application of topical anaesthetic cream.

Botulinum toxin injection is most helpful for those patients with chronic aspiration in whom repeated general anaesthesia may be contraindicated because of chronic pulmonary dysfunction; these patients are often less aware of their surroundings and therefore tolerate injection under local anaesthesia well. The possible side effects may relate to the injection trauma and include pain, haematoma, intraoral bleed, swallowing difficulty associated with swelling of the salivary gland, infection and possible trauma to the facial nerve when injecting the parotid gland. Side effects associated with the botulinum toxin include excessively dry mouth, problems with chewing and swallowing as a result of toxin diffusion to muscles involved in swallowing, facial weakness, recurrent mandibular dislocation and transient fever. The authors believe the dysphagia results from the systemic effect of botulinum toxin, as dysphagia has been described after botulinum toxin injection to the limbs for spasticity and cosmetic facial injection, although it is probably more common after salivary injection. It is important to remember that when severe, dysphagia may necessitate tube feeding for a period of weeks, and parents should be warned against this complication when consenting for botulinum therapy.[1,2,3] Current evidence suggests the medical management of drooling is unsatisfactory, but the administration of botulinum toxin into the salivary glands is perhaps the most effective way of treating drooling.[10]

SURGICAL INTERVENTIONS

Surgery aims to either reduce or remove innervation to the salivary glands, to redirect saliva by rerouting the salivary ducts, to block salivary flow and induce atrophy of the glands through ligation or to eliminate the production of saliva by excising the salivary glands. Surgical intervention can be performed unilaterally or bilaterally and involves a general anaesthetic. In practice, a combination of the surgical procedures is employed to achieve the best outcome for the patient.[11] The surgical interventions can be grouped into those reducing the saliva and those redirecting the salivary flow (Table 69.2).

The sectioning of chorda tympani or tympanic neurectomy works by eliminating the parasympathetic stimulation to the salivary glands. Submandibular and parotid duct ligation works

Table 69.2 Surgical interventions for management of drooling

Reducing the salivary volume	Redirecting the salivary flow
Sectioning of the Chorda tympani	Rerouting of the submandibular gland duct
Tympanic neurectomy	Rerouting of the parotid gland duct
Submandibular gland ligation	
Parotid gland ligation	
Submandibular gland excision	
Sublingual gland excision	

by inducing atrophy of the gland once the duct is tied off. Normally, sublingual gland excision is carried out in combination with submandibular gland excision or when rerouting the submandibular ducts to reduce the risk of rannula formation. Rerouting of the submandibular gland duct involves transferring the submandibular ducts to approximately 1 cm behind the tongue base, just behind the anterior pillar, directing salivary flow posteriorly.

The choice of surgical intervention depends upon the presence or absence of aspiration in a drooling child. If there is any doubt, a videofluoroscopy assessment of swallow should be arranged. For children who aspirate (or where there is any doubt), salivary redirection is unsafe and a bilateral submandibular gland excision with bilateral parotid duct ligation should be performed. However, if there is no aspiration, the most commonly performed procedure is rerouting of the both submandibular ducts.

A recent meta-analysis found that most evidence regarding surgical outcomes of sialorrhea management in children is low-quality and heterogeneous. Despite this, most patients experience a subjective improvement following surgical treatment.[12]

Surgery is a major step for a non–life-threatening condition, and the benefits (one-off treatment with permanent effect and without the risk of dysphagia as compared with botulinum toxin) need to be carefully weighed against the risks and discomforts.[2]

KEY LEARNING POINTS

- Drooling is normal in healthy infants, toddlers and children up to 6 years of age with neuromuscular disorders such as cerebral palsy.
- Drooling with aspiration needs aggressive management to prevent chronic lung damage.
- Detailed history is taken to assess the frequency and severity of drooling.
- Drooling is best managed in a multidisciplinary setting.
- Stepwise approach to management of drooling progresses from behaviour therapy to pharmacotherapy to surgical procedures.

REFERENCES

1. Walshe M, Smith M, Pennington L. Interventions for drooling in children with cerebral palsy. *Cochrane Database of Systematic Reviews*. 2012; Issue 11. Art. No.: CD008624. doi: 10.1002/14651858.CD008624.pub3.
2. Little SA, Kubba H, Hussain SSM. An evidence-based approach to the child who drools saliva. *Clinical Otolaryngology*. 2009 Jun; 34(3): 236–9. doi: 10.1111/j.1749-4486.2009.01917.x.
3. Fairhurst CB, Cockerill H. Management of drooling in children. *Archives of Disease in Childhood – Education and Practice*. 2011 Feb; 96(1): 25–30. doi: 10.1136/adc.2007.129478. Epub 2010 Jul 30.
4. Blasco PA, Allaire JH. Drooling in the developmentally disabled: Management practices and recommendations. Consortium on drooling. 1992; *Developmental Medicine and Child Neurology*. 34: 849–62.
5. Camp-Bruno JA, Winsberg BG, Green-Parsons AR, et al. Efficacy of benztropine therapy for drooling. *Developmental Medicine and Child Neurology* 1989; 31: 309–19.
6. Wong V, Sun JG, Wong W. Traditional Chinese medicine (tongue acupuncture) in children with drooling problems. *Pediatric Neurology*. 2001; 25(1): 47–54.
7. Van der Burg JJ, Didden R, Jongerius PH, Rotteveel JJ. Behavioral treatment of drooling: A methodological critique of the literature with clinical guidelines and suggestions for future research. *Behavior Modification*. 2007 Sep; 31(5): 573–94.
8. Crysdale WS, McCann C, Roske L, et al. Saliva control issues in the neurologically challenged. A 30 year experience in team management. *International Journal of Pediatric Otorhinolaryngology*. 2006; 70: 519–27.
9. Arvedson J, Clark H, Lazarus C, Schooling T, Frymark T. The effects of oral-motor exercises on swallowing in children: An evidence-based systematic review. *Developmental Medicine and Child Neurology*. 2010 Nov; 52(11): 1000–13. doi: 10.1111/j.1469-8749.2010.03707.x.
10. Lakraj AA, Moghimi N, Jabbari B. Sialorrhea: Anatomy, pathophysiology and treatment with emphasis on the role of botulinum toxins. *Toxins (Basel)*. 2013 May 21; 5(5): 1010–31. doi: 10.3390/toxins5051010.
11. Gallagher TQ, Hartnick CJ. Bilateral submandibular gland excision and parotid duct ligation. *Advances in Otorhinolaryngology*. 2012; 73: 70–5. doi: 10.1159/000334319. Epub 2012 Mar 29.
12. Reed J, Mans CK, Brietzke SE. Surgical management of drooling: A meta-analysis. *Archives of Otolaryngology and Head and Neck Surgery*. 2009 Sep; 135(9): 924–31. doi: 10.1001/archoto.2009.110.

SECTION V

Miscellaneous

70

ENT head and neck radiology

THIRU SUDARSHAN

Imaging is often required to confirm a clinical diagnosis, to characterize a lesion or to evaluate the extent of known disease. The last three decades have seen significant improvement both in availability and capability of imaging modalities like ultrasound, computed tomography (CT) and magnetic resonance imaging (MRI). Each modality has its own advantages, and sometimes it may be necessary to do more than one investigation to acquire the required information. Knowledge of capabilities, advantages and disadvantages of an investigation would enable the clinician to tailor the request to address the clinical needs of each patient.

MODALITIES

CONVENTIONAL RADIOGRAPHY

There has been a significant reduction in use of plain x-rays for evaluation of ear, nose and throat (ENT) disorders over the last three decades owing to the development of ultrasound, CT and MRI. While x-rays are cheap and easily available, they also carry the risk of ionizing radiation. Currently the use of x-rays is limited to a small number of indications, such as evaluation of foreign body in neck, assessing position and integrity of cochlear implant electrodes, and so forth.

CONTRAST STUDIES

Barium or water-soluble contrast swallow studies performed under fluoroscopic screening are used to evaluate the structure and motility of the pharynx and oesophagus. These studies can demonstrate pharyngeal webs, pharyngeal pouches, oesophageal diverticula, dysmotility disorders, strictures and mass lesions. These are also used in post-operative patients to evaluate the patency of post-surgical anastomoses.

ULTRASOUND

Ultrasound is one of the most widely used modalities for investigation of ENT disorders. Ultrasound uses high-frequency sound waves and does not have the risks associated with ionizing radiation. It is relatively inexpensive and is widely available. It should be noted that ultrasound is a dynamic examination, and quality of the examination is very much dependent on the skills of the operator. Ultrasound using high-frequency transducers is especially suited for evaluation of the superficial structures of the neck, including parotid and submandibular salivary glands, thyroid gland and cervical lymph nodes. Ultrasound can be used to guide fine-needle aspirations and biopsies.

COMPUTED TOMOGRAPHY

CT scan uses a thin x-ray beam and a row of detectors that rotate around the patient. Based on the intensity of x-rays reaching the detectors, the density of the tissue is calculated and the images are reconstructed by the computer. The current generation of multislice CT scanners has the capability to image at thickness of less than a millimetre. These images, which are acquired as a volume without any gap, can be reconstructed in axial, sagittal and coronal dimensions without any loss of detail.

High density of the bones and low density of surrounding air give natural contrast and help to clearly delineate anatomy and pathologies of the paranasal sinuses and the temporal bones. CT scan with intravenous iodinated contrast is used to evaluate infectious and malignant pathologies affecting the neck.

MAGNETIC RESONANCE IMAGING

MRI involves positioning the patient in a powerful magnet that causes the hydrogen atoms present in water in the body to align along the axis of the magnetic field. The magnetic field is then altered rapidly by switching on radiofrequency coils around the magnet. This causes realignment of the hydrogen atoms with increase in energy. When the radiofrequency coils are switched off, the hydrogen atoms go back to the resting state, releasing the excess energy as photons. The frequency of these released photons varies between tissues. The differences are evaluated by the computer, and images are produced based on these differences.

Excellent soft-tissue resolution of MRI is useful in staging malignancies of the head and neck. It is the investigation of choice in evaluation of the cerebellopontine angle cisterns and internal auditory canals. MRI is also used to characterize lesions in the salivary glands.

MRI is contraindicated in patients with pacemakers, cochlear implants and nerve stimulators.

RADIONUCLIDE IMAGING

Radionuclide imaging can provide anatomical and functional information of the target organ and involves the injection of a radiopharmaceutical tracer and subsequent scanning in a gamma camera. The radiopharmaceutical tracers used usually are technetium pertechnetate or iodine-123 in case of thyroid and technetium-99m sestamibi or technetium-99m tetrofosmin in case of the parathyroid. Iodine-131 is used in the detection and treatment of metastases from thyroid carcinoma.

POSITRON EMISSION TOMOGRAPHY

Positron emission tomography (PET) involves the injection of a radiopharmaceutical. The most commonly used radiopharmaceutical in clinical practice currently is a modified glucose molecule called 18 fluorodeoxyglucose (FDG). FDG in body tissue undergoes decay, releasing a positron that collides with an electron to produce two annihilation photons travelling in opposite directions. These are detected by the scanner and an image is reconstructed. Modern PET scanners are usually hybrid systems with a combination of a PET and CT scanner, able to obtain both anatomical and functional information. In current clinical practice PET-CT is useful in detecting unknown primary lesions in patients who present with metastatic lymph nodes in the neck.

TEMPORAL BONE AND POSTERIOR FOSSA

DEVELOPMENTAL ANOMALIES

External auditory canal and middle ear

Congenital aural dysplasias presenting with deformity of the pinna are often associated with dysplasia of the external auditory canal and middle ear cavity owing to their common development from the brachial apparatus (Figure 70.1). CT demonstrates anomalies of the external auditory canal and middle ear such as vertical angulation of external auditory canal, posterior displacement of temporomandibular joint, fusion of the malleus and incus, dehiscence and inferior displacement of the tympanic segment of the facial nerve and anterior displacement of the mastoid segment of the facial nerve.

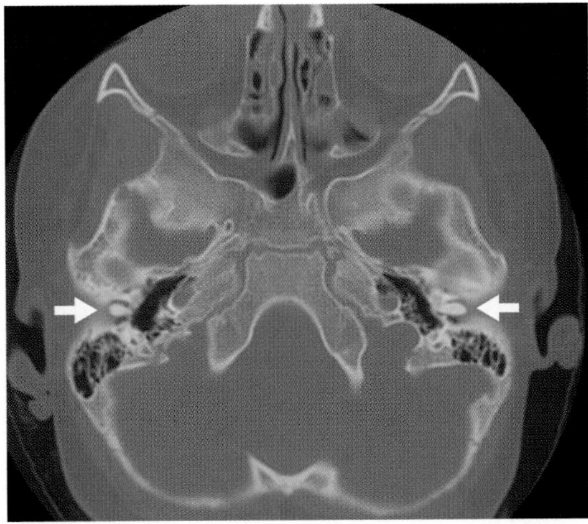

Figure 70.1 Bilateral external auditory canal atresia – Axial CT scan image shows atresia of bilateral external auditory canals with bony spur (arrows) and hypoplastic pinna.

Inner ear

Anomalies of the otic capsule are demonstrated by CT, while abnormal development of the membranous labyrinth can only be visualized by MRI (Figure 70.2). Often a combination of CT and MRI is required to assess suitability for surgery and cochlear implantation. Findings on imaging range from common cystic cavity with complete absence of vestibule and cochlea in case of complete labyrinthine aplasia to varying degrees of hypoplasia of cochlea or semicircular canals, depending on the gestational age at the time of insult to the otic capsule. MRI is used to evaluate the cochlear nerve and to rule out obliteration of the cochlear lumen by fibrous tissue.

TRAUMA

CT is the investigation of choice for evaluation of patients with suspected temporal bone fractures. These patients may present with haemotympanum, hearing loss or cerebrospinal fluid (CSF) otorrhoea. Fractures of the temporal bone are traditionally classified as longitudinal, transverse or mixed. Longitudinal fractures are more common than transverse fractures and run along the long axis of the petrous temporal bone (Figure 70.3).

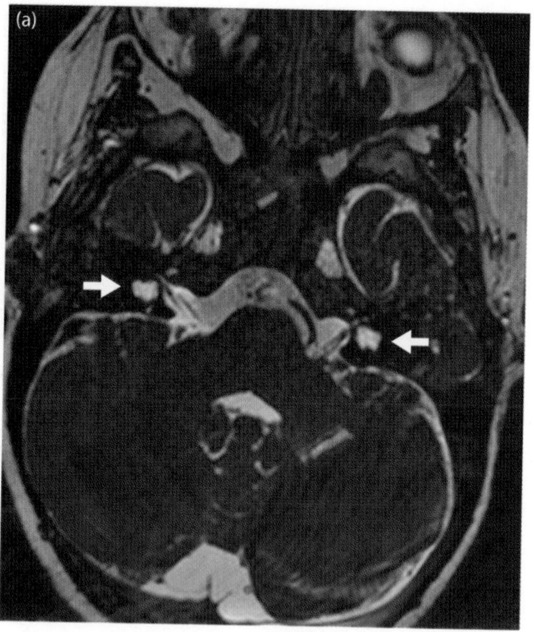

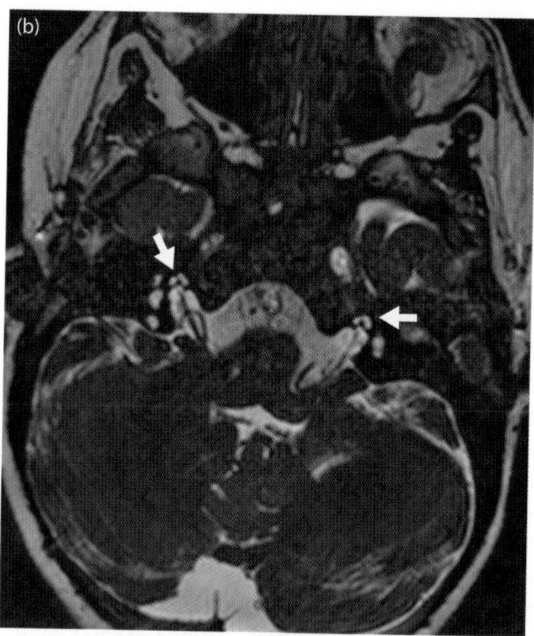

Figure 70.2 Axial T2 MRI images showing bilateral dysplastic vestibule **(a)** and cochlea **(b)**.

Longitudinal fractures are commonly associated with conductive hearing loss owing to ossicular injury and rupture of tympanic membrane. Transverse fractures are perpendicular to the long axis of the petrous temporal bone, and are more commonly associated with sensorineural hearing loss owing to involvement of the

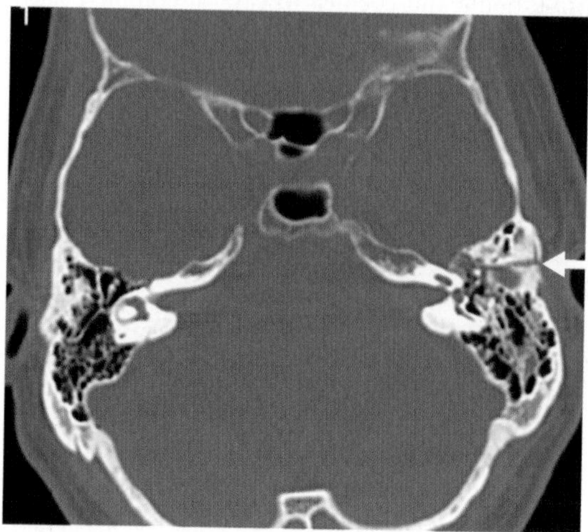

Figure 70.3 Axial CT images show a longitudinal fracture (arrow) involving the epitympanum with subluxation of the malleo-incudal joint.

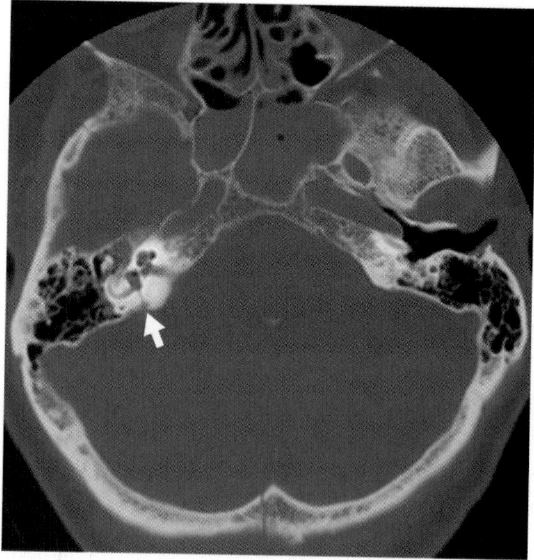

Figure 70.4 Axial CT image shows a transverse fracture (arrow) involving the vestibule that contains a small air pocket. Blood is seen in the epitympanum.

labyrinth (Figure 70.4). Post-traumatic CSF otorrhoea is more likely to be secondary to transverse fractures of the temporal bone involving the tegmen. MRI is useful to rule out the presence of an associated encephalocele in these patients, as encephaloceles show signal characteristics similar to the brain.

INFECTION AND INFLAMMATION

Necrotizing external otitis

Necrotizing external otitis, also called malignant otitis externa, is often seen in diabetic or immunocompromised patients and is usually caused by *Pseudomonas* bacteria. Inflammatory soft-tissue thickening is noted in the external auditory canal. There is often local extension of infection, anteriorly into the temporomandibular joint, inferiorly into the stylomastoid foramen with involvement of the facial nerve and medially into the middle ear. CT is used to identify the presence of bony erosion (Figure 70.5), while MRI delineates the extent of soft-tissue involvement. Gallium scintigraphy is useful in evaluation of the status of infection after treatment.

Acute otomastoiditis and coalescent otomastoiditis

Acute otomastoiditis is very often a clinical diagnosis, and patients are only imaged when there is a suspicion of a complication. CT is the first investigation of choice and shows fluid in the middle ear cavity and mastoid air cells (Figure 70.6). With progression to coalescent otomastoiditis, there is erosion of the mastoid septations. Erosion of the lateral wall of the mastoid cells results in a subperiosteal abscess showing peripheral enhancement on a contrast enhanced CT. Extension of infection posteriorly can cause thinning and erosion of the sinus plate, leading to sigmoid sinus thrombosis, seen as filling defects on a CT or MR venogram. Extension of infection superiorly with erosion of the tegmen tympanum can lead to abscess in the temporal lobe.

Chronic otitis media

CT shows thickening and retraction of the remnant tympanic membrane. There may be complete or partial opacification of the middle ear cavity.

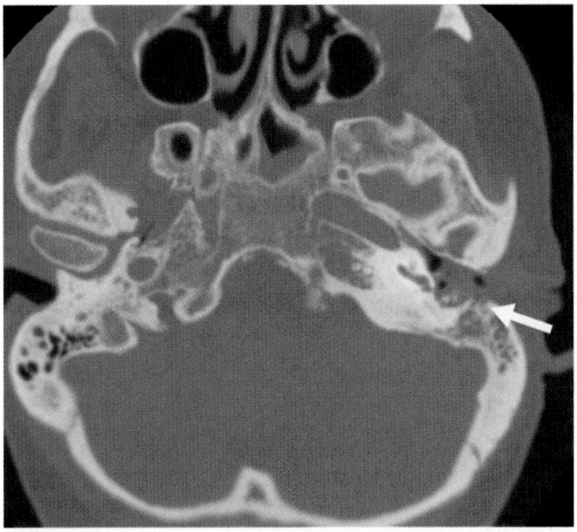

Figure 70.5 Axial CT image shows soft tissue filling the left external auditory canal with erosion of the posterior wall (arrow) of the external auditory canal.

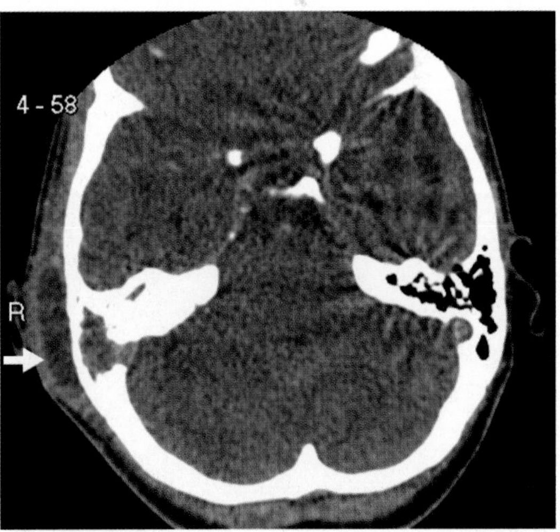

Figure 70.6 Axial image of a contrast-enhanced CT shows fluid in the right mastoid air cells with subperiosteal abscess (arrow) showing peripheral enhancement.

Erosion of the long process of incus is commonly seen. The mastoid air cells are sclerotic. Post-inflammatory calcification (tympanosclerosis) may be seen in the tympanic membrane or within the middle ear cavity.

Cholesteatoma

Pars flaccida cholesteatomas show a soft tissue mass in the Prussak's space, lateral to the head of malleus and body of incus with erosion of the scutum. There is erosion of the anterior aspect of the lateral epitympanic wall.

Pars tensa cholesteatomas arise from the posterosuperior aspect of the tympanic membrane with involvement of sinus tympani and facial nerve recess. Abnormal soft tissue is noted in the middle ear cavity medial to the auditory ossicles.

CT is used to evaluate cholesteatoma as it can delineate the extent of abnormal soft tissue and erosion of bony structures.

Cholesteatomas are associated with erosion of the auditory ossciles, commonly the long process of incus. Erosion of head of malleus and body of incus are also seen (Figure 70.7). Cholesteatomas may extend posterolaterally through the aditus ad antrum into the mastoid air cells, with development of a large cavity filled with soft tissue. Large cholesteatomas can cause erosion and fistula of the lateral semicircular canal, best seen on axial CT images. Erosion of the tympanic segment of the facial nerve canal can be appreciated on coronal CT images. Erosion of the anterior aspect of the tegmen tympanum can result in extension of cholesteatoma into the middle cranial fossa, resulting in temporal lobe abscess. Erosion of the posterosuperior aspect of the tegmen resulting in extension into the posterior fossa leads to septic thrombophlebitis of the sigmoid sinuses and cerebellar abscess. Contrast enhanced CT or MRI are essential to rule out intracranial involvement in large cholesteatomas.

Diffusion-weighted MRI (DWMRI) using non-echo planar imaging sequences has high sensitivity in detecting small foci of residual or recurrent cholesteatomas and is the investigation of choice in post-operative patients before second look surgery. Cholesteatomas show high signal on DWMRI images owing to restricted diffusion.

Appearance on post-operative CT varies with the type of surgery, with visualization of the posterior wall of the external auditory canal anterior to the mastoidectomy cavity in case of canal wall up mastoidectomy, and absence of posterior wall with formation of a single mastoidectomy cavity communicating with the external auditory canal in canal wall down mastoidectomy. Normal post-mastoidectomy cavities appear clear with no debris within the lumen. Filling of the cavity with

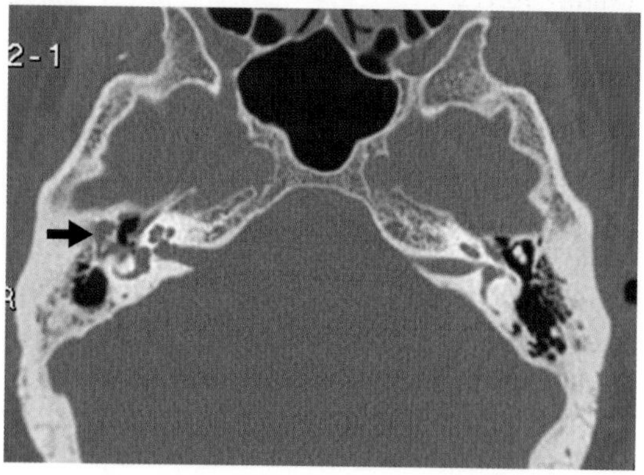

Figure 70.7 Axial CT image shows cholesteatoma in the right epitympanum (arrow) causing erosion of the head of the malleus.

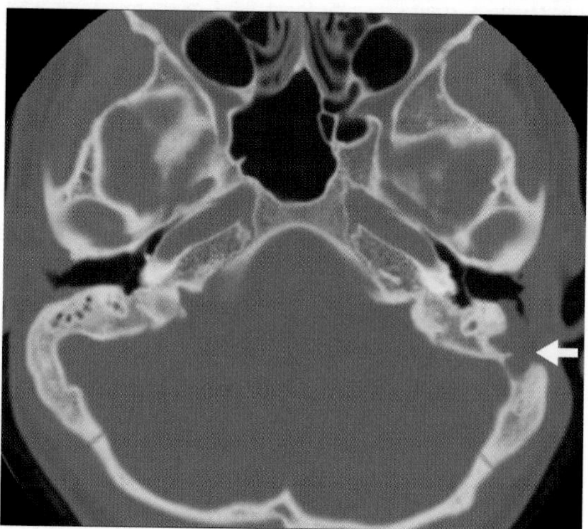

Figure 70.8 Axial CT image shows canal wall down mastoidectomy on the left with recurrent cholesteatoma (arrow).

soft-tissue density could be due to recurrent cholesteatoma or cholesterol granuloma cyst. Recurrent cholesteatomas may cause expansion of the cavity with thinning of the wall, erosion of the tegmen and labyrinthine fistula (Figure 70.8). Cholesterol granuloma cysts have sharply defined margins and show lower density on CT.

Labyrinthitis

Acute labyrinthitis is a clinical diagnosis, and imaging is very rarely performed. Focal enhancement is seen within the labyrinth on the post-contrast T1 MRI images. Chronic labyrinthitis shows blurring of margins and increased density of the lumen of the labyrinth on CT, secondary to osteitis. MRI shows absence of normal high signal within the lumen of the labyrinth.

Facial neuritis

Enhancement of the tympanic and mastoid segments of the facial nerves may be seen normally because of the presence of perineural venous plexus. Post-contrast MRI images may show prominent asymmetrical enhancement of the paralyzed facial nerve in patients with Bell's palsy and Ramsay Hunt syndrome (Figure 70.9). There is enhancement of the canalicular segment, anterior genu, labyrinthine and tympanic segments of the facial nerve in Bell's palsy. There is diffuse enhancement of the facial nerve with involvement of the adjacent vestibulocochlear nerves in Ramsay Hunt syndrome.

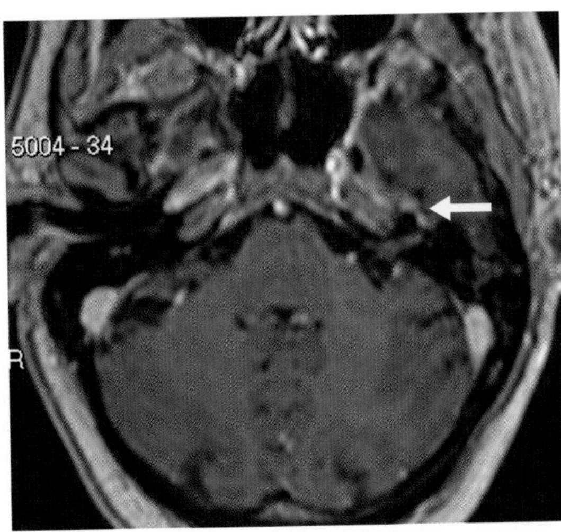

Figure 70.9 Post-contrast T1 MRI axial image shows enhancement of the geniculate ganglion in Ramsay Hunt syndrome.

Otosclerosis

Fenestral otosclerosis is seen on CT as a radiolucent focus in the anterior margin of the oval window. Heaped up new spongiotic bone around the oval window with thickening of the stapes footplate is noted in mature otosclerosis.

Cochlear otosclerosis is seen as an ill-defined focus of low density in the peri-cochlear region on CT (Figure 70.10). Confluent foci of otosclerosis surrounding the cochlea can give rise to double ring effect. Contrast enhancement may be noted on a post-contrast MRI corresponding to active areas of demineralization.

TUMOURS

Exostoses

Exostoses are the most common tumours of the external auditory canal and are more commonly seen in swimmers, surfers and deep-sea divers. These are usually bilateral and are seen on CT as circumferential thickening of the bony wall of the external auditory canal, narrowing the lumen (Figure 70.11).

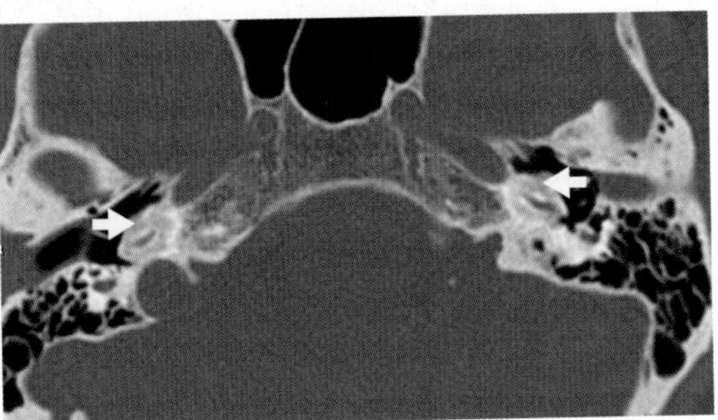

Figure 70.10 Axial CT image shows bilateral cochlear otosclerosis seen as low-density areas (arrows) surrounding the basal turn of cochlea.

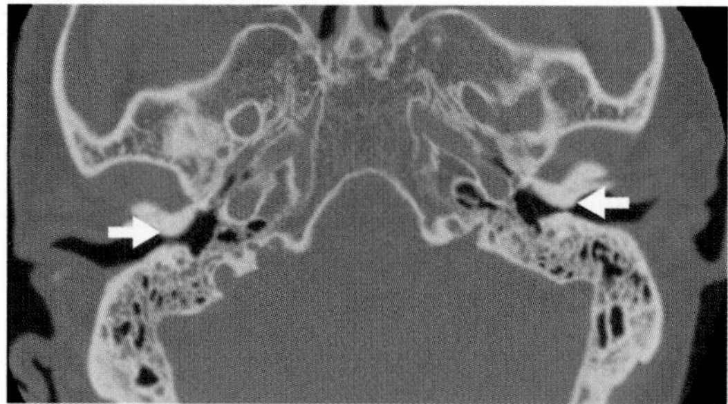

Figure 70.11 Axial CT image shows bilateral exostoses causing marked narrowing of external auditory canals (arrows).

Osteomas

Osteomas are benign lesions that are commonly seen in the external auditory canal. These are visualized as unilateral, well-defined, lobulated bony lesions protruding into the lumen of the bony external auditory canal (Figure 70.12).

Glomus tympanicum

Glomus tympanicum is seen as an enhancing soft-tissue mass on the cochlear promontory (Figure 70.13). Larger lesions fill the middle ear cavity and cause pressure erosion of the auditory ossicles and bony wall. Larger lesions that erode into the jugular fossa cannot be distinguished from glomus jugulare and are called *glomus jugulotympanicum*.

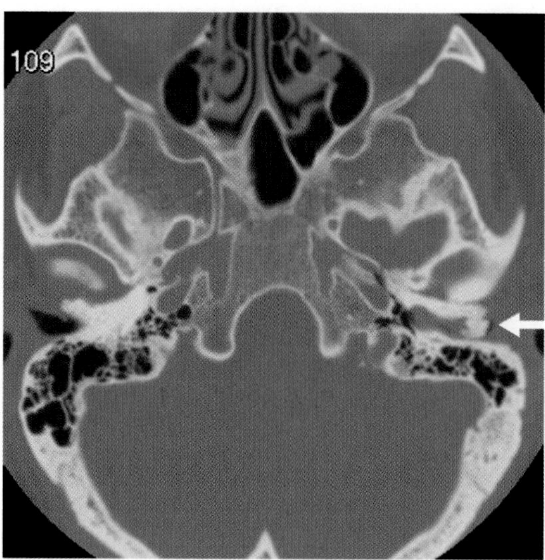

Figure 70.12 Axial CT scan image shows an osteoma (arrow) protruding into the left external auditory canal.

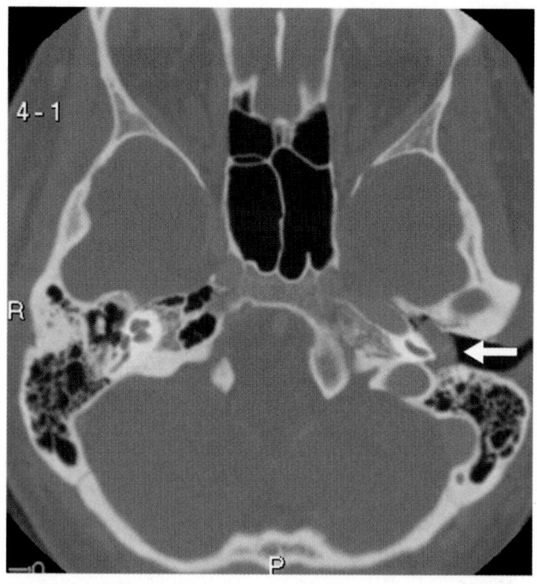

Figure 70.13 Axial CT image shows a lobulated soft-tissue mass at the level of the cochlear promontory encasing the long process of incus.

Pre- and post-contrast CT scans with axial and coronal reformatted images are the investigation of choice for diagnosis and delineation of the extent of glomus tympanicum. MRI is only indicated for larger lesions extending outside the middle ear cavity.

Glomus jugulare

Glomus jugulare fills the jugular foramen with erosion of margins. Erosion of the bony septum between the jugular foramen and the carotid canal may be seen. Glomus jugulare can extend superiorly into the middle ear cavity and medially into the hypoglossal canal and foramen magnum (Figure 70.14). MRI shows characteristic 'salt and pepper' appearance on T1 images. Small foci of haemorrhage within the lesion account for the salt-like appearance, while small foci of flow void caused by the presence of small vessels

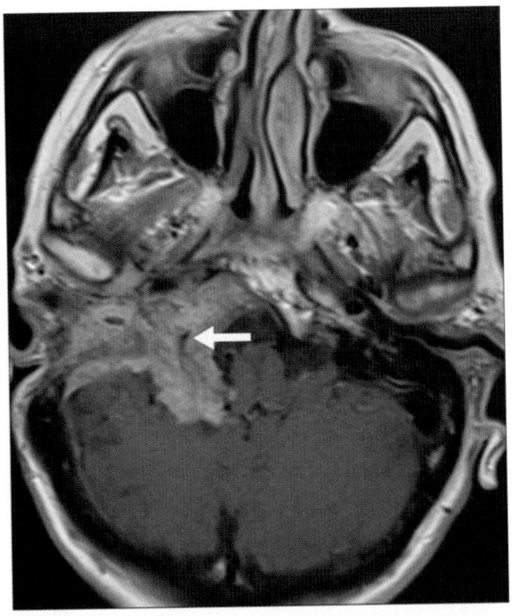

Figure 70.14 Post-contrast MR image shows a large right glomus jugulare (arrow) extending posteriorly into the right hypoglossal canal.

give a pepper-like appearance. Intense contrast enhancement is noted on the post-contrast CT and MRI images. MRI is useful in delineating the tumour extent in the skull base and involvement of the carotid artery, jugular vein and sigmoid sinus.

CEREBELLOPONTINE ANGLE LESIONS

Meningioma

Meningiomas arise from the dura and arachnoid membrane covering the petrous ridge and are seen as well-defined lesions arising outside the brain parenchyma. They are of similar density to the cerebral or cerebellar cortex on the pre-contrast CT images and show intense homogeneous enhancement on the post-contrast images. Foci of calcification within the mass and hyperostosis of the adjacent bone are specific for meningioma. On MRI, meningiomas are seen as well-defined masses showing similar signal to the cerebral or cerebellar cortex on T1 images and high signal on T2 images. Intense homogeneous enhancement

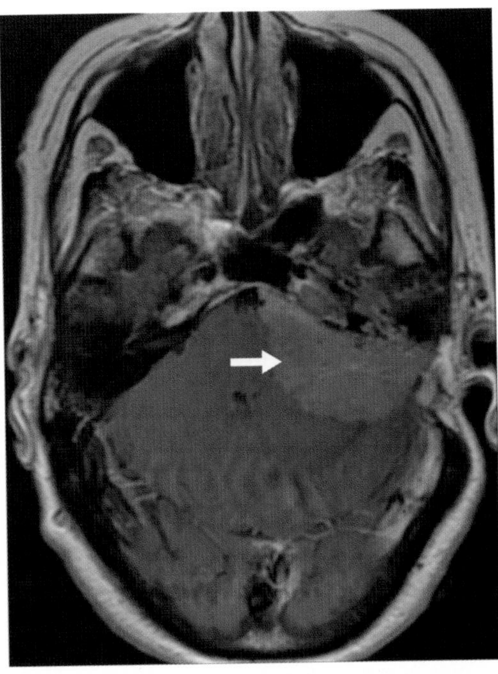

Figure 70.15 Post-contrast T1 MR image shows a meningioma in the left cerebellopontine angle with broad base and homogeneous enhancement.

is seen on the post-contrast T1-weighted images (Figure 70.15). Dural tail sign is seen as linear enhancement in the adjacent dura. *En plaque* meningiomas are usually identified as irregular meningeal thickening on MRI. They may be difficult to identify on a CT scan.

Schwannoma

MRI is the investigation of choice for detection of these tumours. A 3D heavily T2-weighted sequence is useful as a screening test to rule out a mass lesion in the internal auditory canal. Small acoustic schwannomas are seen as rounded dark filling defects within the bright CSF signal on T2 images. They are of intermediate signal on pre-contrast T1 images and show homogenous enhancement on the post-contrast T1 images. Larger tumours may show central areas of necrosis. Erosion of the walls and widening of the internal auditory canal, caused by larger tumours, may be seen on CT. Larger tumours extend into the cerebellopontine angle cistern and can cause encroachment on the brain stem, cerebellum and other cranial nerves. Bilateral acoustic schwannomas are seen in patients with type 2 neurofibromatosis (Figure 70.16).

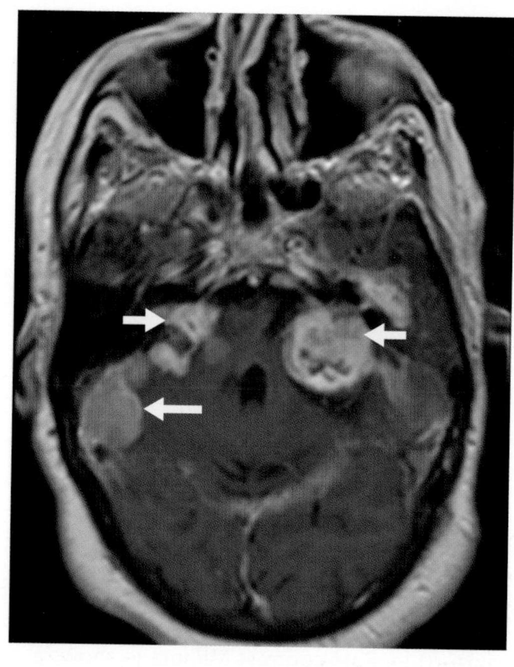

Figure 70.16 Contrast-enhanced axial MR image shows bilateral vestibular schwannomas (small arrows) and right meningioma (arrow) in a patient with type 2 neurofibromatosis.

Arachnoid or epidermoid cyst

These are well-defined lesions showing density similar to cerebrospinal fluid on CT. The cysts show low signal on T1 images and high signal on T2 images. Diffusion-weighted imaging can be used to differentiate these lesions as epidermoid cyst shows high signal due to restricted diffusion (Figure 70.17).

Metastasis

Metastasis in the internal auditory canal or cerebellopontine angle cisterns arises commonly from primary tumours of the breast, bronchus or melanoma. These are usually identified on MRI as small enhancing lesions.

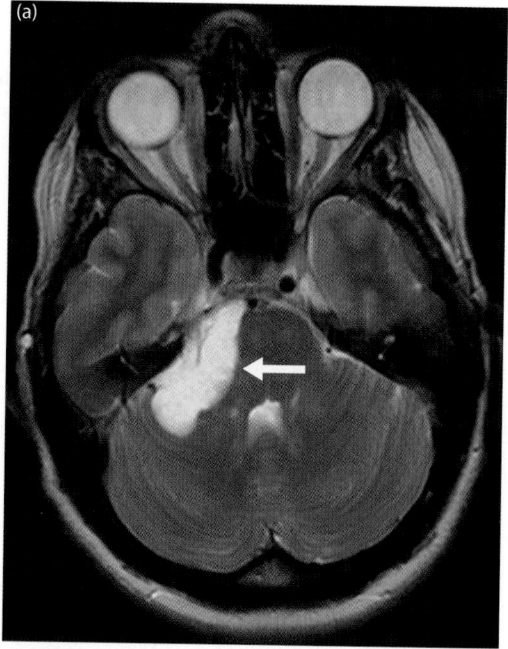

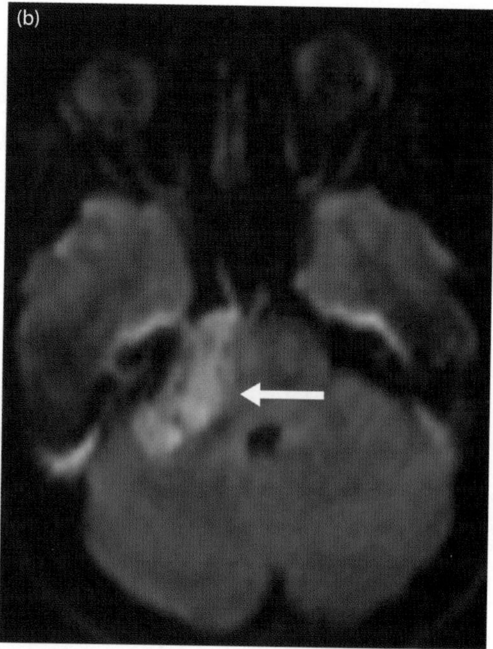

Figure 70.17 Epidermoid in the right cerebellopontine angle showing high signal on axial T2 **(a)** and diffusion-weighted **(b)** images.

NASAL CAVITY, PARANASAL SINUSES AND NASOPHARYNX

DEVELOPMENTAL

Choanal atresia

Choanal atresia is best seen on thin-section CT with multiplanar reconstructions. There is narrowing of the posterior choana with medial bowing of the posterior maxilla. The vomer is thickened and may be fused with the maxilla.

Nasal dermoid

Nasal dermoids are midline subcutaenous tubular lesions that can extend from the columella to the glabella and may communicate with the cranial cavity through the cribriform plate. They contain ectodermal and mesodermal elements and may contain sebaceous material that shows high signal on T1 and T2 MR images (Figure 70.18). Bony defects in the cribriform plate are well seen on CT.

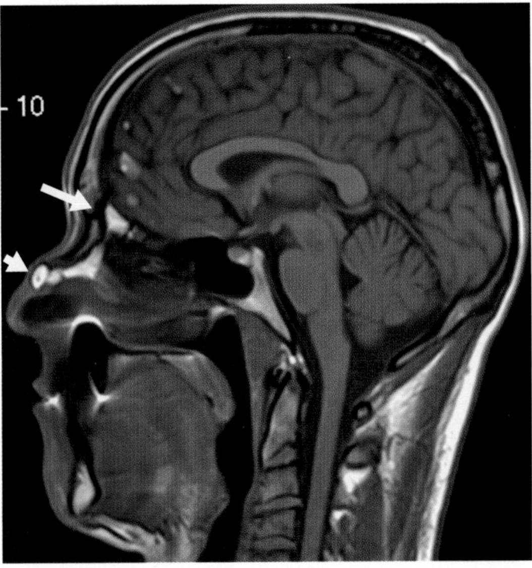

Figure 70.18 T1 sagittal MR image shows a nasal dermoid (small arrow) with intracranial extension (arrow).

Nasal glioma

Nasal glioma is a soft tissue mass of dysplastic neurogenic tissue situated in the dorsal aspect of the nose or within the nasal cavity. This is seen on CT as a well-defined mass of soft-tissue density with erosion of adjacent bone. A bony defect in the cribriform plate may be seen. These lesions show high signal on T2 MR images.

Fronto-ethmoidal encephalocele

Encephaloceles are congenital herniations of brain parenchyma, CSF and meninges through a defect in the base of skull (Figure 70.19). These are seen on CT as soft-tissue density masses with bony defects in the skull base. MRI is the modality of choice for investigation of encephaloceles as it can demonstrate continuity in signal between brain parenchyma and the herniated soft tissue.

Functional endoscopic sinus surgery imaging

CT demonstrates the complex anatomy of the osteomeatal complex in exquisite detail, and is used as a road map for treatment of sinus diseases by functional endoscopic sinus surgery (FESS).

The bony anatomy of the nasal cavity and paranasal sinuses is variable, and there are a number of anatomical variations that have to be recognized from a CT scan before proceeding to FESS. These are usually identified on the coronal images. Variations to look for include

- **Ethmoidal bulla:** This is the largest ethmoidal air cell and drains usually into the hiatus semilunaris in the middle meatus. The ethmoidal bulla can sometimes be made up of a group of cells that may communicate with each other.
- **Concha bullosa:** Aeration of the middle turbinate can cause narrowing of the nasal cavity and also the infundibulum (Figure 70.20).
- **Fovea ethmoidalis:** A low-lying fovea ethmoidalis and cribriform plate have an increased risk of penetration during surgery.
- **Uncinate process:** Position of the superior edge of the uncinate process can be variable. Lateral deviation can cause narrowing of the

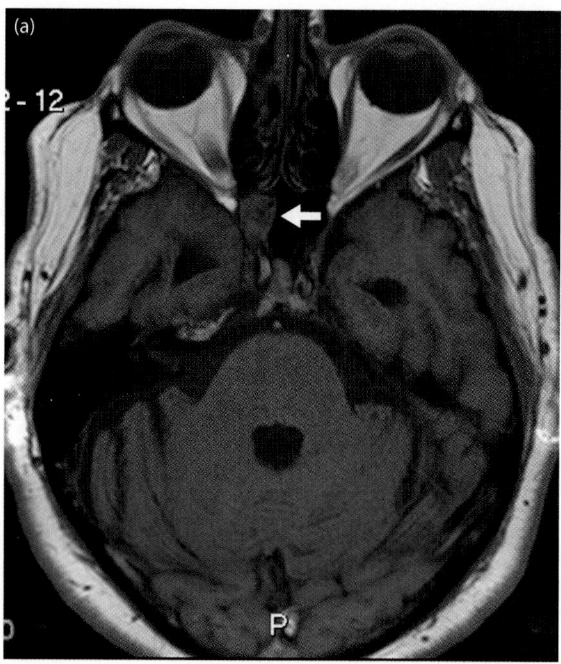

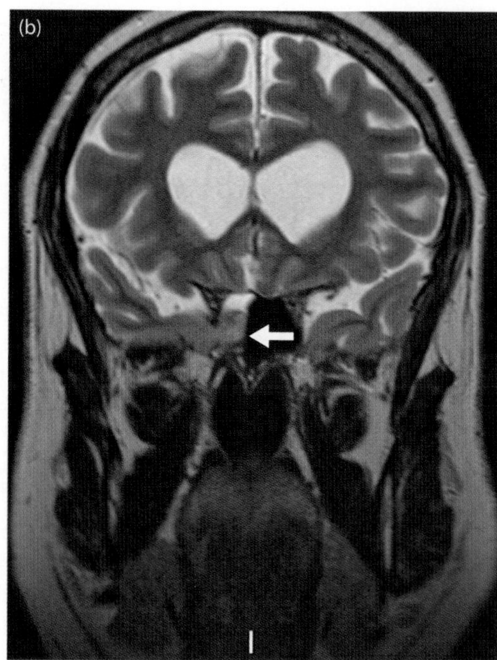

Figure 70.19 T1 axial **(a)** and T2 coronal **(b)** images show an encephalocele (arrow) extending into a right posterior ethmoidal sinus cell.

infundibulum, and medial deviation can cause narrowing of the middle meatus.

- **Haller cells:** These are infraorbital ethmoidal air cells that may cause narrowing of the infundibulum (Figure 70.21).
- **Onodi cell:** This is a pneumatized posterior ethmoidal air cell, encroaching into the sphenoid sinus, which is pushed inferiorly and medially. Presence of the Onodi cell is associated with increased risk of injury to the optic nerve during FESS.
- **Pneumosinus dilatans:** This is characterized by marked aeration and dilatation of the paranasal sinuses with thinning of the bony walls.

INFECTION AND INFLAMMATION

Acute rhinosinusitis

Acute sinusitis is seen on CT or MRI as diffuse mucosal thickening with an air fluid level. Inflamed mucosa shows enhancement on post-contrast CT or MRI, but the central secretions do not enhance.

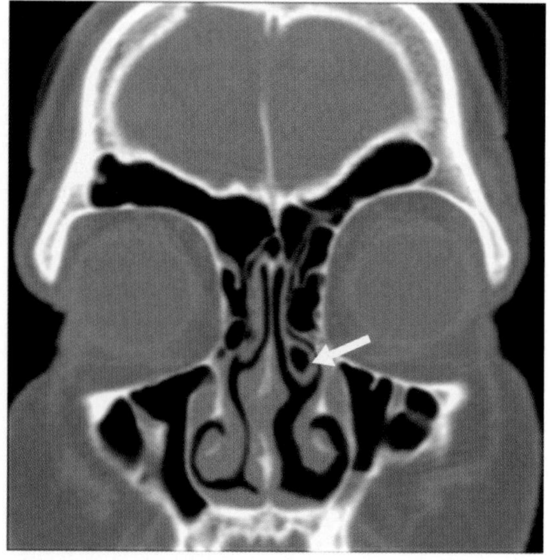

Figure 70.20 Coronal CT image shows aeration of the left middle turbinate in keeping with a concha bullosa (arrow).

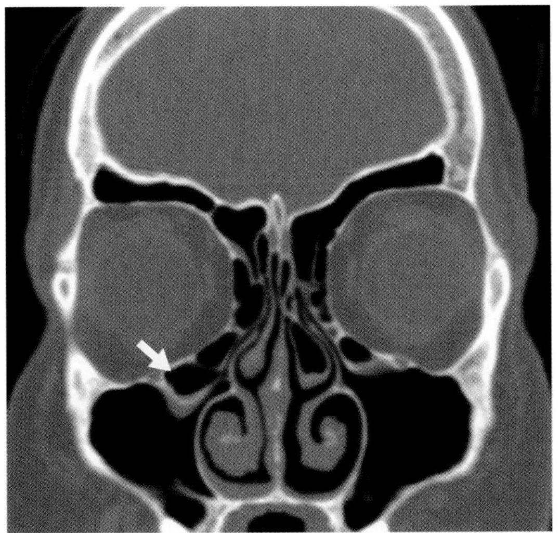

Figure 70.21 Coronal CT image shows a large right Haller cell (arrow) narrowing the infundibulum.

CT or MRI with contrast enhancement is indicated in investigation of suspected complications from acute sinusitis. Complications include orbital periostitis progressing to subperiosteal abscess, seen as a semicircular area of reduced enhancement surrounded by enhancing inflamed periosteum along the lamina papyracea (Figure 70.22). Other complications to look for include meningitis, epidural, subdural and cerebral abscesses, especially in the frontal lobe, cavernous sinus thrombosis and osteomyelitis of the frontal bone.

Chronic rhinosinusitis

Chronic sinusitis is seen on CT as diffuse mucosal thickening with sclerosis and thickening of the sinus walls. Secretions may be of variable density depending on the concentration of protein.

Fungal sinusitis

Fungal sinusitis shows central areas of high density within the sinuses on unenhanced CT (Figure 70.23). These areas of high density are due to the presence of calcium phosphate and sulphate

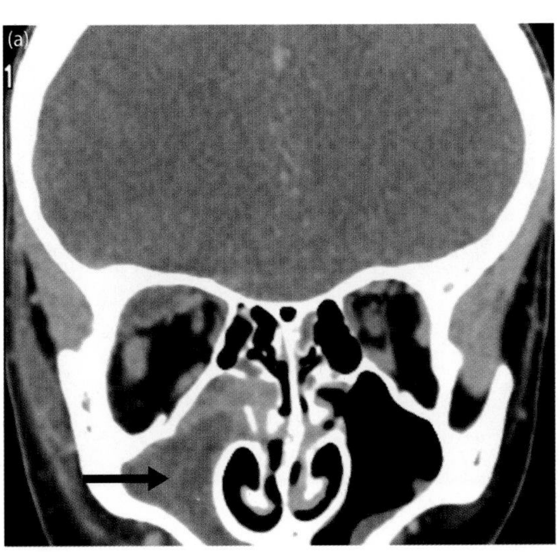

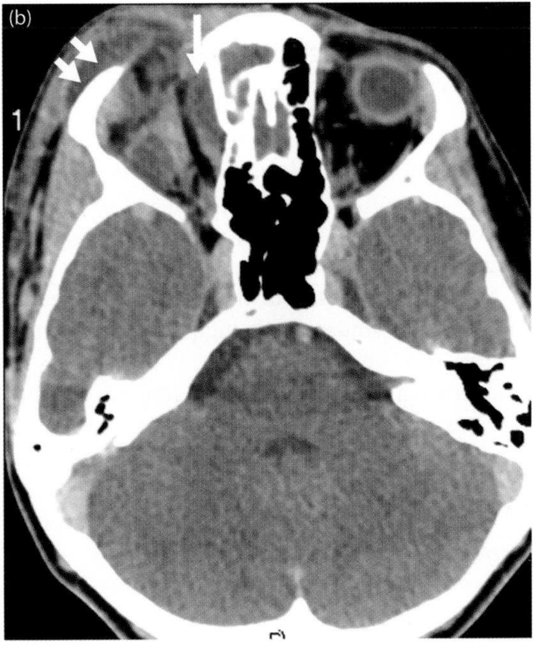

Figure 70.22 Right maxillary sinusitis (arrow) **(a)** with subperiosteal abscess **(b)** in the medial aspect of right orbit (arrow) and a preseptal abscess in the right eyelid (small arrows).

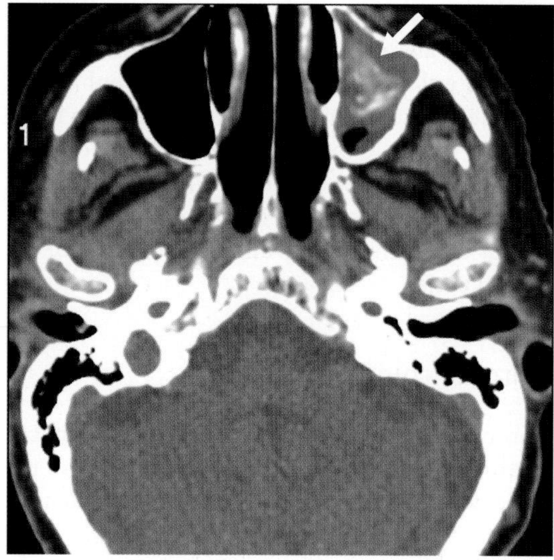

Figure 70.23 Axial CT image shows irregular area of high density in the centre in keeping with fungal sinusitis in the left maxillary sinus.

in the fungal hyphae and appear as areas of low signal on MRI. Thickening and sclerosis of the walls of the sinuses is seen secondary to chronic inflammation.

Invasive fungal sinusitis

Invasive fungal sinusitis occurs in debilitated or immunocompromised individuals. There is rapid extension of infection from the sinus mucosa into the bloodstream, bone and adjacent soft tissue. The disease is characterized by involvement of the nasal cavity, sinuses, orbit and intracranial cavity.

Nodular thickening of the mucosa or opacification of the sinuses with high-density material is often seen on non-contrast CT. Focal areas of bony erosion with infiltration of adjacent soft tissue and muscles are seen on contrast-enhanced CT. Contrast-enhanced MRI is indicated for evaluation of intraorbital and intracranial spread. CT or MR angiography can demonstrate vascular involvement.

Retention cysts

These are usually incidental and are seen as smooth, well-defined dome-shaped areas of fluid density or signal, most commonly in the maxillary or sphenoid sinuses (Figure 70.24).

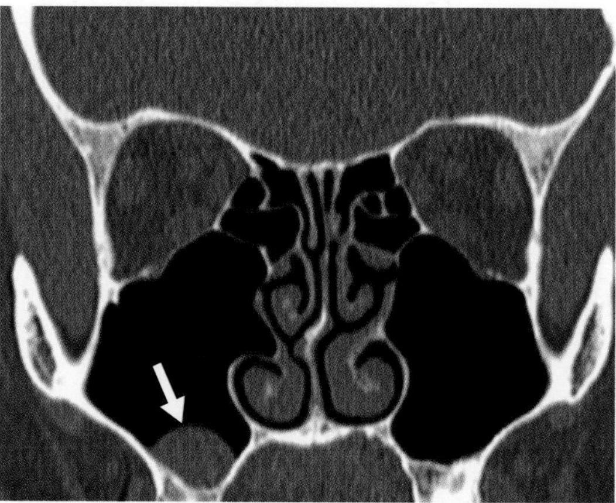

Figure 70.24 Coronal CT image shows a small mucus retention cyst in the right maxillary sinus.

Choanal polyps

Chonal polyps arise from the maxillary antrum and extend through a widened infundibulum into the nasal cavity and nasopharynx. They appear similar to retention cysts, as smooth, well-defined areas of fluid signal, but show peripheral enhancement on contrast-enhanced CT or MRI (Figure 70.25).

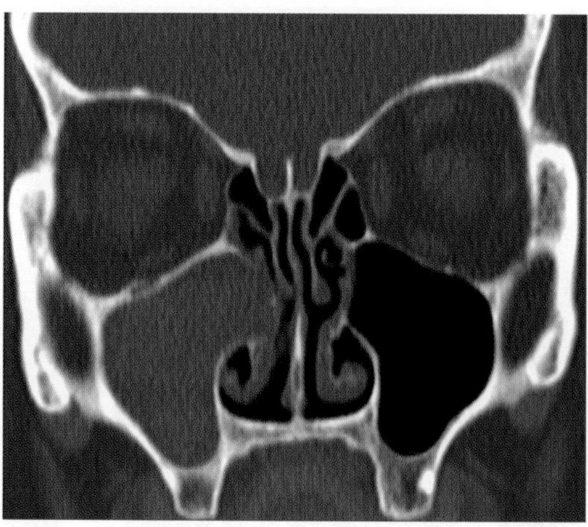

Figure 70.25 Coronal CT image shows a polyp filling the lumen of the right maxillary sinus, extending through the infundibulum into the right nasal cavity.

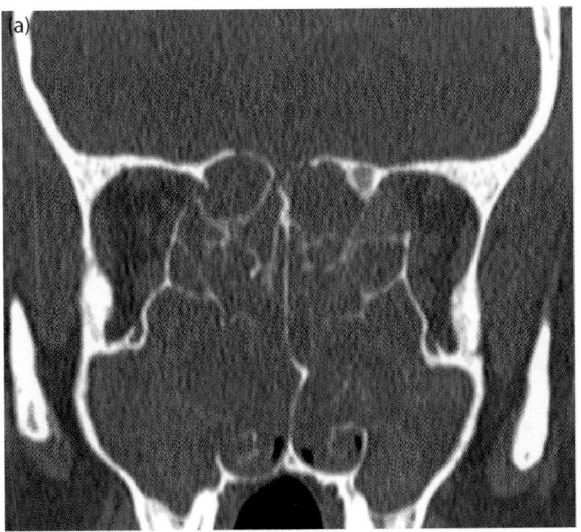

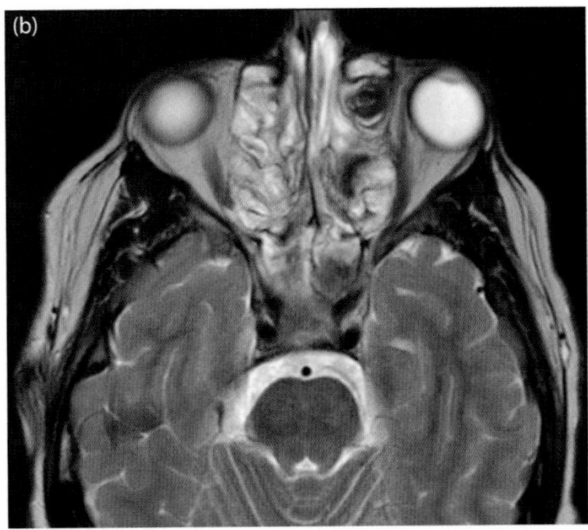

Figure 70.26 CT **(a)** and MR **(b)** images show diffuse polyposis involving bilateral maxillary and ethmoidal sinuses with expansion of air cells and thinning of surrounding bone.

Sinonasal polyposis

Sinonasal polyposis is seen on CT as multiple polypoid soft-tissue masses involving paranasal sinuses and the nasal cavity. Remodelling or erosion of the surrounding bone may be seen, commonly in the ethmoidal air cells in long-standing cases (Figure 70.26). Contrast-enhanced MRI is indicated when there is suspicion of cranial or orbital involvement.

Mucoceles

Mucoceles are commonly seen in the frontal and ethmoidal sinuses, as expansile, fluid-filled air cells with thinning and erosion of the adjacent bony wall on CT (Figure 70.27). Presence of proteinaceous fluid may lead to high signal on T1 images. Peripheral enhancement on contrast-enhanced CT or MRI helps in differentiation from tumours, which usually show diffuse enhancement.

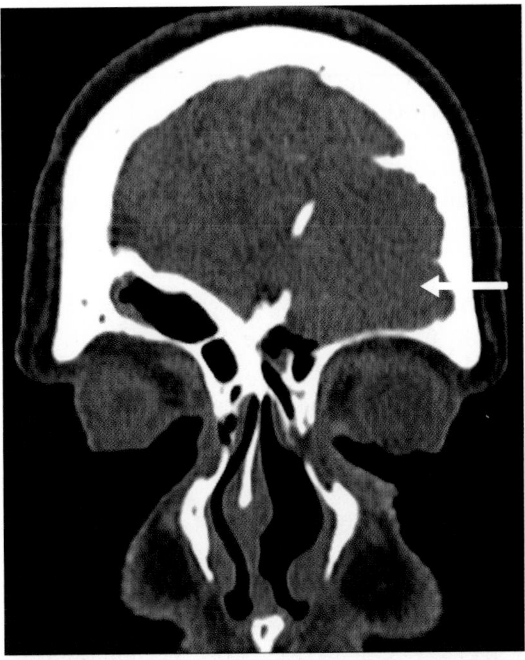

Figure 70.27 Coronal CT image shows a large left frontal sinus mucocoele causing expansion of the sinus and erosion of the superior margin.

Granulatomatosis with polyangiitis (Wegener's granulomatosis)

Granulomatosis with polyangiitis (Wegener's granulomatosis) is a systemic necrotizing granulomatous vasculitis involving the respiratory tract and kidneys. Nodular soft-tissue thickening in the nasal cavity with perforation of the nasal septum is seen on CT (Figure 70.28). Destruction of the lateral wall of the nasal cavity and palate may be seen. Soft-tissue masses tend to show low signal on

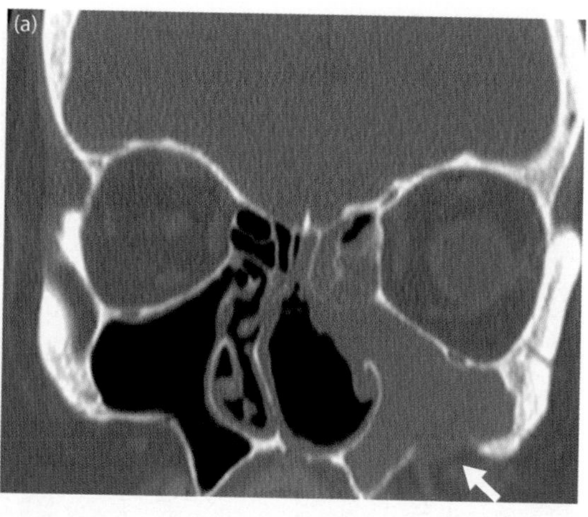

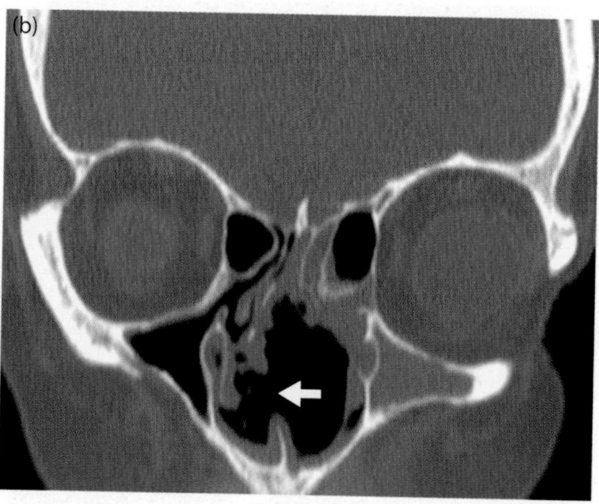

Figure 70.28 Coronal CT images show soft-tissue mass in the left maxillary sinus with erosion of the lateral wall **(a)** and destruction of the nasal septum **(b)**, left middle and inferior turbinates.

T2-weighted images, with enhancement on post-contrast T1 images.

TUMOURS

Osteoma

Osteomas are most commonly seen arising from the wall of the frontal and ethmoid sinuses and are seen as well-defined homogeneous lesions of bone density protruding into the lumen of the sinuses on CT (Figure 70.29).

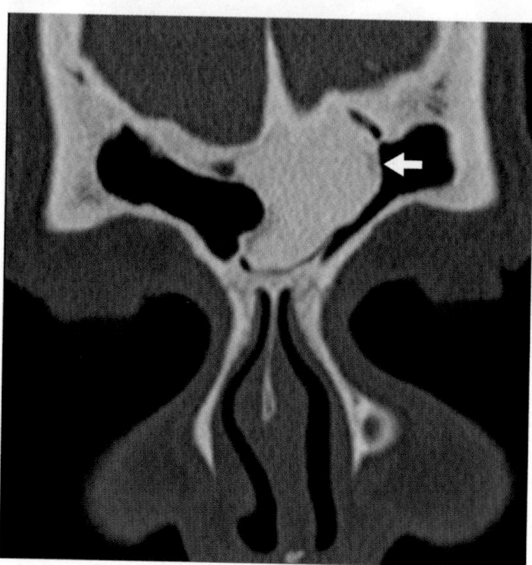

Figure 70.29 Coronal CT image shows an osteoma in the left frontal sinus.

Ossifying fibroma

Ossifying fibromas are seen as well-defined, expansile fibrous lesions with a peripheral rim of ossification on CT. They are of variable signal on MRI and show heterogenous enhancement with contrast. It is not possible to differentiate ossifying fibromas from fibrous dysplasia on imaging.

Inverted papilloma

Inverted papillomas are seen as unilateral enhancing masses arising from the lateral nasal wall at the level of the middle meatus with extension into the maxillary or ethmoidal sinuses as they grow larger (Figure 70.30). They have a characteristic 'cerebriform pattern' on T2-weighted MRI images. It is often not possible on non-contrast CT to differentiate the mass from retained secretions. Close follow-up is required after surgery as there is a high incidence of local recurrence and association with squamous cell carcinoma.

Haemangioma

Capillary haemangiomas are more common than cavernous haemangiomas and are most commonly seen in the anterior aspect of the nasal septum.

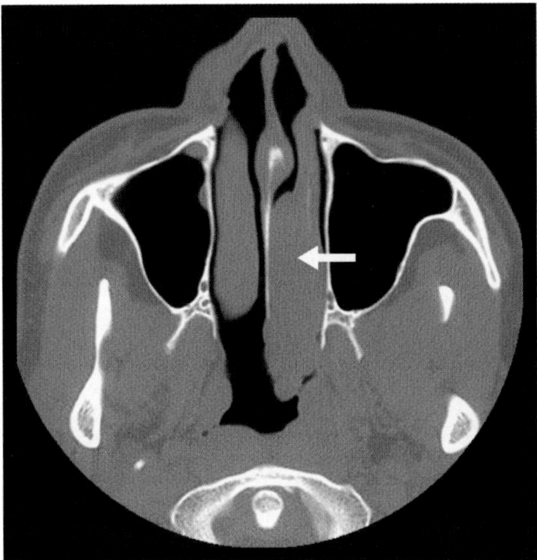

Figure 70.30 Axial CT image shows an inverting papilloma in the left nasal cavity.

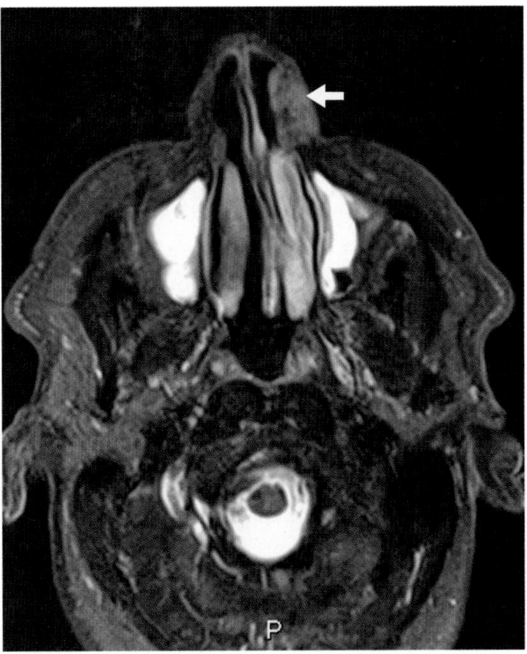

Figure 70.31 T2 axial image shows a haemangioma of the nasal ala showing high signal.

Cavernous haemangiomas occur in the lateral nasal wall and turbinates. These are seen as well-defined soft tissue density masses on CT, causing pressure erosion of the adjacent bone and showing enhancement with contrast. On MRI haemangiomas show intermediate signal on T1, high signal on T2 with enhancement on post-contrast images (Figure 70.31).

Esthesioneuroblastoma

Esthesioneuroblastomas arise from the olfactory epithelium and are seen as dumb-bell–shaped midline tumours extending superiorly into the floor of the anterior cranial fossa and inferiorly into the superior aspect of the nasal cavity (Figure 70.32). CT shows the extent of bone destruction, and contrast-enhanced MRI delineates the extent of the tumour.

Malignant sinus lesion

Squamous cell carcinomas are aggressive soft-tissue mass lesions in the maxillary antrum or ethmoidal sinus with destruction of the surrounding bone and infiltration into the surrounding soft tissue. Involvement of pterygopalatine fossa can lead to

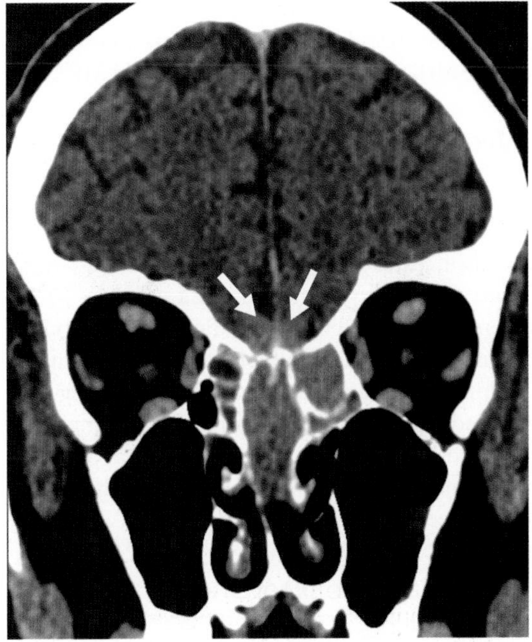

Figure 70.32 Coronal CT image shows esthesioneuroblastoma involving bilateral olfactory fossa (arrows), nasal cavity and ethmoidal sinuses.

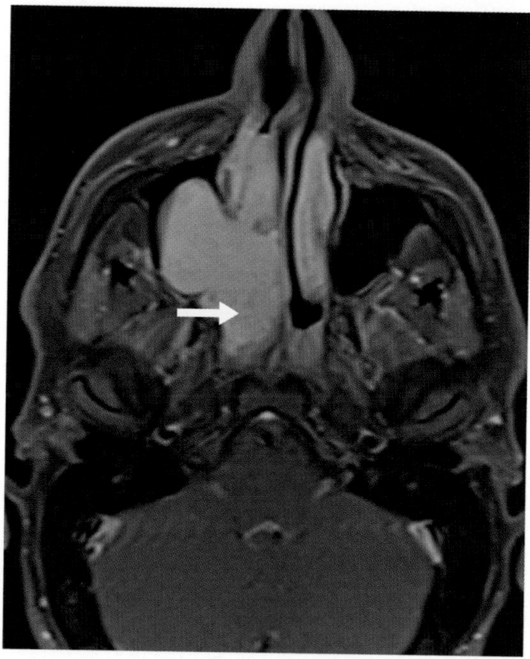

Figure 70.33 Axial MRI image shows a large enhancing nasopharyngeal angiofibroma extending into nasal cavity and right maxillary sinus.

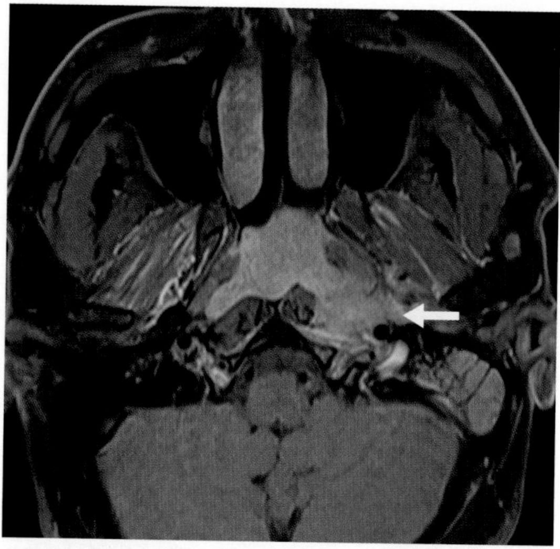

Figure 70.34 Axial MRI shows an enhancing nasopharyngeal carcinoma with infiltration into left parapharyngeal space (arrow).

perineural spread into the cavernous sinus, which can be identified on a contrast-enhanced MRI.

Juvenile angiofibroma

Juvenile angiofibroma is seen as an intensely enhancing soft-tissue mass arising from the sphenopalatine foramen, extending into the nasopharynx, nasal cavity and pterygopalatine fossa (Figure 70.33). There is anterior bowing of the posterior wall of the maxillary sinus. Multiple flow voids are noted within the soft-tissue mass on MRI in keeping with marked vascularity. Preoperative catheter angiography and embolization of the supply from branches of the internal maxillary and ascending pharyngeal artery decrease intraoperative blood loss.

Nasopharyngeal carcinoma

Early nasopharyngeal carcinoma is seen as asymmetrical soft-tissue thickening in the fossa of Rosenmuller. Larger lesions breach the pharyngobasilar fascia with extension into the parapharyngeal and carotid spaces. Destruction of the pterygoid can lead to intracranial extension. Extent of soft-tissue involvement is best delineated by MRI (Figure 70.34). Metastatic cervical lymphadenopathy may be seen even with small lesions. PET-CT may be useful in identifying small primary lesions.

SALIVARY GLANDS

CALCULUS DISEASE

Calculi in submandibular gland or duct are seen on oblique lateral views of the mandible or intra-oral occlusal views by x-ray. Calculi in the parotid gland or duct are seen on anteroposterior or tangential views.

Calculi are seen on ultrasound as focal areas of hyperechogenecity with posterior acoustic shadowing. Dilated intraglandular ductal system can be clearly visualized on ultrasound (Figure 70.35).

Sialography, which involves cannulation and injection of iodinated contrast into the salivary ducts, provides precise anatomical information of the intraglandular salivary ductal system and is useful in investigation of sialectasis, ductal strictures and small intraductal stones.

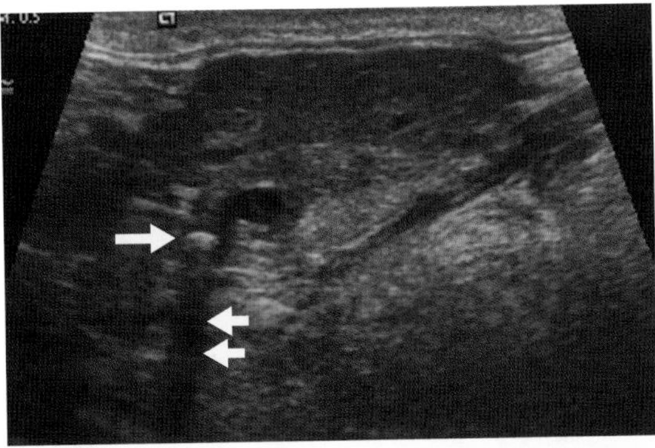

Figure 70.35 Ultrasound image shows a hyperechoic calculus (arrow) in the proximal submandibular duct with acoustic shadowing (small arrows).

CT is the most sensitive method for visualization of calculi in the ducts and salivary glands and is the method of choice for evaluation of post-obstructive inflammation and abscess formation (Figure 70.36).

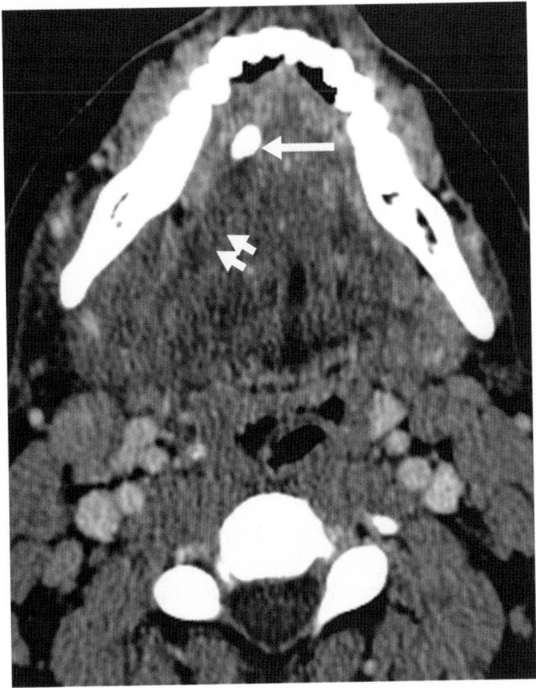

Figure 70.36 Axial CT image shows a right submandibular duct calculus (arrow) with proximal dilatation (small arrows).

MR sialography performed with heavily T2-weighted images is a useful non-invasive method of evaluation of the salivary ductal system.

INFLAMMATION

Sialadenitis

Acute inflammatory sialadenitis is seen as diffuse swelling of the involved gland with inflammation of the surrounding fat. Abscesses in the gland are seen as unilocular or multilocular areas of fluid density showing peripheral enhancement on post-contrast CT or MRI. There is atrophy and scarring of the gland with focal dilatation of the intraglandular ducts in chronic sialadenitis.

Sjogren's syndrome

Multiple well-defined areas of hypoechogenicity are seen in the salivary glands on ultrasound in Sjögren's syndrome. On CT these glands show a honeycomb appearance (Figure 70.37). MRI shows multiple rounded areas of fluid signal thought to be retained saliva. Histological evaluation of solid lesions is important as there is a known association with lymphomas.

Lyphoepithelial lesions

Lymphoeithelial lesions are seen in acquired immune deficiency syndrome (AIDS) patients

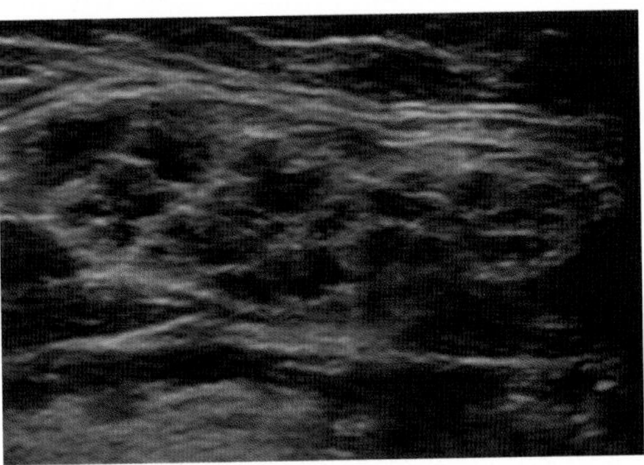

Figure 70.37 Ultrasound image of submandibular gland shows multiple small hypoechoic areas in keeping with Sjögren's syndrome.

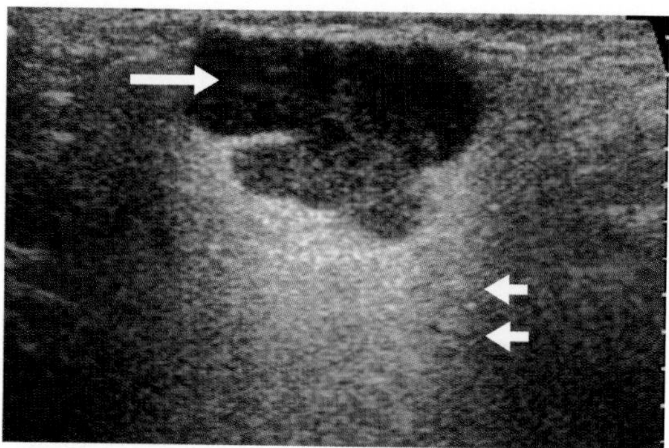

Figure 70.38 Ultrasound image shows a well-defined, lobulated, hypoechoic pleomorphic adenoma (arrow) with posterior acoustic enhancement (small arrows).

and are seen as multiple small, well-defined cystic and solid lesions diffusely distributed in one or both parotid glands. Tonsillar hyperplasia and bilateral cervical lymphadenopathy are often associated.

NEOPLASMS

Pleomorphic adenoma (benign mixed tumour)

Pleomorphic adenomas are more common in the parotid and are seen on ultrasound as well-defined, lobulated, hypoechoic lesions showing posterior acoustic enhancement (Figure 70.38). On MRI they are well-defined, lobulated lesions showing low signal on T1 and heterogenous high signal on T2 images. MRI is used for surgical planning and can demonstrate the involvement of the deep lobe of parotid (Figure 70.39).

Warthin's tumour

Warthin's tumours are usually seen in the tail of the parotid and are identified on ultrasound as well-defined, hypoechoic or cystic lesions. MRI shows well-defined lesions with small areas of cystic change showing high signal and solid components showing intermediate signal on T2 images. Warthin's tumour shows increased uptake of FDG on PET scanning. Warthin's tumour shows increased uptake of 99mTc-pertechnetate.

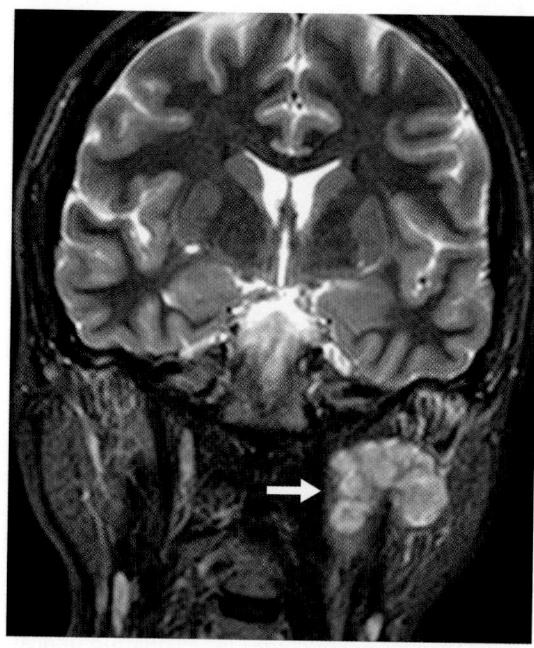

Figure 70.39 Coronal MRI image shows a pleomorphic adenoma (arrow) involving superficial and deep lobes.

Mucoepidermoid carcinoma

Mucoepidermoid carcinomas occur predominantly in the parotid and demonstrate variable appearance on imaging depending on their histological grade (Figure 70.40). Low-grade tumours demonstrate well-defined margins and are cystic, while high-grade tumours are ill-defined, infiltrative, enhancing lesions. Lymphadenopathy is noted within the parotid and in the ipsilateral level 2 group.

Adenoidcystic carcinoma

Adenoidcystic carcinomas have a higher incidence in submandibular, sublingual and minor salivary glands and have a strong tendency for spread by vasculature and lymphatics. Appearances can range from well-defined to ill-defined infiltrating mass lesions. Contrast-enhanced MRI may demonstrate perineural infiltration along the facial nerve.

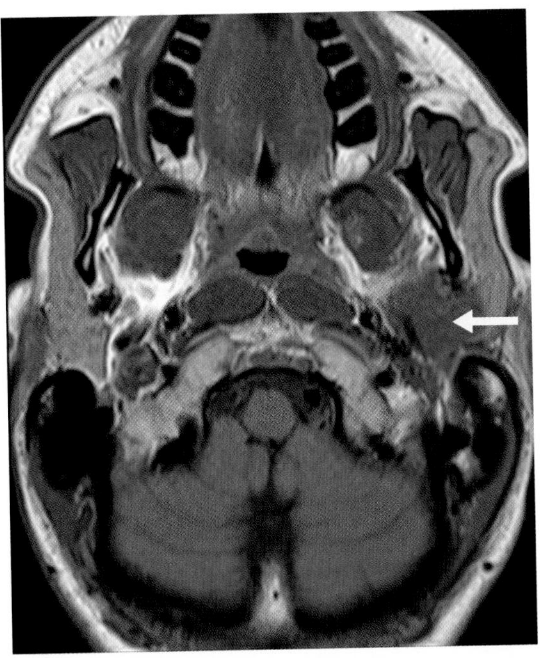

Figure 70.40 Axial T1 MRI image shows an ill-defined mass involving superficial and deep lobes of the left parotid.

Lymphoma

Lymphomas have an increased incidence in patients with Sjögren's syndrome. Lymphomatous lesions of the parotid and submandibular glands are more commonly seen secondary to nodal involvement in the neck.

Metastases

Lymph nodal metastases from cutaneous squamous cell carcinomas and melanomas are the most common cause of intraparotid metastases. Haematogenous metastases may also arise from lung, breast, kidney and prostate tumours.

MANDIBLE

An orthopantomogram is often the first investigation performed to evaluate lesions of the mandible.

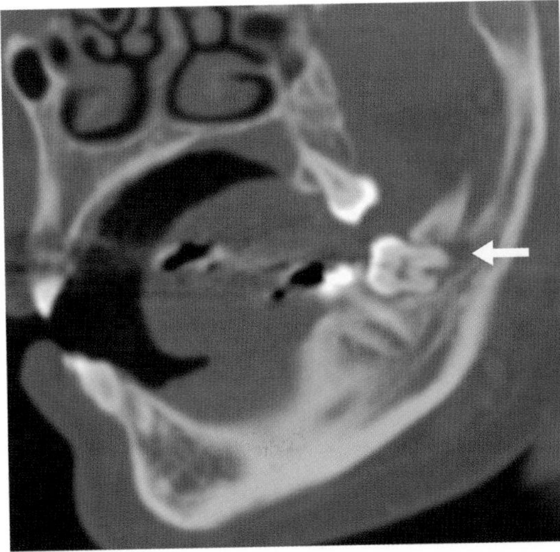

Figure 70.41 Sagittal oblique CT image shows a radicular cyst around the apex of a molar tooth.

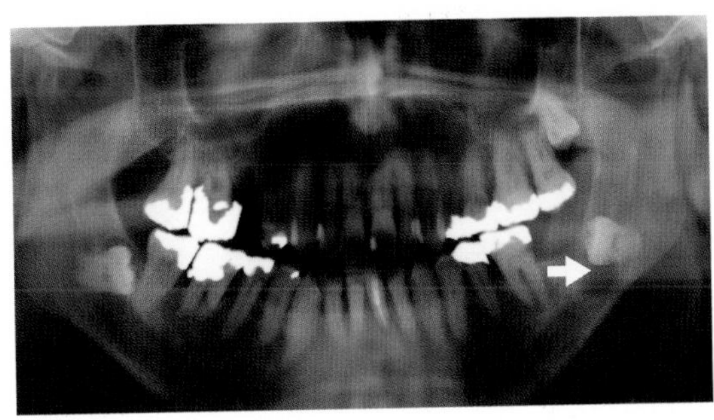

Figure 70.42 Orthopantomogram shows a dentigerous cyst associated with the crown of the unerupted third molar tooth.

Further evaluation with CT or MRI is useful for characterization. Radicular cyst is the most common cyst in the mandible and is seen as a well-defined lucent lesion around the apex of a tooth (Figure 70.41). Dentigerous cysts are seen as well-defined, unilocular cysts related to the crown of an unerupted tooth (Figure 70.42). Odontogenic keratocysts are multilocular, cystic, expansile lesions associated with an unerupted tooth. Ameloblastomas are seen as expansile, multilocular, cystic lesions with thinning of the bony cortex and possible extension into the surrounding soft tissue (Figure 70.43).

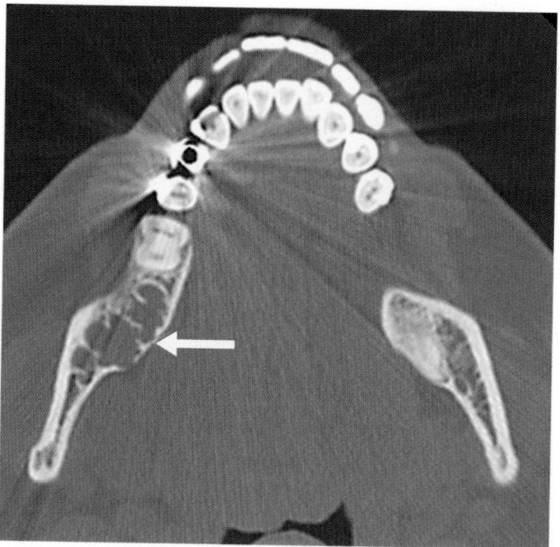

Figure 70.43 Axial CT image of the mandible shows an ameloblastoma seen as an expansile, multiloculated, cystic lesion with bony erosion.

ORAL CAVITY

DEVELOPMENTAL

Lingual thyroid

Ectopic thyroid tissue is often seen in the floor of mouth or base of tongue as a well-defined mass in the midline. It shows high attenuation on non-contrast CT in keeping with high iodine content and shows avid enhancement with contrast. Radionuclide scan with iodine-123 or technetium-99m pertechnetate show increased uptake of tracer by the mass.

Dermoid and epidermoid

These are developmental inclusion cysts containing epithelial elements in case of epidermoid and a mixture of epithelial and dermal elements in case of dermoid. They are commonly seen in the floor of the mouth. Epidermoids are well-defined lesions showing fluid characteristics on CT and MRI. Dermoids are seen as well-defined heterogeneous lesions showing fat, fluid and calcification on CT and MRI (Figure 70.44).

Lymphangioma

Lymphangiomas are unilocular or multilocular cystic lesions involving submandibular or sublingual spaces. They are seen extending across fascial planes without mass effect. While they can be identified on ultrasound as cystic lesions, CT or MRI is usually required to delineate the true extent of the lesion.

Ranula

Ranulas are retention cysts of sublingual salivary gland. They are well-defined and show fluid contents. There is minimal enhancement of the wall with contrast. They may extend posteriorly and inferiorly into the submandibular space when they are called *diving ranulas* (Figure 70.45).

INFLAMMATION

Sublingual and submandibular abscess

Abscesses are seen as ring-enhancing fluid collections. Abscesses involving sublingual space are seen superior and medial to the mylohyoid muscle. Abscesses involving submandibular space are seen inferolateral to the mylohyoid muscle and may cross the midline to form a horseshoe-shaped collection. Infections can cross fascial planes, with involvement of several adjacent spaces in the neck. CT and MRI are helpful in delineating the full extent (Figure 70.46).

Tonsillitis and peritonsillar abscess

Acute and chronic tonsillitis have a non-specific appearance on CT. Peritonsillar abscess is seen as a peripherally enhancing fluid collection adjacent to the tonsils (Figure 70.47). Larger abscesses may extend into the parapharyngeal, masticator and retropharyngeal spaces.

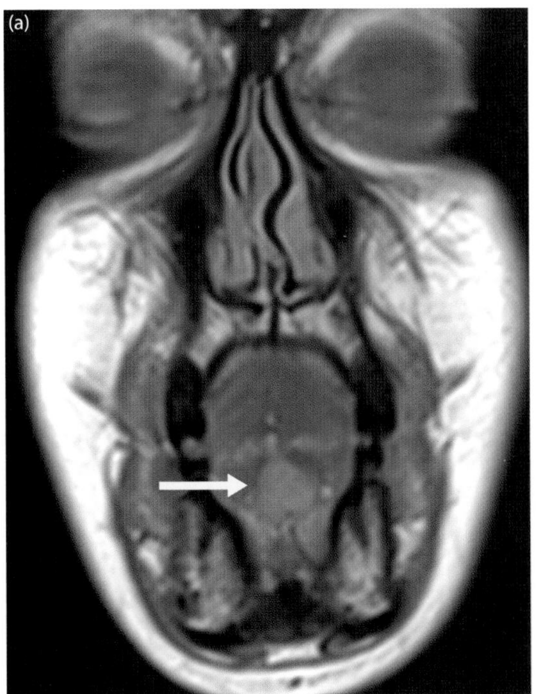

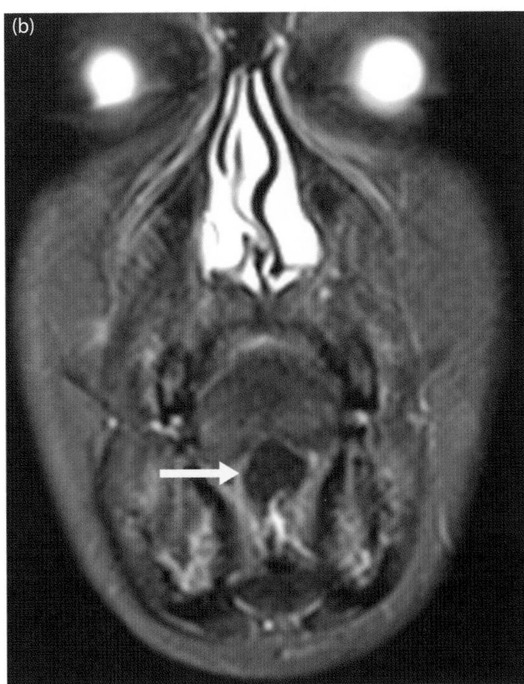

Figure 70.44 Sublingual dermoid showing high signal on coronal T1 MRI image **(a)** with reduction in signal on fat suppressed STIR coronal image **(b)** in keeping with fatty contents.

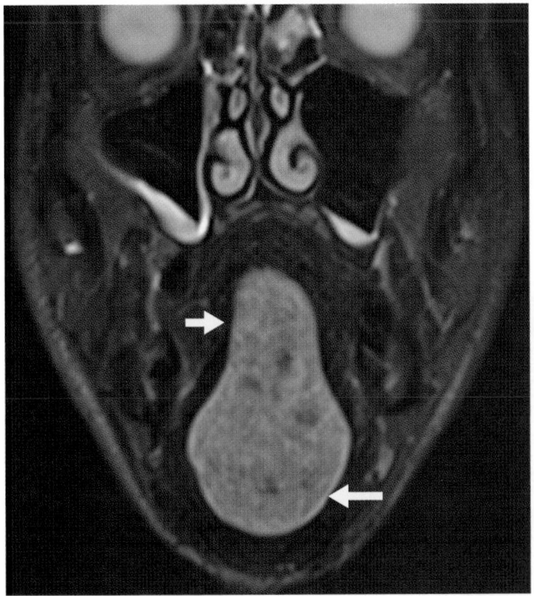

Figure 70.45 Coronal MRI image shows a diving ranula extending into the submandibular space (arrow) from the sublingual space (small arrow).

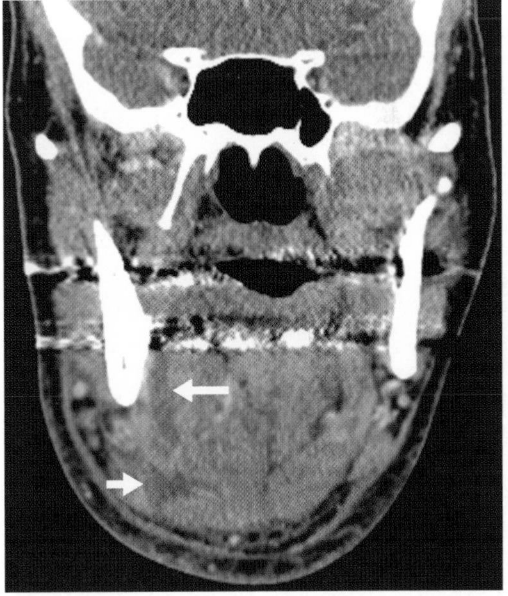

Figure 70.46 Coronal CT scan image shows abscess in the right sublingual space (arrow) and right submandibular space (small arrow).

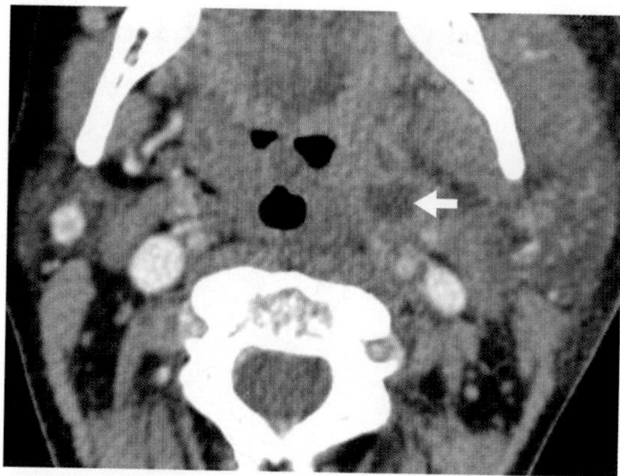

Figure 70.47 Axial CT image shows a left peritonsillar abscess.

Retropharyngeal abscess

CT is the modality of choice for evaluation of retropharyngeal abscess, which is seen as a peripherally enhancing fluid collection pushing the posterior pharyngeal wall anteriorly. Pockets of gas may be seen within the collection. Rupture of the alar fascia in the retropharyngeal space can result in extension of the infection inferiorly into the mediastinum (Figure 70.48). Hence it is important to evaluate the mediastinum in patients with suspected retropharyngeal abscess.

Neoplasm

MRI is the modality of choice for local staging of primary malignancies in the tongue, oral cavity and oropharynx. CT may be useful in the elderly, patients with claustrophobia and patients with contraindications to MRI. Malignant lesions are frequently squamous cell carcinomas from the floor of mouth, tonsillar fossa or the base of tongue (Figure 70.49). They are seen as ill-defined, infiltrative lesions showing high signal on T2 images and enhancement on post-contrast T1 images. Tumour infiltration of the lingual septum, extrinsic muscles and neurovascular bundle can be identified. Tumour extension into the parapharyngeal, carotid and prevertebral spaces is important for staging and can be delineated accurately.

Lymph node metastases, commonly to level 2 nodes, are seen on CT or MRI as enlarged nodes

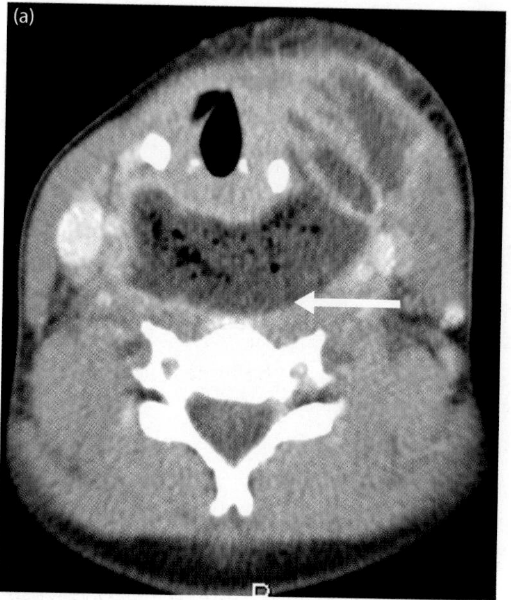

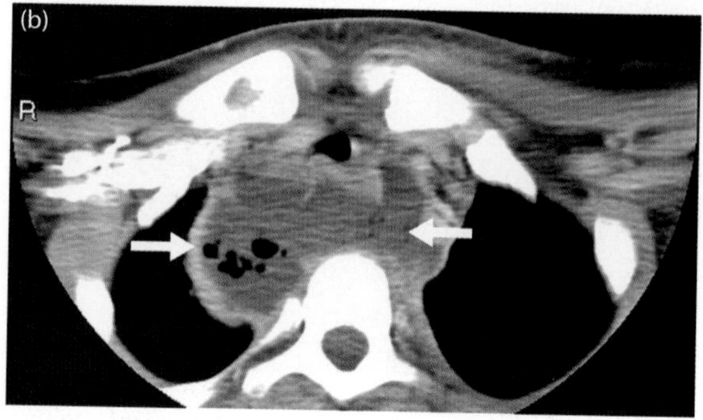

Figure 70.48 Axial CT images show large retropharyngeal abscess **(a)** with extension inferiorly into the mediastinum **(b)**.

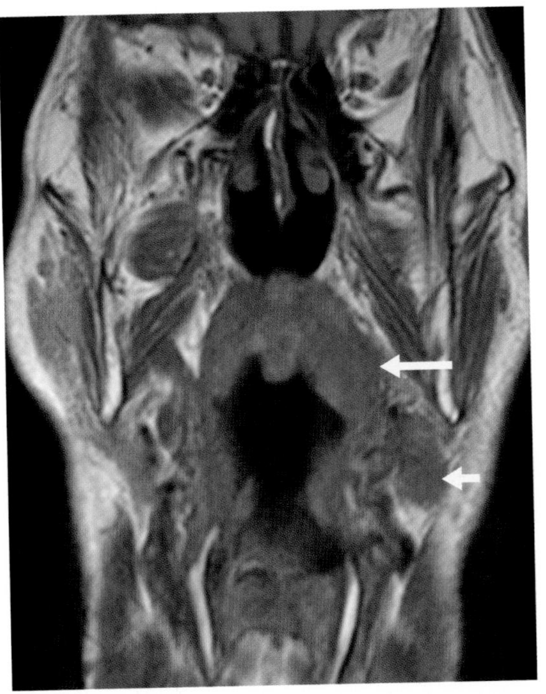

Figure 70.49 Coronal MR image shows a malignant left tonsillar mass (arrow) with a metastatic left cervical node (small arrow).

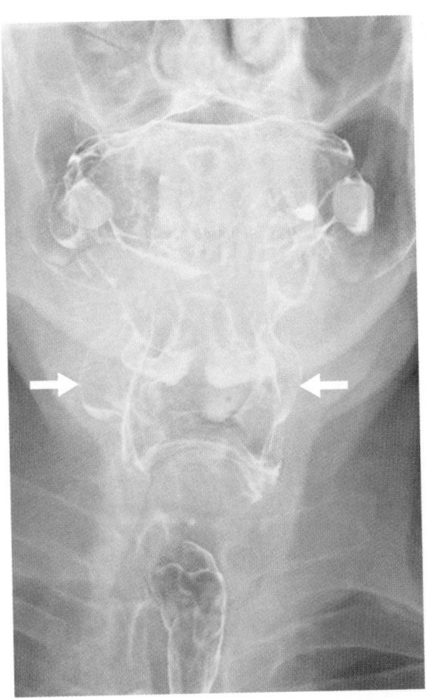

Figure 70.50 Bilateral pharyngoceles (arrows) seen on a barium swallow.

with central areas of necrosis. Ultrasound with high-resolution transducers has a high sensitivity and specificity in characterization of cervical lymph nodes. Metastatic nodes appear hypoechoic with loss of normal fatty hilum on ultrasound. Ultrasound-guided fine-needle aspiration is often used as a problem-solving tool to characterize enlarged lymph nodes that cannot be accurately characterized on CT or MRI.

HYPOPHARYNX

DEVELOPMENTAL

Pharyngocele

Pharyngoceles are mucosal outpouchings from the piriform sinus. They are seen as broad-based outpouchings coated with barium on the frontal view of a barium swallow (Figure 70.50).

Pharyngeal pouch (Zenker's diverticulum)

Pharyngeal pouches are seen as posterior mucosal protrusions identified at the level of the Killian's dehiscence on barium swallow (Figure 70.51). Pooling of barium may be seen in large pouches.

Pharyngeal web

Pharyngeal webs are thin membranes seen arising from the anterior aspect of the hypopharynx, causing narrowing of the lumen. These are best seen on the lateral cine images on barium swallow (Figure 70.52).

Infection and inflammation

Imaging is rarely performed in infectious and inflammatory conditions of the hypopharynx. Thickening of the epiglottis may be seen in epiglottitis on a lateral x-ray of the neck.

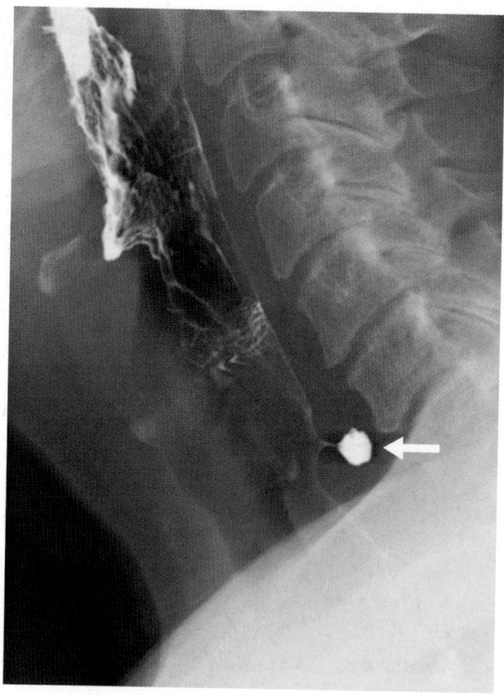

Figure 70.51 Barium swallow showing a pharyngeal pouch (arrow) with a narrow neck.

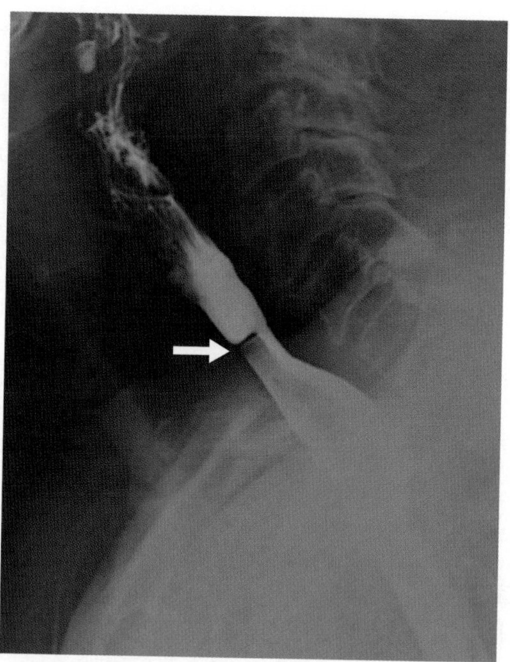

Figure 70.52 Barium swallow showing a pharyngeal web (arrow) causing partial obstruction to the flow of barium.

Malignancy

Hypopharyngeal tumours are most commonly squamous cell carcinomas and may be staged with CT or MRI. Tumours may arise from the piriform sinus, posterior pharyngeal wall or post-cricoid region (Figure 70.53). Tumours can extend into the aryepiglottic fold, paraglottic space or carotid space. Lymph node involvement is often seen at level 2 in the neck on CT and MRI. Equivocal nodes may be evaluated further with ultrasound-guided fine-needle aspiration.

LARYNX

DEVELOPMENTAL

Laryngocele

Laryngoceles are thin-walled areas containing air or fluid communicating with the laryngeal ventricle. They can be identified on axial or coronal images of CT or MRI. Internal laryngoceles are seen in the paraglottic space and are contained laterally by the thyrohyoid membrane. External laryngoceles penetrate the thyrohyoid membrane and extend into the soft tissue of the neck.

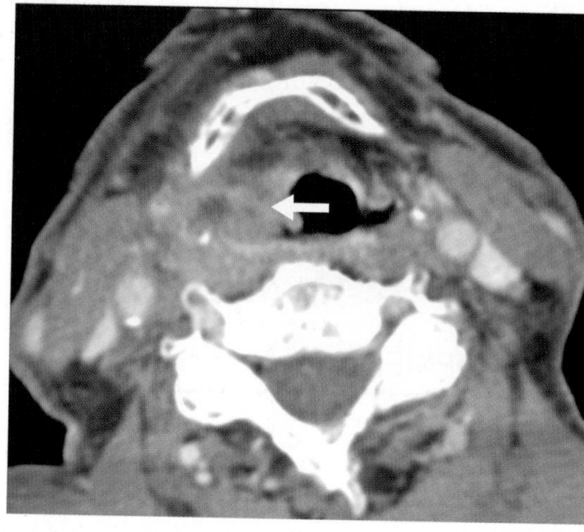

Figure 70.53 Axial CT image shows an enhancing mass lesion in the right piriform sinus.

Laryngeal cyst

Laryngeal cysts are usually seen as incidental abnormalities on CT or MRI. They are well defined and show fluid density on CT. On MRI they show high signal on T2 and low to high signal on T1-weighted images depending on the protein content.

Inflammation

Narrowing of the subglottic lumen (Steeple sign) may be seen on a frontal x-ray of the neck in laryngo-tracheitis. This is seen in less than 50 per cent of patients, and hence x-rays are not routinely performed. CT scan is the modality of choice for investigation of chronic laryngeal or tracheal stenosis secondary to previous inflammation or intervention.

Laryngeal malignancy

Squamous cell carcinomas are the most common tumours in the larynx. While tumours can be staged with CT or MRI, CT is the preferred modality as its shorter examination time reduces artefacts due to swallowing and movement. MRI is more sensitive in detection of early cartilaginous invasion. PET-CT is used in post-surgical patients to differentiate recurrence from post-surgical scarring.

Tumours are seen as enhancing, nodular, infiltrative lesions involving the epiglottis, aryepiglottic fold, true or false cord. Lesions involving the epiglottis may extend anteriorly to involve the pre-epiglottic space, which cannot be evaluated clinically and is best seen on sagittal images on MRI or CT. Infiltration of the paraglottic fat may be seen in tumours of the true or false cord (Figure 70.54). Sclerosis of the arytenoid cartilage on CT is suspicious of infiltration by the tumour. Involvement of anterior commissure and extension into the contralateral side can be identified on axial images of CT or MRI. Superior and inferior extension of the tumour can be identified on coronal images.

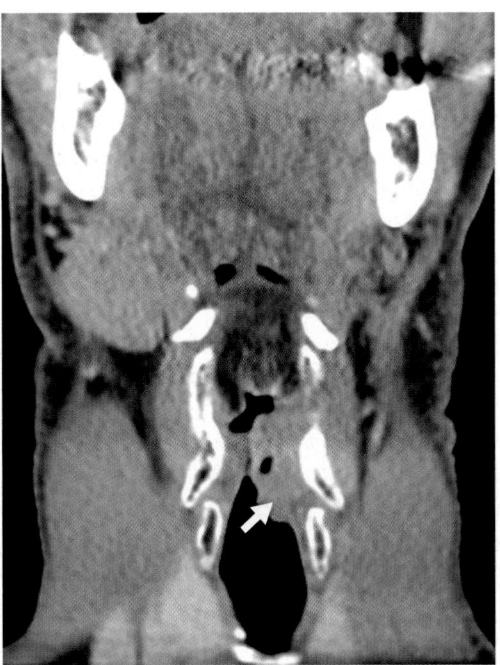

Figure 70.54 Coronal CT image shows a malignant mass involving the left false cord, laryngeal ventricle and left true cord.

Chondrosarcoma of larynx

Chondrosarcomas most commonly arise from the cricoid cartilage and are seen as an expansile soft-tissue mass eroding the cricoid with characteristic popcorn-like chondroid calcification on CT (Figure 70.55).

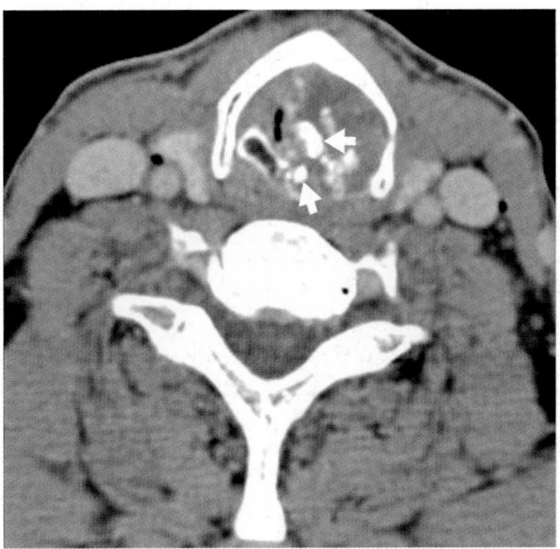

Figure 70.55 Axial CT image shows soft tissue mass causing destruction of the left lateral aspect of the cricoid with chondroid calcification (arrows).

SUPERFICIAL NECK LUMPS

Ultrasound is usually the first choice of investigation for evaluation of neck lumps. Depending on the findings on ultrasound, further evaluation with CT or MRI and ultrasound-guided fine-needle aspiration may be performed for further characterization.

BRANCHIAL CYST

Type 2 branchial cysts are the most commonly identified branchial cleft cysts (Figure 70.56). They can be identified on ultrasound as well-defined, unilocular cysts with clear fluid in the posterior submandibular space, anterior and medial to the sternomastoid. Infected branchial cysts may show echogenic contents. On CT and MRI, a beak pointing medially between the external and internal carotid arteries may be seen, which is pathognomonic. Infected cysts show enhancement of the wall on CT or MRI.

Type 1 branchial cysts are seen as well-defined, unilocular cysts in the preauricular region adjacent to the external auditory canal or in the parotid space. A beak-like projection or sinus may be seen extending posteriorly to the anterior wall of the external auditory canal at the junction of the cartilaginous and bony segments on MRI.

Type 3 branchial cysts are rare and are noted in the posterior triangle as well-defined unilocular cysts. CT or MRI may demonstrate a sinus or fistula extending medially into the piriform sinus.

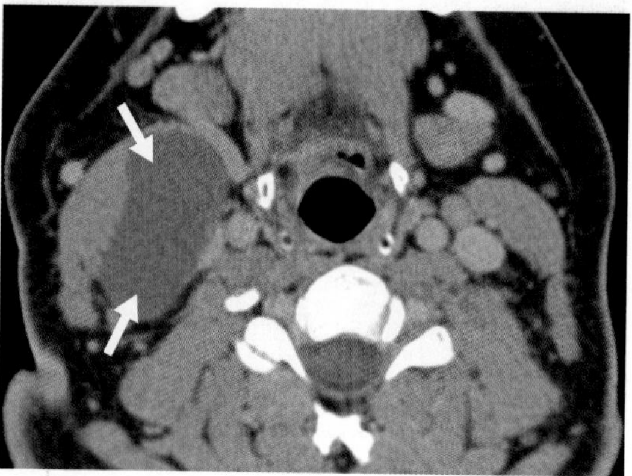

Figure 70.56 Axial CT image shows a right type 2 branchial cyst medial to the sternomastoid muscle.

Type 4 branchial cysts are unilocular thin-walled cysts found in close relation to the left lobe of the thyroid or the thyroid cartilage.

THYROGLOSSAL CYST

Thyroglossal cysts (Figure 70.57) are seen on ultrasound as thin-walled cysts with anechoic or echogenic contents in the midline of the neck extending deep to the strap muscles. Enhancement of the cyst wall is seen on contrast-enhanced CT or MRI in case of infected cysts.

LYMPHANGIOMA

Appearance of lymphangiomas may vary from large, well-defined cystic spaces to the presence of multiple tiny cystic areas. Lymphangiomas are seen to extend across fascial planes with no significant mass effect. While ultrasound is usually the first modality of investigation, MRI is the modality of choice for delineating the true extent of lymphangiomas. Lymphangiomas show high signal on T2-weighted images (Figure 70.58). Lymphangiomas can be differentiated from haemangiomas by the lack of enhancement on post-contrast T1 images.

HAEMANGIOMA

Haemangiomas are seen commonly in the buccal space and masticator spaces as well-defined, lobulated, hypoechoic lesions with variable vascularity on ultrasound. CT can demonstrate the presence of phleboliths and remodelling of adjacent bone. MRI is useful in delineating the extent of haemangiomas showing high signal on T2-weighted images and variable enhancement on the post-contrast images (Figure 70.59).

LYMPH NODAL MASS

Reactive lymphadenitis is the most common cause of lymph nodal enlargement, especially in children. On ultrasound these nodes are enlarged but maintain their normal ovoid shape and show the presence of normal fatty hilum.

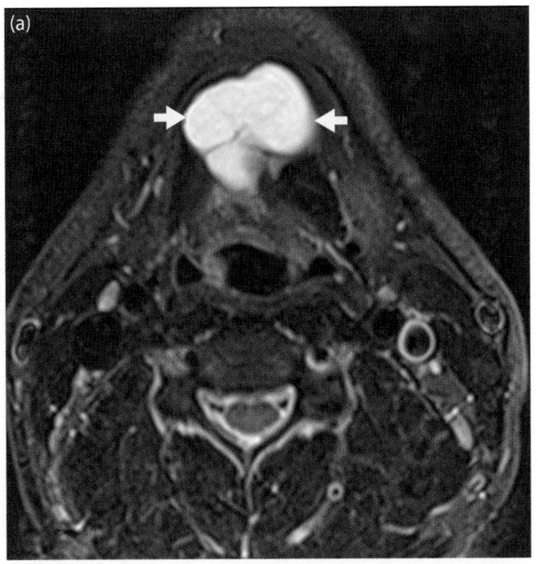

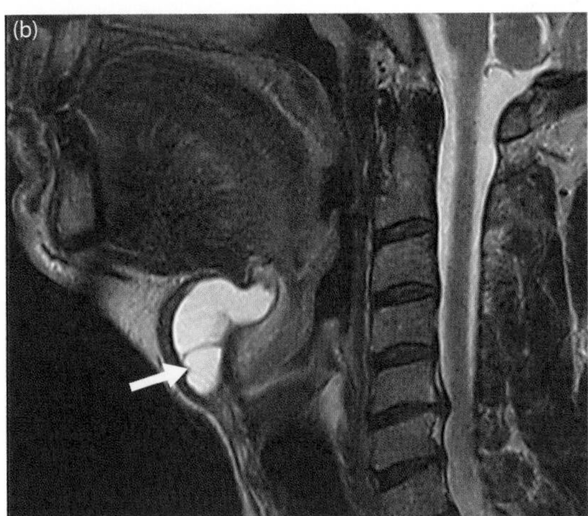

Figure 70.57 Axial **(a)** and sagittal **(b)** MR images show a midline thyroglossal cyst closely related to base of tongue and extending inferiorly.

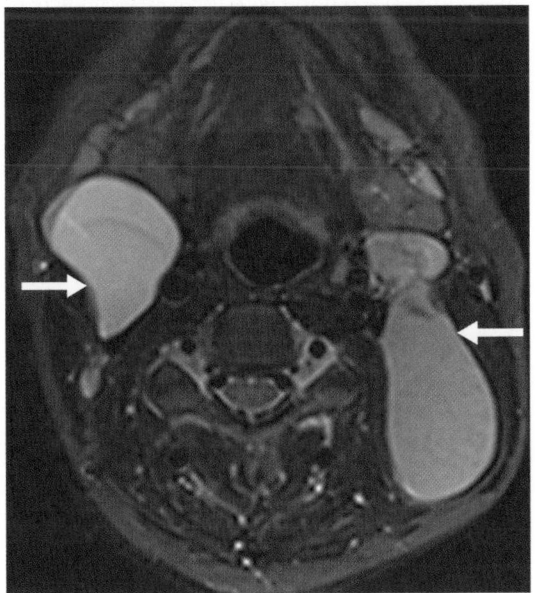

Figure 70.58 Axial T2 MRI image shows bilateral large lymphangiomas showing high signal.

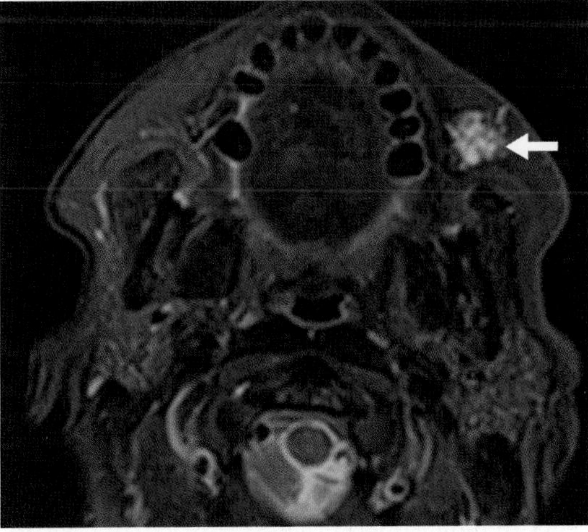

Figure 70.59 Axial T2 STIR image shows a lobulated haemangioma in the left buccal space showing high signal.

Suppurative lymph nodes are seen as enlarged nodes with focal areas of reduced echogenicity in the centre. Confluence or rupture of lymph nodes can lead to development of an abscess. Contrast-enhanced CT or MRI is helpful in delineating the extent of an abscess. The abscess is visualized as central irregular area of fluid density with enhancement of the surrounding wall (Figure 70.60).

Tuberculous lymphadenitis presents as a painless nodal mass in the neck. Findings on ultrasound

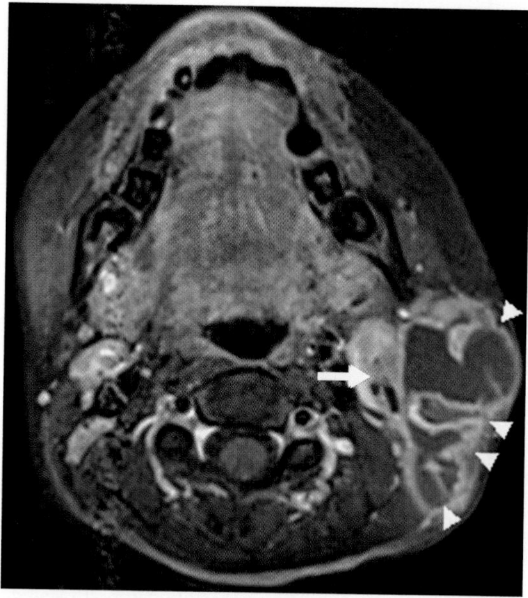

Figure 70.60 Axial post-contrast MRI image shows a confluent left tuberculous abscess with peripheral enhancement (arrowheads) and an enhancing left cervical node (arrow).

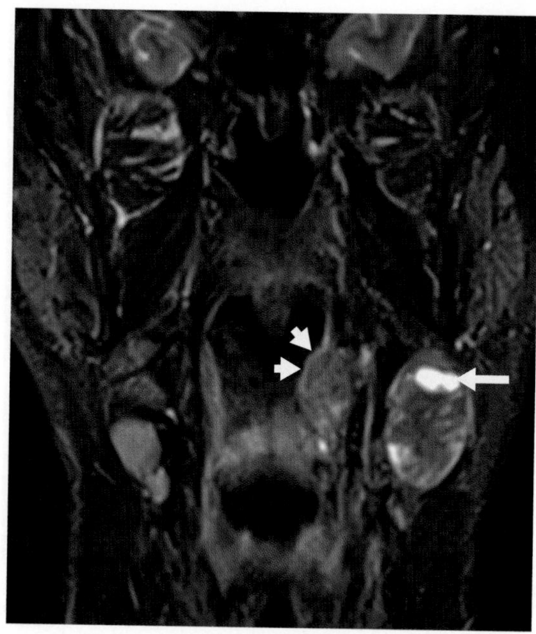

Figure 70.61 Coronal MRI image shows a metastatic left cervical node with focal area of necrosis superiorly (arrow). Primary lesion in the base of tongue is also seen (arrowheads).

or CT include enlarged nodes with central areas of necrosis, abscess formation and presence of multiple foci of calcification. Associated changes in the pulmonary parenchyma may be evident.

Metastatic nodes in the neck arise commonly from primary squamous cell carcinomas involving the pharynx or larynx. On ultrasound, metastatic nodes are enlarged, rounded and diffusely hypoechoic with absence of normal fatty hilum. Contrast-enhanced CT or MRI may show the presence of central areas of necrosis in squamous cell carcinoma metastases (Figure 70.61). Extracapsular spread from metastatic nodes is seen as irregularity of the nodal margins with infiltration of the surrounding fat. Metastatic nodes in the neck are also noted in primary tumours involving the lung, breast, oesophagus and melanoma.

Enlarged nodes in lymphoma are seen on ultrasound as multiple, enlarged, diffusely hypoechoic nodes with no evidence of necrosis. Contrast-enhanced CT or MRI can better delineate the extent of nodal involvement in the neck (Figure 70.62). PET-CT is usually performed for pre-treatment staging and follow-up of lymphoma after chemotherapy.

CAROTID BODY PARAGANGLIOMA

A carotid body tumour is seen on ultrasound as a well-defined solid mass splaying the internal and external carotid arteries at the carotid bifurcation with extensive vascularity (Figure 70.63). Contrast-enhanced CT shows the presence of an intensely enhancing mass lesion at the carotid bifurcation. On MRI, carotid body tumours show serpentine vascular flow voids within the tumour. Intense enhancement is seen on post-contrast T1-weighted images. Preoperative embolization of the tumour can be performed to reduce blood loss during surgery.

THYROID

THYROIDITIS

Thyroiditis is seen on ultrasound as diffuse enlargement of the thyroid with multiple ill-defined foci

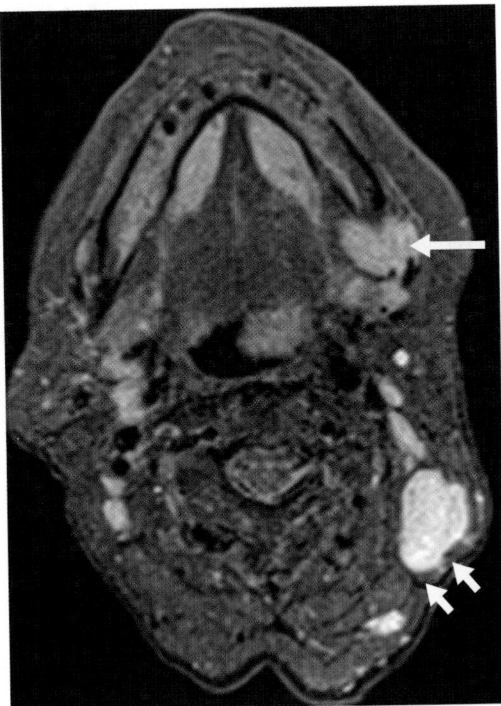

Figure 70.62 Enlarged left submandibular nodes (arrow) and left posterior cervical node (small arrows) in a patient with non-Hodgkin's lymphoma.

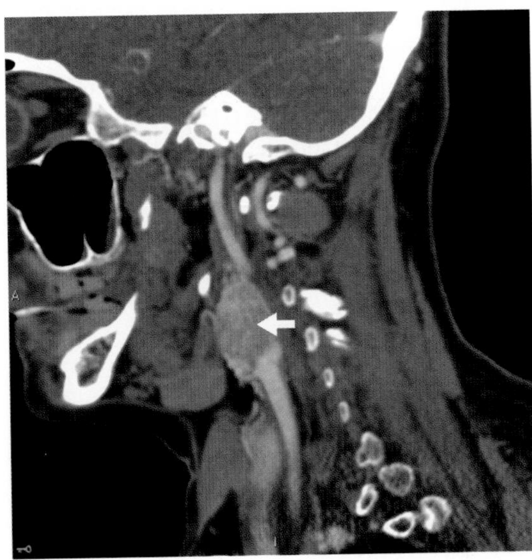

Figure 70.63 Sagittal CT image shows an enhancing carotid body tumour at the carotid bifurcation.

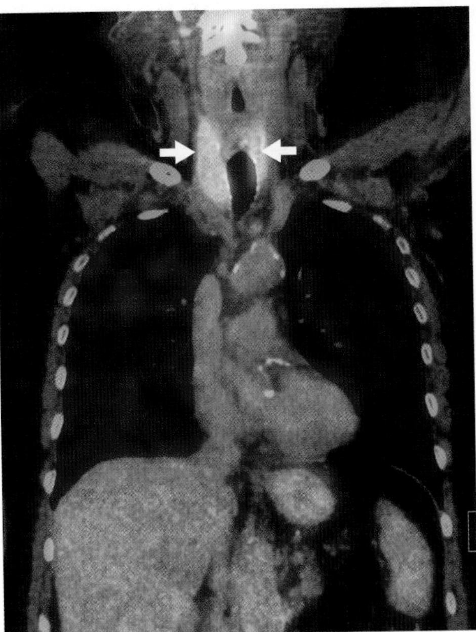

Figure 70.64 Fused PET-CT image shows diffuse fludeoxyglucose uptake in both lobes of thyroid (arrows) in keeping with diffuse thyroiditis.

of hypoechogenicity. Increased vascularity is seen on colour Doppler imaging. It is not possible on ultrasound to differentiate between Hashimoto thyroiditis and Graves' disease. Diffusely increased radionuclide uptake is noted on 99m Tc-pertechnetate and iodine-123 radionuclide imaging. Diffusely increased FDG uptake may also be noted incidentally on PET-CT scans done for other indications (Figure 70.64).

THYROID NODULES

Nodules of the thyroid are very common and are seen in up to 40 per cent of individuals having ultrasound of the thyroid. Up to 10 per cent of nodules in multinodular goitre and around 10 per cent of solitary nodules turn out to be malignant.

Ultrasound is often the initial test used for detection and characterization of thyroid nodules (Figure 70.65). The nodules are evaluated based on their margins, shape, echogenicity, vascularity and calcification. Solid nodules are more likely to be malignant than cystic nodules. Nodules with ill-defined or lobulated margins have a higher

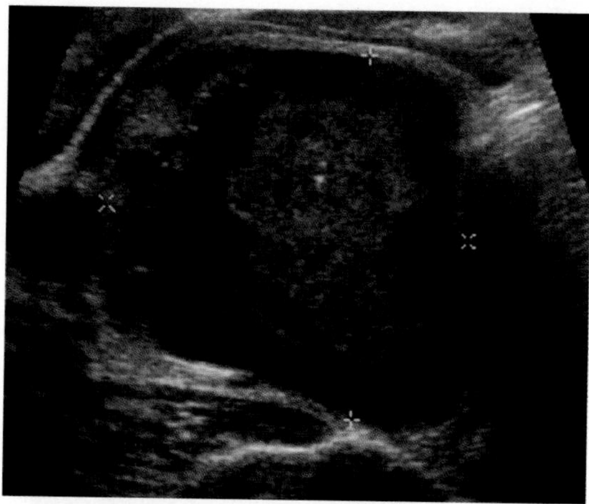

Figure 70.65 Ultrasound image shows a well-defined colloid nodule with areas of cystic degeneration in the periphery.

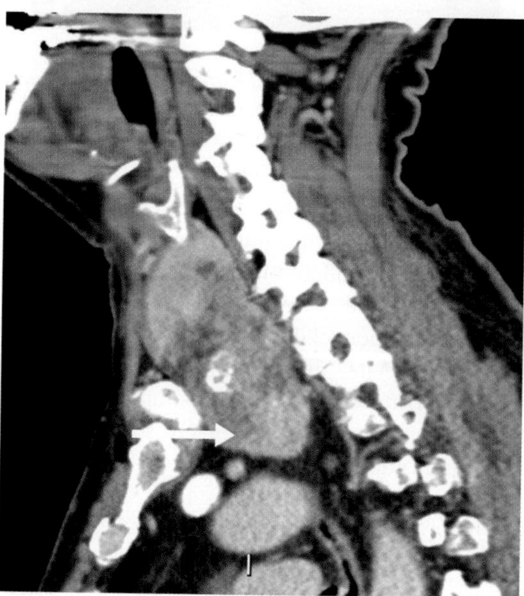

Figure 70.66 Sagittal CT image shows a large thyroid nodule extending inferiorly into the retrosternal space of the mediastinum.

incidence of malignancy. While peripheral calcification is seen in benign nodules, central calcification is associated with an increased incidence of malignancy.

Malignant nodules of the thyroid are more likely to be solid, have ill-defined margins, infiltrate into the surrounding parenchyma and have

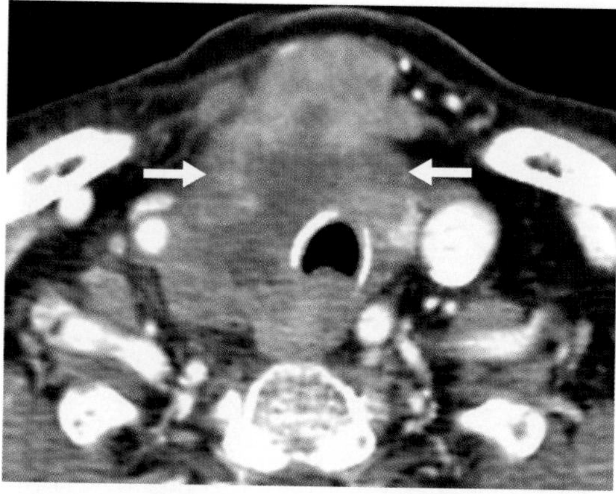

Figure 70.67 Axial CT image shows a malignant thyroid mass with ill-defined margins and central necrosis.

cervical lymphadenopathy. However, the majority of nodules cannot be reliably distinguished as benign or malignant on ultrasound. Hence ultrasound-guided fine-needle aspiration is performed for accurate characterization of nodules.

CT scan may be performed for large multinodular goitres with suspected retrosternal extension before surgery to delineate the full extent (Figures 70.66 and 70.67).

Radionuclide imaging with Tc99m pertechnetate or I123 is used evaluate the functional status of a thyroid nodule. Hot nodules on scintigraphy are more likely to be benign. Medullary thyroid carcinoma takes up octreotide (111-In-pentreotide) or I-131- MIBG (meta iodobenzyl guanidine).

Nodules that are FDG avid on PET-CT scans done for other indications have to be evaluated with ultrasound-guided fine-needle aspiration as the incidence of malignancy in FDG avid nodules is up to 40 per cent.

KEY LEARNING POINTS

- Ultrasound is a very good first investigation for evaluation of pathologies in the superficial organs of the neck.
- CT or MRI is often needed to evaluate the full extent of involvement in infections and tumours.

Index

Note: Page numbers followed by f indicate figures; those followed by t indicate tables.

A

B

E

F

H

I

J

K

N

O

Q

R

S

U

V